# Non-invasive Ventilation and Weaning: Principles and Practice

# Non-invasive Ventilation and Weaning: Principles and Practice


Edited by

**Mark Elliott** MA MB, BChir, MD, FRCP(UK)
Department of Respiratory Medicine,
St James's University Hospital, Leeds, UK

**Stefano Nava** MD
Respiratory Intensive Care Unit,
Fondazione S Maugeri, IRCCS, Pavia, Italy

**Bernd Schönhofer** MD, PhD
Department of Respiratory and Critical Care Medicine,
Klinikum Region Hannover, Oststadt-Heidehaus,
Hannover, Germany


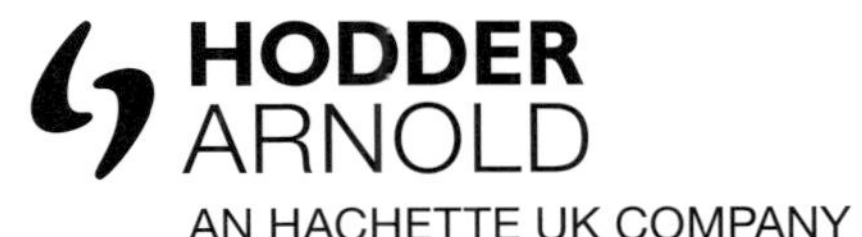

First published in Great Britain in 2010 by
Hodder Arnold, an imprint of Hodder Education,
an Hachette UK Company,
338 Euston Road, London NW1 3BH

**http://www.hodderarnold.com**



Hachette UK's policy is to use papers that are natural, renewable and recyclable products and made from wood grown in sustainable forests. The logging and manufacturing processes are expected to conform to the environmental regulations of the country of origin.



*British Library Cataloguing in Publication Data*
A catalogue record for this book is available from the British Library

*Library of Congress Cataloging-in-Publication Data*
A catalog record for this book is available from the Library of Congress

ISBN 9780340941522

1 2 3 4 5 6 7 8 9 10

Commissioning Editor: Caroline Makepeace
Project Editor: Jane Tod and Stephen Clausard
Production Controller: Kate Harris
Cover Designer: Lynda King
Indexer: Laurence Errington

Typeset in 10/12 pt Minion by MPS Limited,
A Macmillan Company, Chennai, India
Printed and bound in the UK by MPG Books Ltd

# Dedication

To our wives Anna Maria, Nicola and Maria

# Contents

*These appendices are available only in the Vitalsource ebook edition.

# Preface

We have been privileged to have worked through the time during which non-invasive ventilation has been transformed from a niche technique, available in only a few small specialist centres, to become part of the mainstream of respiratory and intensive care medicine. It has been exciting to see how an understanding of basic physiology has underpinned the application of the technique and interaction between industry, engineers, ventilator users and clinicians has lead to innovations and refinements of the equipment, which has been key to its the success.

Non-invasive ventilation is a multidisciplinary endeavour and all the professional groups involved have brought their own perspectives, disciplines and insights. Ventilator users and their carers have played their part, developing ideas and ways around problems, based on their own experience.

None of this would have happened without the vision and enthusiasm of a few individuals. At a personal level we would like to acknowledge the contributions of Dr Margaret Branthwaite and Prof. Dr. Dieter Köhler, who have been pioneers, inspired us and influenced our decision to get involved in this field.

NIV has reached maturity and as such it is sometimes difficult to see how it can be taken further. However, presentations at international meetings and publications in the scientific literature confirm that the prospects for the future remain healthy, with innovations in equipment, application and the extension and refinement of the indications for its use. We are delighted that so many people who have been influential in the field and for the emerging leaders for the future, have agreed to contribute to this book.

Mark Elliott
Stefano Nava
Bernd Schönhofer

# Contributors

**Nicolino Ambrosino**
Chief of Respiratory Section AO Pisana, Cardio-Thoracic Department, Pulmonary Unit, University Hospital of Pisa, and Pulmonary Rehabilitation and Weaning Unit, Auxilium Vitae, Volterra, Italy

**Massimo Antonelli** MD
Professor of Intensive Care and Anesthesiology, and Director, General Intensive Care Unit, Policlinico Universitario A Gemelli, Università Cattolica del Sacro Cuore, Rome, Italy

**Elie Azoulay** MD, PhD
Service de Réanimation Médicale, Groupe de Recherche Respiratoire en Réanimation Onco-hématologique, Groupe de Recherche Famiréa, Hôpital Saint Louis, Université Paris, Paris, France

**Giuseppe Bello** MD
Assistant Professor of Intensive Care and Anesthesiology, General Intensive Care Unit, Policlinico Universitario A Gemelli, Università Cattolica del Sacro Cuore, Rome, Italy

**Joshua O Benditt** MD
Medical Director of Respiratory Care Services, University of Washington Medical Center, Seattle, Washington, USA

**Dominique Benoit** MD, PhD
Department of Intensive Care, Ghent University Hospital, Ghent, Belgium

**Linda L Bieniek**
Advisory Board Member, International Ventilator Users Network, and Retired Certified Employee Assistance Professional, La Grange, Illinois, USA

**Louis Boitano** MS, RPFT, RRT
Respiratory Care Services, University of Washington Medical Center, Seattle, WA, USA

**Jean-Christian Borel** PhD
Hypoxia Pathophysiology Laboratory INSERM ER117, Joseph Fourier University and Physiology Unit, Rehabilitation and Physiology Department, CHU, Grenoble, France

**Stephen C Bourke** MB, BCh (Hons), PhD, FRCP
Consultant Respiratory Physician, Northumbria Healthcare NHS Foundation Trust, and Newcastle University, North Tyneside General Hospital, Newcastle-upon-Tyne, North Shields, UK

**Laurent Brochard**
Medical ICU, AP-HP, Henri Mondor Teaching Hospital, Créteil, University Paris EST, France

**C Burtin** PT, MSc
Respiratory Rehabilitation and Respiratory Division, University Hospitals, Katholieke Universiteit Leuven, and Faculty of Kinesiology and Rehabilitation Sciences, Katholieke Universiteit Leuven, Leuven, Belgium

**Peter M A Calverley** MB, ChB, FRCP, FRCPEd
Professor of Respiratory Medicine and Rehabilitation, School of Clinical Sciences, University of Liverpool, and Aintree Chest Centre, University Hospital Aintree, Liverpool, UK

**Shannon S Carson** MD
Associate Professor, and Associate Director, Medical Intensive Care Unit, and Director, Fellowship Training Program, Pulmonary and Critical Care Medicine, University of North Carolina School of Medicine, North Carolina, USA

**Piero Ceriana**
Pneumologia Riabilitativa E Terapia Subintensiva Respiratoria, IRCCS Fondazione 'S Maugeri', Pavia, Italy

**Gerald Chanques** MD
Assistant Professor of Anesthesiology and Critical Care, Intensive Care Unit, Anesthesia and Critical Care Department B, Saint Eloi Teaching Hospital, Montpellier, France

**Davide Chiumello** MD
U O Anestesia e Rianimazione, Dipartimento di Anestesia, Rianimazione (Intensiva e Subintensiva) e Terapia del Dolore, Milan, Italy

**Enrico M Clini**
Associate Professor, University of Modena, Department of Oncology, Haematology and Pneumology, University of Modena, Modena, Italy

**Giorgio Conti** MD
Professor of Intensive Care and Anesthesia, Pediatric Intensive Care Unit, Catholic University of Rome, Policlinico A Gemelli, Rome, Italy

**Antonio Corrado** MD
Director of Respiratory Intensive Care Unit, Azienda Ospedaliera, Universitaria Careggi, Firenze, Italy

**Borja G Cosio** MD, PhD
Department of Respiratory Medicine, Hospital Universitario Son Dureta, Palma de Mallorca, Spain

**Martin R Cowie** MD, MSc, FRCP, FESC
Professor of Cardiology, National Heart and Lung Institute, Imperial College, London, UK

**Gerard J Criner** MD
Professor of Medicine, Chief of Department of Pulmonary and Critical Care Medicine, Temple University Hospital, Philadelphia, PA, USA

**Ernesto Crisafulli**
Junior Assistant Ospedale Villa Pineta, Pavullo n/F, Ospedale Villa Pineta, Pulmonary Rehabilitation Unit, Pavullo, Modena, Italy

**Antoine Cuvelier**
Professor, Pulmonary and Intensive Care Department, Rouen University Hospital, Rouen, France

**A Craig Davidson** MA, MD, FRCP
Consultant in Respiratory and Intensive Care Medicine, and Director, Lane Fox Respiratory Unit, Guy's and St Thomas' Hospital, London, UK

**Alexandre Demoule**
Medical ICU and Pneumology Department, AP-HP, Pitié-Salpétrière Teaching Hospital, Paris, France

**Pieter Depuydt** MD, PhD
Department of Intensive Care, Universitair Ziekenhuis Gent, Gent, Belgium

**Dan F Dilling** MD
Assistant Professor of Medicine, Loyola University Chicago Stritch School of Medicine, Maywood, Illinois, USA

**Mark Elliott** MA MB BChir MD FRCP (UK)
Department of Respiratory Medicine, St James's University Hospital, Leeds, UK

**Scott K Epstein** MD
Dean for Educational Affairs and Professor of Medicine, Tufts University School of Medicine, Division of Pulmonary, Critical Care and Sleep Medicine, Tufts Medical Center, Boston, USA

**Joan Escarrabill** MD
Director, Master Plan for Respiratory Diseases PDMAR (Health Ministry), Institut d'Estudis de la Salut, Barcelona, Spain

**Antonio M Esquinas Rodriguez** MD, PhD, FCCP
Intensivist, International Fellow AARC, Intensive Care Unit, Hospital Morales Meseguer, Murcia, Spain

**Laura Evans** MD, MSc
Assistant Professor of Medicine, New York University School of Medicine, Bellevue Hospital, New York, USA

**Francesco Fanfulla** MD
Head of Sleep Center, Scientific Institutes of Montescano and Pavia, Salvatore Maugeri Foundation, Pavia, Italy

**Brigitte Fauroux** MD, PhD
Professor of Pediatrics, Paediatric Pulmonary Department and Research Unit INSERM UMR-S 938, AP-HP, Hôpital d'Enfants Armand Trousseau, France

**Ramon Farré** PhD
Biophysics and Bioengineering Unit, School of Medicine, University of Barcelona, IDIBAPS, Barcelona, Spain

**Massimo Ferluga** MD
Department of Perioperative Medicine, Intensive Care and Emergency, Cattinara Hospital, Trieste University School of Medicine, Trieste, Italy

**Miguel Ferrer** MD, PhD
Consultant, Respiratory Intensive and Intermediate Care Unit, Department of Pneumology, Institute of Thorax, Hospital Clinic, IDIBAPS, University of Barcelona, Spain

**Dimitris Georgopoulos** MD, PhD
Professor of Intensive Care Medicine, Department of Intensive Care Medicine, University Hospital of Heraklion, Crete, Greece

**Alicia K Gerke** MD
Associate, Department of Internal Medicine, Division of Pulmonary, Critical Care, and Occupational Medicine, University of Iowa Hospitals and Clinics, Iowa City, Iowa, USA

**G John Gibson** BSc, MD, FRCP, FRCPEd
Emeritus Professor of Respiratory Medicine, Newcastle University, Newcastle-upon-Tyne, UK

**Francisco Javier Gómez de Terreros** MD
Member of Respiratory Research Group, Centro de Investigación Biomédica en Red de Enfermedades Respiratorias, CIBERES, Ministry of Science and Innovation, Madrid, and Attending of Intermediate Respiratory Care Unit, San Pedro de Alcantara Hospital, Cáceres, Spain

**Miguel R Gonçalves**
Senior Respiratory Physiotherapist, Clinical Specialist in Noninvasive ventilation, and University Professor of Respiratory Physiotherapy, Lung Function, Sleep and Ventilation Unit, Pulmonary Medicine Department, Intensive Care Unit, Emergency Department, Faculty of Medicine, University of Porto, University Hospital of S João, Porto, Portugal

**Massimo Gorini** MD
Unità di Terapia Intensiva Respiratoria, Fisiopatologia Toracica, Azienda Ospedaliera, Universitaria Careggi, Firenze, Italy

**Rik Gosselink** PhD, PT
Professor of Rehabilitation Sciences, Dean of Faculty of Kinesiology and Rehabilitation Sciences, Katholieke Universiteit Leuven, Leuven, Belgium

**Alasdair Gray** MB, ChB, MD, FRCS, FCEM
Consultant, Department of Emergency Medicine, Royal Infirmary of Edinburgh, Edinburgh, UK

**Cesare Gregoretti** MD
Director of Anaesthesia and Intensive Care Unit, Adelaide Hospital, Department of Emergency, Adelaide, Turin, Italy

**Gokay Gungor**
Division of Pulmonary and Critical Care Medicine, Loyola University of Chicago Stritch School of Medicine, Illinois, USA, and Sureyyapasa Chest Diseases and Thoracic Surgery Training and Research Hospital, Istanbul, Turkey

**William B Hall** MD
Pulmonary and Critical Care Medicine, University of North Carolina School of Medicine, North Carolina, USA

**Nick Hart** MBBS, BSc (Hons), PhD, MRCP
Clinical Research Consultant, NIHR Comprehensive Biomedical Research Centre, Guy's and St Thomas' NHS Foundation Trust and King's College London, London, UK

**Paul M Haydock** MRCP
Clinical Research Fellow, National Heart and Lung Institute, Imperial College London, London, UK

**Dean R Hess** PhD, RRT
Assistant Director of Respiratory Care, Massachusetts General Hospital, Associate Professor of Anesthesia, Harvard Medical School, Massachusetts General ALS Clinic, Wang Ambulatory Care Center, Boston, USA

**Nicholas S Hill** MD
Professor of Medicine and Chief, Division of Pulmonary Critical Care and Sleep Medicine, Tufts Medical Center, Boston, USA

**David Hilton-Jones**
Clinical Director, Oxford Muscle and Nerve and Myasthenia Centres, Department of Clinical Neurology, John Radcliffe Hospital, Oxford, UK

**Luke Howard** MA, DPhil, FRCP
Consultant Chest Physician, Hammersmith Hospital, and National Pulmonary Hypertension Service, Department of Cardiac Sciences, Hammersmith Hospital, London, UK

**David S C Hui** MD, FRACP, FRCP, FHKCP, FHKAM
Professor, Department of Medicine and Therapeutics, Chinese University of Hong Kong, and Prince of Wales Hospital, Shatin, Hong Kong

**Elini Ischaki** MD
Department of Critical Care and Pulmonary Services, Evangelismos Hospital, University of Athens Medical School, Athens, Greece

**Samir Jaber** MD, PhD
Professor of Anesthesiology and Critical Care Medicine, Department of Anesthesiology and Critical Care (DARB), Saint Eloi University Hospital and Montpellier School of Medicine, Montpellier, France

**Boris Jung** MD
Assistant Professor of Anesthesiology and Critical Care, Intensive Care Unit, Anesthesia and Critical Care Department B, Saint Eloi Teaching Hospital, Montpellier, France

**William J M Kinnear** MD FRCP
Consultant Respiratory Physician, Queens Medical Centre, Nottingham University Hospitals, Nottingham, UK

**Eumorfia Kondili** MD, PhD
Assistant Professor of Intensive Care Medicine, Department of Intensive Care Medicine, University Hospital of Heraklion, Crete, Greece

**Franco Laghi** MD
Professor of Medicine, Division of Pulmonary and Critical Care Medicine, Loyola University Medical Center, Hines, Illinois, USA

**Martin Latham** BSc (Hons), RGN PG Dip
Sleep Service, St James's University Hospital, Leeds, UK

**François Lellouche**
Service de Soins Intensifs de Chirurgie Cardiaque, Centre de Recherche Hôpital Laval, Université Laval, Québec, Canada

**Mitchell M Levy** MD
Professor of Medicine, Warren Alpert Medical School of Brown University, Rhode Island Hospital, Providence, USA

**Patrick Lévy** MD, PhD
Hypoxia Pathophysiology Laboratory INSERM ER117, Joseph Fourier University and Physiology Unit, Rehabilitation and Physiology Department, CHU, Grenoble, France

**Erwan L'Her** MD, PhD
Professeur agrégé sous octroi, Département de Médecine Familiale et Médecine d'Urgence Université Laval, Québec, Canada

**Michael and Alyson Lindley**

**Frédéric Lofaso** MD, PhD
Professor of Physiology, AP-HP, Hôpital Raymond Poincaré, Université Versailles, St Quentin en Yvelines, Physiology Functional Testing and Technological Innovations Centre, Garches, France

**Bruno Louis** PhD
INSERM, Université Paris, Faculté de Médecine, Créteil, Paris, France

**Umberto Lucangelo** MD
Department of Perioperative Medicine, Intensive Care and Emergency, Cattinara Hospital, Trieste University School of Medicine, Trieste, Italy

**Barry Make**
Co-Director, COPD Program, National Jewish Health, and Professor of Medicine, University of Colorado-Denver School of Medicine, National Jewish Medical and Research Center, Denver, Colorado, USA

**Jordi Mancebo**
ICU Medicina Intensiva, Hospital Santa Creu i Sant Pau, Barcelona, Spain

**Juan F Masa** MD
Head of Respiratory Research Group, Centro de Investigación Biomédica en Red de Enfermedades Respiratorias; CIBERES, Ministry of Science and Innovation, Madrid, and Director of Intermediate Respiratory Care Unit, Head of Pulmonary Division, San Pedro de Alcantara Hospital, Cáceres, Spain

**Antonio Messina** MD
Anesthesia and Intensive Care, University Hospital 'Maggiore della Carità' Novara, Università del Piemonte Orientale 'Amedeo Avogadro', Alessandria-Novara-Vercelli, Italy

**Christine Mikelsons** MCSP, BSc, MSc, PGCHE
Consultant Respiratory Physiotherapist, Royal Free Hospital, London, UK

**Jean-François Muir**
Professor and Head, Pulmonary and Respiratory Intensive Care Department, Rouen University Hospital, Rouen, France

**Patrick Murphy** MBBS, BSc (Hons), MRCP
Clinical Research Fellow, Lane Fox Respiratory Unit, Guy's and St Thomas' NHS Trust, King's College London, London, UK

**Matthew T Naughton** MD, FRACP
Head, General Respiratory and Sleep Medicine, Department of Allergy, Immunology and Respiratory Medicine, Alfred Hospital and Monash University, Melbourne, Victoria, Australia

**Stefano Nava** MD
Respiratory Intensive Care Unit, Fondazione S Maugeri, IRCCS, Pavia, Italy

**Paolo Navalesi** MD
Anesthesia and Intensive Care, University Hospital 'Maggiore della Carità' Novara, Università del Piemonte Orientale 'Amedeo Avogadro', Alessandria-Novara-Vercelli, Italy

**Ole Norregaard** MD
Director, Danish Respiratory Center West, Arhus University Hospital, Denmark

**Paolo Pelosi**
Dipartimento Ambiente, Salute E Sicurezza, Universita' Degli Studi Dell'insubria, Varese, Italy

**Jean-Louis Pépin** MD, PhD
Hypoxia Pathophysiology Laboratory INSERM ER117, Joseph Fourier University and Physiology Unit, Rehabilitation and Physiology Department, CHU, Grenoble, France

**Irene Permut** MD
Fellow, Pulmonary and Critical Care, Temple University Hospital, Philadelphia, Pennsylvania, USA

**Marco Piastra** MD
Assistant Professor, Pediatric Intensive Care Unit, Catholic University of Rome, Policlinico A Gemelli, Roma, Italy

**Michael Polkey** MB ChB, PhD, FRCP
National Heart and Lung Institute, Respiratory Biomedical Research Unit, Royal Brompton Hospital, London, UK

**Silvia Pulitanó** MD
Assistant Professor, Pediatric Intensive Care Unit, Catholic University of Rome, Policlinico A Gemelli, Rome, Italy

**Jordi Rigau** PhD
Director of Innovation and Technology, Research, Development and Innovation Department, Sibel Group, Barcelona, Spain

**Dominique Robert**
Professor of Intensive Care, Claude Bernard University Lyon 1, and President, ALLP, Lyon, France

**Roberto Rodríguez-Roisin** MD, FRCPE
Institut del Tòrax (Servei de Pneumologia), Professor of Medicine, Hospital Clinic, Universitat de Barcelona Villarroel, Barcelona, Spain

**Aditi Satti** MD
Assistant Professor of Medicine, Department of Pulmonary and Critical Care Medicine, Temple University School of Medicine, Philadelphia, USA

**Raffaele Scala** MD
Specialist in Respiratory Diseases and Intensive Care Medicine, Ospedale S. Donato, Arezzo, Italy

**Gregory A Schmidt** MD
Professor of Medicine, Department of Internal Medicine, Division of Pulmonary Diseases, Critical Care, and Occupational Medicine, Director, Critical Care Programs, Department of Internal Medicine, University of Iowa Hospitals and Clinics, Iowa City, USA

**Bernd Schönhofer** MD, PhD
Professor of Medicine, Department of Respiratory and Critical Care Medicine, Klinikum Region Hannover, Oststadt-Heidehaus, Hannover, Germany

**Daniel Schuermans** RN
Lung Function Technician, Biomedical Research Unit, University Hospital UZBrussel (VUB), Brussels, Belgium

**J Segers** PT, MSc
Respiratory Rehabilitation and Respiratory Division, University Hospitals, Katholieke Universiteit Leuven, and Faculty of Kinesiology and Rehabilitation Sciences Katholieke Universiteit Leuven, Leuven, Belgium

**Hameeda Shaikh** MD
Division of Pulmonary and Critical Care Medicine, Loyola University of Chicago Stritch School of Medicine, and Edward Hines Jr Veterans Administration Hospital, Hines, Illinois, USA

**John M Shneerson** MA, DM, FRCP, FCCP
Director, Respiratory Support and Sleep Centre, Papworth Hospital, Cambridge, UK

**Anita K Simonds** MD, FRCP
Consultant in Respiratory Medicine, Academic Department of Sleep and Breathing, Royal Brompton and Harefield NHS Foundation Trust, London, UK

**Marcio Soares** MD, PhD
Intensive Care Unit, Instituto Nacional de Câncer, Rio de Janeiro, Brazil

**Renaud Tamisier** MD, PhD
Hypoxia Pathophysiology Laboratory INSERM ER117, Joseph Fourier University and Physiology Unit, Rehabilitation and Physiology Department, CHU, Grenoble, France

**Antoni Torres** MD, PhD
Director of Respiratory, Intensive and Intermediate Care Unit, Department of Pneumology, Institute of Thorax, Hospital Clinic, IDIPAPS, Professor of Medicine, University of Barcelona, Spain

**T Troosters** PT, PhD
Respiratory Rehabilitation and Respiratory Division, University Hospitals, Katholieke Universiteit Leuven, and Faculty of Kinesiology and Rehabilitation Sciences, Katholieke Universiteit Leuven, Leuven, Belgium

**Isabel Utrabo** MD
Attending of Intermediate Respiratory Care Unit, San Pedro de Alcantara Hospital, Cáceres, Spain

**Rosanna Vaschetto** MD
Anesthesia and Intensive Care, University Hospital 'Maggiore della Carità' Novara, Università del Piemonte Orientale 'Amedeo Avogadro', Alessandria-Novara-Vercelli, Italy

**Theodoros Vassilakopoulos** MD
Associate Professor, Department of Critical Care and Pulmonary Services, University of Athens Medical School, Evangelismos Hospital, Athens, Greece

**Lies Verfaillie** MD
Respiratory Division University Hospital, UZ Brussel, Brussels, Belgium

**Michele Vitacca** MD
Respiratory Unit and Weaning Centre, Fondazione Salvatore Maugeri, IRCCS, Lumezzane, Italy

**Paul P Walker** BMed Sci (Hons), BM, BS, MD, FRCP
Consultant in Respiratory Medicine, Aintree Chest Centre, University Hospital Aintree, Liverpool and School of Clinical Sciences, University of Liverpool, Liverpool, UK

**John W H Watt** MB ChB, FRCA, MD
Consultant Anaesthetist, North West Regional Spinal Injuries Centre, Southport Hospital, Southport, England

**Jadwiga A Wedzicha** MA, MD, FRCP
Professor of Respiratory Medicine, Academic Unit of Respiratory Medicine, University College London Medical School, University College London, London, UK

**John P H Wilding** DM, FRCP
Professor of Medicine and Honorary Consultant Physician, Head of Diabetes and Endocrinology Clinical Research Unit, Clinical Sciences Centre, University Hospital Aintree, Liverpool, UK

**João Carlos Winck** PhD
Senior University Professor of Pulmonary Medicine, and Coordinator of the Lung Function, Sleep and Ventilation Unit, Pulmonary Medicine Department, Faculty of Medicine, University of Porto, University Hospital of S João, Porto, Portugal

**Wolfram Windisch** MD, PhD
Professor of Medicine, Department of Pneumology, University Hospital Freiburg, Killianstrasse, Freiburg, Germany

**Bernard Wuyam** MD, PhD
Hypoxia Pathophysiology Laboratory INSERM ER117, Joseph Fourier University and Physiology unit, Rehabilitation and Physiology Department, CHU, Grenoble, France

**Nektaria Xirouchaki** MD, PhD
Department of Intensive Care Medicine, University Hospital of Heraklion, Crete, Greece

# Acknowledgements

For us this book is the culmination of many years of our own work and indirectly of that of many others.

We are grateful to our parents Derek and Barbara, Angelo and Mafalda, Bernhard and Regina for the values they gave us and their support and encouragement throughout our lives.

Our families have shared in our involvement in this field, accepting our absences and distractions; our thanks to Nicola, Ruth, Katherine, Anna Maria, Maria, Felix and Pia.

Much of what we have learnt would not have been possible without the commitment of our colleagues and of learning together with them. Thanks to those who work and have worked in the Sleep and Assisted Ventilation Service and on the Respiratory Wards at St James's University Hospital and Killingbeck Hospital, the Respiratory Intensive Care Unit of Pavia Fondazione S. Maugeri, the Respiratory Intensive care units in Krankenhaus Kloster Grafschaft, Schmallenberg and Klinikum Oststadt-Heidehaus, Hannover.

Mark Elliott
Stefano Nava
Bernd Schönhofer

# Abbreviations

| | |
|---|---|
| ABG | arterial blood gases |
| ACE | angiotensin-converting enzyme |
| ACPE | acute cardiogenic pulmonary oedema |
| ADH | antidiuretic hormone |
| AF | atrial fibrillation |
| AH | absolute humidity |
| AHI | apnoea hypopnoea index |
| AHRF | acute hypoxaemic respiratory failure |
| ALS | amyotrophic lateral sclerosis |
| APAP | auto-titrating positive airway pressure |
| ARDS | acute respiratory distress syndrome |
| ARF | acute respiratory failure |
| ASV | adaptive servo-controlled ventilation |
| ATS | American Thoracic Society |
| AVAPS | average volume assured pressure support |
| BAL | bronchioalveolar lavage |
| BiPAP/BPAP | bi-level positive airway pressure |
| CAP | community-acquired pneumonia |
| CHF | congestive heart failure |
| $CL_{dyn}$ | dynamic compliance |
| $CL_{stat}$ | static compliance |
| CNEP | continuous negative external pressure |
| COPD | chronic obstructive pulmonary disease |
| PEF | peak expiratory flow |
| CPAP | continuous positive airway pressure |
| CRDQ | Chronic Respiratory Disease Questionnaire |
| CRF | chronic respiratory failure |
| CRQ | Chronic Respiratory Questionnaire |
| CRS | compliance of the respiratory system |
| CSA | central sleep apnoea |
| CSAQLI | Calgary Sleep Apnea Quality of Life Index |
| CSR | Cheyne–Stokes respiration |
| CSS | central apnoea syndrome |
| $DA\text{-}aO_2$ | alveolar–arterial gradient |
| DMD | Duchenne muscular dystrophy |
| DMV | domiciliary mechanical ventilation |
| DNI/DNR | 'do not intubate' or 'do not resuscitate' |
| ECG | electrocardiogram |
| EDS | excessive daytime sleepiness |
| EF | ejection fraction |
| ELBG | ear lobe blood gas |
| EMG | electromyography |
| $EMG_{di}$ | diaphragm electromyogram |
| EPAP | expiratory positive airway pressure |
| ERS | European Respiratory Society |
| ET | expiratory time |
| ETI | endotracheal intubation |
| $FEV_1$ | forced expiratory volume in 1 second |
| $FiO_2$ | oxygen inspiratory fraction |
| FRC | functional residual capacity |
| FVC | forced vital capacity |
| GOLD | Global Initiative for Chronic Obstructive Lung Disease |
| GPB | glossopharyngeal breathing |
| HDU | high-dependency unit |
| HFCWO | high-frequency chest wall oscillation |
| HHW | heated humidifier wire |
| HME | heat moisture exchange |
| HMEF | heat and moisture exchanger/filter |
| HMV | home mechanical ventilation |
| HPS | hepatopulmonary syndrome |
| HRQoL | health-related quality of life |
| i:e | inspiratory:expiratory ratio |
| ICU | intensive care unit |
| IL-1 | interleukin 1 |
| IMV | intermittent mandatory ventilation |
| | invasive mechanical ventilation |
| IPAP | inspiratory positive airway pressure |
| IPV | intrapulmonary percussive ventilation |
| ITP | intrathoracic pressure |
| LABD | long-acting bronchodilator |
| LTAC | long-term acute care |
| LTD | long-term dependency |
| LTOT | long-term oxygen therapy |
| LV | left ventricular |
| LVFS | left ventricular fractional shortening |
| MAC | mechanically assisted cough |
| MDI | metered dose inhaler |
| MEP | maximal expiratory pressure |
| MIE | mechanical insufflation-exsufflation |
| MIGET | multiple inert gas elimination |
| MIP | maximal inspiratory pressure |
| MND | motor neurone disease |
| MSNA | muscle sympathetic nerve activity |
| MV | minute volume |
| NAVA | neurally adjusted ventilatory assistance |

| | |
|---|---|
| NAWR | nasal airway resistance |
| n-CPAP | non-invasive CPAP |
| NIV | non-invasive ventilation |
| NMD | neuromuscular disease |
| NIPPV | non-invasive positive pressure ventilation |
| NPSA | National Patient Safety Agency |
| NRD | neural respiratory drive |
| OHS | obesity hypoventilation syndrome |
| OSA | obstructive sleep apnoea |
| PAV | proportional-assist ventilation |
| PCF | peak cough flow |
| PCWP | pulmonary capillary wedge pressure |
| PEEP | positive end-expiratory pressure |
| $PEEP_i$ | intrinsic PEEP |
| PEF | peak expiratory flow |
| PEFR | peak expiratory flow rate |
| PEG | percutaneous endoscopic gastrostomy |
| PMV | prolonged mechanical ventilation |
| $P_{oes}$ | oesophageal pressure |
| PSV | pressure support ventilation |
| QALY | quality-adjusted life-year |
| RAAS | renin–angiotensin–aldosterone system |
| RAW | respiratory airway |
| RCT | randomized controlled trial |
| RH | relative humidity |
| RICU | respiratory intensive care unit |
| RIP | respiratory inductance plethysmography |
| RMS | respiratory muscle strength |
| RV | residual volume |
| SABA | short-acting inhaled $\beta_2$-agonists |
| SABD | short-acting bronchodilator |
| SAMA | short-acting muscarinic antagonist |
| SAOS | sleep apnoea obstructive syndrome |
| SARS | severe acute respiratory syndrome |
| SBT | spontaneous breathing trial |
| SF-36 | Medical Outcome Survey Short Form 36 |
| SGRQ | St George's Respiratory Questionnaire |
| SIMV | synchronized intermittent mandatory ventilation |
| SIP | Sickness Impact Profile |
| SM | sniff manoeuvre |
| SMA | spinal muscle atrophy |
| SNIP | sniff nasal inspiratory pressure |
| SNS | sympathetic nervous system |
| SRI | severe respiratory insufficiency |
| $T_cCO_2$ | transcutaneous carbon dioxide |
| TLC | total lung capacity |
| TMS | transcranial magnetic stimulation |
| TMV | tracheostomy and mechanical ventilation |
| TNF | tumour necrosis factor |
| TV | tidal volume |
| $TwP_{di}$ | twitch transdiaphragmatic pressure |
| SPNS | supramaximal phrenic nerve stimulation |
| VAP | ventilator-associated pneumonia |
| VDU | ventilator-dependent unit |
| VRU | ventilator rehabilitation unit |
| WOB | work of breathing |

# PART I

# EQUIPMENT AND PRACTICE

# 1

# Non-invasive ventilation: from the past to the present

DOMINIQUE ROBERT, BARRY MAKE

## ABSTRACT

Mechanical ventilation – invasive and non-invasive (NIV) – is the most commonly employed life support therapy across multiple settings, and a variety of methods and devices are available to provide effective therapy. In acute care, mechanical ventilation is used during anaesthesia, in critical care units and the emergency department; it is also used in general medical wards in some cases, and in long-term settings including in the home (HMV). Invasive ventilation uses tracheostomy or intubation to deliver intermittent positive pressure ventilation (IPPV). Non-invasive ventilation (NIV) can be provided by devices to deliver intermittent subatmospheric pressure, referred to as intermittent negative pressure ventilation (INPV); INPV is applied using a cylinder (iron lung), shell or poncho to create a space surrounding the patient's thorax and abdomen. Currently NIV is most commonly applied using an interface placed on the face, nose or mouth (nasal, oronasal, full face) to deliver IPPV. The present form of NIV, i.e. NIV-IPPV, was developed in the past 20 years and has provided a stimulus to continued advances in the field of mechanical ventilation. There is now a robust evidence base documenting its efficacy and its role will continue to grow in the armamentarium of respiratory care in both acute and chronic settings.

## HISTORY

The history of non-invasive (NIV) and invasive mechanical (IMV) ventilation is intimately intertwined. The methods to deliver mechanical ventilation were initially described in the early twentieth century and three main periods in the history of mechanical ventilation can be distinguished (Table 1.1).

- **NIV via negative pressure (NIV-INPV) period:** During the first period, from 1928 to 1952, NIV-INPV was exclusively used, peaking with use in patients with poliomyelitis in the 1950s in both acute and chronic care settings.
- **Invasive ventilation period:** From 1953 to 1990, the use of invasive ventilation expanded rapidly and was the most common form of therapy used in acute care. During this period the use of ventilation was established as an important tool in critically ill patients. NIV-INPV was used mostly in the home.
- **NIV via positive pressure breathing/invasive ventilation (NIV-IPPB/invasive ventilation) period:** From 1990 to the present, the use of NIV by IPPV progressively increased in acute care. This technique is used in up to 30–40 per cent of patients in critical care units and up to 90 per cent of patients receiving ventilation in the home.

Insights into the evolution of mechanical ventilation may be a useful starting point for further discussion of the current use and future directions of this therapy.

During the first NIV-INPV period, beginning in the late 1920s, NIV using negative pressure was found to improve survival compared with no ventilator assistance in patients with polio.[1] Many hospitals were equipped with such devices, including in the USA, where President Roosevelt, who was a polio survivor, applied pressure and 'The March of the Dimes' collected public donations. By the 1950s, due to the effectiveness of NIV-INPV, the mortality of the polio patients in specialized centres was about 2 per cent, or

**Table 1.1** The three periods in the history of mechanical ventilation

| Era | NIV via negative pressure (NIV-INPV) | Invasive ventilation (IV) | NIV via positive pressure/invasive ventilation (NIV-IPPV/IV) |
|---|---|---|---|
| **Years** | **1928–52** | **1953–90** | **1990–present** |
| NIV using INPV | *Poliomyelitis* | Rapid decreasing | None |
| NIV using IPPV | None | No or only IPPB | *Increasing. Up to 30–40 per cent of patients in acute setting and 90 per cent at home* |
| Invasive using IPPV | Thoracic surgery | *Used almost exclusively* | Decreasing. Down to 60–70 per cent in acute setting and 10 per cent at home |

Italics represent the most notable feature of the era.
INPV, intermittent negative pressure ventilation; IPPB, intermittent positive pressure breathing; IPPV, intermittent positive pressure ventilation; NIV, non-invasive ventilation.

about 10 per cent of those receiving NIV-INPV.[2,3] This efficacy of NIV-INPV has been underrecognized by healthcare professionals in the modern era. On the other side of the Atlantic, the mortality rate of polio patients needing mechanical ventilation was extremely high, reaching 94 per cent at the beginning of the 1952 polio epidemic in Copenhagen. The explanation for this higher mortality was the lack of availability of ventilators (only one iron lung and six cuirasses in the city). The desperate inability to pursue the conventional use of NIV-INPV led to the necessity of using methods generally only practised during anaesthesia, that is tracheostomy with cuffed tubes and hand-bag ventilation provided continuously for days or months. The success of the use of tracheostomy plus ventilation was immediately evident and mortality decreased to 7 per cent in polio patients receiving mechanical ventilation.[4,5]

The success of tracheostomy plus positive pressure ventilation combined with the ease of caring for the patient compared with treatment with the iron lung explains why the second mechanical ventilation period (invasive ventilation) proceeded rapidly. During the invasive ventilation period tracheostomy or translaryngeal intubation and ventilation with automatic lung ventilator to replace hand-bag ventilation spread rapidly, first in Europe and then in the USA. However, during the same time an alternative form of NIV, namely intermittent positive pressure breathing (NIV-IPPV), was prescribed for other objectives: treatment of pulmonary atelectasis, aerosol delivery and short-term non-invasive ventilator support. But as controversies surfaced, the use of NIV-IPPV as a ventilator support technique fell into disfavour.[6] For chronic ventilator support, NIV-IPPV was confined to use in the home (HMV) for those patients who remained ventilator dependent over the long term;[7] HMV was delivered via tracheostomy and IPPV ventilator not only for polio but also for patients with chronic respiratory insufficiency who remained ventilator dependent after an episode of acute respiratory failure (ARF). Care for these patients was organized not only in intensive care unit (ICU) settings but also in chronic ventilator units leading to discharge.[8] During the invasive ventilation period, although HMV was recognized to significantly prolong life it remained underutilized because of the difficulty in mobility with the iron lung and the invasiveness of tracheostomy.

The transition from the second to the third mechanical ventilation period gradually occurred between 1985 and 1990 and was driven by both the advances in sleep medicine and the practice of HMV. The sentinel event leading to the NIV-IPPV/invasive ventilation period of mechanical ventilation was the description in 1981 of the efficacy of nasal continuous positive airway pressure (CPAP), replacing tracheostomy, in treating obstructive sleep apnoea.[9] Mimicking that experience, some teams working in HMV and to a lesser extent in ICUs began using NIV-IPPV. Treatment with nasal NIV-IPPV of chronic restrictive disorders related to neuromuscular (e.g. Duchenne muscular dystrophy) and chest disease (kyphoscoliosis, sequels of tuberculosis) proved to prevent recurrent hypoventilation.[10–14] Furthermore the non-invasive approach to treating patients with COPD presenting with acute-on-chronic respiratory failure managed in the ICU was successful.[15–17] Other advantages of NIV-IPPV were found to be clinically significant in these patients: fewer nosocomial infections, shorter duration of mechanical ventilation, lower mortality.[18–20] Emphasizing that successful story, other applications were progressively tried with some degree of success: acute pulmonary oedema due to cardiac failure, *de novo* ARF, difficult weaning from invasive ventilation, after surgery in patients at risk of pulmonary complications, and care of the ventilator patient in general ward or emergency room.[21–28] Strong reinforcement for the use of NIV-IPPV came from an increasing number of reports of complications of invasive mechanical ventilation and led to renewed interest in less aggressive, potentially less injurious ventilatory support techniques.[29,30] At the same time small portable ventilators using flow generators (blower, turbine) primarily devised for HMV became available, affording at least comparable if not improved performance compared with ICU ventilators. The advent of algorithms to improve ventilator–patient interaction, especially in case of air leaks, further increased the utility of NIV-IPPV.[31]

## THE PRESENT TIME

### Acute settings

The efficacy of NIV-IPPV has been substantiated over the past 20 years by randomized clinical trials. Based upon these results recommendations can be developed to guide clinicians, even if newer trials will likely modify these in the near future (Box 1.1).

Regardless of the evidence supporting its efficacy in the research setting a number of conditions must be met and important barriers overcome before NIV-IPPV can be used in everyday clinical practice. Results of surveys querying practitioners about their use of NIV and observational studies that document actual utilization in clinical settings can help inform future directions for NIV. There are a few such, peer-reviewed, articles in the literature. The surveys have asked practitioners about their opinions on COPD,[39–41] all patients with ARF[34,42,43] and NIV as a 'ceiling' treatment.[44] Before 2002,[39,40] NIV was available in less than 50 per cent of acute care settings, and the reasons for not using NIV were: lack of equipment due to financial limitations and lack of training. Starting in about 2003, NIV has become available in the majority of hospitals which have been surveyed although marked regional variations in the use of NIV have been found. For example, a large web-based survey collected responses from 2985 intensivists from Europe and the USA (41 per cent in Europe and 19 per cent in the USA).[43] Use of NIV was reported in >25 per cent of cases of ARF by 68 per cent of Europe physicians and 39 per cent of physicians in the USA ($p<0.01$). Sedation was more frequently advocated in the USA than in Europe (41 per cent of respondents compared to 24 per cent, $p<0.01$). The most frequent indications for NIV were COPD exacerbations, heart failure and obesity-hypoventilation. Although surveys can be valuable, a number of shortcomings of such studies need to be pointed out. The reported results are based on only the questionnaires that are returned (which in the studies mentioned above ranged from as high as 100 per cent to as low as 27 per cent), and only reflect limited subsets of healthcare providers. Because surveys report data from individual practitioners and institutions, and are not a randomly chosen sample of all potential respondents, their findings may not be relevant to other clinicians, in different practice settings. And, importantly, these studies can only tell us what the institutions and individuals surveyed say they do, not what they actually do.

Observational studies avoid some of these limitations since they document actual practice in the institutions in which they are performed. The caveats of such studies are that they reflect practice only at the time of the study, for the patients in the cohort and in the clinical setting evaluated. Two such reports are follow-up studies in which more recent NIV use is compared with the results of previous cohorts from the same groups of practitioners.[45–48] They are included in Tables 1.2 and 1.3, which summarize acute-care use of NIV in adult patients, and reported use in the three main disorders in which NIV is commonly used: in acute-on-chronic respiratory failure, congestive heart failure, and hypoxaemic ARF. In Table 1.3 one other observational study is reported.[49] The main findings in these studies were: an increase in NIV use (10.2 per cent to 17 per cent of cases requiring mechanical ventilation); and similar distribution of aetiologies of respiratory failure, primarily in acute-on-chronic failure, and also in ARF. In Table 1.3 the overall failure of NIV (defined as the need for intubation) appears similar across the studies, about 37 per cent. The proportion of patients with acute-on-chronic respiratory failure and ARF treated with NIV is quite similar (about 40 per cent each) but the failure rate is much lower in acute-on-chronic failure (25 per cent) than in ARF (50 per cent). It is important to note that ARF includes many different clinical situations (pneumonia, acute respiratory distress syndrome [ARDS], post-surgical

**Box 1.1 Recommendations for NIV use in clinical settings**

Strong positive evidence from multiple randomized controlled trials:

- exacerbation of COPD[32]
- acute cardiogenic pulmonary oedema[33]
- ARF in immunocompromised patients[32]
- prevention of weaning failure in high-risk patients[34]

Strong negative evidence from multiple randomized controlled trials:

- established extubation failure[34]

Likely positive effect according to case–control series or cohort study and no more than one clinical trial:

- post-operative respiratory failure[35]
- oxygenation prior to endotracheal intubation[36]
- support during endoscopy[37]
- chest trauma[32]

Conflicting findings needing additional studies and clinical trials:

- acute lung injury and acute respiratory distress syndrome[32]
- pneumonia[32]
- extubation failure[34]
- ARF in patients who do not wish to be intubated[34]
- acute severe asthma[38]

**Table 1.2** Epidemiology of mechanical ventilation (MV) and non-invasive ventilation (NIV): multicentre follow-up observational studies conducted with the same methodology in the same environment at 5- and 6-year intervals

| Authors | Study year | MV all | NIV/MV all (%) | Acute-on-chronic (%) | | Cardiogenic pulmonary oedema (%) | | Acute respiratory failure (%) | |
|---|---|---|---|---|---|---|---|---|---|
| | | | | Proportion of all patients on MV | Proportion of patients on NIV | Proportion of all patients on MV | Proportion of patients on NIV | Proportion of all patients on MV | Proportion of patients on NIV |
| Carlucci *et al.*[45] | 1997 | 689 | 16 | 15 | 50 | 7 | 27 | 48 | 14 |
| Demoule *et al.*[46] | 2002 | 1076 | 23 | 16 | 64 | 8 | 43 | 41 | 22 |
| Esteban *et al.*[47] | 1998 | 5183 | 4.4 | 13 | 17 | 10 | NA | 57 | 4 |
| Esteban *et al.*[48] | 2004 | 4968 | 11.1 | 8 | 44 | 6 | NA | 66 | 10 |
| | Before 2000 | 5882 | 10.2 | 14 | 33.5 | 8.5 | NA | 52.5 | 9 |
| | After 2000 | 6044 | 17.5 | 12 | 54 | 7 | NA | 53.5 | 16 |

NA, not applicable.

**Table 1.3** Non-invasive ventilation (NIV) use in respiratory failure and proportion of NIV by cause of respiratory failure

| Authors | Study year | NIV total number | Proportion of NIV use | Acute-on-chronic respiratory failure (%) | | Cardiogenic pulmonary oedema (%) | | Acute respiratory failure (%) | |
|---|---|---|---|---|---|---|---|---|---|
| | | | | Proportion on NIV use | NIV failure | Proportion on NIV | NIV failure | Proportion on NIV | NIV failure |
| Carlucci *et al.*[45] | 1997 | 110 | 40 | 47 | NA | 12 | NA | 42 | NA |
| Demoule *et al.*[46] | 2002 | 247 | 44 | 45 | NA | 15 | NA | 39 | 54 |
| Esteban *et al.*[47] | 1998 | 228 | 31 | 50 | NA | NA | NA | 50 | 37 |
| Esteban *et al.*[48] | 2004 | 551 | 35 | 32 | 26 | NA | NA | 60 | NA |
| Schettino *et al.*[49] | 2001 | 458 | 39 | 27 | 31 | 18 | 16 | 31 | 60 |

NA, not applicable.

respiratory failure) which do not have identical outcomes with NIV. Nevertheless, it is notable that these real-world effectiveness findings roughly confirm those observed in randomized controlled clinical trials in highly selected patients. In addition, data from follow-up studies[45,46] show an increasing use of NIV as the first-line mode for ventilation either before hospital admission (up to 13 per cent of patients receiving mechanical ventilation) or at the time of admission (35 per cent to 52 per cent of patients receiving mechanical ventilation). There are few epidemiological data from observational studies reporting application of NIV as a post-extubation tool,[49] and with NIV as a 'ceiling' approach without the subsequent possibility of invasive ventilation – either at the patient's request (not to be intubated) or as a physician-imposed limitation.

## Home setting

Early limited experience with long-term HMV using either tracheostomy or negative pressure ventilation demonstrated that even patients with essentially no ventilatory function could be continuously supported, whereas individuals who retained partial ventilatory function could benefit from intermittent (e.g. during sleep) ventilatory assistance.[8] Since the 1990s, NIV has progressively obviated the requirement for tracheostomy and has led to the use of long-term HMV in a rapidly growing number of patients.[50] Among home ventilator users are patients presenting with relatively stable neuromuscular diseases or thoracic ventilatory restrictive disorders who gain a long extension of life with quite acceptable quality of life. Although there is no clear benefit in COPD,[51] long-term NIV is frequently prescribed in several countries.[50] In amyotrophic lateral sclerosis (ALS), most notably in those without bulbar involvement, NIV significantly prolongs survival for a few months and improves the quality of life.[52] It is now commonly accepted that in individuals with neuromuscular diseases who become dependent on nearly continuous ventilator assistance, additional techniques to assist coughing are necessary.[53] A large epidemiological survey in Europe has shown an overall incidence of home ventilation use of 10/100 000 people, with huge differences in regional medical practice.[50] Negative pressure ventilation required considerable technical expertise and infrastructure (for example to make custom-built cuirasses, maintain negative pressure ventilators, etc). In the early days of NIV/IPPV there were few masks made by industry, necessitating innovative approaches to customized 'homemade' interfaces, again requiring considerable technical back-up and expertise. These skills were not widely available. Furthermore sleep-disordered breathing was not widely recognized by clinicians. With the increasing recognition of sleep-related abnormalities of breathing and their importance reflected in the training of physicians, the growth of respiratory sleep services and the easy availability of a wide variety of interfaces and ventilators, the provision of home ventilation is now possible from a much wider range of hospitals than was the case in the past. Demand is also rising because of increasing recognition of different groups of patients who might benefit from NIV and improved survival after critical illness but with the patients needing ongoing ventilatory support, and, finally, changes in the population profile, the obesity epidemic and the ageing population. All these factors combined will ensure that NIV will continue to expand in scope, and make its mark as one of the important advances in respiratory medicine in the past 30 years.

## REFERENCES


1. Drinker P, Shaw LA. An apparatus for the prolonged administration of artifical respiration: I. A design for adults and children. *J Clin Invest* 1929; **7**: 229–47.
2. Hodes HL. Treatment of respiratory difficulty in poliomyelitis. In: *Poliomyeliits: papers and discussion presented at the Third International Poliomyelitis Conference.* Philadelphia,1955.
3. Becker LC. *USPHS polio survivors in the US 1915–2000 age distribution data, 2006.* Available at: www.post-polio.org/PolioSurvivorsInTheUS1915-2000.pdf (accessed October 2006).
4. Lassen HCA. The epidemic of poliomyelitis in Copenhagen. *Proc R Soc Med* 1954; **47**: 72–4.
5. Severinghaus JW, Astrup P, Murray JF. Blood gas analysis and critical care medicine. *Am J Respir Crit Care Med* 1998; **157**: 114–22.
6. Murray JF. Review of the state of the art in intermittent positive pressure breathing therapy. *Am Rev Respir Dis* 1974; **110**: 193–9.
7. Splaingard ML, Frates Jr RC, Jefferson LS. Home negative pressure ventilation: report of 20 years of experience in patients with neuromuscular disease. *Arch Phys Med Rehabil* 1985; **66**: 239–42.
8. Robert D, Gerard M, Leger P. Permanent mechanical ventilation at home via a tracheotomy in chronic respiratory insufficiency. *Rev Fr Mal Respir* 1983; **11**: 923–36.
9. Sullivan CR, Berthon-Jones M, Issa FG *et al.* Reversal of obstructive sleep apnea by continuous positive airway pressure applied through the nose. *Lancet* 1981; **i**: 862–5.
10. Ellis ER, Bye PTP, Bruderer JW *et al.* Treatment of respiratory failure during sleep in patients with neuromuscular disease: positive-pressure ventilation through a nose mask. *Am Rev Respir Dis* 1987; **135**: 148–52.
11. Kerby GR, Mayer LS, Pingleton SK. Nocturnal positive-pressure ventilation via nasal mask. *Am Rev Respir Dis* 1987; **135**: 738–40.
12. Bach JR, Alba AS, Mosher R *et al.* Intermittent positive pressure ventilation via nasal access in the management of respiratory insufficiency. *Chest* 1987; **92**: 168–70.

13. Carrol N, Branthwaite MA. Control of nocturnal hypoventilation by nasal intermittent positive pressure ventilation. *Thorax* 1988; **43**: 349–53.
14. Leger P, Jennequin J, Gerard M *et al.* Home positive pressure ventilation via nasal mask for patients with neuromuscular weakness or restrictive lung or chest-wall disease. *Respir Care* 1989; **334**: 73–7.
15. Meduri GU, Conoscenti CC, Menashe P *et al.* Noninvasive face mask ventilation in patients with acute respiratory failure. *Chest* 1989; **95**: 865–70.
16. Brochard L, Isabey D, Piquet J. Reversal of acute exacerbations of chronic obstructive lung disease by inspiratory assistance with a face mask. *N Engl J Med* 1990; **323**: 1523–30.
17. Foglio C, Vitacca M, Quadri A. Acute exacerbations in severe COPD patients. Treatment using positive pressure ventilation by nasal mask. *Chest* 1992; **101**: 1533–8.
18. Bott J, Carroll MP, Conway JH. Randomised controlled trial of nasal ventilation in acute ventilator failure due to chronic obstructive airways disease. *Lancet* 1993; **341**: 1555–7.
19. Brochard L, Mancebo J, Wysocki M. Noninvasive ventilation for acute exacerbations of chronic obstructive pulmonary disease. *N Engl J Med* 1995; **333**: 817–22.
20. Nourdine K, Combes P, Carton MJ. Does noninvasive ventilation reduce the ICU nosocomial infection risk? A prospective clinical survey. *Intensive Care Med* 1999; **25**: 567–73.
21. Mehta S, Jay GD, Woolard RH. Randomized, prospective trial of bilevel versus continuous positive airway pressure in acute pulmonary edema. *Crit Care Med* 1997; **25**: 620–8.
22. Sassoon CSH. Noninvasive positive-pressure ventilation in acute respiratory failure: review of reported experience with special attention to use during weaning. *Respir Care* 1995; **40**: 282–8.
23. Nava S, Ambrosino N, Clini E. Noninvasive mechanical ventilation in the weaning of patients with respiratory failure due to chronic obstructive pulmonary disease: a randomized, controlled trail. *Ann Intern Med* 1998; **128**: 721–8.
24. Joris JL, Sottiuax TM, Chiche JD. Effect of bi-level positive airway pressure nasal ventilation on the postoperative pulmonary restrictive syndrome in obese patients undergoing gastroplasty. *Chest* 1997; **111**: 665–70.
25. Wysocki M, Tric L, Wolff MA. Noninvasive pressure support ventilation in patients with acute respiratory failure. A randomized comparison with conventional therapy. *Chest* 1995; **107**: 761–8.
26. Ferrer M, Esquinas A, Leon M. Noninvasive ventilation in severe hypoxemic respiratory failure: a randomised clinical trial. *Am J Respir Crit Care Med* 2003; **168**: 1438–44.
27. Plant PK, Owen JL, Parrot S. Cost effectiveness of ward based non-invasive ventilation for acute exacerbations of chronic obstructive pulmonary disease: economic analysis of randomized controlled trials. *BMJ* 2003; **326**: 956–60.
28. Craven R, Singletary N, Bosken L. Use of bilevel positive airway pressure in out-of-hospital patients. *Acad Emerg Med* 2000; **7**: 1065–8.
29. Stauffer J, Silvestri RC. Complications of endotracheal intubation, tracheostomy, and artificial airways. *Respir Care* 1982; **27**: 417–34.
30. Tremblay LN, Slutsky AS. Ventilator-induced lung injury: from the bench to the bedside. *Intensive Care Med* 2006; **32**: 24–33.
31. Lofaso F, Brochard L, Hang T. Home versus intensive care pressure support devices. Experimental and clinical comparison. *Am J Respir Crit Care Med* 1996; **153**: 1591–9.
32. Keenan SP, Mehta S. Noninvasive ventilation for patients presenting with acute respiratory failure: The randomized controlled trials. *Respir Care* 2009; **54**: 116–24.
33. Peter JV, Moran JL, Phillips-Huges J. Effect of non-invasive positive pressure ventilation on mortality in patients with acute cardiogenic pulmonary edema: a meta-analysis. *Lancet* 2006; **367**: 1155–63.
34. Burns KE, Adhikari NK, Meade MO. A meta-analysis of noninvasive weaning to facilitate liberation from mechanical ventilation. *Can J Anesth* 2006; **53**: 305–15.
35. Jaber S, Delay JM, Chanques G. Outcomes of patients with acute respiratory failure after abdominal surgery treated with noninvasive positive pressure ventilation. *Chest* 2005; **128**: 2688–95.
36. Baillard C, Fosse JP, Sebbane M. Noninvasive ventilation improves preoxygenation before intubation of hypoxic patients. *Am J Respir Crit Care Med* 2006; **174**: 171–7.
37. Antonelli M, Conti G, Rocco M. Noninvasive positive-pressure ventilation vs conventional oxygen supplementation in hypoxemic patients undergoing diagnostic bronchoscopy. *Chest* 2002; **121**: 1149–54.
38. Medoff BD. Invasive and noninvasive ventilation in patients with asthma. *Respir Care* 2008; **53**: 740–8.
39. Doherty MJ, Greenstone MA. Survey of non-invasive ventilation (NIPPV) in patients with acute exacerbations of chronic obstructive pulmonary disease (COPD) in the UK. *Thorax* 1998; **53**: 863–6.
40. Vanpee D, Delaunois L, Lheureux P. Survey of non-invasive ventilation for acute exacerbation of chronic obstructive pulmonary disease patients in emergency departments in Belgium. *Eur J Emerg Med* 2002; **9**: 217–24.
41. Drummond J, Rowe B, Cheung L. The use of noninvasive mechanical ventilation for the treatment of acute exacerbations of chronic obstructive pulmonary disease in Canada. *Can Respir J* 2005; **12**: 129–33, 135.
42. Maheshwari V, Paioli D, Rothaar R. Utilization of noninvasive ventilation in acute-care hospitals: a regional survey. *Chest* 2006; **129**: 1226–33.
43. Devlin JW, Nava S, Fong JJ. Survey of sedation practices during noninvasive positive-pressure ventilation to treat acute respiratory failure. *Crit Care Med* 2007; **35**: 2298–302.
44. Sinuff T, Cook DJ, Keenan SP. Noninvasive ventilation for acute respiratory failure near the end of life. *Crit Care Med* 2008; **36**: 789–94.

45. Carlucci A, Richard JC, Wysocki M. SRLF collaborative group on mechanical ventilation. Noninvasive versus conventional mechanical ventilation: an epidemiologic survey. *Am J Respir Crit Care Med* 2001; **163**: 874–80.
46. Demoule A, Girou E, Richard JC. Increased use of noninvasive ventilation in French intensive care units. *Intensive Care Med* 2006; **32**: 1747–55.
47. Esteban A, Anzueto A, Frutos F. For the mechanical ventilation international study group. Characteristics and outcomes in adult patients receiving mechanical ventilation. *JAMA* 2002; **287**: 345–55.
48. Esteban A, Ferguson ND, Meade MO. VENTILA Group. Evaluation of mechanical ventilation in response to clinical research. *Am J Respir Crit Care Med* 2008; **177**: 170–7.
49. Schettino G, Altobelli N, Kacmarek RM. Noninvasive positive-pressure ventilation in acute respiratory failure outside clinical trials: experience at the Massachusetts General Hospital. *Crit Care Med* 2008; **36**: 441–7.
50. Lloyd-Owen SJ, Donaldson GC, Ambrosino N *et al.* Patterns of home mechanical ventilation use in Europe: results from the Eurovent survey. *Eur Respir J* 2005; **25**: 1025–31.
51. Wijkstra PJ, Lacasse Y, Guyatt GH *et al.* A meta-analysis of nocturnal noninvasive positive pressure ventilation in patients with stable COPD. *Chest* 2003; **124**: 337–43.
52. Bourke SC, Bullock RE, Williams TL *et al.* Noninvasive ventilation in ALS: indications and effect on quality of life. *Neurology* 2003; **61**: 171–7.
53. International Consensus Conferences in Intensive Care Medicine: noninvasive positive pressure ventilation in acute respiratory failure. *Am J Respir Crit Care Med* 2001; **163**: 283–91.

# SECTION A

# The equipment

# 2

# Positive pressure ventilators

DEAN R HESS

## ABSTRACT

Although any ventilator can be used for non-invasive ventilation (NIV), increasingly ventilators are used that are designed specifically for NIV. Bi-level ventilators are designed specifically for NIV. Intermediate and critical care ventilators increasingly have modes designed specifically for NIV. Bi-level ventilators use a single-limb circuit with a passive exhalation port. This configuration has the potential for rebreathing if the expiratory pressure is set too low. An issue that must be dealt with during NIV is leaks; ventilators for NIV have a variety of features to compensate for leaks and some do this better than others. A number of modes can be used with NIV, and there are advantages and disadvantages of each. Alarms must balance patient safety against annoyance. Ventilators for NIV can be battery powered for safety and increased portability.

## INTRODUCTION

Any ventilator can be attached to a mask or other interface for non-invasive ventilation (NIV), but it is desirable to use one designed specifically for NIV (Box 2.1).[1,2] In this chapter, features of ventilators for NIV will be described. Because there are many different ventilators designed specifically, or in part, for NIV, and because the technical features of these ventilators are constantly changing, a generic approach will be presented.

**Box 2.1 Considerations in the selection of a ventilator for NIV**

- Leak compensation
- Trigger and cycle coupled to patient's breathing pattern
- Rebreathing
- Oxygen delivery (acute care)
- Monitoring
- Alarms (safety vs nuisance)
- Portability (size, weight, battery)
- Tamper-proof
- Cost

## CIRCUITS AND VENTILATORS

### Circuits

For critical care ventilators, dual-limb circuits are used, and these have inspiratory and expiratory valves (Fig. 2.1). The expiratory valve actively closes during the inspiratory phase and the inspiratory valve closes during the expiratory phase. There are separate hoses for the inspiratory gas and the expiratory gas. In this configuration, there is segregation of the inspiratory and expiratory gases. In modern critical care ventilators, the exhalation valve is usually incorporated into the ventilator. For intermediate ventilators (Fig. 2.1), a single-limb circuit is used with an exhalation valve near the patient. The expiratory valve is actively closed during the inspiratory phase to prevent loss of delivered tidal volume. During exhalation, the expiratory valve opens and the inspiratory valve is closed. Because the expiratory valve is near the patient, rebreathing is minimized. For bi-level ventilators, a single-limb circuit is used (Fig. 2.1). A leak port, which serves as a passive exhalation port for the patient, is incorporated into the circuit near the patient or into the interface.

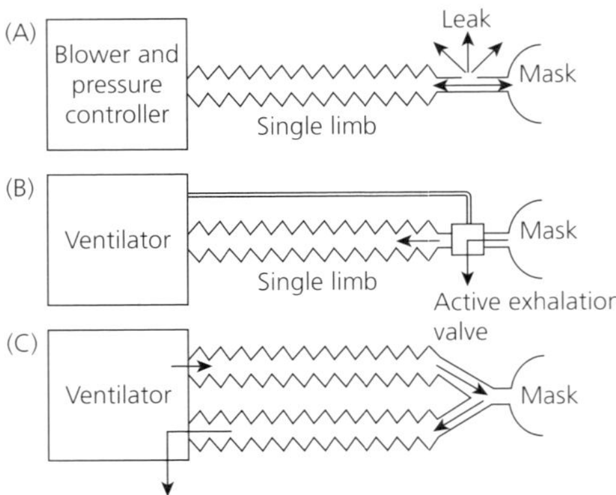


**Figure 2.1** Circuits used with ventilators for non-invasive ventilation. (A) Single-limb circuit with passive exhalation port, such as that used with bi-level ventilators. (B) Single-limb circuit with active exhalation valve, such as that used with intermediate ventilators. (C) Dual-limb circuit with active exhalation valve, such as that used with critical care ventilators.

## Bi-level ventilators

These are blower devices that typically provide pressure support or pressure control ventilation. Pressure applied to the airway is a function of flow and leak. For a given leak, more flow is generated if the pressure setting is increased. They use a single-limb circuit with a passive exhalation port. For a given pressure setting, more flow is required if the leak increases. Some modern bi-level ventilators can generate inspiratory pressures as high as 30–50 cm $H_2O$ and flows >200 L/min. Evaluations of the performance of these ventilators have found that many perform satisfactorily. In terms of gas delivery, some perform as well or better than sophisticated critical care ventilators.[3–13] However, the studies have also shown that the behaviour of bi-level ventilators is variable in response to different simulated efforts and air leaks and this is unpredictable from the operating principles reported in the manufacturers' descriptions. This may be an issue during paediatric applications of NIV.[14] Most of these evaluations have been bench studies, and some caution is necessary in extrapolating such data to the clinical setting.

## Intermediate ventilators

These ventilators are typically used for patient transport or home care ventilation. Many use a single-limb circuit with an active exhalation valve near the patient. Early studies of nocturnal NIV in patients with neuromuscular disease often used these ventilators.[15] Newer generations of these ventilators provide volume controlled, pressure controlled and pressure support ventilation. They vary in their ability to compensate for leaks; some compensate well and some not at all. Some have internal batteries.

## Critical care ventilators

These are sophisticated ventilators with a variety of modes and alarms. They are designed primarily for invasive ventilation, but can be used for NIV. Some early reports of the use of NIV for acute respiratory failure used only critical care ventilators.[16] An issue with the use of critical care ventilators for NIV is that many are leak intolerant, although newer generations feature NIV modes and some compensate well for leaks.[17,18]

## Rebreathing

An issue of concern with the bi-level ventilators is the potential for rebreathing. If the expiratory flow of the patient exceeds the flow capacity of the leak port, it is possible to exhale into the single-limb circuit and rebreathe on the subsequent inhalation. Ferguson and Gilmartin[19] reported that a bi-level positive airway pressure (BiPAP) ventilator configured with the standard passive leak port resulted in no change in $PaCO_2$ in hypercapnic patients. When the ventilator was configured with a valve to minimize rebreathing (e.g. plateau exhalation valve) the $PaCO_2$ decrease was similar to that with a critical care ventilator. Lofaso *et al.*[10,20] reported that, compared with a critical care ventilator, a bi-level ventilator with passive exhalation port was associated with a greater tidal volume, minute ventilation, and work of breathing. Patel and Petrini,[21] however, found no differences in work of breathing, respiratory rate, minute ventilation, or $PaCO_2$ between a bi-level ventilator and a critical care ventilator. This finding is probably related to the higher pressures use by Patel and Petrini[21] compared with Lofaso *et al.*[20]

Although there is a potential for rebreathing with bi-level ventilators, there are several steps that can be taken to minimize that risk. Rebreathing is decreased if the leak port is in the mask rather than the hose,[22,23] if oxygen is titrated into the mask rather than into the hose,[24] with a higher expiratory pressure,[19] and with a plateau exhalation valve.[19] Major determinants of rebreathing are the expiratory time and the flow through the circuit during exhalation. Increasing the expiratory pressure requires greater flow and thus decreases the amount of rebreathing. Thus, the minimum expiratory pressure setting on many bi-level ventilators is 4 cm $H_2O$. Opening the ports on the interface increases leak, which increases the flow through the hose and flushes the hose to decrease rebreathing. Although it effectively decreases rebreathing, the plateau exhalation valve may increase the imposed expiratory resistance.[10] In a study by Hill *et al.*,[25] the plateau exhalation valve was compared with a traditional leak port in seven patients during nocturnal nasal ventilation. The plateau exhalation valve did not improve daytime or nocturnal gas exchange or symptoms compared with a traditional leak port. A nasal mask was used in that study and it is unknown whether the results are applicable to patients using an oronasal mask. Patients found the plateau exhalation valve noisier and less attractive in appearance than the traditional leak port.

## Leak

Ventilators have traditionally been leak intolerant, but leaks are a reality with NIV. The function of bi-level ventilators depends on the presence of a leak. Leaks comprise an intentional leak through the passive exhalation port as well as any unintentional leaks that may be present in the circuit or at the interface. At end-exhalation, the total flow in the patient circuit equals the intentional leak as well as any additional leak related to a poorly fitting interface. If the inhaled tidal volume is greater than the exhaled measured tidal volume, the difference is assumed to be due to unintentional leak. However, the ventilator will underestimate the actual tidal volume if unintentional leak occurs during exhalation.

Some bi-level ventilators allow the user to enter the interface that will used to allow more precise identification of the intentional leak. This approach, however, requires the use of an interface provided by the manufacturer of the ventilator. Other bi-level ventilators allow the user to test the leak port as part of the pre-use procedure. Leak-detection algorithms must adjust for changes in leak with inspiratory and expiratory pressure changes, as well as changes that may occur breath-to-breath due to fit of the interface. Newer generations of bi-level ventilators use redundant leak estimation algorithms. A conservation of mass algorithm computes the average leak for a given pressure and is used when large leak variations are present in the system. A better leak estimate is the parabolic leak algorithm, in which the leak is proportional to the square of the patient pressure, thus adjusting leak estimate to the changing patient pressure.

## Trigger

If the leak is great, the patient may breathe from the leak rather than producing a flow or pressure change that will trigger the start of the breath. On the other hand, the leak could produce a pressure or flow drop that produces auto-trigger. The ability of the ventilator to compensate for leaks thus has an important effect on triggering.

Triggers have traditionally assessed a pressure change or flow change at the proximal airway. Some ventilators are volume triggered, which is a variation on flow triggering. For example, with the Respironics bi-level ventilators, the inspiratory phase is triggered when patient effort generates an inspiratory flow, causing 6 mL of volume to accumulate. The Respironics bi-level ventilators also use a technique called Auto-Trak, in which a shape signal is created by offsetting the actual patient flow by 15 L/min and delaying it for a 300 ms period (Fig. 2.2). A change in patient flow will cross the shape signal, causing the ventilator to trigger to inspiration (or cycle to exhalation). On some ventilators, such as the Respironics bi-level ventilators, the user cannot adjust the trigger sensitivity. On the ResMed bi-level ventilators, the user can choose trigger settings of HI (high), MED (medium) and LO (low), which relate to flow triggers of 2.5 L/min, 4.0 L/min, and 7.5 L/min, respectively. Some use redundant triggering mechanisms to improve sensitivity.

In eight patients recovering from chronic obstructive pulmonary disease (COPD) exacerbations and receiving NIV, Nava *et al.*[26] compared flow triggering and pressure triggering. Minute ventilation, respiratory pattern, dynamic lung compliance and resistance, and changes in end-expiratory lung volume were the same with the two triggering systems. The oesophageal pressure drop during the pre-triggering phase (due to auto-positive end-expiratory pressure [PEEP] and valve opening) was higher with pressure triggering than with flow triggering. Auto-PEEP was lower during flow triggering in the pressure support mode. This not only suggests a benefit from flow triggering but also that triggering issues may often be related to the presence of auto-PEEP.

Borel *et al.*[27] reported that the level of intentional leak in seven commercially available masks ranged from 30 L/min

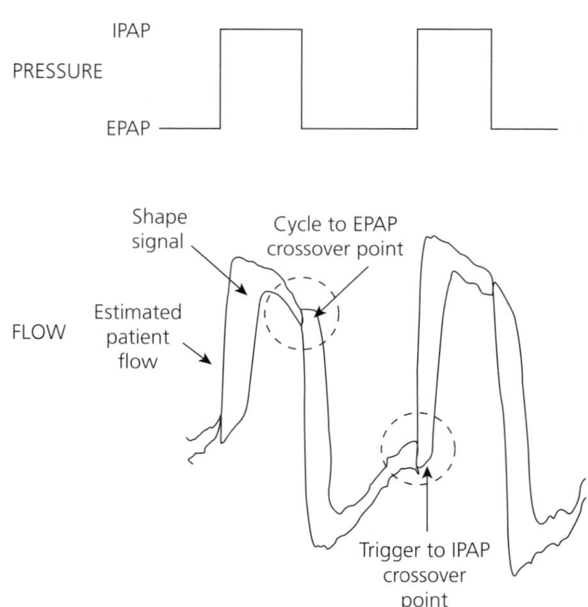


**Figure 2.2** The shape signal used for triggering and cycling with Respironics bi-level ventilators is created by offsetting the signal from the actual patient flow by 15 L/min and delaying it for 300 ms. This intentional delay causes the shape signal to be slightly behind the patient's flow rate. A sudden change in patient flow will cross the shape signal, causing the ventilator to trigger to inspiration or cycle to exhalation. Courtesy of Respironics. EPAP, expiratory positive airway pressure; IPAP, inspiratory positive airway pressure.

to 45 L/min at a pressure of 14 cm $H_2O$, which did not affect the trigger performance of bi-level ventilators. Miyoshi *et al.*[28] reported that bi-level ventilators triggered properly at all levels of unintentional leak (as much as 44 L/min), but uncontrollable auto-triggering occurred in the critical care ventilator when the gas leak was >18 L/min. Others have also reported a tendency for auto-triggering in the presence of leak.[29] Using a lung model, Ferreira *et al.*[17] evaluated the ability of nine critical care ventilators in NIV mode and a bi-level ventilator to function in the presence of leaks. Most ventilators were able to adapt to an increase in the leak to 10 L/min without adjustments, but two of the critical care ventilators auto-triggered when the leak was increased, requiring changes in trigger sensitivity to achieve synchrony. At leaks of as great as 37 L/min, one critical care ventilator and the bi-level ventilators were able to adapt without adjustments. At leaks of 27 L/min and 37 L/min, some the critical care ventilators were unable to synchronize despite changes in trigger sensitivity. Vignaux *et al.*[18] conducted a lung model evaluation of critical care ventilators in NIV mode and found that leaks affected triggering, with marked variations among ventilators.

With neurally adjusted ventilatory assistance (NAVA), the ventilator is triggered by electrical activity of a diaphragm.[30] The electrical activity of the diaphragm is measured by a multiple-array oesophageal electrode, which is amplified to determine the support level (NAVA gain). The cycle-off is commonly set at 80 per cent of peak inspiratory activity. Because the trigger is based on diaphragmatic activity rather than pressure or flow, triggering is not adversely affected in patients with auto-PEEP or large leaks during NIV. It remains to be determined whether this approach will prove useful during NIV. A major drawback to this approach is the need for an oesophageal catheter with the electrodes to measure diaphragmatic activity.

## Tidal volume

Pressure controlled or pressure support ventilation will compensate for leaks better than volume controlled ventilation. With volume control, flow and volume delivery from the ventilator are fixed. Thus, any leak will reduce the inhaled tidal volume. A technique that can be used, with variable success, is to increase the tidal volume setting. However, this is variably successful because increasing the set tidal volume (and the associated pressure in the interface) may increase the leak. The ventilator targets a constant inspiratory pressure for pressure controlled or pressure support ventilation. If a leak occurs, there will be a drop in pressure, at which point the ventilator increases flow to restore the pressure.

In a lung model with leak, Smith and Shneerson[12] reported that the volume delivery of volume controlled ventilators fell by >50 per cent over most of the range of pre-set volumes. This decrease in tidal volume was associated with a fall in pressure of a similar magnitude. However, pressure control and pressure support compensated well for the leak. Mehta *et al.*[29] evaluated the leak compensating abilities of six different ventilators used for NIV in a lung model. Similar to Smith and Shneerson, they found that pressure control and pressure support maintained delivered tidal volume in the presence of leaks better than volume control. Borel *et al.*[26] found that the capacity of bi-level ventilators to achieve and maintain inspiratory positive airway pressure (IPAP) was decreased when intentional leaks increased, but maximum reduction in delivered tidal volume was only 48 mL.

## Cycle

During volume- and pressure-controlled ventilation, the inspiratory phase is time cycled. For these breath types, the presence of a leak will not affect the inspiratory time. However, pressure support is usually flow cycled. If the leak flow is greater than the flow cycle criteria, the inspiratory phase will continue indefinitely.[31] Usually there is a secondary time cycle should this occur, which is fixed on some ventilators (e.g. 3 seconds) but adjustable on others.

If the inspiratory time is prolonged, expiratory time may be shortened, resulting in auto-PEEP. The presence of auto-PEEP makes triggering more difficult. If the patient fails to trigger, expiratory time will be prolonged, the amount of auto-PEEP decreases, and the patient is then able to trigger. The result is variability in the respiratory rate provided by the ventilator. If auto-PEEP increases, the delivered tidal volume for a fixed pressure support setting is less. This results in variability in tidal volume delivery. Hotchkiss *et al.*[32,33] used a mathematical and lung model to explore the issue of leak on ventilator performance. They found that pressure support applied in the context of an inspiratory leak resulted in substantial breath-to-breath variation in the inspiratory phase, resulting in auto-PEEP if the respiratory rate was fixed, or in variability in respiratory rate, inspiratory time and auto-PEEP if the rate was allowed to vary. This was most likely to occur when the respiratory system time constant was long relative to the respiratory rate, as occurs in patients with COPD. A lung model study by Adams *et al.*[34] predicted a relatively narrow range for inspiratory flow cycle that provides adequate ventilatory support without causing hyper-inflation in patients with COPD.

Using an older-generation bi-level ventilator, Mehta *et al.*[29] reported that a large leak interfered with cycling of the ventilator and shortening the expiratory time. Calderini *et al.*[35] compared the effect of time cycled and flow cycled breaths in six patients during NIV. In the presence of leaks, they found that time-cycled breaths provided better synchrony than flow-cycled breaths. Borel *et al.*[27] found that expiratory cycling was not affected by the level of intentional leaks in masks except in COPD conditions. However, Battisti *et al.*[11] reported delayed cycling in the presence of leaks with bi-level ventilators.

Several strategies can be used to address the issue of prolonged inspiration with pressure support. Unintentional leaks should be minimized and use of a ventilator with good leak compensation is ideal. Some bi-level ventilators use redundant measures to determine end of inspiration. For example, the Respironics bi-level ventilators use the shape signal (Fig. 2.2) and a method called spontaneous expiratory threshold. The spontaneous expiratory thres-hold is an electronic signal that rises in proportion to the inspiratory flow rate on each breath; when the spontaneous expiratory threshold and actual patient flow value are equal, the unit cycles to exhalation. The maximum inspiratory time is adjustable on some ventilators and some ventilators allow the flow cycle criteria to be adjusted. Note that the effect of a higher flow cycle as a percentage of peak inspiratory flow translates to a shorter inspiratory time (Fig. 2.3).

## Oxygen delivery

For acute care applications, it is desirable to use a ventilator with a blender allowing precise administration of the fraction of inspired oxygen ($FiO_2$) from 0.21 to 1. Bi-level ventilators used outside the acute care setting generally do not have a blender, but rather provide supplemental oxygen by titration into the circuit or interface. This results in a delivered oxygen concentration that is variable, and only modest concentrations can be achieved (e.g. <60 per cent). With oxygen titration, the $FiO_2$ is affected by the site of the oxygen titration, type of exhalation port, ventilator settings, oxygen flow, breathing pattern and leak. For some bi-level ventilators, oxygen titration can affect the displayed values of tidal volume.

Waugh and Granger[36] reported that with a bi-level ventilator and the leak port in the mask, the $FiO_2$ was higher when oxygen was added at the ventilator outlet instead of the mask and with lower IPAP and expiratory positive airway pressure (EPAP) settings. Thys *et al.*[24] reported that the $FiO_2$ was higher with lower IPAP and when oxygen was added at the mask than when added at the ventilator outlet. They also found that, although the $FiO_2$ was increased with a higher oxygen flow, it was difficult to obtain an $FiO_2$ >0.30 without a very high oxygen flow. Schwartz *et al.*[37] reported that the oxygen concentration was significantly lower with the leak port into the mask, with higher IPAP and EPAP settings, and with lower oxygen flow. With the mask leak port, the oxygen concentration was greater when oxygen was added into the circuit than into the mask, presumably because in the latter much of the oxygen was exhausted out the exhalation port because of the close proximity of the oxygen entrainment site to the port. The highest oxygen concentration was achieved with the leak port in the circuit and oxygen added into the mask using lower IPAP and EPAP values. With a large unintentional leak, Miyoshi *et al.*[28] reported a reduction in $FiO_2$ with a bi-level ventilator and oxygen titration into the circuit. Titration of oxygen into the circuit or interface may affect the monitored values of tidal volume, and high flows (>15 L/min) have the potential to affect ventilator performance.

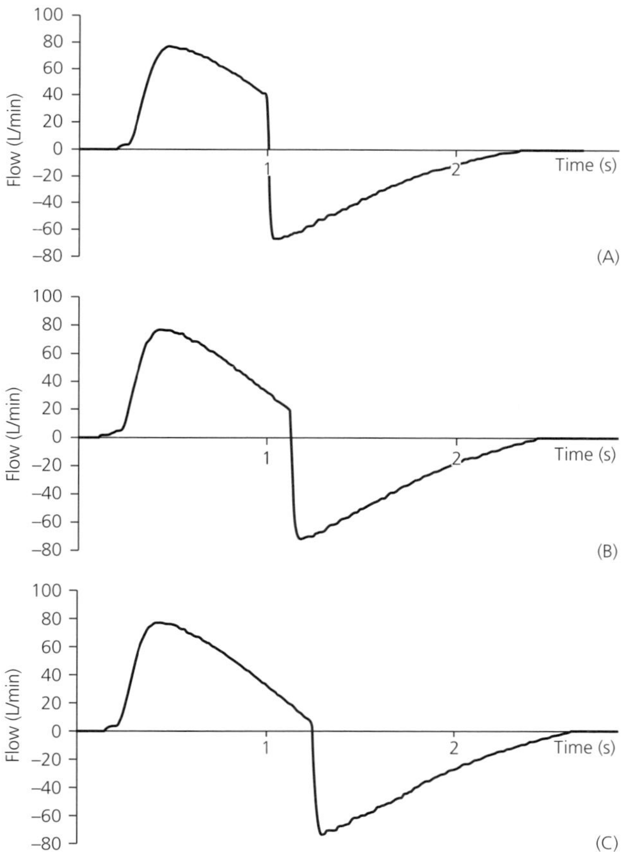


**Figure 2.3** The effect of flow cycle adjustment on the inspiratory time. Note that a higher flow cycle shortens the inspiratory time. A. Flow cycle at 50% of peak inspiratory flow. B. Flow cycle at 25% of peak inspiratory flow. C. Flow cycle at 10% of peak inspiratory flow.

# MODES

## Continuous positive airway pressure

With continuous positive airway pressure (CPAP), no additional pressure is applied during inhalation to assist with delivery of the tidal volume (Fig. 2.4). With NIV, pressure applied to the airway during the inspiratory phase is greater than the pressure applied during exhalation. This provides respiratory muscle assistance, resulting in respiratory muscle unloading and increased tidal volume delivery in proportion to the amount of pressure assist.

## Pressure support ventilation

Pressure support ventilation is used most commonly for NIV.[38,39] With a critical care ventilator, the level of pressure

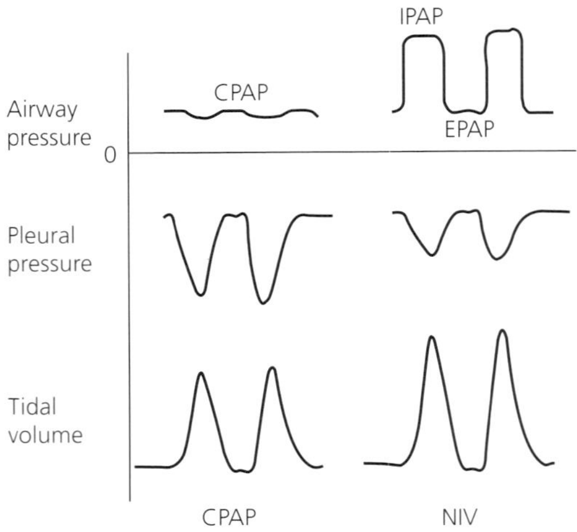


**Figure 2.4** Comparison of continuous positive airway pressure (CPAP) and non-invasive ventilation (NIV). Note that no inspiratory support is provided with CPAP. EPAP, expiratory positive airway pressure; IPAP, inspiratory positive airway pressure.

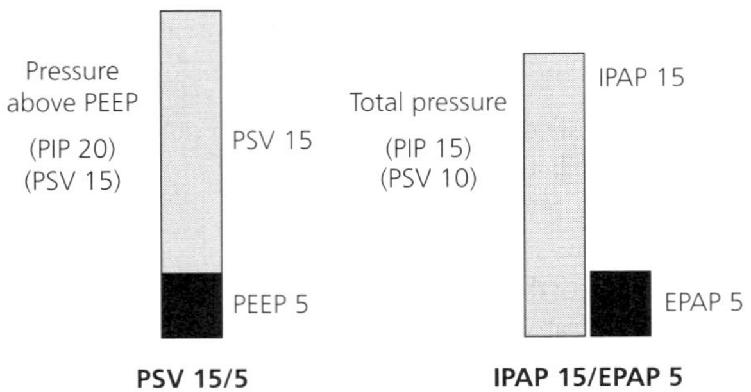


**Figure 2.5** Comparison of pressure support ventilation (PSV), such as with critical care ventilators, and inspiratory positive airway pressure (IPAP) with a bi-level ventilator. Note that the IPAP is the peak inspiratory pressure (PIP) and includes the expiratory positive airway pressure (EPAP), whereas pressure support is provided on top of the positive end-expiratory pressure (PEEP).

support is applied as a pressure above the baseline PEEP. However, the approach is different with bi-level ventilators, where an IPAP and EPAP are set. In this configuration, the difference between the IPAP and EPAP is the level of pressure support (Fig. 2.5). With pressure support, the pressure applied to the airway is fixed for each breath, but there is no back-up rate or fixed inspiratory time (Table 2.1).

Rise time (pressurization rate) is the time required to reach the inspiratory pressure at the onset of the inspiratory phase with pressure support or pressure controlled ventilation.[31] With a fast rise time, the inspiratory pressure is reached quickly, whereas with a slow rise time it takes longer to reach the inspiratory pressure. Rise time has been shown to vary greatly among bi-level ventilators.[3,11] A faster rise time may better unload the respiratory muscles of patients with COPD, but this may be accompanied by substantial air leaks and poor tolerance.[40] In patients with neuromuscular disease, a slower rise time is often better tolerated. Rise time should be set to maximize patient comfort.

In 16 patients with acute respiratory failure, Girault *et al.*[41] reported that both pressure support and volume control provided respiratory muscle rest and similarly improved breathing pattern and gas exchange. These physiologic effects were achieved with a lower inspiratory work load, but at a higher respiratory discomfort, with volume control than with pressure support. Navalesi *et al.*[42] compared pressure support and pressure control in 26 patients with chronic hypercapnic respiratory failure. Compared with spontaneous breathing, NIV provided better ventilation and gas exchange irrespective of the ventilator mode. There were no differences between modes in tolerance of ventilation, gas exchange or breathing pattern. In patients with stable cystic fibrosis, Fauroux *et al.*[43] found that both pressure support and volume control decreased respiratory muscle unloading.

In the spontaneous mode on bi-level ventilators, IPAP and EPAP are set, but there is no back-up rate. With the spontaneous/timed mode, the patient receives pressure support ventilation if the rate is greater than the set rate. However, if the patient becomes apnoeic, the ventilator will deliver flow-cycled or time-cycled breaths at the rate set on the ventilator. For critical care ventilators set for pressure support, back-up ventilation and alarms occur if the patient becomes apnoeic. A back-up rate is important to prevent periodic breathing. Central apnoea was found to be more prevalent with pressure support in normal subjects using a nasal mask,[44] in intubated patients[45] and in patients being evaluated in an outpat-ient sleep laboratory.[46] For these reasons, a back-up rate is recommended during NIV, particularly with nocturnal applications.

**Table 2.1** Comparison of various breath types that can be used during non-invasive ventilation

| | Volume controlled ventilation | Pressure controlled ventilation | Pressure support ventilation | Proportional assist ventilation |
|---|---|---|---|---|
| Tidal volume | Fixed | Variable | Variable | Variable |
| Inspiratory flow | Fixed | Variable | Variable | Variable |
| Airway pressure | Variable | Fixed | Fixed | Variable |
| Inspiratory time | Fixed | Fixed | Variable | Variable |
| Rate | Minimum set | Minimum set | Not set | Not set |

## Pressure controlled ventilation

Pressure controlled ventilation is similar to pressure support, in that the ventilator applies a fixed level of support with each breath. Trigger and rise time are similar between pressure support and pressure control,[47] but there are two differences between the two: there is a back-up rate with pressure control, and the inspiratory time is fixed with pressure control. The back-up rate is beneficial in the setting of apnoea or periodic breathing. The fixed inspiratory time of pressure control is beneficial when the inspiratory phase is prolonged during pressure support due to leak or lung mechanics (e.g. COPD).[32,34] Vitacca *et al.*[48] found no difference in NIV success between volume control and pressure control. Schonhofer *et al.*[49] found that pressure control was successful in the most patients after an initial treatment with volume control. However, a third of the patients who initially did well on volume control failed on pressure control. In chronic stable patients with neuromuscular disease, Chadda *et al.*[50] found that volume control, pressure control and pressure support had similar effects on alveolar ventilation and respiratory muscle unloading. Kirakli *et al.*[51] randomized 35 hypercapnic patients with COPD to 1 hour of pressure support or pressure control. They found that pressure control was as effective and safe as pressure support in carbon dioxide elimination with comparable side effects.

Some bi-level ventilators have a timed mode. With this mode, the ventilator is triggered and cycled by the ventilator at the set rate and inspiratory time. This mode provides little interaction between the patient and the ventilator.

## Proportional assist ventilation

With proportional assist ventilation (PAV), the applied pressure is determined by respiratory drive (i.e. inspiratory flow and tidal volume) and lung mechanics (i.e. resistance and compliance) and the proportion of assist is set by the user. Because respiratory drive varies breath-by-breath and within the breath, the pressure assist also varies. With PAV, there is no back-up rate or set tidal volume (Table 2.1). Proportional assist ventilation has been used effectively with NIV and may improve patient tolerance during acute respiratory failure.[52–55] In patients with chronic respiratory failure due to neuromuscular disease and chest wall deformity, PAV with NIV may also improve patient comfort.[56–58] PAV may also improve sleep quality.[59] It is unclear whether PAV with NIV improves patient outcomes in both acute and chronic care settings.

## Volume controlled ventilation

With volume controlled ventilation, the ventilator delivers a fixed tidal volume and inspiratory flow with each breath (Table 2.2). Usually, the inspiratory time is a function of the tidal volume, inspiratory flow and inspiratory flow pattern selected. However, some ventilators allow tidal volume, inspiratory flow and inspiratory time to be selected independent of one another.

**Table 2.2** Comparison of volume ventilator and bi-level pressure ventilator for non-invasive ventilation (NIV)

| Volume ventilator | Pressure ventilator |
|---|---|
| More complicated to use | Simple to use |
| Wide range of alarms | Limited alarms |
| Constant tidal volume | Variable tidal volume |
| Breath-stacking possible | Breath-stacking not possible |
| No leak compensation | Leak compensation |
| Can be used without positive end-expiratory pressure (PEEP) | PEEP (expiratory positive airway pressure) always present |
| Rebreathing minimized | Rebreathing possible |

Volume control has been used during NIV primarily in the home setting with an intermediate ventilator.[15,60–63] NIV with volume control uses a non-vented interface. It has also been used to provide mouthpiece ventilation.[64–66] A low-pressure alarm is prevented during mouthpiece ventilation by producing enough circuit back pressure with sufficient peak inspiratory flow against the restrictive mouthpiece according to the set tidal volume.[67,68] The ventilator rate is also set at a low level to prevent an apnoea alarm. Breath-stacking manoeuvres can be provided with volume controlled, but not pressure controlled or pressure support ventilation.

## Average volume-assured pressure support and adaptive servo-ventilation

Average volume-assured pressure support (AVAPS) is a feature available on the latest generation of Respironics bi-level ventilators. It maintains a tidal volume equal to or greater than the target tidal volume by automatically controlling the pressure support between the minimum and maximum IPAP settings. The AVAPS averages tidal volume over time and changes the IPAP gradually over several minutes. If patient effort decreases, AVAPS automatically increases IPAP to maintain the target tidal volume. On the other hand, if patient effort increases, AVAPS will reduce IPAP. AVAPS functions much like adaptive support modes such as volume support.

A feature on the ResMed bi-level ventilator is adaptive servo-ventilation (adapt SV). With adapt SV, the algorithm uses three factors to achieve synchronization between pressure support and the patient's breathing: the patient's average respiratory rate; the direction, magnitude and rate of change of the patient's airflow; and a back-up respiratory rate of 15 breaths/min. When central apnoea/hypopnoea occurs, support initially continues to reflect the patient's breathing pattern. If apnoea/hypopnoea persists, the ventilator uses the back-up respiratory rate. When breathing resumes and ventilation exceeds the target, pressure support is reduced to the minimum of 3 cm $H_2O$.

## VENTILATOR OPTIONS TO IMPROVE TOLERANCE

In addition to selection of an appropriate mode, trigger, rise time and expiratory cycle, two other features incorporated into bi-level ventilators to improve patient tolerance are ramp and Bi-Flex.

### Ramp

Ramp reduces the pressure and then gradually increases it to the pressure setting. A ramp has been used primarily in patients receiving CPAP for sleep apnoea to allow the patient to fall asleep more comfortably. The role of a Ramp during NIV is unclear, particularly for acute care applications, where it may be undesirable because it delays application of a therapeutic pressure.

### Bi-Flex

A feature on the Respironics bi-level ventilators, Bi-Flex, inserts a small amount of pressure relief during the later stages of inspiration and the beginning part of exhalation (Fig. 2.6). This feature, when used with CPAP in patients with sleep apnoea, was associated with similar outcomes to standard CPAP, but those with low compliance improved their adherence with this feature.[69] Evidence supporting the use of Bi-Flex with NIV is lacking.

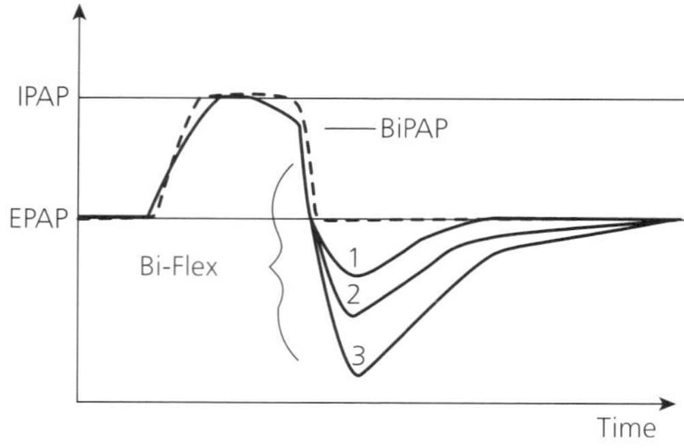


**Figure 2.6** Bi-Flex inserts a small pressure relief during the later stages of inspiration and at the beginning of exhalation. BiPAP, bi-level positive airway pressure; EPAP, expiratory positive airway pressure; IPAP, inspiratory positive airway pressure.

## SAFETY

### Alarms and monitoring

Alarms during NIV are a balance between patient safety and annoyance. The extent of alarms necessary depends on the underlying condition of the patient and the ability of the patient to breathe without support. For example, consider the patient with neuromuscular disease receiving near full support by NIV. This patient is unable to reattach the interface or circuit should it become disconnected. In this case, disconnect alarms and alarms indicating large leaks or changes in ventilation are desirable. Similar alarms are desirable in a patient with acute respiratory failure receiving NIV. On the other extreme, in the case of a patient using daytime mouthpiece ventilation, alarms may be an annoyance and techniques have been described to outsmart these alarms.[68] When a question of the extent of alarms is necessary, one should fault on the side of patient safety. Ventilators for NIV have increasing capability to monitor the patient's breathing. Display of tidal volume, respiratory rate and leak is useful for titrating settings. Many ventilators also display waveforms of pressure, flow and volume. These waveforms can be useful in titrating settings to improve patient–ventilator synchrony.

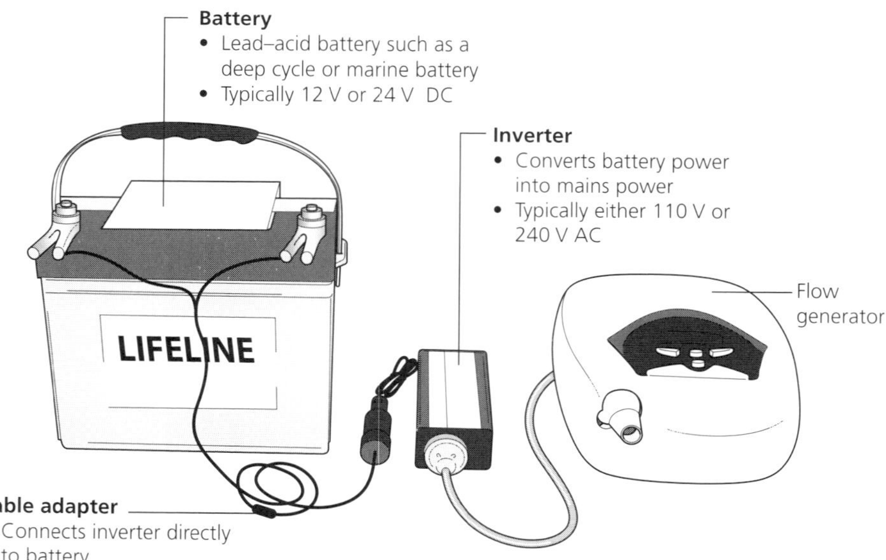


**Figure 2.7** Configuration for use of a bi-level ventilator with a battery and inverter. Courtesy of ResMed.

## Battery power

Ventilators for NIV can be battery powered for safety and portability. Some ventilators for NIV have an internal battery. Others can be powered with a battery or uninterruptable power supply. Many bi-level ventilators can be powered with a direct current (DC) converter. This allows the ventilator to be powered by the auxiliary power source in a vehicle. Bi-level ventilators can also be powered by a lead–acid battery such as a deep cycle or marine battery with an inverter to convert battery power into mains power (Fig. 2.7). The duration of the battery is determined by the size of the battery, ventilator settings, amount of leak, and whether or not a humidifier is used. When using a battery, it is generally best not to use a humidifier to extend the life of the battery. It is also best to avoid use of the humidifier when the bi-level is made portable to avoid accidentally spilling water into the ventilator.

## SUMMARY

A variety of options are available on positive pressure ventilators for NIV. Familiarity with these options allows the clinician to match the ventilator and its features to the needs of the patient who is receiving NIV.

## REFERENCES


1. Chatburn RL. Which ventilators and modes can be used to deliver noninvasive ventilation? *Respir Care* 2009; **54**: 85–101.
2. Scala R, Naldi M. Ventilators for noninvasive ventilation to treat acute respiratory failure. *Respir Care* 2008; **53**: 1054–80.
3. Bunburaphong T, Imanaka H, Nishimura M *et al.* Performance characteristics of bilevel pressure ventilators: a lung model study. *Chest* 1997; **111**: 1050–60.
4. Stell IM, Paul G, Lee KC *et al.* Noninvasive ventilator triggering in chronic obstructive pulmonary disease. A test lung comparison. *Am J Respir Crit Care Med* 2001; **164**: 2092–7.
5. Highcock MP, Morrish E, Jamieson S *et al.* An overnight comparison of two ventilators used in the treatment of chronic respiratory failure. *Eur Respir J* 2002; **20**: 942–5.
6. Highcock MP, Shneerson JM, Smith IE. Functional differences in bi-level pressure preset ventilators. *Eur Respir J* 2001; **17**: 268–73.
7. Richard JC, Carlucci A, Breton L *et al.* Bench testing of pressure support ventilation with three different generations of ventilators. *Intensive Care Med* 2002; **28**: 1049–57.
8. Tassaux D, Strasser S, Fonseca S *et al.* Comparative bench study of triggering, pressurization, and cycling between the home ventilator VPAP II and three ICU ventilators. *Intensive Care Med* 2002; **28**: 1254–61.
9. Vitacca M, Barbano L, D'Anna S *et al.* Comparison of five bilevel pressure ventilators in patients with chronic ventilatory failure: a physiologic study. *Chest* 2002; **122**: 2105–14.
10. Lofaso F, Brochard L, Hang T *et al.* Home versus intensive care pressure support devices. Experimental and clinical comparison. *Am J Respir Crit Care Med* 1996; **153**: 1591–9.
11. Battisti A, Tassaux D, Janssens JP *et al.* Performance characteristics of 10 home mechanical ventilators in pressure-support mode: a comparative bench study. *Chest* 2005; **127**: 1784–92.
12. Smith IE, Shneerson JM. A laboratory comparison of four positive pressure ventilators used in the home. *Eur Respir J* 1996; **9**: 2410–15.
13. Scala R. Bi-level home ventilators for non invasive positive pressure ventilation. *Monaldi Arch Chest Dis* 2004; **61**: 213–21.
14. Fauroux B, Leroux K, Desmarais G *et al.* Performance of ventilators for noninvasive positive-pressure ventilation in children. *Eur Respir J* 2008; **31**: 1300–7.
15. Leger P, Bedicam JM, Cornette A *et al.* Nasal intermittent positive pressure ventilation. Long-term follow-up in patients with severe chronic respiratory insufficiency. *Chest* 1994; **105**: 100–5.
16. Meduri GU, Turner RE, Abou-Shala N *et al.* Noninvasive positive pressure ventilation via face mask. First-line intervention in patients with acute hypercapnic and hypoxemic respiratory failure. *Chest* 1996; **109**: 179–93.
17. Ferreira JC, Chipman DW, Hill NS *et al.* Bilevel vs ICU ventilators providing noninvasive ventilation: effect of system leaks: a COPD lung model comparison. *Chest* 2009; **136**: 448–56.
18. Vignaux L, Tassaux D, Jolliet P. Performance of noninvasive ventilation modes on ICU ventilators during pressure support: a bench model study. *Intensive Care Med* 2007; **33**: 1444–51.
19. Ferguson GT, Gilmartin M. CO2 rebreathing during BiPAP ventilatory assistance. *Am J Respir Crit Care Med* 1995; **151**: 1126–35.
20. Lofaso F, Brochard L, Touchard D *et al.* Evaluation of carbon dioxide rebreathing during pressure support ventilation with airway management system (BiPAP) devices. *Chest* 1995; **108**: 772–8.
21. Patel RG, Petrini MF. Respiratory muscle performance, pulmonary mechanics, and gas exchange between the BiPAP S/T-D system and the Servo Ventilator 900C with bilevel positive airway pressure ventilation following gradual pressure support weaning. *Chest* 1998; **114**: 1390–6.
22. Schettino GP, Chatmongkolchart S, Hess DR *et al.* Position of exhalation port and mask design affect CO2 rebreathing during noninvasive positive pressure ventilation. *Crit Care Med* 2003; **31**: 2178–82.
23. Saatci E, Miller DM, Stell IM *et al.* Dynamic dead space in face masks used with noninvasive ventilators: a lung model study. *Eur Respir J* 2004; **23**: 129–35.


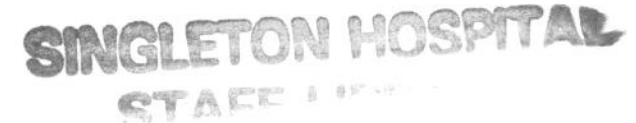

24. Thys F, Liistro G, Dozin O *et al.* Determinants of $FiO_2$ with oxygen supplementation during noninvasive two-level positive pressure ventilation. *Eur Respir J* 2002; **19**: 653–7.
25. Hill NS, Carlisle C, Kramer NR. Effect of a nonrebreathing exhalation valve on long-term nasal ventilation using a bilevel device. *Chest* 2002; **122**: 84–91.
26. Nava S, Ambrosino N, Bruschi C *et al.* Physiological effects of flow and pressure triggering during non-invasive mechanical ventilation in patients with chronic obstructive pulmonary disease. *Thorax* 1997; **52**: 249–54.
27. Borel JC, Sabil A, Janssens JP *et al.* Intentional leaks in industrial masks have a significant impact on efficacy of bilevel noninvasive ventilation: a bench test study. *Chest* 2009; **135**: 669–77.
28. Miyoshi E, Fujino Y, Uchiyama A *et al.* Effects of gas leak on triggering function, humidification, and inspiratory oxygen fraction during noninvasive positive airway pressure ventilation. *Chest* 2005; **128**: 3691–8.
29. Mehta S, McCool FD, Hill NS. Leak compensation in positive pressure ventilators: a lung model study. *Eur Respir J* 2001; **17**: 259–67.
30. Sinderby C, Beck J. Proportional assist ventilation and neurally adjusted ventilatory assist: better approaches to patient ventilator synchrony? *Clin Chest Med* 2008; **29**: 329–42, vii.
31. Hess DR. Ventilator waveforms and the physiology of pressure support ventilation. *Respir Care* 2005; **50**: 166–86; discussion 183–66.
32. Hotchkiss JR Jr, Adams AB, Stone MK *et al.* Oscillations and noise: inherent instability of pressure support ventilation? *Am J Respir Crit Care Med* 2002; **165**: 47–53.
33. Hotchkiss JR, Adams AB, Dries DJ *et al.* Dynamic behavior during noninvasive ventilation: chaotic support? *Am J Respir Crit Care Med* 2001; **163**: 374–8.
34. Adams AB, Bliss PL, Hotchkiss J. Effects of respiratory impedance on the performance of bi-level pressure ventilators. *Respir Care* 2000; **45**: 390–400.
35. Calderini E, Confalonieri M, Puccio PG *et al.* Patient-ventilator asynchrony during noninvasive ventilation: the role of expiratory trigger. *Intensive Care Med* 1999; **25**: 662–7.
36. Waugh JB, Granger WM. An evaluation of 2 new devices for nasal high-flow gas therapy. *Respir Care* 2004; **49**: 902–6.
37. Schwartz AR, Kacmarek RM, Hess DR. Factors affecting oxygen delivery with bi-level positive airway pressure. *Respir Care* 2004; **49**: 270–5.
38. Hess DR. The evidence for noninvasive positive-pressure ventilation in the care of patients in acute respiratory failure: a systematic review of the literature. *Respir Care* 2004; **49**: 810–29.
39. Hess DR. Noninvasive ventilation in neuromuscular disease: equipment and application. *Respir Care* 2006; **51**: 896–911, discussion 911–12.
40. Prinianakis G, Delmastro M, Carlucci A *et al.* Effect of varying the pressurisation rate during noninvasive pressure support ventilation. *Eur Respir J* 2004; **23**: 314–20.
41. Girault C, Richard JC, Chevron V *et al.* Comparative physiologic effects of noninvasive assist-control and pressure support ventilation in acute hypercapnic respiratory failure. *Chest* 1997; **111**: 1639–48.
42. Navalesi P, Fanfulla F, Frigerio P *et al.* Physiologic evaluation of noninvasive mechanical ventilation delivered with three types of masks in patients with chronic hypercapnic respiratory failure. *Crit Care Med* 2000; **28**: 1785–90.
43. Fauroux B, Pigeot J, Polkey MI *et al.* In vivo physiologic comparison of two ventilators used for domiciliary ventilation in children with cystic fibrosis. *Crit Care Med* 2001; **29**: 2097–105.
44. Parreira VF, Delguste P, Jounieaux V *et al.* Effectiveness of controlled and spontaneous modes in nasal two-level positive pressure ventilation in awake and asleep normal subjects. *Chest* 1997; **112**: 1267–77.
45. Parthasarathy S, Tobin MJ. Effect of ventilator mode on sleep quality in critically ill patients. *Am J Respir Crit Care Med* 2002; **166**: 1423–9.
46. Johnson KG, Johnson DC. Bilevel positive airway pressure worsens central apneas during sleep. *Chest* 2005; **128**: 2141–50.
47. Williams P, Kratohvil J, Ritz R *et al.* Pressure support and pressure assist/control: are there differences? An evaluation of the newest intensive care unit ventilators. *Respir Care* 2000; **45**: 1169–81.
48. Vitacca M, Rubini F, Foglio K *et al.* Non-invasive modalities of positive pressure ventilation improve the outcome of acute exacerbations in COLD patients. *Intensive Care Med* 1993; **19**: 450–5.
49. Schonhofer B, Sonneborn M, Haidl P *et al.* Comparison of two different modes for noninvasive mechanical ventilation in chronic respiratory failure: volume versus pressure controlled device. *Eur Respir J* 1997; **10**: 184–91.
50. Chadda K, Clair B, Orlikowski D *et al.* Pressure support versus assisted controlled noninvasive ventilation in neuromuscular disease. *Neurocrit Care* 2004; **1**: 429–34.
51. Kirakli C, Cerci T, Ucar ZZ *et al.* Noninvasive assisted pressure-controlled ventilation: as effective as pressure support ventilation in chronic obstructive pulmonary disease? *Respiration* 2008; **75**: 402–10.
52. Fernandez-Vivas M, Caturla-Such J, Gonzalez de la Rosa J *et al.* Noninvasive pressure support versus proportional assist ventilation in acute respiratory failure. *Intensive Care Med* 2003; **29**: 1126–33.
53. Wysocki M, Richard JC, Meshaka P. Noninvasive proportional assist ventilation compared with noninvasive pressure support ventilation in hypercapnic acute respiratory failure. *Crit Care Med* 2002; **30**: 323–9.
54. Gay PC, Hess DR, Hill NS. Noninvasive proportional assist ventilation for acute respiratory insufficiency. Comparison with pressure support ventilation. *Am J Respir Crit Care Med* 2001; **164**: 1606–11.

55. Rusterholtz T, Bollaert PE, Feissel M *et al.* Continuous positive airway pressure vs. proportional assist ventilation for noninvasive ventilation in acute cardiogenic pulmonary edema. *Intensive Care Med* 2008; **34**: 840–6.
56. Hart N, Hunt A, Polkey MI *et al.* Comparison of proportional assist ventilation and pressure support ventilation in chronic respiratory failure due to neuromuscular and chest wall deformity. *Thorax* 2002; **57**: 979–81.
57. Porta R, Appendini L, Vitacca M *et al.* Mask proportional assist vs pressure support ventilation in patients in clinically stable condition with chronic ventilatory failure. *Chest* 2002; **122**: 479–88.
58. Winck JC, Vitacca M, Morais A *et al.* Tolerance and physiologic effects of nocturnal mask pressure support vs proportional assist ventilation in chronic ventilatory failure. *Chest* 2004; **126**: 382–8.
59. Bosma K, Ferreyra G, Ambrogio C *et al.* Patient–ventilator interaction and sleep in mechanically ventilated patients: pressure support versus proportional assist ventilation. *Crit Care Med* 2007; **35**: 1048–54.
60. Benditt JO. Full-time noninvasive ventilation: possible and desirable. *Respir Care* 2006; **51**: 1005–12; discussion 1012–15.
61. Fauroux B, Boffa C, Desguerre I *et al.* Long-term noninvasive mechanical ventilation for children at home: a national survey. *Pediatr Pulmonol* 2003; **35**: 119–25.
62. Kerby GR, Mayer LS, Pingleton SK. Nocturnal positive pressure ventilation via nasal mask. *Am Rev Respir Dis* 1987; **135**: 738–40.
63. Leger P, Jennequin J, Gerard M *et al.* Home positive pressure ventilation via nasal mask for patients with neuromusculoskeletal disorders. *Eur Respir J Suppl* 1989; **7**: 640s–4s.
64. Bach JR, Alba AS, Bohatiuk G *et al.* Mouth intermittent positive pressure ventilation in the management of postpolio respiratory insufficiency. *Chest* 1987; **91**: 859–64.
65. Bach JR, Alba AS, Saporito LR. Intermittent positive pressure ventilation via the mouth as an alternative to tracheostomy for 257 ventilator users. *Chest* 1993; **103**: 174–82.
66. Toussaint M, Steens M, Wasteels G *et al.* Diurnal ventilation via mouthpiece: survival in end-stage Duchenne patients. *Eur Respir J* 2006; **28**: 549–55.
67. Boitano LJ. Equipment options for cough augmentation, ventilation, and noninvasive interfaces in neuromuscular respiratory management. *Pediatrics* 2009; **123** Suppl 4: S226–30.
68. Boitano LJ, Benditt JO. An evaluation of home volume ventilators that support open-circuit mouthpiece ventilation. *Respir Care* 2005; **50**: 1457–61.
69. Pepin JL, Muir JF, Gentina T *et al.* Pressure reduction during exhalation in sleep apnea patients treated by continuous positive airway pressure. *Chest* 2009; **136**: 490–7.

3

# Negative pressure ventilation

ANTONIO CORRADO, MASSIMO GORINI

ABSTRACT

Evidence now exists that: negative pressure ventilation (NPV) unloads respiratory muscles and improves gas exchange in patients with chronic obstructive pulmonary disease and acute respiratory failure; volume controlled ventilation with continuous negative pressure (CNEP), compared with volume controlled ventilation with positive end-expiratory pressure, increases oxygen delivery and cardiac index in patients with acute lung injury; and iron lung ventilation, in expert hands, is as effective as mask ventilation and invasive ventilation in the treatment of acute-on-chronic respiratory failure. Furthermore, the use of either NPV or mask ventilation may avoid endotracheal intubation and its complications in most of these patients, widening the field of application of non-invasive ventilator techniques.

## INTRODUCTION

Non-invasive mechanical ventilation comprises both negative and positive pressure ventilation. The advantages in using these techniques include the possibility of avoiding endotracheal intubation and associated complications and sedative agents, facilitating communication between patients and care providers, and preserving functions such as swallowing and coughing. Weaning from mechanical ventilation is another important advantage of non-invasive ventilation. In this chapter we discuss the physiological effects and the more recent clinical applications of negative pressure ventilation (NPV).

## NEGATIVE PRESSURE VENTILATION

Negative pressure ventilation works by exposing the surface of the thorax to subatmospheric pressure during inspiration. This pressure causes thoracic expansion and a decrease in pleural and alveolar pressures, creating a pressure gradient for air to move from the airway opening into the alveoli. When the pressure surrounding the thorax increases and becomes equal to or greater than the atmospheric pressure, expiration occurs passively owing to the elastic recoil of the respiratory system. With NPV, the inspiratory changes in pleural and alveolar pressures replicate those that occur during spontaneous breathing.

### Negative pressure ventilators

All negative pressure ventilators have two major components: an airtight, rigid chamber that encloses the rib cage and abdomen, and a pump that generates pressure changes in the chamber. For a recent comprehensive review of negative pressure ventilators see Corrado and Gorini[1] (Fig. 3.1).

Presently, NPV can be delivered in five modes as control or assist-control ventilation:[1]

- intermittent negative pressure (Fig. 3.2)
- negative/positive pressure
- continuous negative pressure (CNEP)
- negative pressure/negative end-expiratory pressure
- external high-frequency oscillation.

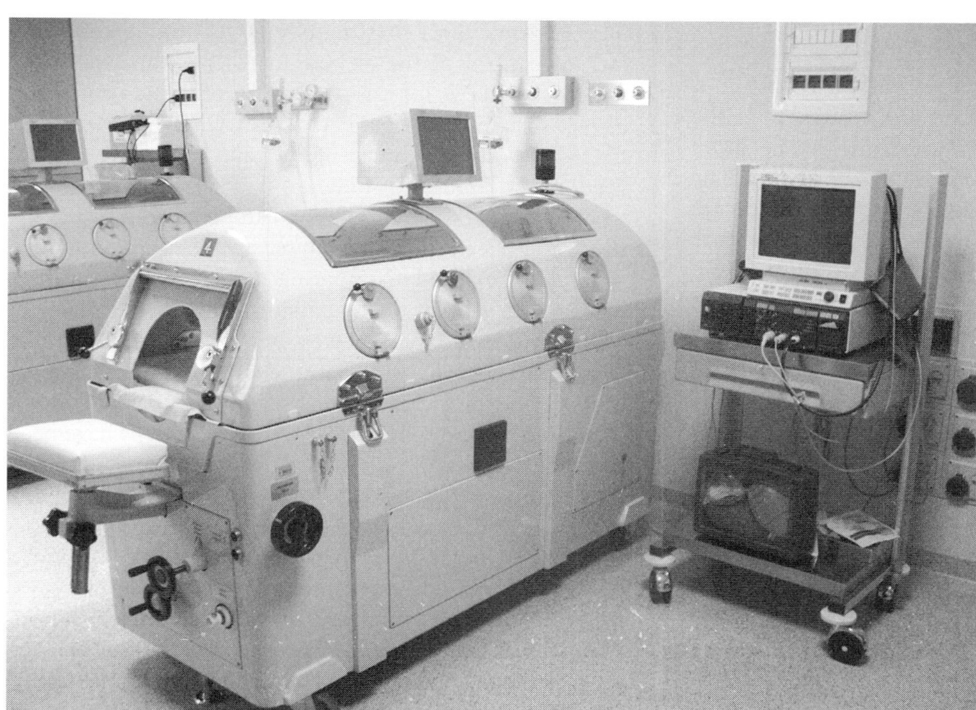

**Figure 3.1** The microprocessor-based iron lung. (Coppa CA 1001, Coppa, Biella, Italy)

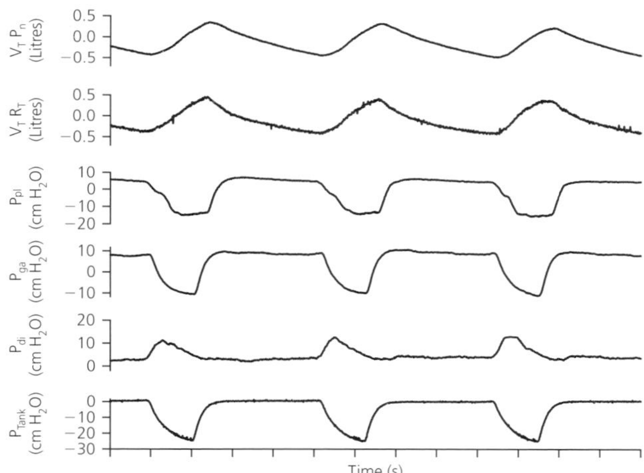


**Figure 3.2** Recordings of rib cage and abdominal displacement, volume ($V_T$ $R_T$), pleural pressure ($P_{pl}$), transdiaphragmatic pressure ($P_{di}$), and tank pressure ($P_{tank}$) in a patient with acute exacerbation of chronic obstructive pulmonary disease during assist negative pressure ventilation provided by an iron lung.

## Physiological effects

### GAS EXCHANGE

The different types of NPV markedly improve ventilatory pattern, arterial blood gases and the pH.[2]

### RESPIRATORY MUSCLES

It has been found that in chronic obstructive pulmonary disease (COPD) patients with acute respiratory failure, compared with spontaneous breathing, CNEP (–5 cm $H_2O$) resulted in a significant decrease in dynamic intrinsic positive end-expiratory pressure (PEEP) and pressure–time product of the diaphragm whereas assist-control NPV caused a significant improvement in the pattern of breathing associated with a marked reduction in both pressure–time product of the diaphragm and electromyographic activity of the parasternal muscles.[2] The application of –5 cm $H_2O$ negative extrathoracic end-expiratory pressure during NPV further slightly decreased the pressure–time product of the diaphragm and improved patient–ventilator interaction by reducing dynamic intrinsic PEEP and non-triggering inspiratory effort.

### UPPER AIRWAYS

Use of NPV during sleep in normal subjects[3] and in patients with chronic respiratory failure secondary to COPD[4] and neuromuscular disorders[5,6] may result in recurrent episodes of apnoea and hypopnoea as well as altered sleep quality. Upper airway obstruction was reported in two of 10 patients with acute-on-chronic respiratory failure during treatment with NPV;[7] it was also the reason for NPV failure in 16 per cent of cases in a large, prospective, cohort study.[8]

## CARDIOVASCULAR SYSTEM

Although the haemodynamic effects of NPV have not been extensively studied,[9] the effects are assumed to be the opposite of those of positive pressure ventilation, i.e. more physiological and more likely to maintain a normal cardiac output. The exposure, however, of the entire body (except for the airway opening) to NPV with tank ventilators has the same haemodynamic effects as with positive pressure ventilation.[10] These effects occur because intrathoracic pressure is actually raised relative to body surface pressure, thus reducing the gradient for venous return. That consequence is not seen when NPV is confined to the thorax and upper abdomen using a cuirass or poncho-wrap ventilator.[11] Unlike tank ventilators, these machines selectively decrease intrathoracic pressure so that right atrial pressure becomes more negative relative to the rest of the body, potentially enhancing the gradient for the venous return. The NPV provided by a cuirass ventilator does not induce adverse haemodynamic effects in stable patients with COPD,[12] whereas a significant reduction in cardiac output has been reported with mask ventilation with PEEP in patients with COPD both when stable[13] and during acute exacerbations.[14] Short-term studies have compared the effects of CNEP provided by cuirass[15] or poncho-wrap[16,17] ventilators with those of PEEP in intubated patients with acute lung injury receiving volume controlled ventilation. CNEP was adjusted to obtain the same change in transpulmonary pressure[17] or functional residual capacity[15] as with PEEP. Compared with volume controlled ventilation with PEEP, the combination of volume controlled ventilation with CNEP resulted in significant increases in oxygen delivery and cardiac index, whereas arterial oxygen content and the $PaO_2/FiO_2$ ratio did not differ between the two modes of ventilation.[15–17]

It has been reported that in coronary artery bypass graft patients the use of a combination of synchronized intermittent mandatory ventilation (SIMV) and CNEP through a cuirass immediately after surgery significantly increased the stroke volume index and cardiac index in comparison to ventilation with SIMV and PEEP. Furthermore, continual negative pressure also reduced venous and wedge pressure.[18]

## EVIDENCE BASE AND CLINICAL APPLICATIONS

### Acute respiratory failure (COPD)

The effectiveness of NPV provided by the iron lung in patients with hypercapnic encephalopathy was retrospectively evaluated in 150 consecutive patients (79 per cent had COPD).[19] The failure rate of NPV (death or need for endotracheal intubation) was 45/150 (30 per cent); the observed mortality rate was 24 per cent versus 67.5 per cent predicted mortality based on APACHE II. Nine patients (6 per cent) required intubation because of a lack of control of the airway. In recent years, the effectiveness of NPV for the treatment of acute-on-chronic respiratory failure in patients with COPD has been confirmed in two case–control studies and in two prospective, randomized controlled studies.[20–23]

Negative pressure ventilation can be used to widen the field of application of non-invasive ventilator techniques. A randomized study comparing mask with conventional mechanical ventilation in patients with exacerbation of COPD who failed medical treatment has shown that mask ventilation helped avoid endotracheal intubation in 48 per cent of patients.[24] Mask ventilation, however, is not without its problems, and failure rates of 7–50 per cent have been reported.[25] Severe respiratory acidosis[26–28] and illness at presentation,[26,29] excessive airway secretions,[29] and inability to minimize the amount of air leakage[29] are major factors associated with failure of this technique. In clinical studies, NPV has been used successfully in patients with severe respiratory acidosis or impaired level of consciousness.[19,20,30] During NPV, unlike positive pressure ventilation, the airway opening is free, and so it is easy to perform bronchial aspiration or fibreoptic bronchoscopy for removal of excessive airway secretions. Finally, NPV can be used in patients who cannot tolerate a mask because of facial deformity, or as a rescue therapy, to avoid endotracheal intubation, in those in whom mask ventilation fails.

Routine implementation of non-invasive positive pressure ventilation in critically ill patients with acute exacerbation of COPD or severe cardiogenic pulmonary oedema has been shown to be associated with improved survival and reduction of nosocomial infection.[31] For these reasons, mask ventilation is recommended as the standard method of ventilator support for exacerbations of COPD, and invasive mechanical ventilation is regarded as second-line rescue therapy when it fails.[32] To bear out the hypothesis that using both non-invasive mask and iron lung ventilation should further reduce the need of endotracheal intubation in patients with acute-on-chronic respiratory failure, a prospective, cohort study was carried out in 258 consecutive patients:[21] 77 per cent of patients were treated exclusively with non-invasive ventilation (40 per cent with NPV, 23 per cent with mask ventilation, and 14 per cent with the sequential use of both), and 14 per cent with invasive ventilation. In patients in whom NPV or mask ventilation failed, the sequential use of the alternative technique allowed a significant reduction in the failure of non-invasive mechanical ventilation (from 23.4 per cent to 8.8 per cent, $p = 0.002$, and from 25.3 per cent to 5 per cent, $p = 0.0001$, respectively). Overall hospital mortality (21 per cent) was lower than that estimated by the APACHE II score (28 per cent). This study showed that use of NPV and mask ventilation mode can avoid endotracheal intubation in the vast majority of unselected patients with acute-on-chronic respiratory disorders needing ventilator support.[8] Another more recent study found that using both modalities of non-invasive ventilation in patients with acute-on-chronic respiratory failure resulted in an overall success rate of 81.6 per cent in avoiding endotracheal intubation.[33]

Two studies have compared the effects of NPV and conventional mechanical ventilation in patients with COPD and severe acute respiratory failure.[22,20] A retrospective case–control study was carried out in 66 patients who underwent NPV or invasive ventilation.[20] The primary endpoints were in-hospital death (for both groups) and the need for endotracheal intubation (in patients treated with NPV). The mortality rate was 23.1 per cent in the NPV group and 26.9 per cent in the group treated with invasive ventilation. The duration of ventilation in survivors was significantly lower with NPV than with invasive ventilation with a median of 22.5 hours (range 2–114) versus 96 hours (range 12–336). Length of hospital stay was similar in both groups. These findings were later confirmed in a prospective, randomized controlled study.[22] Forty-four patients with an exacerbation of COPD and severe respiratory acidosis (mean pH $7.20 \pm 0.04$) were assigned to either iron lung ventilation (22 patients) or invasive ventilation (22 patients). Compared with the baseline, NPV and invasive ventilation induced a similar and significant improvement in $PaO_2/FIO_2$, $PaCO_2$ and pH after 1 hour and at discontinuation of treatment. Four patients treated with NPV (18.2 per cent) needed endotracheal intubation. Major complications tended to be more frequent in patients treated with invasive ventilation than in those treated with NPV (27.3 per cent vs 4.5 per cent), whereas mortality rate was similar (27.3 per cent vs 18.2 per cent). Ventilator-free days and length of hospital stay were significantly lower in the iron lung group than in the invasive ventilation group. This study suggests that iron lung ventilation is as effective as invasive ventilation in improving gas exchange in patients with COPD and acute respiratory failure, and is associated with a tendency towards a lower rate of major complications.

A retrospective case–control study made a direct comparison between the two non-invasive ventilator techniques in the treatment of patients with COPD in acute respiratory failure; 53 pairs of patients were treated with iron lung and mask ventilation.[21] In the NPV group, the rate of treatment failure (death and/or need for endotracheal intubation) was 20.7 per cent whereas it was 24.5 per cent in the mask ventilation group. Duration of mechanical ventilation ($29.6 \pm 28.6$ vs $62.3 \pm 35.7$ hrs) and length of hospital stay ($10.4 \pm 4.3$ vs $15 \pm 5.2$) were significantly lower in patients treated with NPV than in those treated with mask ventilation. These findings suggest that both ventilator techniques are equally effective in avoiding endotracheal intubation and death in patients with COPD in acute respiratory failure. This has been recently confirmed by the results of a multicentre, prospective randomized crossover study[23] carried out in 141 patients (70 assigned to NPV and 71 to mask ventilation). To establish the failure of the technique used as first-line, the major and minor criteria for endotracheal intubation were used. In patients fulfilling the major criteria, endotracheal intubation was promptly established. Patients with at least two minor criteria were shifted from one technique to the other. When used as first line, the success of NPV (87 per cent) was significantly greater ($p = 0.01$) than mask ventilation (68 per cent) owing to the number of patients who met the minor criteria for endotracheal intubation. After patients were shifted, however, the need for endotracheal intubation and hospital mortality was similar in both groups. The overall rate of success using both techniques increased from 77.3 to 87.9 per cent ($p = 0.028$). These data show that when the two techniques are combined, endotracheal intubation can be avoided in a high percentage of patients.

### Neuromuscular disorders

Few uncontrolled studies have investigated the effect of NPV in the treatment of neuromuscular patients with acute respiratory failure. NPV, provided by iron lung[33] or pneumowrap,[34] has been successful in avoiding endotracheal intubation and in facilitating weaning from invasive ventilation in small groups of patients. We have reported in a retrospective study the successful use of NPV provided by iron lung in the treatment of 15 neuromuscular patients with ARF.[35] A retrospective study analysed the outcome of 65 neuromuscular patients with acute respiratory failure who were treated with NPV or mask ventilation.[36] There was no significant difference in mortality rate and need for endotracheal intubation between the two groups, despite more severe clinical conditions on admission in the NPV group than in the mask ventilation group. Although these reports suggest that NPV can be effective in the treatment of acute respiratory failure in patients with neuromuscular diseases, prospective controlled studies are needed to clarify the impact of non-invasive ventilation on clinical outcome in these patients.

## FUTURE RESEARCH

Although physiological studies[15–17] have shown the advantageous haemodynamic effects of NPV applied to the chest wall in patients with acute lung injury, studies on clinical outcomes are still lacking. The absence of this information is particularly relevant because some physiological studies in animals suggest that NPV may result in reduced lung biotrauma[37–41] and atelectasis[42] compared with positive pressure ventilation.

A physiological study[10] showed that NPV by iron lung has the same haemodynamic effects as positive pressure ventilation. Future studies are required to determine whether iron lung ventilation can be applied successfully to patients with cardiogenic pulmonary oedema.

## REFERENCES


1. Corrado A, Gorini M. Negative pressure ventilation. In: Tobin MJ, ed. *Principles and practice of mechanical ventilation*, 2nd edn. New York: McGraw Hill, 2006: 403–18.
2. Gorini M, Corrado A, Villella G *et al.* Physiologic effects of negative pressure ventilation in acute exacerbation of COPD. *Am J Respir Crit Care Med* 2001; **163**: 1614–18.
3. Levy RD, Bradley TD, Newman SL *et al.* Negative pressure ventilation. Effects on ventilation during sleep in normal subjects. *Chest* 1989; **95**: 95–9.
4. Levy RD, Cosio MG, Gibbons L *et al.* Induction of sleep apnoea with negative pressure ventilation in patients with chronic obstructive lung disease. *Thorax* 1992; **47**: 612–15.
5. Hill NS, Redline S, Carskadon MA *et al.* Sleep-disordered breathing in patients with Duchenne muscular dystrophy using negative pressure ventilators. *Chest* 1992; **102**: 1656–62.
6. Bach JR, Penek J. Obstructive sleep apnea complicating negative pressure ventilatory support in patients with chronic paralytic/restrictive ventilatory dysfunction. *Chest* 1991; **99**: 1386–93.
7. Todisco T, Eslami A, Scarcella L *et al.* Flexible bronchoscopy during iron lung mechanical ventilation in nonintubated patients. *J Bronchol* 1995; **2**: 200–5.
8. Gorini M, Ginanni R, Villella G *et al.* Non-invasive negative and positive pressure ventilation in the treatment of acute on chronic respiratory failure. *Intensive Care Med* 2004; **30**: 875–81.
9. Krumpe PE, Zidulka A, Urbanetti J *et al.* Comparison of the effects of continuous negative external chest pressure and positive end-expiratory pressure on cardiac index in dogs. *Am Rev Respir Dis* 1977; **115**: 39–45.
10. Maloney JV, Whittenberger JL. Clinical implication of pressures used in the body respirator. *Am J Med Sci* 1951; **221**: 425–30.
11. Skabursis M, Helal R, Zidulka A. Hemodynamic effects of external continuous negative pressure ventilation compared with those of continuous positive pressure ventilation in dogs with acute lung injury. *Am Rev Respir Dis* 1987; **136**: 886–91.
12. Ambrosino N, Cobelli F, Torbicki A. Hemodynamic effect of negative pressure ventilation in patients with COPD. *Chest* 1990; **97**: 850–6.
13. Ambrosino N, Nava S, Torbicki A *et al.* Haemodynamic effects of pressure support and PEEP ventilation by nasal route in patients with stable chronic obstructive pulmonary disease. *Thorax* 1993; **48**: 523–8.
14. Diaz O, Iglesia R, Ferrer M *et al.* Effects of noninvasive ventilation on pulmonary gas exchange and hemodynamics during acute hypercapnic exacerbations of chronic obstructive pulmonary disease. *Am J Respir Crit Care Med* 1997; **156**: 1840–5.
15. Scholz SE, Knothe C, Thiel A *et al.* Improved oxygen delivery by positive pressure ventilation with continuous negative external chest pressure. *Lancet* 1997; **349**: 1295–6.
16. Torelli L, Zoccali G, Casarin M *et al.* Comparative evaluation of the haemodynamic effects of continuous negative external pressure (CNEP) and positive end-expiratory pressure (PEEP) in mechanically ventilated trauma patients. *Intensive Care Med* 1995; **21**: 67–70.
17. Borelli M, Benini A, Denkevitz T *et al.* Effects of continuous negative extrathoracic pressure versus positive end-expiratory pressure in acute lung injury patients. *Crit Care Med* 1998; **26**: 1025–31.
18. Chaturvedi RK, Zidulka AA, Goldberg P *et al.* Use of negative extrathoracic pressure to improve hemodynamics after cardiac surgery. *Ann Thorac Surg* 2008; **85**: 1355–60.
19. Corrado A, De Paola E, Gorini M *et al.* Intermittent negative pressure ventilation in the treatment of hypoxic hypercapnic coma in chronic respiratory insufficiency. *Thorax* 1996; **5**: 1077–82.
20. Corrado A, Gorini M, Ginanni R *et al.* Negative pressure ventilation versus conventional mechanical ventilation in the treatment of acute respiratory failure in COPD patients. *Eur Respir J* 1998; **12**: 519–25.
21. Corrado A, Confalonieri M, Marchese S *et al.* Iron lung versus mask ventilation in the treatment of acute on chronic respiratory failure in COPD patients: a multicenter study. *Chest* 2002; **121**: 189–95.
22. Corrado A, Ginanni R, Villella G *et al.* Iron lung versus conventional mechanical ventilation in acute exacerbation of COPD. *Eur Respir J* 2004; **23**: 419–24.
23. Corrado A, Gorini M, Melej A *et al.* Iron lung versus mask ventilation in acute exacerbation of COPD: a randomised crossover study. *Intensive Care Med* 2009; **35**: 648–55.
24. Conti G, Antonelli M, Navalesi P *et al.* Noninvasive vs conventional mechanical ventilation in patients with chronic obstructive pulmonary disease after failure of medical treatment in the ward: a randomized trial. *Intensive Care Med* 2002; **28**: 1701–7.
25. Lightowler JVJ, Elliott MW. Predicting the outcome of NIV for acute exacerbations of COPD. *Thorax* 2000; **55**: 815–16.
26. Ambrosino N, Foglio K, Rubini F *et al.* Non-invasive mechanical ventilation in acute respiratory failure due to chronic obstructive pulmonary disease: correlates for success. *Thorax* 1995; **50**: 755–7.
27. Plant PK, Owen JL, Elliott MW. Non-invasive ventilation in acute exacerbations of chronic obstructive pulmonary disease: long term survival and predictors of in-hospital outcome. *Thorax* 2001; **56**: 708–12.
28. Carlucci A, Richard JC, Wysocki M *et al.* Noninvasive versus conventional mechanical ventilation. An epidemiologic survey. *Am J Respir Crit Care Med* 2001; **163**: 874–80.
29. Soo Hoo GW, Santiago S, Williams A. Nasal mechanical ventilation for hypercapnic respiratory failure in chronic obstructive pulmonary disease: determinants of success and failure. *Crit Care Med* 1994; **22**: 1253–61.

30. Corrado A, Gorini M. Negative pressure ventilation: is there still a role? *Eur Respir J* 2002; **20**: 187–97.
31. Girou E, Brun Buisson C, Taille S *et al.* Secular trends in nosocomial infections and mortality associated with noninvasive ventilation in patients with exacerbation of COPD and pulmonary edema. *JAMA* 2003; **290**: 2985–91.
32. Elliott MW. Non-invasive ventilation in acute exacerbations of chronic obstructive pulmonary disease: a new gold standard? *Intensive Care Med* 2002; **28**: 1691–3.
33. Todisco T, Baglioni S, Eslami A *et al.* Treatment of acute exacerbations of chronic respiratory failure. *Chest* 2004; **125**: 2217–23.
34. Libby BM, Briscoe WA, Boyce B *et al.* Acute respiratory failure in scoliosis or Kyphosis. *Am J Med* 1982; **73**: 532–8.
35. Braun SR, Sufit RL, Giovannoni R *et al.* Intermittent negative pressure ventilation in the treatment of respiratory failure in progressive neuromuscular disease. *Neurology* 1987; **37**: 1874–5.
36. Corrado A, Gorini M, De Paola E. Alternative techniques for managing acute neuromuscular respiratory failure. *Semin Neurol* 1995; **15**: 84–9.
37. Corrado A, Vianello A, Arcaro G *et al.* Noninvasive mechanical ventilation for the treatment of acute respiratory failure in neuromuscular diseases. *Eur Respir J* 2000; **16**: 542s.
38. Uhlig S. Ventilation-induced lung injury and mechanotransduction: stretching it too far? *Am J Physiol Lung Cell Mol Physiol* 2002; **282**: L892–6.
39. Culver BH, Butler J. Mechanical influence on the pulmonary microcirculation. *Ann Rev Physiol* 1980; **42**: 187–98.
40. Koyama S, Hildebrandt J. Air interface and elastic recoil affect vascular resistance in three zone of rabbit lung. *J Appl Physiol* 1991; **70**: 2422–31.
41. Von Bethmann AN, Brasch F, Nusing R *et al.* Hyperventilation reduces release of cytokines from perfused mouse lung. *Am J Respir Crit Care Med* 1998; **157**: 263–72.
42. Grasso F, Engelberts D, Helm E *et al.* Negative pressure ventilation. Better oxygenation and less lung injury. *Am J Respir Crit Care Med* 2008; **177**: 412–18.
43. Helm E, Talakoub O, Grasso F *et al.* Use of dynamic CT in acute respiratory distress syndrome (ARDS) with comparison of positive and negative pressure ventilation. *Eur Radiol* 2009; **19**: 50–7.

# 4

# Continuous positive airway pressure

A CRAIG DAVIDSON


## ABSTRACT

The non-specialist often confuses continuous positive airway pressure (CPAP) with non-invasive ventilation (NIV). This is because both employ some sort of mask as an interface rather than an endotracheal or tracheostomy tube; CPAP, however, has a different purpose to NIV, it can be used domestically in the treatment of obstructive sleep apnoea and is also employed when weaning from invasive mechanical ventilation. This chapter concentrates on its use non-invasively in acute type I respiratory failure.


## INTRODUCTION

Continuous positive airway pressure (CPAP) involves the application of positive pressure throughout the respiratory cycle in a spontaneously breathing patient. It can be provided by an endotracheal or tracheostomy tube during weaning from invasive ventilation, but it is most commonly delivered using a non-invasive interface, such as a full face mask or helmet.

The primary indication for CPAP is hypoxaemia that is refractory to high-concentration oxygen therapy, i.e. severe type I respiratory failure. This is in distinction from the use of non-invasive pressure support (ventilation) used to increase effective alveolar ventilation and reduce the increased $PaCO_2$ seen in type II respiratory failure. Conventionally, the term non-invasive ventilation (NIV) is now synonymous with non-invasive positive pressure ventilation (NIPPV), although NIV can be used to encompass NIPPV, CPAP, negative pressure (cuirasse, tank) ventilation and even physical methods such as the rocking bed. Further confusion of CPAP with NIPPV arises because both usually involve a close fitting face mask. Finally, CPAP may be successfully used in hypercapnic patients, notably cardiogenic pulmonary oedema (see Chapter 30).

In this chapter, we will consider the use of CPAP in acute respiratory illness and not its domiciliary use to treat obstructive sleep apnoea.

## RATIONALE FOR CONTINUOUS POSITIVE AIRWAY PRESSURE

Acute hypoxaemia arises because of a reduction in the number of normally functioning alveolar units, the site of gas exchange between fresh inspired gas entering the alveolus and blood circulating around the air space within the alveolar capillary.

Hypoxaemia most commonly arises because of infection and/or alveolar flooding caused by either cardiogenic or non-cardiogenic oedema. More proximal disturbance of ventilation may result from airway obstruction, such as in bronchopneumonia or asthma, and obstruction of the pulmonary vasculature as in pulmonary embolism. A third factor may be chest wall disease, such as a flail segment of the chest wall (trauma) or because of diaphragm dysfunction (pain, abdominal tamponade) following abdominal surgery. Continuous positive airway pressure may be effective in countering any of the mechanisms involved in producing hypoxaemia and arterial oxygenation will improve with any increase in the number of functioning alveolar units (recruitment).

In many cases, recruitment occurs by re-expansion of poorly ventilated lung in the dependent areas where airway opening is late in inspiration or fails to occur.[1] Continuous positive airway pressure leads to an increase in end-expiratory residual volume (RV) and in doing so also improves pulmonary mechanics. The increase in RV may also be associated with more effective clearance of secretions from the larger airways. By limiting intrinsic positive end-expiratory pressure (PEEP) and providing a (mild) degree of inspiratory support, CPAP also reduces the work of breathing,[2] especially when there is diffuse airway obstruction as is typically seen in an acute exacerbation of COPD. This effect will be the more obvious when airway collapse during expiration arises because of lack of support of the small airways (emphysema) than when airway obstruction arises because of airway inflammation or remodelling (chronic bronchitis). With relief of hypoxaemia, respiratory rate may fall (reduced hypoxic drive) and this, along with improved respiratory mechanics, will lead to better alveolar gas mixing, increased alveolar ventilation, a fall in $PCO_2$ when elevated and relief of dyspnoea. Finally, CPAP will counter any tendency to upper airway obstruction caused by neck flexion or airflow limitation resulting from laryngeal oedema that may become apparent following extubation.

## TECHNICAL CONSIDERATIONS

### Equipment

As the primary indication for CPAP is hypoxaemia, the driving gas will need to have a high oxygen concentration. It also needs to be at a high flow rate. Domiciliary CPAP or NIV machines are unsuitable for delivering acute CPAP therapy. The immediate increase in $SaO_2$ often observed with initiation of CPAP may partially result from the high $FiO_2$ delivered by CPAP in comparison with conventional supplementary oxygen. Wall-mounted oxygen mixers that employ the Venturi principle rarely achieve an $FiO_2$ approaching 60 per cent (despite this being set on the device) as air is necessarily entrained at the interface during early inspiration. Only non-rebreathe high-flow masks that employ a reservoir bag reliably achieve the delivery of an $FiO_2$ of 60 per cent or higher.

Flow generators capable of delivering >100 L/min are required to achieve positive airway pressure throughout the respiratory cycle. A close-fitting face mask is employed either with an integral CPAP exhalation valve mounted on the front of the mask or, more commonly, attached to the distal limb of a short section of ventilator tubing. CPAP valves are available in 2.5 increments from 5.0 cm $H_2O$ to 20 cm $H_2O$. It is conventional to start at 5 or 7.5 and monitor the response. The author rarely uses >10 cm $H_2O$ as high pressures are uncomfortable, with expiration being noticed as limiting. It is also difficult to get a good seal at higher pressures. While there is marked dissipation of pressure within the airways, intrathoracic pressure will be increased by the set CPAP with a resulting reduction in right ventricular preload. This is also more of a risk with CPAP >10 cm $H_2O$. In the volume-depleted patient, especially in atrial fibrillation (loss of atrial kick), CPAP may cause a fall in cardiac output and symptomatic hypotension. When setting up CPAP, the operator needs to adjust the flow rate to the patient to ensure that the exhalation valve is in the open position throughout the respiratory cycle. If this is not the case then pressure in the mask will necessarily fall and may give a sense of 'air-hunger' to the patient.

Two flow generators are most commonly employed. In one (Downs CPAP generator, Vital Signs, Barnham, UK) piped high-pressure oxygen provides the power. By adjusting oxygen flow, and its dilution by air entrained by the Venturi effect (Fig. 4.1), the desired flow rate and oxygen concentration can be achieved. In its simplest form no measure of gas flow or other monitoring information is provided to the operator. As it does not require an electricity supply, it is portable and 'low tech' but, of course, does not have electronic alarms. More sophisticated generators include alarms and monitors of airway pressure, oxygen concentration and flow rate (for instance, Whisper Flow with Caradyne Criterion monitor). The main disadvantage with Venturi-based flow generators is the noise generated by turbulent flow of air at the air inlet.

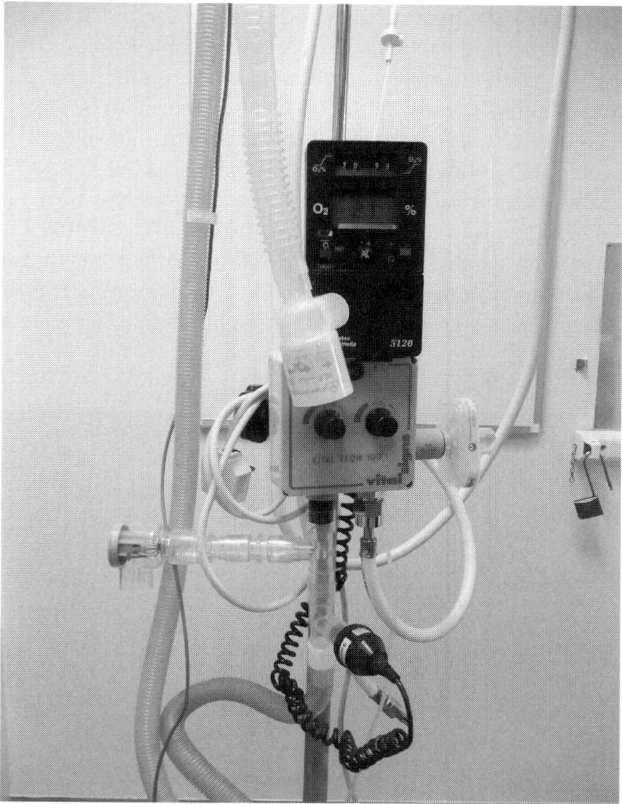


**Figure 4.1** Vital Signs' continuous positive airway pressure (CPAP) generator. Air is entrained by the Venturi effect. The filter acts to prevent particulate entrainment. The safety CPAP valve has a higher pressure ring than the treatment valve, which is mounted downstream of the CPAP mask (not shown). Oxygen analyser in circuit. Courtesy Vital Signs.

A bacterial filter can be attached at the inlet to prevent particulate matter from being entrained and this helps to reduce noise. The danger is that several filters in series are employed by staff wishing to further silence the device with a resulting failure to generate sufficient flow.

Another type of flow generator commonly used (Drager CF800, Lubeck, Germany) requires both compressed piped air and oxygen. Rotameters are individually adjusted to provide an approximate $FiO_2$ using preset formulae. The expandable reservoir bag (Fig. 4.2) ensures that high peak inspiratory flows result in only a minor drop in mask pressure. Theoretically this type of device will be less costly to operate (less use of oxygen) and, being quieter, these devices are often better tolerated by both patient and staff. With both flow generators, an oxygen analyser in the inspiratory circuit is required to allow precise control and monitoring of $FiO_2$. Some CPAP generators have integral oxygen analysers and other monitoring available.

Although the CPAP circuit is simple to construct from individual components, there is the potential risk of barotrauma, especially when used across a cuffed endotracheal or tracheostomy tube. This can occur if the CPAP valve is mounted in reverse. Of the reports with CPAP sent to the National Patient Safety Agency (NPSA) in the UK, incorrect alignment of the CPAP valve is the most serious and has led to the introduction of preassembled circuits that do not allow incorrect orientation of the CPAP valve. An additional safeguard is provided by inserting a higher-rated CPAP valve (20 cm) proximal to the patient. This will then be the maximum pressure applied in the case of failure of the exhalation valve. Modern flow generators also have an internal pressure relief safety valve, usually also 20 cm $H_2O$.

A consequence of both types of flow generator is that it is not possible to deliver an $FiO_2$ <33 per cent. This is usually of no significance but may be important in patients at risk of hypercapnia with high concentration oxygen, such as those with chronic respiratory failure from neuromuscular or chest wall disease or COPD. Such patients should be treated with non-invasive pressure support. If CPAP is being used to wean such patients from invasive ventilation, it is probably better to employ the intensive care unit (ICU) ventilator so that $FiO_2$ can be controlled.

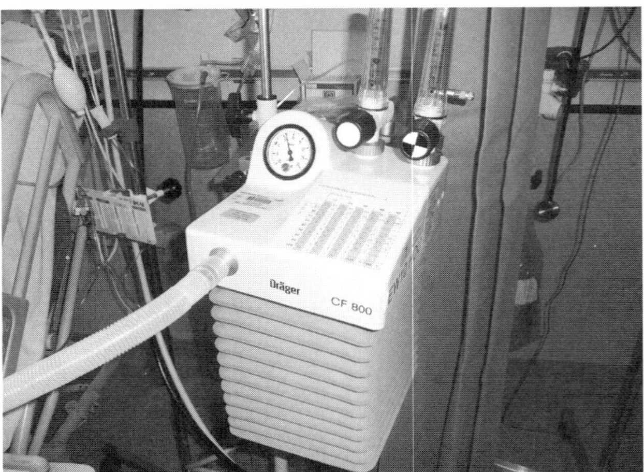


**Figure 4.2** Drager's bellows-type continuous positive airway pressure (CPAP) generator. Guide to flow rates of air and oxygen, adjusted by rotameters, to produce required $FiO_2$ and CPAP pressure monitor. Courtesy Drager.

## Interfaces

The most commonly used CPAP mask covers both nose and mouth. In the case of the helmet, the whole head is contained within the interface (see below). A soft silicone seal is adjusted to avoid significant leak, especially into the eyes, by tightening the slings of the head harness. Overtightening will result in patient discomfort and may result in ulceration because of ischaemic necrosis of the skin on the bridge of the nose. This rarely occurs with short-term use, e.g. cardiogenic pulmonary oedema, but some skin trauma is inevitable with prolonged CPAP use. We routinely employ GranuFLEX cushions over the bridge of the nose and cheeks when CPAP therapy is likely to be required for more than a few hours. The high $FiO_2$ employed with CPAP also causes mucosal drying, particularly of the mouth, and humidification is usually necessary with prolonged CPAP. A heated humidifier can be employed in the circuit with, or without, heated circuits depending on whether 'rain out' is occurring.

A nasogastric tube should be inserted if there is a risk of gastric paresis, e.g. diabetic ketoacidosis or other risk for vomiting. The author favours its insertion routinely. Not only can it be left on free drainage to limit the effect of air swallowing but it is also then available to aspirate prior to intubation if this proves necessary. It will also allow early enteral feeding if CPAP is successful.

# CLINICAL APPLICATIONS

## Tolerance of CPAP

Patient acceptability will be dependent on mask comfort, the noise associated by the flow generator and the potential respiratory distress caused by applying a close-fitting mask in a breathless patient. On the other hand, relief of hypoxaemia and improved pulmonary mechanics will aid patient comfort. Short-term tolerance is usually good if physiological benefit is obvious. If it is not, this may signal the need to consider intubation or a trial of a higher pressure exhalation valve. It is, of course, vital that nursing staff, and others, provide sufficient explanation to the competent patient. Profound breathlessness is a very uncomfortable sensation and strong reassurance as to the benefit of CPAP can be both therapeutic as well as good practice. It is also important to allow treatment breaks for mouth care, communication and to encourage secretion

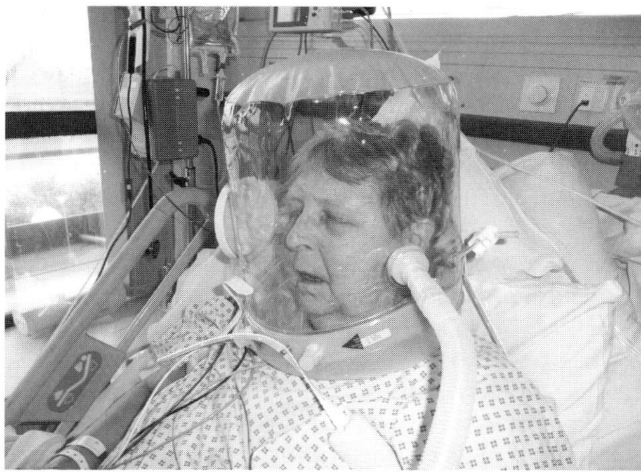

**Figure 4.3** Continuous positive airway pressure helmet.

clearance. Occasionally, it is both necessary and therapeutic to give opiates, e.g. morphine 2.5–5 mg or an anxiolytic such as lorazepam 0.5–1 mg.

Continuous positive airway pressure helmets (e.g. Starmed Castar Helmet-Miranodola, Italy, see Fig. 4.3) are increasingly being employed because of the significant failure (10 per cent +) with prolonged use of mask CPAP. Helmets rely on a flexible membrane around the inside of the helmet that expands and seals around the neck, ties under the arms limiting the caudal displacement of the helmet. The high dead space (9–15 L) causes re-breathing of exhaled carbon dioxide unless higher inspiratory flow rates than normal are used to flush out exhaled air.[3,4] The helmet appears to reduce the sense of claustrophobia associated with a CPAP mask and is well tolerated once applied. Initially the helmet looks a more daunting prospect to patients. It is not possible to humidify the gas flow as otherwise the patient disappears from view as condensation occurs within the helmet. Mucosal drying is less of an issue, presumably because airflow around the upper airway has a lower velocity and so causes less drying. In one comparative study, tolerance was no different from a CPAP mask but the use of the helmet allowed longer use without skin complications.[5] Interestingly, the noise inside the helmet is greater than with mask CPAP (>100 dB) but can be reduced by attaching a bacterial or a heat moisture exchange (HME) filter to the inlet and outlet ports.[6] The main problem is the cost of the helmet which is up to 10 times the cost of disposable CPAP masks.

## Contraindications to CPAP, patient monitoring and place of therapy

The absolute contraindications to CPAP are similar to the use of non-invasive methods of augmenting spontaneous breathing: an inability to maintain or protect the upper airway (including depressed consciousness), facial trauma, significant risk of aspiration or recent oesophageal surgery, gastrointestinal ileus or a history of vomiting, and the presence of copious secretions.

Relative contraindications include significant agitation and hypotension, particularly shock unresponsive to fluid challenge. Nevertheless, in cases of left ventricular failure with pulmonary oedema, CPAP may be beneficial by reducing both preload and afterload.[7] For a full discussion of the place of CPAP and NIV in acute cardiogenic pulmonary oedema, see Chapter 30.

The likelihood of disease progression is the most important aspect to consider when deciding on a trial of CPAP versus proceeding to intubation. Even if initially successful, there is the danger of exposing the patient to risk when rapid recovery cannot be expected, such as pneumonia or acute lung injury. In one evaluation of CPAP versus standard oxygen therapy,[8] CPAP was associated with more serious adverse events than usual oxygen therapy although intubation was reportedly not delayed by its use. Of 62 patients randomized to CPAP, 21 were intubated because of disease progression, i.e. CPAP failure. Four of these patients had cardiac arrest because of profound and sudden hypoxaemia at the time of intubation on CPAP removal. Another four subsequently developed gastrointestinal haemorrhage. At the initiation of CPAP, it is a 'trial of therapy' and progression to a need for intubation and invasive mechanical ventilation means that CPAP should only be started in clinical areas where access to intubation is immediately available.[9] This effectively means the emergency department, critical care (ICU or respiratory high-dependency unit [HDU]) and in theatre recovery areas. Nevertheless, the NPSA in the UK has received many descriptions of inexperienced staff attempting to use CPAP in non-critical care areas with an attendant increase in adverse events.

Monitoring the inspired oxygen concentration and the resulting patient saturation by oximetry is clearly essential but other indicators of the benefit of CPAP will include a fall in respiratory and heart rate and in systolic blood pressure when elevated. Commonly, an arterial line will be available to allow monitoring of pH and $PCO_2$.

## In what conditions is CPAP indicated?

Potentially any cause of type I respiratory failure could be managed by CPAP. As with all therapy, it is the balance of risks and benefits in comparison with alternative treatments. These include the conventional treatment appropriate to the condition – antibiotics for pneumonia, nitrates and diuretics for cardiogenic pulmonary oedema or haemofiltration in the context of renal failure – and treatment aimed at the life-threatening hypoxaemia by either high-concentration oxygen or intubation. Although the benefits of NIV in hypercapnic acute exacerbation of COPD has repeatedly been demonstrated, the evidence for the effectiveness of CPAP in *all-cause* acute respiratory failure is uncertain. Keenan *et al.*

carried out a systematic review of NIV in non-cardiogenic type I acute respiratory failure.[10] The headline findings were an absolute reduction in the need for intubation (23 per cent) and reduced length of ICU stay (2 days) but a less certain mortality reduction (17 per cent). The trials included in the analysis were, however, significantly heterogeneous, suggesting that effectiveness was dependent on patient selection and the underlying disease process. No such meta-analysis is available for CPAP. Although clinical experience demonstrates its effectiveness in improving oxygenation, it is unlikely that CPAP would be as effective as NIV in the more important outcomes of preventing intubation or reducing mortality. Two randomized trials deserve mention at this point. One was in post-surgical cases and was positive and the other in acute lung injury and was negative.

Following abdominal surgery, hypoxaemia develops in 30–50 per cent and leads to a reintubation rate of 8–10 per cent.[11] Squadrone *et al.*[12] report a comparison of CPAP with standard oxygenation therapy in 209 patients (16 per cent of all abdominal surgery cases screened) who developed a $PaO_2/FiO_2$ <300 and who were randomized to oxygen or CPAP (initially at 7.5 cm) using helmet CPAP. Therapy was continued for a mean of 19 hours. There were no CPAP failures because of patient intolerance. The intubation rate was 10 per cent in the control group and 1 per cent with CPAP ($p < 0.005$) with a reduced incidence of pneumonia and shortened length of ICU stay in the CPAP group.

Declaux *et al.*[8] compared CPAP by face mask with oxygen in patients with lung infiltrates and a $PaO_2/FiO_2$ <300. Acute lung injury was suspected in 81 per cent, with infection as the precipitant in 60 per cent and a contribution from cardiogenic pulmonary oedema in 30 per cent. There was a significant improvement in oxygenation index at 1 hour ($p < 0.001$) but no difference in overall intubation rate (30 per cent) or ICU mortality (20 per cent). Adverse events were significantly greater in the CPAP group (23 per cent vs 8 per cent, $p < 0.01$) with evidence, mentioned above, of major risk at the point of intubation and possibly an increased incidence of stress-induced gastrointestinal haemorrhage.

Smaller randomized controlled trials have been performed following abdominal aortic surgery[13] and chest wall trauma,[14] and in other conditions such as respiratory failure in immunosuppressed patients. These support the use of CPAP in reducing the need for intubation or reintubation. One study is notable in being performed out of hospital.[15] This unblinded but randomized trial in 71 emergency service callouts for acute respiratory distress involved management either conventionally or with the addition of CPAP in the immediate resuscitation of the patient. Fifty per cent of usual care patients were intubated against 20 per cent CPAP-treated cases ($p < 0.005$) giving a number needed to treat (NNT) of only 3. Mortality was also significantly less (14 per cent vs 35 per cent). Further trials in the out-of-hospital setting are clearly indicated. For further detailed discussion in individual patient populations see Chapters 41–48.

### CPAP IN WEANING FROM INVASIVE VENTILATION

Continuous positive airway pressure is commonly employed in the ICU during the weaning process. Unassisted breathing through an endotracheal or tracheostomy tube is used as part of the spontaneous breathing trial performed prior to extubation. In these circumstances, CPAP counteracts the resistance to flow by the tube and simulates the expiratory 'break' provided by the upper airway, which acts to preserve end-expiratory lung volume. As cuffed tubes are involved, high flows are not required. The normal double lumen ventilator tube is used with the patient remaining attached to the ICU ventilator. Pressure is generated by the ventilator rather than by using a CPAP valve in the expiratory limb. This is mostly for the convenience of switching back to mechanical ventilation but also allows monitoring of respiratory variables. Modern ICU ventilators can, of course, be used in the NIV mode but may not be suitable for use with helmet CPAP.[3] For further details of CPAP during weaning see Chapter 59.

### CPAP AND DIAGNOSTIC BRONCHOSCOPY

Continuous positive airway pressure and NIV reduce the need for invasive mechanical ventilation in the septic immunocompromised patient. One advantage of intubation in these circumstances is the ability to safely obtain diagnostic specimens, particularly when there has been failure of initial antibiotic and antifungal therapy. While not for the faint hearted, bronchioalveolar lavage may be performed through the CPAP mask[16] or helmet. For further consideration of this topic see Chapter 52.

### CPAP AND THE PHYSIOTHERAPIST

A number of methods may be used by therapy staff to promote lung re-expansion. These include CPAP,[17] although methods that combine CPAP followed by coughing, such as the cough in-exsufflator, are gaining in popularity. This topic is covered further in Chapter 62.

## SUMMARY AND CONCLUSIONS

While widely employed in acute care, the evidence for CPAP is surprisingly limited. Anyone with experience of working in the ICU or HDU will have witnessed the immediate improvement in $PaO_2/FiO_2$ ratio that commonly occurs after application of CPAP. This leads the clinician, understandably, to feel that CPAP must be benefiting the patient. The evidence on outcome is, however, mixed and there are no reliable and/or specific indicators that will predict the eventual need for intubation (when CPAP could be described as 'delaying the inevitable') versus cases where success with CPAP actually prevents intubation. As with NIV, there is the danger of exposing the patient to the risk of further physiological decline or of simply 'improving the numbers' for a short period.

When the benefit of avoiding intubation is high, such as in the immunocompromised or post-surgical case, the risk of delaying intubation is outweighed by this gain. Similarly, when a 'holding measure' is required, while awaiting effective therapy such as diuretics, CPAP is justified as the risk of progression to intubation in such circumstances is low. When, however, the patient trajectory is of progressive decline and/or the aetiological ca use for respiratory failure will take days to resolve, intubation should not, in the author's opinion, be delayed by a trial of CPAP and certainly not in an area where intubation is not safely and immediately available.

## REFERENCES


1. Linder KH, Lotz P, Ahnefeld FW. Continuous positive airway pressure effect on functional residual capacity, vital capacity and its subdivisions. *Chest* 1987; **92**: 66–70.
2. Katz, JA, Marks JD. Inspiratory work with and without continuous positive airway pressure in patients with acute respiratory failure. *Anesthesiology* 1985; **63**: 598–607.
3. Taccone P, Hess D, Caironi P, Bigatello M. Continuous positive airway pressure delivered with a helmet: effects on carbon dioxide re-breathing. *Crit Care Med* 2004; **32**: 2090–6.
4. Patroniti N, Foti G, Manfio A *et al.* Head helmet v facemask for non-invasive continuous positive airway pressure: a physiological study. *Intensive Care Med* 2003; **29**: 1680–7.
5. Tonnelier JM, Prat G, Nowak E *et al.* Non-invasive continuous positive airway pressure ventilation using a new helmet interface: a case control prospective pilot study. *Intensive Care Med* 2003; **29**: 2077–80.
6. Cavaliere F, Conti G, Costa R *et al.* Noise exposure during non-invasive ventilation with a helmet, a nasal mask and a facial mask. *Intensive Care Med* 2004; **30**: 1755–60.
7. Mehta S, Liu P, Fitzgerald F *et al.* Effects of continuous positive airway pressure on cardiac volumes in patients with ischaemic and dilated cardiomyopathy. *Am J Respir Crit Care Med* 2000; **161**: 128–34.
8. Declaux C, L'Here, Alberti C *et al.* Treatment of acute hypoxaemic non-hypocapneic respiratory insufficiency with continuous positive airway pressure delivered by a facemask: a randomised controlled trial. *JAMA* 2000; **284**: 2352–60.
9. Evans TW. International consensus conference in intensive care medicine: non-invasive positive pressure ventilation. In: Acute respiratory failure. *Intensive Care Med* 2001; **27**: 166–78.
10. Keenan SP, Sinuff T, Cook DJ *et al.* Does noninvasive positive pressure ventilation improve outcome in acute hypoxaemic respiratory failure? A systematic review. *Crit Care Med* 2004; **32**: 2516–23.
11. O'Donohue WJ. National survey of the usage of lung expansion modalities for the prevention and treatment of postoperative atelectasis following abdominal and thoracic surgery. *Chest* 1985; **87**: 76–80.
12. Squadrone V, Coha M, Cerutti *et al.* Continuous positive airway pressure for treatment of post-operative hypoxaemia: a randomised controlled trial. *JAMA* 2005; **293**: 589–95.
13. Kindgen-Milles D, Muller E, Buhl R *et al.* Nasal-continuous positive pressure reduces pulmonary morbidity and length of stay following thoracoabdominal aortic surgery. *Chest* 2005; **128**: 821–8.
14. Gunduz M, Unlugenc H, Ozalevi M *et al.* A comparative study of continuous positive airway pressure (CPAP) and intermittent positive pressure ventilation (IPPV) in patients with flail chest. *Emerg Med J* 2005; **22**: 325–9.
15. Thompson J, Petrie DA, Ackroyd-Stolarz S *et al.* Out-of-hospital continuous positive airway pressure ventilation versus usual care in acute respiratory failure. *Ann Emerg Med* 2008; **52**: 232–41.
16. Maitre B, Jaber S, Maggiore S *et al.* Continuous positive airway pressure during fibre optic bronchoscopy in hypoxaemic patients: a randomised double-blind study using a new device. *Am J Respir Crit Care Med* 2000; **162**: 1063–7.
17. Placidi G, Cornacchia M, Polese G *et al.* Chest physiotherapy with positive airway pressure: a pilot study of short term effects on sputum clearance in patients with cystic fibrosis and severe airway obstruction. *Respir Care* 2006; **51**: 1145–53.

# 5

# Emerging modes for non-invasive ventilation

PAOLO NAVALESI, ROSANNA VASCHETTO, ANTONIO MESSINA

## ABSTRACT

A variety of modes can be used to deliver non-invasive ventilation (NIV). Pressure support ventilation (PSV) is the most commonly used mode for NIV. New features to improve PSV application have been recently proposed, such as the algorithms for leak compensation, and adjustment of cycling-off threshold and rate of pressurization. In the past few years, some new modes have been introduced into clinical practice, which can also be used for NIV. Proportional assist ventilation (PAV) and neurally adjusted ventilatory assistance (NAVA) aim to improve patient–ventilator interaction by matching the ventilator support with the neural output of the respiratory centres. Average volume-assured pressure support (AVAPS) aims to guarantee an adequate tidal volume regardless of clinical variations over time.

## INTRODUCTION

New modes of ventilation generally introduce novel approaches to support delivery.[1] Non-invasive ventilation (NIV) can be considered a specific technique, in which the tracheal tube is replaced by an external interface, such as a mask, mouthpiece or helmet. Although, in principle, NIV can be applied using the same ventilator equipment as is used for invasive ventilation, several features make NIV a unique technique. As for mechanical ventilation through an endotracheal tube, the primary reasons for applying NIV are improving gas exchange and reducing inspiratory effort. Although intubated patients commonly receive continuous sedative infusion, those undergoing NIV are awake or only mildly sedated, so that patient comfort becomes a key issue for NIV success. In fact, poor tolerance is not infrequently reported as the primary reason for NIV failure.[2,3] In contrast to invasive ventilation, NIV is characterized by almost constant air leaks,[4] which interfere with support delivery, causing patient–ventilator mismatch, adding to patient discomfort, and, overall, impairing NIV tolerance.[2]

Although the use of controlled mechanical ventilation during NIV has been reported,[4] NIV is commonly applied using forms of partial support, where the ventilator recognizes the onset of the patient's effort to breathe through the triggering function. Once triggered, the mechanical breath is delivered either as volume targeted or pressure targeted. With volume targeted breaths, so-called volume-targeted assist-control, a preset inspiratory volume is delivered with a flow rate that depends on the predetermined inspiratory time. Flow rates that do not match the patient's demand and are either excessive or insufficient cause patient discomfort; moreover, in the case of leaks, the amount of inspiratory volume actually delivered to the patient is decreased.[5]

Pressure-targeted modes of support are the most widely utilized for NIV application. With these modes, the ventilator delivers a constant pressure for a time that either is preset (pressure-targeted assist-control) or depends on the drop of inspiratory flow below a threshold, so-called pressure support ventilation (PSV). As the pressure in the mask is limited due to its square profile, for the same delivered tidal volume, air leaks are reduced; furthermore, because the preset pressure is kept constant throughout insufflation, irrespective of the presence of leaks, an adequate tidal volume is more likely to be achieved.[5,6]

Unfortunately, however, PSV may fail to achieve optimal patient–ventilator interaction, resulting in poor patient comfort.[2] For these reasons, several additional features have been introduced in the recent years by many ventilator manufacturers in the attempt to facilitate patient–ventilator interaction. A further challenging approach to improve patient–ventilator interaction would be to match ventilator support with the neural output of the respiratory centres.

Two modes, proportional assist ventilation (PAV)[7] and neurally adjusted ventilatory assistance (NAVA),[8] have been developed for this purpose. Maintaining an adequate tidal volume, regardless of clinical variations over time, is another clinical goal. In PSV the preset pressure does not vary in the presence of modifications of the respiratory system impedance, secondary to changes in airway resistance and pulmonary and/or chest wall compliance, so that alveolar hypoventilation may occur. To overcome this drawback, average volume-assured pressure support (AVAPS) has been proposed.[9,10]

## NEW FEATURES OF PRESSURE SUPPORT VENTILATION

The combination of PSV and positive end-expiratory pressure (PEEP) is the most common form of assistance for NIV application. When PEEP is applied to PSV, the preset inspiratory pressure is intended as an addition to PEEP and the actual pressure applied during inspiration is the sum of inspiratory and expiratory preset pressures. When turbine-driven bi-level ventilators are used, the terms EPAP (expiratory positive airway pressure) and IPAP (inspiratory positive airway pressure) are generally used; in this latter case, IPAP is the total pressure applied during inspiration and, therefore, the inspiratory support is the difference between IPAP and EPAP.

Invasive and non-invasive applications of PSV have been proved to have comparable physiological and clinical benefits, improving gas exchange and reducing dyspnoea and diaphragm energy expenditure.[11] This holds true, however, only when NIV is well tolerated by the patients. Air leaks may alter patient–ventilator matching, primarily by interfering with cycling-off of ventilator insufflation. In PSV, in fact, the machine cycles from inspiration to expiration when the flow drops below a preset threshold, which is in general a percentage of the peak inspiratory flow achieved at the onset of inspiration. Leaks through the interface delay, and sometimes prevent, the attainment of that threshold and cause remarkable asynchronies, leading to NIV failure.[2] Air leaks may also affect inspiratory trigger function.[12] Nowadays it is generally accepted that ventilators capable of detecting and compensating for leaks are more likely to achieve successful NIV.

Beside the presence of leaks, the cycling-off threshold plays an important role in determining the quality of patient–ventilator synchrony and the patient's comfort during NIV. Many ventilators offer a specific function that allows modifying this threshold value, which should be set, in principle, in a manner to match as close as possible the patient's own (neural) end of inspiration. When the ventilator stops the mechanical insufflations before the end of the patient's effort, the inspiratory muscles continue to contract during the expiratory phase, causing double triggering and an increase in the work of breathing (WOB).[13] In contrast, prolonging mechanical insufflation into neural expiration may worsen dynamic hyperinflation by reducing the time available for lung emptying, causing ineffective inspiratory efforts, recruiting expiratory muscles, and, overall, leading to patient discomfort.[14]

In two studies in patients with acute lung injury a cycling-off threshold anticipating mechanical insufflation with respect to neural inspiration caused a reduction in tidal volume, with an increase in respiratory rate and WOB.[15,16] In contrast, two other studies performed in chronic obstructive pulmonary disease (COPD) patients found that anticipating the cycling-off threshold reduced dynamic hyperinflation and WOB.[17,18] During non-invasive ventilation, the presence of air leaks further complicate this complex interplay.[2]

In the past, most ventilators applied the inspiratory support with a fixed, usually the fastest, rate of pressurization. Nowadays, most ventilators permit varying the rate of rise of airway pressure to match patient demand and improve patient comfort. A faster rate of pressurization generally corresponds to a higher and earlier peak inspiratory flow. Prinianakis *et al.* studied 15 COPD patients recovering from an episode of hypercapnic acute respiratory failure (ARF), who underwent four trials of non-invasive PSV with different rates of pressurization applied in random order.[19] The authors found that increasing the rate of pressurization progressively decreased inspiratory effort; at the same time, however, air leaks increased and patient tolerance to NIV worsened. Noteworthy, arterial blood gases were not significantly affected by the different settings. This study confirms that individual titration of this specific setting may help achieve the best results with respect to WOB and patient comfort during NIV.

## PROPORTIONAL ASSIST VENTILATION

During partial support, the overall pressure applied to the respiratory system is contributed by the respiratory muscles and the ventilator. While during PSV, a constant pressure is applied throughout inspiration regardless of the intensity of the patient's drive to breathe, with proportional assist ventilation (PAV) the ventilator generates pressure in proportion to the patient's effort.[7] With PAV, in fact, the ventilator instantaneously delivers positive pressure throughout inspiration in proportion to patient-generated flow, flow assist (FA) expressed in $cmH_2O/L/s$, and volume assist (VA) in $cmH_2O/L$. Consequently, an augmented ventilatory output (i.e. flow and volume), secondary to an increase in patient demand and effort, corresponds to a higher amount of support delivery. The patient retains control of both timing and size of the breath and there are no preset pressure, flow or volume targets.

In comparison with PSV, PAV aims to improve patient–ventilator interaction. Good patient–ventilator synchrony implies that onset and end of the patient's neural inspiration are properly detected, and that mechanical assistance is delivered in synchrony with the patient's effort. With both modes, however, ventilator support is triggered by pneumatic signals (airway pressure, flow or volume) and the ability to trigger the ventilator is equally impaired in the presence of intrinsic PEEP (PEEPi), a threshold load that the patient has to overcome before the preset negative airway pressure and/or inspiratory flow are generated,[20] which makes it necessary to apply external PEEP to reduce patient effort and trigger delay.[21]

Proper adjustment of PAV settings necessitates knowledge of the mechanical characteristics of the respiratory system.[1,22] This drawback has been overcome by a further development of PAV, so-called PAV+, where resistance and elastance are constantly monitored through a non-invasive technique, and FA and VA are accordingly automatically adjusted;[23,24] this technique, however, requires a closed system and is not applicable for NIV. Moreover, in the presence of air leaks expiration is hampered because the ventilator keeps providing positive pressure related to the leaked volume and flow, and therefore the application of PAV through a non-invasive interface necessitates the use of ventilators with specific algorithms to recognize and compensate for leaks.[25]

The effects of PAV have been investigated in patients with ARF and chronic respiratory failure (CRF). It has been found that in patients with stable hypoxaemic and hypercapnic CRF secondary to COPD or restrictive chest wall disease, PAV delivered through a nasal mask is well tolerated and improves arterial blood gases,[26] and decreases WOB.[27] Porta *et al.* compared the short-term physiological effects of NIV delivery by PSV and PAV in clinically stable patients with CRF secondary to COPD and restrictive chest wall disease.[28] Compared with spontaneous unassisted breathing, there was no difference in the improvement in breathing pattern and reduction in inspiratory muscle effort between PSV and PAV.[28] Serra *et al.* studied the acute physiological response to NIV delivered by PSV and PAV, set according to patient comfort, in 12 patients with severe cystic fibrosis and chronic hypercapnia.[29] They found that short-term application of NIV with both modes had positive effects on minute ventilation, gas exchange and diaphragmatic effort, although with PAV these results were achieved at lower mean inspiratory pressure.

Non-invasive PAV has also been shown to increase exercise tolerance during constant power submaximal exercise in severe COPD with CRF.[30,31] In a crossover study by Wysocki *et al.*, 12 patients with ARF due to COPD exacerbation underwent NIV with both PAV and PSV.[25] Compared to PSV, PAV was equally effective in unloading the respiratory muscles and improved NIV tolerance. Gay *et al.* compared PAV with PSV in a randomized pilot study including patients with mild to moderate ARF receiving NIV.[32] They found that PAV was feasible and, compared with PSV, was associated with a more rapid improvement in a few physiological variables and resulted in better patient tolerance. A major limitation of this study was that PAV and PSV were delivered using two different ventilators, only one of which (PAV) incorporated algorithms for air leak compensation. A randomized controlled trial compared NIV with PSV and PAV in 117 patients with ARF of varied aetiologies.[33] The primary endpoints were rate of death and intubation, and the secondary outcomes were gas exchange, respiratory rate, haemodynamics, dyspnoea, comfort and length of intensive care unit (ICU) and hospital stay. Mortality and intubation rate were not different. Among the secondary outcome variables, only dyspnoea and comfort were significantly improved with PAV as opposed to PSV, with no other significant differences. Rusterholtz *et al.* compared PAV added to 5 cm $H_2O$ of continuous positive airway pressure (CPAP) with CPAP 10 cm $H_2O$ in the treatment of 36 patients with acute cardiogenic pulmonary oedema causing unresolving dyspnoea, tachypnoea and hypoxaemia despite maximal standard treatment. PAV was not superior to CPAP with respect to either efficacy or tolerance.[34]

In conclusion, compared with PSV, PAV may improve patient comfort during NIV to some extent, but this extent of this improvement and its overall clinical benefit seems to be rather small and not quite clinically relevant.

## NEURALLY ADJUSTED VENTILATORY ASSISTANCE

Neurally adjusted ventilatory assistance was developed in an attempt to overcome some of the limitations of PAV while maintaining part of its potential advantages.[8] With NAVA, triggering, cycling-off and assist profile are regulated by the electrical activity of the diaphragm ($EA_{di}$), whereas the amount of assistance depends on a user-controlled gain factor (NAVA level); $EA_{di}$, obtained by transoesophageal electromyography, is the best achievable index of the neural respiratory drive.[8,35] The electrodes used to measure $EA_{di}$ are mounted on a nasogastric feeding tube routinely used in critically ill patients. Because the ventilator is directly triggered by $EA_{di}$, with NAVA the synchrony between neural and mechanical inspiratory time is guaranteed both at the onset and at the end of inspiration, regardless of the mechanical properties of the respiratory system, presence of dynamic hyperinflation and PEEPi, variations in muscle length or contractility, and occurrence of air leaks.[8] As long as the respiratory centres, phrenic nerves and neuromuscular junctions are intact, and the ventilatory drive is not entirely suppressed by sedative drugs, the amount of support provided instantaneously corresponds to the ventilatory demand[8] (Fig. 5.1). In a series of critically ill patients with ARF of varied aetiologies, compared with PSV, NAVA had similar effects on gas exchange and improved patient–ventilator synchrony, irrespective of the amount of support provided.[36]

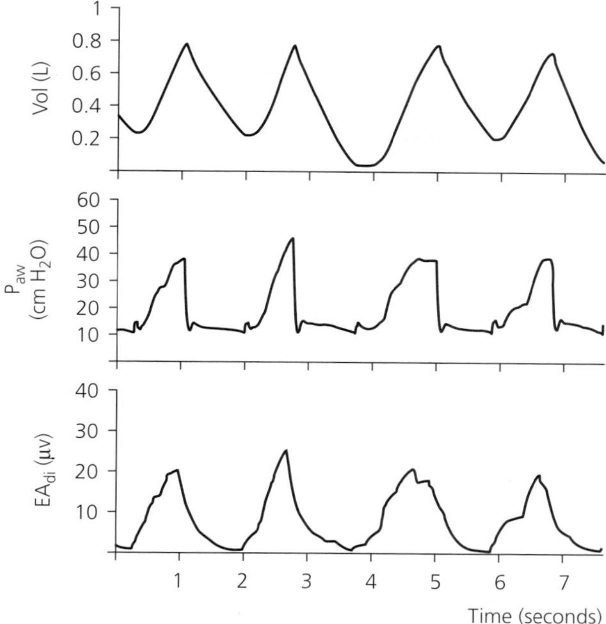


**Figure 5.1** Volume, airway pressure ($P_{aw}$) and electrical activity of the diaphragm ($EA_{di}$) tracings from a patient receiving neurally adjusted ventilatory assistance (NAVA). Note the precise synchronization between patient effort ($EA_{di}$) and ventilator assistance ($P_{aw}$).

Few studies have evaluated the use of NAVA to deliver NIV. Beck *et al.* demonstrated in an animal model of acute lung injury that the application of NAVA through a leaky non-invasive interface was effective in unloading the respiratory muscles while maintaining good subject–ventilator synchrony.[37] The efficacy of NIV delivery was ensured also in the presence of large leaks.[37] Moerer *et al.* compared the use of $EA_{di}$ with a conventional pneumatic signal in healthy subjects for cycling on and off the ventilator during PSV via helmet.[38] Subject–ventilator synchrony, triggering effort and breathing comfort were significantly less impaired at increasing levels of support and breathing frequency with $EA_{di}$ as opposed to the conventional pneumatic signal. A physiological study has been recently conducted to compare the short-term effects of PSV and NAVA in delivering NIV through a helmet in patients with acute hypoxaemic respiratory failure.[39] There were no significant differences with regard to gas exchange, respiratory rate and neural effort between the two modes, while patient–ventilator synchrony was significantly improved with NAVA as opposed to PSV.[39] Although NAVA has the potential to improve patient–ventilator interaction during NIV, regardless of the amount of air leaks, further physiological and clinical studies are necessary to confirm its efficacy in the clinical setting. Because a nasogastric tube is necessary to apply NAVA, its use will likely be limited to the most severe patients in ICU.

## AVERAGE VOLUME-ASSURED PRESSURE SUPPORT

This is a novel form of non-invasive support that associates a tidal volume target to PSV by means of an algorithm estimating the patient's tidal volume over several breaths and calculating the variation in IPAP necessary to achieve the target tidal volume. AVAPS has been designed to adapt the amount of IPAP to changes in respiratory impedance, with the aim of improving patient comfort and safety. The algorithm progressively varies IPAP by 0.5–1 cm $H_2O$ every minute to guarantee the preset target tidal volume.

Using a crossover design, Storre *et al.* studied 10 mildly hypercapnic patients with obesity–hypoventilation syndrome who failed to respond to nocturnal CPAP (8.9 ± 1.0 mbar).[10] Patients were randomized to undergo 6 weeks of nocturnal NIV either in conventional bi-level mode (IPAP 14.7 ± 2.4 mbar, EPAP 6.1 ± 1.1 mbar) or AVAPS (IPAP 16.4 ± 3.9 mbar, EPAP 5.4 ± 1.2 mbar) and then switched to 6 further weeks of NIV with the complementary mode.[10] Compared with pretreatment baseline, sleep quality and health-related quality of life were improved with both modes (CPAP not evaluated); furthermore, AVAPS, but not CPAP and bi-level ventilation, ameliorated transcutaneous carbon dioxide tension.[10] Another recent study comparing NIV delivered with PSV and AVAPS in 28 patients with CRF of varied aetiologies found no difference between the two modes with regard to sleep efficiency; AVAPS resulted in higher minute ventilation in the lateral decubitus, but not in the supine position.[9] Studies evaluating the use of AVAPS in acute patients are lacking.

The paucity of data and the relatively small differences found between AVAPS and PSV do not prove so far any clear advantage of this novel approach over the conventional pressure-targeted NIV modes.

## REFERENCES


1. Navalesi P, Costa R. New modes of mechanical ventilation: proportional assist ventilation, neurally adjusted ventilatory assist, and fractal ventilation. *Curr Opin Crit Care* 2003; **9**: 51–8.
2. Calderini E, Confalonieri M, Puccio PG *et al.* Patient-ventilator asynchrony during noninvasive ventilation: the role of expiratory trigger. *Intensive Care Med* 1999; **25**: 662–7.
3. Squadrone E, Frigerio P, Fogliati C *et al.* Noninvasive vs invasive ventilation in COPD patients with severe acute respiratory failure deemed to require ventilatory assistance. *Intensive Care Med* 2004; **30**: 1303–10.
4. Mehta S, Hill NS. Noninvasive ventilation. *Am J Respir Crit Care Med* 2001; **163**: 540–77.
5. Mehta S, McCool FD, Hill NS. Leak compensation in positive pressure ventilators: a lung model study. *Eur Respir J* 2001; **17**: 259–67.

6. Highcock MP, Smith IE, Shneerson JM. The effect of noninvasive intermittent positive-pressure ventilation during exercise in severe scoliosis. *Chest* 2002; **121**: 1555–60.
7. Younes M. Proportional assist ventilation, a new approach to ventilatory support. Theory. *Am Rev Respir Dis* 1992; **145**: 114–20.
8. Sinderby C, Navalesi P, Beck J *et al.* Neural control of mechanical ventilation in respiratory failure. *Nat Med* 1999; **5**: 1433–6.
9. Ambrogio C, Lowman X, Kuo M *et al.* Sleep and non-invasive ventilation in patients with chronic respiratory insufficiency. *Intensive Care Med* 2009; **35**: 306–13.
10. Storre JH, Seuthe B, Fiechter R *et al.* Average volume-assured pressure support in obesity hypoventilation: A randomized crossover trial. *Chest* 2006; **130**: 815–21.
11. Vitacca M, Ambrosino N, Clini E *et al.* Physiological response to pressure support ventilation delivered before and after extubation in patients not capable of totally spontaneous autonomous breathing. *Am J Respir Crit Care Med* 2001; **164**: 638–41.
12. Miyoshi E, Fujino Y, Uchiyama A *et al.* Effects of gas leak on triggering function, humidification, and inspiratory oxygen fraction during noninvasive positive airway pressure ventilation. *Chest* 2005; **128**: 3691–8.
13. Vignaux L, Vargas F, Roeseler J *et al.* Patient-ventilator asynchrony during non-invasive ventilation for acute respiratory failure: a multicenter study. *Intensive Care Med* 2009; **35**: 840–6.
14. Younes M, Kun J, Webster K *et al.* Response of ventilator-dependent patients to delayed opening of exhalation valve. *Am J Respir Crit Care Med* 2002; **166**: 21–30.
15. Chiumello D, Pelosi P, Carlesso E *et al.* Noninvasive positive pressure ventilation delivered by helmet vs. standard face mask. *Intensive Care Med* 2003; **29**: 1671–9.
16. Tokioka H, Tanaka T, Ishizu T *et al.* The effect of breath termination criterion on breathing patterns and the work of breathing during pressure support ventilation. *Anesth Analg* 2001; **92**: 161–5.
17. Chiumello D, Polli F, Tallarini F *et al.* Effect of different cycling-off criteria and positive end-expiratory pressure during pressure support ventilation in patients with chronic obstructive pulmonary disease. *Crit Care Med* 2007; **35**: 2547–52.
18. Tassaux D, Gainnier M, Battisti A *et al.* Impact of expiratory trigger setting on delayed cycling and inspiratory muscle workload. *Am J Respir Crit Care Med* 2005; **172**: 1283–9.
19. Prinianakis G, Delmastro M, Carlucci A *et al.* Effect of varying the pressurisation rate during noninvasive pressure support ventilation. *Eur Respir J* 2004; **23**: 314–20.
20. Appendini L, Patessio A, Zanaboni S *et al.* Physiologic effects of positive end-expiratory pressure and mask pressure support during exacerbations of chronic obstructive pulmonary disease. *Am J Respir Crit Care Med* 1994; **149**: 1069–76.
21. Appendini L, Purro A, Gudjonsdottir M *et al.* Physiologic response of ventilator-dependent patients with chronic obstructive pulmonary disease to proportional assist ventilation and continuous positive airway pressure. *Am J Respir Crit Care Med* 1999; **159**: 1510–17.
22. Navalesi P, Hernandez P, Wongsa A *et al.* Proportional assist ventilation in acute respiratory failure: effects on breathing pattern and inspiratory effort. *Am J Respir Crit Care Med* 1996; **154**: 1330–8.
23. Younes M, Kun J, Masiowski B *et al.* A method for noninvasive determination of inspiratory resistance during proportional assist ventilation. *Am J Respir Crit Care Med* 2001; **163**: 829–39.
24. Younes M, Webster K, Kun J *et al.* A method for measuring passive elastance during proportional assist ventilation. *Am J Respir Crit Care Med* 2001; **164**: 50–60.
25. Wysocki M, Richard JC, Meshaka P. Noninvasive proportional assist ventilation compared with noninvasive pressure support ventilation in hypercapnic acute respiratory failure. *Crit Care Med* 2002; **30**: 323–9.
26. Ambrosino N, Vitacca M, Polese G *et al.* Short-term effects of nasal proportional assist ventilation in patients with chronic hypercapnic respiratory insufficiency. *Eur Respir J* 1997; **10**: 2829–34.
27. Polese G, Vitacca M, Bianchi L *et al.* Nasal proportional assist ventilation unloads the inspiratory muscles of stable patients with hypercapnia due to COPD. *Eur Respir J* 2000; **16**: 491–8.
28. Porta R, Appendini L, Vitacca M *et al.* Mask proportional assist vs pressure support ventilation in patients in clinically stable condition with chronic ventilatory failure. *Chest* 2002; **122**: 479–88.
29. Serra A, Polese G, Braggion C *et al.* Non-invasive proportional assist and pressure support ventilation in patients with cystic fibrosis and chronic respiratory failure. *Thorax* 2002; **57**: 50–4.
30. Bianchi L, Foglio K, Pagani M *et al.* Effects of proportional assist ventilation on exercise tolerance in COPD patients with chronic hypercapnia. *Eur Respir J* 1998; **11**: 422–7.
31. Dolmage TE, Goldstein RS. Proportional assist ventilation and exercise tolerance in subjects with COPD. *Chest* 1997; **111**: 948–54.
32. Gay PC, Hess DR, Hill NS. Noninvasive proportional assist ventilation for acute respiratory insufficiency. Comparison with pressure support ventilation. *Am J Respir Crit Care Med* 2001; **164**: 1606–11.
33. Fernandez-Vivas M, Caturla-Such J, Gonzalez de la Rosa J. Noninvasive pressure support versus proportional assist ventilation in acute respiratory failure. *Intensive Care Med* 2003; **29**: 1126–33.

34. Rusterholtz T, Kempf J, Berton C *et al.* Noninvasive pressure support ventilation (NIPSV) with face mask in patients with acute cardiogenic pulmonary edema (ACPE). *Intensive Care Med* 1999; **25**: 21–8.
35. Beck J, Gottfried SB, Navalesi P *et al.* Electrical activity of the diaphragm during pressure support ventilation in acute respiratory failure. *Am J Respir Crit Care Med* 2001; **164**: 419–24.
36. Colombo D, Cammarota G, Bergamaschi V *et al.* Physiologic response to varying levels of pressure support and neurally adjusted ventilatory assist in patients with acute respiratory failure. *Intensive Care Med* 2008; **34**: 2010–18.
37. Beck J, Brander L, Slutsky AS *et al.* Non-invasive neurally adjusted ventilatory assist in rabbits with acute lung injury. *Intensive Care Med* 2008; **34**: 316–23.
38. Moerer O, Beck J, Brander L *et al.* Subject-ventilator synchrony during neural versus pneumatically triggered non-invasive helmet ventilation. *Intensive Care Med* 2008; **34**: 1615–23.
39. Cammarota G, Costa R, Blando C *et al.* Non invasive ventilation (NIV) by helmet for treatment of hypoxemic acute respiratory failure (ARF): pressure support (PS) vs. neurally adjusted ventilatory assist (NAVA). *Intensive Care Med* 2009; **35**: 9.

# 6

# Interfaces

CESARE GREGORETTI, DAVIDE CHIUMELLO

ABSTRACT

Non-invasive ventilation (NIV) has an important role in the treatment of acute respiratory failure (ARF) and in stable chronic hypercapnic respiratory failure. The success of NIV depends on several factors, such as the patient population, the setting in which the treatment is provided, presence of a well-trained and motivated team, rigorous monitoring, type of ventilator and, most importantly, the type of interface used. Practically, a full face mask or a total full face mask should be the first-line strategy in the initial management of hypercapnic acute respiratory failure with NIV. However, if NIV has to be prolonged, switching to a nasal mask may improve comfort by reducing face mask complications. In contrast, in mild ARF a nasal mask should be tried first, which is better tolerated, or nasal pillows, which are less likely to cause skin damage. Helmet ventilation may also offer an appealing approach. However, physicians must know the physical and mechanical properties of the helmets, to obtain effective carbon dioxide clearance and downloading of the patient's muscles.

## INTRODUCTION

Non-invasive ventilation (NIV) has an important role in the treatment of acute respiratory failure (ARF)[1–12] and in stable chronic hypercapnic respiratory failure.[13–15] The choice of interface is a major determinant of NIV success or failure, mainly because the interface strongly affects patient comfort.[16–18] As a consequence patient comfort is crucial for NIV success in both acute[19,20] and chronic[21] settings. Patient comfort may be affected by the interface with respect to many factors, such as air leaks, claustrophobia, facial skin erythema, acneiform rash, eye irritation and skin breakdown.[17,18,22–35]

In a survey of over 3000 home care patients ventilated with continuous positive airway pressure (CPAP), Meslier *et al.*[36] found that only about half of the patients classified their interface fit as 'good' or 'very good'. Although nasal masks are more comfortable for stable chronic patients undergoing long-term domiciliary NIV,[18] in patients with ARF, who breathe through both the nose and the mouth, a face mask is preferred.[37]

A review of studies using NIV showed that in ARF, the face mask is the most commonly used interface (63 per cent) followed by nasal mask (31 per cent), nasal pillow, and mouthpiece.[18] Recent data[38] from a web-based survey of about 300 intensive care units and respiratory wards throughout Europe confirmed that oronasal masks are the most commonly used interfaces for ARF, followed by nasal masks, full face masks and helmets.

In chronic respiratory failure the most common interface used is the nasal mask (73 per cent) followed by nasal pillow, face masks and mouthpieces.[31]

## CHARACTERISTICS, ADVANTAGES, AND DISADVANTAGES OF THE VARIOUS NON-INVASIVE VENTILATION INTERFACES

Box 6.1 summarizes the characteristics of an ideal NIV interface.

Air leak minimization and comfort depend on the complex interplay between the patient (underlying disease, face contour and claustrophobia), the ventilator settings (mode of ventilation, inspiratory–expiratory applied pressures, and inspiratory–expiratory trigger thresholds), the interface (type, size, material, and shape) and the securing system (sites of attachment and tension).[31–39] NIV is now considered by most critical care physicians as an effective treatment for selected forms of ARF because of the continuous development of new materials and designs which have increased the availability of interfaces and therefore

**Box 6.1 Characteristics of an ideal NIV interface and securing system**

Interface and securing system

- Ideal interface
- Leak-free
- Good stability
- Non-traumatic
- Light-weight
- Long-lasting
- Non-deformable
- Non-allergenic material
- Low resistance to airflow
- Minimal dead space (when needed)
- Low cost
- Easy to manufacture (for the moulded interfaces)
- Available in various sizes

Ideal securing system

- Stable (to avoid interface movements or dislocation)
- Easy to put on or remove
- Non-traumatic
- Light and soft
- Breathable material
- Available in various sizes
- Washable, for home care
- Disposable, for hospital use

Modified from Nava *et al.*[31]

**Box 6.2 Classes of non-invasive ventilation interfaces**

- Oral interfaces: mouthpiece placed between the patient's lips and held in place by lip seal or the teeth
- Nasal mask: covers the nose but not the mouth
- Nasal pillows: plugs inserted into the nostrils
- Oronasal: covers the nose and mouth
- Full face: covers the mouth, nose and eyes
- Helmet: covers the whole head and all or part of the neck

enhanced the use of NIV.[39,40] The classes of NIV interface are shown in Box 6.2.

Interfaces include standard commercially available ready-to-use models in various sizes (neonatal, paediatric, and adult small, medium, and large) or custom-fabricated, moulded directly on the patient or from a moulded cast previously obtained.[24–26] Depending on the model, the time required to custom-fabricate a mask ranges from 10 minutes to 30 minutes for a skilled operator,[27,28] so custom-fabricated masks are probably not indicated for critically ill patients in ARF.

Many commercially available masks consist of two parts: a cushion of soft material (polyvinyl chloride, polypropylene, silicone, silicone elastomer or hydrogel), which forms the seal against the patient's face, and a frame of stiff material (polyvinyl chloride, polycarbonate or thermoplastic), which in many models is transparent. There are four types of face-seal cushion: transparent non-inflatable, transparent inflatable, full hydrogel and full foam. The mask frame has several attachment points (e.g. prongs) to anchor the headgear. The higher the number of attachment points, the higher is the probability of obtaining the best fit and the ability to target the point of maximum pressure.[29] Many types of strap assemblies are available.[17] Straps secure the mask with hooks or Velcro. Some interfaces have one or more holes in the frame to prevent rebreathing (so-called 'vent system') (Fig. 6.1). Such a mask should not be used with a circuit that has separate inspiratory and expiratory limbs or with an expiratory valve or other external device for carbon dioxide clearance (e.g. the Respironics Plateau valve).[31]

A tube adapter allows insertion of a nasogastric tube and prevents the air leak and facial skin damage that could occur if the nasogastric tube was tucked under the seal of a conventional mask.[17–22] Chin straps, lips seals, and mouth taping have also been proposed as means to prevent air leaks.[16,17] Reducing the risk of skin damage is one of the major goals (Box 6.3).

Gregoretti *et al.*[22] performed a multicentre randomized study to evaluate patient comfort, skin breakdown and eye irritation in patients ventilated with different face masks in the acute setting. Interestingly they found that 10 patients presented a certain amount of skin breakdown after only 24 hours.

So far, the most important strategy to prevent skin damage is to avoid an excessively tight fit.[31] A simple method to avoid this risk is to leave enough space to allow two fingers to pass beneath the headgear.[29] A small amount of air leak is acceptable and should not strongly affect patient–ventilator

**Box 6.3 Reducing skin breakdown during NIV**

- Rotate various types of interfaces
- Proper harness and tightening
- Skin and mask hygiene
- Nasal-forehead spacer (to reduce the pressure on the bridge of the nose)
- Forehead pads (to obtain the most comfortable position on the forehead)
- Cushioning system between mask prong and forehead
- Remove patient's dentures when making impression for a moulded mask
- In home care, replace the mask according to the patient's daily use
- Skin pad or woundcare dressing

Modified from Nava *et al.*[31]

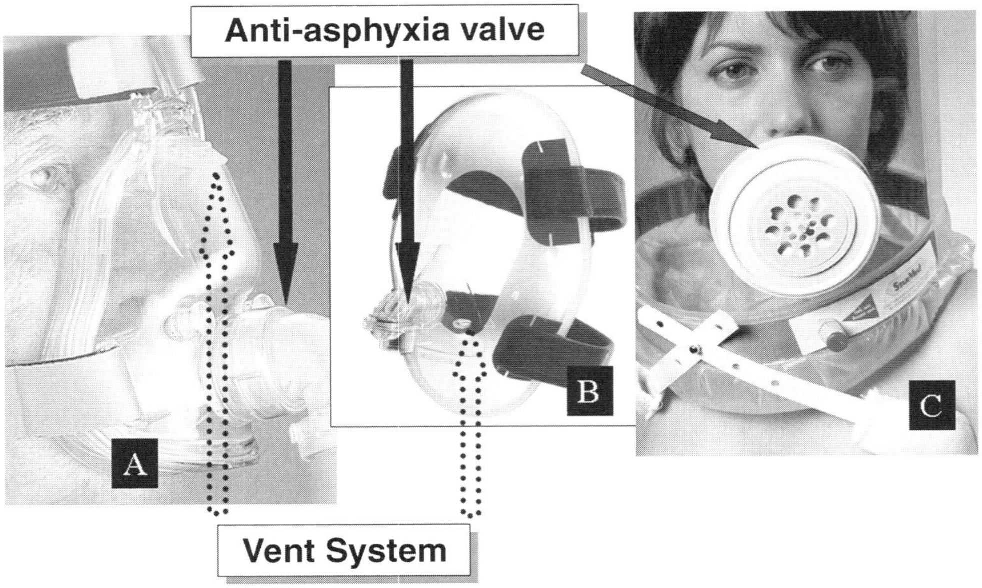

**Figure 6.1** Anti-asphyxia and vent systems. (A, B) Vent system (dotted arrows) of a full face and of a total full face. (C) An anti-asphyxia valve (thick arrows) of a total full face mask and of a helmet respectively. Courtesy of the manufacturers.

**Box 6.4 Reducing air leaks in NIV**

- Proper interface type and size
- Proper securing system
- Mask-support ring
- Comfort flaps
- Adapter for feeding tube
- Hydrogel or foam seals
- Chin strap
- Lips seal or mouth taping

Modified from Nava *et al.*[31]

interaction.[41] Woundcare dressing has also been used to limit or treat skin damage.[42] Long-term use of tight-fitting headgear retards facial skeletal development in children.[43,44]

## PHYSIOLOGICAL ASPECTS

### Air leaks

Air leaks may reduce the efficiency of NIV and patient tolerance, increase patient–ventilator asynchrony (through loss of triggering sensitivity) and cause awakenings and fragmented sleep.[45,46] Several methods have been proposed to reduce air leaks (Box 6.4).

During pressure support ventilation (PSV), leaks can hinder achievement of the inspiration termination criterion.[41,47] Vignaux *et al.*[48] conducted a prospective multicentre observational study to determine the prevalence of patient–ventilator asynchrony in patients receiving NIV for ARF. They found that ventilator asynchrony due to leaks is quite common in patients receiving NIV. Borel *et al.*[32] measured intentional leaks in seven different industrial masks to determine whether higher leaks could modify ventilator performance and quality of ventilation. The level of intentional leaks in the seven masks ranged from 30 L/min to 45 L/min for an inspiratory pressure level of 14 cm $H_2O$. The capacity to achieve and maintain the set inspiratory pressure was significantly decreased with all ventilators and in all simulated lung conditions when intentional leaks increased.

In patients with neuromuscular disorders receiving nocturnal NIV, leaks are also associated with daytime hypercapnia.[49] Schettino *et al.*[50] evaluated air leaks and mask mechanics and estimated the pressure required to seal the mask to the skin and prevent leaks (mask–face seal pressure) as the difference between the airway pressure and the mask pressure against the face. Higher mask pressure against the face decreases air leaks, as does decreasing the airway pressure applied by the ventilator.

### Dead space and carbon dioxide rebreathing

The dead space added by the interface is also recognized as a major problem, in particular, for the treatment of hypercapnic patients, because it may reduce NIV effectiveness in correcting respiratory acidosis.[51,52]

Bench studies have suggested that carbon dioxide rebreathing is significantly increased with masks having a large internal volume,[51] and conversely decreased with masks having a built-in exhalation port, as designed for use with single-circuit bi-level ventilators.[51,52]

Navalesi *et al.*[23] measured the differences in apparatus dead space between a nasal mask and a full face mask. Although the *in vitro* difference was substantial (205 mL vs 120 mL with full face mask and nasal mask, respectively), the *in vivo* results (which took into account anatomical structures) were similar (118 mL vs 97 mL with full face mask and nasal mask, respectively). Nasal pillows add very little dead space and can be as effective as face masks in reducing arterial carbon dioxide and increasing pH, but are less tolerated by patients.[23]

Different flow patterns and pressure waveforms may also influence the apparatus dead space. Saatci *et al.*[51] found that a face mask increased dynamic dead space from 32 per cent to 42 per cent of tidal volume above physiological dead space, during unsupported breathing. Other investigators have confirmed the importance of the site of the exhalation ports on carbon dioxide rebreathing.[53] Cuvelier *et al.*[35] conducted a randomized controlled study to compare the clinical efficacy of a cephalic mask versus an oronasal mask in 34 patients with acute hypercapnic respiratory failure. Compared with values at inclusion, pH, arterial carbon dioxide, encephalopathy score, respiratory distress score and respiratory frequency improved significantly and were similar with both masks.

Fraticelli *et al.*[34] evaluated the physiological effects of four interfaces with different internal volumes in patients with hypoxaemic or hypercapnic ARF receiving NIV through ICU ventilators. Three face masks with very high (977 mL), high (163 mL) and moderate (84 mL) internal volume, and a mouthpiece having virtually no internal volume were tested. NIV decreased inspiratory effort and improved gas exchange with no significant difference between the four interfaces. An increased rate of air leaks and asynchrony, and reduced comfort were observed with the mouthpiece, as opposed to all three face masks. The leakage around the mask could act as a bias flow resulting in mask carbon dioxide washout, which could minimize the possible differences in dead space.[34]

In patients undergoing NIV for ARF, the addition of a dead space through a heat and moisture exchanger was shown to reduce the efficacy of NIV, by increasing arterial carbon dioxide,[54] respiratory rate, minute ventilation[54,55] and the work of breathing.[55]

The helmet has a much larger volume than any of the other NIV interfaces (always larger than tidal volume), and it behaves as a semi-closed environment, in which the increase in inspired partial pressure of carbon dioxide is an important issue. Similar to a pressurized aircraft,[56] the inspired partial pressure of carbon dioxide in a semi-closed environment depends on the amount of carbon dioxide produced by the subject(s) and the flow of fresh gas that flushes the environment (with a helmet this is called the 'helmet ventilation'). Taccone *et al.*[57] found in a bench study with a lung model and helmets of various sizes that a 33 per cent reduction in helmet volume had no effect on the amount of carbon dioxide rebreathing at steady state. During either CPAP or NIV, the helmet affects carbon dioxide clearance.[38,58–71] High gas flow (40–60 L/min) is required to maintain a low inspired partial pressure of carbon dioxide during helmet CPAP.[58,59,65] In contrast, when they delivered CPAP with a ventilator, Taccone *et al.*[57] found considerable carbon dioxide rebreathing.

The effect of a helmet on carbon dioxide during NIV was also evaluated in two physiological studies.[64,65] In both the studies the inspired partial pressure of carbon dioxide was significantly higher with helmet PSV than with mask PSV. However, a recent study[34] of two full face masks found no significant negative effect of dead space on gas exchange or patient effort. In contrast, studies of masks versus helmets found a helmet less efficient in unloading the respiratory muscles[67], especially in the presence of a resistive load[65] and higher likelihood of patient–ventilator asynchrony. This may be explained by the longer time required to reach the target pressure, because part of the gas delivered by the ventilator is used to pressurize the helmet.[62,64,65] Some portion of inspiratory effort is unassisted because of greater inspiratory-trigger and expiratory-trigger delay.[65–67]

Vargas *et al.*[72] in a prospective crossover study evaluated the ventilatory setting (PSV plus PEEP and pressurization rate) in 11 patients at risk for respiratory distress, undergoing in a random order face mask, helmet and helmet ventilation with specific setting (50 per cent increases in both PSV and with the highest pressurization rate). Compared with the face mask, the helmet with the same settings worsened patient–ventilator synchrony, as indicated by longer triggering-on and cycling-off delays.

## ORAL INTERFACES

Figure 6.2 shows the oral NIV interfaces, and these are of two types: standard narrow mouthpieces with various degrees of flexion, which are held by the patient's teeth and lips; and custom-moulded bite-plates. Oral interfaces are used for long-term ventilation of patients with severe chronic respiratory failure due to neuromuscular disease.[73,74]

In subjects who required several hours of ventilatory support, Bach *et al.*[73] reported the sequential use of a narrow flexed mouthpiece during the day time and a nasal mask overnight. They suggested the possible use of a standard mouthpiece with lip seal retention or custom-moulded orthodontic bites for overnight use.[73] One study used mouthpieces in patients with cystic fibrosis and acute or chronic respiratory failure.[75] A recent study suggested that a mouthpiece is as effective as a full face mask in reducing inspiratory effort in patients receiving NIV for ARF.[34]

Mouthpieces may elicit the gag reflex, salivation or vomiting. Long-term use can also cause tooth and jaw deformities. Vomit aspiration is another potential complication, though so far that risk has only been theoretical.[73]

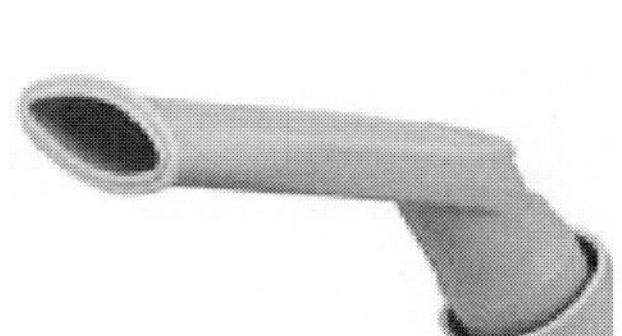
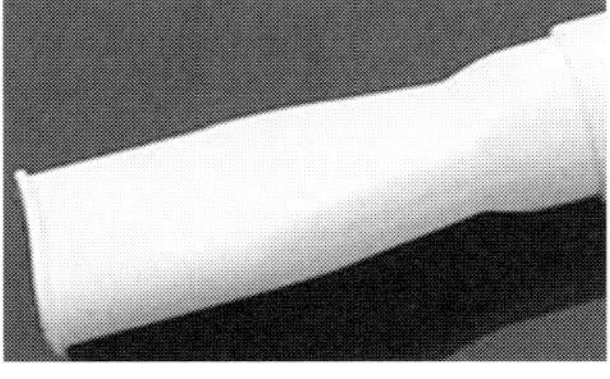

**Figure 6.2** Oral interfaces from Respironics. Courtesy of the manufacturer.

Mouth air leaks may be controlled with a tight-fitting lip seal. Nasal pledges or nose clips can be used to avoid air leak through the nares.[73]

## NASAL MASKS AND PILLOWS

Although nasal masks are the first choice for long-term ventilation they have also been used for acute hypercapnic[1,2,9,76–82] and hypoxaemic[80,83–91] respiratory failure. Nasal masks are shown in Figure 6.3, and Box 6.5 summarizes the reported advantages of and contraindications to nasal masks.

Preliminary studies with normal adults suggested that nasal ventilation is of limited effectiveness when nasal resistance exceeds 5 cm $H_2O$.[92]

The two types of nasal mask are:

- full nasal mask: covers the whole nose
- external nostril mask (also called nasal slings): applied externally to the nares.

Nasal pillows (Fig. 6.4), like nasal slings, have less dead space than face masks, are less likely to produce claustrophobia, and allow the patient to wear glasses.[17] They offer advantages similar to those of nasal masks; they allow expectoration, food intake, and speech without removing the mask. Nasal pillows potentially also allow the user to wear glasses for reading.

With nasal pillows and masks, the presence of expiratory air leak makes tidal volume monitoring unreliable.[20] Nasal

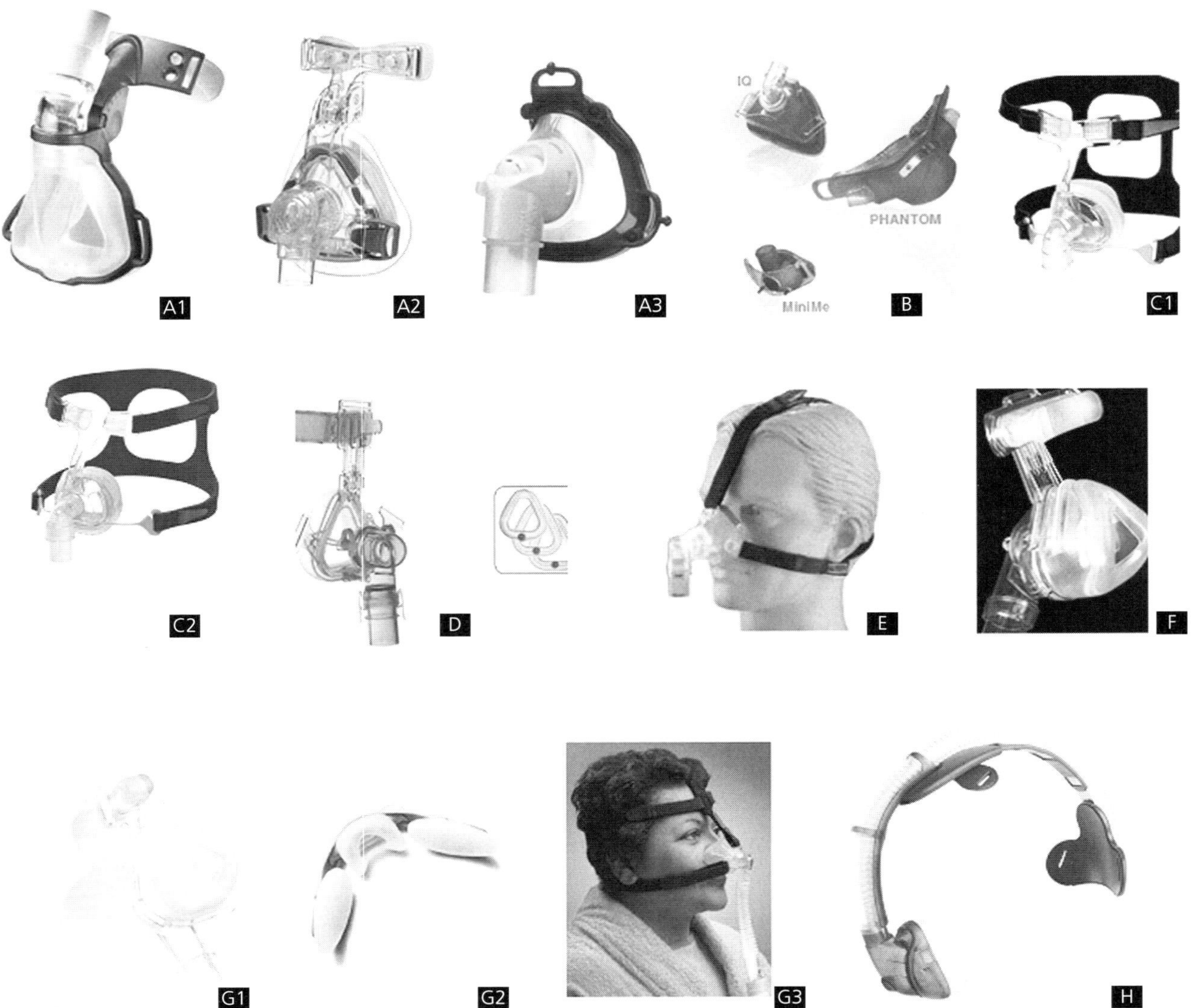


**Figure 6.3** Nasal masks. ResMed: (A1) Papillon, (A2) Activa, (A3) Mirage Micro, (B) SleepNet IQ, Phantom, and MiniMe. Fisher and Paykel: (C1) HC407. (C2) Zest Clear Cut (D) Koo Deluxe. (E) Hans Rudolph Nasal Alizes 7800. (F) CareFusion Standard Series Nasal Mask. Respironics: (G1) Comfort Classic, (G2) Comfort Curve, (G3) Simplicity, (H) Covidien Breeze DreamSeal. (Courtesy of the manufacturers).

**Box 6.5 Advantages of and contraindications to nasal masks for non-invasive ventilation**

Advantages

- Less interference with speech and eating
- Allows cough
- Less danger with vomiting
- Claustrophobia uncommon
- No risk of asphyxia in case of ventilator malfunction
- Less likely to cause gastric distension

Relative contraindications

- Edentulism
- Leaks from the mouth during sleep

Absolute contraindications

- Respiration from the mouth or unable to breath through the nose
- Oronasal breathing in severe acute respiratory failure
- Surgery of the soft palate

Modified from Nava *et al.*[31]

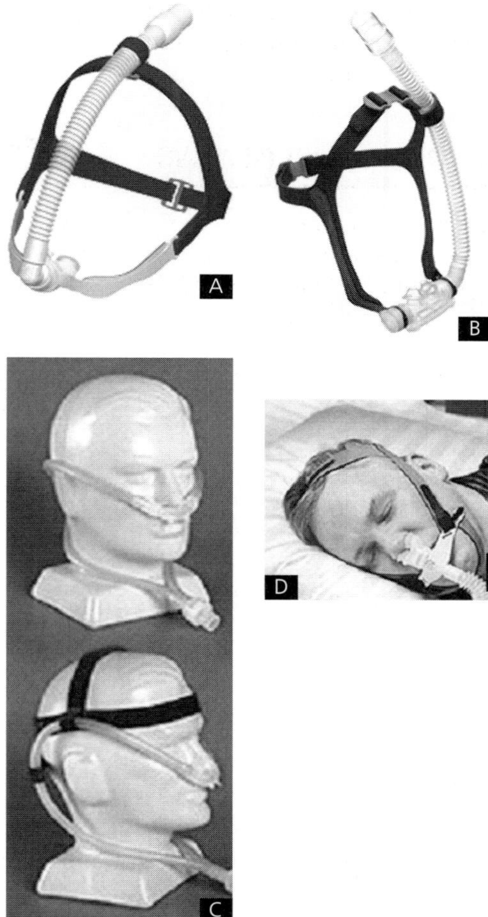

**Figure 6.4** Nasal Pillows. (A) Fisher and Paykel. (A) New Opus; ResMed: (B) Mirage Swift II, (C) InnoMed Nasal-Airell. Respironics: (D) OptiLife (Courtesy of the manufacturers).

pillows can be alternated with oronasal and nasal masks to minimize friction and pressure on the skin, at least for a few hours, which could improve tolerance of NIV and therefore allow more hours of ventilation per day.

## ORONASAL AND FULL FACE MASKS

It is a common belief that oronasal masks are preferred for patients with ARF, because those patients generally breathe through the mouth to bypass nasal resistance.[77] Kwok *et al.*[37] studied a heterogeneous population of 35 patients with congestive heart failure, sepsis, acute lung injury, asthma, pneumonia, and COPD. Although both masks performed similarly with regard to improving vital signs and gas exchange and avoiding intubation, the nasal mask was less tolerated than the oronasal mask in patients with ARF.

Girault *et al.*,[33] in patients with hypercapnic ARF due to acute COPD with mixed aetiology, compared the initial choice of face mask and nasal mask and its clinical effectiveness and tolerance. Patients randomized to nasal NIV had significant mask failure (75 per cent), occurring within 6 hours of NIV therapy, mainly due to buccal air leak (94 per cent), necessitating a switch to a face mask. None in the face NIV group needed mask change. In the nasal NIV group, no intubation was required among those who did not require a mask change, but in those who needed a change of mask, 18 per cent needed intubation and mechanical ventilation. There were, however, no significant differences in intubation rate, intensive care unit length of stay and intensive care unit mortality. However, studies comparing two different interfaces cannot be blinded and it is impossible to eliminate bias. The decision to change masks is based on subjective opinion by the attending physician and not based on objective criteria, and the use of different ventilators to deliver NIV could cause variations in outcome.[9] Figure 6.5 shows some types of oronasal mask.

One mask is a combination of a nasal pillow and an oral interface. Interestingly, it also skips the nasal bridge once fitted to the patient, thus avoiding nasal skin breakdown (Fig. 6.5 D1). A cephalic mask (total full face mask or integral mask) has a soft cuff that seals around the perimeter of the face, so there is no pressure on areas that an oronasal mask contacts[25,34] (Fig. 6.6). The frame of the total full face mask may include an anti-asphyxia valve that automatically opens to room air in case of ventilator malfunction when airway pressure falls below 3 cm $H_2O$ (Fig. 6.1B). Compared with a full face mask, a cephalic

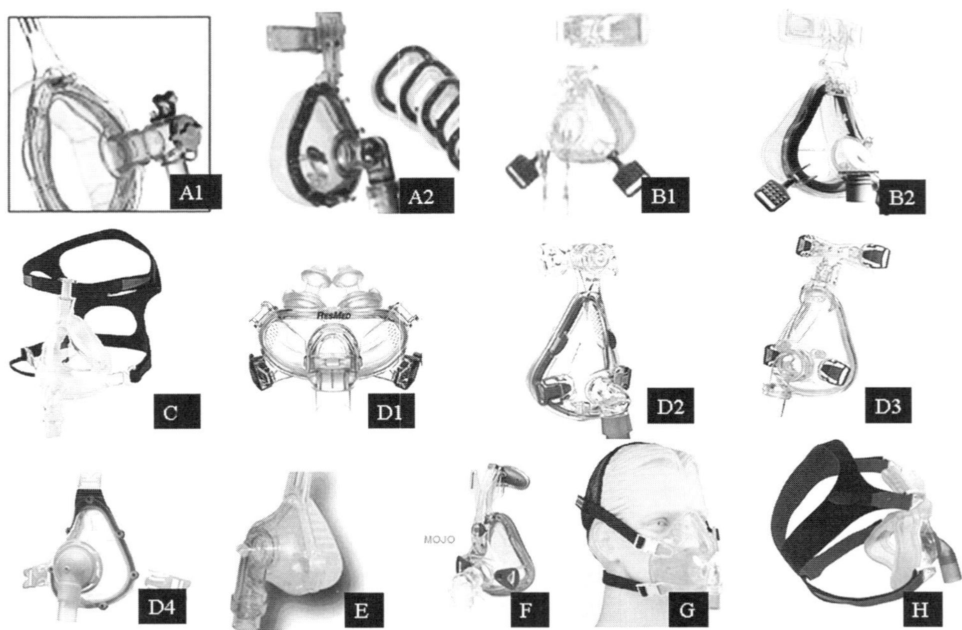


**Figure 6.5** Full face masks. Koo: (A1) Blustar, (A2) Blustar Plus. Respironics: (B1) Comfort Fusion, (B2) Comfort Gel; (C) Fisher and Paykel HC431. ResMed: (D1) Mirage Quattro, (D2) Liberty, (D3) Mirage, (D4) Hospital Mirage; (E) Viasys; (F) SleepNet Mojo; (G) Hans Rudolph VIP 75/76; (H) Weinmann Joyce. Courtesy of the manufacturers.

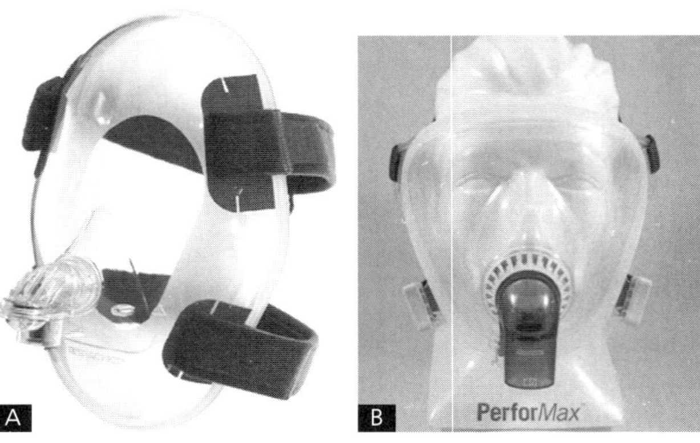


**Figure 6.6** Total full face masks. Respironics: (A) Total, (B) PerforMax. Courtesy of Respironics.

mask has a larger inner volume because it covers the entire anterior surface of the face. Its main advantage is that it limits the risk of deleterious cutaneous side effects during NIV.[22,25,34–35] This mask also is of potential interest as an alternative to conventional masks for patients with skin breakdown or morphologic characteristics hindering adaptation to other interfaces.[34]

Fraticelli *et al.*[34] found that nose comfort was better with the mouthpiece and the cephalic mask. Cuvelier *et al.*[35] when comparing cephalic mask versus an oronasal mask, found that in spite of its larger inner volume, the cephalic mask has the same clinical efficacy and requires the same ventilatory settings as the oronasal mask during ARF. Tolerance of the oronasal mask was improved at 24 hours and further. However, one patient with the cephalic mask had claustrophobia, but this did not lead to dropping out from the study.

Box 6.6 gives the advantages of and contraindications to oronasal and full face masks.

**Box 6.6 Advantages of and contraindications to oronasal and full face masks for NIV**

Advantages (compared with nasal mask)

- Fewer air leaks with more stable mean airway pressure, especially during sleep
- Less patient cooperation required

Relative contraindications

- Tetraparetic patients with severe impairment in arm movement

Absolute contraindications

- Vomiting
- Claustrophobia

Modified from Nava *et al.*[31]

## HELMETS

A helmet has a transparent hood and soft (polyvinyl chloride or silicone) collar that contacts the body at the neck and/or shoulders (Fig. 6.7). A helmet has at least two ports: one through which gas enters, and another from which gas exits. The helmet is secured to the patient by armpit straps. All the available helmets are latex-free and available in multiple sizes. Helmets were originally used to deliver a precise oxygen concentration during hyperbaric oxygen therapy. The United States Food and Drug Administration has not approved any of the available helmets, but they have been approved in some other

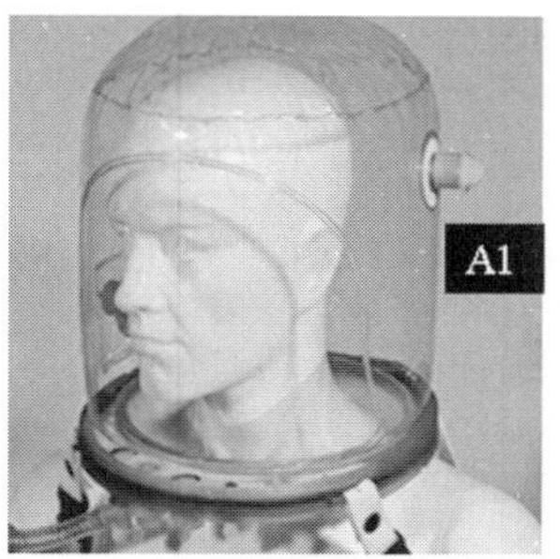

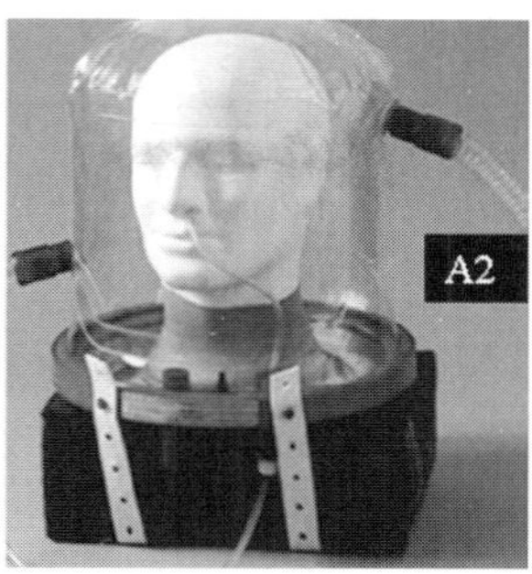

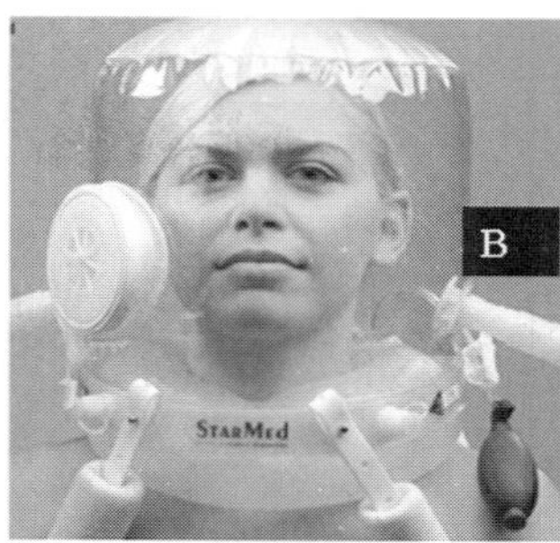


**Figure 6.7** Helmets. Harol: (A1) NIV10201, (A2) NIV10301/X; (B) StarMed Castar R. Courtesy of the manufacturers.

**Box 6.7 Advantages of and contraindications to helmets**

Advantages (compared with oronasal mask)

- Less resistance to flow
- Can be applied regardless of the facial contour, facial trauma or edentulism
- Allows coughing
- Less need for patient cooperation
- Better comfort
- Less interference with speech
- Less likelihood of causing skin damage

Relative contraindications

- Need for monitoring of volumes
- Likelihood of difficult humidification

Absolute contraindications

- Claustrophobia
- Tetraplegia

Modified from Nava *et al.*[31]

countries.[38,40,57–67,69,94–103] The helmet, which covers the head of the patient entirely, is particularly indicated in the presence of skin breakdown.[104]

Box 6.7 lists the advantages of and contraindications to helmets.

## CONCLUSIONS

Practically, a full face mask or a total full face mask should be the first-line strategy in the initial management of hypercapnic acute respiratory failure with NIV. The internal volume of the mask seems not to be a major problem in terms of arterial blood gases and patient effort.[34] However, if NIV has to be prolonged, switching to a nasal mask may improve comfort by reducing face mask complications. In contrast, in mild ARF we recommend trying a nasal mask first, which is better tolerated,[23,31] or nasal pillows, which are less likely to cause skin damage.[31]

Helmet CPAP with continuous flow devices may also offer an appealing approach, taking into account the physical properties of the helmet and the problems related to carbon dioxide clearance.[58] However, physicians must bear in mind that, when switching from CPAP to intermittent positive ventilation, the mechanical properties of the helmet must be considered to achieve effective downloading of the patient's muscles.[72]

## REFERENCES

1. Bott J, Carroll MP, Conway JH *et al.* Randomised controlled trial of nasal ventilation in acute ventilatory failure due to chronic obstructive airways disease. *Lancet* 1993; **341**: 1555–7.
2. Kramer N, Meyer TJ, Meharg J *et al.* Randomized, prospective trial of noninvasive positive pressure ventilation in acute respiratory failure. *Am J Respir Crit Care Med* 1995; **151**: 1799–806.
3. Brochard L, Mancebo J, Wysochi M *et al.* Noninvasive ventilation for acute exacerbation of chronic obstructive pulmonary disease. *N Engl J Med* 1995; **333**: 817–22.
4. Celikel T, Sungur M, Cayhan B *et al.* Comparison of non-invasive positive pressure ventilation with standard medical therapy in hypercapnic acute respiratory failure. *Chest* 1998; **114**: 1636–42.
5. Plant PK, Owen JL, Elliot MW. Early use of non-invasive ventilation in acute exacerbation of chronic obstructive pulmonary disease on general respiratory wards: a multicentre randomised controlled trial. *Lancet* 2000; **335**: 1931–5.
6. Antonelli M, Conti G, Bufi M *et al.* Noninvasive ventilation for treatment of acute respiratory failure in patients undergoing solid organ transplantation: a randomized trial. *JAMA* 2000; **283**: 235–41.
7. Confalonieri M, Potena A, Carbone G *et al.* Acute respiratory failure in patients with severe community acquired pneumonia. A prospective randomised evaluation of non-invasive ventilation. *Am J Respir Crit Care Med* 1999; **160**: 1585–91.
8. Hilbert G, Gruson D, Vargas F *et al.* Noninvasive ventilation in immunosuppressed patients with pulmonary infiltrates, fever, and acute respiratory failure. *N Engl J Med* 2001; **344**: 481–7.
9. Martin TJ, Hovis JD, Costantino JP *et al.* A randomized, prospective evaluation of non-invasive ventilation for

acute respiratory failure. *Am J Respir Crit Care Med* 2000; **161**: 807–13.
10. Antonelli M, Conti G, Rocco M *et al.* A comparison of noninvasive positive-pressure ventilation and conventional mechanical ventilation in patients with acute respiratory failure. *N Engl J Med* 1998; **339**: 429–35.
11. Nava S, Ambrosino N, Clini E *et al.* Noninvasive mechanical ventilation in the weaning of patients with acute respiratory failure due to chronic obstructive pulmonary disease: a randomized controlled trial. *Ann Intern Med* 1998; **128**: 721–8.
12. Girault C, Daudenthun I, Chevron V *et al.* Noninvasive ventilation as a systematic extubation and weaning technique in acute-on-chronic respiratory failure: a prospective, randomized controlled study. *Am J Respir Crit Care Med* 1999; **160**: 86–92.
13. Meecham-Jones DJ, Paul EA, Jones PW *et al.* Nasal pressure support ventilation plus oxygen compared with oxygen therapy alone in hypercapnic COPD. *Am J Respir Crit Care Med* 1995; **152**: 538–44.
14. Clini E, Sturani C, Rossi A *et al.* Rehabilitation and Chronic Care Study Group, Italian Association of Hospital Pulmonologists (AIPO). The Italian multicentre study on noninvasive ventilation in chronic obstructive pulmonary disease patients. *Eur Respir J* 2002; **20**: 529–38.
15. Casanova C, Celli BR, Tost L *et al.* Long-term controlled trial of nocturnal nasal positive pressure ventilation in patients with severe COPD. *Chest* 2000; **118**: 1582–90.
16. Meduri GU. Noninvasive positive pressure ventilation in patients with acute respiratory failure. *Clin Chest Med* 1996; **17**: 513–53.
17. Mehta S, Hill NS. Noninvasive ventilation. *Am J Respir Crit Care Med* 2001; **163**: 540–77.
18. Schönhofer B, Sortor-Leger S. Equipment needs for non-invasive mechanical ventilation. *Eur Respir J* 2002; **20**: 1029–36.
19. Antonelli M, Conti G, Moro ML *et al.* Predictors of failure of noninvasive positive pressure ventilation in patients with acute hypoxemic respiratory failure: a multicenter study. *Intensive Care Med* 2001; **27**: 1718–28.
20. Squadrone E, Frigerio P, Fogliati C *et al.* Noninvasive vs invasive ventilation in COPD patients with severe acute respiratory failure deemed to require ventilatory assistance. *Intensive Care Med* 2004; **30**: 1303–10.
21. Criner GJ, Brennan K, Travaline JM *et al.* Efficacy and compliance with noninvasive positive pressure ventilation in patients with chronic respiratory failure. *Chest* 1999; **116**: 667–75.
22. Gregoretti C, Confalonieri M, Navalesi P *et al.* Evaluation of patient skin breakdown and comfort with a new face mask for non-invasive ventilation: a multicenter study. *Intensive Care Med* 2002; **28**: 278–84.
23. Navalesi P, Fanfulla F, Frigerio P *et al.* Physiologic valuation of noninvasive mechanical ventilation delivered with three types of masks in patients with chronic hypercapnic respiratory failure. *Crit Care Med* 2000; **28**: 1785–90.
24. Tsuboi T, Ohi M, Kita H *et al.* The efficacy of a custom-fabricated nasal mask on gas exchange during nasal intermittent positive pressure. *Eur Respir J* 1999; **13**: 152–6.
25. Criner GJ, Travaline JM, Brennan KJ *et al.* Efficacy of a new full face mask for non-invasive positive pressure ventilation. *Chest* 1994; **106**: 1109–15.
26. McDermott I, Bach JR, Parker C *et al.* Custom fabricated interfaces for intermittent positive pressure ventilation. *Int J Prosthodontics* 1989; **2**: 224–33.
27. Bach JR, Sotor SM, Saporito LR. Interfaces for non-invasive intermittent positive pressure ventilatory support in North America. *Eur Respir Rev* 1993; **3**: 254–9.
28. Cornette A, Mougel D. Ventilatory assistance via the nasal route: mask and fitting. *Eur Respir Rev* 1993; **3**: 250–3.
29. Meduri GU, Spencer SE. Noninvasive mechanical ventilation in the acute setting. Technical aspects, monitoring and choice of interface. *Eur Respir Mon* 2001; **16**:106–24.
30. Navalesi P, Frigerio P, Gregoretti C. Interfaces and humidification in the home setting *Eur Respir Mon* 2008; **41**: 338–49.
31. Nava S, Navalesi P, Gregoretti C Interfaces and humidification for noninvasive mechanical ventilation. *Respir Care* 2009; **54**: 71–84.
32. Borel JC, Sabil A, Janssens JP *et al.* Intentional leaks in industrial masks have a significant impact on efficacy of bilevel noninvasive ventilation: a bench test study. *Chest* 2009; **135**: 669–77.
33. Girault C, Briel A, Benichou J *et al.* Interface strategy during noninvasive positive pressure ventilation for hypercapnic acute respiratory failure. *Crit Care Med* 2009; **37**: 124–31.
34. Fraticelli AT, Lellouche F, L'her E *et al.* Physiological effects of different interfaces during noninvasive ventilation for acute respiratory failure. *Crit Care Med* 2009; **37**: 939–45.
35. Cuvelier A, Pujol W, Pramil S *et al.* Cephalic versus oronasal mask for noninvasive ventilation in acute hypercapnic respiratory failure. *Intensive Care Med* 2009; **35**: 519–26.
36. Meslier N, Lebrun T, Grillier-Lanoir V *et al.* A French survey of 3,225 patients treated with CPAP for obstructive sleep apnoea: benefits, tolerance, compliance and quality of life. *Eur Respir J* 1998; **12**: 185–92.
37. Kwok H, McCormack J, Cece RM *et al.* Controlled trial of oronasal versus nasal mask ventilation in the treatment of acute respiratory failure. *Crit Care Med* 2003; **31**: 468–73.
38. Crimi C, Noto A, Esquinas A *et al.* Non-invasive ventilation practices: a European web-survey. *Eur Respir J* 2010; 14 January (published ahead of print).
39. Navalesi P. Internal space of interfaces for noninvasive ventilation: dead, but not deadly. *Crit Care Med* 2009; **37**:1146–7.
40. Antonelli M, Conti G, Pelosi P *et al.* New treatment of acute hypoxemic respiratory failure: non-invasive pressure support ventilation delivered by helmet: a pilot controlled trial. *Crit Care Med* 2002; **30**: 602–8.

41. Calderini E, Confalonieri M, Puccio PG *et al.* Patient-ventilator asynchrony during noninvasive ventilation: the role of expiratory trigger. *Intensive Care Med* 1999; **25**: 662–7.
42. Li KK, Riley RW, Guilleminault C. An unreported risk in the use of home nasal continuous positive airway pressure and home nasal ventilation in children: mid-face hypoplasia. *Chest* 2000; **117**: 916–18.
43. Callaghan S, Trapp M. Evaluating two dressings for the prevention of nasal bridge pressure sores. *Professional Nurse* 1998; **13**: 361–4.
44. Fauroux B, Lavis JF, Nicot F *et al.* Facial side effects during noninvasive positive pressure ventilation in children. *Intensive Care Med* 2005; **31**: 965–9.
45. Meyer TJ, Pressman MR, Benditt J *et al.* Air leaking through the mouth during nocturnal nasal ventilation: effect on sleep quality. *Sleep* 1997; **20**: 561–9.
46. Bach JR, Robert D, Leger P *et al.* Sleep fragmentation in kyphoscoliotic individuals with alveolar hypoventilation treated by NIPPV. *Chest* 1995; **107**: 1552–8.
47. Mehta S, McCool FD, Hill NS. Leak compensation in positive pressure ventilators: a lung model study. *Eur Respir J* 2001; **17**: 259–67.
48. Vignaux L, Vargas F, Roeseler J *et al.* Patient–ventilator asynchrony during non-invasive ventilation for acute respiratory failure: a multicenter study. *Intensive Care Med* 2009; **34:** 1416-25.
49. Gonzalez J, Sharshar T, Hart N *et al.* Air leaks during mechanical ventilation as a cause of persistent hypercapnia in neuromuscular disorders. *Intensive Care Med* 2003; **29**: 596–602.
50. Schettino GP, Tucci R, Sousa R *et al.* Mask mechanics and leak dynamics during noninvasive pressure support ventilation: a bench study. *Intensive Care Med* 2001; **27**: 1887–91.
51. Saatci E, Miller DM, Stell IM *et al.* Dynamic dead space in face masks used with noninvasive ventilators: a lung model study. *Eur Respir J* 2004; **23**: 129–35.
52. Schettino GP, Chatmongkolchart S, Hess DR, *et al.* Position of exhalation port and mask design affect CO2 rebreathing during noninvasive positive pressure ventilation. *Crit Care Med* 2003; **31**: 2178–82.
53. Ferguson GT, Gilmartin M. CO2 rebreathing during BiPAP ventilatory assistance. *Am J Respir Crit Care Med* 1995; **151**: 1126–35.
54. Jaber S, Chanques G, Matecki S *et al.* Comparison of the effects of heat and moisture exchangers and heated humidifiers on ventilation and gas exchange during non-invasive ventilation. *Intensive Care Med* 2002; **28**: 1590–4.
55. Lellouche F, Maggiore SM, Deye N *et al.* Effect of the humidification device on the work of breathing during noninvasive ventilation. *Intensive Care Med* 2002; **28**: 1582–9.
56. Lumb A. High altitude and flying. In: Nunn JF, ed. *Applied respiratory physiology*, 5th edn. Philadelphia: Butterworth-Heinemann Medical; 2000: 357–74.
57. Taccone P, Hess D, Caironi P *et al.* Continuous positive airway pressure delivered with a 'helmet': effects on carbon dioxide rebreathing. *Crit Care Med* 2004; **32**: 2090–6.
58. Patroniti N, Foti G, Manfio A *et al.* Head helmet versus face mask for non-invasive continuous positive airway pressure: a physiological study. *Intensive Care Med* 2003; **29**: 1680–7.
59. Patroniti N, Saini M, Zanella A *et al.* Danger of helmet continuous positive airway pressure during failure of fresh gas source supply. *Intensive Care Med* 2007; **33**: 153–7.
60. Tonnelier JM, Prat G, Nowak E *et al.* Noninvasive continuous positive airway pressure ventilation using a new helmet interface: a case-control prospective pilot study. *Intensive Care Med* 2003; **29**: 2077–80.
61. Squadrone V, Coha M, Cerutti E *et al.* Piedmont Intensive Care Units Network (PICUN). Continuous positive airway pressure for treatment of postoperative hypoxemia: a randomized controlled trial. *JAMA* 2005; **293**: 589–95.
62. Chiumello D, Pelosi P, Severgnini P *et al.* Performance of a new 'helmet' versus a standard face mask. *Intensive Care Med* 2003; **29**: 1671–9.
63. Antonelli M, Pennisi MA, Pelosi P *et al.* Noninvasive positive pressure ventilation using a helmet in patients with acute exacerbation of chronic obstructive pulmonary disease: a feasibility study. *Anesthesiology* 2004; **100**: 16–24.
64. Costa R, Navalesi P, Antonelli M *et al.* Physiologic evaluation of different levels of assistance during noninvasive ventilation delivered through a helmet. *Chest* 2005; **128**: 2984–90.
65. Racca F, Appendini L, Gregoretti C *et al.* Effectiveness of mask and helmet interfaces to deliver noninvasive ventilation in a human model of resistive breathing. *J Appl Physiol* 2005; **99**: 1262–71.
66. Moerer O, Fischer S, Hartelt M *et al.* Influence of two different interfaces for noninvasive ventilation compared to invasive ventilation on the mechanical properties and performance of a respiratory system: a lung model study. *Chest* 2006; **129**: 1424–31.
67. Navalesi P, Costa R, Ceriana P *et al.* Non-invasive ventilation in chronic obstructive pulmonary disease patients: helmet versus facial mask. *Intensive Care Med* 2007; **33**: 74–81.
68. Conti G, Cavaliere F, Costa R *et al.* Noninvasive positive-pressure ventilation with different interfaces in patients with respiratory failure after abdominal surgery: a matched control study. *Respir Care* 2007; **52**: 1463–71.
69. Foti G, Sangalli F, Berra L *et al.* Is helmet CPAP first line pre-hospital treatment of presumed severe acute pulmonary edema? *Intensive Care Med* 2009; **35**: 656–62.
70. Bellani G, Patroniti N, Greco M *et al.* The use of helmets to deliver non-invasive continuous positive airway pressure in hypoxemic acute respiratory failure. *Minerva Anestesiol* 2008; **74**: 651–6.
71. Racca F, Appendini I, Gregoretti C *et al.* Helmet ventilation and carbon dioxide rebreathing: effects of adding a leak at the helmet ports *Intensive Care Med* 2008; **34**: 1461–8.

applications for which a ventilator can be used.[8,9] Consequently, the manufacturer of the ventilator must analyse the potential risks that the technology poses to the patient or user based on its intended use. However, the equipment used during NIV comprises not only the ventilator device but also the patient interface (mask) and the tubing connecting the ventilator's outlet with the mask, as well as filters and valves. Each part plays a role in the correct functioning of the system and should be kept in good condition to ensure a correct application of the treatment.[3] These components must therefore also be taken into account in quality control procedures.

Some of the risks associated with NIV therapy are related to the ventilator and its accessories. Incidents such as device failure or malfunction, power cuts, misuse by the patient or user or incorrect maintenance of the equipment can generate adverse events of varying degrees of severity, such as incorrect treatment, infections, serious injuries or even the patient's death.[4] All these potential incidents should be identified and minimized, paying special attention to those with potentially life-threatening consequences. Thus, healthcare professionals – as well as patients and other agents involved in the application of NIV – should be trained in the basic principles of the treatment and maintenance of the equipment and be familiar with the characteristics and potential associated risks.[4]

This chapter focuses on the current situation with regard to quality control procedures for NIV. Several issues will be discussed: clinically relevant differences in the characteristics and performance of mechanical ventilators, current procedures for the service and maintenance of NIV equipment and the control of infections related to mechanical ventilation. Finally, the various phases and agents involved in the quality control of NIV will be addressed in the light of the regulations for medical devices.

## CHARACTERISTICS AND PERFORMANCE OF MECHANICAL VENTILATORS

Like all other medical devices, mechanical ventilators are subjected to regulations issued by government authorities. These regulations vary in accordance with the country in which the medical device is commercially available, e.g. the European Directives 93/42/CEE on Medical Devices amended by Directive 2007/47/EC in Europe and the Code of Federal Regulations Title 21 (CFR 21) of the Food and Drug Administration (FDA) in the USA market.[8–10] The main aim of these regulations is to guarantee the safety of the patients, users and third parties by minimizing the occurrence and effects of potential risks, and to ensure the device performs in accordance with the manufacturer's intentions.[8,9] To this end, the regulations define a number of essential requirements that medical devices have to satisfy before they can be put on the market or into service. These requirements are related to issues such as risk assessment and management, chemical, physical, electrical and biological properties, infection and microbiological contamination and protection against radiation.

To facilitate compliance with the regulations, a manufacturer can voluntarily adhere to harmonized standards that provide a presumption of conformity with the relevant essential requirements.[8] However, these essential requirements do not provide any rules or recommendations on how to design or manufacture a medical device, a strategy that allows for the development of new technical improvements. The current international standards for lung ventilators define basic requirements for some of the fundamental variables (tidal volume, inspiratory pressure, etc.), but other important issues such as inspiratory waveform and trigger sensitivity are not defined.[11] Consequently, the mechanical ventilation market offers a number of different modes for controlling artificial breathing, cycling from inspiration to expiration and starting inspiration, as well as a great variety of flow and pressure profiles and modes of ventilation.[12,13] Although these unrestricted technological developments have improved mechanical ventilation by overcoming specific problems or fulfilling needs for different pathologies and scenarios, the variability of the commercially available ventilators and their different characteristics sometimes makes it difficult to choose the correct ventilator for a specific patient.[14] Furthermore, the undemanding requirements imposed by harmonized standards make the level of device performance entirely dependent on the manufacturer. The regulations do not specify any minimum performance requirements or provide any indications on how to assess the correct functioning of devices.[8,9] Accordingly, the ventilators that are now available commercially offer a wide range of performance levels. In fact, several studies have analysed the functioning of mechanical ventilators from various viewpoints related to the main parameters of ventilatory support, revealing clinically relevant differences between devices.[15–19]

## SERVICE AND MAINTENANCE OF HOME MECHANICAL VENTILATION

The main advantages of mechanical ventilation in the home, as opposed to the hospital, are reductions in hospital-acquired infections, increased mobility, improved nutritional status, patient empowerment and lower healthcare costs.[3,20] However, since HMV is usually administered without the permanent supervision of specialized staff, there is an increased risk of adverse events or suboptimal treatment, which can be minimized with adequate service and maintenance procedures. The use of HMV has increased rapidly in recent decades, albeit in the absence of any standardized criteria and guidelines for implementing this therapy in clinical practice.[21,22] The lack of evidence about the best HMV procedures for the different patient groups, the complexity of HMV prescription, supply and follow-up logistics and the limited experience in the application of this relatively new therapy in many centres were some of the probable reasons for the application of many different non-standardized procedures for HMV, including the quality control of ventilators.[6] Between 2001 and 2002, a detailed survey of HMV use, called Eurovent, was carried out in Europe as part of a Concerted Action of the European Commission entitled 'The role of home respiratory ventilators in the management of chronic respiratory failure'.[22] This survey analysed HMV in 16 European countries to identify patterns of use in different countries and settings, on the basis of data from 329 HMV centres, representing around 21 500 HMV patients. Eurovent showed that quality control procedures varied considerably between the various HMV providers.[6] Indeed, although the servicing of home ventilators (including maintenance, repair and delivery of spare parts) was mainly undertaken by an external company, considerable differences were found between countries in the percentage of centres servicing HMV through an external company and in the mean regularity of routine servicing.

The variety of quality control procedures in different centres and countries may lead to inadequate treatment of patients in their homes. In effect, a survey of 300 patients using HMV reported that a non-negligible number of ventilators exhibited significant discrepancies between the actual measured main ventilator variables (minute ventilation or inspiratory pressure) and the corresponding values prescribed by the physician.[5] These differences were due in part to the inadequate performance of the ventilator and to inconsistencies between the values set in the ventilator control panel and the settings prescribed by the physician. It is important to note that the patient and the prescriber also have roles in equipment maintenance that are relevant in the quality control of HMV, as inadequate cleaning and maintenance of the ventilator at home has been associated with an increased risk of equipment contamination and patient colonization.[23] The education of patients, families and caregivers is a key aspect of any homecare programme, as it helps them to use the equipment confidently and safely and to promptly identify simple problems, and encourages them to seek help or advice when necessary.[4]

Current data show that there is room for improvement in HMV quality control procedures. In contrast to the ICU setting, where professionals involved in NIV treatment work in a well-coordinated way in the same facility following protocols defined by the centre, the different partners involved in the treatment at home make HMV quality control a complex process (Fig. 7.1). The role played by each agent (prescriber, patient/caregiver, home ventilation provider, funding agency and vigilance system) and their interaction are crucial in ensuring good treatment outcomes at home.[6] The agency funding HMV (a national health service or insurance company) regulates the kind of ventilator that can be prescribed to each patient and the procedures for servicing the equipment that the provider must follow. On the one hand, the prescriber should have a structured discharge plan adapted to the patient. The prescriber should provide adequate training to the patient/caregiver, including written instructions, to allow them to correctly operate and maintain the ventilator and solve basic technical problems.[4] It is also important to train caregivers in the recognition of early signs of clinical deterioration, basic

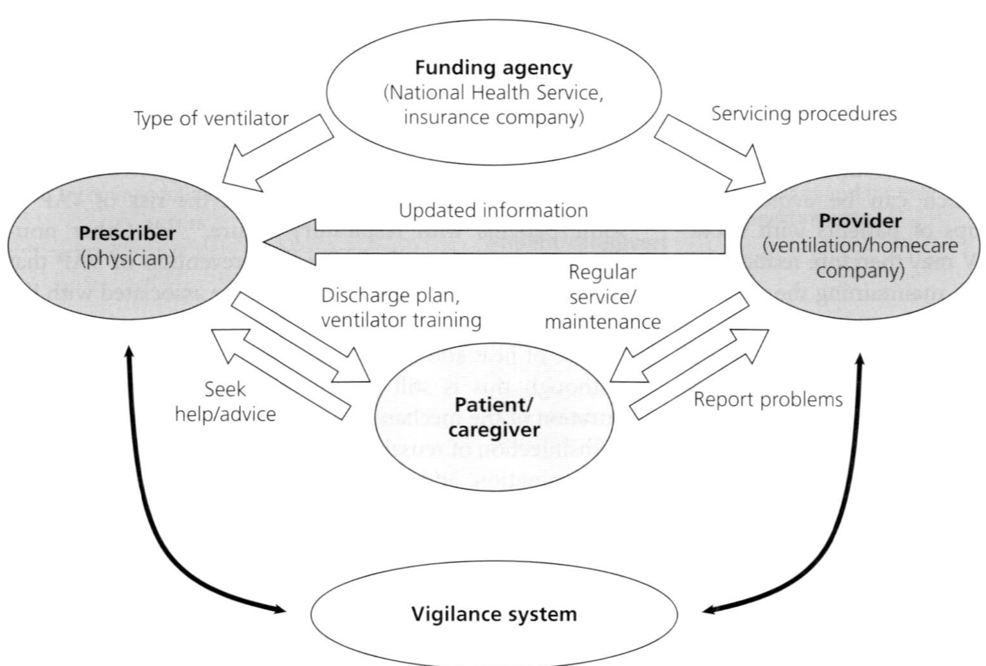


**Figure 7.1** Roles of the different actors involved in the quality control process in home mechanical ventilation.

of bronchodilator drugs. During an acute phase, the ventilatory pattern, high flow as well as peripheral mask leaks will continue to influence the selection of nebulization versus MDI.

## REFERENCES


1. Miyoshi E. Effects of gas leak on triggering function, humidification, and inspiratory oxygen fraction during noninvasive positive airway pressure ventilation. *Chest* 2005; **128**: 3691–8.
2. Duong M, Jayaram L, Camfferman D *et al.* Use of heated humidification during nasal CPAP titration in obstructive sleep apnoea syndrome. *Eur Respir J* 2005; **26**: 679–85.
3. Richards GN, Cistulli PA, Ungar RG *et al.* Mouth leak with nasal continuous positive airway pressure increases nasal airway resistance. *Am J Respir Crit Care Med* 1996; **154**: 182–6.
4. Martins De Araújo MT, Vieira SB, Vasquez EC *et al.* Heated humidification or face mask to prevent upper airway dryness during continuous positive airway pressure therapy. *Chest* 2000; **117**: 142–7.
5. Tuggey JM, Delmastro M, Elliott MW. The effect of mouth leak and humidification during nasal non-invasive ventilation. *Respir Med* 2007; **101**: 1874–9.
6. Hayes M, McGregor F, Roberts D *et al.* Continuous nasal positive airway pressure with a mouth leak: effect on nasal mucosal blood flux and geometry. *Thorax* 1995; **50**: 1179–82.
7. Esquinas A, Escobar C, Chavez A *et al.* Noninvasive mechanical ventilation and humidification in acute respiratory failure. A morpho histological and clinical study of side effects. *Am J Respir Crit Care Med* 2002; **165**: A-385.
8. Wood KE, Flaten AL, Backes WJ. Inspissated secretions: a life threatening complication of prolonged noninvasive ventilation. *Respir Care* 2000; **45**: 491–3.
9. Esquinas A, Nava S, Scala R *et al.* Humivenis working group. Humidification and difficult endotracheal intubation in failure of noninvasive mechanical ventilation (NIV). Preliminary results. *Am J Respir Crit Care Med* 2008; **177**: A644.
10. Mador MJ, Krauza M, Pervez A *et al.* Effect of heated humidification on compliance and quality of life in patients with sleep apnea using nasal continuous positive airway pressure. *Chest* 2005; **128**: 2151–8.
11. Chanques G, Constantin JM, Sauter M *et al.* Discomfort associated with underhumidified high-flow oxygen therapy in critically ill patients. *Intensive Care Med* 2009; **35**: 996–1003.
12. Wiest GH, Foerst J, Fuchs FS *et al.* Heated humidifiers used during CPAP-therapy for obstructive sleep apnea under various environmental conditions. *Sleep* 2001; **24**: 435–40.
13. Nava S, Cirio S, Fanfulla F *et al.* Comparison of two humidification systems for long-term noninvasive mechanical ventilation. *Eur Respir J* 2008; **32**: 460–4.
14. Massie CA, Hart RW, Peralez K *et al.* Effects of humidification on nasal symptoms and compliance in sleep apnea patients using continuous positive airway pressure. *Chest* 1999; **116**: 403–8.
15. Nava S, Navalesi P, Gregoretti C. Interfaces and humidification for noninvasive mechanical ventilation. *Respir Care* 2009; **54**: 71–84.
16. Fischer Y, Keck T. Measurements were taken in a climatic chamber and relative humidity. *Sleep Breath* 2008; **12**: 353–7.
17. Severgnini P, D'Onofrio D, Frigerio A *et al.* A rationale basis for airways conditioning: too wet or not too wet? *Minerva Anestesiol* 2003; **69**: 297–301.
18. Wenzel M, Wenzel G, Klauke M *et al.* Characteristics of several humidifiers for CPAP-therapy invasive and non-invasive ventilation and oxygen therapy under standardised climatic conditions in a climatic chamber. *Pneumologie* 2008; **62**: 324–9.
19. Chiumello D. Effect of a heated humidifier during continuous positive airway pressure delivered by a helmet. *Crit Care* 2008; **12**: R55.
20. Poulton TJ, Downs JB. Humidification of rapidly flowing gas. *Crit Care Med* 1981; **9**: 59–63.
21. Wiest GH, Fuchs FS, Brueckl WM *et al.* In vivo efficacy of heated and non-heated humidifiers during nasal continuous positive airway pressure (nCPAP)-therapy for obstructive sleep apnoea. *Respir Med* 2000; **94**: 364–8.
22. Holland AE, Denehy L, Buchan CA *et al.* Efficacy of a heated passover humidifier during noninvasive ventilation: a bench study. *Respir Care* 2007; **52**: 38–44.
23. Esquinas A, Carrillo A, González G. Humivenis working group. Absolute humidity variations with a variable inspiratory oxygenation fraction in noninvasive mechanical ventilation (NIV). A pilot study. *Am J Respir Crit Care Med* 2008; **177**: A644.
24. Schumann S, Stahl CA, Mäller K *et al.* Moisturizing and mechanical characteristics of a new counter-flow type heated humidifier. *Br J Anaesthesiol* 2007; **98**: 531–8.
25. Randerath WJ, Meier J, Genger H *et al.* Efficiency of cold passover and heated humidification under continuous positive airway pressure. *Eur Respir J* 2002; **20**: 183–6.
26. Jaber S, Chanques G, Matecki S *et al.* Comparison of the effects of heat and moisture exchangers and heated humidifiers on ventilation and gas exchange during non-invasive ventilation. *Intensive Care Med* 2002; **28**: 1590–4.
27. Carter BG, Whittington N, Hochmann M *et al.* The effect of inlet gas temperatures on heated humidifier performance. *J Aerosol Med* 2002; **15**: 7–13.
28. Campbell RS, Davis K Jr, Johannigman JA *et al.* The effects of passive humidifier dead space on respiratory variables in paralyzed and spontaneously breathing patients. *Respir Care* 2000; **45**: 306–12.
29. Lellouche F. Effect of the humidification device on the work of breathing during noninvasive ventilation. *Intensive Care Med* 2002; **28**: 1582–9.

30. Lellouche F. Water content of delivered gases during non-invasive ventilation in healthy subjects. *Intensive Care Med* 2009; **35**: 987–95.
31. Lellouche F, Lellouche F, Taillé S *et al.* Humidification performance of 48 passive airway humidifiers: comparison with manufacturer data. *Chest* 2009; **135**: 276–86.
32. Dhand R. Aerosol bronchodilator therapy during noninvasive positive-pressure ventilation. *Respir Care* 2005; **50**: 1621–2.
33. Hess D. The mask for noninvasive ventilation: principles of design and effects on aerosol delivery. *J Aerosol Med* 2007; **20** Suppl 1: S85–98.
34. Chatmongkolchart S, Schettino GP, Dillman C *et al.* In vitro evaluation of aerosol bronchodilator delivery during noninvasive positive pressure ventilation: effect of ventilator settings and nebulizer position. *Crit Care Med* 2003; **30**: 2515–19.
35. Dhand R, Tobin MJ. Inhaled bronchodilator therapy in mechanically ventilated patients. *Am J Respir Crit Care Med* 1997; **156**: 3–10.
36. Fink JB. Aerosol delivery from a metered-dose inhaler during mechanical ventilation. An in vitro model. *Am J Respir Crit Care Med* 1996; **154**: 382–7.
37. Dolovich M. Influence of inspiratory flow rate, particle size, and airway caliber on aerosolized drug delivery to the lung. *Respir Care* 2000; **45**: 597–608.
38. Branconnier MP, Hess DR. Albuterol delivery during noninvasive ventilation. *Respir Care* 2005; **50**: 1649–53.
39. Parkes SN, Bersten AD. Aerosol kinetics and bronchodilator efficacy during continuous positive airway pressure delivered by face mask. *Thorax* 1997; **52**: 171–5.
40. Newhouse MT, Dolovich MB. Control of asthma by aerodilator. *N Engl J Med* 1986; **315**: 870–3.
41. Pollack CV Jr, Fleisch KB, Dowsey K. Treatment of acute bronchospasm with beta-adrenergic agonist aerosols delivered by a nasal bilevel positive airway pressure circuit. *Ann Emerg Med* 1995; **26**: 552–7.
42. Brandao DC, Lima VM, Filho VG *et al.* Reversal of bronchial obstruction with bi-level positive airway pressure and nebulization in patients with acute asthma. *J Asthma* 2009; **46**: 356–61.
43. Nava S, Karakurt S, Rampulla C *et al.* Salbutamol delivery during non-invasive mechanical ventilation in patients with chronic obstructive pulmonary disease: a randomized controlled study. *Intensive Care Med* 2001; **27**: 1627–35.
44. Laube BL, Links JM, LaFrance ND *et al.* Homogeneity of bronchopulmonary distribution of 99mTc aerosol in normal subjects and in cystic fibrosis patients. *Chest* 1989; **95**: 822–30.
45. Miller DD, Amin MM, Palmer LB *et al.* Aerosol delivery and modern mechanical ventilation: in vitro/in vivo evaluation. *Am J Respir Crit Care Med* 2003; **168**: 1205–9.
46. Diot P, Morra L, Smaldone GC. Albuterol delivery in a model of mechanical ventilation: comparison of metered-dose inhaler and nebulizer efficiency. *Am J Respir Crit Care Med* 1995; **152**: 1391–4.
47. Reychler G. Effect of continuous positive airway pressure combined to nebulization on lung deposition measured by urinary excretion of amikacin. *Respir Med* 2007; **101**: 2051–5.
48. Mercer TT. Production of therapeutic aerosols. Principles and techniques. *Chest* 1981; **80**: 813–18.

success rate keeping all other factors (staff, equipment, environment) constant.[12] Girou *et al.*[13] attributed the reduction in ventilator-associated pneumonia and in mortality rate of a French ICU over 7 years to the 'learning effect' after a routine use of NIV. These data are negatively mirrored by a Spanish 'real-world' study[14] showing that the greater rate of NIV failure reported in a general versus a respiratory ward was due to poorer staff training.

Concerning the workload, initially considered to be a time-consuming technique,[31] NIV has been shown to require a shorter application time once the team improved its 'physiologic learning curve'.[32] An ICU study demonstrated quite low nursing assistance time in chronic obstructive pulmonary disease (COPD) patients, which dropped from 25 per cent to 15 per cent of the time on NIV after the first 24 hours.[33] In the RHDCU setting, nurses, RTs,[27,34] and MD time consumption[28] to manage COPD exacerbations was similar for NIV versus both medical therapy and invasive ventilation, with a significant reduction of NIV workload after the first hours of ventilation.[27,34]

The impact of NIV on time consumption depends on the location as well, especially outside ICU, where nurses have responsibility for a larger number of patients. In two ward-based RCTs in the UK,[30,35] nursing NIV patients was not different from the controls despite the inclusion of a supernumerary NIV research staff in one study.[35] However, there were no data regarding either the care of other non-ventilated patients or whether the outcome would have been better if nurses had spent more time with ventilated patients.[7]

## Location

The 'ideal environment' for starting NIV[7] should have expert staff in adequate numbers for 24-hour cover, facilities for monitoring, rapid access to ETI and invasive ventilation and reasonable cost (Table 9.1). The ICU fits all these criteria except for the cost; moreover, there is an imbalance between ICU beds and patients requiring NIV.

One of the most innovative aspects of NIV in ARF is the possibility of successful application of ventilatory support outside ICU due to the lack of need for sedation, and the early intervention.[1,2,5–7,30,36,37] Initiating NIV outside ICU has the advantage of treating less severe patients with a similar success but at lower costs than in ICU,[38] avoiding a potential distressing experience.[7] However, the lower level of care provided in some areas might increase the risk that patient deterioration will not be promptly recognized and treated.

The question of where to start NIV has generated much debate since there are no studies that have clearly addressed this question. Part of the reason for this is the large heterogeneity of the different settings capable of delivering NIV and of step-down and/or step-up pathways even within the same hospital. In 'the real-life' North American scenario,[15,18–20,39] NIV is started more often in ICU (almost half of cases) than in the emergency department and in wards (between a third and fifth of cases) with fewer cases managed in RHDCUs. As the model of hospital care varies from country to country, ICU, RHDCU and wards may have different characteristics and, therefore, it may happen

**Table 9.1** Advantages and disadvantages of starting non-invasive ventilation (NIV) in different settings to treat acute respiratory failure (ARF)

| Location | Advantages | Disadvantages |
|---|---|---|
| Prehospital | Early application | Limited equipment/monitoring<br>Difficulty in corrected diagnosis<br>No evidence |
| Emergency department | Early application<br>Adequate monitoring | Short-stay<br>Usually no experience with NIV<br>Low-level evidence |
| Intensive care unit | Highest monitoring capabilities and nurse/patient ratio<br>Usually, dedicated RTs<br>Suitable for high-risk patients | Highest costs<br>Limited bed availability<br>Distressing experience |
| RHDCU | Central monitoring<br>Specialized NIV skills<br>Often dedicated RTs<br>Cost-effective for ARF in chronic diseases | Limited bed availability<br>Nurse/patient ratio from 1:2 to <1:4<br>Medical doctor not available 24/24 hours in all units<br>Heterogeneity of care |
| General ward | Higher bed availability<br>Lowest costs<br>Suitable for low-risk patients | Lowest monitoring capabilities and nurse/patient ratio<br>Usually inadequate experience with NIV<br>Usually no dedicated RTs<br>Risk of delay in intubation |

RHDCU, respiratory high-dependency care unit; RT, respiratory therapist.

that the same patient who requires ICU admission in one institution may be appropriately treated in the RHDCU or even the ward in another institution.[5]

The most important factors that should be considered in the choice of where to start NIV are the patient's need for monitoring, the unit's monitoring capabilities, staff experience, and time-response to NIV. The first two variables are strictly linked as the greater the severity of ARF, the likelihood of NIV failure (Box 9.1), then the higher the need for monitoring and the availability of treatment escalation.[1,2,26] Patients with ARF with a cause in which the role of NIV is uncertain, such as pneumonia, acute lung injury/acute respiratory distress syndrome (ALI/ARDS), and asthma should only be treated in the ICU, where immediate ETI is available.[21] One exception is when NIV is applied in 'do not intubate' or 'do not resuscitate' (DNI)/DNR) context, when the goal is palliation of symptoms.[11] Fast-responding diseases such as acute cardiogenic pulmonary oedema (ACPE) may be appropriately ventilated in short-stay settings.[5]

### Box 9.1 Predictors of NIV failure in ARF

Hypercapnic ARF

- Before NIV
  - Low body mass index (BMI)
  - Poor pre-ARF status
  - Pneumonia
  - Excessive secretions
  - Colonization with non-fermenting Gram-negative bacilli
  - Respiratory rate ≥30 breaths/min
  - pH <7.25
  - KMS >3
  - APACHE II score ≥29
- During NIV
  - No improvement within 2 hours in pH/respiratory rate/$PaCO_2$/APACHE II score/KMS
  - Late failure
  - Inability to minimize leak
  - Patient–ventilator asynchrony
  - Poor compliance

Hypoxaemic ARF

- Before NIV
  - ARDS or pneumonia
  - Age >40 years
  - Systolic blood pressure <90 mm Hg
  - pH <7.25
  - SAPS II score ≥35
- During NIV
  - Inability to improve $PaO_2/FiO_2$ over 175 after 1 hour
  - SAPS II score >34

KMS, Kelly-Mattahy score; APACHE, Acute Physiology And Chronic Health Evaluation; ARDS, acute respiratory distress syndrome; SAPS, Simplified Acute Physiology Score

## PREHOSPITAL

Even though monitoring and diagnostic capabilities are limited, prehospital treatment is feasible in rapidly evolving conditions, typically ACPE, for which a delay in initiating NIV may increase the need for ETI.[5] In a French RCT,[40] the immediate prehospital therapy with full face mask continuous positive airway pressure (CPAP) relieved dyspnoea more rapidly and lowered ETI and hospital mortality rates versus the same therapy delayed by 15 minutes in 124 patients with suspected ACPE.

Conversely, the feasibility of starting NIV before hospital arrival needs to be ascertained. In one RCT, prehospital application of NIV to treat ACPE did not show any benefit even though important biases (higher doses of nitrates and better pH in control arm; low pressures in NIV arm) may have favoured the control arm.[41]

## EMERGENCY DEPARTMENT

Starting NIV in adequately equipped emergency departments may be advantageous because it avoids the delay in initiating ventilation especially for 'rapid solving' diseases and DNR/DNI status.[5] The emergency department may be a good location for starting NIV in 'real-life' situations with clinical findings suggesting but not proving a DNR status in order to 'buy time' for obtaining further information or letting the patient recover to the point where he or she can make a choice.[7]

There are some concerns in starting NIV in the emergency department. First, given the emergency department short-stay, unstable patients should be rapidly moved to other NIV services; consequently, the emergency department is not the ideal setting for 'slow solving' disorders under NIV (i.e. COPD exacerbations, pneumonia, ALI/ARDS). Second, a substantial proportion of ARF patients quickly improve after optimized medical therapy. In a UK study,[42] in 25 per cent of patients admitted to the emergency department for an acidotic COPD exacerbation, the pH had completely corrected by the time of arrival onto the ward suggesting that, in at least some patients, respiratory acidosis had been precipitated by high-flow oxygen therapy administered in the ambulance. A recent emergency department Australian study[43] showed that the injudicious use of oxygen therapy in COPD exacerbations increased the need for NIV, ETI and RHDCU/ICU admission. Third, the experience of the emergency department's staff in NIV may not be adequate due to the heterogeneity of the disorders admitted, most of them unrelated with ARF, and to the short stay of patients submitted to NIV.

Two RCTs investigating[22,44] the use of NIV in emergency department have reported inconsistent findings; however, several biases were criticised. A recent retrospective study[45] showed that a 'NIV trial strategy' in which ventilation was started in emergency department and then continued in RHDCU reduced in-hospital mortality and length of stay in ICU/RHDCU for most patients admitted with ARF. In this context, easy predictors of success may be useful to 'push' NIV in emergency department such as improvement in pH and $PaCO_2$ within the first 30 minutes.[46]

#### INTENSIVE CARE UNIT

Since ICU offers the highest care level, this is the appropriate location for starting NIV in the sickest patients for whom an immediate ventilatory support is mandatory.[47,48] Careful selection of patients admitted to ICU for initiating NIV is needed to reduce costs. This process is dependent on the hospital model: for example the existence of an RHDCU is likely to reduce ICU admission for delivering NIV in COPD patients.[6,38]

Recently, an Italian ICU group[49] reported its experience with NIV outside ICU (mainly emergency department/general ward) to treat 129 ARF patients (mostly COPD, ACPE, pneumonia) for whom ETI was not immediately needed or appropriate. The overall success of 77.5 per cent was obtained with a high workload but without clinically relevant complications. Since the efficacy and safety of this model are strongly dependent on hospital organization, its generalized adoption cannot be recommended.

#### RESPIRATORY HIGH-DEPENDENCY CARE UNIT

The term RHDCU refers to heterogeneous specialized units for patients who require an intermediate level of care between ICU and the ward.[6,37] RHDCU may work as 'step-down unit' for stabilized patients transferred from ICU and as 'step-up unit' for cases not responding to medical therapy in emergency departments or wards.

A European survey identified three levels of RHDCUs based on equipment, staff and typology of patients.[6] The key feature of these units is their high experience in NIV and, for few centres, in iron lung ventilation as well;[50] moreover, some RHDCUs are capable of providing invasive monitoring and ETI, managing invasively ventilated patients and prolonged weaning.[37] Starting NIV in RHDCU gives the chance of successfully treating ARF in chronic respiratory disorders[50] with similar efficacy[51] and lower costs than in ICU.[38] Unfortunately, in several countries, the number of these units is still lower than required,[5] as shown by a recent Italian survey.[52]

#### WARDS

General/respiratory wards vary considerably in their ability to manage patients on NIV. Wards that have nursing staff experienced with NIV, readily available skilled RTs and central telemetry may deliver NIV safely to selected acute patients provided that prompt intubation is available. Conversely, NIV is unlikely to be successful on wards with low nursing numbers and other ill patients requiring considerable care.[5,7,30] Monitoring patients at risk of sudden deterioration on general wards is usually not adequate, so it would not be appropriate to start NIV in these unstable patients. Emphasizing this point is a UK multicentre RCT,[30] which did not show any clinical benefit with NIV in more severe COPD exacerbations (i.e. pH <7.30) which might have been better managed in RHDCU/ICU. However, in the UK, as in other countries with a shortage of ICU beds, the only option for COPD exacerbations requiring NIV may be the ward.

## Selection of patients

Several points should be considered when starting NIV (Fig. 9.2).

First, clinicians should be aware of the aims of NIV:[9] to prevent an impending ARF or post-extubation failure; to prevent further clinical-physiological deterioration and ETI when ARF is already established but ventilatory support is not mandatory; as an alternative to invasive ventilation in more advanced ARF when ventilatory support is mandatory or to facilitate weaning from invasive ventilation; and as a palliative care in DNI/DNR patients with end-stage chronic respiratory or neoplastic diseases.[11] The aim strongly influences when and where to start NIV, as well as what to do in case of failure. Concerning the timing, NIV should be started early because a delay may permit further deterioration and increase the likelihood of failure (Box 9.2).[2] However, there is no point in starting NIV too early in patients with mild ARF.[29] This issue is discussed in another chapter.

Second, the clinician has to identify the type of acute disease to be first-line treated with NIV. Several RCTs, meta-analyses and reviews[1,2,21] have been helpful in identifying the aetiology of ARF that is more likely to be successfully managed with NIV. In this context, a first distinction should be made between hypercapnic ARF – mostly occurring in patients with pre-existent chronic respiratory disorders (i.e. COPD, chest-wall deformities, neuromyopathies) – and hypoxaemic or '*de novo*' ARF – occurring in patients without pre-existent cardio-respiratory diseases (i.e. ALI/ARDS), the former being more responsive to NIV.[1,2] The use of NIV in these conditions is discussed elsewhere in this book.

Third, care should be taken to exclude patients with contraindications from a NIV trial (Box 9.3). With the exception of cardiorespiratory arrest requiring emergency intubation, other contraindications have not been proved but are derived from exclusion criteria used in RCTs.[1,2] For instance, NIV is considered to be contraindicated in encephalopathy based on the concern that it would increase the risk of pulmonary aspiration and reduce patient

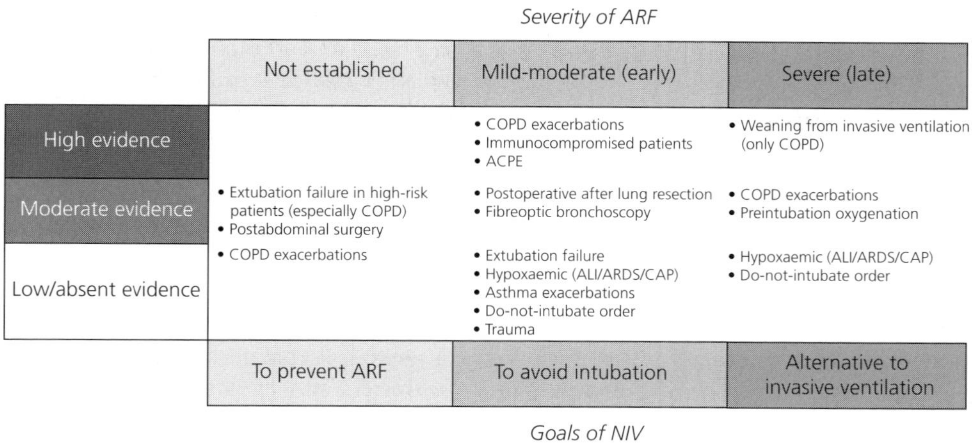

| | *Severity of ARF* | | |
|---|---|---|---|
| | Not established | Mild-moderate (early) | Severe (late) |
| High evidence | | • COPD exacerbations<br>• Immunocompromised patients<br>• ACPE | • Weaning from invasive ventilation (only COPD) |
| Moderate evidence | • Extubation failure in high-risk patients (especially COPD)<br>• Postabdominal surgery | • Postoperative after lung resection<br>• Fibreoptic bronchoscopy | • COPD exacerbations<br>• Preintubation oxygenation |
| Low/absent evidence | • COPD exacerbations | • Extubation failure<br>• Hypoxaemic (ALI/ARDS/CAP)<br>• Asthma exacerbations<br>• Do-not-intubate order<br>• Trauma | • Hypoxaemic (ALI/ARDS/CAP)<br>• Do-not-intubate order |
| | To prevent ARF | To avoid intubation | Alternative to invasive ventilation |
| | *Goals of NIV* | | |

**Figure 9.2** Flowchart showing steps in selection of patients for non-invasive ventilation (NIV) according to the level of literature evidence, the severity of acute respiratory failure (ARF) and the goals to be achieved with NIV. ACPE, acute cardiogenic pulmonary oedema; ALI, acute lung injury; ARDS, acute respiratory distress syndrome; CAP, community-acquired pneumonia. Modified from Nava *et al.*[9]

**Box 9.2 Indication to start NIV in ARF**

- Clinical signs
  - Moderate-to-severe dyspnoea
  - Respiratory rate >25 breaths/min
  - Accessory muscles use and paradoxical breathing
- Blood gases
  - pH <7.35 and $PaCO_2$ >45 mm Hg
  - $PaO_2/FiO_2$ <200

**Box 9.3 Contraindications to starting NIV in ARF**

- Cardiac/respiratory arrest
- Severe encephalopathy
- Agitation requiring sedation
- Severe gastrointestinal bleeding
- Bowel obstruction
- Multiple comorbidities
- Severe haemodynamic instability and/or unstable cardiac angina
- Facial surgery /trauma
- Fixed upper-airway obstruction
- High-risk aspiration
- Inability to clear secretions
- Untreated pneumothorax

cooperation. This is not true for moderate-to-severe hypercapnic encephalopathy. This may be 'safely' treated with NIV,[51,53] which has been found to be associated with a similar short- and long-term survival and fewer nosocomial infections than invasive ventilation.[51] Another example is the feasibility of NIV to successfully treat ARF patients with retention of secretions and depressed cough thanks to an integrated mechanical management of secretions.[54,55]

The use of predictive factors may be useful in the selection process even though those with a greater predictive value are available after a trial of NIV.[26] Non-invasive ventilation being considered as '*ars medica*', there is no 'magic formula' that will forecast the outcome of patients started on this 'miracle machine'. So, for instance, if ETI is not appropriate, there is nothing to be lost by a trial of NIV.[11]

## Equipment

This topic is covered elsewhere in this book. Here, some issues dealing with the choice of interface and ventilator to start NIV will be discussed.

### INTERFACES

The interface used to start NIV in ARF is crucial to its success as excessive air leaks, poor tolerance and skin lesions are predictors of failure.[18,56] The 'ideal interface' should be comfortable, stable, easy and quick to apply, inexpensive, and either disposable or reusable; it should fit as many face sizes and shapes as possible while reducing leaks, claustrophobia and skin damage. Given the fact that it is difficult to have such an interface, the most rational approach is to have a variety of interfaces, with different types and sizes, to ensure that the mask used best fits the patient's facial anatomy. The spectrum of available interfaces is large and a strategy incorporating the sequential utilization of different interfaces may be useful to improve tolerance and efficacy of NIV.[57]

Although nasal masks have the advantages over full face masks of greater comfort, less likelihood of claustrophobia, and easier speech and expectoration, their main limitation is the risk of leakage of air through the mouth, especially in severely dyspnoeic patients.[1,2] Even if chinstraps may reduce this problem, this device is likely to fail in case of excessive leaks. Few studies have specifically examined the influence of interface on effectiveness and tolerance of NIV in ARF.

Furthermore, the findings obtained in CRF cannot be transposed to acute patients.[58] In the two published RCTs in acute patients,[59,60] both nasal and full face mask equally improved physiologic parameters and avoided intubation, but the nasal mask was less well tolerated because of mouth leaks; conversely, after 2 days of ventilation, the comfort level worsened with more frequent skin and ENT problems occurring with full face mask.[60] Accordingly, full face mask should be the first-line strategy in starting acutely NIV, while in stabilized patients requiring prolonged NIV, the switch to nasal mask may improve comfort. In the practical field, these findings cannot be generalized due to the differences between available masks and the variable experience gained by the staff in using masks.

The total-face mask seals around the perimeter of the face and may enhance tolerance and minimize skin breakdown. Despite its larger volume,[61] dynamic dead space of the total-face mask is not larger compared with the full face mask, probably because of exhalation ports located within it, which prevent $CO_2$ rebreathing. No significant differences emerged in terms of clinical-physiological improvement, ventilatory setting and comfort within the first day of NIV between full face and total-face mask in hypercapnic ARF.[62] If a clinician decides to start NIV with this interface, a single-limb circuit bi-level ventilator must be used. The total-face mask which is available in one size, requires staff with experience in order to fit quickly without substantial air leaks. Recently, a new model has been produced having a lower volume, in two available sizes, and is easier to use.

The helmet has the advantage of reducing discomfort, skin damage, eye irritation and gastro-distension.[1,2] However, some mechanical characteristics of the helmet (i.e. large volume and highly compliant soft collar) are associated with clinical-physiological disadvantages compared with full face mask such worse patient–ventilator interaction, unloading of respiratory muscles and $CO_2$ clearance.[63–65] The helmet is not a first-line interface compared with full face mask in hypercapnic ARF but, if 'handled with care', this interface is useful in severely hypoxaemic patients needing prolonged NIV.[66]

The mouthpiece shows a limited acute application in NIV because, despite a similar efficacy in improving gas exchange, it is associated with greater discomfort, leaks, patient–ventilator asynchrony and nurse workload compared with full face mask.[67] Unlike in CRF,[58] nasal pillows have been occasionally used in ARF.

### VENTILATORS

Even if any ventilator can be used to start NIV in ARF, success is more likely if the ventilator is able to: adequately compensate for leaks; let the clinician continuously monitor patient–ventilator synchrony and ventilatory parameters due to a display of pressure-flow-volume waveforms and a double-limb circuit; adjust the fraction of inspired oxygen with a blender to assure stable oxygenation; and adjust inspiratory trigger sensitivity and expiratory cycling as an aid to manage patient–ventilator asynchronies.[17,68]

Non-invasive ventilation is usually delivered either by bi-level or by ICU ventilators. Even if able to efficiently compensate for air leaks, traditional bi-level ventilators have some technical limitations ($CO_2$ rebreathing due to their single-limb circuit in non-vented masks; inadequate monitoring; lack of alarms and $O_2$ blending), which have been largely overcome by the newer generations of machines.[68,69] Conversely, conventional ICU ventilators are not able to cope with leaks but allow good monitoring of ventilatory parameters and of flow-pressure-volume waves as well as a fine setting of $FiO_2$ and of ventilation.[68] The newest ICU ventilators efficiently assist acute patients with NIV thanks to the option of leak compensation, which allows partial or total correction of air leaks.[70]

Even if no study has shown greater NIV clinical success for one type of ventilator than another, some points should be clear when starting ventilation. First, as excessive air leaks are correlated with treatment failure,[56] clinicians should choose ventilators designed for NIV with leak compensation (i.e. bi-level and new ICU ventilators). Moreover, the chance of setting several parameters and looking at flow-volume-pressure waveforms with newer ventilators may help in improving patient–ventilator synchrony, comfort and, hopefully, clinical outcome.[1,68]

Second, the choice of ventilator should be tailored to the pathophysiology and the severity of ARF. In hypoxaemic patients, ventilators with an oxygen blender are recommended while, in those with hypercapnia, ventilators with a dual-limb circuit have an advantage in lowering $PaCO_2$. In mild COPD exacerbations, home ventilators may be appropriate, particularly if the patient is already on home NIV; by contrast, patients with life-threatening ARF at risk of ETI should be treated with more sophisticated machines.[68]

Third, the selection of a ventilator should take into account costs and staff experience. The more sophisticated a ventilator is, the longer is the training required for clinicians. Owing to the tremendous growth of the ventilator market in terms of complexity, some of the new bi-level ventilators are not user friendly.[71] The smaller the variety of devices used, the greater the likelihood that all team members will acquire enough experience in NIV set-up, with positive effects on costs and workload.[68]

Whatever ventilator is used, it is essential that all staff know the correct circuit and expiratory valve to use, how to set ventilatory parameters and alarms, how to administer oxygen, how to monitor ventilation, and how often a technical check is needed.

## Practical issues

Even though NIV has been successfully applied with both volume- and pressure-cycled modes,[57] pressure support ventilation (PSV) with positive end-expiratory pressure (PEEP) is mostly used in acute NIV because, despite a similar clinical-physiological improvement, it is better tolerated.[57,68] Lack of clear advantages and need of expertise have prevented the routine use of other modalities.[1,68]

All staff should understand that the levels of pressure support and PEEP to start NIV are not standardized but should be titrated in each case, and then dynamically adjusted depending on interface fitting, tolerance, and clinical-physiological response. It is advisable to start with low pressures while the mask is held to the face, ideally by the patient, to gain the patient's confidence especially once they realize that NIV improves dyspnoea.[17] As the patient accepts NIV, the mask may be fixed and pressure support increased (usually 8–20 cm $H_2O$/hPa) according to expiratory tidal volume (6–10 mL/kg), respiratory rate (<25 breaths/min), leaks, comfort and blood gases.[57] Peak pressures above the lower oesophageal sphincter opening pressure (25–30 cm $H_2O$) should be avoided to minimize the risk of gastric distension with vomiting.

Clinicians should bear in mind that, when PEEP is used with bi-level ventilators, the inspiratory positive airway pressure (IPAP) setting depends on whether the device works with an algorithm for true pressure support, so it is possible to set pressure support without taking into account PEEP, or that the IPAP setting is the maximum inspiratory pressure and the clinician has to set it at a value which is the sum of the chosen pressure support plus PEEP.[68] Concerning the interface, it is recommended not to tighten it excessively or weakly, since an excessive pressure can cause skin breakdown, while a poor seal will facilitate air leaks and patient–ventilator asynchronies.[21,72]

Monitoring the patient in the first hours of NIV is mandatory to verify its clinical-physiological efficacy through a periodic evaluation of respiratory distress, haemodynamic status, sensorium, and gas exchange.[17,57] Even if clinical-physiological response after 1–2 hours of NIV is a predictor of success, 'late failures' may occur in 20 per cent of cases.[73]

Continuous observation is needed to ensure that the patient does not remove the mask and leaks are minimized. Even if the patient tolerates the mask there is a tendency for the Velcro straps of the headgear to loosen gradually at high pressures and for mask leaks to develop. Although allowing the identification of major mask leaks, clinical detection has a low sensitivity and does not allow quantification of leakage. Non-invasive methods for accurate and early detection of leaks are: to monitor the difference between inspired and expired tidal volumes with double-tube circuit ventilators; to carefully examine flow-pressure-volume waveforms, which may identify and solve most of leak-induced asynchronies even without electromyographic and/or transdiaphragmatic pressure traces.[57,72] Recently,[72] severe asynchrony was observed in 43 per cent of 60 acute patients receiving NIV and was predicted by pressure support level and leak amount. A common phenomenon is the mismatching between ventilator and patient inspiratory time caused by air leaks during PSV because the flow threshold required to cycle into expiration cannot be achieved by the ventilator whose inspiration is prolonged. Several strategies can be adopted to solve this problem: to reduce pressure support or PEEP; to adjust the flow threshold above the leak flow rate; to switch to pressure controlled ventilation mode.[74] The measurement of respiratory rate may be helpful to detect asynchronies, such as ventilator auto-triggering (ventilator RR > patient RR) and ineffective efforts (ventilator RR < patient RR).

In the context of improving patient comfort, special care should be taken to prevent skin ulceration, which may occur after prolonged NIV use, particularly over the nasal bridge.[21] So far there are only limited data on the effectiveness of protective dressings. In a recent RCT, the occurrence of earlier pressure ulcers was significantly lower in 'protected' groups versus controls.[75]

Adherence to NIV may be improved by providing suitable humidification in patients with a dry throat and/or thick secretions. Heated humidifiers (HH) show greater clinical-physiological advantages versus heat-moisture exchangers (HME).[76–78] This issue is discussed in Chapter 8. Finally, since NIV failures may be due to refusal of treatment, in expert hands, patient comfort, patient–ventilator synchrony and likelihood of success may be improved by 'safe' sedation.[79,80] Although this strategy is feasible, the risk of oversedation and ETI has prevented extensive clinical application.[81]

## HOW TO START NON-INVASIVE VENTILATION IN CHRONIC RESPIRATORY FAILURE

### Education

Many of the issues that affect the use of NIV in ARF are equally applicable to CRF. Some long-term conditions (Table 9.2) expose patients to the risk of developing CRF and it is also understood that the progression into hypercapnic ventilatory failure is often predictable.[2,4,,82,83] This predictability of the progression into CRF offers the unique opportunity to the clinician of preparing the patient in advance for the eventuality that they may require NIV.[84] Preparing the patient, their family and caregivers about NIV should therefore begin before the need to start NIV arises. Educating those involved has been shown to be fundamental for the effective management of long-term conditions.[85] Several patient organisations produce excellent leaflets[86–89] detailing the signs and symptoms of CRF, as well as the treatment options. Some specifically discuss the need for NIV, explaining what is involved and give advice on troubleshooting. It is useful to signpost patients to these available resources.

**Table 9.2** Long-term conditions that cause chronic respiratory failure (CRF) leading to non-invasive ventilation (NIV)

| Type of condition | Examples |
|---|---|
| Musculoskeletal | Scoliosis |
| | Kyphoscoliosis |
| | Thoracoplasty |
| Neuromuscular | Duchenne and other dystrophies |
| | Amyotrophic lateral sclerosis |
| | Myotonic dystrophy |
| | Spinal muscular atrophy |
| | Post-polio syndrome |
| | Myopathies |
| | Charcot–Marie–Tooth syndrome |
| | Diaphragmatic paralysis |
| | Cervical spinal cord injury |
| | Myasthenia gravis |
| | Multiple sclerosis |
| | Polyneuropathies |
| Neurological | Congenital central hypoventilation syndrome |
| | Brainstem stroke |
| Obesity | Obesity–hypoventilation syndrome |
| | Severe obstructive sleep apnoea syndrome |
| | Prader–Willi syndrome |
| Pulmonary parenchymal or vascular | Chronic obstructive pulmonary disease |
| | Cystic fibrosis |
| | Fibrosing alveolitis |
| | Primary pulmonary hypertension |
| | Cheynes–Stokes ventilation with heart failure |
| | Bridge to lung transplantation |
| Idiopathic | Idiopathic non-obstructive alveolar hypoventilation |

## Timing

The rationale of NIV in CRF is discussed elsewhere in this book.[90] Non-invasive ventilation is usually started once the patient begins to develop signs and symptoms of diurnal ventilatory failure or has symptomatic nocturnal hypoventilation[3,4,10,91,92] (Table 9.3). When to assess and monitor those patients at risk of developing CRF is covered in another chapter.

The question of timing the start of NIV needs to be considered in the light of the natural history of the underlying disease process. Patients with a rapidly progressive disease such as amyotrophic lateral sclerosis may only have a short survival time from the onset of CRF; this could be a matter of only a few weeks which leaves little time to start NIV.[93] Patients with rapidly progressive diseases should be educated in the signs and symptoms of CRF and monitored closely so that the clinical evolution is identified rapidly and acted upon.[4] When starting this group on NIV, there is the need to titrate the patients on to the effective treatment quickly against a background of a dynamic process of deterioration, which can be quite challenging.

**Table 9.3** Signs and symptoms related to chronic respiratory failure (CRF)

| Group | Signs and symptoms |
|---|---|
| Sleep | Sleep fragmentation |
| | Frequent arousals |
| | Excessive daytime sleepiness |
| | Nocturnal hypoventilation |
| Respiratory | Severe orthopnoea |
| | Vital capacity <50 per cent of predicted value |
| | Daytime hypercapnia |
| Neurological | Excessive fatigue |
| | Impaired cognitive function |
| | Morning headaches |
| Muscular | Respiratory muscular weakness |
| | Reduced exercise tolerance |
| Metabolic | Failure to thrive |

Patients with a chronically stable condition such as a kyphoscoliosis will deteriorate more gently than those with a rapidly progressive condition, so the clinical evolution is more subtle and often missed by the patient.[3,4] Many times the patients will ascribe the excessive daytime fatigue to the ageing process rather than to sleep fragmentation. Depending on the severity of the presenting CRF, the imperative to rapidly achieve effective treatment is not so great in this group. Where the CRF is mild then titration to effective treatment may take several weeks or months depending on the methods used. There is, however, evidence[94] that, in the absence of signs and symptoms of CRF or nocturnal hypoventilation, commencing NIV too early is not protective and may be counterproductive.

## Location

The location for initiating NIV in CRF will depend on the individual circumstances of the providing organization but there is a wide variety of options that can be tailored to suit the needs of the patient, family and caregivers (Table 9.4).

Where a rapid acclimatization to NIV is required then an inpatient stay may be more appropriate. However if they have complex care needs provided for by caregivers in a specially adapted home environment, then it may be less traumatic for the patient to be started on NIV in that location rather than being brought into hospital.

**Table 9.4** Locations for starting non-invasive ventilation (NIV) in chronic respiratory failure (CRF)

| Location | Advantages | Disadvantages |
|---|---|---|
| Home | Familiar environment especially for patients with complex needs<br>Using NIV *in situ* | Clinical staff should operate away from hospital<br>Portable equipment |
| Outpatient department (1–2 hours) | Shorter appointment for patient<br>All equipment available | Time constraints<br>Unable to titrate ventilation with need of multiple visits and follow-up to solve problems<br>Large volume of information for patient/caregivers to assimilate in a short time |
| Day case (up to 8 hours) | More time to acclimatize to ventilation than outpatients<br>Patient can use a bed<br>Caregivers can stay | May still require multiple visits and follow-up to solve problems<br>No overnight titration |
| Overnight stay (up to 30 hours) | Able to titrate ventilation overnight<br>More time to acclimatize to ventilation and problem solve | Unfamiliar environment<br>Equipment patient usually uses not available<br>Problems may only become apparent once home<br>Caregivers may not be able to stay |
| Inpatient stay (several days and nights) | Able to titrate ventilation accurately<br>Plenty of time to acclimatize to ventilation<br>Problems more likely to become apparent and solved | Unfamiliar environment<br>Equipment patient usually uses not available<br>Time-consuming for patient and provider<br>Caregivers may not be able to stay |

Patients with a chronically stable condition may prefer outpatient or daycase initiation as this has less impact on work and home life. A recent study[8] suggests that there is an equivalent outcome whether patients were initiated as outpatients compared with inpatients in terms of improvement in ventilatory failure and ventilator usage compliance. What is key to success irrespective of the location chosen to initiate NIV is the need to have staff who are fully competent in the techniques of starting and maintaining NIV.[5]

## Equipment

### INTERFACE

Like in ARF, there is currently a wide range of interfaces available for the chronic setting. It cannot be emphasized how important a good selection of masks is in achieving success in starting NIV in CRF.[95] All the available options should be discussed with the patient, as ultimately they are going to have to wear the mask during sleep and possibly longer. There are many components to choosing the right interface, as each particular mask has its own advantages and disadvantages, which may steer a patient towards a particular choice. For example, a patient who likes to read in bed may prefer an interface that allows the wearing of spectacles, such as nasal pillows, so that their field of vision is not impaired. Another patient may prefer the stability that a mask with a forehead support offers as they are a restless sleeper. Similar to ARF, by giving the chronic patient as much choice as possible and providing ample opportunity to try out the different types of mask the clinician can improve the compliance with the interface chosen. Acclimatization to mask wearing may take a considerable time.

### VENTILATOR

Just as there are many masks there are also many ventilators, and choosing which one to use depends on a number of factors. Conditions where respiratory drive is good (i.e. COPD) could use a simple ventilator that works in a spontaneous mode whereas those in whom the respiratory drive is absent must have mandatory back-up rate. Patients with neuromuscular disorders who may progress to more than 12 hours a day ventilator use will need battery back-up and possibly wheelchair mounting.[96] Some individuals, especially those with neuromuscular disease, may find it difficult to cope with PEEP at first as they cannot speak easily or keep their mouth closed when wearing nasal masks and may benefit from intermittent positive pressure ventilation (IPPV) during the acclimatization period; IPPV ventilation means that the ventilator only blows during inhalation and this can be easier to cope with compared with bi-level ventilation. Conditions where the patient generates intrinsic PEEP, such as in COPD, may benefit from bi-level ventilation as the addition of PEEP can reduce the work of breathing.[3,90]

Generally at the start the pressures can be kept low, which will help with compliance, and then increased to achieve a therapeutic effect.[90] The duration of this titration upwards of pressures depends on the underlying condition and location where NIV is started; titration may be done overnight or over several weeks (Table 9.4).

Where time constrains allow and the patients are starting NIV mainly at home, they may prefer to acclimatize to NIV during the day, gradually increasing use until they are able to cope with NIV for at least an hour, then switching to night-time use. Ventilators that have a ramp facility to build up the pressures may also be useful where the patient is having difficulty coping with ventilation. It is important to explain to the patient that initially they may not experience any symptomatic relief if they are starting with subtherapeutic pressures and that the aim is to build compliance first, and to increase pressures to achieve symptomatic relief, which is the main catalyst in ensuring continued use. There are a couple of considerations when starting with low pressures: the work of breathing could be increased if IPAP is too low; and carbon dioxide rebreathing may occur depending on the mask if PEEP is below 4 cm $H_2O$.[69]

## Practical issues

Starting NIV in CRF is a complex process with many subtle factors at play, so preparing individuals fully and giving them as much choice as possible are key factors in ensuring success. Early and timely problem solving is key to maintaining NIV once it has been started. By far, the most common problems are related to the interface and are often because of poor fit. The second most common group of problems relate to the drying effects of NIV: many patients experience dryness of the nose and mouth, which can be rectified with the addition of adequate humidification. Heated humidifiers are efficient at delivering warm moist air with some manufacturers producing ventilators with integral humidifiers. Heat and moisture exchange can also be used but produces some resistance to the flow of gas in the ventilator circuit,[78,77] which increases the more moist they become.

Other problems that may be faced include noise related to the ventilator or mask. Careful positioning of the ventilator may help reduce noise. Often ventilators are placed on the bedside table which is at ear level, so placing the ventilator lower than the bed surface may reduce the noise disturbance significantly. Finally the clinician must not forget bed partners. Noise disturbance affects partners too and they may need to use earplugs. Care must also be taken when setting the alarms on the ventilator to ensure that they will only function when a genuine need arises, as frequent spurious alarms can significantly disturb sleep, especially that of the partner.

## REFERENCES


1. Ambrosino N, Vagheggini G. Noninvasive positive pressure ventilation in the acute care setting: where are we? *Eur Respir J* 2008; **31**: 874–86.
2. Nava S, Hill N. Non-invasive ventilation in acute respiratory failure. *Lancet* 2009; **374**: 250–9.
3. Ozsancak A, D'Ambrosio C, Hill NS. Nocturnal noninvasive ventilation. *Chest* 2008; **133**: 1275–86.
4. Annane D, Orlikowski D, Chevret S *et al.* Nocturnal mechanical ventilation for chronic hypoventilation in patients with neuromuscular and chest wall disorders. *Cochrane Database Syst Rev* 2007; CD001941.
5. Hill NS. Where should noninvasive ventilation be delivered? *Respir Care* 2009; **54**: 62–70.
6. Corrado A, Roussos C, Ambrosino N *et al.* Respiratory intermediate care units: a European survey. *Eur Respir J* 2002; **20**: 1343–50.
7. Miller SDW, Latham M, Elliott MV. Where to perform NIV. *Eur Respir Mon* 2008; **41**: 189–99.
8. Chatwin M, Nickol AH, Morrell MJ *et al.* Randomised trial of inpatient versus outpatient initiation of home mechanical ventilation in patients with nocturnal hypoventilation. *Respir Med* 2008; **102**: 1528–35.
9. Nava S, Navalesi P, Conti G. Time of non-invasive ventilation. *Intensive Care Med* 2006; **32**: 361–70.
10. Fauroux B, Lofaso F. Non-invasive ventilation: when to start for what benefit? *Thorax* 2005; **60**: 979–80.
11. Scala R, Nava S. NIV and palliative care. *Eur Respir Mon* 2008; **41**: 287–306.
12. Carlucci A, Delmastro M, Rubini F *et al.* Changes in the practice of non-invasive ventilation in treating COPD patients over 8 years. *Intensive Care Med* 2003; **29**: 419–25.
13. Girou E, Brun-Buisson C, Taillé S *et al.* Secular trends in nosocomial infections and mortality associated with noninvasive ventilation in patients with exacerbation of COPD and pulmonary edema. *JAMA* 2003; **290**: 2985–91.
14. Lopez-Campos JL, Garcia Polo C, Leon Jimenez A Staff *et al.* training influence on non-invasive ventilation outcome for acute hypercapnic respiratory failure. *Monaldi Arch Chest Dis* 2006; **65**: 145–51.
15. Schettino G, Altobelli N, Kacmarek RM. Noninvasive positive-pressure ventilation in acute respiratory failure outside clinical trials: experience at the Massachusetts General Hospital. *Crit Care Med* 2008; **36**: 441–7.
16. Goldring J, Wedzicha J. Home NIV: results and lessons from a European survey. *Eur Respir Mon* 2008; **41**: 392–9.
17. Kacmarek RM. Noninvasive positive-pressure ventilation: the little things do make the difference! *Respir Care* 2003; **48**: 919–21.
18. Sinuff T, Kahnamoui K, Cook DJ *et al.* Practice guidelines as multipurpose tools: a qualitative study of noninvasive ventilation. *Crit Care Med* 2007; **35**: 776–82.

19. Maheshwari V, Paioli D, Rothaar R *et al.* Utilization of noninvasive ventilation in acute care hospitals: a regional survey. *Chest* 2006; **129**: 1226–33.
20. Burns KE, Sinuff T, Adhikari NK *et al.* Bilevel noninvasive positive pressure ventilation for acute respiratory failure: survey of Ontario practice. *Crit Care Med* 2005; **33**: 1477–83.
21. BTS Standards of Care Committee. Non-invasive ventilation in acute respiratory failure. *Thorax* 2002; **57**: 192–211.
22. Wood KA, Lewis L, Von Harz B *et al.* The use of noninvasive positive pressure ventilation in the emergency department: results of a randomized clinical trial. *Chest* 1998; **113**: 1339–46.
23. Demoule A, Girou E, Richard JC *et al.* Benefits and risks of success or failure of noninvasive ventilation. *Intensive Care Med* 2006; **32**: 1756–65.
24. Evans T, Elliott MW, Ranieri M *et al.* Pulmonary medicine and (adult) critical care medicine in Europe. *Eur Respir J* 2002; **19**: 1202–6.
25. Vianello AM, Arcaro GM, Braccioni FS *et al.* Management of tracheal intubation in the respiratory intensive care unit by pulmonary physicians. *Respir Care* 2007; **52**: 26–30.
26. Confalonieri M, Garuti G, Cattaruzza MS *et al.* A chart of failure risk for noninvasive ventilation in patients with COPD exacerbation. *Eur Respir J* 2005; **25**: 348–55.
27. Nava S, Evangelisti I, Rampulla C *et al.* Human and financial costs of noninvasive mechanical ventilation in patients affected by COPD and acute respiratory failure. *Chest* 1997; **111**: 1631–8.
28. Norrenberg M, Vincent JL. A profile of European intensive care unit physiotherapists. *Intensive Care Med* 2000; **26**: 988–94.
29. Keenan SP, Powers CE, McCormack DG. Noninvasive positive-pressure ventilation in patients with milder chronic obstructive pulmonary disease exacerbations: a randomized controlled trial. *Respir Care* 2005; **50**: 610–16.
30. Plant PK, Owen JL, Elliott MW. Early use of non-invasive ventilation for acute exacerbations of chronic obstructive pulmonary disease on general respiratory wards: a multicentre randomised controlled trial. *Lancet* 2000; **355**: 1931–5.
31. Chevrolet JC, Jolliet P, Abajo B *et al.* Nasal positive pressure ventilation in patients with acute respiratory failure. Difficult and time-consuming procedure for nurses. *Chest* 1991; **100**: 775–82.
32. Jolliet P, Abajo B, Pasquina P *et al.* Non-invasive pressure support ventilation in severe community-acquired pneumonia. *Intensive Care Med* 2001; **27**: 812–21.
33. Hilbert G, Gruson D, Vargas F *et al.* Noninvasive ventilation for acute respiratory failure. Quite low time consumption for nurses. *Eur Respir J* 2000; **16**: 710–16.
34. Kramer N, Meyer TJ, Meharg J *et al.* Randomized, prospective trial of noninvasive positive pressure ventilation in acute respiratory failure. *Am J Respir Crit Care Med* 1995; **151**: 1799–806.
35. Bott J, Carroll MP, Conway JH *et al.* Randomised controlled trial of nasal ventilation in acute ventilatory failure due to chronic obstructive airways disease. *Lancet* 1993; **341**: 1555–7.
36. Bolton R, Bleetman A. Non-invasive ventilation and continuous positive pressure ventilation in emergency departments: where are we now? *Emerg Med J* 2008; **25**: 190–4.
37. Confalonieri M, Gorini M, Ambrosino N *et al.* Respiratory intensive care units in Italy: a national census and prospective cohort study. *Thorax* 2001; **56**: 373–8.
38. Bertolini G, Confalonieri M, Rossi C *et al.* Costs of the COPD. Differences between intensive care unit and respiratory intermediate care unit. *Respir Med* 2005; **99**: 894–900.
39. Paus-Jenssen ES, Reid JK, Cockcroft DW *et al.* The use of noninvasive ventilation in acute respiratory failure at a tertiary care center. *Chest* 2004; **126**: 165–72.
40. Plaisance P, Pirracchio R, Berton C *et al.* A randomized study of out-of-hospital continuous positive airway pressure for acute cardiogenic pulmonary oedema: physiological and clinical effects. *Eur Heart J* 2007; **28**: 2895–901.
41. Sharon A, Shpirer I, Kaluski E *et al.* High-dose intravenous isosorbide-dinitrate is safer and better than Bi-PAP ventilation combined with conventional treatment for severe pulmonary edema. *J Am Coll Cardiol* 2000; **36**: 832–7.
42. Plant PK, Owen JL, Elliott MW. One year period prevalence study of respiratory acidosis in acute exacerbations of COPD: implications for the provision of non-invasive ventilation and oxygen administration. *Thorax* 2000; **55**: 550–4.
43. Joosten SA, Koh MS, Bu X *et al.* The effects of oxygen therapy in patients presenting to an emergency department with exacerbation of chronic obstructive pulmonary disease. *Med J Aust* 2007; **186**: 235–8.
44. Barbé F, Togores B, Rubí M *et al.* Noninvasive ventilatory support does not facilitate recovery from acute respiratory failure in chronic obstructive pulmonary disease. *Eur Respir J* 1996; **9**: 1240–5.
45. Tomii K, Seo R, Tachikawa R *et al.* Impact of noninvasive ventilation (NIV) trial for various types of acute respiratory failure in the emergency department; decreased mortality and use of the ICU. *Respir Med* 2009; **103**: 67–73.
46. Poponick JM, Renston JP, Bennett RP *et al.* Use of a ventilatory support system (BiPAP) for acute respiratory failure in the emergency department. *Chest* 1999; **116**: 166–71.
47. Conti G, Antonelli M, Navalesi P *et al.* Noninvasive vs. conventional mechanical ventilation in patients with chronic obstructive pulmonary disease after failure of medical treatment in the ward: a randomized trial. *Intensive Care Med* 2002; **28**: 1701–7.
48. Squadrone E, Frigerio P, Fogliati C *et al.* Noninvasive vs invasive ventilation in COPD patients with severe acute respiratory failure deemed to require ventilatory assistance. *Intensive Care Med* 2004; **30**: 1303–10.

49. Cabrini L, Idone C, Colombo S *et al.* Medical emergency team and non-invasive ventilation outside ICU for acute respiratory failure. *Intensive Care Med* 2009; **35**: 339–43.
50. Corrado A, Gorini M, Melej R *et al.* Iron lung versus mask ventilation in acute exacerbation of COPD: a randomised crossover study. *Intensive Care Med* 2009; **35**: 648–55.
51. Scala R, Nava S, Conti G *et al.* Noninvasive versus conventional ventilation to treat hypercapnic encephalopathy in chronic obstructive pulmonary disease. *Intensive Care Med* 2007; **33**: 2101–8.
52. Scala R, Corrado A, Confalonieri M *et al.* The second National survey of Italian respiratory high dependency units: changes from 1996 to 2006. *Eur Respir J* 2008: **32** Suppl 52: 331s.
53. Scala R, Naldi M, Archinucci I *et al.* Noninvasive positive pressure ventilation in patients with acute exacerbations of COPD and varying levels of consciousness. *Chest* 2005; **128**: 1657–66.
54. Vianello A, Corrado A, Arcaro G *et al.* Mechanical insufflation-exsufflation improves outcomes for neuromuscular disease patients with respiratory tract infections. *Am J Phys Med Rehabil* 2005; **84**: 83–8.
55. Vargas F, Bui HN, Boyer A *et al.* Intrapulmonary percussive ventilation in acute exacerbations of COPD patients with mild respiratory acidosis: a randomized controlled trial. *Crit Care* 2005; **9**: R382–9.
56. Carlucci A, Richard JC, Wysocki M *et al.* Noninvasive versus conventional mechanical ventilation. An epidemiologic survey. *Am J Respir Crit Care Med* 2001; **163**: 874–80.
57. Maggiore SM, Mercurio G, Volpe C. NIV in the acute setting: technical aspects, initiation, monitoring and choice of interface. *Eur Respir Mon* 2008; **41**: 173–88.
58. Navalesi P, Fanfulla F, Frigerio P *et al.* Physiologic evaluation of noninvasive mechanical ventilation delivered with three types of masks in patients with chronic hypercapnic respiratory failure. *Crit Care Med* 2000; **28**: 1785–90.
59. Kwok H, McCormack J, Cece R *et al.* Controlled trial of oronasal versus nasal mask ventilation in the treatment of acute respiratory failure. *Crit Care Med* 2003; **31**: 468–73.
60. Girault C, Briel A, Benichou J *et al.* Interface strategy during noninvasive positive pressure ventilation for hypercapnic acute respiratory failure. *Crit Care Med* 2009; **37**: 124–31.
61. Saatci E, Miller DM, Stell IM *et al.* Dynamic dead space in face masks used with noninvasive ventilators: a lung model study. *Eur Respir J* 2004; **23**: 129–35.
62. Cuvelier A, Pujol W, Pramil S *et al.* Cephalic versus oronasal mask for noninvasive ventilation in acute hypercapnic respiratory failure. *Intensive Care Med* 2009; **35**: 519–26.
63. Navalesi P, Costa R, Ceriana P *et al.* Non-invasive ventilation in chronic obstructive pulmonary disease patients: helmet versus facial mask. *Intensive Care Med* 2007; **33**: 74–81.
64. Antonelli M, Pennisi MA, Pelosi P *et al.* Noninvasive positive pressure ventilation using a helmet in patients with acute exacerbation of chronic obstructive pulmonary disease: a feasibility study. *Anesthesiology* 2004; **100**: 16–24.
65. Nava S, Navalesi P. Helmet to deliver noninvasive ventilation: 'Handle with care'. *Crit Care Med* 2009; **37**: 2111–13.
66. Antonelli M, Conti G, Pelosi P *et al.* New treatment of acute hypoxemic respiratory failure: noninvasive pressure support ventilation delivered by helmet – a pilot controlled trial. *Crit Care Med* 2002; **30**: 602–8.
67. Schneider E, Dualé C, Vaille JL *et al.* Comparison of tolerance of facemask vs. mouthpiece for non-invasive ventilation. *Anaesthesia* 2006; **61**: 20–3.
68. Scala R, Naldi M. Ventilators for noninvasive ventilation to treat acute respiratory failure. *Respir Care* 2008; **53**: 1054–80.
69. Lofaso F, Brochard L, Touchard D *et al.* Evaluation of carbon dioxide rebreathing during pressure support ventilation with airway management system (BiPAP) devices. *Chest* 1995; **108**: 772–8.
70. Vignaux L, Tassaux D, Jolliet P. Performance of noninvasive ventilation modes on ICU ventilators during pressure support: a bench model study. *Intensive Care Med* 2007; **33**: 1444–51.
71. Gonzalez-Bermejo J, Laplanche V, Husseini FE *et al.* Evaluation of the user-friendliness of 11 home mechanical ventilators. *Eur Respir J* 2006; **27**: 1236–43.
72. Vignaux L, Vargas F, Roeseler J *et al.* Patient-ventilator asynchrony during non-invasive ventilation for acute respiratory failure: a multicenter study. *Intensive Care Med* 2009; **35**: 840–6.
73. Moretti M, Cilione C, Tampieri A *et al.* Incidence and causes of non-invasive mechanical ventilation failure after initial success. *Thorax* 2000; **55**: 819–25.
74. Calderini E, Confalonieri M, Puccio PG *et al.* Patient-ventilator asynchrony during noninvasive ventilation: the role of expiratory trigger. *Intensive Care Med* 1999; **25**: 662–7.
75. Weng MH. The effect of protective treatment in reducing pressure ulcers for non-invasive ventilation patients. *Intensive Crit Care Nurs* 2008; **24**: 295–9.
76. Lellouche F, Maggiore SM, Deye N *et al.* Effect of the humidification device on the work of breathing during noninvasive ventilation. *Intensive Care Med* 2002; **28**: 1582–9.
77. Jaber S, Chanques G, Matecki S *et al.* Comparison of the effects of heat and moisture exchangers and heated humidifiers on ventilation and gas exchange during non-invasive ventilation. *Intensive Care Med* 2002; **28**: 1590–4.
78. Tuggey JM, Delmastro M, Elliott MW. The effect of mouth leak and humidification during nasal non-invasive ventilation. *Respir Med* 2007; **101**: 1874–9.
79. Constantin JM, Schneider E, Cayot-Constantin S *et al.* Remifentanil-based sedation to treat noninvasive

ventilation failure: a preliminary study. *Intensive Care Med* 2007; **33**: 82–7.

80. Akada S, Takeda S, Yoshida Y *et al.* The efficacy of dexmedetomidine in patients with noninvasive ventilation: a preliminary study. *Anesth Analg* 2008; **107**: 167–70.
81. Devlin JW, Nava S, Fong JJ *et al.* Survey of sedation practices during noninvasive positive-pressure ventilation to treat acute respiratory failure. *Crit Care Med* 2007; **35**: 2298–302.
82. Casey KR, Cantillo KO, Brown LK. Sleep-related hypoventilation/hypoxemic syndromes. *Curr Opinion Pulm Med* 2007; **131**: 1936–48.
83. Dhand UK, Dhand R. Sleep disorders in neuromuscular diseases. *Curr Opinion Pulm Med* 2006; **12**: 402–8.
84. Gilgoff I, Prentice W, Baydur A. Patient and family participation in the management of respiratory failure in Duchenne's muscular dystrophy. *Chest* 1989; **95**: 519–24.
85. Henderson Y. Understanding the benefits of pulmonary rehabilitation. *Nursing Times* 2004; **100**: 53.
86. Motor Neurone Disease Association. *Information sheet P14A: Understanding how MND may affect breathing.* Northampton: Motor Neurone Disease Association, 2007. Available at: www.mndassociation.org/life_with_mnd/getting_more_information/publications/publications_.html (accessed 23 June 2009).
87. Motor Neurone Disease Association. *Information sheet P14B: Ventilation in MND.* Northampton: Motor Neurone Disease Association, 2007. Available at: www.mndassociation.org/life_with_mnd/getting_more_information/publications/publications_.html (accessed 23 June 2009).
88. Motor Neurone Disease Association. *Information sheet P14D: Troubleshooting problems when using non-invasive ventilation (NIV).* Northampton: Motor Neurone Disease Association, 2007. Available at: www.mndassociation.org/life_with_mnd/getting_more_information/publications/publications_.html (accessed 23 June 2009).
89. Simonds AK. *Factsheet making breathing easier.* London: Muscular Dystrophy Campaign, 2008. Available at: www.muscular-dystrophy.org/how_we_help_you/care_publications/factsheets/656_making_breathing_easier.html (accessed 28 June 2009).
90. Turkington PM, Elliott MW. The rationale for the use of non-invasive ventilation in chronic ventilatory failure. *Thorax* 2000; **55**: 417–23.
91. ATS Consensus Conference. Respiratory care of the patient with Duchenne muscular dystrophy. *Am J Respir Crit Care Med* 2004; **170**: 456–65.
92. Ward S, Chatwin M, Heather S *et al.* Randomised controlled trial of non-invasive ventilation for nocturnal hypoventilation in neuromuscular and chest wall disease patients with daytime normocapnia. *Thorax* 2005; **60**: 1019–24.
93. Bourke SC, Bullock RE, Williams TL *et al.* Noninvasive ventilation in ALS, indications and effect on quality of life. *Neurology* 2003; **61**: 171–7.
94. Raphael JC, Chevret S, Chastang C *et al.* Randomised trial of preventative nasal ventilation in Duchenne muscular dystrophy. *Lancet* 1994; **343**: 1600–4.
95. Elliott MW. The interface: crucial for successful non-invasive ventilation. *Eur Respir J* 2004; **23**: 7–8.
96. Jardine E. Wallis C. Core guidelines for the discharge home of the child on long term assisted ventilation in the United Kingdom. *Thorax* 1998; **53**: 762–7.

# SECTION B

# The practice: acute non-invasive ventilation

# 10

# How to set up an acute non-invasive ventilation service

ALICIA K GERKE, GREGORY A SCHMIDT

## ABSTRACT

With mounting evidence for the use of non-invasive ventilation (NIV) in acutely ill patients, healthcare practitioners are recognizing the need to set up acute NIV services in the hospital setting. In certain populations, the use of NIV can obviate the need for invasive ventilation, decrease nosocomial infections and improve mortality in a cost-effective manner. Setting up an acute NIV service requires forethought and planning. The charge should be led by a 'champion' who can provide the organizational leadership to incorporate multiple hospital departments and administration. In setting up the service, consideration must be given to the hospital infrastructure, location of use, equipment, training, protocols, and methods for quality measurement and assurance. Challenges and obstacles should be anticipated when instituting change in the organization. Continuing education and feedback are vital to the setting up and ongoing success of a NIV programme.

## INTRODUCTION

Indications for use of non-invasive ventilation (NIV) are increasing, based on improved outcomes (compared with invasive ventilation) and reduced risks (such as fewer nosocomial infections). At the same time, NIV has made it possible to support or palliate patients who have elected to forego more invasive life-sustaining measures, such as endotracheal intubation. Despite evidence that NIV can prevent intubations or improve mortality, especially in COPD exacerbations, cardiogenic pulmonary oedema and immunocompromised patients with hypoxaemic respiratory failure, underutilization is widespread. Some hospitals miss opportunities to provide NIV because they lack expertise, fail to invest the necessary resources, have no champions, or resist change. Although NIV is becoming more common, it could be used more extensively. Therefore, we emphasize a multidisciplinary team approach to building the competencies necessary for an institution to succeed at providing NIV safely to those most likely to benefit.

Starting a NIV service is a complex process that relies on multiple factors for its success, related to both the clinicians and the organizational structure of the healthcare setting. These factors include the practice, beliefs and attitudes of clinicians, expectations of the patients, clinicians or administrators, the organizational context of the hospital including resources and current care processes, and public policy or legislation that can influence practice.[1,2] Each of these factors is vital to a successful new paradigm and must be addressed. In this chapter, we present methods and suggestions on how to set up an acute NIV unit in the hospital setting. Issues include identification of appropriate use opportunities, the setting of use, training and types of personnel, necessary infrastructure and barriers to acceptance (Box 10.1). Although a comprehensive approach to implementing and maintaining a NIV service is presented, marked differences in healthcare settings and practices across regions and the world contribute to the challenge of change.

## WHY A NON-INVASIVE VENTILATION SERVICE?

Current data suggest that NIV is underutilized despite growing evidence of its success in decreasing the need for

**Box 10.1 Key ingredients in starting a non-invasive ventilation programme**

- Identify a 'champion' to lead the process
- Assemble a multidisciplinary team with training and experience in NIV
- Incorporate hospital administration, departmental leaders, clinical providers into initial set-up decision-making
- Decide on a location for NIV and/or mobile service
- Establish monitoring methods and assemble equipment
- Create protocols including initiation, training, and maintenance of NIV
- Establish quality management strategies and outcomes monitoring
- Anticipate resistance to change and establish strategies to overcome barriers

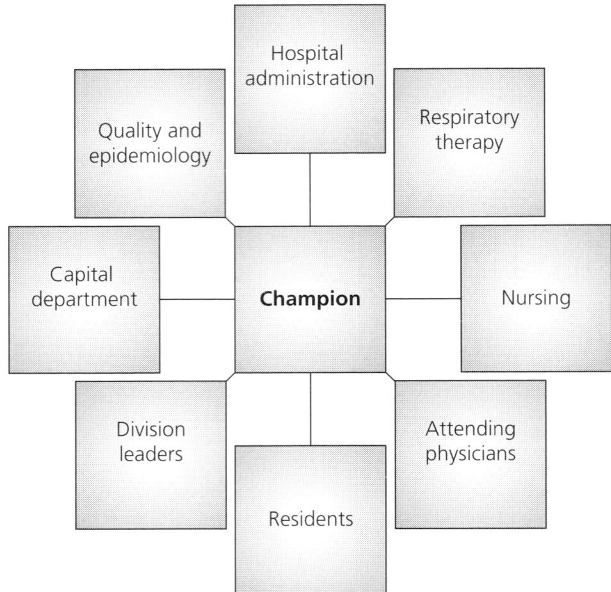


**Figure 10.1** The role of the champion.

initiation of mechanical ventilation, preventing failure of extubation, and decreasing nosocomial pneumonias. For instance, in one utilization study, two-thirds of intensive care unit (ICU) patients who had an admitting diagnosis of COPD or cardiogenic pulmonary oedema and fulfilled criteria for use of NIV were intubated without a trial.[3] Maheshwari studied utilization practices in north-eastern USA and found marked variation in utilization rates (0 to greater than 50 per cent), noting that the two main perceived barriers to utilization were lack of physician knowledge and inadequate equipment.[4] Undoubtedly, the reasons behind this variability are more complex. However, this study highlights the necessity for increased education and visibility of this technique to aid in widespread safe and effective use.

Next, lack of a structured service and inexperience with the technique can also lead to misuse of NIV and suboptimal care. For instance, in a review of 91 patients in whom NIV was initiated, physician orders were missing for 15 per cent of the NIV trials, cardiorespiratory monitoring was not explicitly ordered in any patient, and documentation of equipment was lacking.[5] Further, experience of operators is particularly important in severely ill patients. A review of the outcomes of patients on NIV over a 7-year period of time found that increased experience with NIV may allow increasingly severely ill patients to be treated without compromising the rate of success.[6]

## A MULTIDISCIPLINARY TEAM

It is important to have one clinician or a small group of clinicians who serve as 'champions' or leaders of the process (Fig. 10.1).[2] The champion should be available to answer questions, troubleshoot, and maintain momentum of the process. This person must remain flexible to problems and suggestions, implementing changes in protocols and processes where needed. To be the most effective, leaders also need to maintain knowledge of the latest technologies and evidence regarding NIV, and maintain collaborations with other institutions for advice and consultation. Having a champion increases awareness and knowledge, and promotes an evidence-based culture, thereby increasing appropriate utilization.

The champion should be integrally involved in both the planning and implementation phases of the acute NIV service, serving to bridge this gap. Planning will involve a different group of team members than the actual implementation team. In planning, hospital administration, a member of the capital department and division leaders should be involved in cost analyses, resource allocation, logistics and public relations. On the other hand, the implementation team involves educators, clinical care providers, hospital epidemiology and quality control members. These team members should include caregivers who are trained and experienced in NIV. In the USA, these are often respiratory therapists, but can also be nurses, respiratory physiologists, physicians' assistants or nurse practitioners. The prevalence of each of these caregivers varies regionally and internationally, and the make-up of the implementation team depends on local availability. Overall, it is important to involve different types of caregiver as each brings a different expertise to the forefront of care, all inherent to patient success.

## THE LOCATION FOR NIV

An acute NIV service can be located in a particular ward or unit in a hospital, or can be defined more broadly to include a team that administers NIV in various locations within the hospital. Currently, NIV is used in a variety of places. One study showed that the primary site of initiation of NIV in the hospital was the emergency department although the ICU and the clinical teaching unit incorporated the most total hours of NIV.[5] Other reviews confirm that the emergency department, ICU and general wards are the most common sites of initiation.[4,7] Clinical teaching units that use NIV most frequently are internal medicine, pulmonology and cardiology. More recently, successful use of NIV has been shown in the post-operative care units,[8] particularly in treating acute respiratory failure after lung resection.[9] Outside of the hospital, NIV started in-home and upon transport has been shown to be a feasible and effective method to improve the emergency management of patients with pulmonary oedema[10] and may become increasingly used for other causes.[11,12]

Factors influencing the location of NIV use include monitoring capabilities of the unit, ICU bed capacity, convenience if intubation is required, nurse-to-patient ratio, respiratory therapy availability, cost-effectiveness, and clinician experience.[13] While it is often recommended that candidates for NIV be treated in an ICU for reasons of safety (especially in North America), this is not always possible because such beds are often in short supply. At the same time, costly ICU beds may not be necessary for appropriately selected patients. Experience is critically important in judging which patients can be managed safely outside the ICU. Key factors include the type and severity of illness, respiratory parameters, mental status, and ability to clear secretions, in combination with the type of equipment needed and ward infrastructure, when deciding on a location for NIV initiation (Box 10.2). Level of consciousness should be taken into account as decreased levels have been associated with worse outcomes in multiple studies.[5,14] Nevertheless, obtundation is not a contraindication to NIV. Finally, the decision on where to monitor should take into account the experienced clinician's subjective judgement regarding the severity of illness and potential for deterioration.

### Box 10.2 Patients who can be managed outside an ICU

The ideal candidate

- COPD exacerbation
- Haemodynamically stable
- Alert, cooperative and able to remove the mask themselves when appropriate
- Capable of tolerating brief periods off NIV
- Adequate cough with no excessive secretions
- Shows improvement of pH and respiratory rate during first 1–2 hours of therapy
- Staff are experienced in NIV use

Higher risk of NIV failure

- Acute respiratory failure of undetermined aetiology
- Hypoxaemic respiratory failure not due to cardiogenic pulmonary oedema
- Agitation or poor mask tolerance
- Greater overall illness severity
- Tolerance off NIV unproved
- Excessive or tenacious secretions or poor cough
- Not clearly improving after initial trial of therapy
- Staff less experienced in recognizing respiratory deterioration, troubleshooting NIV, or facilitating endotracheal intubation

## EMERGENCY WARD

The emergency department is an important venue as it is one of the earliest opportunities to institute NIV to prevent intubation, with the impetus that NIV has a higher success rate if started early.[15] Initiating NIV in the emergency department may also decrease the need for ICU admission,[16–17] and thereby reduce ICU costs.[18] Careful application in this setting is imperative, as use for inappropriate indications or lack of appropriate monitoring can delay life-saving care in some cases.[19] Challenges in the emergency department include the tentative nature of the respiratory failure diagnosis, high risk of intubation need in the first hours of NIV, staff inexperience in the longitudinal management of NIV, and lack of continuity with the team that will manage the subsequent hospital care. Moreover, NIV success benefits from time taken to engage the patient, troubleshoot the equipment, titrate the settings and judge the impact – an approach that sometimes contradicts a goal of securing the airway and transferring to a ward. A NIV service can provide education for emergency department physicians and staff with regard to how to maximize success. Guidelines regarding use should be enforced to prevent adverse events in a hectic emergency department where monitoring and communication may be difficult. Posted protocols can help provide an easy reference regarding selection of patients, instructions on who to call for placement of NIV, monitoring requirements, and how to recognize a failing patient. Often, a separate consult service can help alleviate strain on the emergency department personnel.

Success and ease of use in the emergency department setting are important, as many potential patients are seen. However, perceived failures or lack of ease of use can lead to frustration and scepticism on the part of emergency department staff. Failure rates can also appear higher in this setting given the heterogeneity of patients and potential for inappropriate use. Last, it should be emphasized that NIV is most often a bridge to admission and continuation of NIV, as a majority of patients require more than a few hours of use. Nevertheless, there is some experience with using

NIV to improve vital signs and acid/base parameters, followed by an assessment for immediate discharge to an unmonitored general ward. For example, following an initial 90-minute period of NIV for acute cardiogenic pulmonary oedema, 43 of 58 patients who tolerated 15 minutes of NIV removal without dyspnoea or haemodynamic instability were treated on a general ward.[16] None of these patients subsequently died, was intubated or required ICU transfer. Overall, in light of these complexities, a NIV service can be of particular importance to the emergency department environment in order to capture patients who would benefit, alleviate a considerable time and effort burden off emergency department personnel, and potentially improve outcomes in a cost-effective process.

### GENERAL WARD

Similarly, NIV can be used on general wards in certain patients depending on severity of illness. Intense monitoring standards must be applied, as well as proper education and training of nurses, as NIV cannot be applied universally on wards without these factors in place. Furthermore, high concern for patient selection based on current evidence should be implemented. For example, one study shows that early use of NIV in COPD patients with mild or moderate acidaemia on general wards resulted in fewer intubations and decreased in-hospital mortality.[20] Therefore, NIV may be reasonable in these cases. Also, institutions highly experienced with NIV have treated an increasing fraction of moderately ill patients (COPD exacerbation and pH >7.28) on a general medical ward without compromising safety.[6] Alternatively, studies have shown that patients in hypercapnic coma can be treated with NIV.[21,22] However, these studies were performed in controlled, well monitored ICUs or respiratory monitoring units, and therefore, these patients should not be placed on a regular ward. Patients on the ward should be awake enough to take off the mask in case of vomiting or able to press a call button for a nurse. It has been suggested that patients should be capable of breathing spontaneously for 1 hour without NIV.[7] In addition, documentation of monitoring and checks is essential to ensure identification of a failing patient in need of more specialized care. We believe that use of NIV on general wards in non-COPD respiratory failure (such as hypoxaemic failure or pulmonary oedema) is rarely appropriate, unless there has been a clear decision to limit life-sustaining treatments.

### RESPIRATORY INTERMEDIATE CARE UNIT

In those patients with more potential for failure, a specialized NIV ward can be utilized with similar monitoring to an ICU. These wards may be less stressful for patients than the ICU atmosphere and contribute to increased sleep, comfort, and improved experience for the patient. A number of studies have suggested that these units can be cost-effective and successful.[13,23–26] Elpern and colleagues found that using a non-invasive ventilatory unit for specialty care of mechanically ventilated patients was a cost-saving measure primarily due to savings from ICU time.[23] Use of an intermediate respiratory unit can free up vital ICU resources and decrease nursing requirements. The number of beds can vary according to the needs and resources of different institutions, and therefore, assessment of patient population, bed utilization and overall need is necessary prior to setting up this type of ward. The size often ranges from four to ten beds.[27] It is also important that the institution have at least a minimum number of patients, not only for cost structuring but also to maintain the experience of the teams involved in patient care. This type of ward can often be the most efficient place for NIV and offer high-quality care, given the specialization.

The Intensive Care Assembly of the European Respiratory Society Task Force has adopted criteria defining a respiratory intermediate care unit which includes criteria for admission, type of intervention and equipment, and staffing.[27] Criteria for admission are single organ failure, acute respiratory failure requiring monitoring (but not mechanical ventilation) or tracheostomy-ventilated patients coming from the ICU. The unit should have NIV, availability of conventional ventilators and monitoring equipment. Staffing should be a ratio of four or fewer patients to every one nurse, a respiratory physiotherapist, and a doctor with the same profile as the senior doctor (training in pneumology and NIV) immediately available 24 hours per day.

### INTENSIVE CARE UNIT

The ICU provides the highest standard of monitoring, with high ratios of nurses and dedicated respiratory therapists. It is important to note that a majority of the evidence regarding NIV efficacy and safety is derived from ICU environments. If NIV is used only in the ICU, however, there is likely to be underutilization of NIV. On the other hand, if NIV is used anywhere, there may be overutilization, sacrificing patient safety. We believe it is prudent to treat most respiratory failure patients who are candidates for NIV in an ICU or dedicated NIV unit, whenever such beds are readily available. One of the functions of a NIV service should be to balance these issues of utilization and patient safety, taking into account the capabilities of the individual institution.

## MONITORING

Monitoring is essential to the successful use of NIV and should be available (for further details, see Chapter 11). Experienced personnel, preferably including a physician, should be available on a 24-hour basis. Monitoring the patient in the first hours after initiation is particularly intensive and vital to patient safety (Box 10.3).

**Box 10.3 Tasks in the first hours of NIV**

- Educate and reassure the patient
- Assess mask fit, comfort, and tolerance
- Seek and correct leaks
- Determine synchrony of patient and ventilator
- Titrate inspiratory positive airway pressure (IPAP) and expiratory positive airway pressure (EPAP)
- Monitor heart rate, respiratory rate, accessory muscle use and level of consciousness
- Judge cough adequacy and secretions
- Consider the role for judicious sedation
- Analyse arterial blood gas values at 1 hour
- Actively estimate the probability of failure and re-evaluate the level of monitoring
- Diagnose and treat the underlying cause of respiratory failure

Utilization reviews show that intubation rate and death are higher in hospital settings outside of clinical trials, and may be partially due to unsystematic monitoring.[5] Communication between the ICU teams, wards, and during shift changes can also be standardized to improve patient safety. Correct interpretation of monitoring data to guide decision-making is crucial, and therefore, training in this area is important.

## SET-UP AND EQUIPMENT

Obtaining and maintaining equipment needed for the NIV service requires the efforts of hospital administration, the capital department, champion physicians, and the respiratory therapists and nurses who administer the equipment. This is important, as one of the main barriers to usage has been lack of adequate equipment.[4] Further, a greater number of ventilators has been associated with increased NIV usage.[28] Therefore, an assessment of projected usage is important to ensure cost-effectiveness, balanced by adequate resources for all patients in whom a trial of NIV is indicated (for further details, refer to Part 1, Section A).

## TRAINING

Protocols for training can be implemented across a variety of healthcare professionals to ensure safe and effective utilization of NIV (Box 10.4). In a survey of NIV use in the UK, the two primary reasons for lack of utilization were lack of consultant training and lack of other staff training.[29] The best practices on how to train physicians and healthcare professionals on NIV are currently unclear. However, it is likely that a combination of methods is effective. The training also depends on the type of practitioner involved. A survey of 242 physicians who used NIV revealed that the most common method of learning about NIV was from physician and respiratory therapy colleagues, rather than from educational conferences or direct examination of the evidence.[28] Elliott *et al.* support this premise of preceptorship when they found that clinician experience, and not necessarily training, led to increased use of NIV on the wards.[13]

In general, physicians, nurses and other ward personnel should be educated on the indications for NIV, since any of these groups can help identify appropriate candidates and initiate NIV. This includes residents and physicians in all areas of the hospital. For the same reason, signs and symptoms of failure of NIV should be taught to all of those involved in order to maintain safe use. This can be accomplished through conferences, didactic sessions, or direct teaching by champions and leaders during rounds and patient care. Furthermore, training and education directed towards the entire healthcare team may be necessary to improve guideline awareness and increase comfort with recommended practices.[30]

**Box 10.4 Training goals for the NIV programme***

Theory

- Practical theory of mechanical ventilation
- Evidence base supporting NIV

Equipment

- How to initiate NIV
- Mask fit, headgear, comfort, and leak detection
- Machines and modes
- Titration of pressures and settings
- Troubleshooting alarms
- Standards of monitoring
- Maintaining and stocking equipment

Patient care

- Identification of appropriate candidates for NIV
- Coaching the patient
- Interpreting arterial blood gases during NIV
- Symptoms and signs of NIV failure
- Indications for intubation

*The ideal programme includes simulation, case-based learning, and preceptorship during real patient care. Programmes that reinforce learning at regular intervals, such as twice yearly, are more likely to effect long-lasting change.

More targeted training regarding the technical aspects of machine specifics and mask application should be directed to those healthcare professionals directly involved in initiating and placing NIV on a patient. This mainly includes respiratory therapists, but can also be nurses or physicians, particularly in regions where respiratory therapists do not exist. The training is best done with hands-on workshops with demonstrations of masks, tubing, and ventilators, but also can include some lectures or didactics. Simulation sessions can also be very helpful, such as mask applications practised on classmates. Last, shadowing and preceptorship with clinical rotations accompanying those who place the masks and initiate ventilation should be incorporated to train healthcare professionals with actual patients.

The training material of those directly involved in initiating the ventilator and monitoring the patient should include how to put on equipment, provide facial care, titrate pressures, troubleshoot alarms and monitor. The complexity of the technical training is often based on the type of ventilator utilized. At a minimum, this education includes basic ventilatory mechanics and theory. Further focus should be placed on routine patient assessment, coaching of the patient, and identifying a failing patient. Problem solving and case-based learning can simulate true ward situations. These training objectives should be documented and ongoing routine training on a biannual or annual basis should be enforced. This ongoing training requirement is particularly important in teaching hospitals where resident and practitioner turnover is high.

One university teaching hospital accounted its success to training and orientation of caretakers.[7] They incorporated a 4-hour training session for respiratory therapy on application of NIV to patients, while nurses received classroom orientation and bedside instruction by respiratory therapy.

Certification may also be helpful for a variety of reasons. First, certifications can help to assure standardized training amongst different groups. Second, certifications can be useful to track outcomes as they relate to training, which can reveal a cause or contributory factor to increased failure rate.

## QUALITY MANAGEMENT

Review of utilization, successes, and failures of a NIV service is integral to its maintenance and continuous improvement strategy. Mortality, reintubation rate according to location, costs, use for appropriate indications, infection rates and adherence to documentation should be assessed on a regular basis. It is important to realize that there is an inherent failure rate of NIV even when used strictly according to the evidence. Review of one's own care practices, as well as others, can help implement important quality and safety measures to ensure ongoing success. It is important to share these results with colleagues, hospital administration, and community in order to increase buy-in and support for NIV.

## INSTITUTING CHANGE

Mechanical ventilation practices are changing internationally, based on evolving evidence.[31] Instituting organizational change can be a challenge, and knowledge of organizational change models can be helpful. In one study assessing change-avid respiratory therapy departments it was found that the main differences between change-avid and non-change-avid departments was the presence of a vision for change, effective leadership, engaging employees in the change effort, celebrating wins and assuring the sustainability of the change.[32] Conversely, the least desirable traits included an authoritative culture, passive leadership and limited communication with respiratory therapy staff. These concepts highlight the important role of having a champion of the effort, leading change and promoting a clear vision and effective plan.

Involvement of those personnel on the 'front lines' is imperative to successful change. This involves communication with respiratory therapists or nurses who will be responsible for implementing the service. The champion should be open and available to listen to suggestions and input. Furthermore, empowering this group to take responsibility is often desirable for both the physicians and the respiratory therapists, and may even translate to improved care of the patient. Multiple studies have shown that implementation of respiratory care protocols by non-physician healthcare professionals can improve outcomes for critically ill patients.[33–35] Increasing the roles and involvement of the therapists encourages internal change and ownership of the plan. Empowerment has been effective in other realms, and is accomplished by appropriate delegation of work, guidelines and protocols.

Implementing a change is the first battle – however, sustaining change is equally important. First, success should be acknowledged in a global sense. Second, the champions should commend individuals for efforts and successes. It is important to recognize the programme and individuals on a continuing basis in order to maintain motivation and ongoing positive change. This is also where it is important to be conservative at the onset of the service, as to decrease the likelihood of an early failure which can be a considerable setback to the morale of the programme. For instance, it may be prudent to focus initial implementation in one or two key locations in the hospital. Growth to other venues can then occur as the service becomes more accepted and successes become obvious to all stakeholders. Recognition of efforts sets the stage for forward growth and continuous improvement.

When instituting change, resistance should always be expected. In one evaluation assessing the difficulties in instituting infection control practices, active resistance was present in 14/14 sites, primarily by attending physicians or competing authorities. Mid- to high-level administration also created barriers with ambivalence, passive resistance or active blocking of an initiative.[36] This leads to poor morale and frustration at an organizational level. Suggested solutions to overcome the 'active resister' and 'organizational constipator' include regular feedback, effective champions, participation in collaborative efforts, improving communication with executives, and working around or excluding individuals who are barriers to change.[36]

## 'SELLING YOUR SERVICE': NEEDS ASSESSMENT AND HOSPITAL BUY-IN

The implementation of an NIV service will involve 'buy in' by a number of groups, including hospital administration, physician colleagues in multiple specialties, and ward personnel who care for the patient. Often, this involves education on the evidence behind the benefits of a successful programme such as patient safety, improved outcomes and increased patient satisfaction. Furthermore, financial justification is becoming an increasingly important problem that the champion will encounter.

In the planning phase, the champion must argue that the NIV service is worth the input of resources by the hospital, personnel and colleagues. A careful assessment of the projected need based on patient admissions and missed opportunity for NIV is necessary. Resources must be allocated towards purchase of equipment and training of the staff. Importantly, time and effort of the team must not be overlooked. For instance, Kramer and co-authors found that respiratory therapy may spend up to an hour of time in the first 8 hours of initiation of NIV,[37] and the time involved by staff in care of NIV may be similar to invasive ventilation. Overall, these resources must be enacted in entirety, as a programme lacking in any one of the components, whether it is time, equipment or enthusiasm, is increasingly likely to fail.

Improved outcome and patient safety should be one of the primary reasons to implement NIV service. This is supported by multiple reports of decreased mortality and improved outcomes. For instance, implementing routine use of NIV in critically ill patients with acute exacerbation of COPD or severe pulmonary oedema was associated with improved survival and reduction of nosocomial infections in a French population.[38] Long-term benefits in appropriate patients include fewer readmissions and greater 1-year survival.[39–41] NIV use has also been associated with decrease in ventilator associated pneumonia[42] and reduced antibiotic use.[43]

Cost-effectiveness of NIV will be an important argument for overall buy-in. Multiple studies have demonstrated that, if implemented correctly, NIV can be a cost-saving measure. Keenan and colleagues found that using NIV in COPD exacerbations is not only more effective, but less expensive.[24] A similar analysis in the UK hospital system indicated that providing a NIV service will avoid six deaths and three to nine admissions to ICUs per year, with an associated cost reduction of £12 000–53 000 per year.[25] Furthermore, the use of NIV for COPD and acute respiratory failure of other causes doubled from 1998 to 2004, coinciding with a 50 per cent reduction in the overall numbers of patients in the ICU with a primary diagnosis of COPD or cardiogenic pulmonary oedema.[31] This aspect is important when considering the investment in equipment and personnel which may initially seem prohibitive.

## PROBLEMS AND OBSTACLES

In any institution, problems and obstacles to implementation are expected to occur as with introduction of many new devices or protocols. First, the effects on other departments or services should not be minimized. A NIV service may be perceived as an effort to limit another service's privileges or infringement upon their independence to provide care. This is where the champion can make a concerted effort to educate all services on the known benefits and confer support, rather than dominance, with the technique. At times, finding collaborators in different departments to relay information to his or her colleagues or subordinates can be useful. It is also important to circulate success rates and 'advertising' to build support and visibility among the departments.

Logistics can be an issue, particularly if the service is not confined to one ward. This includes not only the ability of the NIV team physically to reach a patient but also the ability to monitor, the availability of emergency response, and proximity to more intensive care. Placing a patient in a room closer to a nursing station, incorporating emergency carts in each location and having immediate availability of personnel to help in more emergent situations (such as a 'rapid response team') can help to alleviate some of these concerns.

Staffing will also be an important issue that should be first addressed in the planning phase. A 24-hour service staffed with trained and experienced personnel requires availability and cooperation of the team. Hospital administration should be involved in the investment of resources towards this goal, and team members must be willing to provide care for patients, including night coverage. Furthermore, nursing coverage, particularly on a specialized NIV ward service, should include a group of experienced and trained nurses who can provide continuity of care. Large numbers of 'floating' nurses through this area should be avoided to ensure that appropriate specialized care is provided. A mobile team should be formed to provide NIV and aid in care of patients on general wards.

## USE OF PROTOCOLS

Protocols can improve practice, help implement evidence-based strategies, reduce errors, and ensure uniformity and quality of care. Essential to adherence to guidelines in the intensive care setting are effective leadership and positive interprofessional team dynamics, education tailored to the learning preferences of different groups, repeated education, and feedback.[44] Using guidelines and protocols can lead to an increase in NIV utilization, although the question of whether this equates to improved mortality outcomes is still unproven.[45] However, evidence on the use of non-physician implemented protocols is gaining momentum in the care of critically ill patients, improving outcomes and allocation of respiratory care services.[34]

The creation of new protocols or modification of existing ones should involve multidisciplinary input from physicians, respiratory therapy and nursing. This collaboration can serve to decrease obstacles and problems in implementation and increase confidence towards usage. Preprinted orders or computerized order entry order sets can be useful for fast, uniform implementation, as are pocket cards for care personnel with algorithms, guidelines, and troubleshooting (Fig. 10.2). Protocols must be concrete, explicit, and easy to follow. Complicated algorithms will lead to lack of acceptance by hospital caregivers.

Due to the complexity of care of a patient with NIV, multiple protocols or guidelines may be necessary (Box 10.5). For example, protocols may be necessary for initiation of NIV and maintenance and assessment of the patient currently on NIV. These may also differ or include information based on the type of respiratory failure or unit (ICU, step-down unit, or ward). Protocols may be written or implemented for titration of NIV or how to identify and treat the failing patient. All protocols must be reassessed regularly to ensure their effectiveness and use. Published protocols may be used, but often need modification depending on institutional infrastructure and personnel.

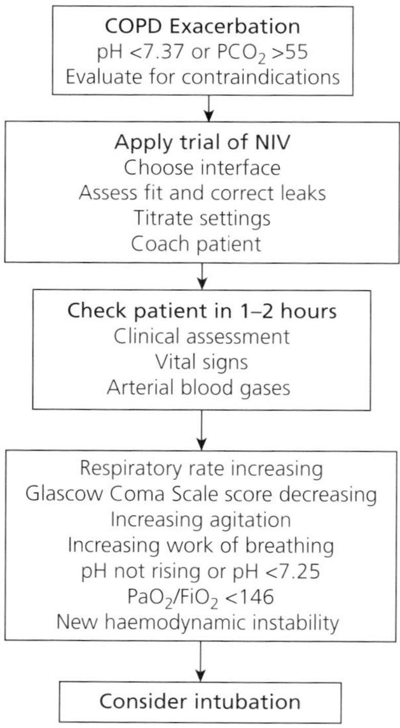


**Figure 10.2** Example guideline for care of a chronic obstructive pulmonary disease (COPD) patient. NIV, non-invasive ventilation.

> **Box 10.5 Types of protocols for NIV**
>
> - Indications for NIV
> - Applying NIV
> - Monitoring
> - Titrating NIV
> - Identifying the failing patient
> - Intubation

Implementation of protocols can also meet resistance, particularly from physicians who may feel a lack of control over patients. In this respect, attention to education on the evidence supporting protocols, monitoring of compliance and maintaining feedback can help to facilitate the process.[34] Furthermore, it should be reinforced that protocols are second to a clinician's judgement, and should serve as guidelines rather than strict rules to a decision-making process.

## CONCLUSIONS

With increased use of NIV and the emergence of new indications, there is now an increasing need for acute NIV services in hospitals. Creation of a service requires intense planning and the cooperation of physicians, hospital administration, nursing, and respiratory therapists. Problems such as generalized acceptance, logistics and resource allocation must be expected. Of the utmost importance to a programme's success is the training and education of the caregivers. Despite these complexities, a successful acute NIV service can provide better outcomes, improved patient experience, and a cost-effective system.

## REFERENCES

1. Grol R, Grimshaw J. Evidence-based implementation of evidence-based medicine. *Joint Comm J Q Improve* 1999; **25**: 503–13.
2. Hess DR. How to initiate a noninvasive ventilation program: bringing the evidence to the bedside. *Respir Care* 2009; **54**: 232–43; discussion 43–5.
3. Sweet DD, Naismith A, Keenan SP *et al.* Missed opportunities for noninvasive positive pressure ventilation: a utilization review. *J Crit Care* 2008; **23**: 111–17.
4. Maheshwari V, Paioli D, Rothaar R *et al.* Utilization of noninvasive ventilation in acute care hospitals: a regional survey. *Chest* 2006; **129**: 1226–33.
5. Sinuff T, Cook D, Randall J *et al.* Noninvasive positive-pressure ventilation: a utilization review of use in a teaching hospital. *CMAJ* 2000; **163**: 969–73.

6. Carlucci A, Delmastro M, Rubini F *et al.* Changes in the practice of non-invasive ventilation in treating COPD patients over 8 years. *Intensive Care Med* 2003; **29**: 419–25.
7. Schettino G, Altobelli N, Kacmarek RM. Noninvasive positive-pressure ventilation in acute respiratory failure outside clinical trials: experience at the Massachusetts General Hospital. *Criti Care Med* 2008; **36**: 441–7.
8. Jhanji S, Pearse RM. The use of early intervention to prevent postoperative complications. *Curr Opin Crit Care* 2009; **15**: 349–54.
9. Auriant I, Jallot A, Herve P *et al.* Noninvasive ventilation reduces mortality in acute respiratory failure following lung resection. *Am J Respir Crit Care Med* 2001; **164**: 1231–5.
10. Weitz G, Struck J, Zonak A *et al.* Prehospital noninvasive pressure support ventilation for acute cardiogenic pulmonary edema. *Eur J Emerg Med* 2007; **14**: 276–9.
11. Bruge P, Jabre P, Dru M *et al.* An observational study of noninvasive positive pressure ventilation in an out-of-hospital setting. *Am J Emerg Med* 2008; **26**: 165–9.
12. Duchateau FX, Beaune S, Ricard-Hibon A *et al.* Prehospital noninvasive ventilation can help in management of patients with limitations of life-sustaining treatments. *Eur J Emerg Med* 2010; **17**: 7–9.
13. Elliott MW, Confalonieri M, Nava S. Where to perform noninvasive ventilation? *Eur Respir J* 2002; **19**: 1159–66.
14. Ambrosino N, Foglio K, Rubini F *et al.* Non-invasive mechanical ventilation in acute respiratory failure due to chronic obstructive pulmonary disease: correlates for success. *Thorax* 1995; **50**: 755–7.
15. Celikel T, Sungur M, Ceyhan B *et al.* Comparison of noninvasive positive pressure ventilation with standard medical therapy in hypercapnic acute respiratory failure. *Chest* 1998; **114**: 1636–42.
16. Giacomini M, Iapichino G, Cigada M *et al.* Short-term noninvasive pressure support ventilation prevents ICU admittance in patients with acute cardiogenic pulmonary edema. *Chest* 2003; **123**: 2057–61.
17. Soroksky A, Stav D, Shpirer I. A pilot prospective, randomized, placebo-controlled trial of bilevel positive airway pressure in acute asthmatic attack. *Chest* 2003; **123**: 1018–25.
18. Huang DT. Clinical review: impact of emergency department care on intensive care unit costs. *Crit Care* 2004; **8**: 498–502.
19. Wood KA, Lewis L, Von Harz B *et al.* The use of noninvasive positive pressure ventilation in the emergency department: results of a randomized clinical trial. *Chest* 1998; **113**: 1339–46.
20. Plant PK, Owen JL, Elliott MW. Early use of non-invasive ventilation for acute exacerbations of chronic obstructive pulmonary disease on general respiratory wards: a multicentre randomised controlled trial. *Lancet* 2000; **355**: 1931–5.
21. Diaz GG, Alcaraz AC, Talavera JC *et al.* Noninvasive positive-pressure ventilation to treat hypercapnic coma secondary to respiratory failure. *Chest* 2005; **127**: 952–60.
22. Scala R, Naldi M, Archinucci I *et al.* Noninvasive positive pressure ventilation in patients with acute exacerbations of COPD and varying levels of consciousness. *Chest* 2005; **128**: 1657–66.
23. Elpern EH, Silver MR, Rosen RL *et al.* The noninvasive respiratory care unit. Patterns of use and financial implications. *Chest* 1991; **99**: 205–8.
24. Keenan SP, Gregor J, Sibbald WJ *et al.* Noninvasive positive pressure ventilation in the setting of severe, acute exacerbations of chronic obstructive pulmonary disease: more effective and less expensive. *Crit Care Med* 2000; **28**: 2094–102.
25. Plant PK, Owen JL, Parrott S *et al.* Cost effectiveness of ward based non-invasive ventilation for acute exacerbations of chronic obstructive pulmonary disease: economic analysis of randomised controlled trial. *BMJ* 2003; **326**: 956.
26. Carrera M, Marin JM, Anton A *et al.* A controlled trial of noninvasive ventilation for chronic obstructive pulmonary disease exacerbations. *Am J Repir Crit Care Med* 2009; **179**: 533–41.
27. Corrado A, Roussos C, Ambrosino N *et al.* Respiratory intermediate care units: a European survey. *Eur Respir J* 2002; **20**: 1343–50.
28. Burns KE, Sinuff T, Adhikari NK *et al.* Bilevel noninvasive positive pressure ventilation for acute respiratory failure: survey of Ontario practice. *Crit Care Med* 2005; **33**: 1477–83.
29. Doherty MJ, Greenstone MA. Survey of non-invasive ventilation (NIPPV) in patients with acute exacerbations of chronic obstructive pulmonary disease (COPD) in the UK. *Thorax* 1998; **53**: 863–6.
30. Sinuff T, Kahnamoui K, Cook DJ *et al.* Practice guidelines as multipurpose tools: a qualitative study of noninvasive ventilation. *Crit Care Med* 2007; **35**: 776–82.
31. Esteban A, Ferguson ND, Meade MO *et al.* Evolution of mechanical ventilation in response to clinical research. *Am J Respir Crit Care Med* 2008; **177**: 170–7.
32. Stoller JK, Kester L, Roberts VT *et al.* An analysis of features of respiratory therapy departments that are avid for change. *Respir Care* 2008; **53**: 871–84.
33. Kollef MH, Shapiro SD, Silver P *et al.* A randomized, controlled trial of protocol-directed versus physician-directed weaning from mechanical ventilation. *Crit Care Med* 1997; **25**: 567–74.
34. Ely EW, Meade MO, Haponik EF *et al.* Mechanical ventilator weaning protocols driven by nonphysician health-care professionals: evidence-based clinical practice guidelines. *Chest* 2001; **120**: 454S–63S.
35. Marelich GP, Murin S, Battistella F *et al.* Protocol weaning of mechanical ventilation in medical and surgical patients by respiratory care practitioners and nurses: effect on weaning time and incidence of ventilator-associated pneumonia. *Chest* 2000; **118**: 459–67.

36. Saint S, Kowalski CP, Banaszak-Holl J *et al.* How active resisters and organizational constipators affect health care-acquired infection prevention efforts. *Joint Comm J Q Patient Safety/Joint Comm Resources* 2009; **35**: 239–46.
37. Kramer N, Meyer TJ, Meharg J *et al.* Randomized, prospective trial of noninvasive positive pressure ventilation in acute respiratory failure. *Am J Respir Crit Care Med* 1995; **151**: 1799–806.
38. Girou E, Brun-Buisson C, Taille S *et al.* Secular trends in nosocomial infections and mortality associated with noninvasive ventilation in patients with exacerbation of COPD and pulmonary edema. *JAMA* 2003; **290**: 2985–91.
39. Confalonieri M, Parigi P, Scartabellati A *et al.* Noninvasive mechanical ventilation improves the immediate and long-term outcome of COPD patients with acute respiratory failure. *Eur Respir J* 1996; **9**: 422–30.
40. Vitacca M, Clini E, Rubini F *et al.* Non-invasive mechanical ventilation in severe chronic obstructive lung disease and acute respiratory failure: short- and long-term prognosis. *Intensive Care Med* 1996; **22**: 94–100.
41. Bardi G, Pierotello R, Desideri M *et al.* Nasal ventilation in COPD exacerbations: early and late results of a prospective, controlled study. *Eur Respir J* 2000; **15**: 98–104.
42. Guerin C, Girard R, Chemorin C *et al.* Facial mask noninvasive mechanical ventilation reduces the incidence of nosocomial pneumonia. A prospective epidemiological survey from a single ICU. *Intensive Care Med* 1997; **23**: 1024–32.
43. Girou E, Schortgen F, Delclaux C *et al.* Association of noninvasive ventilation with nosocomial infections and survival in critically ill patients. *JAMA* 2000; **284**: 2361–7.
44. Sinuff T, Cook D, Giacomini M *et al.* Facilitating clinician adherence to guidelines in the intensive care unit: A multicenter, qualitative study. *Crit Care Med* 2007; **35**: 2083–9.
45. Sinuff T, Cook DJ, Randall J *et al.* Evaluation of a practice guideline for noninvasive positive-pressure ventilation for acute respiratory failure. *Chest* 2003; **123**: 2062–73.

# 11

# Monitoring during acute non-invasive ventilation

EUMORFIA KONDILI, NEKTARIA XIROUCHAKI, DIMITRIS GEORGOPOULOS

## ABSTRACT

Non-invasive mechanical ventilation (NIV) has been shown to be an effective therapy for patients with respiratory failure of various causes in both the acute and chronic setting. Monitoring is essential to evaluate the efficacy of NIV and to identify patients who will fail on this technique. During the first few hours of NIV, monitoring is mainly performed by a continuous evaluation of the patient's clinical status and arterial blood gases to assess the initial response to the treatment. More advanced monitoring is important to optimize the efficacy of therapy. This should include monitoring of air leakage, patient–ventilator asynchrony and sleep quality.

## INTRODUCTION

Several studies have shown that non-invasive mechanical ventilation (NIV) represents an effective treatment for acute respiratory failure. This technique has been applied in patients with acute exacerbation of chronic obstructive pulmonary disease (COPD), cardiogenic pulmonary oedema and hypoxaemic respiratory failure due to various causes.[1–17] In addition, NIV has been also used in post-extubation respiratory failure and as a weaning tool mainly in patients with COPD.[18–23] Monitoring is essential to evaluate the efficacy of NIV and to identify patients who will fail on this technique. During the first few hours of NIV monitoring is mainly performed by a continuous evaluation of the patient's clinical status and arterial blood gases to assess the initial response to this treatment.[1,6,7,15,16,24–28] More advanced monitoring is important in order to optimize the efficacy of therapy. This should include monitoring of air leakage, patient–ventilator asynchrony and sleep quality. Box 11.1 summarizes the monitoring requirements during NIV.

The intensive care (ICU) or high-dependency (HDU) unit is the best environment of applying NIV.[29,30] These locations offer many capabilities and close monitoring of the patients is feasible. Nevertheless due to shortage of ICU or HDU beds, many patients receive NIV in wards.[2,5,6,15,16] In this case the intensity of monitoring should be determined by the severity of the respiratory failure and particularly by the risk of NIV

### Box 11.1 Monitoring during acute non-invasive ventilation

Essential:

- Regular clinical evaluation:
  - comfort (mask and ventilator settings)
  - breathing effort: accessory muscle use; paradoxical breathing
  - synchrony: triggering; expiratory asynchrony
  - air leaks
  - agitation
  - delirium
  - secretion clearance
  - complications: nasal erythema, ulceration; conjunctivitis; gastric distension
- Continuous recording of heart rate and breathing frequency with continuous pulse oximetry
- Arterial blood gases 1–4 hours after non-invasive positive pressure ventilation (NIPPV) and after 1 hour of any change in ventilator settings or $FiO_2$

Desirable:

- Electrocardiogram
- Objective quantification of leaks
- Graphical display to monitor patient–ventilator asynchrony
- Invasive monitoring for patients with haemodynamic instability
- Sleep evaluation

failure. The latter is probably the most important determinant of the intensity of monitoring. Therefore risk factors for NIV failure should be carefully sought and identified[1,6,7,15,16,24–28] (see Boxes 12.1 and 12.2, p. 108). A patient with multiple risk factors should be closely monitored in the ICU or HDU.[30,31]

## CLINICAL EVALUATION

Bedside clinical evaluation is essential, particularly during the first few hours of treatment where the majority of failures occur. Clinical evaluation should include monitoring of patient comfort, work of breathing, and neurological and mental status.

### Patient comfort

Several studies have shown that poor tolerance to this technique and thus discomfort is an independent risk factor of NIV failure.[32,33] It follows that patient comfort should be closely monitored. Of the various scales that quantify the patient's comfort, the most common is the visual analogue scale (VAS) which has been validated in mechanically ventilated patients.[34] In addition to patient comfort, attention should be paid to the mask. It is important to make sure that the mask is of an appropriate size with the correct headgear and correctly positioned. Also, attention should be paid to the mask pressures.[1,29,35,36] Excessive mask pressures lead to discomfort and skin damage whereas a weak mask sealing may facilitate air leakage.[36]

### Work of breathing

One of the main goals of NIV is to minimize the patient's work of breathing. Although precise estimation of work of breathing necessitates the placement of an oesophageal balloon, there are clinical signs that may serve as indirect indices of increased work of breathing. The use of accessory muscles during inspiration, paradoxical abdominal motion and active expiratory efforts is a reliable sign of excessive work of breathing. Other signs are tachycardia, increased respiratory rate and diaphoresis.[7,29,31,32,37,38] All these signs should be recorded and carefully monitored. Increased work of breathing is also associated with dyspnoea, which, however, is a highly subjective symptom. It is important for patient monitoring to quantify the dyspnoea sensation, as quantitative measurements of dyspnoea provide a baseline to assess the efficacy of NIV. There are several dyspnoea scales that can be easily used in clinical practice and permit the quantification of dyspnoea and monitor change.[34,39,40]

### Evaluation of mental and neurological status

This task is essential especially in patients with acute hypercapnic respiratory failure. The Glasgow Coma Scale should be used to evaluate neurological impairment.[30–32,41] Although in the past, coma has been considered a contraindication for NIV, recent studies have shown high success rate of NIV in patients with hypercapnic coma.[28,42] In addition to neurological status, another important aspect that should be monitored is delirium. Several studies have now confirmed that delirium occurs in 60–80 per cent of mechanically ventilated patients and in up to 50 per cent of non-intubated critically ill patients.[43–46] Delirium is an independent risk factor for increased morbidity and mortality.[44,46] Although data are lacking regarding the incidence of delirium in patients during NIV, these patients are theoretically prone to this complication since risk factors of delirium are usually present in this population.[47,48] The occurrence of delirium may significantly affect the patient's tolerance to this treatment. In this regard, we suggest that patients on NIV should be carefully monitored for delirium and treated accordingly. The delirium status can be assessed several times during the day using a well validated and highly reliable instrument: the Confusion Assessment Method for the ICU (CAM-ICU)[43] (Fig. 11.1).

### Conventional vital signs

Heart rate and breathing frequency should be monitored, preferably continuously.[30,49,50] A decrease in breathing frequency and heart rate within 1 hour of NIV is a sign of success.[1,7,27] In patients without haemodynamic instability arterial blood pressure may be recorded non-invasively. Urine output should be also measured. Patients with acute hypoxaemia and/or persistent respiratory acidosis, or whose condition is deteriorating, require a higher level of monitoring, which includes central venous access, arterial line and urine catheter.[30,49,50] This is particularly true in patients with haemodynamic instability in whom the rate of failure on NIV is very high.[30,49,50]

### Gas exchange

Improving the gas exchange defects (hypoxaemia and/or hypercapnia) is a priority during NIV. The most commonly used method to access oxygenation is the continuous arterial oxygen saturation ($SaO_2$), which is feasible by continuous pulse oximetry at the bedside ($SpO_2$).[29–31,49,50] All patients should be monitored with pulse oximetry. We should note that the addition of oxygen during NIV may occasionally worsen the hypercapnia, particularly in patients with high $PaCO_2$ and rapid shallow breathing pattern.[51] If patients have COPD or other risk factors for hypercapnic respiratory failure, a saturation of 88–92 per cent

**The Confusion Assessment Method for the Intensive Care Unit (CAM-ICU)**

| Features and descriptions | Absent | Present |
|---|---|---|
| **I. Acute onset or fluctuating course** | | |
| A. Is there evidence of an acute change in mental status from the baseline?<br>B. Or, did the (abnormal) behaviour fluctuate during the past 24 hours, that is, tend to come and go or increase and decrease in severity as evidenced by fluctuations on the Richmond Agitation Sedation Scale (RASS) or the Glasgow Coma Scale? | | |
| **II. Inattention** | | |
| Did the patient have difficulty focusing attention as evidenced by a score of less than 8 correct answers on either the visual or auditory components of the Attention Screening Examination (ASE)? | | |
| **III. Disorganized thinking** | | |
| Is there evidence of disorganized or incoherent thinking as evidenced by incorrect answers to 3 or more of the 4 questions and inability to follow the commands?<br>Questions<br>1. Will a stone float on water?<br>2. Are there fish in the sea?<br>3. Does 1 pound weigh more than 2 pounds?<br>4. Can you use a hammer to pound a nail?<br>Commands<br>1. Are you having unclear thinking?<br>2. Hold up this many fingers. (Examiner holds 2 fingers in front of the patient.)<br>3. Now do the same thing with the other hand (without holding the 2 fingers in front of the paient).<br>(If the patient is already extubated from the ventilator, determine whether the patient's thinking is disorganized or incoherent, such as rambling or irrelevent conversation, unclear or illogical flow of ideas, or unpredictable switching from subject to subject.) | | |
| **IV. Altered level of consciousness** | | |
| Is the patient's level of consciousness anything other than alert, such as being vigilant or lethargic or in a stupor, or coma?<br>Alert: spontaneously fully aware of environment and interacts appropriately<br>Vigilant: hyperalert<br>Lethargic: drowsy but easily aroused, unware of some elements in the environment or not spontaneously interacting with the interviewer; becomes fully aware and appropriately interactive when prodded minimally<br>Stupor: difficult to arouse, unaware of some or all elements in the environment or not spontaneously interacting with the interviewer; becomes incompletely aware when prodded strongly; can be aroused only by vigorous and repeated stimuli and as soon as the stimulus ceases, stuporous subject lapses back into unresponsive state<br>Coma: unarousable, unaware of all elements in the environment with no spontaneous interaction or awareness of the interviewer so that the interview is impossible even with maximal prodding | | |
| **Overall CAM-ICU Assessment (Features I and II and either Feature III or IV): Yes___No___** | | |

**Figure 11.1** The Confusion Assessment Method for the Intensive Care Unit. Reproduced from Ely *et al.*[43] with permission.

is recommended that should be adjusted to 94–98 per cent if the $PaCO_2$ is normal (unless there is a history of respiratory failure requiring NIV or invasive positive pressure ventilation).[52] Blood gases should be rechecked after 30–60 minutes.[52]

Assessment of the $PaCO_2$ remains the gold standard for the evaluation of alveolar ventilation. The opportunity to assess $PaCO_2$ continuously and non-invasively is desirable particularly in patients receiving NIV on a ward. There are two different techniques for non-invasive $PaCO_2$ monitoring, the end-tidal carbon dioxide and the transcutaneous $PCO_2$ measurements.[53,54] However, both methods are limited in patients receiving NIV and should only be used as a trend monitor.

Blood gases should be obtained on admission and after 1–4 hours.[29–31,49] Several studies have shown that changes in arterial blood gases and acid–base status after a short period of NIV application predict the successful outcome.[1,7,27,55] Ventilator settings should be adjusted based on results of arterial blood gases obtained within 1 hour and as necessary at 2–4 hours intervals.[1,7,27,29–31]

## MONITORING OF LEAKS

Non-invasive ventilation is a semi-open system, and thus air leaks are inherent to its design. Leaks commonly occur through the mouth (with nasal masks) or around the interface. These are termed non-intentional leaks. Leaks may also occur through expiratory ports or valves that are placed in the circuit close to or directly on the mask (intentional leaks). An important characteristic of a ventilator delivering NIV is its ability to recognize and compensate for leaks in the system. Ideally, leak compensation should automatically affect the triggering and cycling off functions to maintain optimum ventilator performance. Even though most of the modern ICU ventilators and bi-level devices may compensate for

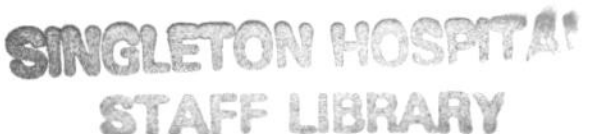

leakage, this ability is significantly compromised in the presence of excessive leaks.[12,35,56–59] In addition marked differences have been observed between ventilators as far as the ability to compensate for leaks is concerned.[12,35,56–59]

Excessive non-intentional leaks have a detrimental effect on the efficiency of NIV. With all modes of mechanical ventilation, air leaks reduce the efficiency of NIV by altering the actual tidal volume that the patient receives and impairing the triggering and cycling-off functions of the ventilator (see below).[12,35,56–59] Furthermore excessive leaks may cause the patient discomfort, arousal and sleep fragmentation.[12,35,56–60] In addition to non-intentional leaks, intentional leaks may also affect ventilator performance and the quality of ventilation.[56] In this regard, independently of their origin air leaks should be monitored. Gross air leaks can be easily assessed at bedside. Vibration of lips or other structures around the airway is indicative of air leaks. Less obvious leaks can be detected by tactile means, i.e. by placing hands near the mouth or seal and feeling for air; however, this method has low sensitivity and it does not allow for quantification of the amount of air leakage. In some ventilators, the expired volume is continuously monitored and leaks can be calculated by subtracting expired volume from the corresponding inspiratory volume. In some new-generation bi-level positive airway pressure (BiPAP) devices, leaks are automatically estimated with sophisticated algorithms and are displayed on the screen of the ventilator breath by breath. Even with these systems, estimates of the quantity of leakage may be inaccurate. Inspection of the pressure volume and flow waveform provided by the new-generation ventilators on a breath-by-breath basis may be helpful for identifying leakage. Greater area under the inspiratory flow curve than that under the expiratory flow is indicative of air leaks. In addition, identification of leak-associated asynchronies such as auto-triggering and prolonged inspiration (see below) allow the detection of air leaks. Since leaks may affect both the function of the ventilator and patient comfort every effort should be made to minimize these (Fig. 11.2).

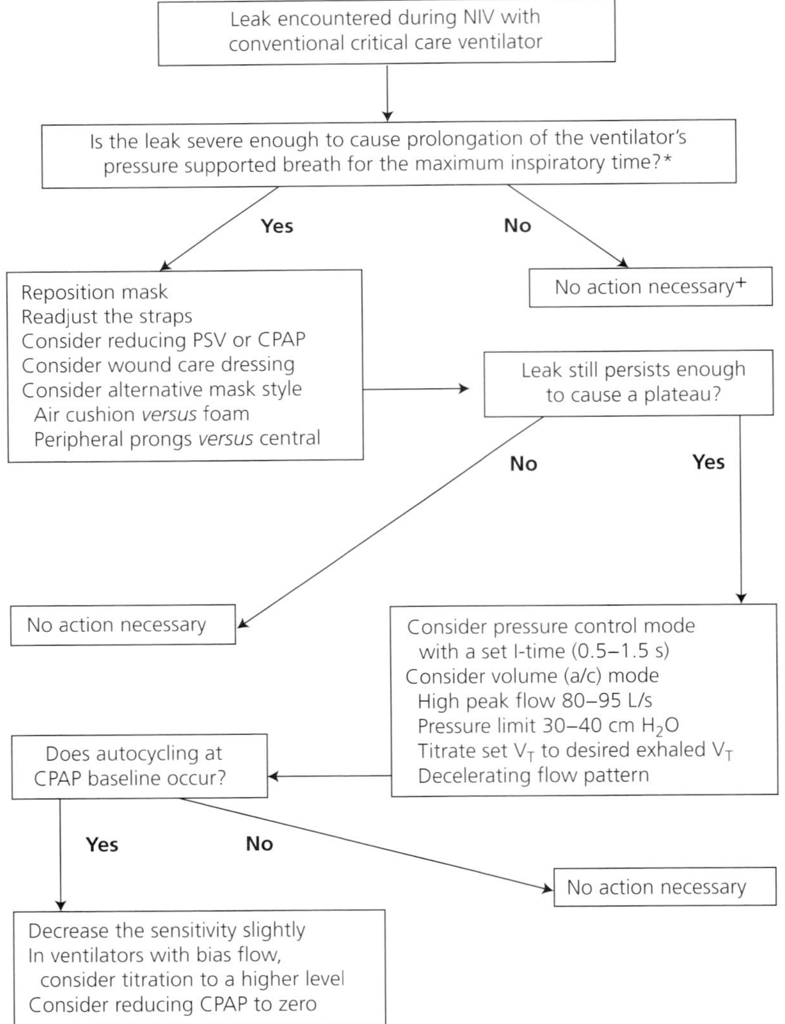


**Figure 11.2** Approach in patients with significant air leakage while receiving continuous positive airway pressure and pressure support. *: this can reduce respiratory rate, cause air trapping and increase work of breathing. +: tidal volume ($V_T$) remains constant as long as the leak does not cause an inspiration plateau. From Meduri[26] with permission.

## MONITORING PATIENT–VENTILATOR ASYNCHRONY

Asynchrony is defined as the uncoupling of ventilator-delivered inspiratory flow from the patient's ventilatory demands in terms of either timing or drive.[61,62] In intubated patients the mode of ventilation, ventilator settings and respiratory system mechanics are the main factors that determine both the incidence and the severity of asynchrony.[61,62] During NIV there are two additional factors that modify the patient on ventilator asynchrony. These are the presence of air leaks, and the type of interface. These factors complicate the issue of patient–ventilator synchrony during NIV. The prevalence of patient–ventilator asynchrony during NIV was recently evaluated in a multicentre study by Vignaux *et al*,[63] who studied a group of 60 patients receiving NIV for acute respiratory failure and found that 43 per cent of the patients exhibited severe asynchrony. The most frequent asynchrony was prolonged insufflation, which was present in 23 per cent of the patients. This was followed by double triggering (15 per cent), auto-triggering (13 per cent), ineffective efforts (13 per cent) and premature cycling (12 per cent).[63]

Patient–ventilator asynchrony can be assessed at bedside by the interpretation of ventilator waveforms.[62,64] In most of the new-generation ICU and portable ventilators, pressure, flow and volume waveforms are continuously displayed on the screen on a breath-by-breath basis. This non-invasive approach is a valuable tool that allows the physician to recognize patient–ventilator asynchrony and take the appropriate action.[62,64] However, it should be noted that significant information can be provided by clinical observation. The physician should focus on the expansion of both the rib cage and the abdomen while listening for the timing and coordinated triggering of the ventilator.

Non-invasive methods such as impedance plethysmography and magnetometry may also be helpful for identifying patient ventilatory asynchrony; however, currently both methods are mainly used for research proposes and not for everyday clinical practice. More detailed monitoring, such as estimation of various indices of respiratory neural and motor output, requires complex methods such as evaluation of diaphragmatic EMG and calculation of transdiaphragmatic pressure and instantaneous pressure output of the respiratory muscles. These approaches, however, necessitate the placement of oesophageal electrodes and oesophageal and gastric catheters.

Recently, three new technologies for automatic detection of patient–ventilator asynchrony have been introduced aiming to monitor and improve patient–ventilator interaction.[65–67] The effectiveness of these systems in intubated patients in terms of identifying triggering delay, ineffective effort and expiratory asynchrony has been clinically evaluated and recently reported.[65–67] It should be noted, however, that data are lacking regarding the accuracy of these systems during NIV, in which the occurrence of leaks is a common phenomenon.

### Identifying patient–ventilator asynchrony during the triggering phase

#### AUTO-TRIGGERING

Auto-triggering occurs when the ventilator is triggered in the absence of inspiratory muscle contraction.[62,64] It may be caused by a low triggering threshold, excessive leaks, the presence of water in the circuit and/or cardiogenic oscillation.[62,64] During NIV, air leaks represent by far the most significant factor leading to auto-triggering. With pressure triggering, an absence of the initial pressure drop below the end-expiratory pressure is indicative of auto-triggering.[62,64] A short cycle during PSV with different flow-time waveform than previous breaths is also indicative of auto-triggering (Fig. 11.3). Cycles triggered by signals that do not come from the patient may cause among other complications, discomfort, and should be corrected.[62,64]

#### EXCESSIVE TRIGGERING DELAY AND INEFFECTIVE EFFORT

During NIV, air leaks and excessive ventilator support are the most important causes of triggering delay and ineffective effort. A recent clinical study showed a significant correlation between the magnitude of leaks and the number of ineffective efforts.[63] Although most of the modern ventilators compensate for air leaks by automatically adjusting the triggering threshold, this capability is significantly affected by the presence of large intentional or non-intentional leaks.[57–59,68] Furthermore, clinical studies have demonstrated that the type of interface may also affect patient–ventilator asynchrony during the triggering phase.[35,69–71] Ineffective efforts and triggering delays can be detected with accuracy through the inspection of flow-time and/or airway pressure–time waveforms (Fig. 11.3).[62,64]

### Identifying patient–ventilator asynchrony during the pressure delivery phases

Ineffective efforts during the pressure delivery phase represent a common form of asynchrony during NIV.[63] It is mainly promoted by high ventilator assistance which, during pressure support, is associated with prolonged inspiration due to increased air leaks.[63] Ineffective efforts during insufflation can be identified using the flow or $P_{aw}$ (airways pressure) waveform depending on the mode of support.[62,64] With assist volume control ineffective efforts are mainly presented as a transient $P_{aw}$ distortion, although this distortion is not always easy to recognize. With pressure support, ineffective efforts are mainly observed during prolonged insufflations as an abrupt increase in inspiratory flow.[62,64]

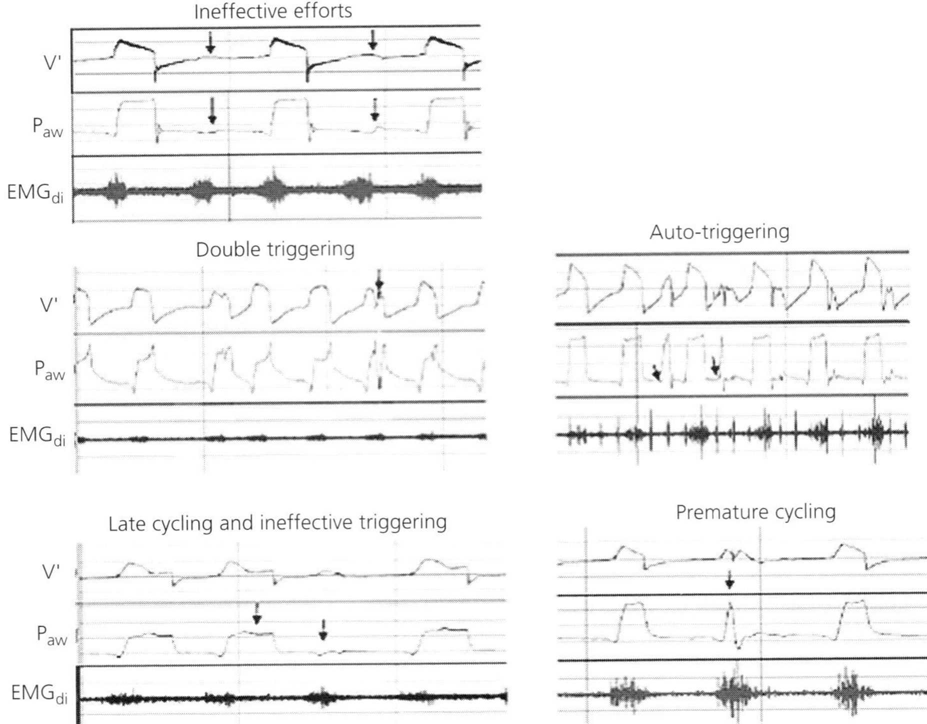


**Figure 11.3** Flow (V'), airway pressure ($P_{aw}$) and diaphragmatic electromyography ($EMG_{di}$), in a patient ventilated on pressure support during non-invasive ventilation. *Ineffective efforts:* Observe the flow distortion during expiration (arrows), which is not followed by a mechanical breath, signifying the presence of ineffective efforts. Note also that the signal of flow distortion is much clearer than the corresponding $P_{aw}$ change. *Double triggering:* Note that in the sixth breath (arrow), one inspiratory effort triggered the ventilator twice. *Auto-triggering:* Observe that the third and the fifth breath (arrows) are triggered in the absence of the patient's inspiratory effort (no EMG activity). Note also that auto-triggering results in a distortion in flow waveform (arrows). *Premature cycling:* Note that in the second breath $EMG_{di}$ activity continues far beyond the end of the ventilatory inspiratory time. Also note that in this breath the premature opening of the exhalation valve is indicated by an abrupt drop in $P_{aw}$ from peak pressure to baseline (arrow). *Late cycling and ineffective triggering:* Note that in all breaths due the presence of leaks, the ventilator continues to insufflate far beyond the end of $EMG_{di}$ activity (arrow). Under this circumstance the time available for expiration is reduced, resulting in the presence of an ineffective effort. Modified from Vignaux *et al.*[63] with permission.

In some of the new-generation ventilators, the pressurization rate with PS (defined as the incremental increase in $P_{aw}$ per time unit) is adjustable in order to optimize patient–ventilator synchrony. Prinianakis *et al.* observed that a rapid pressurization rate was associated with a reduction in the pressure–time product, an index of oxygen consumption of the diaphragm. However, this resulted in increased air leakage[72] (Fig. 11.4). Since both leaks and patient discomfort may modify the effectiveness of NIV, the pressurization rate should not be set to very high.[72]

Finally the caregiver should check whether the demands of the patient are being met by the ventilator-delivered flow.[64] By observing the contour of $P_{aw}$ during assist volume control and that of flow during PS, the caregiver may have an estimate of the patient respiratory effort.[64] Nevertheless we should note that the presence of leaks may interfere with this technique and monitoring this type of asynchrony is not always easy.

## Identifying patient–ventilator asynchrony during the cycling-off phase (expiratory asynchrony)

Two types of expiratory asynchrony have been recognized: premature opening of the expiratory valve, in which the end of mechanical inflation precedes the end of neural inspiration; and delayed opening of the expiratory valve, in which the end of mechanical inflation follows the end of neural inspiration.[62,64]

### PREMATURE OPENING OF THE EXHALATION VALVE

During assisted modes of support, premature opening of the exhalation valve is evidenced by the presence of zero or small inspiratory flow for some time immediately after $P_{aw}$ decreases to the positive end-expiratory pressure (PEEP) level,[62,64] and a sharp decline in the peak expiratory flow that lasts a few milliseconds and is followed by an increase

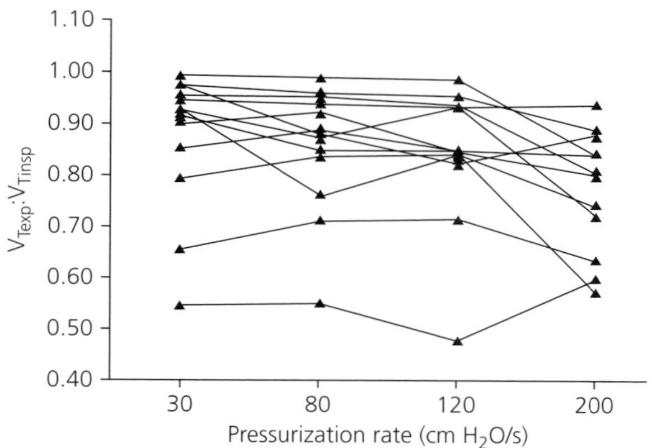


**Figure 11.4** Amount of air leaks through the mask, as assessed by the ratio between expiratory ($V_{Texp}$) and inspiratory tidal volume ($V_{Tinsp}$) for the different values of pressurization rate for each patient. From Prinianakis *et al.*[72] with permission.

and then a gradual decrease to zero at the end of expiration (Fig. 11.3).[62,64] In the $P_{aw}$ waveform, premature expiratory opening is indicated by an abrupt drop from peak pressure to baseline rather than the expected gradual decay because of the finite resistance of the expiratory ventilator circuit.[62,64]

In some breaths, inspiratory effort after opening of the exhalation valve reverses the expiratory flow to an inspiratory flow (in-flow triggering system); in addition, inspiratory effort can reduce $P_{aw}$ to below the PEEP and thereby initiate the triggering process. In this case, one inspiratory effort triggers the ventilator twice (or even more) (see Fig. 11.3).[62,64] Expiratory asynchrony due to premature opening of the valve may be minimized by actions that increase the mechanical inflation time or decrease the neural inspiratory time. The latter is particularly important in patients with prolonged inspiratory efforts due to excessive administration of opioids. On the other hand, in order to increase the mechanical inflation time the mode of support should be taken into consideration. In patients ventilated with pressure mode, mechanical inflation time may be increased by decreasing the flow threshold for cycling off, increasing the pressure support level or decreasing the rising time. With pressure or volume control modes the increase in mechanical inflation may be easily achieved by proper adjustment of ventilator setting (i.e. inspiratory time, pause time, inspiratory flow).

### DELAYED OPENING OF THE EXHALATION VALVE

The ventilator permits transition from inspiration to expiration according to a predetermined cycling-off criterion. The most commonly used criterion is the decrease of inspiratory flow to a predetermined percentage of peak inspiratory flow. During NIV, the presence of leaks may lead to a prolonged mechanical inspiration because the delivered flow remains above the flow threshold for cycling off. Under this circumstance the time available for expiration is reduced and the patient is at risk of triggering delay and ineffective efforts (Fig. 11.3). The frequency of delayed cycling and ineffective efforts correlates with the magnitude of the leaks.[63] Prolonged mechanical inspiration can be eliminated by reducing either the leaks or the ventilator inspiratory time.[63,73] Calderini *et al.* demonstrated that patient–ventilator synchrony is improved and patient effort is reduced with cycling time compared to flow cycling[73] (Fig. 11.5). In patients ventilated with PS, the continuation of mechanical inflation into neural expiration is evidenced by a rapid decrease in inspiratory flow followed by an exponential decline toward the end of mechanical inspiration, and a small spike (increase) in airway pressure ($P_{aw}$) near the end of the breath.[62,64]

## SLEEP EVALUATION

Clinical studies using both polysomnographic data and patients' perceptions have shown a poor quality of sleep among mechanically ventilated patients.[74–77] Although data are lacking regarding the sleep quality of patients during NIV, it is unlikely to be better than those on invasive mechanical ventilation in acute settings, considering the significant sleep disruptions that are caused by the frequent mask readjustments required to prevent air leakage, the air leak *per se* and the significant sleep deprivation.[78–80] Detailed sleep evaluation is only feasible through overnight polysomnography studies. Considering the difficulty of performing polysomnography studies in acute settings and the absence of data supporting the necessity of routine sleep evaluation, we do not recommend sleep studies in this population. Evaluation of sleep might be done using clinical criteria, which, however, are not accurate.

## MONITORING OF COMPLICATIONS

Complications that should be monitored during NIV are skin necrosis particularly over the bridge of the nose (with masks), carbon dioxide retention (with helmet), retention of secretions, abdominal distension and upper airway obstruction.[31,36,81]

## CONCLUSIONS

During NIV, close monitoring is important in order to optimize therapy and minimize complications as well as the risk of treatment failure. The intensity of monitoring depends on the patient's condition and the location where NIV is applied. Essential monitoring should include regular clinical evaluation, and continuous pulse oximetry. In the last two decades, significant technical advances in

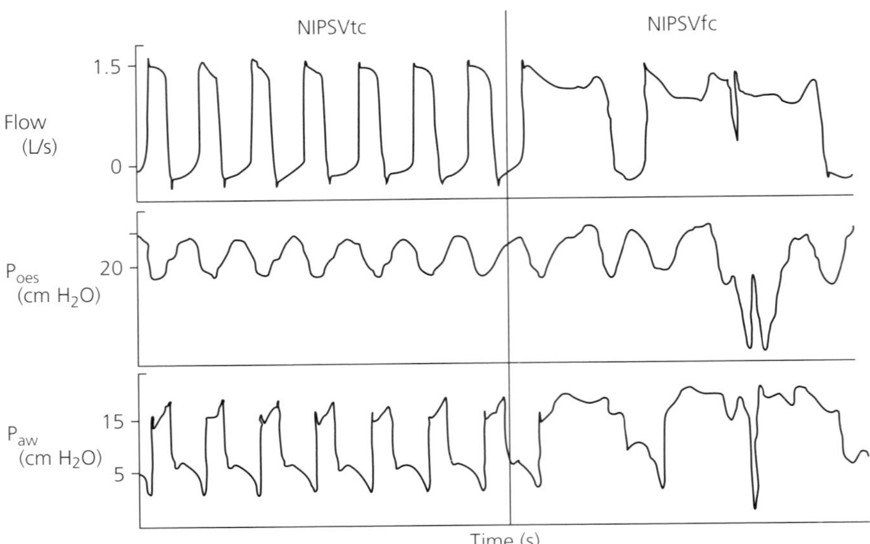


**Figure 11.5** A representative experimental record in a patient treated with NIV using time and conventional flow percentage as cycling off criterion. Notice the perfect synchronization between patient and machine during time cycling off criterion. With flow cycling off criterion, the prolonged mechanical assist into the neural expiratory time results into wasted next inspiratory effort, as evident by the following negative deflections on the $P_{oes}$ curve. From Calderini *et al.*[73] with permission.

ventilators and interfaces have allowed detailed monitoring which may guide the caregiver to take actions to reduce leaks and improve the patient–ventilator synchrony, crucial obstacles during this modality of ventilatory support. It should, however, be emphasized that advanced monitoring is not a substitute for detailed clinical evaluation. In addition, advanced monitoring effectiveness depends on adequate data interpretation, a task that is not always easy, necessitating background knowledge and skills.

## REFERENCES


1. Ambrosino N, Foglio K, Rubini *et al.* Non-invasive mechanical ventilation in acute respiratory failure due to chronic obstructive pulmonary disease: correlates for success. *Thorax* 1995; **50**: 755–7.
2. Angus RM, Ahmed AA, Fenwick LJ *et al.* Comparison of the acute effects on gas exchange of nasal ventilation and doxapram in exacerbations of chronic obstructive pulmonary disease. *Thorax* 1996; **51**: 1048–50.
3. Antonelli M, Conti G, Bufi M *et al.* Noninvasive ventilation for treatment of acute respiratory failure in patients undergoing solid organ transplantation: a randomized trial. *JAMA* 2000; **283**: 235–41.
4. Antonelli M, Conti G, Rocco M *et al.* A comparison of noninvasive positive-pressure ventilation and conventional mechanical ventilation in patients with acute respiratory failure. *N Engl J Med* 1998; **339**: 429–35.
5. Barbe F, Togores B, Rubi M *et al.* Noninvasive ventilatory support does not facilitate recovery from acute respiratory failure in chronic obstructive pulmonary disease. *Eur Respir J* 1996; **9**: 1240–5.
6. Bott J, Carroll MP, Conway JH *et al.* Randomised controlled trial of nasal ventilation in acute ventilatory failure due to chronic obstructive airways disease. *Lancet* 1993; **341**: 1555–7.
7. Brochard L, Mancebo J, Wysocki M *et al.* Noninvasive ventilation for acute exacerbations of chronic obstructive pulmonary disease. *N Engl J Med* 1995; **333**: 817–22.
8. Confalonieri M, Potena A, Carbone G *et al.* Acute respiratory failure in patients with severe community-acquired pneumonia. A prospective randomized evaluation of noninvasive ventilation. *Am J Respir Crit Care Med* 1999; **160**: 1585–91.
9. Hilbert G, Gruson D, Vargas F *et al.* Noninvasive ventilation in immunosuppressed patients with pulmonary infiltrates, fever, and acute respiratory failure. *N Engl J Med* 2001; **344**: 481–7.
10. Lightowler JV, Wedzicha JA, Elliott MW *et al.* Non-invasive positive pressure ventilation to treat respiratory failure resulting from exacerbations of chronic obstructive pulmonary disease: Cochrane systematic review and meta-analysis. *BMJ* 2003; **326**: 185.
11. Masip J, Betbese AJ, Paez J *et al.* Non-invasive pressure support ventilation versus conventional oxygen therapy in acute cardiogenic pulmonary oedema: a randomised trial. *Lancet* 2000; **356**: 2126–32.
12. Mehta S, Jay GD, Woolard RH *et al.* Randomized, prospective trial of bilevel versus continuous positive airway pressure in acute pulmonary edema. *Crit Care Med* 1997; **25**: 620–8.
13. Peter JV, Moran JL, Phillips-Hughes J *et al.* Effect of non-invasive positive pressure ventilation (NIPPV) on mortality in patients with acute cardiogenic pulmonary oedema: a meta-analysis. *Lancet* 2006; **367**: 1155–63.
14. Peter JV, Moran JL, Phillips-Hughes J *et al.* Noninvasive ventilation in acute respiratory failure – a meta-analysis update. *Crit Care Med* 2002; **30**: 555–62.
15. Plant PK, Owen JL, Elliott MW. Early use of non-invasive ventilation for acute exacerbations of chronic

obstructive pulmonary disease on general respiratory wards: a multicentre randomised controlled trial. *Lancet* 2000; **355**: 1931–5.

16. Wood KA, Lewis L, Von Harz B *et al.* The use of noninvasive positive pressure ventilation in the emergency department: results of a randomized clinical trial. *Chest* 1998; **113**: 1339–46.
17. Ferrer M, Esquinas A, Leon M *et al.* Noninvasive ventilation in severe hypoxemic respiratory failure: a randomized clinical trial. *Am J Respir Crit Care Med* 2003; **168**: 1438–44.
18. Ferrer M, Esquinas A, Arancibia F *et al.* Noninvasive ventilation during persistent weaning failure: a randomized controlled trial. *Am J Respir Crit Care Med* 2003; **168**: 70–6.
19. Ferrer M, Valencia M, Nicolas JM *et al.* Early noninvasive ventilation averts extubation failure in patients at risk: a randomized trial. *Am J Respir Crit Care Med* 2006; **173**: 164–70.
20. Girault C, Daudenthun I, Chevron V *et al.* Noninvasive ventilation as a systematic extubation and weaning technique in acute-on-chronic respiratory failure: a prospective, randomized controlled study. *Am J Respir Crit Care Med* 1999; **160**: 86–92.
21. Keenan SP, Powers C, McCormack DG *et al.* Noninvasive positive-pressure ventilation for postextubation respiratory distress: a randomized controlled trial. *JAMA* 2002; **287**: 3238–44.
22. Nava S, Ambrosino N, Clini E *et al.* Noninvasive mechanical ventilation in the weaning of patients with respiratory failure due to chronic obstructive pulmonary disease. A randomized, controlled trial. *Ann Intern Med* 1998; **128**: 721–8.
23. Nava S, Gregoretti C, Fanfulla F *et al.* Noninvasive ventilation to prevent respiratory failure after extubation in high-risk patients. *Crit Care Med* 2005; **33**: 2465–70.
24. Confalonieri M, Garuti G, Cattaruzza MS *et al.* A chart of failure risk for noninvasive ventilation in patients with COPD exacerbation. *Eur Respir J* 2005; **25**: 348–55.
25. Lightowler JV, Elliott MW. Predicting the outcome from NIV for acute exacerbations of COPD. *Thorax* 2000; **55**: 815–16.
26. Meduri GU. Noninvasive positive-pressure ventilation in patients with acute respiratory failure. *Clin Chest Med* 1996; **17**: 513–53.
27. Meduri GU, Abou-Shala N, Fox RC *et al.* Noninvasive face mask mechanical ventilation in patients with acute hypercapnic respiratory failure. *Chest* 1991; **100**: 445–54.
28. Scala R, Naldi M, Archinucci I *et al.* Noninvasive positive pressure ventilation in patients with acute exacerbations of COPD and varying levels of consciousness. *Chest* 2005; **128**: 1657–66.
29. Elliott MW, Confalonieri M, Nava S. Where to perform noninvasive ventilation? *Eur Respir J* 2002; **19**: 1159–66.
30. Hill NS. Where should noninvasive ventilation be delivered? *Respir Care* 2009; **54**: 62–70.
31. Nava S, Hill N. Non-invasive ventilation in acute respiratory failure. *Lancet* 2009; **374**: 250–9.
32. Demoule A, Girou E, Richard JC *et al.* Benefits and risks of success or failure of noninvasive ventilation. *Intensive Care Med* 2006; **32**: 1756–65.
33. Demoule A, Girou E, Richard JC *et al.* Increased use of noninvasive ventilation in French intensive care units. *Intensive Care Med* 2006; **32**: 1747–55.
34. Mahler DA. Dyspnea: diagnosis and management. *Clin Chest Med* 1987; **8**: 215–30.
35. Fraticelli AT, Lellouche F, L'Her E *et al.* Physiological effects of different interfaces during noninvasive ventilation for acute respiratory failure. *Crit Care Med* 2009; **37**: 939–45.
36. Kwok H, McCormack J, Cece R *et al.* Controlled trial of oronasal versus nasal mask ventilation in the treatment of acute respiratory failure. *Crit Care Med* 2003; **31**: 468–73.
37. Chiumello D, Conti G, Foti G *et al.* Non-invasive ventilation outside the Intensive Care Unit for acute respiratory failure. *Minerva Anestesiol* 2009; **75**: 459–66.
38. Garpestad E, Brennan J, Hill NS. Noninvasive ventilation for critical care. *Chest* 2007; **132**: 711–20.
39. Borg GA. Psychophysical bases of perceived exertion. *Med Sci Sports Exerc* 1982; **14**: 377–81.
40. Mahler DA, Weinberg DH, Wells CK *et al.* The measurement of dyspnea. Contents, interobserver agreement, and physiologic correlates of two new clinical indexes. *Chest* 1984; **85**: 751–8.
41. Nava S, Navalesi P, Carlucci A. Non-invasive ventilation. *Minerva Anestesiol* 2009; **75**: 31–6.
42. Diaz GG, Alcaraz AC, Talavera JC *et al.* Noninvasive positive-pressure ventilation to treat hypercapnic coma secondary to respiratory failure. *Chest* 2005; **127**: 952–60.
43. Ely EW, Inouye SK, Bernard GR *et al.* Delirium in mechanically ventilated patients: validity and reliability of the confusion assessment method for the intensive care unit (CAM-ICU). *JAMA* 2001; **286**: 2703–10.
44. Ely EW, Shintani A, Truman B *et al.* Delirium as a predictor of mortality in mechanically ventilated patients in the intensive care unit. *JAMA* 2004; **291**: 1753–62.
45. Ely EW, Stephens RK, Jackson JC *et al.* Current opinions regarding the importance, diagnosis, and management of delirium in the intensive care unit: a survey of 912 healthcare professionals. *Crit Care Med* 2004; **32**: 106–12.
46. Thomason JW, Shintani A, Peterson JF *et al.* Intensive care unit delirium is an independent predictor of longer hospital stay: a prospective analysis of 261 non-ventilated patients. *Crit Care* 2005; **9**: R375–81.
47. Girard TD, Pandharipande PP, Ely EW. Delirium in the intensive care unit. *Crit Care* 2008; **12** Suppl 3: S3.
48. Maldonado JR. Delirium in the acute care setting: characteristics, diagnosis and treatment. *Crit Care Clin* 2008; **24**: 657–722, vii.
49. International Consensus Conferences in Intensive Care Medicine: noninvasive positive pressure ventilation in

acute respiratory failure. *Am J Respir Crit Care Med* 2001; **163**: 283–91.

50. Hill NS, Brennan J, Garpestad E *et al.* Noninvasive ventilation in acute respiratory failure. *Crit Care Med* 2007; **35**: 2402–7.
51. Stradling JR. Hypercapnia during oxygen therapy in airways obstruction: a reappraisal. *Thorax* 1986; **41**: 897–902.
52. O'Driscoll BR, Howard LS, Davison AG. BTS guideline for emergency oxygen use in adult patients. *Thorax* 2008; **63** Suppl 6: vi1–68.
53. Cox M, Kemp R, Anwar S *et al.* Non-invasive monitoring of $CO_2$ levels in patients using NIV for AECOPD. *Thorax* 2006; **61**: 363–4.
54. Storre JH, Steurer B, Kabitz HJ *et al.* Transcutaneous $PCO_2$ monitoring during initiation of noninvasive ventilation. *Chest* 2007; **132**: 1810–16.
55. Meduri GU, Fox RC, Abou-Shala N *et al.* Noninvasive mechanical ventilation via face mask in patients with acute respiratory failure who refused endotracheal intubation. *Crit Care Med* 1994; **22**: 1584–90.
56. Borel JC, Sabil A, Janssens JP *et al.* Intentional leaks in industrial masks have a significant impact on efficacy of bilevel noninvasive ventilation: a bench test study. *Chest* 2009; **135**: 669–77.
57. Ferreira JC, Chipman DW, Hill NS *et al.* Bilevel vs ICU ventilators providing noninvasive ventilation, effect of system leaks: A COPD lung model comparison. *Chest* Published online before print 8 May 2009, doi: 10.1378/chest.08-3018.
58. Miyoshi E, Fujino Y, Uchiyama A *et al.* Effects of gas leak on triggering function, humidification, and inspiratory oxygen fraction during noninvasive positive airway pressure ventilation. *Chest* 2005; **128**: 3691–8.
59. Vignaux L, Tassaux D, Jolliet P. Performance of noninvasive ventilation modes on ICU ventilators during pressure support: a bench model study. *Intensive Care Med* 2007; **33**: 1444–51.
60. Wysocki M, Richard JC, Meshaka P. Noninvasive proportional assist ventilation compared with noninvasive pressure support ventilation in hypercapnic acute respiratory failure. *Crit Care Med* 2002; **30**: 323–9.
61. Kondili E, Prinianakis G, Georgopoulos D. Patient-ventilator interaction. *Br J Anaesth* 2003; **91**: 106–19.
62. Kondili E, Xirouchaki N, Georgopoulos D. Modulation and treatment of patient-ventilator dyssynchrony. *Curr Opin Crit Care* 2007; **13**: 84–9.
63. Vignaux L, Vargas F, Roeseler J *et al.* Patient-ventilator asynchrony during non-invasive ventilation for acute respiratory failure: a multicenter study. *Intensive Care Med* 2009; **35**: 840–6.
64. Georgopoulos D, Prinianakis G, Kondili E. Bedside waveforms interpretation as a tool to identify patient-ventilator asynchronies. *Intensive Care Med* 2006; **32**: 34–47.
65. Chen CW, Lin WC, Hsu CH *et al.* Detecting ineffective triggering in the expiratory phase in mechanically ventilated patients based on airway flow and pressure deflection: feasibility of using a computer algorithm. *Crit Care Med* 2008; **36**: 455–61.
66. Mulqueeny Q, Ceriana P, Carlucci A *et al.* Automatic detection of ineffective triggering and double triggering during mechanical ventilation. *Intensive Care Med* 2007; **33**: 2014–18.
67. Younes M, Brochard L, Grasso S *et al.* A method for monitoring and improving patient:ventilator interaction. *Intensive Care Med* 2007; **33**: 1337–46.
68. Mehta S, Hill NS. Noninvasive ventilation. *Am J Respir Crit Care Med* 2001; **163**: 540–77.
69. Navalesi P, Costa R, Ceriana P *et al.* Non-invasive ventilation in chronic obstructive pulmonary disease patients: helmet versus facial mask. *Intensive Care Med* 2007; **33**: 74–81.
70. Racca F, Appendini L, Gregoretti C *et al.* Effectiveness of mask and helmet interfaces to deliver noninvasive ventilation in a human model of resistive breathing. *J Appl Physiol* 2005; **99**: 1262–71.
71. Vargas F, Thille A, Lyazidi A *et al.* Helmet with specific settings versus facemask for noninvasive ventilation. *Crit Care Med* 2009; **37**: 1921–8.
72. Prinianakis G, Delmastro M, Carlucci A *et al.* Effect of varying the pressurisation rate during noninvasive pressure support ventilation. *Eur Respir J* 2004; **23**: 314–20.
73. Calderini E, Confalonieri M, Puccio PG *et al.* Patient-ventilator asynchrony during noninvasive ventilation: the role of expiratory trigger. *Intensive Care Med* 1999; **25**: 662–7.
74. Cooper AB, Thornley KS, Young GB *et al.* Sleep in critically ill patients requiring mechanical ventilation. *Chest* 2000; **117**: 809–18.
75. Parthasarathy S. Sleep during mechanical ventilation. *Curr Opin Pulmon Med* 2004; **10**: 489–94.
76. Parthasarathy S, Tobin MJ. Effect of ventilator mode on sleep quality in critically ill patients. *Am J Respir Crit Care Med* 2002; **166**: 1423–9.
77. Parthasarathy S, Tobin MJ. Sleep in the intensive care unit. *Intensive Care Med* 2004; **30**: 197–206.
78. Gonzalez J, Sharshar T, Hart N *et al.* Air leaks during mechanical ventilation as a cause of persistent hypercapnia in neuromuscular disorders. *Intensive Care Med* 2003; **29**: 596–602.
79. Gonzalez MM, Parreira VF, Rodenstein DO. Non-invasive ventilation and sleep. *Sleep Med Rev* 2002; **6**: 29–44.
80. Meyer TJ, Pressman MR, Benditt J *et al.* Air leaking through the mouth during nocturnal nasal ventilation: effect on sleep quality. *Sleep* 1997; **20**: 561–9.
81. Gregoretti C, Confalonieri M, Navalesi P *et al.* Evaluation of patient skin breakdown and comfort with a new face mask for non-invasive ventilation: a multi-center study. *Intensive Care Med* 2002; **28**: 278–84.

# 12

# Troubleshooting non-invasive ventilation

NICHOLAS S HILL

ABSTRACT

Problems arising with non-invasive ventilation (NIV) use are best avoided or dealt with promptly by selecting appropriate patients and monitoring them closely. Selection of patients for NIV depends on the presence of an appropriate diagnosis, need for ventilatory assistance and absence of contraindications. Successful NIV requires a systematic approach to management of frequently encountered problems that predispose to failure. This includes taking into consideration environmental/caregiver team factors (lack of skilled, experienced caregiver team, poor patient selection and lack of adequate monitoring), patient-related factors (mask problems, agitation, excessive secretions, inability to protect airway, progression of underlying disease), and technical factors (inadequate equipment, failure to ventilate, failure to oxygenate, patient–ventilator asynchrony, air leaks). Intolerance is one of the most commonly cited reasons for NIV failure; this may be because of an inappropriately applied interface, incorrect ventilator settings, etc. In other words the fault may lie with the operator rather than the patient. A correctly sized mask together with the correct head gear is vital. Ventilator settings should be chosen to reduce respiratory distress, improve gas exchange and, most importantly, to achieve synchrony between the ventilator and the patient. Patient intolerance of NIV or failure to improve physiologically should prompt a review of the way in which NIV is being applied. Caregivers should have a strategy to deal with agitated patients including the use of sedative drugs. In a proportion of cases, failure is unavoidable due to the progression of the underlying cause. Prompt efforts to reverse treatable risk factors for failure and to optimize medical therapy are mandatory.

## INTRODUCTION

Non-invasive ventilation (NIV) has assumed an important role in the management of respiratory failure, with recent surveys indicating that it comprises 20–40 per cent of initial ventilator starts in acute care hospitals in Europe and North America.[1,2] Strong evidence now supports the use of NIV as the ventilator modality of first choice to treat respiratory failure due to chronic obstructive pulmonary disease (COPD) exacerbations,[3] acute cardiogenic pulmonary oedema[4] and immunocompromised states,[5] with numerous other potential applications.[6] Yet, NIV can be very challenging to administer, with failure rates (need for intubation or death, mainly in do-not-intubate patients) exceeding 40 per cent in some studies.[7,8] This high failure rate underlines the importance of troubleshooting for reversible factors contributing to the high failure rates and strategies for managing them. The following presents a systematic approach to management of problems frequently encountered during use of NIV that predispose to failure and is meant to serve as a troubleshooting guide for clinicians aiming to optimize success rates. The focus will be on the acute care setting, but some principles discussed will be relevant to the long-term setting as well.

## PREDICTORS OF NON-INVASIVE VENTILATION FAILURE

A number of investigations have identified factors associated with NIV success or failure, as summarized in Boxes 12.1 and 12.2. These can be useful in informing clinicians on identifying potentially modifiable factors as well as avoiding patients at high risk of failing NIV so that success rates can be improved.

A fairly consistent picture emerges from these studies to assess the risk of NIV failure. Patients with an inability to cooperate with the technique or coordinating their breathing with the ventilator, unable to handle their secretions, excessive air leaking or a high severity of acute

**Box 12.1 Predictors of failure: NIV for hypercapnic respiratory failure**

- Advanced age
- Higher acuity of illness (APACHE score)
- Uncooperative
- Poor neurological score
- Unable to coordinate breathing with ventilator
- Large air leaks
- Edentulous
- Tachypnoea (>35/min)
- Acidaemia (pH <7.18)
- Failure to improve pH, heart and respiratory rates or Glasgow Coma Score within the first 2 hours*

*Most powerful predictor

Adapted from Soo Hoo *et al.*,[9] Ambrosino *et al.*[10] and Confalonieri *et al.*[11]

**Box 12.2 Predictors of failure: NIV for hypoxaemic respiratory failure**

- Diagnosis of acute respiratory distress syndrome (ARDS) or pneumonia
- Simplified Acute Physiology Score (SAPS) ≥ 35
- Lower $PaO_2/FIO_2$ (low 100s or below)
- Low pH
- Age >40 years
- Septic shock
- Multiorgan system failure
- Failure to improve $PaO_2/FIO_2$ >146 within first hour

Adapted from Antonelli *et al.*[13] and Rana *et al.*[14]

illness, especially with multiorgan system failure, fare poorly with NIV. Greater severity of the oxygenation defect is also a risk factor for failure, but not so for greater carbon dioxide retention, which correlates with success in some studies. Furthermore, the failure to manifest an early favourable response to NIV is a strong predictor of a poor outcome.

## REASONS FOR NON-INVASIVE VENTILATION FAILURE

Predictors of NIV failure permit clinicians to estimate the risk of failure in a given candidate being considered for NIV, but specific reasons for failure can be identified only after failure has occurred. Thus, a major goal of NIV management is to anticipate problems likely to arise during NIV use and address them before they lead to NIV failure. Common specific reasons for NIV failure are listed in Box 12.3.[16] Considerable overlap exists between the categories, so it is difficult to accurately determine the occurrence of the specific reasons for failure. For example, patients who fail to improve their ventilation on NIV may be unable to tolerate adequate inspiratory pressure or to synchronize with the ventilator, or have excessive air leaking or airway secretions or some combination of these factors. Investigators analysing reasons for failure attempt to categorize patients according to primary reasons for failure, but these categorizations are open to interpretation. Nonetheless, these categories assist clinicians in identifying situations that may lead to failure and lead to strategies for dealing with them. The following will address each of these reasons commonly cited for NIV failure and discuss possible approaches to alleviating them.

**Box 12.3 Common reasons for NIV failure**

Environmental/caregiver team factors

- Lack of skilled, experienced caregiver team
- Poor patient selection
- Lack of adequate monitoring

Patient-related factors

- Intolerance
- Mask problems: discomfort; poor fit; skin ulceration; claustrophobia
- Agitation
- Excessive secretions, inability to protect airway
- Progression of underlying disease

Technical factors

- Inadequate equipment
- Failure to ventilate
- Failure to oxygenate
- Patient–ventilator asynchrony
- Air leaks

### Environmental/caregiver team factors in non-invasive ventilation failure

In order to avoid problems with NIV and promptly deal with those that arise, NIV must be administered in an appropriate environment by a knowledgeable, skilled team in well-selected patients. The importance of developing a skilled, experienced team to optimize the delivery of mechanical ventilation is discussed in more detail in Chapter 10.

## Selection of appropriate patients for non-invasive ventilation

Regardless of the specific reason for NIV failure, selection of patients at very high risk of NIV failure will lead to high failure rates. Thus, one of the most important ways to avoid problems with the administration of NIV is to select appropriate recipients and avoid those at very high risk. Patient selection is a key responsibility of the physician and should be based on evidence from the medical literature, available guidelines, knowledge of risk factors for NIV failure (as discussed above) and clinical judgement.

As evidence regarding the use of NIV has accumulated,[17] it has become clear that certain forms of respiratory failure, such as that due to COPD exacerbations or cardiogenic pulmonary oedema, are well suited for it.[3,18] These entities are usually characterized by intact upper airway function and prompt reversibility with medical therapy, usually within hours for cardiogenic pulmonary oedema and within days for COPD. Other forms of acute respiratory failure that may benefit from NIV include that occurring in immunocompromised patients, who are at very high risk of healthcare-acquired pneumonias and other infections that are avoided by NIV.[19,20] Non-invasive ventilation may be tried in many other forms of acute respiratory failure but the evidence to support these applications is weaker, and such patients should be monitored closely to optimize success.

An assessment of risk factors for NIV failure is also important when deciding on whether a patient should receive NIV. The risk factors listed in Boxes 12.1 and 12.2 are helpful in stratifying risk for patients with hypercapnic and hypoxaemic respiratory failure, respectively, and should be considered before initiating NIV. Patients deemed at excessively high risk for NIV failure should forego a trial entirely and those at high risk might undergo a cautious trial in a closely monitored ICU setting with plans to intubate if there is no clear evidence of improvement within the first hour or two.

The decision to initiate NIV, though, must often be made quickly at the bedside with little information other than that gleaned from direct observation of the patient. Thus, it must be based on simple observations and measurements, often before arterial blood gas results are known, because loss of valuable time initially can predispose to failure later. The first step in selection is to assess the need for ventilatory assistance (Box 12.4) based on the presence of at least moderate dyspnoea, evidence of increased work of breathing and an appropriate cause of respiratory failure. Such patients are at risk of needing intubation if NIV is not initiated promptly.

The second step is to ascertain that there are no contraindications to NIV that would render its use excessively risky (Box 12.5). Some of these are absolute, such as a respiratory arrest, but most are relative, such as excessive agitation or secretions, and require assessment based on experience. Once again, when in doubt, the clinician can either intubate upfront or initiate a trial of NIV in a closely monitored setting and proceed to intubation if there is no improvement.

### Box 12.4 Selection guidelines for NIV in the acute setting

- Appropriate diagnosis with potential reversibility (i.e. COPD or congestive heart failure [CHF])
- Establish need for ventilatory assistance
  - Moderate to severe respiratory distress

  and

  - tachypnoea (>24 for COPD, >30 for CHF)
  - Accessory muscle use or abdominal paradox
  - Blood gas derangement: pH <7.35, $PaCO_2$ >45, or $PaO_2/FiO_2$ <300*

*Awaiting return of blood gas results is discouraged in very dyspnoeic patients to avoid delays in initiation

### Box 12.5 Contraindications to NIV

- Respiratory or cardiac arrest
- Too unstable (e.g. hypotensive shock, myocardial infarction requiring intervention, uncontrolled ischaemia or arrhythmias, uncontrolled upper gastrointestinal bleed, unevacuated pneumothorax)
- Unable to protect airway*
  - Excessive secretions
  - Poor cough
  - Impaired swallowing
- Aspiration risk*
  - Distended bowel; obstruction or ileus
  - Frequent vomiting
- Uncooperative or agitated*
- Unable to fit mask
- Recent upper airway or oesophageal surgery
- Multiorgan system failure (more than 2)

*Relative contraindications

## Proper monitoring of non-invasive ventilation

Effective troubleshooting of NIV is impossible without adequate monitoring. Unless detected and addressed promptly, problems arising with the administration of NIV can precipitate NIV failure. Selection of a proper location for administration of NIV is important, based on the patient's need for monitoring and the capabilities of the unit.[21] Patients deemed at higher risk of NIV failure, such as those with greater gas exchange derangement, increased airway secretions, impaired cough, severe respiratory distress, marginal vital signs or altered mental status, should be monitored in a more closely observed setting such as an ICU or respiratory step-down unit. One potentially useful method for establishing the patient's need for monitoring is to temporarily remove the NIV mask and determine the length of time before deterioration occurs and NIV must be reinitiated.[22] If this occurs within minutes, a closely monitored setting would be mandatory. Alternatively, if the patient can tolerate more than 20 or 30 minutes without needing NIV and is capable of calling for help if necessary, location on a regular hospital ward might be appropriate. Erring on the side of caution is prudent, however, with patients placed in a higher intensity setting until it is clear that they have stabilized.

Potential complications should be anticipated and prevented, if possible, such as the routine use of artificial skin or other protective coverings at the first sign of skin redness over the bridge of the nose. The value of monitoring by a skilled and experienced team cannot be overestimated. For further information about monitoring during NIV see Chapter 11.

## PATIENT-RELATED FACTORS CONTRIBUTING TO NON-INVASIVE VENTILATION FAILURE

Problems may arise during NIV because of patient-related factors such as inability to tolerate NIV or agitation that often precipitate NIV failure unless promptly addressed. Sometimes these occur in a particularly anxious patient or are related to progression of the underlying process rendering NIV failure inevitable, but these may be reversible if recognized and managed early enough. A strategy to deal with intolerance/agitation is depicted in Figure 12.1.

### Intolerance of non-invasive ventilation

Intolerance is one of the most commonly cited reasons for NIV failure but is not precisely defined. In a general sense, it describes a patient who becomes uncomfortable or agitated and demands that the mask be removed or removes it themselves. Specific reasons for intolerance include mask discomfort, the sensation of claustrophobia and discomfort related to excessive pressure from the ventilator. Respiratory distress and associated anxiety causing agitation also contribute to the problem.

### Mask discomfort

Many patients find the interfaces used for NIV uncomfortable and this is one of the most common reasons for intolerance of NIV. Some discomfort occurs in most patients using NIV and the aim should be to make the mask tolerable. Patients with respiratory distress initially may feel a sense of suffocation when the mask is first strapped on and need reassurance. Giving cooperative patients a sense of control by having them hold the mask in place may facilitate initiation.

An ill-fitting mask, a mask type that is unacceptable to the patient, or excessively tightened straps may also contribute to mask intolerance. A properly fitting mask is essential to NIV tolerance. Some masks come with gauges to assist with fitting. Usually, the smallest mask that just accommodates the nose and mouth is the best choice;

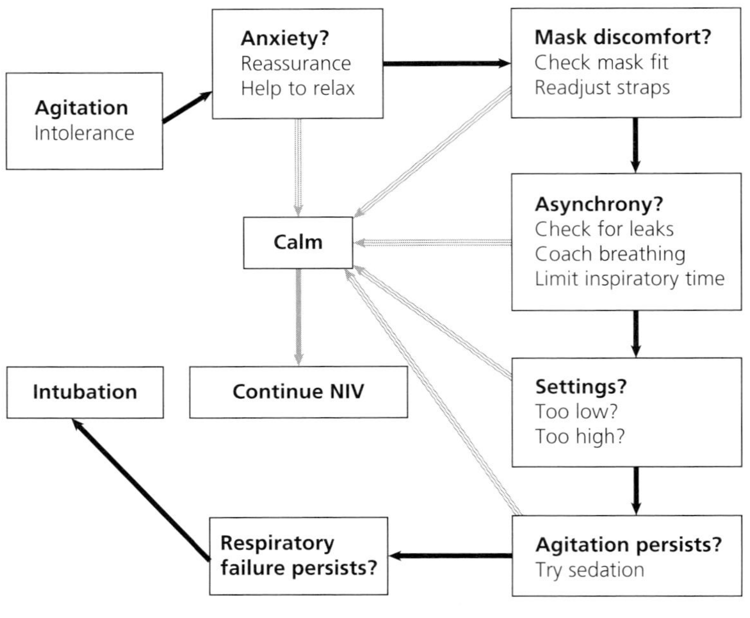


**Figure 12.1** Schematic suggesting an approach to the agitated/intolerant patient using non-invasive ventilation (NIV). Black solid arrows indicate persisting agitation despite intervention and striped arrows indicate that the patient is becalmed so that NIV can continue. According to the schema, the first step is to see if anxiety responds to reassurance. Failing that, readjust the mask, eliminate asynchrony and check the ventilator settings. If those fail, try chemical sedation. If the patient remains agitated and in respiratory failure, perform intubation.

excessively large masks can contribute to air leaking and may necessitate more tightening of the straps to control the leaks.

Patients also differ markedly in their preferences for mask types. In the acute setting, oronasal masks that cover both the nose and mouth are better tolerated than nasal masks as the initial mask choice, largely because of better control of mouth leaks.[23] In the long-term setting, however, nasal masks are rated by patients as more comfortable than oronasal.[24] Thus, switching to a nasal mask after initial oronasal mask use may be desirable for some patients who are to be continued on NIV after the first days or so of use. Also, patients who are claustrophobic or are expectorating frequently may fare better with the nasal mask for initiation. If a nasal mask is used, however, the patency of the nasal passages should be assured.

Many mask types besides the typical nasal or oronasal ones are now available that may be more comfortable for some patients because they are larger and seal around the perimeter of the face, avoiding the nose and mouth. Nasal prongs may be useful in patients developing nasal ulcers because they seal in the nares and not on the bridge of the nose. These and 'hybrid' masks that combine nasal prongs with a mask that fits over the mouth are more often used in the long-term setting. The 'helmet', used mainly in certain European centres,[25] seals over the neck and shoulders using straps secured under the axillae and may offer a more comfortable alternative for some patients. However, cost and noise (related to the high gas flow rates needed to minimize rebreathing) may be barriers to more widespread use.[26] As mentioned above, the capability of quickly trying different mask types may enhance tolerance in the acute setting, so having a 'mask bag' containing a number of different choices attached to the non-invasive ventilator can be advantageous.

## Other mask-related problems

In the past, ulceration on the bridge of the nose has been reported to occur in up to 40 per cent of patients using certain kinds of masks,[27] but should be an infrequent occurrence today because of advances in mask technology and heightened awareness of the problem. Newer masks have soft silicone seals that are less apt to traumatize the face, and some have forehead spacers that help to relieve tension on the nose. In addition, artificial skin should be applied over the bridge of the nose either routinely or at the first sign of nasal skin irritation as indicated by redness over the bridge of the nose.

## Claustrophobia

Claustrophobic reactions commonly lead to NIV intolerance. Many patients feel panic when a mask is tightly strapped over their nose or nose and mouth, especially when they are sensing respiratory distress. These patients have a natural desire to remove the mask, but may respond to verbal reassurance. Giving them control over the mask during initiation by having them hold it in place may also help. Using a mask that covers less of the face such as a nasal mask or nasal prongs instead of an oronasal mask may help, but many patients require sedation (see below). Sometimes, though, the claustrophobic reaction and aversion to the mask are so intense that NIV failure is unavoidable.

## Intolerance of ventilator settings

Suboptimal adjustment of ventilator settings may also contribute to intolerance. Excessively high pressures contribute to discomfort, not only via direct effects on the ears and sinuses causing burning and pain, but also because they promote air leaks and necessitate greater tightening of the mask straps. Insufficient pressures may contribute to intolerance because of inadequate alleviation of respiratory distress. An excessively high backup rate or rise in inspiratory pressure 'rise time' may also contribute to ventilator asynchrony and intolerance. (See later section on ventilator asynchrony for a more extensive discussion.)

## Agitation

Agitation is another commonly cited reason for NIV intolerance and failure. It refers to a state of high anxiety, usually associated with uncooperativeness, with the patient grabbing at and removing the mask, and unable to coordinate breathing with the ventilator. The term is non-specific and may be precipitated by claustrophobia or mask discomfort. It may also be associated with underlying delirium, referring to a state of inattention and disorientedness, which becomes manifest when the patient is stressed by having to use NIV. Agitation contributes to NIV failure because the patient is unable to relax and let the ventilator assist with the breathing load.

Strategies to deal with agitation should first focus on non-pharmacological measures such as verbal reassurance, efforts to enhance comfort, giving the patient control over the mask or, if the respiratory insufficiency is not too severe, frequent 'vacations' from NIV (Fig. 12.1). Often, however, sedation is necessary to calm the patient. Most pulmonary and critical care physicians in North America and Europe are reluctant to use sedation because of the perceived risks of interfering with ability to protect the airway or depressing respiratory drive.[28] If sedation is used, however, the preferred agents are small doses of benzodiazepines (midazolam or lorazepam) and/or narcotics (morphine sulphate or fentanyl) to enhance tolerance of NIV. If the patient is closely monitored while doses are titrated to achieve calmness and cooperativeness, these drugs can be safely administered without significant blunting of respiratory drive, especially if given while the patient is receiving ventilatory assistance. Other agents such as haloperidol (often used for delirious patients),[29] dexmedetomidine[30] and propofol,[31] have been used to calm patients receiving NIV. Dexmedetomidine and propofol have relatively short half-lives, rendering them suitable for intravenous infusion and providing easier titration of the level of sedation than with longer-acting drugs, but patients receiving propofol must be observed carefully for the potential depression of respiratory drive.[31] Dexmedetomidine has little respiratory depressant effect and combines sedation with analgesia, which alleviate mask comfort, but it is expensive and, as with most of the other agents, its use with NIV is only anecdotal.[30]

### Excessive secretions

Excessive secretions or the inability to adequately cough or swallow are listed as contraindications to NIV. However, these are relative, because many patients succeed with NIV despite the presence of secretions or cough or swallowing impairment. Thus, a clinical judgement must be made in these patients as to whether the problems are so severe as to preclude the use of NIV. Sometimes, patients with mild or moderate impairment of airway protection undergo a trial of NIV under close observation and preparedness to intubate if they fail to respond favourably.

While these patients are under observation, some interventions may be helpful. Clinicians should ascertain that hydration is adequate and provide humidification of inhaled gas to avoid desiccation of mucus. Mucolytics such as acetylcysteine should also be considered, although this may provoke bronchospasm in patients with airway hyperreactivity. In some patients, chest physiotherapy sometimes coupled with postural drainage can help. Vest-like devices that vibrate the chest can also help to dislodge mucus, although they appear to be of greatest help in patients with bronchiectasis or cystic fibrosis.[33] For patients with weakened cough muscles, cough inexsufflators can be sufficiently effective in facilitating cough to avoid intubation.[34] They are used most often in outpatients with neuromuscular disease,[35] but may have applications in the acute setting as well.

### Progression of the underlying process

Non-invasive ventilation may succeed initially yet fail after the first 24 or 48 hours because of progression of the underlying disease.[36] This is a particular concern in patients with severe hypoxaemic respiratory failure and underlying pneumonia or ARDS who may succumb to excessive secretions, progressive hypoxaemia or multiorgan system failure, conditions that overwhelm the capabilities of NIV and necessitate intubation. Antonelli *et al.*[13] found that in a cohort of 354 patients with hypoxaemic respiratory failure treated with NIV, inability to correct hypoxaemia was the most common cause of NIV failure between 24 and 48 hours after initiation of therapy, while inability to manage secretions or to correct dyspnoea were distant second and third causes. Comorbidities at presentation such as severe hyperglycaemia or significant functional impairment predict late NIV failure.[36] Considering that unanticipated emergency intubations add to the morbidity and mortality of these patients and are to be avoided, patients deemed to be at risk of NIV failure due to progression of the underlying disease (i.e. severe hypoxaemic respiratory failure, airway secretions or significant comorbidities) must be monitored closely in a general or respiratory ICU and intubated promptly when deemed necessary to avoid a respiratory arrest and its attendant morbidity and mortality.

## TECHNICAL FACTORS CONTRIBUTING TO NON-INVASIVE VENTILATION FAILURE

Non-invasive ventilation failure may sometimes be related to inadequate equipment, inability to reverse hypoventilation or hypoxaemia, asynchrony or inadequately controlled air leaks.

### Proper equipment for non-invasive ventilation

The skill to properly apply equipment is probably more important than the equipment itself. But proper equipment can make a difference, particularly masks. As discussed above in the section on intolerance, having familiarity with the many mask choices available and a mask bag containing a variety of types and sizes of masks attached to the ventilator is strongly recommended.

No studies have convincingly demonstrated the superiority of one ventilator type over another. For acute applications of NIV, newer 'bi-level positive pressure devices' have advantages over older bi-level devices in that they have much improved monitoring and alarm systems, better graphic displays, oxygen blenders, sophisticated algorithms to limit inspiratory time and enhance synchrony, and an internal battery to facilitate transport. These factors, especially the oxygen blender, can make the difference between success and failure in patients with hypoxaemic respiratory failure. Most other 'bi-level ventilators' were designed to deliver NIV at home and not to ventilate challenging hypoxaemic patients. They lack an oxygen blender and even when oxygen is supplemented into a 'T' connector in the ventilator tubing or directly into the mask, maximal fraction of inhaled oxygen concentration ($FiO_2$) reaches only 45–50 per cent.[37]

Many manufacturers have been adding 'NIV' modes to their 'critical care ventilators' that enhance leak compensation, silence 'nuisance' alarms and limit inspiratory time.

Few have been tested clinically but bench studies indicate that these do not all function the same.[38,39] In the face of air leaks, caregivers must be prepared to make additional adjustments on most of these ventilators,[39] but they appear to function better at delivering NIV than traditional pressure support modes that were used in the past. Despite the advantages of the newer ventilators, it is important to keep in mind that many ventilator types, including both 'bi-level' and 'critical care', can be adjusted to deliver NIV successfully. The lack of newer, sophisticated ventilators is no reason to avoid using NIV unless a patient with hypoxaemic respiratory failure cannot be adequately oxygenated.

## Failure to ventilate

A commonly cited reason for NIV failure, failure to adequately assist ventilation, is encountered most often in patients with acute hypercapnic respiratory failure, most of whom have COPD. Reported NIV success rates among patients with acute hypercapnic respiratory failure are high, usually above 70 per cent[13,17,30] and sometimes even exceeding 90 per cent.[31] Nonetheless, failures to improve ventilation do occur, often associated with other factors that interfere with the effectiveness of NIV, including intolerance or agitation, patient–ventilator asynchrony or excessive air leaks.

Obviously, a major aim in treating acute or acute-on-chronic respiratory acidosis is to lower $PaCO_2$ and raise pH. For this reason, clinicians are encouraged to obtain baseline arterial blood gases for comparison with a repeat test after the first hour or two of therapy. If $PaCO_2$ rises substantially during this interim (>10 mm Hg, for example), intubation should be contemplated. However, the drop in $PaCO_2$ is often gradual,[17] and as long as other aims are being achieved (decreased respiratory rate and dyspnoea in a haemodynamically stable patient) a rise in $PaCO_2$ might be tolerated initially without resorting to intubation.

Nonetheless, reasons for lack of improvement in $PaCO_2$ should be sought, even if intubation is not deemed urgent, to reduce the eventual need. Intolerance, refusal to wear the mask and asynchrony with the ventilator can be addressed as discussed above and air leaks are discussed in more detail below. Failure to adequately ventilate can also be caused if the ventilator is set inappropriately and the driving pressure or 'pressure support' that assists each patient breath is too small. Low inspiratory (8–10 cm $H_2O$) and expiratory (4–5 cm $H_2O$) pressures are often used to facilitate patient tolerance initially, but unless the difference between inspiratory and expiratory pressure – the 'driving' pressure or pressure support – is promptly increased, many patients will derive too little ventilatory assistance to improve ventilation. As with the use of pressure support in an intubated patient, the pressure support level should be increased until the patient's tidal volume reaches 6–7 mL/kg and respiratory rate decreases, ideally, to the low 20s.[40] These targets may not be achievable if the increase in inspiratory pressure causes too much discomfort, but the highest tolerable inspiratory pressure should be used. Arterial blood gases, vital signs and subjective adaptation should be monitored closely in an ICU or intermediate care environment until stability is assured.

## Failure to oxygenate

With the exception of cardiogenic pulmonary oedema, failure rates for NIV are higher for hypoxaemic than for hypercapnic failure, approaching or even exceeding 50 per cent in some studies.[41,42] Also, most non-cardiogenic oedema patients with hypoxaemic respiratory failure are poor candidates for NIV and selection of appropriate candidates with hypoxaemic respiratory failure is challenging. Nonetheless, there may be subgroups of patients with hypoxaemic respiratory failure whose outcomes would be improved by use of NIV (see above).[15] Although multiple reasons contribute to the higher NIV failure rate, including mask intolerance and failure to correct dyspnoea, the most commonly cited reason in these patients is failure to oxygenate.[13]

Strategies to deal with persistent hypoxaemia during NIV include assurance that a mask that covers the nose and mouth is being used. In a prospective, randomized trial, Kwok *et al.*[23] found that the oronasal mask was better tolerated initially than nasal masks because of fewer mouth leaks and associated desaturation episodes. In addition, hypoxaemic patients must be watched closely in an intensive care unit (ICU) until stabilized because mask dislodgement can precipitate severe desaturations that lead to NIV failure unless detected and corrected promptly. Furthermore, as discussed above, the ventilator must be capable of delivering high $FiO_2$s, generally by means of an oxygen blender, and sufficient $FIO_2$ must be delivered to maintain a target $O_2$ saturation, usually greater than 90 per cent.

Once the appropriateness of the mask and ventilator to treat hypoxaemic patients is assured, ventilator adjustments may be helpful to enhance oxygenation. Just as positive end-expiratory pressure (PEEP) is helpful to maintain oxygenation in invasively ventilated patients, so increases in expiratory pressure are helpful in oxygenating patients on NIV. However, increases are limited because of patient intolerance and the tendency of high mask pressures to increase air leaks. Also, to maintain the pressure support level, the inspiratory pressure must be raised in tandem with the expiratory pressure, something that can heighten intolerance. Thus, during acute applications of NIV to treat oxygenation failure, the maximum tolerated expiratory pressure is usually in the range of 8–10 cm $H_2O$.

In a group of patients with hypoxaemic respiratory failure, L'Her *et al.*[43] found that, as might be anticipated, increases in pressure support to as high as 15 cm $H_2O$

improved ventilation and reduced dyspnoea. On the other hand, increases in PEEP to 10 cm $H_2O$ improved oxygenation, but at the expense of reduced patient comfort. They recommended titration to arrive at a compromise, enhancing oxygenation without sacrificing too much comfort.

Patients with respiratory failure due to pneumonia or ARDS are at risk for progression of the underlying process over a period of hours or days after initiation of NIV. For this reason, NIV for oxygenation failure may still fail even after 24–48 hours of ventilation.[13] The need to watch these patients in a closely monitored setting and to avoid delays in needed intubation cannot be overemphasized. Also, a chest radiograph should be obtained routinely in patients with failure to ventilate or oxygenate because progression of pneumonia, worsening CHF and pneumothoraces are possible contributors.

Unanticipated respiratory arrests and the need for emergency intubation in these patients greatly add to morbidity and mortality and should be avoided by anticipating the need for intubation before it becomes emergent. Also, if PEEP levels of 10 cm $H_2O$ or below are insufficient to adequately oxygenate patients with hypoxaemic respiratory failure or if sophisticated ventilatory techniques such as pressure release ventilation or high-frequency oscillation are needed, then intubation and invasive ventilator management should be performed without delay.

## Patient–ventilator asynchrony

In the ideal situation, the ventilator should precisely follow the patient's neural output from the respiratory centre, as signified by neural activity of the phrenic nerves, assisting or replacing the action of the diaphragm. Patients breathing asynchronously with the ventilator cannot take full advantage of the pressure increase meant to be delivered in time with diaphragmatic activity and thus do not realize the benefits of reduced inspiratory work of breathing or improved gas exchange. Furthermore, the asynchrony contributes to discomfort and agitation as the patient exhales against the higher inspiratory pressure or inhales when the ventilator is providing insufficient airflow. Thus, patient–ventilator asynchrony is a significant cause of NIV failure.

Intermittent patient–ventilator asynchrony is virtually universal among patients receiving NIV and need not be cause for concern as long as the large majority of breaths are synchronous and the patient is reasonably comfortable. But as more breaths become asynchronous, the efficacy of NIV becomes more compromised and NIV failure more likely. Thus, prompt attention to the problem of patient–ventilator synchrony is a key to NIV success.

Asynchrony can be related to many potentially reversible factors during NIV use. Patients must learn how to adjust their breathing pattern to benefit from NIV when first starting, and coaching from an experienced caregiver with instructions like 'try to breathe slower and let the respirator breathe for you' can be very helpful. Many patients become anxious and uncomfortable during initiation of NIV, causing them to breathe asynchronously, and may respond to reassurance or, if these non-pharmacological interventions fail, judicious doses of anxiolytics and/or analgesics. Mask discomfort or inappropriate ventilator settings (too high contributing to discomfort or too low failing to relieve respiratory distress) may also contribute to agitation and thereby asynchrony.

Pressure support modes commonly have problems synchronizing with the breathing pattern of COPD patients, whether ventilated invasively or non-invasively. Auto-PEEP occurs commonly during exacerbations, increasing the inspiratory effort required to initiate the next breath and leading to failure to trigger (initiate the next ventilator breath). Also, inspiratory flow may not drop rapidly at the end of inspiration related to lack of lung recoil causing the ventilator to continue inspiratory pressure in the face of the patient's attempt to exhale, referred to as failure to cycle or 'expiratory asynchrony'.[44] The inspiration can be quite prolonged, as some ventilator algorithms permit a maximal inspiratory phase of up to 3 seconds.[39]

Excessive expiratory asynchrony contributes to patient discomfort and loss of ventilator efficacy.[39,44] Strategies to alleviate these types of asynchrony include reducing the level of pressure support to lower tidal volume and thereby auto-PEEP, and raising the cycling threshold so that it triggers at higher inspiratory flow.[45] Limiting inspiratory time[46] and minimizing air leaks that can also contribute to these forms of asynchrony (see below) are also effective strategies.

Other avenues for improving the matching of ventilator output and patient effort include adjustments in inspiratory flow or 'rise time' (found on some 'bi-level' ventilators to permit adjustments in the time to reach target inspiratory pressure),[45] adaptive servoventilation, proportional-assist ventilation (PAV) and neurally adjusted ventilatory assistance (NAVA). COPD patients tend to prefer relatively rapid inspiratory flow rates (in the range of 60 L/min).[47] Such flow rates reduce inspiratory work compared with lower flow rates, but excessively rapid rates can add to patient discomfort.[48]

## Air leaks

Air leaks are virtually universal during NIV because the system is open. 'Bi-level' positive pressure ventilators have intentional leaks in the mask or ventilator tubing, of course, because they use single circuit tubing and must have a fixed exhalation port to minimize $CO_2$ rebreathing. Although some earlier studies raised concern about the possibility of rebreathing contributing to NIV failure during use of 'bi-level' devices,[49] this has never been demonstrated in a clinical setting and seems unlikely as long as expiratory pressure is kept at 4 cm $H_2O$ or higher to maintain a sufficiently high bias flow. Interfaces like the helmet may be more susceptible to rebreathing and require high air flows that are associated with loud noise levels.[50–52]

Other contributors to leak include nasal as opposed to oronasal masks because of leakage through the mouth.[23] Yet, even when properly fitted masks are applied using 'critical care ventilators' with dual limb circuits that do not require fixed intentional leaks, some leakage occurs under the mask seal, because of the irregularity of the facial contour and the laxity of the mandible. Air leaking is intensified by poorly fitted masks and high ventilator pressures.

The consequences of air leaks depend on the severity of the leak. Smaller leaks, in the range of 30 L/min or less, are generally well compensated by the ventilators and do not interfere with ventilator function. Large leaks (>60 L/min) wreak havoc, contributing to patient discomfort and agitation, patient–ventilator asynchrony, diminished tidal volumes and NIV failure. Leaks in between these limits cause problems depending on the location of the leak, the capability of the ventilator to compensate and synchronize and the patient's level of tolerance.[53]

Air leaks under the mask seal can be noisy and frightening to patients. Leaks not uncommonly occur along the sides of the nose, sometimes flowing into the eyes and causing conjunctivitis. During the use of nasal masks, leaks through the mouth cause increased air flow through the nose as the ventilator compensates by increasing and prolonging inspiratory flow. This can cause nasal dryness or congestion as well as nasal mucosal cooling which can increase nasal resistance.[54] Some air can leak into the oesophagus, causing gastric insufflation and distension, which can occasionally interfere with ventilation. But the most concerning consequences of leak are patient–ventilator asynchrony and NIV failure.

As mentioned in the section on asynchrony above, the high airflow rates associated with leak make it difficult for ventilators to sense the onset of inspiration and exhalation, leading to delayed and sometimes totally asynchronous ventilator inspiratory triggering as well as cycling.[46] Some ventilators respond to excessive leak by auto-cycling as their triggering function mistakes the leak for the patient's inspiratory flow.[53] Others delay cycling into expiration for more than 2 seconds as they permit total inspiratory durations of up to 3 seconds. At the extreme, excessively large leaks interfere with delivery of target pressure or volume leading to NIV failure.

The first step in managing air leaks is to monitor for them with the aim of detecting and managing them before adverse consequences occur. Some ventilators provide digital displays of leak flow rate that can be early indicators. Others have graphic displays of inspiratory flow that show the increases associated with leak. Most will alarm when target pressure or volume are not being reached. Once a leak is detected and is deemed large enough to cause problems, it should be located. Often the patient is aware of the leak, but the fingers can be used to detect leaks as well, moving them around the perimeter of the mask seal, keeping in mind that, during bi-level ventilation, some of the leaks are intentional.

Once detected, attempts are made to eliminate the leak or at least minimize it. Often, the initial reflex is to tighten the mask straps, sometimes intensifying discomfort and raising the risk of facial ulcers. Rather, the first step should be to pull the mask away from the face to reposition the mask and reseat the seal, which sometimes eliminates the problem. Next, straps should be adjusted, always attempting to use the minimal tension necessary to control the leak. When patients are using nasal masks, verbal instructions to close the mouth may help and chin straps may be helpful. But more often, switching to an oronasal or other larger mask may be necessary. When leaks are happening repeatedly, humidification of air may be helpful to avoid desiccation of mucosa and to enhance comfort. (See Figure 11.2, p. 100, for an algorithm for recognizing and dealing with leaks.) Gastric insufflation may be treated with agents such as simethicone or, in the unusual circumstance that it interferes with ventilation, nasogastric suction. Lowering inspiratory pressure or tidal volume is also an effective strategy to reduce air leaking, but may also intensify respiratory distress if lowered too much. Humidification of inspired gas may also help to alleviate mucosal drying, enhance comfort and alleviate work of breathing.[55]

## SUMMARY AND CONCLUSIONS

Over the past 20 years, NIV has occupied a growing role in the treatment of acute respiratory failure due to COPD exacerbations, acute cardiogenic pulmonary oedema and in association with immunocompromised states. It is also the ventilatory modality of first choice for chronic respiratory failure associated with neuromuscular disease or obesity, but its role in stable COPD remains to be defined. Although it is generally well tolerated, adverse effects are not uncommon and it suffers from a failure rate approaching 40 per cent in some series in the acute setting. Problems arising with NIV use are best avoided or dealt with promptly by selecting appropriate patients and monitoring them closely as long as they are acutely ill. Intolerance is a common problem related to mask discomfort, agitation or inappropriate ventilator settings. Using the right equipment delivered by a skilled, experienced staff helps to optimize outcomes. When there is a failure to ventilate or oxygenate, clinicians should rapidly assess the situation for reversible contributing factors, but be prepared to intubate without undue delay if rapid reversal cannot be achieved. A systematic approach to troubleshooting can help assure the best possible NIV outcomes.

## REFERENCES


1. Demoule A, Girou E, Richard JC *et al.* Increased use of noninvasive ventilation in French intensive care units. *Intensive Care Med* 2006; **32**: 1747–55.
2. Ozsancek A, Alkana P, Khodabandeh A *et al.* Increasing utilization of non-invasive positive pressure ventilation in acute care hospitals in Massachusetts and Rhode Island. *Am J Resp Crit Care Med* 2008; **177**: A283.
3. Lightowler JV, Wedjicha JA, Elliot MW *et al.* Non-invasive positive pressure ventilation to treat respiratory failure resulting from exacerbations of chronic obstructive pulmonary disease: Cochrane systematic review and meta-analysis. *BMJ* 2003; **326**: 185–9.
4. Masip J, Roque M, Sanchez B *et al.* Noninvasive ventilation in acute cardiogenic pulmonary edema. *JAMA* 2005; **294**: 3124–30.
5. Hilbert G, Gruson D, Vargas F *et al.* Noninvasive ventilation in immunosuppressed patients with pulmonary infiltrates, and acute respiratory failure. *N Engl J Med* 2001; **344**: 481–7.
6. Nava S, Hill N. Non-invasive ventilation in acute respiratory failure. *Lancet* 2009; **374**: 250–9.
7. Schettino G, Altobelli N, Kacmarek RM. Noninvasive positive pressure ventilation reverses acute respiratory failure in selected 'do-not-intubate' patients. *Crit Care Med* 2005; **33**: 1976–82.
8. Levy M, Tanios MA, Nelson D *et al.* Outcomes of patients with do-not-intubate orders treated with noninvasive ventilation. *Crit Care Med* 2004; **32**: 2002–7.
9. Soo Hoo GW, Santiago S, Williams AJ. Nasal mechanical ventilation for hypercapnic respiratory failure in chronic obstructive pulmonary disease: determinants of success and failure. *Crit Care Med* 1994; **22**: 1253–61.
10. Ambrosino N, Foglio K, Rubini F *et al.* Non-invasive mechanical ventilation in acute respiratory failure due to chronic obstructive pulmonary disease: correlates for success. *Thorax* 1995; **50**: 755–7.
11. Confalonieri M, Garuti G, Cattaruzza MS *et al.* Italian noninvasive positive pressure ventilation (NPPV) study group. A chart of failure risk for noninvasive ventilation in patients with COPD exacerbation. *Eur Respir J* 2005; **25**: 348–55.
12. Gonzalez Diaz G, Carillo A, Perez P *et al.* Noninvasive positive-pressure ventilation to treat hypercapnic coma secondary to respiratory failure. *Chest* 2005; **127**: 952–60.
13. Antonelli M, Conti G, Moro ML *et al.* Predictors of failures of noninvasive positive pressure ventilation in patients with acute hypoxemic respiratory failure: a multi-center study. *Intensive Care Med* 2001; **27**: 1718–28.
14. Rana S, Hussam J, Gay P *et al.* Failure of non-invasive ventilation in patients with acute lung injury: observational cohort study. *Crit Care* 2006; **10**: R79.
15. Antonelli M, Conti G, Esquinas A *et al.* A multiple-center survey on the use in clinical practice of noninvasive ventilation as a first-line intervention for acute respiratory distress syndrome. *Crit Care Med* 2007; **35**: 18–25.
16. Nava S, Ceriana P. Causes of failure of noninvasive mechanical ventilation. *Resp Care* 2004; **49**: 295–303.
17. Carlucci A, Delmastro M, Rubini F *et al.* Changes in the practice of non-invasive ventilation in treating COPD patients over 8 years. *Intensive Care Med* 2003; **29**: 419–25.
18. Keenan SP, Sinuff T, Cook DJ, *et al.* Which patients with acute exacerbation of chronic obstructive pulmonary disease benefit from noninvasive positive-pressure ventilation? A systematic review of the literature. *Ann Intern Med* 2003; **138**: 861–70.
19. Rocco M, Dell'Utri D, Morelli A, *et al.* Noninvasive ventilation by helmet or face mask in immunocompromised patients: a case-control study. *Chest* 2004; **126**: 1508–15.
20. Nourdine K, Combes P, Carton MJ *et al.* Does noninvasive ventilation reduce the ICU nosocomial infection risk? A prospective clinical survey. *Intensive Care Med* 1999; **25**: 567–573.
21. Hill NS. Where should noninvasive ventilation be delivered? *Respir Care* 2009; **54**: 62–70.
22. Giacomini M, Iapichino G, Cigada M *et al.* Short-term noninvasive pressure support ventilation prevents ICU admittance in patients with acute cardiogenic pulmonary edema. *Chest* 2003; **123**: 2057–61.
23. Kwok H, McCormack J, Cece R *et al.* Controlled trial of oronasal versus nasal mask ventilation in the treatment of acute respiratory failure. *Crit Care Med* 2003; **31**: 468–73.
24. Navalesi P, Fanfulla F, Frigerio P *et al.* Physiologic evaluation of noninvasive mechanical ventilation delivered by three types of masks in patients with chronic hypercapnic respiratory failure. *Crit Care Med* 2000; **28**: 1785–90.
25. Navalesi P, Costa R, Ceriana P *et al.* Non-invasive ventilation in chronic obstructive pulmonary disease patients: helmet versus facial mask. *Intensive Care Med* 2007; **33**: 74–81.
26. Cavaliere F, Conti G, Costa R *et al.* Noise exposure during noninvasive ventilation with a helmet, a nasal mask, and a facial mask. *Intensive Care Med* 2004; **30**: 1755–60.
27. Gregoretti C, Confalonieri M, Navalesi P *et al.* Evaluation of patient skin breakdown and comfort with a new face mask for non-invasive ventilation: a multi-center study. *Intensive Care Med* 2002; **28**: 278–84.
28. Devlin JW, Nava S, Fong JJ *et al.* Survey of sedation practices during noninvasive positive-pressure ventilation to treat acute respiratory failure. *Crit Care Med* 2007; **35**: 2298–302.
29. Salluh JI, Dal-Pizzol F, Mello PV *et al.* Delirium recognition and sedation practices in critically ill patients: a survey on the attitudes of 1015 Brazilian critical care physicians. *J Crit Care* 2009; **24**: 556–62.
30. Akada S, Takeda S, Yoshida Y *et al.* The efficacy of dexmedetomidine in patients with noninvasive ventilation: a preliminary study. *Anesth Analg* 2008; **107**: 167–70.
31. Iwama H, Suzuki M. Combined local-propofol anesthesia with noninvasive positive pressure ventilation in a

vasectomy patient with sleep apnea syndrome. *J Clin Anesth* 2003; **15**: 375–7.

32. Ferreira JC, Chipman DW, Hill NS *et al.* Bi-level vs. ICU ventilators providing noninvasive ventilation, effect of system leaks: a lung model comparison. *Chest* 2009; **136**: 448–56.
33. Arens R, Gozal D, Omlin KJ. Comparison of high frequency chest compression and conventional chest physiotherapy in hospitalized patients with cystic fibrosis. *Am J Respir Crit Care Med* 1994; **150**: 1154–7.
34. Tzeng AC, Bach JR. Prevention of pulmonary morbidity for patients with neuromuscular disease. *Chest* 2000; **118**: 1390–6.
35. Simonds AK. Recent advances in respiratory care for neuromuscular disease. *Chest* 2006; **130**: 1879–86.
36. Moretti M, Cilione C, Tampieri A *et al.* Incidence and causes of non-invasive mechanical ventilation failure after initial success. *Thorax* 2000; **55**: 819–25.
37. Schwartz AR, Kacmarek RM, Hess DR. Factors affecting oxygen delivery with bi-level positive airway pressure. *Respir Care* 2004; **49**: 270–5.
38. Brochard L, Mancebo J, Wysocki M *et al.* Noninvasive ventilation for acute exacerbations of chronic obstructive pulmonary disease. *N Engl J Med* 1995; **333**: 817–22.
39. Mehta S, McCool FD, Hill NS. Leak compensation in positive pressure ventilators: a lung model study. *Eur Respir J* 2001; **17**: 259–67.
40. Abou-Shala N, Meduri U. Noninvasive mechanical ventilation in patients with acute respiratory failure. *Crit Care Med* 1996; **24**: 705–15.
41. Schettino G, Altobelli N, Kacmarek RM. Noninvasive positive-pressure ventilation in acute respiratory failure outside clinical trials: experience at the Massachusetts General Hospital. *Crit Care Med* 2008; **36**: 441–7.
42. Jolliet P, Abajo B, Pasquina P *et al.* Non-invasive pressure support ventilation in severe community-acquired pneumonia. *Intensive Care Med* 2001; **27**: 812–21.
43. L'Her E, Deye N, Lellouche F *et al.* Physiologic effects of noninvasive ventilation during acute lung injury. *Am J Respir Crit Care Med* 2005; **172**: 1112–18.
44. Parthasarathy S, Jubran A, Tobin MJ. Cycling of inspiratory and expiratory muscle groups with the ventilator in airflow limitation. *Am J Respir Crit Care Med* 1998; **158**: 1471–8.
45. Hess DR. Ventilator waveforms and the physiology of pressure support ventilation. *Respir Care* 2005; **50**: 166–86.
46. Calderini E, Confalonieri M, Puccio PG *et al.* Patient-ventilator asynchrony during noninvasive ventilation: the role of expiratory trigger. *Intensive Care Med* 1999; **25**: 662–7.
47. Bonmarchand G, Chevron V, Chopin C *et al.* Increased initial flow rate reduces inspiratory work of breathing during pressure support ventilation in patients with exacerbation of chronic obstructive pulmonary disease. *Intensive Care Med* 1996; **22**: 1147–54.
48. Prinianakis G, Delmastro M, Carlucci A. Effect of varying the pressurization rate during noninvasive pressure support ventilation. *Eur Respir J* 2004; **23**: 314–20.
49. Vignaux L, Tassaux D, Jolliet P. Performance of noninvasive ventilation modes on ICU ventilators during pressure support: a bench model study. *Intensive Care Med* 2007; **33**: 1444–51.
50. Ferguson GT, Gilmartin M. $CO_2$ rebreathing during BiPAP ventilatory assistance. *Am J Respir Crit Care Med* 1995; **151**: 1126–35.
51. Lofaso F, Brochard L, Touchard D *et al.* Evaluation of carbon dioxide rebreathing during pressure support ventilation with BiPAP devices. *Chest* 1995; **108**: 772–8.
52. Schettino GPP, Chatmongkolchart S, Hess D *et al.* Position of exhalation port and mask design affect CO2 rebreathing during noninvasive positive pressure ventilation. *Crit Care Med* 2003; **31**: 2178–82.
53. Cavaliere F, Conti G, Costa R, *et al.* Noise exposure during noninvasive ventilation with a helmet, a nasal mask, and a facial mask. *Intensive Care Med* 2004; **30**: 1755–60.
54. Richards GN, Cistulli PA, Ungar RG *et al.* Mouth leak with nasal continuous positive airway pressure increases nasal airway resistance. *Am J Respir Crit Care Med* 1996; **154**: 182–6.
55. Lellouche F, Maggiore SM, Deye N *et al.* Effect of the humidification device on the work of breathing during noninvasive ventilation. *Intensive Care Med* 2002; **28**: 1582–9.

# 13

# Timing of non-invasive ventilation

STEFANO NAVA, PAOLO NAVALESI

## ABSTRACT

Non-invasive ventilation (NIV) is a safe, versatile and effective technique that can avoid the side effects and complications associated with endotracheal intubation. The success of NIV relies on several factors including the type and severity of acute respiratory failure, underlying disease, location of treatment, and experience of the team. Timing is also an important factor. NIV is primarily used: to prevent the occurrence of impending (but not established) acute respiratory failure; at an early stage, when respiratory failure is already established, to avoid the need for endotracheal intubation; as an alternative to invasive ventilation at a more advanced stage of acute respiratory failure; if the patient has required intubation to prevent the development of respiratory failure once extubated; to treat established post-extubation respiratory failure; and to facilitate the process of weaning from mechanical ventilation. The chapter analyses, compares and discusses the results of studies in which NIV was applied at various times during the evolution of acute respiratory failure.

## INTRODUCTION

The timing of non-invasive ventilation (NIV) application is important. If, on the one hand, the chances of successful application of NIV are increased when it is initiated early to avert excessive progression of the underlying disorder, on the other hand, if it started too early, when the patient's condition is such that ventilatory assistance is not truly needed, they are more likely to develop mask intolerance. Finally, there are those situations in which the patient is already admitted to the hospital in a critical condition, and mandatory and rapid application of mechanical ventilation is required. Even in these circumstances, a cautious NIV attempt may be considered, especially for some specific pathologies, but only if prompt intubation may be provided in the case of NIV failure. Clearly, the timing of NIV institution affects duration and intensity of NIV.[1]

As summarized in Figure 13.1, NIV may be used at different times, which in this chapter are classified as:

- to prevent the occurrence of impending (but not established) acute respiratory failure (ARF)
- at an early stage, when respiratory failure is already established, to avert the need for endotracheal intubation
- as an alternative to invasive ventilation at a more advanced stage of ARF
- if the patient has required intubation to prevent the development of respiratory failure once extubated
- to treat established post-extubation respiratory failure and
- to facilitate the process of weaning from mechanical ventilation.

## NON-INVASIVE VENTILATION TO PREVENT ACUTE RESPIRATORY FAILURE

### Exacerbation of chronic obstructive pulmonary disease and hypercapnic respiratory failure

Very few studies have so far assessed the efficacy of NIV in preventing the occurrence of ARF, and all of those that have done have included patients with a mild exacerbation of chronic obstructive pulmonary disease (COPD). Bardi *et al.*[2] randomized 30 patients, the large majority of whom had a pH >7.35, to early NIV or medical therapy alone. No significant reduction was found in mortality, or improvement in need for endotracheal intubation or time spent in hospital. In a similar population, Keenan *et al.*[3]

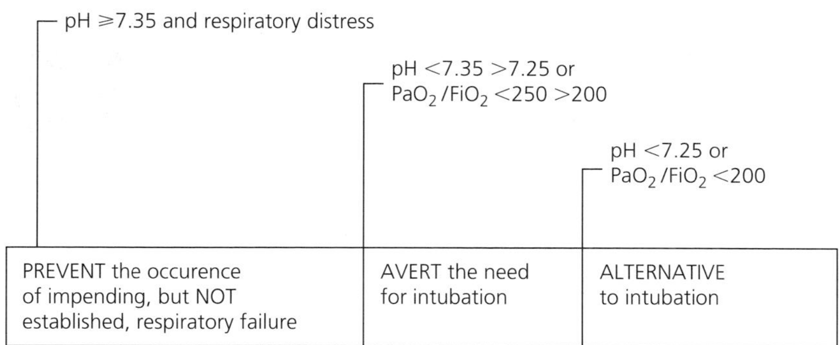


**Figure 13.1** Use of non-invasive ventilation at different times in the patient journey.

reported no difference in any clinical outcome, but a significant reduction in dyspnoea with NIV, although mask ventilation was found to be very poorly tolerated. Conversely Pastaka *et al.*[4] found that patients with a pH >7.35 receiving NIV demonstrated good tolerance to the technique and, in contrast to those in the control group who received the sole medical treatment, had faster improvement in arterial blood gases and shorter length of hospital stay. According to these studies, anticipating the use of NIV in patients with an exacerbation of COPD to prevent, rather than to treat, respiratory distress and ventilatory failure may be futile, and would therefore be an unnecessary waste of resources.

### Cardiogenic pulmonary oedema

Some studies performed on cardiogenic pulmonary oedema did not include as a primary enrolment criterion the presence of ARF. For example Park *et al.*[5] studied those patients with acute onset of respiratory distress (breathing rate >25 breaths/min), associated tachycardia and diaphoresis, and findings of pulmonary congestion on physical examination, and similar criteria were used by Crane *et al.*[6] All these investigations showed overall a more rapid improvement of gas exchange, dyspnoea and, in one study, a reduction in intubation rate, using either continuous positive airway pressure (CPAP) or pressure support with the addition of CPAP versus oxygen therapy alone. Indeed Crane *et al.* also demonstrated a statistically higher hospital survival rate but only in the CPAP group.

The results of these two studies suggest a possible role of this technique as a means to prevent the occurrence of ARF during an episode of cardiogenic pulmonary oedema with respiratory distress.

### *De novo* hypoxic respiratory failure

There are no studies on the use of NIV to prevent an episode of ARF in this condition.

## NON-INVASIVE VENTILATION TO AVERT THE NEED OF ENDOTRACHEAL INTUBATION AND REINTUBATION

### Chronic obstructive pulmonary disease exacerbation and hypercapnic respiratory failure

The patients who benefit most from NIV are those with acute respiratory acidosis caused by an exacerbation of COPD.[7] In the past decade, several randomized controlled trials (RCTs) have shown that the addition of NIV to medical treatment relieves dyspnoea, improves vital signs and gas exchange, prevents endotracheal intubation, reduces complications, lowers mortality and shortens the time spent in hospital.[8–12] Brochard *et al.*[9] however, found that the benefits of NIV over standard treatment vanished when only those patients in whom treatment failed and those who required intubation were considered.

Notwithstanding a general consensus on the value of NIV, resulting from this large body of evidence, some aspects still deserve consideration. For example, one randomized trial[13] found that adding NIV to standard treatment in hypercapnic COPD patients admitted to a respiratory ward with very mild ARF did not produce further advantages; the success rate, however, was 100 per cent for both NIV and standard treatment. In a large multicenter trial, Plant *et al.*[8] found that rate of intubation and mortality were overall reduced when NIV was added to the standard medical therapy; a subgroup analysis, however, indicated that the improvement was limited to those patients who had a pH ≥7.30. The authors surmised that the patients with pH <7.30 might have fared better in the intensive care unit (ICU) rather than in the ward.

Surprisingly there are no RCTs assessing the use of NIV in those patients with hypercapnic respiratory failure related to restrictive thoracic disorders, despite the clinical use in this condition is relatively wide. The only retrospective study[14] performed in restrictive thoracic disorders showed that the effectiveness of NIV for acute decompensation is less in patients with chronic restrictive pulmonary disease as compared with those with COPD.

In conclusion, considering the strong evidence of efficacy and the relatively low risk of failure, to avoid intubation in COPD patients with mild to moderate ARF NIV is considered the ventilatory therapy of first choice and can be safely administered in appropriately monitored and staffed areas outside the ICU. Patients with a lower pH are still candidates for NIV, but transfer to a more closely monitored location is strongly advised.

## Cardiogenic pulmonary oedema

Non-invasive ventilation has been used to avoid intubation during an episode of ARF in patients with cardiogenic pulmonary oedema.[15–18] Several meta-analyses[19,20] have concluded that the addition to the standard medical therapy of non-invasive CPAP (n-CPAP) with or without addition of inspiratory support reduces the rate of intubation. These conclusions have been recently challenged by the results of a large multicentre trial comparing oxygen therapy alone, n-CPAP and NIV.[18] The authors concluded that although the clinical and physiological improvement was faster with CPAP and NIV, compared with oxygen alone, there was no significant difference between the groups with respect to rate of intubation and mortality. The quite low rate of intubation in this study (<3 per cent) has raised questions as to whether the patient population was comparable with that of other studies.

In conclusion, the results of several RCTs indicated that both CPAP and NIV may effectively reduce the rate of intubation and in some instances mortality, when compared with oxygen therapy.

## *De novo* hypoxic respiratory failure

Several clinical trials have evaluated NIV as a means to prevent intubation in patients with mild to moderate hypoxaemic ARF (i.e. $PaO_2/FiO_2 \geq 200$) of varied aetiology. The results have been controversial.

Wysocki *et al.*[21] showed that, compared with standard therapy, NIV reduced the need for endotracheal intubation, shortened the duration of ICU stay and decreased mortality rate only in the subgroup of patients with associated hypercapnia, and produced no advantage in purely hypoxaemic patients. In contrast, in a similar group of patients Martin *et al.*[22] found that NIV reduced the rate of intubation. Ferrer and co-workers[23] randomized a group of 105 patients with hypoxaemic ARF to receive either NIV or high oxygen concentration alone. NIV reduced the need for endotracheal intubation, incidence of septic shock, ICU mortality and 90-day mortality.

One of the major confounders in these studies was the marked variability of the case mix; patients with different underlying disorders and patho-physiological pathways were included under the same generic definition of having hypoxaemia. Confalonieri *et al.*[24] evaluated NIV in patients with ARF ($PaO_2/FiO_2$ <250) consequent to community acquired pneumonia, including patients both with and without COPD. Compared with standard treatment alone, NIV produced a significant reduction in respiratory rate, need for endotracheal intubation and ICU stay. However, a subgroup analysis showed that the benefits of NIV occurred only in the subgroup of COPD patients.

Major surgery is sometimes complicated by the occurrence of atelectasis and pneumonia, which lead to hypoxaemia and respiratory distress during the early post-operative period. A randomized study[25] showed that n-CPAP delivered through a helmet decreases atelectasis and prevents pneumonia more effectively than standard therapy alone during an episode of mild respiratory failure after upper abdominal surgery; another study showed that NIV significantly ameliorates gas exchange and pulmonary function abnormalities after gastroplasty in obese patients.[26]

NIV may be used in the early treatment of ARF secondary to lung resection, a fatal complication in up to 80 per cent of cases. Auriant *et al.*[27] showed that NIV is safe and effective in reducing the need for intubation and improving survival. Early NIV application may be extremely helpful in immunocompromised patients, in whom intubation greatly increases the risk of pneumonia, infections and ICU mortality.

Antonelli *et al.*[28] compared NIV with standard therapy in solid organ transplant recipients with hypoxaemic ARF. Within the first hour of treatment, $PaO_2/FiO_2$ improved in 70 per cent of patients in the NIV group and in only 25 per cent of patients receiving medical therapy alone. NIV was associated with a significant reduction in the rate of intubation, complications, mortality and duration of ICU stay among survivors. In patients with immunosuppression secondary to haematological malignancies, transplantation or human immunodeficiency virus infection, Hilbert *et al.*[29] compared early NIV with standard treatment. All patients had fever, bilateral pulmonary infiltrates and hypoxaemia. Fewer patients in the NIV group required intubation, had serious complications or died in the ICU or in the hospital.

The use of NIV for severe acute respiratory syndrome (SARS) and other airborne diseases has generated debate. Two observational studies from China[30,31] found no evidence of viral spread to caregivers who took appropriate precautions. In the event of a flu pandemic, ventilator resources are likely to be severely strained, and NIV may offer a means of supporting some of the afflicted, mainly those with initial respiratory failure. However, some consider NIV contraindicated in respiratory failure from communicable respiratory airborne diseases unless it is used within a negative pressure isolation room and strict precautions are taken.

Patients with severe irreversible chronic medical diseases often eschew invasive mechanical ventilation when they present with ARF and/or distress and it may even be medically inappropriate when they are in terminal stages of their disease. NIV may be seen as an intermediate step for relieving symptoms as well as for achieving hospital survival in some cases. Two large US-based studies[32,33] on patients with ARF and do not intubate (DNI) order observed that about half of the patients treated with NIV survived and were discharged from the hospital. The underlying disease was an important determinant of survival; patients with congestive heart failure (CHF) and COPD had better survival rates than those with pneumonia or cancer. Observational studies have also reported that NIV may be effective in relieving respiratory distress in patients admitted to either a respiratory unit[34] or a palliative care unit.[35]

In conclusion, the outcome of NIV in patients with hypoxaemic ARF for whose endotracheal intubation is not mandatory yet, depends primarily on the type and evolution of the underlying disorder. The high rate of failure of NIV in community-acquired pneumonia and acute respiratory distress syndrome suggests for these patients a cautious approach consisting of early treatment and avoidance of delay of needed intubation. A trial of NIV is advisable in immunosuppressed patients (in whom intubation is, *per se*, a strong predictor of mortality), after lung resection and major abdominal surgery. Patients with CHF or COPD with DNI orders respond well to NIV, but use for other diagnoses as well as for palliation, although appealing, requires further study.

## NON-INVASIVE VENTILATION AS AN ALTERNATIVE TO INVASIVE VENTILATION

### Exacerbations of chronic obstructive pulmonary disease

Only one RCT has compared NIV with invasive ventilation in COPD patients with severe ARF in whom ventilatory support was deemed necessary.[36] The average pH on study entry was 7.20 for both groups, indicating that these patients had more severe ARF than those enrolled in the clinical trials in which NIV was used at an earlier stage. In the NIV group, treatment failed in 12 patients (52 per cent), who were thus intubated to receive invasive mechanical ventilation. The authors found no significant differences between the two groups in ICU and hospital mortality, overall complications, duration of mechanical ventilation and ICU stay. The patients in the NIV group had a lower rate of sepsis and septic shock and showed a trend toward a lower incidence of nosocomial pneumonia during their time in the ICU. In addition, at a 12-month follow-up, the rate of hospital readmissions and the number of patients on long-term oxygen therapy were lower in the NIV group.

These results were confirmed by a subsequent case–control clinical trial[37] including 64 consecutive COPD patients with severe ARF caused by exacerbation or community-acquired pneumonia. The average pH in the patients and controls on entry into the study was 7.18. Non-invasive ventilation failed in 40 patients (62 per cent) who were intubated. The mortality rate, duration of mechanical ventilation, time spent in the ICU and duration of post-ICU hospitalization were similar in the two groups; however, patients in the NIV group had fewer complications and showed a trend toward a lower probability of remaining on mechanical ventilation after 30 days. Apart from confirming the results obtained by Conti *et al.*,[36] the large sample of patients and high rate of NIV failures allowed a subgroup analysis that showed that the outcomes of the 40 patients in whom NIV failed and of the 64 controls were no different, while the 24 patients in whom NIV was successful had better outcomes.

In all the aforementioned studies NIV was used in an ICU and the study protocols had predefined criteria for NIV failure which led in all cases to a prompt intubation, when required.

In conclusion, in patients with COPD deemed severe enough to require ventilatory support, the use of NIV at a more advanced stage of ARF is more likely to fail. A NIV trial before proceeding to intubation and invasive ventilation does not, however, harm the patient and may be cautiously attempted, while closely monitoring the patient in an ICU and avoiding excessive delay of the required intubation.

### Cardiogenic pulmonary oedema

There are no studies formally assessing the use of NIV as a real alternative to intubation for cardiogenic pulmonary oedema, despite the only randomized trial[38] that has so far evaluated the use of NIV in hypoxaemic patients considered sufficiently ill to require mandatory ventilatory assistance, which enrolled about 20 per cent of patients with this pathology. Interestingly, four of seven patients in the NIV group did not require intubation, so that it may be suggested that a cautious NIV trial may be performed even in the presence of severe ARF due to cardiogenic pulmonary oedema.

### *De novo* hypoxic respiratory failure

Antonelli *et al.*[38] compared NIV with conventional ventilation through an endotracheal tube in selected patients with hypoxaemic ARF. Sixty-four consecutive patients were enrolled. After 1 hour of mechanical ventilation, the $PaO_2/FiO_2$ ratio had improved in both groups. Ten patients in the NIV group required intubation. Patients randomized to conventional ventilation more frequently developed serious complications and, in particular, infections secondary to endotracheal intubation. Among survivors, the duration of mechanical ventilation and ICU stay was shorter in patients randomized to NIV. It should, however, be kept in mind that this single study was conducted in selected patients in one well-experienced centre.

A study performed in three European ICUs having expertise with NIV clarifies the issue of the 'real life' use of NIV in these conditions.[39] It was shown that 'only' 16.5 per cent of the patients admitted with acute respiratory distress syndrome may be successfully treated with this technique. In two years time, 479 patients were admitted and the large majority of these patients (69 per cent) were already intubated at admission, so that only 147 were eligible for this study. NIV improved gas exchange and avoided intubation in 54 per cent of this subset of patients, leading to an overall success rate <20 per cent. This was associated with less ventilator-associated pneumonia and lower ICU mortality rate (6 per cent versus 53 per cent). In summary, the use of NIV as an alternative to invasive ventilation in severely hypoxaemic patients is not generally advisable and should be limited to haemodynamically stable patients who can be closely monitored in an ICU.

## NON-INVASIVE VENTILATION TO PREVENT EXTUBATION FAILURE IN THOSE PATIENTS PREVIOUSLY INTUBATED

Postextubation failure is a major clinical problem in ICUs since extubation attempts may fail in as many as 23.5 per cent of patients and the in-hospital mortality of these patients may approach 30–40 per cent.[40] The cause of extubation failure and the time elapsed before reintubation are independent predictors of outcome.[41]

Two randomized trials have been performed to assess whether NIV is effective in preventing the occurrence of post-extubation failure in patients at risk.[42,43] Both studies, which adopted similar criteria to define patients at risk and had comparable study designs, showed that the groups treated with NIV had a lower rate of reintubation than the groups in which standard therapy was used; furthermore, in one of the two studies a *post-hoc* analysis showed that ICU mortality was also reduced in the subgroup of hypercapnic patients treated with NIV.[43] A more recent RCT performed in this specific condition has confirmed this important result.[44]

Obesity is an epidemic health and socioeconomic problem in many countries and predisposes to chronic alveolar hypoventilation and/or respiratory problem in the post-extubation period. El-Solh *et al.*[45] showed in a case–control study that NIV may be effective in averting respiratory failure in severely obese patients when applied preventively. In the subgroup of hypercapnic patients, NIV also conferred a survival benefit.

In conclusion, promptly initiated use of NIV for at least 48 hours in selected patients 'at risk' may prevent post-extubation respiratory failure, especially in those patients with persistent hypercapnia.

## NON-INVASIVE VENTILATION TO TREAT ESTABLISHED POST-EXTUBATION RESPIRATORY FAILURE OR DISTRESS

The use of NIV has been suggested in an attempt to avoid reintubation in patients who show signs of 'incipient' or even overt respiratory failure following extubation.[41] In one RCT, NIV was applied to patients who developed ARF within 48 hours after extubation and compared with standard medical therapy.[46] The patients were randomized to standard therapy alone or to NIV. The authors did not find any difference in reintubation rate, hospital mortality rate, ICU and hospital stay, despite there being a trend to a shorter duration of hospital stay in the NIV group.

Esteban *et al.*[47] conducted a large multicentre, randomized trial to evaluate the effect of NIV on mortality in this clinical setting. Patients who had respiratory failure were randomly assigned within the subsequent 48 hours to either NIV (114 patients) or standard medical therapy (107 patients). There was no difference between the two groups in the need for reintubation, but ICU mortality was higher in the NIV group (25 per cent vs 14 per cent; relative risk = 1.78); the median time from respiratory failure to reintubation was longer in the NIV group, raising the doubt that this delay in reintubation may have influenced the negative results. The authors concluded that NIV does not prevent the need for reintubation or reduce mortality in unselected patients who have respiratory failure after extubation. It is noteworthy that NIV was used as a 'rescue' therapy in the patients who failed standard therapy and the rate of success was much higher than in the NIV group.

In summary, in spite of the early promising data from non-randomized studies, NIV does not prevent the need for reintubation or reduce mortality in unselected patients with established post-extubation respiratory failure.

## NON-INVASIVE VENTILATION TO FACILITATE THE PROCESS OF WEANING FROM INVASIVE VENTILATION

In the majority of cases withdrawal of mechanical ventilation and extubation are possible immediately after resolution of the underlying problems responsible for ARF. However, there is a group of ventilated patients who require more gradual and longer withdrawal of mechanical ventilation. NIV is theoretically able to counteract several physiological mechanisms associated with weaning failure or difficulties. In ventilator-dependent COPD patients NIV has been shown to be as effective as invasive ventilation in reducing inspiratory effort and improving arterial blood gases.[48] The first RCT of this strategy was performed in severely ill COPD patients ventilated through an endotracheal tube.[49] Patients who failed the T-piece trial were randomized to either extubation, with immediate application of NIV, or to continued weaning with the endotracheal tube in place. Overall, this study showed that when NIV is used as a weaning technique the likelihood of weaning success is increased, whereas the duration of mechanical ventilation and ICU stay are decreased.

A second RCT was conducted on patients with chronic respiratory disorders, intubated for an episode of ARF.[50] This study also found a shorter duration of invasive mechanical ventilation in the groups weaned non-invasively, although no differences were found in ICU or hospital stay or 3-month survival. In a third RCT, patients who failed spontaneous breathing trials on 3 consecutive days were randomized to either extubation and NIV or remaining intubated and continuing a conventional weaning protocol.[51] Most of the patients had hypercapnic respiratory failure. The duration of conventional mechanical ventilation, time spent in the ICU and the duration of hospitalization were significantly reduced in the NIV group. Patients treated with NIV also had lower rates of nosocomial pneumonia and septic shock and better 90-day survival.

A recent study randomized unselected patients who failed a spontaneous breathing T-piece to extubation and NIV or traditional weaning trial during invasive ventilation.[52] The percentage of complications in the NIV group was lower, with lower incidences of pneumonia and tracheostomy. Length of stay in the intensive care unit and mortality were not statistically different when comparing the groups. Further studies are clearly needed to assess the real benefits of NIV in weaning in other forms of respiratory failure, such as acute respiratory distress syndrome, post-surgical complications or cardiac impairment.

In conclusion, in accord with the results of a recent meta-analysis,[53] NIV may be safely and successfully used in ICU to shorten the process of liberation from mechanical ventilation in stable patients recovering from an episode of hypercapnic ARF who had previously failed a weaning trial.

## CONCLUSIONS

Following on from a 'pioneering era', NIV is currently a therapeutic strategy that belongs to the real world of clinical practice. It should primarily be used for the early treatment of established episodes of ARF, in order to avoid further deterioration and intubation, and eventually to shorten the duration of invasive mechanical ventilation in COPD patients. Depending on the type and severity of the episode of ARF, on the prognosis of the underlying disease, on the setting where it is applied, and on the level of expertise of the team involved, NIV may be profitably applied at different timings. To paraphrase from a famous song, 'time is on NIV's side'.[54]

## REFERENCES


1. Nava S, Navalesi P, Conti G. Time of non-invasive ventilation *Intensive Care Med* 2006; **32**: 361–70.
2. Bardi G, Pierotello R, Desideri M *et al.* Nasal ventilation in COPD exacerbations: early and late results of a prospective, controlled study. *Eur Respir J* 2000; **15**: 98–104.
3. Keenan SP, Powers CE, McCormack DG. Noninvasive positive-pressure ventilation in patients with milder chronic obstructive pulmonary disease exacerbations: a randomized controlled trial. *Respir Care* 2005; **50**: 610–16.
4. Pastaka C, Kostikas K, Karetsi E *et al.* Non-invasive ventilation in chronic hypercapnic COPD patients with exacerbation and a pH of 7.35. *Eur J Intern Med* 2007; **18**: 524–30.
5. Park M, Sangean MC, Volpe MS *et al.* Randomized, prospective trial of oxygen, continuous positive airway pressure, and bilevel positive airway pressure by face mask in acute cardiogenic pulmonary edema. *Crit Care Med* 2004; **32**: 2407–15.
6. Crane SD, Elliott MW, Gilligan P *et al.* Randomised controlled comparison of continuous positive airways pressure, bilevel non-invasive ventilation, and standard treatment in emergency department patients with acute cardiogenic pulmonary edema. *Emerg Med J* 2004; **21**: 155–61.
7. Lightowler JV, Wedzicha JA, Elliott MW *et al.* Non-invasive positive pressure ventilation to treat respiratory failure resulting from exacerbations of chronic obstructive pulmonary disease: Cochrane systematic review and meta-analysis. *BMJ* 2003; **326**: 185.
8. Plant PK, Owen JL, Elliot MW. A multicentre randomised controlled trial of the early use of non-invasive ventilation in acute exacerbation of chronic obstructive pulmonary disease on general respiratory wards. *Lancet* 2000; **335**: 1931–5.
9. Brochard L, Mancebo J, Wysochi M *et al.* Noninvasive ventilation for acute exacerbation of chronic obstructive pulmonary disease. *N Engl J Med* 1995; **333**: 817–22.
10. Bott J, Carrol MP, Conway JH *et al.* Randomised controlled trial of nasal ventilation in acute ventilatory failure due to chronic obstructive airways disease. *Lancet* 1993; **341**: 1555–7.
11. Kramer N, Meyer TJ, Meharg J *et al.* Randomized, prospective trial of noninvasive positive pressure ventilation in acute respiratory failure. *Am J Respir Crit Care* 1995; **151**: 1799–806.
12. Celikel T, Sungur M, Cayhan B *et al.* Comparison of noninvasive positive pressure ventilation with standard medical therapy in hypercapnic acute respiratory failure. *Chest* 1998; **114**: 1636–42.
13. Barbè F, Togores B, Rubi M *et al.* Noninvasive ventilatory support does not facilitate recovery from acute respiratory failure in chronic obstructive pulmonary disease. *Eur Respr J* 1996; **9**: 1240–5.
14. Robino C, Faisy C, Dieh JL *et al.* Effectiveness of non-invasive positive pressure ventilation differs between decompensated chronic restrictive and obstructive pulmonary disease patients. *Intensive Care Med* 2003; **29**: 603–10.
15. Mehta S, Jay GD, Woolard RH *et al.* Randomized, prospective trial of bilevel versus continuous positive

airway pressure in acute pulmonary edema. *Crit Care Med* 1997; **25**: 620–8.
16. Masip J, Betbese AJ, Paez J *et al.* Non-invasive pressure support ventilation versus conventional oxygen therapy in acute cardiogenic pulmonary oedema: a randomised trial. *Lancet* 2000; **356**: 26–32.
17. Nava S, Carbone G, Dibattista N *et al.* Noninvasive ventilation in cardiogenic pulmonary edema: a multicenter, randomized trial. *Am J Respir Crit Care Med* 2003; **168**: 1432–7.
18. Gray A, Goodacre S, Newby DE *et al.* Noninvasive ventilation in acute cardiogenic pulmonary edema. *N Engl J Med* 2008; **359**: 142–51.
19. Masip J, Rocha M, Sanchez B *et al.* Non invasive ventilation in acute pulmonary edema. Systematic review and meta-analysis. *JAMA* 2005; **294**: 3124–30.
20. Peter JV, Moran JL, Phillips-Hughes J *et al.* Effect of non-invasive positive pressure ventilation on mortality in patients with acute cardiogenic pulmonary oedema: a meta-analysis. *Lancet* 2006; **367**: 1155–63.
21. Wysocki M, Tric L, Wolff MA *et al.* Noninvasive pressure support ventilation in patients with acute respiratory failure. A randomized comparison with conventional therapy. *Chest* 1995; **107**: 761–8.
22. Martin TJ, Hovis JD, Costantino JP *et al.* A randomized, prospective evaluation of noninvasive ventilation for acute respiratory failure. *Am J Respir Crit Care Med* 2000; **161**: 807–13.
23. Ferrer M, Esquinas A, Leon M *et al.* Noninvasive ventilation in severe hypoxemic respiratory failure: a randomised clinical trial. *Am J Respir Crit Care Med* 2003; **168**: 1438–44.
24. Confalonieri M, Della Porta R, Potena A *et al.* Acute respiratory failure in patients with severe community-acquired pneumonia: a prospective randomized evaluation of noninvasive ventilation. *Am J Respir Crit Care Med* 1999; **160**: 1585–91.
25. Squadrone V, Coha M, Cerutti E *et al.* Continuous positive airway pressure for treatment of postoperative hypoxemia. *JAMA* 2005; **293**: 589–95.
26. Joris JL, Sottiaux TM, Chiche JD *et al.* Effect of bi-level positive airway pressure nasal ventilation on the postoperative pulmonary restrictive syndrome in obese patients undergoing gastroplasty. *Chest* 1997; **111**: 665–70.
27. Auriant I, Jallot A, Herve P *et al.* Noninvasive ventilation reduces mortality in acute respiratory failure following lung resection. *Am J Respir Crit Care Med* 2001; **164**: 1231–5.
28. Antonelli M, Conti G, Bufi M *et al.* Noninvasive ventilation for treatment of acute respiratory failure in patients undergoing solid organ transplantation: a randomized trial. *JAMA* 2000; **283**: 235–41.
29. Hilbert G, Gruson D, Vargas F *et al.* Noninvasive ventilation in immunosuppressed patients with pulmonary infiltrates, fever, and acute respiratory failure. *N Engl J Med* 2001; **344**: 481–7.
30. Cheung TMT, Lau CWA, Poon E *et al.* Effectiveness of noninvasive positive pressure ventilation in the treatment of acute respiratory failure in severe acute respiratory syndrome. *Chest* 2004; **126**: 845–50.
31. Zaho Z, Zhang F, Xu M *et al.* Description and clinical treatment of an early outbreak of severe acute respiratory syndrome (SARS) in Guangzhou, PR China. *J Med Microbiol* 2003; **52**: 715–20.
32. Levy M, Tanios MA, Nelson D *et al.* Outcomes of patients with do-not-intubate orders treated with noninvasive ventilation. *Crit Care Med* 2004; **32**: 2002–7.
33. Schettino G, Altobelli N, Kacmarek RM. Noninvasive positive pressure ventilation reverses acute respiratory failure in selected 'do-not-intubate' patients. *Crit Care Med* 2005; **33**: 1976–82.
34. Nava S, Sturani C, Hartl S *et al.* ERS Task Force. End-of-life decision-making in respiratory intermediate care units: a European survey. *Eur Respir J* 2007; **30**: 156–64.
35. Cuomo A, Conti G, Delmastro M *et al.* Noninvasive mechanical ventilation as a palliative tretment of acute respiratory failure in patients with end-stage solid cancer. *Palliat Med* 2004; **18**: 602–10.
36. Conti G, Antonelli M, Navalesi P *et al.* Noninvasive vs. conventional mechanical ventilation in patients with chronic obstructive pulmonary disease after failure of medical treatment in the ward: a randomized trial. *Intensive Care Med* 2002; **28**: 1701–7.
37. Squadrone E, Frigerio P, Fogliati C *et al.* Noninvasive vs invasive ventilation in COPD patients with severe acute respiratory failure deemed to require ventilatory assistance. *Intensive Care Med* 2004; **30**: 1303–10.
38. Antonelli M, Conti G, Rocco M *et al.* A comparison of noninvasive positive-pressure ventilation and conventional mechanical ventilation in patients with acute respiratory failure. *N Engl J Med* 1998; **339**: 429–35.
39. Antonelli M, Conti G, Esquinas A *et al.* A multiple-center survey on the use in clinical practice of noninvasive ventilation as a first-line intervention for acute respiratory distress syndrome. *Crit Care Med* 2007; **35**: 18–25.
40. Epstein SK, Ciubataru RL, Wong JB. Effect of failed extubation on the outcome of mechanical ventilation. *Chest* 1997; **112**: 186–92.
41. Espstein SK, Ciubotaru RL. Independent effects of etiology of failure and time of reintubation on outcome for patients failing extubation. *Am J Respir Crit Care Med* 1998; **158**: 489–93.
42. Nava S, Gregoretti C, Fanfulla F *et al.* Noninvasive ventilation to prevent respiratory failure after extubation in high risk patients. *Crit Care Med* 2005; **33**: 2465–70.
43. Ferrer M, Valencia M, Nicolas JM *et al.* Early non-invasive ventilation averts extubation failure in patients at risk: a randomized trial. *Am J Respir Crit Care Med* 2006; **173**: 164–70.
44. Ferrer M, Sellarés J, Valencia M *et al.* Non-invasive ventilation after extubation in hypercapnic patients with chronic respiratory disorders: randomised controlled trial. *Lancet* 2009; **374**: 1082–8.

45. El-Solh AA, Aquilina A, Pineda L *et al.* Noninvasive ventilation for prevention of post-extubation respiratory failure in obese patients. *Eur Respir J* 2006; **28**: 588–95.
46. Keenan SP, Powers C, McCormack DG *et al.* Noninvasive positive-pressure ventilation for postextubation respiratory distress. *JAMA* 2002; **287**: 3238–44.
47. Esteban A, Frutos-Vivar F, Ferguson ND *et al.* Non-invasive positive pressure ventilation for respiratory failure after extubation. *N Engl J Med* 2004; **350**: 2452–60.
48. Vitacca M, Ambrosino N, Clini E *et al.* Physiological response to pressure support ventilation delivered before and after extubation in patients not capable of totally spontaneous autonomous breathing. *Am J Respir Crit Care Med* 2001; **164**: 638–41.
49. Nava S, Ambrosino N, Clini E *et al.* Noninvasive mechanical ventilation in the weaning of patients with respiratory failure due to chronic obstructive pulmonary disease. A randomized, controlled trial. *Ann Intern Med* 1998; **128**: 721–8.
50. Girault C, Daudenthun I, Chevron V *et al.* Noninvasive ventilation as a systematic extubation and weaning technique in acute-on-chronic respiratory failure. A prospective, randomized controlled study. *Am J Respir Crit Care Med* 1999; **160**: 86–92.
51. Ferrer M, Esquinas A, Arancibia F *et al.* Noninvasive ventilation during persistent weaning failure: a randomized controlled trial. *Am J Respir Crit Care Med* 2003; **168**: 70–6.
52. Trevisan CE, Vieira SR. Research group in mechanical ventilation weaning. Noninvasive mechanical ventilation may be useful in treating patients who fail weaning from invasive mechanical ventilation: a randomized clinical trial. *Crit Care* 2008; **12**: R51.
53. Burns KEA, Adhikari NK, Keenan SP *et al.* Use of non-invasive ventilation to wean critically ill adults off invasive ventilation: meta-analysis and systematic review. *BMJ* 2009; **338**: b1574.
54. Winding K and his orchestra. *Time is on my side.* Verve Records, 1963.

# 14

# Why non-invasive ventilation works in acute respiratory failure

MIQUEL FERRER, ANTONI TORRES


## ABSTRACT

Non-invasive ventilation (NIV) is an effective support for severe acute respiratory failure (ARF) with different etiologies. The pathophysiology of these conditions includes an imbalance between increased mechanical load of the respiratory system and decreased capacity of the respiratory muscles, worsening of pulmonary gas exchange, and inappropriate cardiovascular function with increased ventricle preload and afterload. Non-invasive ventilation is effective in unloading the respiratory muscles and decreasing the work of breathing (WOB) by applying inspiratory positive pressure. In obstructive lung disease, intrinsic positive end-expiratory pressure (PEEPi) further increases the mechanical load of the respiratory muscles. Patients adopt a rapid and shallow breathing pattern that helps in decreasing dyspnoea but contributes to further deterioration of hypercapnia and development of respiratory acidosis. Non-invasive ventilation is effective in decreasing the WOB and correcting the abnormal breathing pattern, hence contributing to reverse respiratory acidosis. Adding external PEEP to inspiratory positive pressure further unloads the respiratory muscles by counterbalancing PEEPi. Similar mechanisms may help in advancing extubation of ventilator-dependent patients with chronic respiratory disorders. In patients with cardiogenic pulmonary oedema, positive pressure either with NIV and PEEP or continuous positive airway pressure (CPAP) can increase intrathoracic pressure and decrease venous return, hence reducing right ventricle preload and left ventricle afterload. Moreover, positive pressure results in recruiting collapsed alveolar units and increased lung volumes, with further improvement in arterial oxygenation and lung compliance. Patients with severe acute hypoxaemic respiratory failure often have collapsed lung tissue and increased respiratory muscle effort. In these patients CPAP is effective in improving oxygenation but fails to unload the respiratory muscles. Non-invasive ventilation with appropriate levels of inspiratory positive pressure and PEEP are needed to unload the respiratory muscles and relieve dyspnoea. Avoidance of intubation or shortening the period of intubation in difficult weaning with NIV is associated with reduced incidence of hospital-acquired infections, particularly pneumonia.


## INTRODUCTION

Non-invasive ventilation (NIV) has been used in various clinical settings of patients with severe acute respiratory failure (ARF). The clearest evidence for favourable use has been shown in severe exacerbation of chronic obstructive pulmonary disease (COPD), facilitating weaning and extubation in COPD patients, cardiogenic pulmonary oedema and immunosuppressed patients.[1] A constant finding in all clinical settings of ARF is that patients who benefit from using NIV have intermediate severity of respiratory failure: not severe enough so as to need life-support measures such as intubation and invasive mechanical ventilation (IMV) in addition to the specific treatment, but severe enough so that oxygen therapy is not sufficient support for ARF. This is the concept of the 'window of opportunity' (Fig. 14.1).

This chapter will review the physiological effects of NIV, the mechanisms of action in the clinical indications for NIV in ARF and the role of NIV in reducing the incidence of hospital-acquired infections.

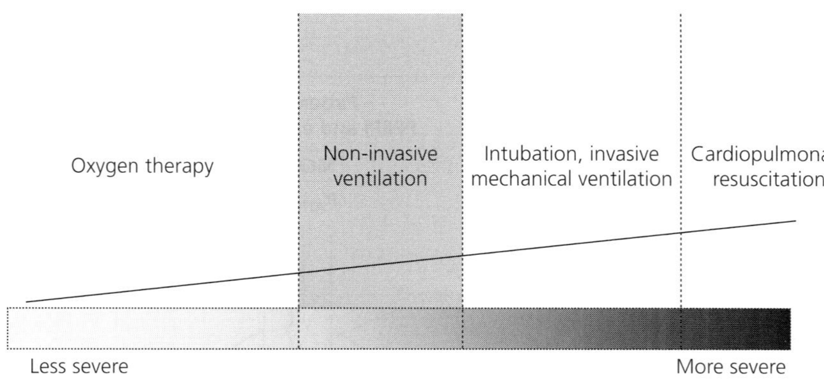


**Figure 14.1** Ventilatory support in acute respiratory failure: the 'window of opportunity'.

## EFFECTS OF NON-INVASIVE VENTILATION ON RESPIRATORY MECHANICS

Appropriate ventilation requires overcoming the elastic and resistive characteristics of the respiratory system. During spontaneous breathing, the pressure applied to the respiratory system during inspiration is generated by the respiratory muscles, while during mechanical ventilation positive inspiratory pressure is provided by the ventilator (Fig. 14.2).

Applying positive pressure to the respiratory system results in increased functional residual capacity (FRC). This may improve alveolar collapse and gas exchange by decreasing intrapulmonary shunt and ventilation–perfusion ($V_A/Q$) mismatching in patients with alveolar oedema or exudates. Alternatively, particularly in patients with airways disease, it may worsen pulmonary hyperinflation and increase dead space, thereby worsening $V_A/Q$, as well as flattening the diaphragm and reducing the inspiratory muscle strength.

Dynamic hyperinflation is mainly caused by worsening of chronic airflow limitation during an episode of COPD exacerbation. Thus, pressure in lung parenchyma at end-expiration remains positive, namely intrinsic positive end-expiratory pressure (PEEPi). In the presence of dynamic hyperinflation, the lung compliance decreases as the lung volume increases. Moreover, the diaphragm is flattened, with shortening of the muscle fibres. The disadvantaged inspiratory muscles have then to overcome this increased elastic workload, and an additional workload superimposed by PEEPi to initiate inspiration.[2]

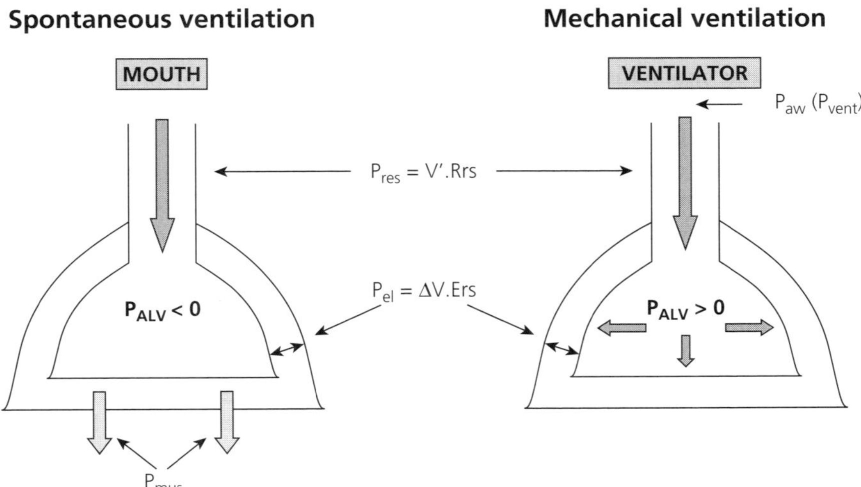


**Figure 14.2** Schematic representation of pressures acting on the respiratory system during spontaneous and mechanical ventilation. During spontaneous ventilation, pressure generated by inspiratory muscles ($P_{mus}$) overcomes the resistive ($P_{res}$) and elastic ($P_{el}$) pressures, resulting in negative alveolar pressure ($P_{ALV}$). $P_{res}$ depends on the inspiratory flow (V') and respiratory system resistance (Rrs), and $P_{el}$ on respiratory system elastance (Ers) and changes in lung volume ($\Delta V$). During mechanical ventilation the pressure generated by the ventilator ($P_{vent}$) increases airway pressure ($P_{aw}$), drives inspiratory flow into the lungs and increases $P_{ALV}$, which is opposed by $P_{res}$ and $P_{el}$ pressures.

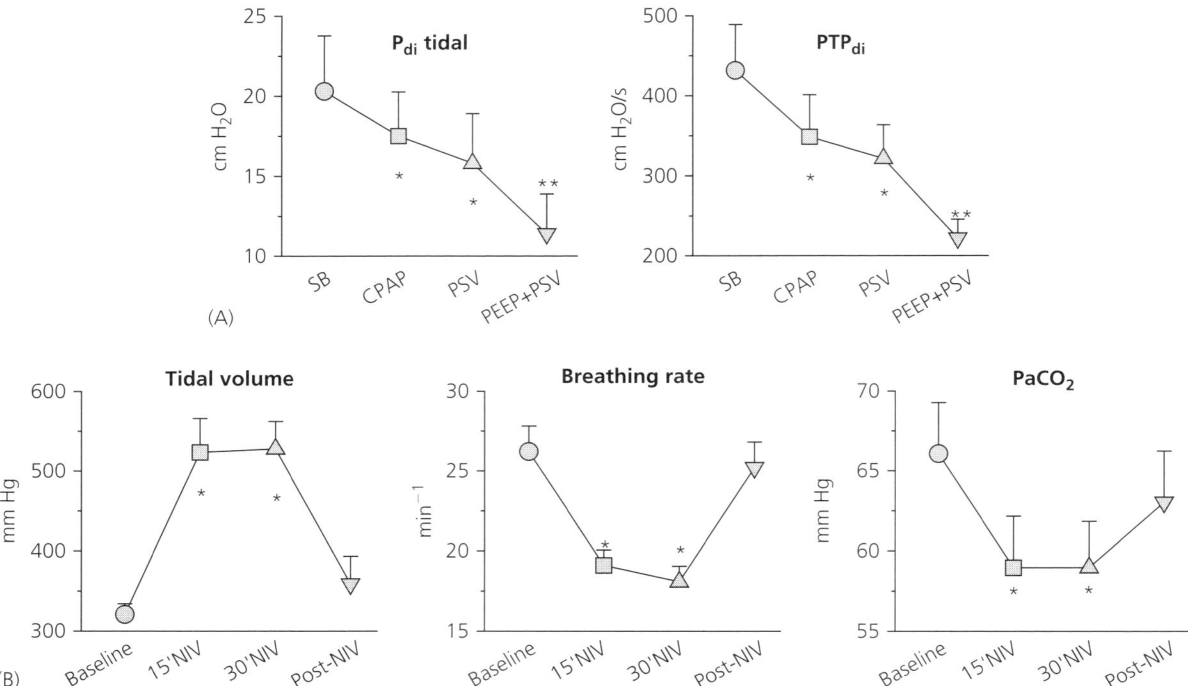


**Figure 14.5** (A) Mean ± SEM values for tidal transdiaphragmatic pressure ($P_{di}$ tidal) and pressure-time product of the diaphragm ($PTP_{di}$) during spontaneous breathing (SB), continuous positive airway pressure (CPAP), pressure support ventilation (PSV) and PSV with positive end-expiratory pressure (PEEP) in patients with chronic obstructive pulmonary disease (COPD) exacerbation. *Differences compared with SB. **Differences with CPAP and PSV alone. Adapted from Appendini *et al.*[11] (B) Mean ± SEM values for tidal volume, breathing frequency and arterial $CO_2$ tension ($PaCO_2$) at baseline in spontaneous breathing, after 15 and 30 minutes of non-invasive ventilation (NIV), and again in spontaneous breathing 15 minutes after withdrawal of NIV. *Differences compared with baseline. Adapted from Diaz *et al.*[12]

### Box 14.1 Pathophysiological basis of weaning failure during transition from positive pressure ventilation to spontaneous breathing

- Rapid and shallow breathing pattern
- Increased workload of the respiratory muscles:
  - increased PEEPi
  - increased elastance and resistance of the respiratory system
  - increased work of breathing
  - increased effective inspiratory impedance
  - increased load/capacity balance
- Inappropriate cardiovascular response:
  - increased venous return to right ventricle
  - increased negative deflections in intrathoracic pressure
  - increased left ventricular afterload
  - fall of mixed venous $P_VO_2$ and $S_VO_2$
- Impaired neurological status

$P_VO_2$, mixed venous oxygen tension; $S_VO_2$, mixed venous oxygen saturation.

Conversely, mixed venous oxygen tension or saturation remains unchanged or increased during a successful spontaneous breathing trial compared with positive pressure ventilation.[25–27]

## Effects of non-invasive ventilation during unsuccessful weaning (Box 14.2)

The rationale for using NIV to facilitate weaning is based on its ability to offset several pathophysiological mechanisms associated with unsuccessful weaning. The effects of NIV on respiratory mechanics and gas exchange in non-intubated COPD patients with acute hypercapnia also apply in intubated patients with difficult weaning.[11,12]

Similarly, intubated patients with chronic respiratory disorders not ready to breathe spontaneously after recovery from the acute episode have been studied, while they were still intubated, in PSV and spontaneously breathing through a T-piece. Afterwards, they were extubated and studied in non-invasive PSV and spontaneous breathing with an oxygen mask[28] (Fig. 14.6). Invasive and non-invasive PSV were equally effective in

**Box 14.2 Physiological effects of non-invasive positive pressure ventilation**

- Effect on respiratory mechanics:
  - decreased negative deflections of intrathoracic pressure
  - decreased WOB
  - additive effects of positive pressure ventilation and external PEEP
- Effects on gas exchange:
  - reduction in hypoxaemia and hypercapnia secondary to slower and deeper breathing pattern
  - no effects on $V_A/Q$ mismatch

reducing the WOB and improving arterial blood gases, compared with spontaneous breathing. In addition, NIV improved better the breathing pattern and the efficacy of the respiratory pump, with better tolerance than invasive PSV.[28] Therefore, the physiological changes in NIV observed in non-intubated COPD patients persist during the weaning period.

## NON-INVASIVE VENTILATION IN HEART FAILURE

The effects of NIV in heart failure are extensively discussed in Chapter 31. Changes in intrathoracic pressure during the respiratory cycle are transmitted to the heart; therefore, the pressure gradients for both systemic venous return (right ventricle preload) and systemic arterial outflow (left ventricular afterload) also change.[29]

The decrease of pleural pressure during spontaneous inspiratory efforts can become extremely negative in heart failure.[30,31] When positive inspiratory pressure is applied and the respiratory muscles are unloaded, the negative swings of pleural pressure during inspiration decrease. Furthermore, both PEEP and CPAP increase pleural pressure during expiration.[30,32]

The most relevant physiological effects of CPAP or NIV in patients with heart failure are: decreased venous return and ventricular preload related to increased right atrial pressure;[33,34] decreased left ventricle afterload related to attenuation of the exaggerated negative swings of pleural pressure during inspiration (Fig. 14.7);[31,33–35] decreased WOB and oxygen consumption of the respiratory muscles

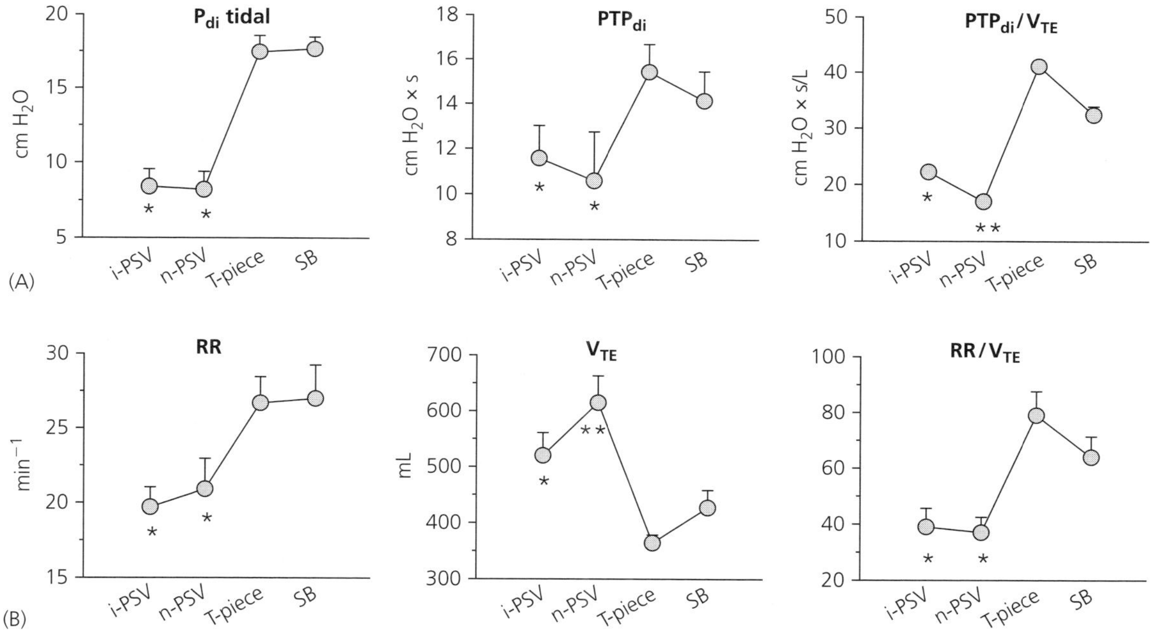


**Figure 14.6** Physiologic effects of non-invasive ventilation in the weaning from invasive mechanical ventilation in ventilator-dependent patients with chronic respiratory disorders. Sequential measurements were done, prior to extubation, during a T-piece trial (T-piece) and invasive pressure support ventilation (i-PSV), and later after extubation, in spontaneous breathing (SB) with oxygen mask and non-invasive PSV (n-PSV). (A) Mean ± SEM values for tidal transdiaphragmatic pressure ($P_{di}$ tidal), pressure-time product of the diaphragm ($PTP_{di}$) and the efficacy of the respiratory pump, assessed by the ratio of $PTP_{di}$ and the expired tidal volume ($V_{TE}$). (B) Mean ± SEM values for respiratory rate (RR), $V_{TE}$ and rapid shallow breathing index ($RR/V_{TE}$). *Differences between i-PSV and n-PSV versus T-piece and SB. **Differences between n-PVS versus i-PSV. Adapted from Vitacca *et al.*[28]

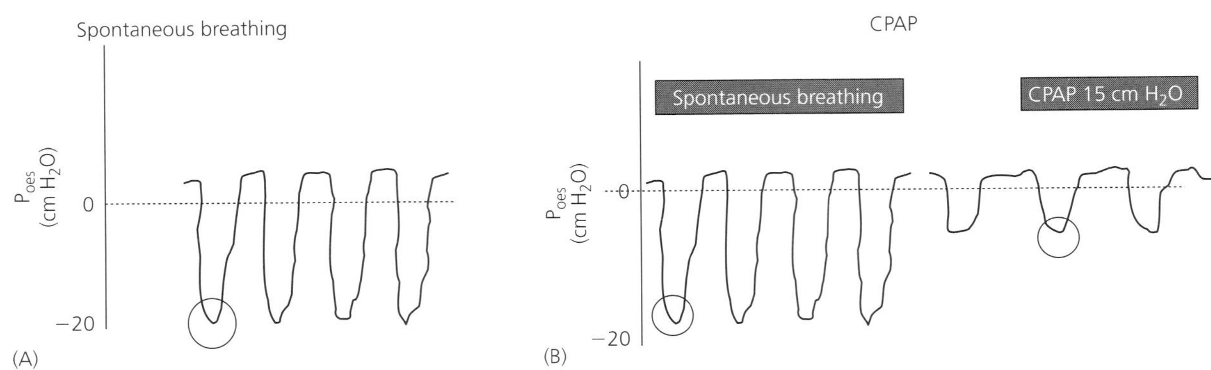


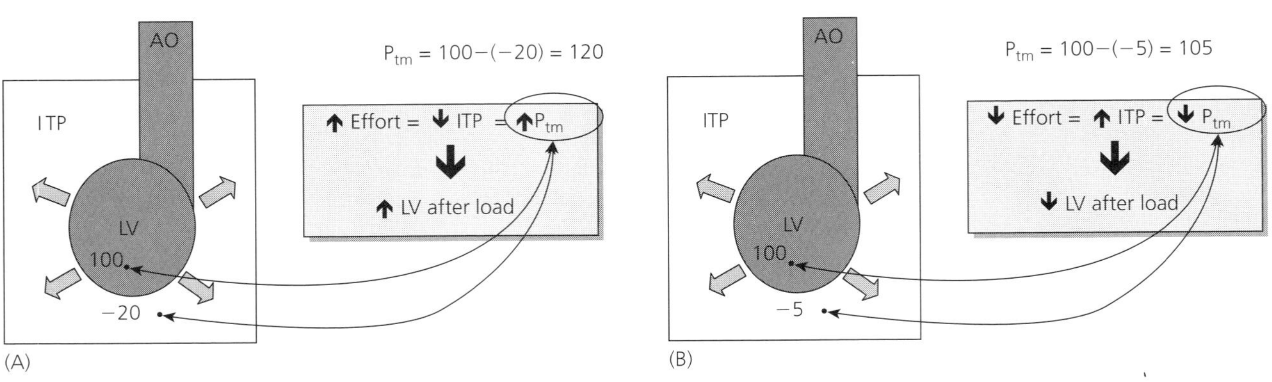


**Figure 14.7** Schematic representation of the effects of continuous positive airway pressure (CPAP) on the negative inspiratory deflections of pleural pressure and left ventricle (LV) afterload in a patient with cardiogenic pulmonary oedema (CPO). Upper panel (A) Pleural pressure during spontaneous breathing. The exaggerated negative swings of pleural pressure, assessed by oesophageal pressure ($P_{oes}$), may reach up to −20 cm $H_2O$. Lower panel (A) The transmural pressure ($P_{tm}$) represents the pressure needed by the LV to overcome both the aortic (AO) and the negative intrathoracic pressure (ITP). Due to the highly negative ITP, the increased $P_{tm}$ of the LV results in increased LV afterload. Upper panel (B) Pleural pressure while breathing with CPAP. The negative swings of pleural pressure are attenuated by the increase in pleural pressure induced by CPAP. Lower panel (B) As a result of the decreased negative deflection of ITP, $P_{tm}$ of the LV decreases, which results in decreased LV afterload. Courtesy of Dr Stefano Nava (Pavia, Italy).

by unloading the respiratory muscles,[30] thus increasing oxygen delivery to other organs, mixed venous and arterial oxygen saturation, and decreasing lactic acidosis;[36] and variable effects on right ventricle afterload due to the possible combination of reverting hypoxic pulmonary vasoconstriction due to recruitment of collapsed lung areas by applying positive pressure, and induction of pulmonary hyperinflation due to excessive pressure level.

## NON-INVASIVE VENTILATION IN ACUTE HYPOXAEMIC RESPIRATORY FAILURE

In selected patients with acute hypoxaemic respiratory failure (AHRF), early institution of NIV may help in reversing the acute episode and reduce the need for endotracheal intubation.[37] However, switching to invasive ventilation is required in more than 40–50 per cent of hypoxaemic patients receiving NIV in observational studies.[38–41]

### Effects of continuous positive airway pressure

Applying PEEP to the airway opening may increase alveolar recruitment, lessen the reduction in FRC and improve respiratory mechanics and gas exchange.[42] These data have led physicians to use CPAP in order to prevent subsequent clinical deterioration and reduce the need for endotracheal intubation.[43,44] Nevertheless, using CPAP alone in patients with acute lung injury is not strongly supported by clinical data.[45]

The inspiratory effort expended by patients with ARF is approximately four to six times the normal value and can be brought down near the normal range by careful selection of ventilator settings.[46] Non-invasive CPAP, which is the simplest way to apply positive pressure to the respiratory system, raises intrathoracic pressure and reduces the transpulmonary WOB in intubated patients, indicating an improvement in respiratory mechanics, decreases intrapulmonary shunting, and may improve oxygenation and reduce dyspnoea.[43] Few studies have compared the respiratory effects of non-invasive PSV versus CPAP in non-cardiological patients with AHRF. A physiological study in patients ventilated by endotracheal intubation[47] suggested that PSV might be superior to CPAP alone in terms of the clinical response and/or decrease in respiratory effort.

The short-term physiological effects of two combinations of PSV above PEEP and CPAP alone have been studied in patients with AHRF who were treated with NIV to distinguish the physiological reasons that may underlie the discrepancies in terms of clinical outcome between these two modalities of positive pressure.[48] The study showed that PSV at two different levels reduced neuromuscular drive, unloaded the inspiratory muscles, and improved dyspnoea. When used alone in this setting, CPAP was unable to reduce inspiratory effort. The maximal improvement in arterial oxygenation was achieved at a PEEP level of 10 cm $H_2O$, either with CPAP or PSV. Finally, the greatest improvement in dyspnoea was obtained with the highest level of PSV in this study.[48] The absence of an effect of CPAP on the respiratory effort, as demonstrated in this study, may explain the failure of non-invasive CPAP to provide clinical benefits in patients with AHRF.[45] These results also emphasize that improving oxygenation, as with CPAP alone, should not be the sole objective, because it is not always associated with a decrease in respiratory effort. Figure 14.8 shows the most relevant findings of this study.[48]

The lack of beneficial effects of CPAP in patients with AHRF observed in this study[48] does not rule out potential clinical benefits for CPAP in other populations. For instance, in the post-operative period, loss of lung volume, atelectasis and oxygenation impairment are frequent, and may be the main pathophysiologic pathways of respiratory complications.[49–52] In post-operative thoracic and abdominal surgery patients, CPAP increases arterial oxygenation and reduces respiratory rate[53] and may help in preventing worsening of oxygenation during the post-operative period.[54] These effects may explain the usefulness of CPAP in this setting.[55]

## Effects of non-invasive ventilation

As stated above, the changes in respiratory muscle effort observed during NIV with PSV in one physiological

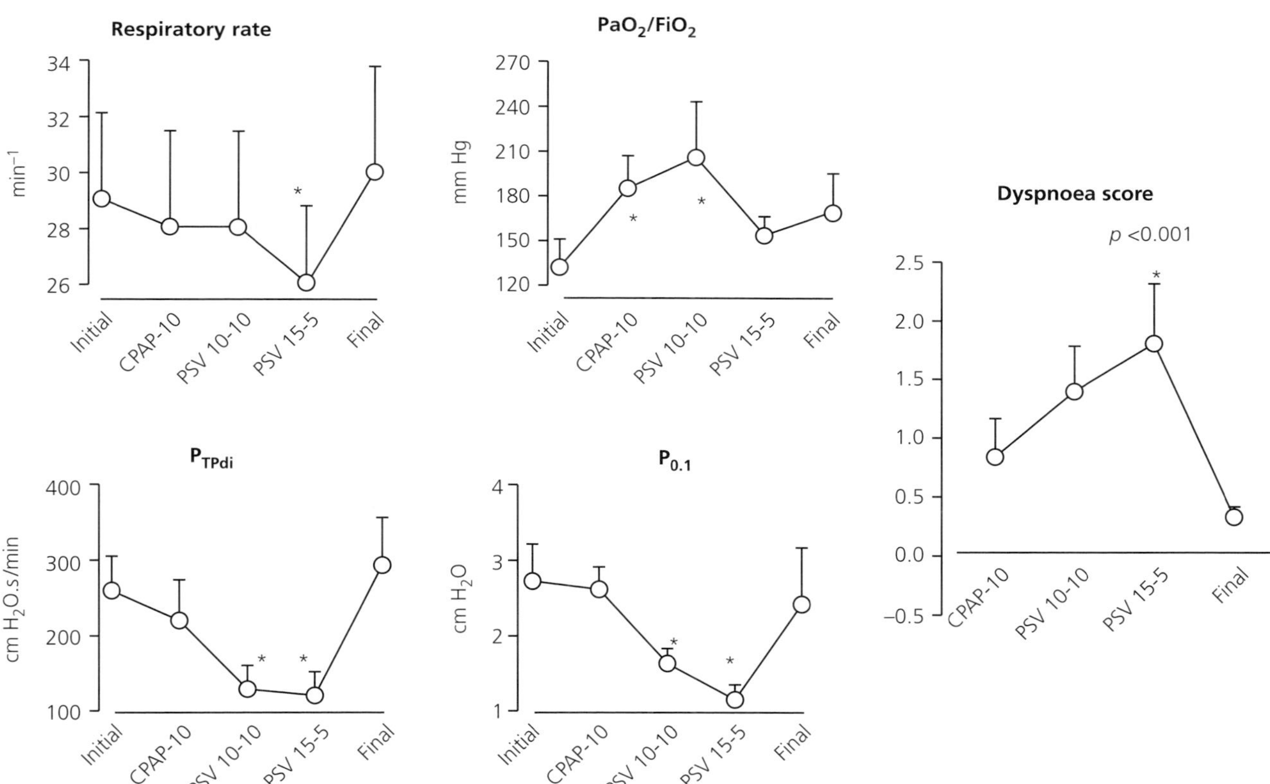


**Figure 14.8** Summary of the most relevant physiological effects of non-invasive ventilation (NIV) in patients with acute hypoxaemic respiratory failure (AHRF) under spontaneous breathing (initial and final part of the study), during continuous positive airway pressure (CPAP) 10 cm $H_2O$, and during two combinations of pressure support ventilation (PSV) and positive end-expiratory pressure (PEEP) 10–10 cm $H_2O$ and 15–5 cm $H_2O$. $PTP_{di}$, pressure-time product of the diaphragm; $P_{0.1}$, neuromuscular drive, assessed by the oesophageal pressure decrease after 0.1 seconds. Changes in dyspnoea were assessed on the following scale: +2, marked improvement; +1, slight improvement; 0, no change; −1, slight deterioration; and −2, marked deterioration. Adapted from L'Her *et al.*[48]

study[48] (Fig. 14.8) are in accordance with previous data obtained in intubated patients[47,56] and with clinical studies suggesting clinical beneficial effects of NIV in selected patients with AHRF.[57–61] On balance, these results suggest that adding PSV to PEEP may be indispensable in patients with AHRF treated with NIV. Indeed, rather than refractory hypoxaemia, the most frequent feature at the time of intubation in these patients was signs of exhaustion.[57]

The main goals of NIV in patients with parenchymal lung disease and AHRF are improving oxygenation, unloading the respiratory muscles and relieving dyspnoea. The first goal can usually be achieved by using PEEP, often at levels of 10 cm $H_2O$ or above, in order to recruit and stabilize previously collapsed lung tissue. The lack of significant improvement in arterial oxygenation using 5 cm $H_2O$ PEEP in the physiological study[48] suggests that improving oxygenation with NIV requires sufficient PEEP levels. However, leakage and poor tolerance by the patient usually limit the end-inspiratory level of pressure during NIV. Therefore, clinicians must seek the best compromise, at a given end-inspiratory pressure, between increasing the PEEP level to improve oxygenation, and increasing the PSV level above PEEP to relieve dyspnoea and diminish respiratory muscle effort.

## NON-INVASIVE VENTILATION IN PREVENTING HOSPITAL-ACQUIRED INFECTIONS

Ventilation-associated pneumonia (VAP) is a frequent and severe infection with important morbidity, mortality and economic cost.[62,63] Therefore, the identification of risk factors for developing VAP is important in the implementation of preventive measures.

Invasive mechanical ventilation is a major risk factor for developing hospital-acquired pneumonia. The impairment of local defences to infection secondary to intubation with abnormal airway colonization, and the aspiration to the lower airway of contaminated secretions pooled above the endotracheal tube cuff, are important pathogenic mechanisms of increased risk for respiratory infections in patients with IMV.[64] The most relevant pathogenic mechanisms of VAP related to IMV are associated with: endotracheal tubes, including direct mucosal injury, elimination of cough reflex, pooling of contaminated secretions above the endotracheal tube cuff, biofilm formation, the nasotracheal route of intubation, and reintubation; nasogastric tubes and enteral nutrition, including gastro-oesophageal reflux and the aspiration to lower airways of contaminated gastric contents; and contamination of the ventilator circuit and respiratory therapy equipment.

Among different strategies, NIV may potentially prevent the development of VAP by avoiding the need for tracheal intubation and IMV.

### Microbial airway colonization among patients with invasive and non-invasive ventilation

Abnormal airway colonization in patients needing IMV is considered a first step to developing hospital-acquired pneumonia, and this could be potentially avoided using NIV. However, a prospective cohort study investigating the microbial airway colonization in exacerbated COPD patients needing NIV and IMV showed that previous airway colonization by non-fermenting Gram-negative bacilli, mainly *Pseudomonas aeruginosa*, was strongly associated with NIV failure.[65] Interestingly, because these pathogens were acquired before intubation, this appeared to be a marker, and not only a consequence of NIV failure needing intubation.[65]

### Preventing or shortening intubation with NIV and hospital-acquired pneumonia

There is increasing evidence that using NIV to avoid intubation may reduce the incidence of hospital-acquired infections, particularly pneumonia. An observational cohort study showed that NIV was associated with a lower incidence of VAP and other hospital-acquired infections than IMV.[66] Similarly, a matched case–control study in patients with hypercapnic respiratory failure secondary to COPD exacerbations or cardiogenic pulmonary oedema showed lower rates of hospital-acquired pneumonia and other infections, less use of antibiotics to treat these infections, and lower length of ICU stay and mortality among patients treated with NIV compared with those needing IMV.[67] The same group observed a significant increase of NIV use and a concomitant decrease in mortality and ICU-acquired infection rates in similar patients over an 8-year period.[68] The authors found NIV independently linked with a reduced risk of death, while high severity scores and the occurrence of hospital-acquired infection were independent predictors of death.

The randomized clinical trials published on NIV have been focused on preventing intubation, facilitating difficult weaning and treating or avoiding extubation failure. A few studies have reported lower rates of hospital-acquired pneumonia in patients treated with NIV[57,58,69–71] (Table 14.1). In these cases, the use of NIV was associated with either decreased need for intubation or shorter duration of IMV. Since most cases of hospital-acquired pneumonia in these studies occurred in patients who needed intubation[57,58,69] or underwent prolonged weaning,[70,71] the reduction in the need for, or the duration of, intubation with NIV may reduce the risk of infection. On the other hand, the observed association of non-fermenting Gram-negative bacilli in airway secretions and increased need for intubation in COPD exacerbations treated with NIV[65] suggests that patients with infection are more likely to fail. Conversely, when NIV failed to avoid

**Table 14.1** Summary of the randomized clinical trials on non-invasive ventilation (NIV) with reported incidence of hospital-acquired pneumonia (HAP)

| Authors | Year | Patient types | Comparator | Subjects | | Incidence of HAP | | *p* Value |
|---|---|---|---|---|---|---|---|---|
| | | | | NIV | Control | NIV (per cent) | Control (per cent) | |
| *NIV in acute respiratory failure* | | | | | | | | |
| Brochard *et al.*[69] | 1995 | Acute COPD | Oxygen therapy | 42 | 43 | 2 (5) | 7 (17) | 0.088 |
| Ferrer *et al.*[57] | 2003 | Severe hypoxaemia | Oxygen therapy | 51 | 54 | 5 (10) | 13 (24) | 0.093 |
| Antonelli *et al.*[58] | 1998 | Severe hypoxaemia | Invasive mechanical ventilation | 32 | 32 | 1 (3) | 8 (25) | 0.026 |
| *NIV in weaning failure* | | | | | | | | |
| Nava *et al.*[70] | 1998 | COPD, early weaning failure | Conventional weaning | 25 | 25 | 0 (0) | 7 (28) | 0.001 |
| Ferrer *et al.*[71] | 2003 | Persistent weaning failure | Conventional weaning | 21 | 22 | 5 (24) | 13 (59) | 0.042 |
| *NIV in the treatment or prevention of extubation failure* | | | | | | | | |
| Keenan *et al.*[72] | 2002 | Extubation failure | Oxygen therapy | 39 | 42 | 16 (41) | 17 (40) | 0.61 |
| Ferrer *et al.*[73] | 2006 | Risk for extubation failure | Oxygen therapy | 79 | 83 | 18 (23) | 27 (33) | 0.23* |
| Ferrer *et al.*[74] | 2009 | Risk for extubation failure | Oxygen therapy | 54 | 52 | 3 (6) | 9 (17) | 0.12 |

*Incidence of all intensive care unit (ICU)-acquired infections.
COPD, chronic obstructive pulmonary disease.

clinical trial. *Am J Respir Crit Care Med* 2003; **168**: 1438–44.

58. Antonelli M, Conti G, Rocco M *et al.* A comparison of noninvasive positive-pressure ventilation and conventional mechanical ventilation in patients with acute respiratory failure. *N Engl J Med* 1998; **339**: 429–35.
59. Antonelli M, Conti G, Bufi M *et al.* Noninvasive ventilation for treatment of acute respiratory failure in patients undergoing solid organ transplantation. *JAMA* 2000; **283**: 235–41.
60. Hilbert G, Gruson D, Vargas F *et al.* Noninvasive ventilation in immunosuppressed patients with pulmonary infiltrates, fever, and acute respiratory failure. *N Engl J Med* 2001; **344**: 481–7.
61. Martin T, Hovis J, Costantino J *et al.* A randomized, prospective evaluation of noninvasive ventilation for acute respiratory failure. *Am J Respir Crit Care Med* 2000; **161**: 807–13.
62. American Thoracic Society. Guidelines for the management of adults with hospital-acquired, ventilator-associated, and healthcare-associated pneumonia. *Am J Respir Crit Care Med* 2005; **171**: 388–416.
63. Chastre J, Fagon JY. Ventilator-associated pneumonia. *Am J Respir Crit Care Med* 2002; **165**: 867–903.
64. Kollef MH. The prevention of ventilator-associated pneumonia. *N Engl J Med* 1999; **340**: 627–34.
65. Ferrer M, Ioanas M, Arancibia F *et al.* Microbial airway colonization is associated with noninvasive ventilation failure in exacerbation of chronic obstructive pulmonary disease. *Crit Care Med* 2005; **33**: 2003–9.
66. Nourdine K, Combes P, Carton MJ *et al.* Does noninvasive ventilation reduce the ICU nosocomial infection risk? A prospective clinical survey. *Intensive Care Med* 1999; **25**: 567–73.
67. Girou E, Schortgen F, Delclaux C *et al.* Association of noninvasive ventilation with nosocomial infections and survival in critically ill patients. *JAMA* 2000; **284**: 2361–7.
68. Girou E, Brun-Buisson C, Taille S *et al.* Secular trends in nosocomial infections and mortality associated with noninvasive ventilation in patients with exacerbation of COPD and pulmonary edema. *JAMA* 2003; **290**: 2985–91.
69. Brochard L, Mancebo J, Wysocki M *et al.* Noninvasive ventilation for acute exacerbations of chronic obstructive pulmonary disease. *N Engl J Med* 1995; **333**: 817–22.
70. Nava S, Ambrosino N, Clini E *et al.* Noninvasive mechanical ventilation in the weaning of patients with respiration failure due to chronic obstructive pulmonary disease. A randomized, controlled trial. *Ann Intern Med* 1998; **128**: 721–8.
71. Ferrer M, Esquinas A, Arancibia F *et al.* Noninvasive ventilation during persistent weaning failure. A randomized controlled trial. *Am J Respir Crit Care Med* 2003; **168**: 70–6.
72. Keenan SP, Powers C, McCormack DG *et al.* Noninvasive positive-pressure ventilation for postextubation respiratory distress: a randomized controlled trial. *JAMA* 2002; **287**: 3238–44.
73. Ferrer M, Valencia M, Nicolas JM *et al.* Early noninvasive ventilation averts extubation failure in patients at risk: a randomized trial. *Am J Respir Crit Care Med* 2006; **173**: 164–70.
74. Ferrer M, Sellares J, Valencia M *et al.* Non-invasive ventilation after extubation in hypercapnic patients with chronic respiratory disorders: randomised controlled trial. *Lancet* 2009; **374**: 1082–8.

# SECTION C

# The practice: chronic non-invasive ventilation

# 15

# The chronic ventilator service

JEAN-FRANÇOIS MUIR, ANTOINE CUVELIER

## ABSTRACT

The way in which a chronic ventilator service is organized will vary from institution to institution. The following key components must however be addressed: titration (initiation and set-up of non-invasive ventilation [NIV]); monitoring (what is involved will depend on the individual and their disease process); rehabilitation (this is a key component in the management of patients with chronic respiratory disability and will often run alongside home ventilation); and equipment provision. An experienced multidisciplinary team is needed and should include: medical staff, nurses, respiratory physiotherapists, pulmonary physiologists and ventilator technicians. Access to other care professionals such as dieticians, social workers and occupational therapists should also be available. All team members and other staff require training, not just in the practical application of NIV but also the theory and rationale behind it. The patient and their family or caregivers must all be trained in the practical aspects of NIV including emergency measures, and 24-hour telephone support should be available for emergencies. The equipment and the support that the patient will need will depend on the aetiology of their respiratory failure and their degree of ventilator dependence. The patient who can maintain prolonged periods of spontaneous ventilation and who retains a high degree of functional independence requires little, whereas the patient with complex neurological disability who is ventilator dependent will require a very different package of care. The potential consequences of equipment failure must always be considered and catered for. Monitoring again will vary from patient to patient. In the early stages of acclimatization to domiciliary ventilation, monitoring will be required more frequently than when patients are well established on ventilation. Monitoring should always include an assessment of clinical status, particularly symptoms of nocturnal hypoventilation or of complications associated with NIV. Patients will require assessment of arterial blood gas tensions by day with particular focus on $PaCO_2$ and bicarbonate and some form of overnight monitoring, depending on the patient's clinical status.

## INTRODUCTION

Domiciliary mechanical ventilation (DMV) delivered either in a non-invasive way or via a tracheostomy is the key treatment for patients with chronic respiratory failure (CRF) and hypercapnia. Domiciliary mechanical ventilation decreases the frequency of acute hypercapnic respiratory failure (AHRF) episodes, improves survival, clinical symptoms and health status in patients with restrictive pulmonary disorders (neuromuscular diseases, thoracic deformities, obesity-hypoventilation syndrome). In obstructive pulmonary diseases (chronic obstructive pulmonary disease [COPD], bronchiectasis, cystic fibrosis, etc.) neither NIV nor tracheostomy and mechanical ventilation (TMV) improve overall survival when compared with long-term oxygen therapy alone but they reduce dyspnoea and the number of hospitalizations for AHRF and allow organizing surgical treatments, such as pulmonary transplantation in cystic fibrosis. In all of the abovementioned medical conditions, NIV has progressively replaced TMV, although TMV still has some specific indications especially in the course of difficult weaning.

The overall prevalence of DMV in Europe is around 6.6/100 000, but this varies greatly between countries.[1] The increasing incidence of COPD, severe obesity and adult neuromuscular diseases, and also the increasing lifespan of the general population, points to a major increase in the incidence and the medical load associated with CRF in the next 10 years. The development of NIV by chest physicians during the early 1990s has considerably popularized this technique and facilitated the development of centres delivering NIV to patients with CRF or AHRF. The wide variations between local organizations, from the technical, administrative or economic point of view, including the variable investment of chest physicians in the field of CRF and the relationship with the local intensive care unit (ICU), has progressively led to differences in management of CRF patients in the various centres. The need to rationalize healthcare costs and the development of more sophisticated technological tools progressively imposes the obligation to better structure the steps in the management of patients with chronic ventilatory assistance, beginning with titration and long-term monitoring and also including rehabilitation and management of ARF episodes.[2] Clinical research in CRF patients is difficult to perform but we can take advantage of the experience from sleep laboratories, where clinicians have developed (for a slightly different scenario) a rational management structure and there has been productive research on ventilator assistance titration and monitoring.

In this chapter, we describe a chronic ventilator service (CVS) that we set up in our university hospital in the early 1990s. This very structured network manages around 200 new CRF patients each year, in connection with a non-profit provider for domiciliary management. This way of working is probably not valuable for all healthcare organizations but is an example of how to rationalize the management of CRF patients. This chapter will describe the two components of a CVS: the specific activities provided in the hospital and the support provided at home.

## THE CHRONIC VENTILATOR SERVICE IN THE HOSPITAL

Creation of a CVS first requires a sustained collaboration between chest physicians and the hospital administration, beginning with the identification of the number of NIV or TMV patients who may enter the CVS active file. This calculation clearly influences the subsequent choices about the location, the medical and nursing staffing requirements, and the technical armamentarium required to run the CVS. Our experience is that offering such a CVS immediately leads to an increase in the number of patients utilizing such a service compared with the predicted needs. The different components of a CVS may be schematized as shown in Figure 15.1.

It is not known if CVS improves the management of chronic and disabled patients as compared with conventional management in the ward. Its impact will have to be assessed through objective indicators such as the mean length of stay to initiate domiciliary ventilation, long-term compliance with the treatment and efficacy (reflected in the potential decrease of AHRF episodes or unplanned hospitalizations). It is plausible that a CVS has

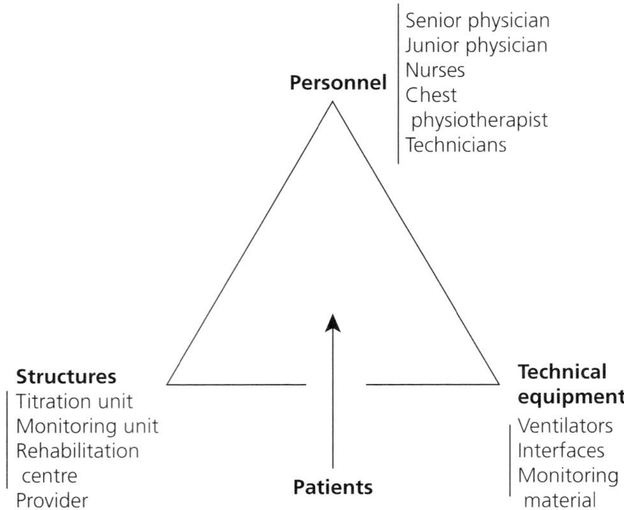


**Figure 15.1** Organizational structure of a chronic ventilator unit.

some economic justifications because of the likely consequences on healthcare costs despite the numbers of medical and nursing staff required to run it and the complexity of the involved technologies.

### Organization

The CVS is integrated into a network of departments of different competencies (Fig. 15.2). The heart of the CVS is the place where patients are first received and routinely assessed in the hospital. New patients enter the CVS through the *titration unit*, where the planned domiciliary ventilation may be installed and titrated. The titration unit organizes planned hospitalizations, usually after a pulmonary consultation or after referral from a sleep laboratory. The relationship with the sleep laboratory is crucial since a large number of CRF patients receive their diagnosis after investigations for a sleep apnoea syndrome for instance. Non-invasive ventilation is therefore initiated in between two and five consecutive days. Beds in an intermediate respiratory care unit or even the pneumology ward may be utilized for this aim but we do not recommend this option because of the need for dedicated nursing staff and specific equipment. In most centres, the expertise in invasive or non-invasive ventilation is available in the intensive care unit, and one of the challenges for the CVS is to take advantage of this expertise for patients with CRF on a long-term basis.

Also in the heart of the organization is the associated component of the CVS, the *monitoring unit*. This unit is dedicated to scheduled and sometimes unplanned long-term assessments of CRF patients having NIV or TMV at home. These assessments are performed at regular intervals that vary according to the aetiology of the CRF; in some situations the assessments may be also be performed

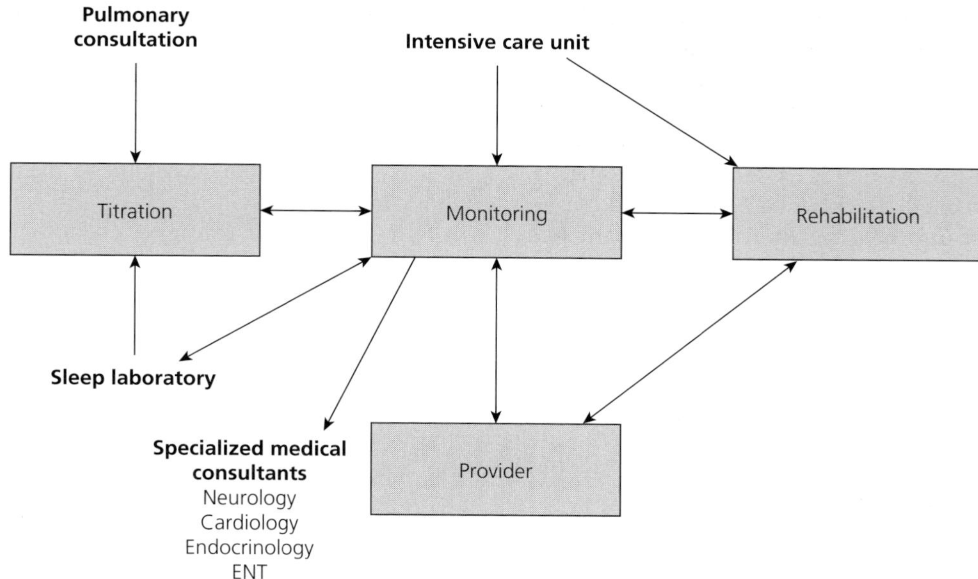


**Figure 15.2** Network organization of the clinical management of patients with chronic respiratory failure requiring domiciliary ventilator assistance. The network is organized around the chronic ventilator unit and its collaborative units.

irregularly, owing to unpredictable clinical evolution, for instance if DMV becomes less tolerated or less efficient. It is probably better if the monitoring unit is localized at the same place as the titration unit, and both units may even actually be just one unit. However, both units are very different in their operational functioning, especially regarding the duration of patient stay. The titration unit usually accepts patients from 48 hours to 5 days and the monitoring unit should be organized to accept patients for not only 6–8 hour-long assessments but also for one to several consecutive nights if there is a requirement to assess or to change the ventilator settings. Presently, there is no evidence recommending performance of night-time ventilatory assessments in chronically ventilated patients. Some of these nocturnal assessments are presently performed at home through the provider, but there has not been any large study to validate such an approach. The recent development of polysomnography under NIV will probably modify the nature of assessments and may lead to a larger number of one-night hospitalizations in selected patients.

A high proportion of patients treated with NIV or TMV are introduced to their ventilatory treatment in the context of an AHRF episode, managed in an intensive care or an intermediate care unit. Therefore, these patients enter the CVS via the monitoring unit and are subsequently managed like all other CRF patients. The monitoring unit can be located within the same infrastructure as the titration unit but it receives patients following a much shorter period of time, sometimes less than 24 hours. This unit should be accessible to patients with reduced mobility. It should also be organized to receive input from various professionals such as non-respiratory physicians, dieticians, occupational therapists, social services, etc. The multidisciplinary approach is key to the success of such a programme, for instance for patients with neuromuscular diseases or severely obese patients. Regular reports from the monitoring unit should be sent to the patients' general practitioners (GPs), the nurses and the chest physiotherapists in the community.

The third component of the CVS is the *rehabilitation unit*. Pulmonary rehabilitation is a major issue in the management of COPD patients, even in those with severe disease (categorized Global Initiative for Chronic Obstructive Lung Disease [GOLD] IV for these patients).[3] Today, pulmonary rehabilitation may also improve the clinical symptoms and quality of life in patients with CRF of other aetiologies such as restrictive pulmonary diseases, severe obesity and cystic fibrosis.[4,5] In the CVS, rehabilitation may be organized in the hospital or in the home and always delivered by dedicated staff, usually a chest physiotherapist who can visit the patients in their homes.

Finally, the last component of the CVS is the *provider*, which should be well integrated into the activities of the centre, in order to provide and manage the ventilatory equipment at home. The quality of the coordination between the CVS and the provider will be detailed later.

## Staffing

The success of a CVS largely depends on the availability of dedicated medical, nursing and physiotherapist staff. The ratio of patients and staff varies largely between centres and between different healthcare organizations. In any case, the nursing staff should be distinct from the staff on the pulmonary ward and should have competencies in mechanical ventilation initiation and monitoring, not only during the day but also during sleep. Medical staff and the physiotherapists should be trained in the management of these patients but need not be exclusively dedicated to the CVS. In fact it is cost-effective to use these resources in other areas of management of CRF patients, such as in the intensive care unit or the pulmonary ward. Staff also include the technician staff supplied by the provider, who should help establish the link between the centre and the home. Their role begins as soon as the titration is finished and they should participate in monitoring of the ventilator and the supply and renewal of various pieces of equipment, as well as all notifications and alerts about the medical devices.

## Staff training

The success of a CVS largely depends on the progressively increasing competence of its medical and nursing staff. The best training, in our view, is the medical teaching at bedside and is largely dependent on the number of managed patients and resolved clinical situations. This competence is also improved by knowledge of the theory of mechanical ventilation and by regular handling of domiciliary ventilators during bench tests. This is particularly true for learning how to set a ventilator and manipulate the interfaces, the ventilatory circuits and the humidification devices. A low training level will decrease the efficiency of the whole healthcare team and affect the overall short- and long-term therapeutic benefits for the patient. Also, all the components of training should be regularly reinforced, probably twice a year, but there is no consensus at present regarding the schedule of learning. Training for physicians should be organized in a similar way but they should also keep abreast of the medical literature, current technological advances and availability, and the various guidelines that may be published by health agencies. These guidelines should be adopted after being suitably adapted for the local needs by all the actors of the CVS. Finally, it is recommended that the physicians involved in a CVS should have basic knowledge about intensive care and should be able to perform an endotracheal intubation as quickly as possible. In the context of AHRF, the barriers to the development of a NIV service have been clearly identified as a low prevalence of patients, little medical practice in the field and also inappropriate equipment. These factors impact on the clinical results of the treatment and subsequently accelerate the demotivation of the entire team.

Thus, ventilation training, which should be organized for and tailored to the needs of all the different staff in the CVS team, may also include a good level of theoretical knowledge about ventilatory physiology, ventilatory modes and the indications and contraindications of domiciliary ventilatory assistance. It should also include practising not only clinical skills in order to enable examination of patients but also some technical skills in order to set and interpret the different ventilatory modes and settings, especially during sleep. These competencies should be complemented by appropriate communication skills for communicating with the patient and their family, in order to make the treatment acceptable to them and to achieve high compliance. Training should also aim to develop the capacity for clinical reasoning and problem solving, for instance intolerance of long-term NIV, patient–ventilator asynchrony, persistent nocturnal hypoxaemia or diurnal hypercapnia.

## Equipment

The third component of a CVS is the updated equipment to titrate and monitor NIV and TMV, either during the day or while sleeping.

### VENTILATORS (SEE ALSO CHAPTER 2)

An active CVS inventory should consist of almost all the available domiciliary ventilators on the market and the staff should be trained to use them. Bench tests have shown great performance variability between different domiciliary ventilators, for instance with regard to triggering, cycling off and airways pressurization.[6,7] Moreover, a recent paper has shown that the same ventilator may behave differently when applied to patients with different mechanical ventilatory conditions[8] and the comfort under a ventilator may also vary greatly according to the machine.[9] The large number of available ventilators may be perceived as a barrier to the training of physicians, nurses and physiotherapists. This is not the case in our experience, especially for people who are already familiar with one type of ventilator and if some theoretical knowledge about triggering, cycling and pressurization has been acquired. Although most ventilators present differently, their manipulation is rather similar. Careful attention should be paid to the teaching of ventilatory modes and the associated nomenclature, which can be very heterogeneous from one machine to another.[10]

The CVS should have titration ventilators, which are sometimes more sophisticated than domiciliary ventilators. These titration machines usually have monitoring capacities, for instance the capacity to display the minute ventilation, unintentional leaks variations, and/or nocturnal desaturations, owing to built-in software. They can also incorporate external data coming from a transcutaneous carbon dioxide monitor or a ventilatory polygraph. The drawback is the transfer of the titration parameters from the titration machine to the domiciliary ventilator since the two machines may have different technical and performance characteristics. The physician will therefore have to titrate the patient using a domiciliary ventilator, with the better bi-level ventilators having a central turbine to act as a flow generator rather than a piston or a bellow. With regard to batteries, French legislation obliges the physician to prescribe a domiciliary ventilator with an inner or an outer battery once the prescribed ventilation is ≥ 12 hours/day. This clearly limits the number of potential ventilators for the home, but again, the increasing number of patients with CRF will require management with most, if not all, the available ventilators on the market.

#### INTERFACES (SEE ALSO CHAPTER 6)

The situation for interfaces, which is another factor influencing the efficacy and compliance with the treatment, is largely the same as for the ventilators as discussed in the previous section. If moulded interfaces still have a place in the treatment of children, the large number of masks that are available today (nasal masks, face masks and nasal plugs) allows management of almost all adult patients. Seventy-five per cent of all our domiciliary ventilated patients are treated with only two models of nasal or facial interface. The difficulty therefore arises in the case of the minority of patients in whom several interfaces should be tested to get a balance between tolerance and efficacy. This phenomenon is still poorly understood because of the various related factors such as the amount of intentional leaks according to the delivered pressure, the configuration of intentional leaks on the mask or the circuit and the gas trajectory into the interface.[11,12] Also, an additional psychological factor cannot be excluded. Any attempt by the medical administration to standardize the interfaces on offer in some centres is therefore futile for around 25 per cent of the patients, and all types of interface should therefore be available in the CVS, both in the titration and the monitoring units and also with the provider. At all of these three steps, staff should be able to detect any complication related to the interface and to suggest a solution to the patient and their family, not only in the form of counselling, but also trying out another interface or optimization of the humidification devices. All these issues about interfaces are different for TMV patients since tracheostomy tubes have roughly similar technical characteristics and their clinical performance is not influenced by the ventilatory modalities.

### Monitoring

The third technical component of a CVS is the monitoring capacity, whose importance is progressively increasing in the long-term management of CRF, especially at night. Routine follow-up is not based solely on nocturnal oximetry and repeated arterial blood gases but on other devices that may help to identify the efficacy of the nocturnal ventilation and its impact on sleep quality. Titration now includes routine initial polygraphy or polysomnography to identify potential sleep breathing disorders and hypoventilation during the different sleep stages. Transcutaneous capnography may also have a role.[13]

Other monitoring tools to use in a CVS include the software embedded in some domiciliary and titration ventilators. This software can provide a record of the evolution of nocturnal saturation in parallel with conventional parameters from the pneumotachograph (minute delivered ventilation, respiratory frequency), and an estimated value of the unintentional leaks. These data can be acquired in real time or uploaded afterwards but they have never been validated prospectively in a cohort of non-selected patients. One of the pitfalls of this software is that it can acquire data with low acquisition frequency and provide calculated and estimated values rather than measured values like in a numeric acquisition system. To display correct estimations of unintentional leaks, the software needs to know the value of the intentional leaks, which vary between the interfaces. When these factors are taken into account, the validity of the leak measure seems to be quite good, at least on bench tests;[14] but, again, this tool needs clinical validation.

Ventilatory polygraphy and polysomnography are very powerful techniques for domiciliary ventilation titration and long-term monitoring. All CVS should now have access to these techniques, either by collaborating with a sleep laboratory or by using ambulatory polygraphs. Data issued from polysomnography under domiciliary ventilation are numerous and help to identify central apnoeas and patient–ventilator asynchrony that may be the consequence of poor ventilator titration, especially during triggering and cycling. By juxtaposing ventilatory events with microarousals and sleep stages the impact of the ventilatory events on nocturnal $SaO_2$ and sleep quality may be evaluated. This objective approach may therefore help to improve the quality of ventilator titration and may help to understand why some patients do not tolerate long-term nocturnal ventilation.

Nocturnal long-term monitoring of patients at home is clearly the weak link for the management of CRF patients and is now one of the challenges for all researchers in this field. Hospitalizing a patient for one night in the monitoring unit or the sleep laboratory is a possible alternative but is subjected to the 'first night effect', which modifies the usual sleep. There is a clear need for non-invasive simple tools that can monitor the patients during several consecutive nights at home and this activity would be a new development for the provider.

## THE CHRONIC VENTILATOR SERVICE IN THE COMMUNITY

### Definition and goals

The role of the respiratory home care service (RHCS) is to provide health services to patients and caregivers at home (Fig. 15.3), to restore and maintain an acceptable clinical status and to minimize the effects of respiratory failure and disability,[15] leading to a potential prevention of further episodes of ARF. When they are discharged from the in-hospital CVS, and thus are considered as clinically

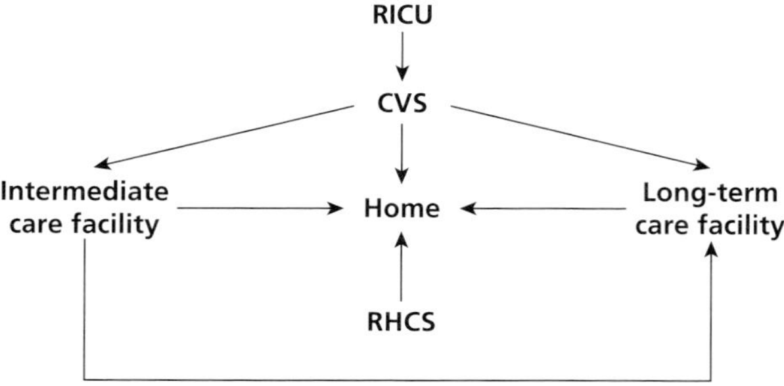


**Figure 15.3** Integration of home care into out-of-hospital facilities. CVS, chronic ventilatory service; RHCS, respiratory home care service; RICU, respiratory intensive care unit.

stable, patients on long-term mechanical ventilation need an adequate environment in which to continue their treatment.[16] They may be orientated towards either a long-term in-hospital facility, or more often home. At home, they need a structure at least able to provide the equipment and its monitoring and maintenance. As CRF patients are becoming older and more and more frail, with frequent comorbidities, they must be under the charge of not only respiratory technicians for their equipment, but also polyvalent home care services as they are frequently dependent within their environment.

Thus RHCS organizations represent a complex set of medical, ethical and social issues that involve multiple interest groups:[17] ventilator-assisted individuals; those who are completely dependent upon assisted ventilation for life support, those frequently needing tracheostomy (generally neurological or neuromuscular patients, or severe end-of-life COPD patients), and partially dependent patients with varying degrees of severity and aetiology (neuromuscular diseases, chest wall disorders, primary and secondary hypoventilation, tuberculosis sequelae, and more and more obese patients)[1] generally treated by NIV.

## Transition to home (see also Chapters 17 and 18)

The transition between the CVS and home is a crucial period. It is important that the first days at home are successful as they will impact on the long-term acceptance of the ventilatory treatment by the patient. The keys for success are discussed below.

### CONTINUUM OF THE IN-HOSPITAL EDUCATION PROGRAMME FOR THE PATIENT AND THEIR FAMILY

Discharge from the CVS to home must be anticipated by in-hospital education involving a dedicated team consisting of physicians, nurses, respiratory therapists and social workers on one hand, and technicians and nurses of the RHCS, who made contact with the patient in hospital[18] on the other hand. According to the aetiology of CRF, other professionals should be consulted, such as psychologists, dieticians and speech pathologists. Prior to the discharge, the RHCS team should meet the patient and their family, and perform a home visit to plan the installation of the equipment and discuss potential improvement of the home setting in order to optimize the transfer and settling in of the patient.[19]

The training period is begun as soon as possible with the patient and their family during the stay in hospital and is continued after the patient has returned home.[20] The home nursing staff (who are directly involved in the day-to-day care of the patient) have the task to demonstrate and repeat, as needed, the instructions to the patient and their caregivers on medication and nasal/face mask use.[21] Another important item is to ask the RHCS technician to check, at home, the level of knowledge of the patient and their family with regard to not only the equipment for its 'chronic' use but also the equipment and procedures to be used at home in case of an emergency (self-inflating manual resuscitator) for the most severe of them.

The follow-up scheme and the 24-hour free telephone line must be explained as well as the therapeutic protocol indicating the timing and duration of night ventilation, and daytime oxygen therapy, sometimes interrupted by NIV sessions. The follow-up scheme must be planned with adequate frequency of follow-up. It is also important to ensure a 24-hour free helpline for emergency telephone calls. A physician should be contactable concerning any information about treatment or other management problems. This same arrangement should also be in place for contacting the device manufacturing companies and technicians.

Finally, the patient should be made aware that the main goals of RHC are: to enhance their quality of life; to reduce hospital admissions, and so be cost-beneficial; and to supervise patients' compliance with therapy. These goals are achieved by ensuring that the clinical and physiological functions (mainly adequate ventilation) and the patient's safety are maintained.

### SOCIAL CONSIDERATIONS

An important factor for success is to coordinate the social assistance that will be available at home.[22] The spectrum ranges from the simplest case where the patient has numerous, motivated, available family members to where there are no relatives in proximity. If the patient wants to go back home and if their clinical status permits it, collaboration with social workers must be organized according to the financial possibilities of the society and the social network; in France for instance, patients with established CRF benefit from 100 per cent reimbursement for their healthcare costs; social services have budgets that are supported by the social charges (*cotisations*; similar to the National Insurance in the UK) paid by workers and their employers that are used to pay for social workers at home or for home hospitalization services, which can care for the most severely dependent patients, as for instance a tracheostomized tetraplegic patient with 24-hour dependence on a respirator.

### The home care setting

The home equipment for ventilator-assisted individuals depends on the aetiology of the CRF, the degree of impairment, the upper airway function, and the mode of ventilatory support.[17,23] A middle-aged patient on non-invasive night-time mechanical ventilation, who is clinically stable, in general does not need a large amount of equipment. Usually the standard equipment (i.e. a ventilator with the circuit and filters, and mask [nasal or face]) is sufficient. This type of patient does not need a humidifier system, oxygen, and sometimes no supplemental oxygen on the respirator, and not even a secondary battery. Additional elements are needed for patients on long-term oxygen therapy (LTOT) or for those with diaphragmatic impairment or neurological diseases. In these cases the patient, if supine, often cannot maintain spontaneous breathing; so when the ventilator fails it is essential to have another device or manual resuscitator bag. Ventilator-dependent individuals should always have a back-up ventilator and an emergency power source. This would include a battery, and in areas where power failures are frequent, a generator. Local police and fire departments should also be made aware of these individuals.

Several types of small-sized respirator are available nowadays;[6,10] the choice made during the in-hospital CVS stay is followed up at home by the RHCS and depends on the preference of the prescriber and the availability in the RHCS. Pressure cycled respirators are increasingly used for long-term NIV as they are easier to set and synchronize compared with classic volume cycled respirators.[1,24] An important item is also the choice of the connection between the patient and the respirator: this will depend on the anatomy and tolerance of the patient, and at the lowest level of leaks.

## RESPIRATORY HOME CARE SERVICES: OBLIGATIONS AND ORGANIZATION

### Obligations

An RHCS must ensure for its patients a 24-hour service with facilities for on-call intervention at home by skilled technicians, nurses[25] or other qualified employees. When the size of the RHCS is important, the availability of a physician who is a part- or full-time employee of the organization ensures a superior quality of home care performance.

In parallel, the RHCS also works with technicians who get involved either at home to ensure optimal maintenance of the equipment as well as education and motivation of the patient and their family, or in the maintenance workshop generally located in the headquarters of the RHCS. Such technicians provide a regular daytime service and are also on duty during the night or weekend. The frequency of the daytime visits varies according to the therapeutic scheme. In France, the reimbursements to the RHCS are also different, depending on the type of respiratory home care provided to the patients. Specific contracts stating a precise frequency of visits and the obligations of the RHCS may be submitted for reimbursement.

Respiratory physiotherapists also have a role to provide chest physiotherapy in patients with bronchial hypersecretion, and pulmonary rehabilitation. The availability of an on-call secretary is vital to provide answers to patients who call for information and sometimes in emergency situations as well as for a technical problem. An RHCS also needs a well-planned administrative structure to manage the financial budget, which is important in terms of deciding future investments and purchase of equipment.[26]

The criteria and procedures for homologation set by the national health service and/or quality control commissions vary widely between different countries.

### Organization

The early national public health services that historically initiated home care services have largely been replaced by the trend towards parity between public and private organizations. In some countries, all the home care is supplied by private companies; in others, the public health service still has a monopoly.

In France, the *Association Nationale pour les Traitements à Domicile, l'Innovation et la Recherche* (ANTADIR) initiated a large public network in the beginning of the 1980s that created a federation of 33 regional associations devoted to home respiratory care.[27] At the beginning these non-profit (ruled by '1901 law') associations were intended to treat home patients with CRF and a need for oxygen therapy and/or ventilatory assistance. They were funded by the French social security to ensure delivery and maintenance of the equipment as no reimbursement was factored in to permit CRF patients with such equipment to go back home. This system largely developed alone nearly without any challenge from the private health service during the first 10 years; following an improvement to the reimbursement of the contracts, private health services became more and more interested by this type of package. Nowadays in France, home respiratory care service (HRCS) (including nasal continuous positive airway pressure [CPAP] for sleep apnoea syndrome) is shared between the association network (35 per cent) and private companies (65 per cent). Generally, the most severe patients (i.e. those who are discharged by the public hospitals) are managed by the association network and patients treated in private practice, who are less severe, are managed by the private HRCS network.

With the increasing demand, HRCS is looking to manage not only respiratory care but the whole package for health

Table 15.1 Monitoring the patient on home mechanical ventilation over 24 months

| ITEM | M1 | M3 | M6 | M9 | M12 | M18 | M24 |
|---|---|---|---|---|---|---|---|
| Clinical evaluation | × | × | × | × | × | × | × |
| Chest X-ray | × | | | | × | | × |
| Electrocardiogram | × | | | | × | | × |
| Biology | × | | | | × | | × |
| Arterial blood gases | × | × | × | × | × | × | × |
| Compliance recording | × | × | × | × | × | × | × |
| Pulmonary function tests | × | | | | × | | × |
| Respiratory monitoring (software of the machine) | × | × | × | × | × | × | × |
| Equipment maintenance | × | × | × | × | × | × | × |

maintenance at home (medical beds installation, artificial feeding, home perfusion treatments, subcutaneous insulin, wheelchair location) and social worker management.

## Costs of home care

Several studies[26,28–30] show that home care is less expensive than in-hospital treatment, either in acute care hospitals or in other long-term facilities. Non-invasive ventilation is efficient in maintaining the clinical stability of patients with CRF and reducing the need for further hospitalizations. If the natural history of CRF is a non- or slowly progressive disease, such as post-polio or kyphoscoliosis, with good long-term prognosis,[31] the cost of the equipment, its maintenance, and the possible need for supplemental oxygen constitute the major economic burden. The decision whether to purchase or rent a ventilator should be made in the light of the prognosis of the disease and economic convenience in the contract with the local dealer (accessories, maintenance, other services) and varies from one country to another[32,33] according to the organization of services and healthcare. In most European countries, a national policy regarding prescription modalities, reimbursement, assistance and medical supervision if it exists, does not provide complete coverage, even if the costs of LTOT and the ventilator are usually reimbursed by the national health service or an insurance company. In France, social security covers the costs of installation, maintenance and medical and technical supervision of patients with CRF under respiratory assistance at home, through specific contracts designed according to the kind of respiratory assistance which has been prescribed. Patients are reimbursed at a 100 per cent rate for all their other specific costs (medications, chest physiotherapy). Indirect costs must also be considered (Table 15.1). French social security is increasingly assisted by private insurances' finances for these contacts through the regional association network that is mainly regulated by ANTADIR,[27] with its public philosophy, and also through private networks that have strongly increased their presence in this field during the past 10 years. When the severity of the disease increases, the cost of respiratory assistance cannot be separated from the cost of chronic care, as in neuromuscular patients, who usually have a variably progressive disorder, and severe COPD, where NIV is most often a step before the use of more invasive techniques towards progressive ventilator-dependence. Caregivers in Europe are usually family members with a progressively increasing need for external medical-social help from social workers for cooking, bathing and toileting. A home care programme that includes these 'social' needs is obviously desirable, but funding and organization needs are usually a major obstacle as patients have to pay for a part of the care.

## MONITORING THE PATIENT ON HOME MECHANICAL VENTILATION (BOX 15.1)

Patients on long-term mechanical ventilation require regular follow-up on a clinical basis by their general practitioner, in collaboration with the pulmonologist and the CVS. The frequency of visits is greater during the first year of follow-up, or if the status of the patient is unstable; it is more convenient for the patient to come to a daytime hospital where there is time to control the clinical status and the equipment in collaboration with the RHCS, and to perform routine investigations (chest X-ray, electrocardiogram, arterial blood gases under room air, and/or under oxygen therapy and under mechanical ventilation). The RHCS may provide on request computed data obtained from the internal memory of the respirator, which help refine the monitoring of respiratory behaviour of the patient under the machine.

## FUTURE CONSIDERATIONS

In parallel with the constant improvement in respiratory assistance, which should not slow down in the coming years, the development of telemonitoring should in part

**Box 15.1 Components of home care costs[33]**

- Direct costs:
  - physician fees
  - formal services purchased by family
  - hospital and skilled nursing facility inpatient days
  - medications
  - equipment rental
  - oxygen
  - ambulance
  - medical supplies
  - extra utility charges
  - major one-time purchases or remodelling
- Indirect costs:
  - alterations in employment
  - lost wages resulting from caregiving

reduce the cost of human presence, which, however, will often be mandatory for the most severe patients. A further decrease of costs could be achieved by more closely involving the general practitioner in the medical supervision of the patient to screen for decompensations and thus prevent them. Governments have already to cope with an impressive increase in medical-social demand because of the increase in lifespan and its consequence, physical dependence. A solution is to favour development of home medico-social assistance that is not only focused as it was 30 years ago on the availability of a set of equipment but also on organizing a network of medico-social assistance involving family and relatives assisted by social workers and home care services run by technicians and nurses. It is the way that several national public and private organizations have already opted to go to meet this major challenge.

## REFERENCES


1. Lloyd-Owen SJ, Donaldson GC, Ambrosino N *et al.* Patterns of home mechanical ventilation use in Europe: results from the Eurovent survey. *Eur Respir J* 2005; **25**: 1025–31.
2. Haute Autorité de Santé. *Practical aspects of long-term noninvasive positive pressure ventilation at home in neuromuscular disease.* Clinical practice guidelines. 2006. Available at: www.has-sante.fr/portail/jcms/c_334439 (accessed 22 July 2009).
3. Carone M, Patessio A, Ambrosino N *et al.* Efficacy of pulmonary rehabilitation in chronic respiratory failure (CRF) due to chronic obstructive pulmonary disease (COPD): The Maugeri Study. *Respir Med* 2007; **101**: 2447–53.
4. Borel JC, Wuyam B, Chouri-Pontarollo N *et al.* During exercise non-invasive ventilation in chronic restrictive respiratory failure. *Respir Med* 2008; **102**: 711–19.
5. Bradley J, Moran F: Physical training for cystic fibrosis. *Cochrane Database Syst Rev* 2008: CD002768.
6. Battisti A, Tassaux D, Janssens JP *et al.* Performance characteristics of 10 home mechanical ventilators in pressure-support mode: a comparative bench study. *Chest* 2005; **127**: 1784–92.
7. Bunburaphong T, Imanaka H, Nishimura M *et al.* Performance characteristics of bilevel pressure ventilators: a lung model study. *Chest* 1997; **111**: 1050–60.
8. Fauroux B, Leroux K, Desmarais G *et al.* Performance of ventilators for noninvasive positive-pressure ventilation in children. *Eur Respir J* 2008; **31**: 1300–7.
9. Vitacca M, Barbano L, D'Anna S *et al.* Comparison of five bilevel pressure ventilators in patients with chronic ventilatory failure: a physiologic study. *Chest* 2002; **122**: 2105–14.
10. Gonzalez-Bermejo J, Laplanche V, Husseini FE *et al.* Evaluation of the user-friendliness of 11 home mechanical ventilators. *Eur Respir J* 2006; **27**: 1236–43.
11. Schettino GP, Chatmongkolchart S, Hess DR *et al.* Position of exhalation port and mask design affect CO2 rebreathing during noninvasive positive pressure ventilation. *Crit Care Med* 2003; **31**: 2178–82.
12. Schettino GP, Tucci MR, Sousa R *et al.* Mask mechanics and leak dynamics during noninvasive pressure support ventilation: a bench study. *Intensive Care Med* 2001; **27**: 1887–91.
13. Cuvelier A, Grigoriu B, Molano LC *et al.* Limitations of transcutaneous carbon dioxide measurements for assessing long-term mechanical ventilation. *Chest* 2005; **127**: 1744–8.
14. Rabec C, Georges M, Kabeya NK *et al.* Evaluating NIV using a monitoring system coupled to a ventilator: a bench to bedside study. *Eur Respir J*, published online before print March 26, 2009 as doi:doi:10.1183/09031936.00170508
15. Donner C, Zaccaria S, Braghiroli A *et al.* Organization of home care in patients receiving home mechanical ventilation. *Eur Respir Monograph* 1988; **3**: 380–99.
16. Make BJ, Gilmartin ME. Mechanical ventilation in the home. *Crit Care Clin* 1990; **6**: 785–96.
17. Gilmartin ME. Transition from the intensive care unit to home: patient selection and discharge planning. *Respir Care* 1994; **39**: 456–80.
18. Findeis A, Larson JL, Gallo A *et al.* Caring for individuals using home ventilators: an appraisal of family caregivers. *Rehabil Nurs* 1994; **19**: 6–11.
19. Muir JF. *Architecture intérieure et handicap respiratoire,* vol. 1. Paris: Margaux Orange, 2007:182.
20. Fischer DA, Prentice WS. Feasibility of home care for certain respiratory dependent restrictive or obstructive lung disease patients. *Chest* 1982; **82**: 739–43.
21. Haddock KS. Collaborative discharge planning: nursing and social services. *Clin Nurse Spec* 1994; **8**: 248–52.
22. Zaccaria S, Zaccaria E, Spada EL *et al.* How is the family to be prepared? *Eur Respir Rev* 1992; **10**: 413–15.
23. AARC Clinical Practice Guideline. Discharge planning for the respiratory care patient on long-term invasive

mechanical ventilation in the home. *Respir Care* 1995; **40**: 1308–20.

24. Farre R, Lloyd-Owen SJ, Ambrosino N *et al.* Quality control of equipment in home mechanical ventilation: a European survey. *Eur Respir J* 2005; **26**: 86–94.
25. American Thoracic Society. Standards of nursing care for adult patients with pulmonary dysfunction. *Arn Rev Respir Dis* 1991; **144**: 231–6.
26. Sivak ED, Cordasco EM, Gipson WT. Pulmonary mechanical ventilation at home: a reasonable and less expensive alternative. *Respir Care* 1983; **28**: 42–9.
27. Stuart M, Weinrich M. Integrated health system for chronic disease management: lessons learnt from France. *Chest* 2004; **125**: 695–703.
28. Goldberg AJ. Home care for life-supported persons: is a national approach the answer? *Chest* 1986; **90**: 744–8.
29. Fields A, Rosenblatt A, Pollak M *et al.* Home care cost-effectiveness for respiratory technology-dependent children. *Ani J Dis Child* 1991; **145**: 729–33.
30. Bach J, Intitola P, Alba A *et al.* The ventilator-assisted individual: cost analysis of institutionalization vs rehabilitation and in-home management. *Chest* 1992; **101**: 26–30.
31. Criner GJ, Kreimer DT, Tomaselli M *et al.* Financial implications of noninvasive positive pressure ventilation. *Chest* 1995; **108**: 475–81.
32. Fauroux B, Howard P, Muir JE. Home treatment for chronic respiratory insufficiency: the situation in Europe in 1992. *Eur Respir* 1994; **7**: 1721–6.
33. Downes JJ, Parra MM. Costs and reimbursement issues in long-term mechanical ventilation of patients at home. In: Hill NS, ed. *Long-term mechanical ventilation*, vol. 1. New York: Marcel Dekker, 2001:556, 353–74.

# 16

# Diagnostic tests in the assessment of patients for home mechanical ventilation

PATRICK MURPHY, MICHAEL POLKEY, NICHOLAS HART

## ABSTRACT

A range of measurements must be undertaken when selecting patients for domiciliary non-invasive ventilation (NIV). Daytime hypercapnia is detected by arterial blood gas sampling. It is the result of alveolar hypoventilation and its presence indicates advanced disease. Ideally, the onset of ventilatory failure should be anticipated before this arises, allowing forward planning of the initiation of NIV outside of an acute deterioration (an otherwise unexplained elevation of the standardised bicarbonate concentration is an earlier indicator and is also available from an arterial blood gas sample). Although vital capacity is widely available, the non-linear relationship between volume and pressure makes it a poor predictor of respiratory muscle weakness. However, a vital capacity less than 50% predicted should raise suspicion of the possibility of nocturnal hypoventilation. Other tests are available to measure respiratory muscle strength, the most useful of which is the sniff nasal test; it is simple and quick to perform requiring no coaching and is rapidly mastered by the patient. It can be used in patients with bulbar dysfunction. It correlates closely with respiratory failure and prognosis in neuromuscular diseases and should be considered mandatory in the follow-up of these patients. Patients with respiratory muscle weakness are at risk of acute deterioration because of sputum retention and subsequent infection. A cough is a complex action involving the inspiratory and expiratory muscles as well as coordinated bulbar function. Objective measurement of cough peak expiratory flow (cough PEF) helps in the prediction of patients who are unable to clear their secretions. Nocturnal hypoventilation precedes diurnal ventilatory failure. While it is rarely necessary to perform full polysomnography-limited sleep studies using oximetry, measurement of carbon dioxide tension and markers of respiratory effort aid in the diagnosis of sleep disordered breathing and the optimization of ventilatory support.

## INTRODUCTION

The respiratory system maintains oxygen and carbon dioxide homeostasis, which cannot be achieved without repetitive cyclical neural activation of the respiratory muscles. This neural respiratory drive (NRD) results in the activation of the respiratory muscles, which causes an increase in intrathoracic volume, and consequent decrease in intrathoracic pressure, which generates a pressure gradient causing airflow into the lungs. The efficiency of this respiratory muscle system is dependent on the strength and endurance of the respiratory muscles (respiratory muscle capacity) working against the resistance and compliance of the airways, lung and chest wall (respiratory muscle load). Respiratory failure arises due to an imbalance in the relationship between neural respiratory drive, respiratory muscle capacity and respiratory muscle load (Fig. 16.1). Non-invasive ventilation (NIV) is commonly used to augment alveolar ventilation during acute and chronic ventilatory failure.

While superficially it could be imagined that the evaluation of patients with chronic respiratory failure (CRF) necessitating home mechanical ventilation (HMV) requires no more than measurement of blood gas tensions, in practice detailed physiological assessment of these key areas is often appropriate. This not only ensures the correct diagnosis for the cause of CRF is made but also can enhance patient adherence by maximizing therapeutic benefit and optimizing comfort. As with all patient care, history and clinical examination should be

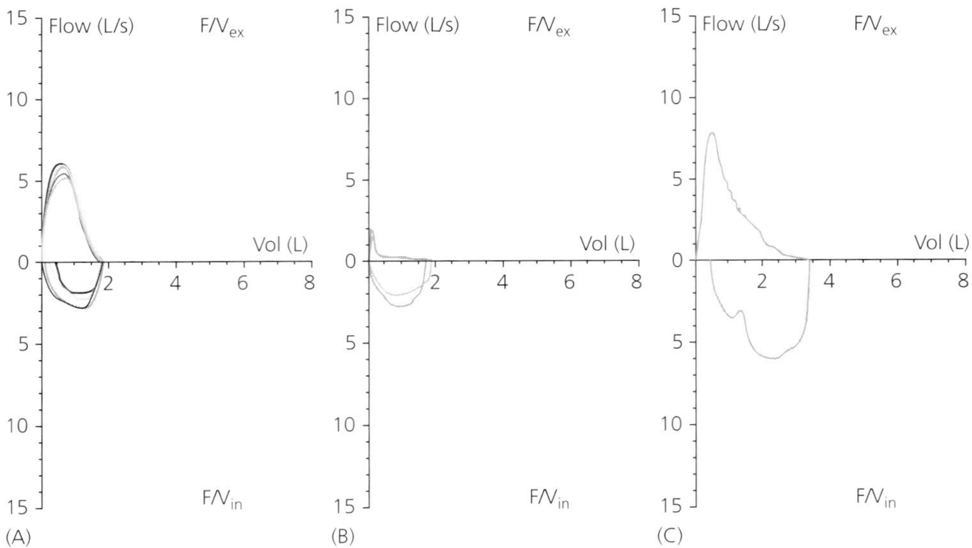


**Figure 16.2** Flow-volume loops from patients with: (A) neuromuscular disease (myotonic dystrophy), showing reduced lung volumes and without airway obstruction; (B) chronic obstructive pulmonary disease, showing a typical concave expiratory loop indicating airways obstruction; and (C) obesity, revealing mildly reduced lung volumes with some concavity of the expiratory loop consistent with early airway closure.

abnormalities found in COPD, obesity and neuromuscular disease summarized in Table 16.2 and Figure 16.2.

## Lung volumes

The pattern of change of lung volumes depends on the underlying disease with hyperinflation occurring in COPD and reduced lung volumes in obesity and restrictive thoracic disorders, such as chest wall disease and neuromuscular disease. Functional residual capacity (FRC) is the point at which outward elastic recoil of the chest wall balances inward recoil of the lungs. A change in FRC may move the patient to an inefficient position on the pressure–volume curve, increasing work of breathing.[4,5] A number of techniques can be used to measure FRC, including helium dilution and nitrogen washout, and arithmetically from whole body plethysmography. Each technique has potential advantages and disadvantages but, in clinical practice, the methods produce similar results except when there are large areas of unventilated lung as is the case in some patients with bullous emphysema.[6] Usually the differences are only important when conducting research or considering specialized therapies such as lung volume reduction surgery. It is important to recognize that true FRC can only be measured with the respiratory muscles relaxed. This may not be the case in patients with advanced COPD in whom measured FRC may be falsely elevated.

Basic spirometry, used to measure forced expiratory volume in 1 second ($FEV_1$) and forced vital capacity (FVC), is the most commonly encountered measure of pulmonary mechanics and is used to monitor progression of a range of diseases including COPD and is useful in predicting survival in neuromuscular disease, including amyotrophic lateral sclerosis.[7] A fall in FVC of greater than 20 per cent from sitting to supine is abnormal and may indicate significant diaphragmatic weakness.[8,9] However, because of the non-linear relationship between volume and pressure, tests of respiratory muscle strength (RMS) that measure the pressure generated by the respiratory muscles are a more sensitive marker of declining respiratory function than the measurement of lung volumes.[10] In clinical practice, this will include sniff inspiratory nasal pressure (SNIP) and maximal inspiratory pressures (MIP) measured at the mouth, which are discussed in the 'Respiratory muscle testing' section of this chapter.

## Advanced physiological measurements

The detailed measurement of pulmonary mechanics requires the use of specialist equipment and skills, but it is increasingly feasible in the clinical arena (Fig. 16.3). The basic mechanics of the respiratory system involve the action of respiratory muscles to produce negative intrathoracic pressure changes that result in airflow. To study this phenomenon requires the measurement of pressure changes throughout the system and the flow generated. This is most commonly achieved with the use of differential pressure transducers and a pneumotachograph; the signals from these devices are amplified and converted from analogue to digital signals and presented by commercially available software packages. Once digitized, the signals can

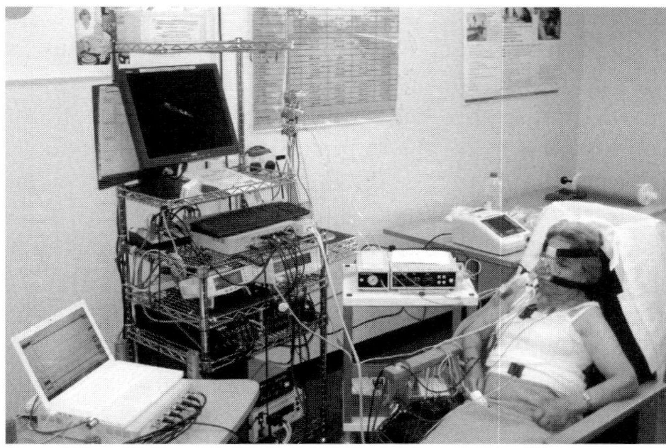

**Figure 16.3** Range of equipment needed for specialist invasive testing of a patient attending for physiological evaluation including measurement of respiratory muscle strength, neural respiratory drive and pulmonary mechanics on and off non-invasive ventilation.

be later manipulated and studied to measure pulmonary mechanics. As pleural pressure cannot be measured directly, mid-oesophageal pressure is used as a surrogate marker and is measured with an oesophageal balloon catheter inserted per nasally.[11] Pressure measurements are also acquired from gastric balloon catheters, to determine transdiaphragmatic pressure, and at the mouth, in order to calculate pressures across the system as a whole. The use of oesophageal catheters also allows the measurement of the diaphragm electromyogram ($EMG_{di}$) without the disadvantages of poor signals acquired from surface electrodes.[12] Despite initial concern with regard to changes in $EMG_{di}$ signal with changes in lung volume, recent studies have shown the reliability and reproducibility of this technique using multi-pair recording electrodes.[13,14]

## Compliance

Compliance of the respiratory system ($C_{rs}$) reflects the ease at which pressure changes produced by the respiratory muscles change the volume of the lung. It is defined as the change in lung volume per unit change in pressure across the respiratory system. In obese patients, for example, the $C_{rs}$ can be reduced thus meaning the lungs are more difficult to inflate and such patients require higher levels of pressure support to ensure adequate ventilation.[15–18] Patients with neuromuscular disease often have a normal or slightly reduced lung and chest wall compliance[19–21] due to the loss of muscle mass, and thus the overall compliance of the respiratory system is preserved. Therefore these patients can usually be ventilated easily at lower pressures.

Compliance may be measured as a static or dynamic measure, each providing useful physiological data and both having advantages and disadvantages. The measurement of static compliance ($C_{Lstat}$) requires the use of specialized equipment, including a body box for plethysmography, and relies on the ability of the patient to completely relax their respiratory muscles and make no respiratory effort as the measurements are taken at zero flow to exclude airway resistance. This is, in practice, difficult to achieve in spontaneously breathing patients. Although modified techniques exist to measure $C_{Lstat}$, such as rapid airway occlusion, these are still limited in the clinical setting.[22] However, dynamic compliance ($C_{Ldyn}$) can be achieved easily in spontaneously breathing patients, although like $C_{Lstat}$ measurements, it does require the insertion of a balloon catheter to measure oesophageal pressure ($P_{oes}$) and rests on the assumption that the respiratory muscles are inactive at the point of zero flow. The patient simply performs resting breathing through a pneumotachograph with an oesophageal balloon *in situ*. The integration of the flow from the pneumotachograph provides a value for $V_T$ and this is divided by the pressure change between end inspiration to end expiration ($\Delta P_{oes}$). Values are averaged over five to ten stable breaths. The pressure changes are taken from zero flow at end-inspiration and end-expiration as this should represent points of complete relaxation of the respiratory muscles. During inspiration, a proportion of the pressure produced by the respiratory muscles is to overcome surface tension and airways resistance and thus $C_{Ldyn}$ is measured in the relaxed expiratory phase. The main limitation of $C_{Ldyn}$ is that it can be inaccurate in obstructive lung disease as there remains intrapulmonary airflow at end of inspiration. Furthermore, the value is falsely reduced in patients with tachypnoea.

## Positive end-expiratory oesophageal pressure

True intrinsic positive end-expiratory pressure (PEEPi) occurs due to airflow limitation resulting from the narrowing of airways with resultant residual positive pressure in the alveolus (and so also the pleura) at the end of expiration. This results in an increase in the work of breathing and has a negative impact on ventilator triggering. Although it is not often measured in the HMV population and is more pertinent in acute ventilation in critical care, knowledge of the concept can enhance patient set-up for HMV. The presence of PEEPi can occur due to a range of processes including:

- insufficient expiratory time to allow pressure equalization across lung units due to airway obstruction, e.g. COPD[23]
- dynamic airway collapse causing flow limitation, e.g. emphysema or obesity[24]
- pulmonary oedema due to cardiac dysfunction.

Both static and dynamic PEEPi can be measured and requires the use of oesophageal balloon catheter and a pneumotachograph, similar to the measurement of compliance. For the measurement of static PEEPi airway occlusion is required at the end of passive expiration. The resultant plateau pressure represents the average PEEPi across the whole lung and may vary considerably between lung units in disease processes associated with profound heterogeneity, e.g. emphysema. Active expiration will cause a falsely high value and patients should be coached to avoid this phenomenon.[25] Dynamic PEEPi can be measured in the spontaneously breathing patient without the need for airway occlusion. The $P_{oes}$ at the end of expiration at the point of zero flow represents the lowest level of PEEPi within the lung that is required to be overcome in order to instigate flow. This can therefore be substantially lower than static PEEPi, most notably in those with airflow obstruction. If active expiration occurs this can be partly compensated for by subtracting the change in gastric pressure ($\Delta P_{ga}$) from the value of PEEPi calculated.[17,23] In the clinical setting failure to correctly titrate EPAP high enough to match the patient's intrinsic PEEP can lead to increased work of breathing, discomfort and triggering problems, especially in the acute setting.[26] Equally an expiratory positive airway pressure (EPAP) set too high can worsen gas trapping and again lead to patient–ventilator asynchrony. PEEPi depends on underlying disease and, in general, it is usually absent in neuromuscular disease, but can be a significant problem in patients with both obstructive airways disease and obesity.[27] Significant PEEP occurs in obese patients in the supine position due to the pressure exerted by the abdominal contents and therefore the position of the patient during measurements must be taken into consideration when interpreting measured PEEP values and setting EPAP.[24] It must also be noted that EPAP is used to abolish upper airway obstruction and maintain airway patency if there is coexistent obstructive sleep apnoea.

### Work of breathing

In the normal state, the respiratory system consumes a small proportion of the total oxygen consumption, typically less than 5 per cent, but in illness this can rapidly escalate to more than 30 per cent of the total. Although rarely measured in a clinical setting, unloading the respiratory muscles and reducing work of breathing has been shown to be associated with improved ventilator comfort and can be used to compare the effectiveness of modes of ventilation.[28] Again, measurements are taken during spontaneous breathing using a balloon catheter to measure $P_{oes}$ and a pneumotachograph with the integration $\Delta P_{oes}$ between points of zero flow generating the pressure-time product, which correlates with oxygen consumption and metabolic work of breathing.[29] This technique can show changes in work of breathing against changes in respiratory load, but with the addition of assisted ventilation it can be difficult to interpret as the changes in $P_{oes}$ represent, in part, the work performed by the ventilator rather than respiratory muscles.[28] To accurately measure changes in work of the respiratory muscles during ventilation, either change in oxygen consumption from spontaneous breathing to assisted breathing can be measured or the respiratory muscle activity can be measured using the $EMG_{di}$. These methods allow the physiological effects of modes of ventilation to be compared in detail as well as providing insights into the pathological processes involved in patients requiring HMV. Patients with high work of breathing during spontaneous respiration include those with COPD and obesity due to the high load on the respiratory system imposed by either airflow obstruction and hyperinflation or low chest wall and abdominal compliance. Patients with neuromuscular disease, if no other disease process is present, have a low work of breathing and consequently require lower levels of respiratory support.

## RESPIRATORY MUSCLE TESTING

Respiratory muscle weakness can be a cause of unexplained breathlessness with classical symptoms of diaphragm paralysis including orthopnoea, breathlessness in water and breathlessness on exercise.[30,31] Although routine imaging techniques may raise the suspicion of diaphragm paralysis the sensitivity and specificity of these tests are poor and should not be relied upon to make a diagnosis.[32] Profound respiratory muscle weakness initially leads to nocturnal hypoventilation prior to diurnal hypercapnia becoming established and this may be used as an early detector of need for nocturnal ventilatory support in at-risk populations.[33,34] Tests of RMS (respiratory muscle strength) are used in the diagnosis of unexplained hypercapnic respiratory failure and abnormalities require further testing to ascertain whether there is a generalized systemic neuromuscular problem or whether it is isolated to the diaphragm. The latter can often be a consequence of neuralgic amyotrophy. Although either isolated unilateral or bilateral diaphragm weakness may produce sleep-disordered breathing, a further pathological process is usually required to cause respiratory failure necessitating treatment with NIV.[9,35,36]

### Non-invasive tests

A simple test of RMS is change in ventilatory capacity from sitting to supine. However, other more specific tests, including SNIP and MIP, are available that better predict the presence of sleep-disordered breathing and need for NIV, particularly in patients with neuromuscular disorders.[33,37] Both these pressure measurements can be performed using handheld devices with a nasal bung or mouth piece, respectively. SNIP and MIP reflect overall respiratory muscle strength and are generally performed from functional residual capacity (FRC). Although the early literature reported that MIP testing should be performed from residual volume (RV)[3,8] more recent work has shown that it is reasonable to simplify the procedure by measuring peak pressure from FRC.[39] Previous work has shown good correlation between airway pressure and $P_{oes}$ during sniff manoeuvres in patients without significant airways obstruction.[40] Due to wide normal range of MIP values and the technical difficulty some patients have with performing the procedure, particularly those with bulbar dysfunction, SNIP may provide a better method of excluding significant respiratory muscle weakness without the need for invasive testing.[41] However, multiple tests to assess RMS are required to exclude weakness in symptomatic patients.[42,43] Details on the test protocols can be found in the European Respiratory Society and American Thoracic Society statement on respiratory muscle testing.[44]

Due to the passive nature of expiration normally the focus of respiratory muscle testing is usually on the inspiratory muscles. Expiratory muscle function may be assessed non-invasively using maximum expiratory pressure (MEP) with pressure measured at the mouth in an analogous fashion to MIP during a forced expiration (from total lung capacity [TLC]) manoeuvre. It is important to prevent the subject from using buccal manoeuvres to increase the mouth pressure. As with MIPs, MEPs have a wide normal range, meaning low readings should be interpreted within a clinical evaluation. Another simple and commonly used test of expiratory muscles is the cough peak expiratory flow (cough PEF). This can be performed using a standard peak flow meter attached to a face mask and usually requires little or no coaching to produce acceptable technique. It must be realized that although this test indicates expiratory muscle performance the pressure and force generated depends on lung volumes and coordinated bulbar function to rapidly open and close the glottis during cough pressure generation and release. Therefore, values obtained will be reduced in patients with inspiratory muscle weakness due to inability to perform deep inspiration prior to cough initiation and in those patients with bulbar dysfunction as well as those with true expiratory muscle weakness.[45] Patients with a cough PEF <180 mL/min have been shown to be unable to independently clear secretions.[46] These patients can augment cough response with manual physiotherapy and using insufflation-exsufflation devices[47] and this augmented cough level is associated with improved prognosis independent of vital capacity or breathing pattern.[46]

The normal ranges for voluntary respiratory manoeuvres are provided in Table 16.3.

**Table 16.3** Normal ranges for voluntary respiratory muscle manoeuvres. Units given as cm $H_2O$ and are mean (SD)[41,48]

| | Male | Female |
|---|---|---|
| $Sniff_{Pdi}$ | 148 (24) | 122 (25) |
| $Sniff_{na}$ | 105 (24.5) | 94 (21) |
| MIP (FRC) | 106 (22) | 87 (21) |
| MIP (RV) | 114 (27) | 88 (18) |

FRC, functional residual capacity; MIP, maximum static inspiratory pressure; $Sniff_{na}$, sniff nasal pressure; $Sniff_{Pdi}$, transdiaphragmatic sniff pressure; RV, residual volume.

## Invasive tests

As both SNIP and MIP are volitional tests, a low value does not necessarily indicate inspiratory muscle weakness but could represent inadequacy in performing the test. Therefore, if the non-invasive testing value is equivocal or a more accurate assessment is needed, invasive respiratory muscle testing can be performed. These require both a technically skilled operator as well as more specialized, but commercially available, equipment. For these reasons, these tests are usually performed in tertiary specialist units. They require the insertion of oesophageal catheters to measure $P_{oes}$ and $EMG_{di}$ and a gastric catheter to measure $P_{ga}$.

Voluntary manoeuvres are performed – maximal sniff efforts ($Sniff_{Poes}$ and $Sniff_{Pdi}$) and maximal cough effort ($Cough_{Pga}$) (Fig. 16.4). The pressures generated will, in part, be affected by lung volumes and this should be taken into account when analysing the results. These tests produce a measure of global respiratory muscle strength but to assess diaphragm function in isolation phrenic nerve stimulation must be performed. Currently, this is performed using magnetic rather than electrical phrenic nerve stimulation as it is better tolerated and easier to perform.[49,50] The measurement of transdiaphragmatic pressure following supramaximal phrenic nerve stimulation (twitch transdiaphragmatic pressure [$TwP_{di}$]) is the gold standard for demonstrating unilateral or bilateral diaphragm weakness (Fig. 16.5); normal ranges for phrenic nerve stimulation are provided in Table 16.4. Furthermore, diaphragm activation can be stimulated centrally via transcranial magnetic stimulation (TMS).[53–55] This allows accurate measurement of nerve conduction time, central and peripheral diaphragm fatigue, $EMG_{di}$ latency and amplitude as either compound muscle action potential (CMAP) or motor evoked potential. These measurements are generally used as research tools, although these detailed assessments are required when evaluating patients for intramuscular diaphragmatic pacer insertion.[56]

The use of an oesophageal electrode to measure $EMG_{di}$ during tidal breathing can be normalized to the maximum $EMG_{di}$ produced during voluntary manoeuvres.[13] This can provide an index of NRD, which is the proportion of maximum muscle activation required to perform tidal breathing. This provides insights into the physiological reserve in the respiratory system to cope with increased demand, e.g. during pulmonary infection; NRD can now be performed non-invasively utilizing the electrical activity of the second intercostal space parasternal muscles.[24]

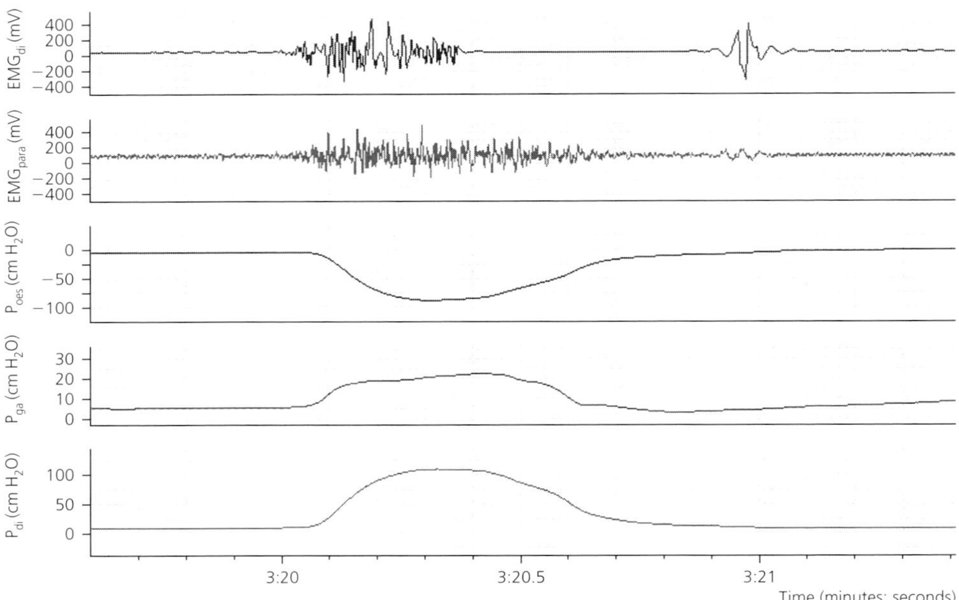


**Figure 16.4** Trace showing a maximum sniff manoeuvre in a healthy volunteer with coordinated activity of diaphragm and parasternal muscles preceding respiratory system pressure changes. Figure shows diaphragm EMG ($EMG_{di}$), parasternal EMG ($EMG_{para}$), oesophageal pressure ($P_{oes}$), gastric pressure ($P_{ga}$) and transdiaphragmatic pressure ($P_{di}$). All pressure traces are shown in cm $H_2O$ and EMG traces in mV after amplification (× 1000).

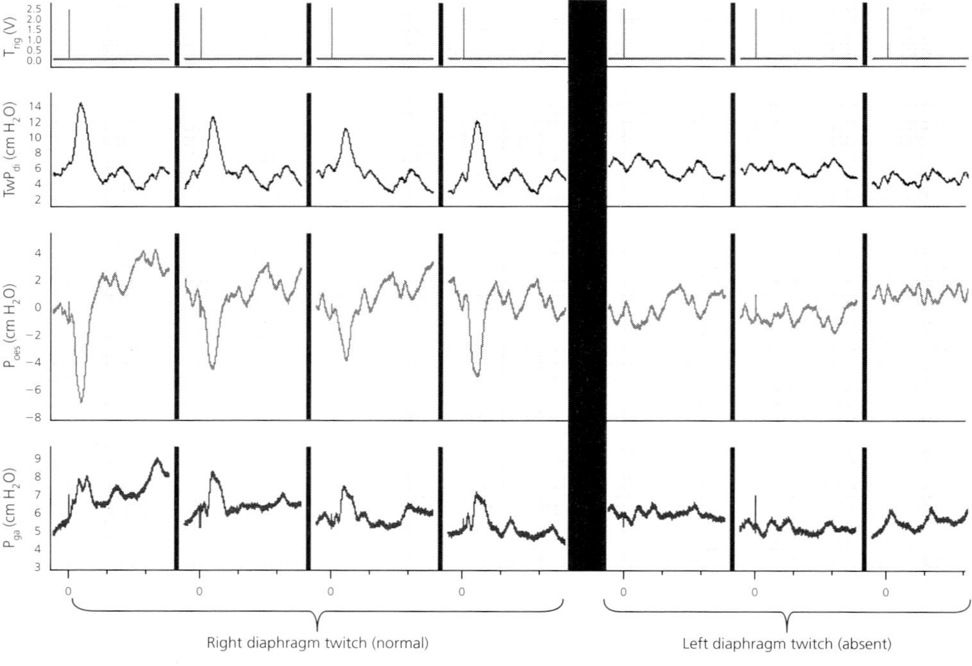


**Figure 16.5** Left hemidiaphragm paralysis on invasive muscle testing. Traces show time of magnetic discharge ($T_{rig}$), transdiaphragmatic pressure ($TwP_{di}$), oesophageal pressure ($P_{oes}$) and gastric pressure ($P_{ga}$). All pressure traces are shown in cm $H_2O$.

These may be a useful tool in the future for assessing patient–ventilator interaction by allowing investigation of unloading of the respiratory muscles and neuroventilator coupling (Fig. 16.6). Respiratory drive is also assessed using $P_{0.1}$, representing the pressure developed during the first 100 ms of inspiration as this is believed to be relatively free of voluntary control.[57] While initially thought to accurately reflect respiratory motor output and

**Table 16.4** Normal ranges for $TwP_{di}$ performed by magnetic stimulation. Units given as cm $H_2O$ and are mean (SD)[51,52]

| | Pressure |
|---|---|
| Bilateral $TwP_{di}$ | 31 (6) |
| Left $TwP_{di}$ | 16 (3) |
| Right $TwP_{di}$ | 12 (4) |

$TwP_{di}$, twitch transdiaphragmatic pressure.

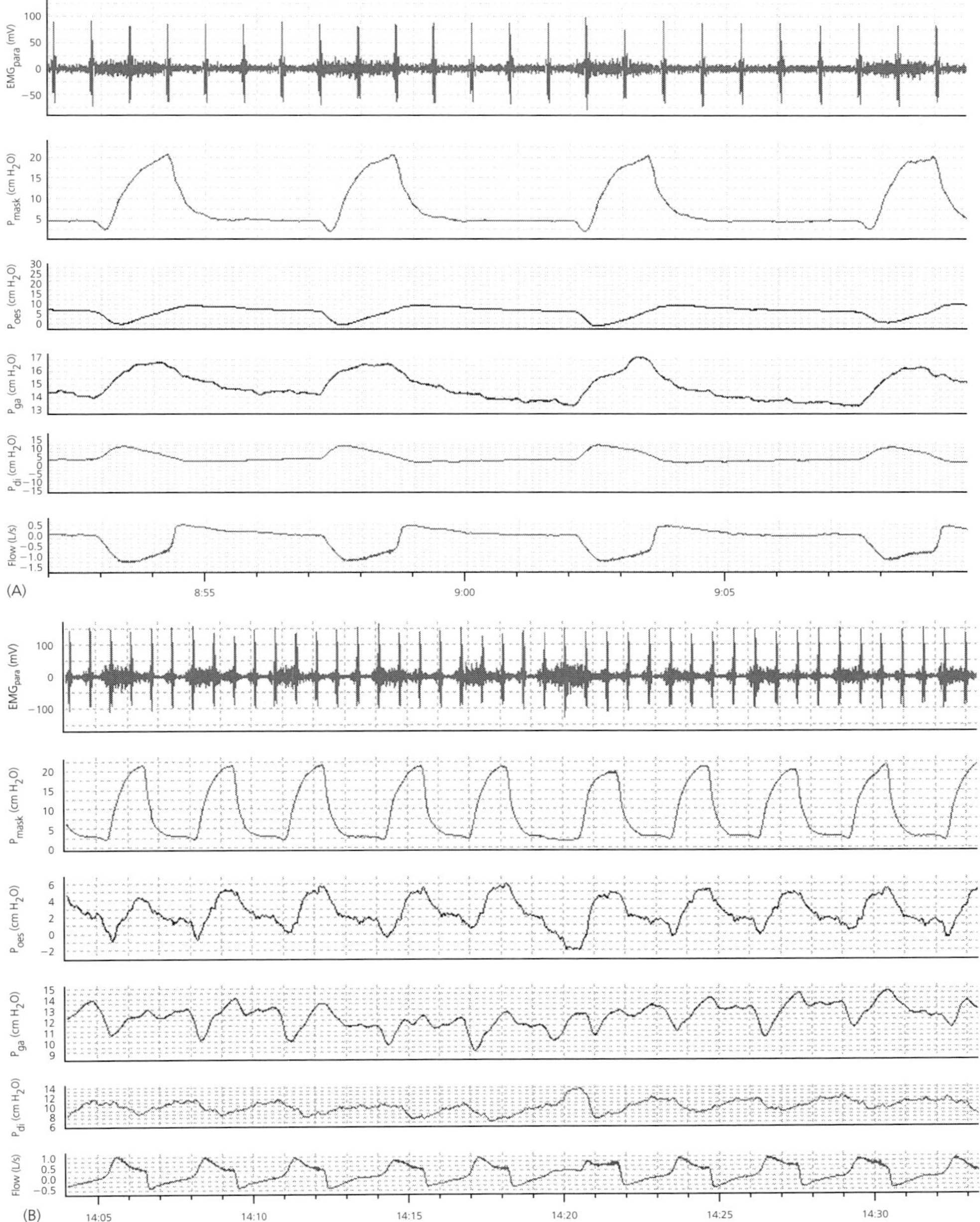


**Figure 16.6** Section of physiological monitoring during a patient study examining patient–ventilator interaction showing parasternal EMG ($EMG_{para}$), mask pressure ($P_{mask}$), oesophageal pressure ($P_{oes}$), gastric pressure ($P_{ga}$), transdiaphragmatic pressure ($P_{di}$) and flow. The use of $EMG_{para}$ allows neuroventilator coupling to be investigated. (A) Period of ventilation with pressure control ventilation and adequate trigger with inspiratory activity (indicated by $EMG_{para}$) resulting in ventilator activation and augmented ventilation. (B) Poor patient–ventilator interaction with inspiratory activity (indicated by $EMG_{para}$), failing to cause ventilator activation and resulting in wasted patient effort.

be unaffected by pulmonary mechanics or respiratory pattern, it is now appreciated that it can be affected by altering the force-length relationship of the diaphragm, such as in hyperinflation.[58] It is therefore often considered using a ratio of the $P_{0.1}$ during tidal breathing to that produced during a maximum inspiratory manoeuvre ($P_{0.1}$:$P_{0.1\ max}$). Unlike metabolic changes, pulmonary mechanics or respiratory muscle strength, changes in $P_{0.1}$ have been shown to explain the variance in dyspnoea in individual patients with COPD during hypercapnic ventilatory response and exercise testing,[59] demonstrating the importance of respiratory drive on the perception of breathlessness.

## PATIENT–VENTILATOR INTERACTION

The principal areas that should be addressed during the consultation include:

- *interface* – mask leak, mouth leak, mask seal, head gear, mask and head gear age and skin pressure areas
- *trigger efficiency* – inspiratory and expiratory synchronization, frequency of auto-cycling, frequency of prolonged inspiratory support (Figs 16.7 and 16.8)
- *pressurization* – symptoms of daytime hypersomnolence and headache, worsening breathlessness, continued snoring and signs of cor pulmonale, excess or inadequate pressure delivered.

Sufficient time must be allowed during the initial set-up of NIV to individualize the ventilator settings. Furthermore, regular follow-up must be undertaken to assess adherence to, and efficacy of, HMV, as a failure to improve gas exchange or poor compliance may represent patient–ventilator asynchrony, progression of the underlying disease or ventilator malfunction. The use of physiological targeted set-up has been reported by some investigators to improve patient comfort and enhances patient–ventilator interaction.[26,28] Although some patient–ventilator interactions can be assessed clinically others require the use of more invasive physiological testing to assess a problem. We find the use of a questionnaire useful to address problems of patient–ventilator asynchrony in the clinical setting. For more on monitoring patient–ventilator asynchrony and how to deal with it, see Chapters 11 and 12.

## OVERNIGHT PHYSIOLOGICAL MONITORING

The investigations discussed so far in this chapter allow the physician to understand the interaction between respiratory muscle load, respiratory muscle capacity and neural respiratory drive. However, this is directed to daytime measurements in the awake state for diagnosis of the clinical problem. The assessment of the respiratory physiological changes occurring during sleep that alter the load, capacity, drive relationship are required to assess for nocturnal

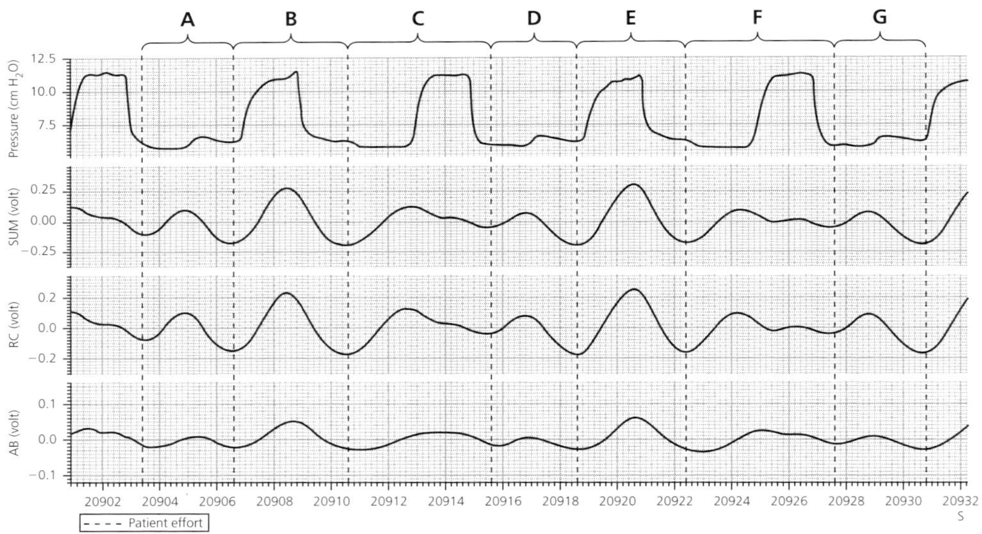


**Figure 16.7** Section of respiratory monitoring on a patient initiating non-invasive ventilation showing, from the top trace, mask pressure, respiratory inductance plethysmography total (RIP sum), thoracic component (RIP RC) and abdominal component (RIP AB). The tracing shows poor synchronization with ventilator pressurization not responding to patient effort. Breaths B and E are synchronized with patient effort and ventilator pressurization occurring together. Breaths A, E and G show patient effort without ventilator response with small rise in mask pressure during expiration. Breaths C and F show respiratory effort unrewarded by pressure support with auto-cycling during expiration.

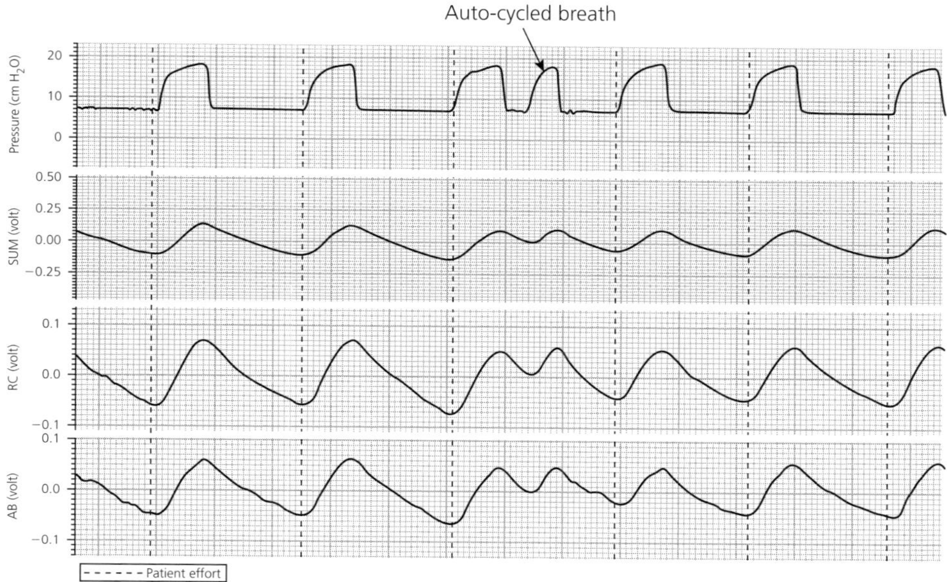


**Figure 16.8** Section of respiratory monitoring on a patient initiating pressure control ventilation showing, from the top trace, mask pressure, respiratory inductance plethysmography total (RIP sum), thoracic component (RIP RC) and abdominal component (RIP AB). The trace shows an auto-cycled breath occurring during patient expiration.

ventilatory support. There are a range of home and hospital systems, from simple to advanced, and these are used to:

- diagnose sleep-disordered breathing
- assess the severity of the problem
- monitor efficacy of treatment.

## Oximetry

Overnight oximetry offers a simple, non-invasive and robust measure of nocturnal oxygenation and is a useful screening test in patients for the presence of sleep-disordered breathing. Due to its ease and low cost it has been used extensively in obstructive sleep apnoea but is insufficiently sensitive to exclude a diagnosis in that condition.[60] The use of oximetry in the assessment of HMV can provide the clinician with valuable insights into the severity of disease and efficacy of treatment without requiring the patient to be admitted into hospital for full physiological monitoring studies, and an experienced analyst can use these simple studies to diagnose a range of more complex sleep-disordered breathing (Fig. 16.9). Computerized scoring systems provide automated analysis producing oxygen desaturation index, time spent with oxygen saturations <90 per cent and heart rate variability that allow an indication of hypoxic load. There is limited evidence available to set a standard lower level of nocturnal oxygenation, although clinical practice would aim for an oxygen saturation levels greater than 88 per cent. Although these devices have widespread availability, the user should appreciate their limitations. This is most noticeable when patients are receiving nocturnal oxygen therapy, resulting in a relatively normal oximetry trace as the hypoventilation and/or upper airways obstruction may result in minimal changes in oxygen saturations.

## Transcutaneous capnography

The hallmark of hypoventilation is an increase in $PaCO_2$. Previously monitoring changes in $CO_2$ used either intermittent arterial sampling or end tidal monitoring; the former is invasive and the latter unreliable in obstructive airways disease and during treatment with NIV. The advent of robust and reliable transcutaneous $CO_2$ ($T_cCO_2$) monitoring has allowed for improved analysis of nocturnal breathing disorders. $T_cCO_2$ is measured electrochemically using a Severinghuas pH electrode to quantify the potentiometric difference between a reference and a measuring electrode. The resultant potential difference is proportional to the negative logarithm of $PaCO_2$. The technical constraints of the technique must be realized along with the appreciation that it is transcutaneous and not arterial values that are being measured. The measurements are taken using a heated electrode, allowing increased permeability of the skin to carbon dioxide facilitating measurement. The temperature settings will vary between systems but are usually in the order of 40–42 °C. This elevation in temperature causes an increase in the local $PaCO_2$, and combined with the fact that the skin is a metabolically active tissue, consuming oxygen and producing carbon dioxide, further increases the recorded value. The commercially available systems correct for this with an automated algorithm that incorporates these factors and produces a value that should reflect $PaCO_2$.

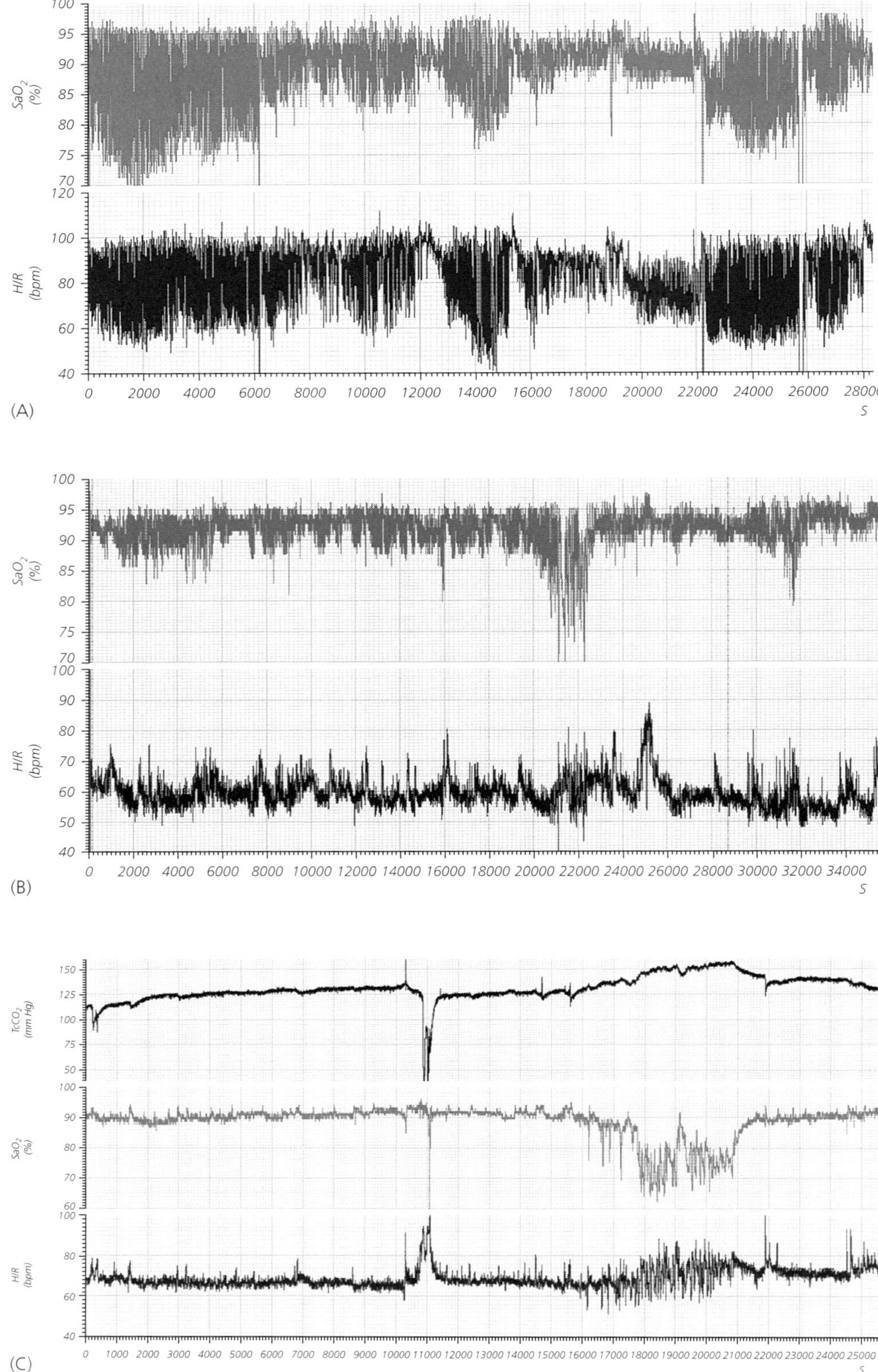


**Figure 16.9** Examples of overnight oximetries, demonstrating patterns of common sleep-disordered breathing. (A) Oximetry showing tight repetitive desaturations with heart rate variability consistent with obstructive sleep apnoea. (B) These traces show features of both hypoventilation and obstructive apnoeas with prolonged deep desaturations superimposed on rapid repetitive desaturations. This pattern is classical of obesity-hypoventilation syndrome with obstructive sleep apnoea. (C) These traces show a prolonged period of sleep state or positional deep desaturation suggestive of hypoventilation.

Clinical studies have shown $T_cCO_2$ to reliably and reproducibly reflect $PaCO_2$ in a range of clinical situations and conditions including critical care and acute NIV as well as in sleep-disordered breathing and obesity.[61–64] The introduction of combined pulse oximeter and $T_cCO_2$ sensors has further increased the usefulness of these devices simplifying the amount of monitoring equipment necessary to study respiratory disorders during sleep. The sensors need to be intermittently 're-membraned' and calibrated at the beginning and end of use to ensure accuracy.

## Advanced sleep studies

Full polysomnography is rarely required in the management of HMV, although it can be useful if it is desired to elucidate the cause of persistent sleepiness despite therapy[65] but the use of transcutaneous carbon dioxide, nasal flow and respiratory inductance plethysmography (RIP) allows full assessment of patients prior to initiation and during follow-up. These modalities allow full respiratory sleep studies to be performed and the appropriate identification of complex sleep-disordered breathing, differentiating obstructive from central apnoeas and documenting hypoventilation (Fig. 16.10) as well as diagnosing periodic breathing abnormalities, such as Cheyne–Stokes respiration. Differentiation of obstructive from central events is made by the absence of respiratory effort in the latter. This is routinely performed by RIP to measure abdominal and thoracic excursion. The technique is widely accepted and is well tolerated by patients and easy to perform, however it may over diagnose central events.[66] Respiratory sleep studies are also helpful in initial titration of NIV settings and diagnosing synchronization issues between the patient

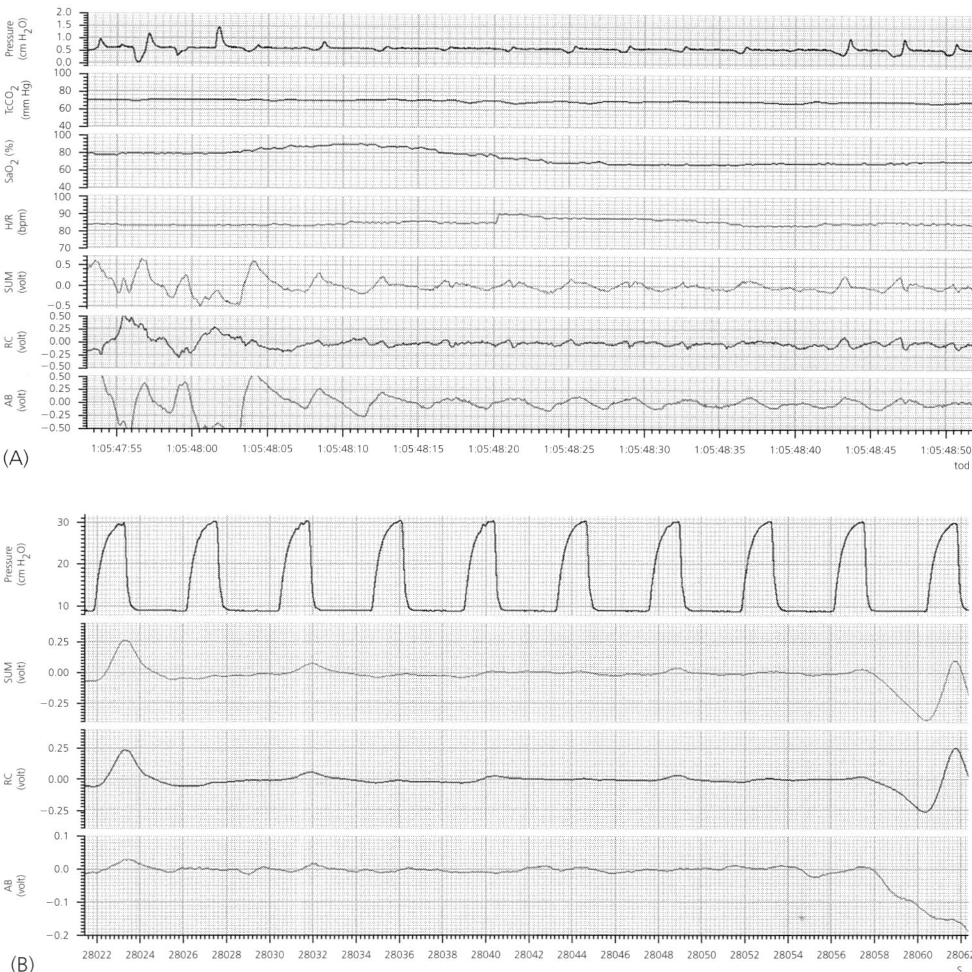


**Figure 16.10** (A) Section of a diagnostic sleep study with recording of nasal pressure, transcutaneous carbon dioxide ($CO_2$), heart rate, oxygen saturations, respiratory inductance plethysmography (RIP) sum, RIP thorax and RIP abdomen. Shows obstructive hypopnoea with chest wall paradox. (B) Section of respiratory sleep study on patient initiating ventilation for obesity-hypoventilation syndrome. Shows central apnoea/hypopnoea with absent/reduced respiratory effort and cycling of the ventilator at the back-up without respiratory movement suggesting upper airways obstruction preventing transmission of pressure.

and the ventilator as well as identifying common events such as ventilator auto-cycling and trigger delay.

## CONCLUSION

The management of patients receiving HMV requires a detailed knowledge of the respiratory physiology with a clear understanding of the relationship between respiratory muscle load, respiratory muscle capacity and neural respiratory drive. In addition to the respiratory physiological changes that occur during sleep, the assessment of patients receiving HMV requires the clinician to have an integrated advanced knowledge of ventilator technology and the issues that are common to specific underlying disease processes. In order to achieve this, a coordinated team approach involving physicians, physiological technicians and specialist nurses is required.

See Appendix A: Invasive respiratory muscle studies in the Vitalsource ebook edition.

## REFERENCES


1. Dar K, Williams T, Aitken R *et al.* Arterial versus capillary sampling for analysing blood gas pressures. *BMJ* 1995; **310**: 24–5.
2. Sauty A, Uldry C, Debetaz L-F *et al.* Differences in pO2 and pCO2 between arterial and arterialised earlobe samples. *Eur Respir J* 1996; **9**: 186–9.
3. Nocturnal Oxygen Therapy Trial Group. Continuous or nocturnal oxygen therapy in hypoxemic chronic obstructive lung disease: a clinical trial. *Ann Intern Med* 1980; **93**: 391–8.
4. O'Donnell DE, Flüge T, Gerken F *et al.* Effects of tiotropium on lung hyperinflation, dyspnoea and exercise tolerance in COPD. *Eur Respir J* 2004; **23**: 832–40.
5. Biring MS, Lewis MI, Liu JT *et al.* Pulmonary physiologic changes of morbid obesity. *Am J Med Sci* 1999; **318**: 293–7.
6. Clayton N. Lung function made easy. *Chron Respir Dis* 2007; **4**: 151–7.
7. Baumann F, Henderson RD, Morrison SC *et al.* Use of respiratory function tests to predict survival in amyotrophic lateral sclerosis. *Amyotrophy Lateral Sclerosis* 2009; **18**: 1–9.
8. Allen SM, Hunt B, Green M. Fall in vital capacity with posture. *Br J Dis Chest* 1985; **79**: 267–71.
9. Steier J, Jolley CJ, Seymour J *et al.* Sleep-disordered breathing in unilateral diaphragm paralysis or severe weakness. *Eur Respir J* 2008; **32**: 1479–87.
10. De Troyer A, Borenstein S, Cordier R. Analysis of lung volume restriction in patients with respiratory muscle weakness. *Thorax* 1980; **35**: 603–10.
11. Mead J, McIlroy MB, Selverstone NJ *et al.* Measurement of intraesophageal pressure. *J Appl Physiolol* 1955; **7**: 491–5.
12. Luo YM, Moxham J, Polkey MI. Diaphragm electromyography using an oesophageal catheter: current concepts. *Clin Sci (Lond)* 2008; **115**: 233–44.
13. Jolley CJ, Luo YM, Steier J *et al.* Neural respiratory drive in healthy subjects and in COPD. *Eur Respir J* 2009; **33**: 289–97.
14. Luo YM, Lyall RA, Harris ML *et al.* Effect of lung volume on the oesophageal diaphragm EMG assessed by magnetic phrenic nerve stimulation. *Eur Respir J* 2000; **15**: 1033–8.
15. Kallet RH, Diaz JV. The physiologic effects of noninvasive ventilation. *Respir Care* 2009; **54**: 102–15.
16. Heinemann F, Budweiser S, Dobroschke J *et al.* Non-invasive positive pressure ventilation improves lung volumes in the obesity hypoventilation syndrome. *Respir Med* 2007; **101**: 1229–35.
17. Appendini L, Patessio A, Zanaboni S *et al.* Physiologic effects of positive end-expiratory pressure and mask pressure support during exacerbations of chronic obstructive pulmonary disease. *Am J Respir Crit Care Med* 1994; **149**: 1069–76.
18. Parameswaran K, Todd DC, Soth M. Altered respiratory physiology in obesity. *Can Respir J* 2006; **13**: 203–10.
19. Hart N, Cramer D, Ward SP *et al.* Effect of distribution and severity of respiratory muscle weakness on gas transfer and lung volumes. *Eur Respir J* 2002; **20**: 996–1003.
20. Estenne M, Heilporn A, Delhez L *et al.* Chest wall stiffness in patients with chronic respiratory muscle weakness. *Am Rev Respir Dis* 1983; **128**: 1002–7.
21. Gibson G, Pride N, Newsom-Davis J *et al.* Pulmonary mechanics in patients with respiratory muscle weakness. *Am Rev Respir Dis* 1977; **115**: 389–95.
22. D'Angelo E, Robatto FM, Calderini E *et al.* Pulmonary and chest wall mechanics in anesthetized paralyzed humans. *J Appl Physiol* 1991; **70**: 2602–10.
23. Kyroussis D, Polkey MI, Hamnegard CH *et al.* Respiratory muscle activity in patients with COPD walking to exhaustion with and without pressure support. *Eur Respir J* 2000; **15**: 649–55.
24. Steier J, Jolley CJ, Seymour J *et al.* Neural respiratory drive in obesity. *Thorax* 2009; **64**: 719–25.
25. Purro A, Appendini L, Patessio A *et al.* Static intrinsic PEEP in COPD patients during spontaneous breathing. *Am J Respir Crit Care Med* 1998; **157**: 1044.
26. Fanfulla F, Delmastro M, Berardinelli A *et al.* Effects of different ventilator settings on sleep and inspiratory effort in patients with neuromuscular disease. *Am J Respir Crit Care Med* 2005; **172**: 619–24.
27. Ozsancak A, D'Ambrosio C, Hill NS. Nocturnal noninvasive ventilation. *Chest* 2008; **133**: 1275–86.
28. Fauroux B, Pigeot J, Polkey MI *et al.* In vivo physiologic comparison of two ventilators used for domiciliary ventilation in children with cystic fibrosis. *Crit Care Med* 2001; **29**: 2097–105.

29. Thomas AM, Turner RE, Tenholder MF. Esophageal pressure measurements in cardiopulmonary exercise testing. *Chest* 1997; **112**: 829–32.
30. Schonhofer B, Koehler D, Polkey MI. Influence of immersion in water on muscle function and breathing pattern in patients with severe diaphragm weakness. *Chest* 2004; **125**: 2069–74.
31. Hart N, Nickol AH, Cramer D *et al.* Effect of severe isolated unilateral and bilateral diaphragm weakness on exercise performance. *Am J Respir Crit Care Med* 2002; **165**: 1265–70.
32. Chetta A, Rehman AK, Moxham J *et al.* Chest radiography cannot predict diaphragm function. *Respir Med* 2005; **99**: 39–44.
33. Lyall RA, Donaldson N, Polkey MI. Respiratory muscle strength and ventilatory failure in amyotrophic lateral sclerosis. *Brain* 2001; **124**: 2000–13.
34. Ward S, Chatwin M, Heather S *et al.* Randomised controlled trial of non-invasive ventilation (NIV) for nocturnal hypoventilation in neuromuscular and chest wall disease patients with daytime normocapnia. *Thorax* 2005; **60**: 1019–24.
35. Bennett JR, Dunroy HMA, Corfield DR *et al.* Respiratory muscle activity during REM sleep in patients with diaphragm paralysis. *Neurology* 2004; **62**: 134–7.
36. Mier-Jedrzejowicz A, Brophy C, Moxham J *et al.* Assessment of diaphragm weakness. *Am Rev Respir Dis* 1988; **137**: 877–83.
37. Soliman MG, Higgins SE, El-Kabir DR *et al.* Non-invasive assessment of respiratory muscle strength in patients with previous poliomyelitis. *Respir Med* 2005; **99**: 1217–22.
38. Black LF, Hyatt RE. Maximal respiratory pressures: normal values and relationship to age and sex. *Am Rev Respir Dis* 1969; **99**: 696–702.
39. Windisch W, Hennings E, Sorichter S *et al.* Peak or plateau maximal inspiratory mouth pressure: which is best? *Eur Respir J* 2004; **23**: 708–13.
40. Koulouris N, Vianna LG, Mulvey DA *et al.* Maximal relaxation rates of esophageal, nose, and mouth pressures during a sniff reflect inspiratory muscle fatigue. *Am Rev Respir Dis* 1989; **139**: 1213–17.
41. Miller JM, Moxham J, Green M. The maximal sniff in the assessment of diaphragm function in man. *Clin Sci (Lond)* 1985; **69**: 91–6.
42. Steier J, Kaul S, Seymour J *et al.* the value of multiple tests of respiratory muscle strength. *Thorax* 2007; **62**: 975–80.
43. Hart N, Polkey MI, Sharshar T *et al.* Limitations of sniff nasal pressure in patients with severe neuromuscular weakness. *J Neurol Neurosurg Psychiatry* 2003; **74**: 1685–7.
44. American Thoracic Society/European Respiratory Society. ATS/ERS statement on respiratory muscle testing. *Am J Respir Crit Care Med* 2002; **166**: 518–624.
45. Polkey MI, Lyall RA, Green M *et al.* Expiratory muscle function in amyotrophic lateral sclerosis. *Am J Respir Crit Care Med* 1998; **158**: 734–41.
46. Bach JR. Amyotrophic lateral sclerosis: predictors for prolongation of life by noninvasive respiratory aids. *Arch Phys Med Rehabil* 1995; **76**: 828–32.
47. Chatwin M, Ross E, Hart N *et al.* Cough augmentation with mechanical insufflation/exsufflation in patients with neuromuscular weakness. *Eur Respir J* 2003; **21**: 502–8.
48. Uldry C, Fitting J-W. Maximal values of sniff nasal inspiratory pressures in healthy subjects. *Thorax* 1995; **50**: 371–5.
49. Luo YM, Johnson LC, Polkey MI *et al.* Diaphragm electromyogram measured with unilateral magnetic stimulation. *Eur Respir J* 1999; **13**: 385–90.
50. Mills GH, Kyroussis D, Hamnegard CH *et al.* Bilateral magnetic stimulation of the phrenic nerves from an anterolateral approach. *Am J Respir Crit Care Med* 1996; **154**: 1099–105.
51. Hamnegard C-H, Wragg SD, Mills GH *et al.* Clinical assessment of diaphragm strength by cervical magnetic stimulation of the phrenic nerves. *Thorax* 1996; **51**: 1239–42.
52. Mills GH, Kyroussis D, Hamnegard CH *et al.* Unilateral magnetic stimulation of the phrenic nerve. *Thorax* 1995; **50**: 1162–72.
53. Murphy K, Mier A, Adams L *et al.* Putative cerebral cortical involvement in the ventilatory response to inhaled CO2 in conscious man. *J Physiol* 1990; **420**: 1–18.
54. Barker AT, Jalinous R, Freeston IL. Non-invasive magnetic stimulation of human motor cortex. *Lancet* 1985; **1**: 1106–7.
55. Sharshar T, Ross E, Hopkinson NS *et al.* Effect of voluntary facilitation on the diaphragmatic response to transcranial magnetic stimulation. *J Appl Physiol* 2003; **95**: 26–34.
56. National Institute for Health and Clinical Excellence. Intramuscular diaphragm stimulation for ventilator-dependent chronic respiratory failure due to neurological disease. 2009.
57. Whitelaw WA, Derenne JP, Milic-Emili J. Occlusion pressure as a measure of respiratory center output in conscious man. *Respir Physiol* 1975; **23**: 181–99.
58. Milic-Emili J. Recent advances in clinical assessment of control of breathing. *Lung* 1982; **160**: 11–17.
59. Marin JM, Carrizo SJ, Gascon M *et al.* Inspiratory capacity, dynamic hyperinflation, breathlessness, and exercise performance during the 6-minute-walk test in chronic obstructive pulmonary disease. *Am J Respir Crit Care Med* 2001; **163**: 1395–9.
60. Williams AJ, Yu G, Santiago S *et al.* Screening for sleep apnea using pulse oximetry and a clinical score. *Chest* 1991; **100**: 631–5.
61. Maniscalco M, Zedda A, Faraone S *et al.* Evaluation of a transcutaneous carbon dioxide monitor in severe obesity. *Intensive Care Med* 2008; **34**: 1340–4.
62. Senn O, Clarenbach CF, Kaplan V *et al.* Monitoring carbon dioxide tension and arterial oxygen saturation by a

single earlobe sensor in patients with critical illness or sleep apnea. *Chest* 2005; **128**: 1291–6.

63. Rodriguez P, Lellouche F, Aboab J *et al.* Transcutaneous arterial carbon dioxide pressure monitoring in critically ill adult patients. *Intensive Care Med* 2006; **32**: 309–12.
64. Storre JH, Steurer B, Kabitz HJ *et al.* Transcutaneous PCO2 monitoring during initiation of noninvasive ventilation. *Chest* 2007; **132**: 1820–6.
65. Meyer TJ, Pressman MR, Benditt J *et al.* Air leaking through the mouth during nocturnal nasal ventilation: effect on sleep quality. *Sleep* 1997; **20**: 561–9.
66. Luo YM, Tang J, Jolley C *et al.* Distinguishing obstructive from central sleep apnea events: diaphragm electromyogram and esophageal pressure compared. *Chest* 2009; **135**: 1133–41.

# 17

# Patient and caregiver education

OLE NORREGAARD, JOAN ESCARRABILL

## ABSTRACT

It is important to define the respective responsibilities of the ventilator user, caregivers and of the hospital/HMV centre. The educational programme should address both theoretical and practical issues. There needs to be instruction, assisted and supervised performance, independent performance, and signed confirmation of each specified competence. While the primary focus will be on the ventilator user, the needs of the caregiver should also be addressed. Travel should be discussed and planning for any trip should start early. Whether supplementary oxygen will be needed during air travel should be determined before flights are booked as airlines vary greatly in their provision of oxygen. Regardless of the mode of travel there are a number of things that should be considered. When crossing borders be aware of possible changes in standards and regulations including voltage and connections for ventilators, oxygen concentrators and other equipment. Check the availability of healthcare facilities at destination. Distances within airports can be considerable; book assistance if needed.

## INTRODUCTION

Home mechanical ventilation (HMV) has a long history dating back to the 1930s and was utilized in particular in the 1950s during the poliomyelitis epidemic. The major expansion, however, took place during the past couple of decades, especially in western Europe and North America.[1–4] The overall goal is to improve quality of life, to improve survival and to save money. Data indicate that the cost of HMV is in the range of 20–50 per cent of the cost of stay at an intensive care unit (ICU).[5] The cost associated with HMV is mainly related to wages of the caregivers, in some studies amounting to around two-thirds.[6]

The practice of HMV includes, among various issues, achieving a balance between quality of life[7–9] and the level of risk.[10] Although data on adverse events are scarce and may be underreported, cases have been documented.[11] To what extent the risks are associated with poorly trained caregivers is not clear. However, caregivers are obviously an integral part of HMV. Without attendants in some form, the practice of HMV would be close to non-existing, at least for the most severely disabled patients, and the recent expansion in HMV would not have been possible.

Caregiving is managed in ways that vary a great deal from place to place. In some countries the task is performed primarily by family members and relatives, while in others it is handled by professional healthcare personnel or trained lay individuals.[12,13] There is no agreed standard for minimal requirements for caregivers and even more recent guidelines almost do not even comment on the issue.[14] To what extent that is a problem is not very well known, but studies have documented that attendants express the desire and need for formal training,[15] and that parents who care for their medically complex children in the home, although they express satisfaction, also 'report challenges, including health impacts on the primary care giver(s)'.[16,17] They may feel that they are the lifeline of the child.[18] In a group of well-educated North American mothers caring for ventilator-assisted children at home, 45 per cent had a score indicating depression.[19] Recently the ventilator users themselves[20,21] have expressed 'significant concerns about the risk of ventilator failure or mucous plugging', or fear that the ventilator hose will pop off the tracheostomy tube.[22]

The stress and strain associated with the unassisted responsibility for an individual on HMV can lead to exhaustion, anxiety and depression and thus obviously to a compromised quality of life. Ventilator users have hoped that properly trained attendants/personal support workers could at least partly ameliorate problems[22] and it has been reported that 'competence and continuity of healthcare personnel are factors for success'.[23]

## LEGAL AND ETHICAL ISSUES

To our knowledge, there is no legal framework to specifically regulate HMV and caregivers' work, much less any common international regulation of the area. In the absence/paucity of legal regulations, ethical standards may help to guide the practice of HMV. The Appleton Consensus[24] stated more than 20 years ago the four principles of ethics:

- beneficence (do good)
- non-maleficence (do not do bad)
- autonomy (self-determination)
- distributive justice.

Recently it seems there has been a trend towards giving higher priority to the principle of autonomy, often translated to patient autonomy, to some extent at the cost of the other three principles. This has in some countries resulted in the patient's right to choose or not to choose a specific treatment, and also to choose to terminate this treatment, even if this will result in the (immediate) death of the patient. Translated into the area of HMV this means that patients in some countries can ask for termination of life-sustaining ventilator treatment.

When it comes to the caregivers' rights, almost no attention has been given to them. However, caregivers' rights and responsibilities should be an area of interest. In the absence of legal regulations the caregiver may be left lost and unprotected, in some cases not even with a centre for HMV or a similar institution to rely on. Funding also varies tremendously, ranging from state-financed arrangements including attendants, equipment, modifications of the home and a vehicle as is the case in some of the Nordic countries, to scenarios where funding is very limited (in parts of the world it is non-existent), and the financial burden is placed largely on the family members, who may experience life as a struggle for economic support.

## EDUCATION

### Purpose

The overall purpose of HMV should be addressed, and it should be made clear to the ventilator-assisted individual and to the attendants that an active, self-directed life based on independency is a core issue in HMV. If that is not an option in specific cases, for instance because of an advanced malignant condition, it should be made clear that palliation with HMV is the setting, so attendants do not develop a sense of guilt when the ventilator-assisted individual expires.

It is important that acceptance of common goals is in place, as motivation is a critical element in the learning process, in addition to reinforcement and retention.[25] A structured learning process should be the aim, and it has been reported that formal training programmes for caregivers have documented an improvement in caregivers' skills as well as in their satisfaction with the educational programme.[26] In addition, evidence is emerging that patient self-management is associated with improved patient satisfaction and outcome,[27] underlining the importance of involvement of the ventilator-assisted individual. This involvement could preferably also include participation in training for HMV, to the extent that the ventilator-assisted individual can participate.

### Setting

Education of the ventilator-assisted individual and of attendants/relatives where they are a part of the arrangement, will usually take place in hospital, preferably in a centre for HMV if such is available, or depending on how extensively the ventilator user is disabled, possibly in the patient's home or in an alternative outpatient setting.

The actual educational process can optimally, before admission to the hospital, be preceded by thorough information and adjustment of expectations through talks with hospital staff, as well as with individuals already on HMV. This service should be facilitated by the hospital clinic. The experience is that the more realistic expectations the ventilator-assisted individual has in advance, the smoother will be the educational and discharge processes.

Education could initially, during a common session with all involved parties present, clarify the responsibilities of each of these parties:

- The responsibility of the ventilator user can vary from being totally self-reliant to – where attendants and/or relatives are involved – being the employer who can direct, hire and fire the attendants, and further to – in case of severe disability – an individual with very limited competencies and more or less totally dependent on the attendants.
- The responsibility of the caregiver would typically be to behave in a professional manner including respect for the ventilator user's autonomy and individual requirements and needs, and to practise the skills and attitudes acquired during the training programme – and in principle no further. It is advisable to make the limits of responsibility clear to the attendant as well as to the ventilator-assisted individual.
- The responsibility of the hospital/HMV centre is obviously to educate, to treat medical and technical problems, to secure discharge planning and subsequently back-up through, for instance, a 24-hour hotline and regular follow-up visits to the hospital and/or in the ventilator-assisted individual's living site.

It is important that adequate time is allowed for the process to unfold. Depending on the local programme, usually 2–5 days are needed for the establishment of non-invasive ventilation, and 2–6 weeks for implementing complex invasive HMV. Ideally a programme should be so organized that the process is advancing without wasting time, to the benefit of the individual ventilator user and to the optimal use of various resources and of the facility, enabling the individual facility to maximize the number of ventilator-assisted individuals it can accommodate.

**Box 17.1 Content of a theoretical educational programme for a ventilator-assisted individual and their caregiver(s)**

General knowledge

1. The rationale for long-term non-invasive and invasive ventilation
2. Basic anatomy and physiology of the airways
3. The working principles of the ventilator(s) the individual ventilator user will be using in their home
4. The principles and differences between alarms activated by either a change of flow or by a change in pressure. Specifically, a decrease in the circuit pressure indicates a leakage, whereas a decrease in flow indicates obstruction, and vice versa. This point should be particularly clarified
5. Importance of appropriate humidification

Non-invasive ventilation

6. The rationale for choosing different types of masks
7. The adverse effects of non-invasive ventilation, in particular leakage, irritation to mucous membranes and the eyes, gastrointestinal inflation, skin lesions, and importantly – pressure-induced malformation of the facial bony structures in children

Invasive ventilation

8. The rational for choosing different types of tracheostomy tubes, in particular cuffed versus uncuffed and fenestrated versus non-fenestrated types and the significance and risk of cuff pressure
9. The adverse effects of invasive ventilation, in particular leakage around the tube via the stoma during uncuffed ventilation, pneumothorax during cuffed ventilation, mucous plugging, pneumonia, lesions to the tracheal mucous membrane, tracheal scarring, tracheal stenosis and tracheomalacia
10. The risk of accidental disconnection from the ventilator
11. The risk of accidental extubation and the reinsertion procedure, possibly using a smaller tube and/or using a suctioning catheter as a guidewire during intubation
12. The fundamental importance of preserving and optimizing speech, whenever the ventilator-assisted individual's pathology is compatible with that goal

## Methodology

The learning atmosphere should not be stressful, but supportive and encouraging, and learning objectives should be clear to promote original learning and to facilitate subsequent retention of skills.[25] The learning process should preferably be **goal directed** and **competence based**.

The educational programme could be divided into a **theoretical** and a **practical** part. The theoretical part will, depending on the specific equipment the individual ventilator-assisted individual will be using, explain the necessary background knowledge in a step-by-step way (Box 17.1).

If the ventilator-assisted individual poses other problems that need theoretical attention, this should be included in the programme. For the more disabled users, attention should possibly be paid to nutritional support typically via a percutaneous endoscopic gastrostomy (PEG) tube, to pressure sores and contractures and to communication equipment and techniques.

The practical part can be structured in three steps:

1. instruction by the staff
2. assisted and supervised performance by the ventilator-assisted individual and/or attendant (Fig. 17.1)
3. independent performance by the attendant and signed approval by the staff of each specified competence.

When requirements to competences are outlined in detail it will to a large extent be possible to:

- document progress and thus stimulate motivation and self-assurance of the attendant (and of the ventilator-assisted individual)
- verify that the required knowledge and practical skills are retained.

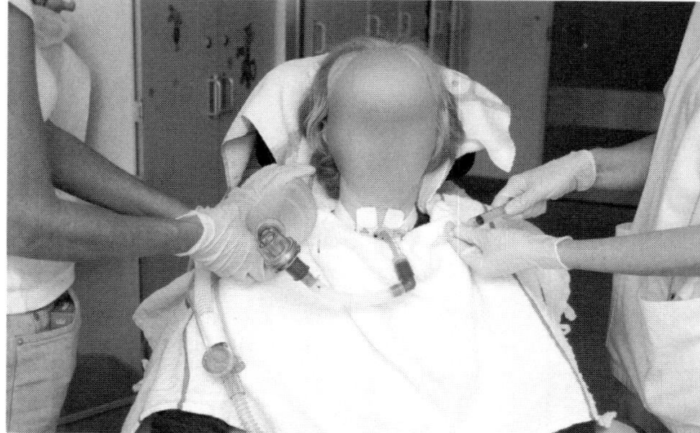

**Figure 17.1** Lay attendant (left) learning to manage manual ventilation for tracheostomized patient while being supervised by a nurse (right).

Documentation and quality assurance are important aspects that easily make up another component of this method, which in addition provides a structured framework that is accessible for stepwise adjustments as techniques and equipment change and develop over time.

The acquisition of practical skills is best done at the bedside. The details of a typical list of practical skills is given in Box 17.2.

## Box 17.2 Practical skills that should be acquired during the educational process

### General

- Recognition of signs of infection of the airways and elsewhere
- Hygienic precautions when dealing with ventilator user and equipment (masks, cannulas, hoses, humidifiers, ventilators and disposable items)
- Understanding ventilator settings and troubleshooting up to some defined level, understanding alarms and the ability to take proper action in response, in particular to understand the significance of low-pressure alarms versus high-pressure alarms
- Assemble and disassemble relevant equipment such as masks, the ventilator circuit and the humidifier
- Knowledge about whom to call and what to do in an emergency
- Patient care, including helping with personal hygiene, dressing, handling special beds, handling lifts to ensure safe transfer from bed to wheelchair, driving the ventilator-assisted individual's vehicle
- In some cases additional skills including handling a PEG tube, catheterization of the urinary bladder, working with computer-assisted communication, physical exercises to mobilize limbs
- Handle specific needs in the technology-dependent neonate or child (and its parents) including familiarity with downscaled interfaces, downscaled equipment generally, low functional residual capacity leading to low oxygen reserves and short response time in hypoxaemic conditions, delicate balance with respect to fluids and nutrition, possibly tension and anxiety in parents
- Resuscitation skills are sometimes included. At our institution, we have chosen not to include this responsibility in the attendant's curriculum. However, if an attendant already possesses resuscitation skills, they are allowed to resuscitate when needed

### Non-invasive ventilation

- Selection of mask, positioning of mask, securing an unobstructed airway and, especially in children, awareness of the fact that even small displacements can partly occlude the nostrils, selection of headgear and the balanced tightening that will on the one hand prevent or minimize leaks and on the other hand exert minimal pressure on the face (Fig. 17.2)
- Forced expiration technique, breath-stacking using a one-way valve, cough assist via a mask

### Invasive ventilation

- Suctioning procedures via the tracheostomy tube using either a suctioning catheter or a cough assist, changing of inner cannula and in some cases of the tracheostomy tube itself; tracheostomy tube cleaning and maintenance, assessment and cleaning of the stoma
- Manual ventilation with a self-inflating ventilation bag, typically in relation to suctioning procedures in the invasively ventilated patient

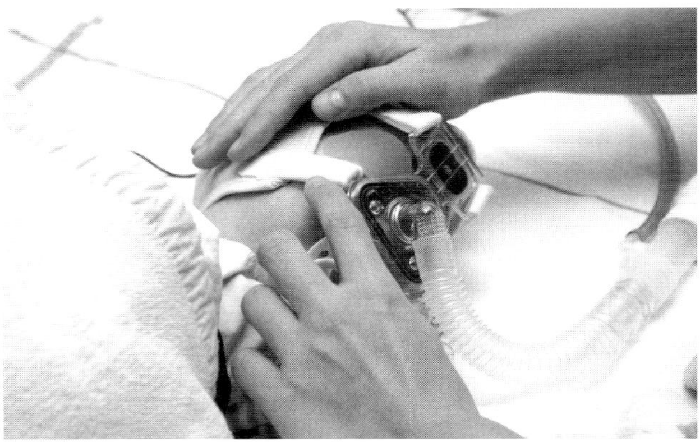

**Figure 17.2** Mounting hood and nasal mask for non-invasive ventilation in an infant.

This range of skills and competences should be tailored to fit the ventilator-assisted individual's requirements. Some of the individual issues that may require modification of the standard educational programme are listed in Box 17.3.

When one further takes into account the physiological differences between different conditions such as amyotrophic lateral sclerosis (ALS), cystic fibrosis, chronic obstructive pulmonary disease (COPD), neuromuscular diseases (Duchenne, Limb-Girdle, SMA-II), quadriplegia and obesity-hypoventilation syndrome, it is intuitively clear that the generic plan for caregiver training has to be modified – sometimes quite vigorously – to the individual case.

The practical outline and format of the training programme will also vary from place to place, depending on economic, cultural, geographic and other factors.

**Box 17.3 Ventilator-assisted individual-dependent issues that may require modification of the educational programme**

- Level of mental and cognitive competence and also presence of a complex psychological profile
- Ventilator-assisted individual's ability (or not) to communicate
- Their degree of bulbar and general motor weakness, sometimes in combination with marked obesity
- Presence of comorbidities (cardiac issues, nutritional problems, urinary and faecal incontinence, skin lesions, painful contractures of limbs and the jaw, spasms and more)
- Other issues such as speaking a foreign language, religious beliefs and habits, family characteristics, strain or crisis caused by the disease or failed expectations, 'invisible' siblings while the technology-dependent child gets all attention, and divorce

## SPECIFIC ISSUES

### Caregivers

It may not come as a surprise that the rest of the world will focus on the health of the ventilator user (sometimes with visible physical disabilities) and not on the health of the caregiver, but caregivers themselves often neglect their own health and even may experience a decline in health over time as a caregiver.[28,29] The explanation seems straightforward across a series of different disabilities where caregivers report depression,[30,31] overload and burden.[32] The rate of some degree of depression among caregivers has at times been reported to exceed 50 per cent, and studies have found that 6 months after discharge 15 per cent of caregivers were classified as having symptoms consistent with severe depression. This again may be explained on the basis of or triggered by social isolation[17,33] and a heavy work load of 12–14 hours a day.[34] Thirty per cent of caregivers working with patients with advanced ALS have rated their quality of life as lower than that of their patient, and 60 per cent of them left their jobs. If the caregiver at the same time is also a parent or a spouse of the ventilator user, it is conceivable that the strain may be even stronger.[17,33] It is a paradox that even today the interest in the health of caregivers is so small,[35] considering the crucial role they play in supporting the whole system of HMV. As mentioned before, caregivers themselves express a desire for training, and the cost of HMV is easily competitive to that of a stay in hospital.

Considering the above premises, it is not difficult to propose that securing reasonable training and working conditions for caregivers may be the best and cheapest way to secure survival and quality of life in this vulnerable population of patients. This is to some extent already in place in some countries, and has recently been suggested in a Canadian report on chronic ventilation, accompanied with proposals for improving the supporting community network of healthcare professionals and allied partners.[36]

### Travel

Travel is increasingly popular, and to longer distances in particular by air. This has increased to a level where 50 million passengers are passing through one of the major European airports every year and worldwide the estimate is around two billion passengers annually. Older data[37] reported that around 5 per cent of travellers were 'ambulatory patients'. The number of air passengers on some sort of long-term mechanical ventilation is not known, but it is known to clinicians that even severely physically disabled individuals on long-term mechanical ventilation take short- and long-distance flights, and in many cases successfully.

It is also known that in travelling by air, one will be – depending on flight altitude – exposed to conditions that will bring the $PaO_2$ of a healthy passenger down to 7.0–8.5 kPa; exposed to lowered humidity (also in people with difficulty clearing secretions); exposed to an increase in body gas volumes by roughly a third (also in people with muscular dystrophy with decreased gastrointestinal mobility and in people with emphysematous bullae); predisposed to venous thrombosis; and possibly increased risk for acquiring an infection.[38]

There is not much hard evidence to back suggestions on what to do if one is on long-term mechanical ventilation and for instance has a neuromuscular disease and the person plans to travel by air. Most is commonsense, but there is some information available online, especially for people with COPD (see reference 39). However, for attendants it has not been possible to identify suggestions, let alone guidelines.

One important suggestion is to start planning the trip very early and in detail and with the caregivers, if they will be participating in the trip. This will increase the chances of taking the necessary precautions. Overall, it should be recommended that individuals on long-term mechanical ventilation or ventilator support should undergo a preflight assessment and fill in a medical information form (available at www.iata.org/medical manual) and check with the airline whether one can be accepted as a passenger, and if yes, on what conditions. A detailed list of specific recommendations that should be followed is given in Box 17.4.[38]

Good advice in general whether travelling on ground, water or by air includes:[42]

- disabled people should be seated near toilet and exit
- get information about healthcare facilities at airport(s) and at destination
- acquire permission for transportation at transit airport – distances within airports can be considerable

**Box 17.4 Preflight precautions for individuals on long-term ventilator support**

- If $SaO_2$ is below 92 per cent or below 95 per cent associated with a risk factor, which long-term mechanical ventilation obviously is, the ventilator user should be exposed to a hypoxic challenge test (HCT). A recent study[40] in neuromuscular patients documented that even patients with a resting $SaO_2$ >95 per cent who desaturated during a HCT met the criteria suggested by the British Thoracic Society Standards of Care Committee for inflight oxygen[41]
- For individuals with cystic fibrosis or other chronic lung diseases with lowered forced expiratory volume in one second ($FEV_1$), in particular if below 50 per cent, a HCT should be performed
- People with pneumothorax should not undertake air travel until 6 weeks after resolution is confirmed by a chest radiograph
- People with asthma should carry bronchodilators.
- Individuals with ventilators should bring only dry batteries and external lithium ion batteries with capacity <160 Wh
- People with history of thromboembolism should be started on anticoagulation
- Medication in original packing is accepted maximally for 1 year in the European Union (EU) for EU citizens and for others only for 3 months

- acquire permission from hotel/accommodation at destination
- when crossing borders be aware of possible changes in standards and regulations including voltage and connections for ventilators, oxygen concentrators and other equipment.

## SUMMARY

The importance of proper education of a ventilator-assisted individual and, if needed, also of their caregivers is increasingly recognized as vital for a successful life with the ventilator at home. This field is not very well documented and even less well regulated. Both ventilator-assisted individuals and caregivers often do express a desire for better education to alleviate the burden of HMV.

The education should follow a well-structured programme that includes provision of theoretical knowledge and practical skills with clarified goals and checklists. It is important to verify that the ventilator-assisted individual, and if needed also the caregivers, have acquired the necessary competences to secure proper safety and risk management as a platform for a good quality of life.

Travelling, also by air, is increasingly an integral part of the life of ventilator-assisted individuals, and professional planning, paying attention to the recommended precautions, should be the rule.

Whenever caregivers or relatives are a part of the ventilator-assisted individual's life, attention to their working conditions and often huge burden of responsibility should be recognized.

## REFERENCES

1. Duiverman ML, Bladder G, Meinesz AF *et al.* Home mechanical ventilatory support in patients with restrictive ventilatory disorders: a 48 year experience. *Respir Med* 2006; **100**: 56–65.
2. Lloyd-Owen SJ, Donaldson GC, Ambrosino N *et al.* Patterns of home mechanical ventilation use in Europe: results from the Eurovent survey. *Eur Respir J* 2005; **25**: 1025–31.
3. Jeppesen J, Green A, Steffensen BF *et al.* The Duchenne muscular dystrophy population in Denmark, 1977–2001: prevalence, incidence and survival in relation to the introduction of ventilator use. *Neuromuscul Disord* 2003; **13**: 804–12.
4. Laub M, Berg S, Midgren B. Swedish Society of Chest Medicine. Home mechanical ventilation in Sweden – inequalities within a homogenous health care system. *Respir Med* 2004; **98**: 38–42.
5. Final report of the Ontario Chronic Ventilation Strategy Task Force. 2006; 54–6.
6. Dranove D. What impact did the programs have on the costs of care for ventilator assisted children? In: Aday LA, Aitken MJ, Wegener DH, eds. *Pediatric home care: results of a national evaluation of programs for ventilator assisted children.* Chicago: Pluribus Press, University of Chicago, 1988; 295–321.
7. Lumeng JC, Warschausky SA, Nelson VS *et al.* The quality of life of ventilator-assisted children. *Pediatric Med* 2001; **4**: 21–7.
8. Moss AH, Oppenheimer EA, Casey P *et al.* Patients with amyotrophic lateral sclerosis receiving long-term mechanical ventilation. Advance care planning and outcome. *Chest* 1996; **110**: 249–55.
9. Bourke CB, Tomlinson M, Williams TL *et al.* Effects of non-invasive ventilation on survival and quality of life in patients with amyotrophic lateral sclerosis: a randomized controlled trial. *Lancet Neurol* 2006; **5**: 140–7.
10. Srinivasan S, Doly SM, White TR *et al.* Frequency, causes and outcomes of home ventilator failure. *Chest* 1998; **114**: 1363–7.
11. Lechtzin N, Weiner CM, Clawson L. A fatal complication of noninvasive ventilation. *N Engl J Med* 2001; **344**: 533.
12. Brooks D, Gibson B, DeMatteo D. Perspectives of personal support workers and ventilator-users on training needs. *Patient Educ Couns* 2008; **71**: 244–50.

13. Norregaard O. *Home mechanical ventilation in Denmark.* Paper presented at the 43rd Nordic Lung Congress, Uppsala, Sweden, May 2007.
14. Wallgren-Pettersson C, Bushby K, Mellies U *et al.* 117th ENMC workshop: ventilatory support in congenital neuromuscular disorders – congenital myopathies, congenital muscular dystrophies, congenital myotonic dystrophies and SMA (II). 4–6 April 2003 Naarden, The Netherlands. *Neuromuscul Disord* 2004; **14**: 56–69.
15. Yamada K, Sugai K, Fukumizu M *et al.* The parents'assessment and needs for home mechanical ventilation in patients with pediatric neurologic disorders. *No To Hattatsu* 2003; **35**: 147–52.
16. Wang K-W K, Bernard A. Technology-dependent children and their families: a review. *J Adv Nurs* 2004; **45**: 36–46.
17. Carnevale FA, Alexander E, Davis M *et al.* Daily living with distress and enrichment: the moral experience of families with ventilator-assisted children at home. *Pediatrics* 2006; **117**: e48–e60.
18. Mah JK, Tannhauser JE, McNeil DA *et al.* Being the lifeline: the parent experience of caring for a child with neuromuscular disease on home mechanical ventilation. *Neuromuscul Disord* 2008; **18**: 983–8.
19. Kuster PA, Badr LK. Mental health of mothers caring for ventilator-assisted children at home. *Issues Ment Health Nurs* 2006; **7**: 817–35.
20. Gibson BE, Upshur REG, Young NL *et al.* Disability, technology and place: social and ethical implications on long-term dependency on medical devices. *Ethics Place Environ* 2007; **10**: 7–28.
21. Gibson BE, Upshur REG, Young NL *et al.* Men on the marg. Bourdiesian examination of living into adulthood with muscular dystrophy. *Social Sci Med* 2007; **65**: 505–17.
22. Sarvey SI. Living with a machine: The experience of the child who is ventilator dependent. *Ment Health Nurs* 2008; **29**: 179–86.
23. Ballangrud R, Bogsti WB, Johansson IS. Clients' experiences of living at home with a mechanical ventilator. *J Adv Nurs* 2009; **65**: 425–34.
24. Stanley JM. The Appleton Consensus: suggested international guidelines for decisions to forego medical treatment. *J Med Ethics* 1989; **15**: 129–36.
25. Lieb S. *Principles of adult learning.* Arizona Department of Health Services. South Mountain Community College. Vision. 1991.
26. Tearl DK, Hertzog JH. Home discharge of technology-dependent children: evaluation of a respiratory-therapist driven family education program. *Respir Care* 2007; **52**: 171–6.
27. Holman H, Lorig K. Patient self-management: a key to effectiveness and efficiency in care of chronic disease. *Public Health Rep* 2004; **119**: 239–43.
28. Douglas SL, Daly BJ. Caregivers of long-term ventilator patients: physical and psychological outcomes. *Chest* 2003; **123**: 1073–81.
29. Sexton DL, Munro BH. Impact of a husband's chronic illness (COPD) on the spouse's life. *Res Nurs Health* 1985; **8**: 83–90.
30. Miller B, Townsend A, Carpenter E *et al.* Social support and caregiver stress: a replication analysis. *J Gerontol B Psychol Sci Soc Sci* 2001; **56**: S249–56.
31. Pilisuk M, Parks SH. Caregiving: where families need help. *Soc Work* 1988; **33**: 436–40.
32. Pearlin LI, Mullan JT, Semple SJ *et al.* Caregiving and the stress process: an overview of concepts and their measures. *Gerontologist* 1990; **30**: 583–94.
33. Ibañez M, Aguilar JJ, Maderal MA *et al.* Sexuality in chronic respiratory failure: coincidences and divergences between patient and primary caregiver. *Respir Med* 2001; **95**: 975–9.
34. Kaub-Wittemer D, Steinbüchel N, Wasner M *et al.* Quality of life and psychosocial issues in ventilated patients with amyotrophic lateral sclerosis and their caregivers. *J Pain Symptom Manage* 2003; **26**: 890–6.
35. Talley RC, Crews JE. Framing in the public health of caregiving. *Am J Public Health* 2007; **97**: 224–8.
36. Final report of the Ontario Chronic Ventilation Strategy Task Force. 2006; 72.
37. Coker R. *Air travel and respiratory disease.* Paper presented at 14th Annual Congress of the European Respiratory Society. Glasgow, Scotland, September 2004.
38. Coker RK, Shiner RJ, Partridge MR. Is air travel safe for those with lung disease? *Eur Respir J* 2007; **30**: 1057–63.
39. British Thoracic Society. Air travel guidelines. Available at: http://www.brit-thoracic.org.uk/clinical-information/air-travel/air-travel-guideline.aspx (accessed 15 February 2010).
40. Mestry N, Thirumaran M, Tuggey JM *et al.* Hypoxic challenge flight assessment in patients with severe chest wall deformity or neuromuscular disease at risk for nocturnal hypoventilation. *Thorax* 2009; **64**: 532–4.
41. British Thoracic Society Standards of Care Committee. Managing passengers with respiratory disease planning air travel: British Thoracic Society recommendations. *Thorax* 2002; **57**: 289–304.
42. Edvardsen A. Practical aspects of travel. Paper presented at the 19th Annual Congress of the European Respiratory Society. Vienna, Austria, September 2009.

# 18

# Discharging the patient on home ventilation

JOAN ESCARRABILL, OLE NORREGAARD

## ABSTRACT

Discharge of a patient is a process that usually takes a few days or, in the case of a patient with very complex needs, can be extended over a few months. The first hours at home are crucial for adaptation and it is preferable that the patient can connect directly with the care team if there is a problem (weekends are usually best avoided). The needs of caregivers (family, relatives and friends) must always be considered; it is a significant event for them also. Discharge is not a one-way journey – if things are not going well the patient can return to hospital. A multitude of players can be involved and need to be coordinated. A care manager is someone who: builds patient and caregiver confidence; assures specific competence of everyone involved; is a single point of contact in case of problems; helps to ensure that all issues have been addressed; and ensures efficient use of resources. Patient safety is very important and a key component of this is the transfer of information to all members of the care team; a patient with a chronic disease can see many different specialists in a year. All need to be aware of the issues that are relevant to them.

## THE D-DAY IN DISCHARGE PLANNING

Discharge of a patient is a process that may take a few days (in most cases) or can be extended even to a few months (in the case of complex patients with long stays in the intensive care unit [ICU]). Generally, we speak of 'discharge plan' if it develops a strategy that allows the patient to adapt to a new treatment outside the hospital setting (in this case a treatment involving ventilatory support). The purpose of the discharge plan is to achieve maximum independence for the patient using therapeutic resources and technology to suit their needs, taking into account the efficacy and safety of treatment. Broadly speaking, we can distinguish four types of discharge plans:

- from hospital to home
- from hospital to a more or less complex health facility (from hospital to a community hospital or hospice, for example)
- for outpatient initiation of home mechanical ventilation (HMV)[1,2]
- for patients on HMV admitted to the hospital for an acute exacerbation or to regulate the ventilatory settings.

In all these circumstances, discharge should be planned carefully. The discharge plan is not formulated just once at the time of establishment of HMV and is never 'final'. It must be revisited whenever circumstances lead to change in the ventilatory requirements: worsening of the disease, weight gain or loss or change of device.

In their classic article on the discharge of patients, Bertoye *et al.*[3] described how a patient with sequelae of polio began the process of transfer from hospital to the patient's home. Patients require a short period of adaptation and in this case a temporary transfer was made from the hospital to the patient's home, but the patient quickly decided to stay home with the ventilator. As illustrated in this classic experience, return home is possible if there is an agreement between the caregiver, patient and the care team. It is essential that the caregiver is competent and he or she accepts the workload of caring for a patient with HMV; finally, the home conditions should be adequate for this kind of therapy. Technical support should cover emergencies around the clock, with a short response time. At the time of discharge, the recommendations concerning the use of the ventilator must be clearly written down, including the patient monitoring scheme.[4]

In the discharge plan, there is a 'D-Day', which is agreed between the patient and caregiver and case manager. It is imperative to take time to decide the 'D-Day', especially in patients who have been admitted in the hospital for a long period of time. In such patients, it is not reasonable to plan the discharge on a weekend. The first hours at home are crucial for adaptation and it is preferable that the patient can communicate directly with the care team if there is any problem.

Moreover, the discharge plan is not a journey without return. The patient should be assured that the return to the previous situation is possible (though in most cases it will not be necessary or desired by the patient or caregiver).

## DISCHARGE PLANNING

It has been recognized for many years that without a discharge plan in place the risk for failure is imminent.[5] Discharge planning should start as early as possible, and is best started at the beginning of the educational stay. The plan should be comprehensible and ideally include all needs and actors in the often very complex scenario that the education of a HMV candidate with attendants constitutes. At the same time it is advisable to try to make things as simple as possible.

It is recommended to organize the planning in each case as a matrix including all involved parties, and carried out in a well-defined temporal sequence with clearly defined actions, and to appoint a case manager for the job. This will increase chances that all relevant questions are addressed, minimum time is wasted and the whole process will be seen as forward moving and experienced more satisfactorily by all parties including the ventilator user, his or her attendants and the staff. This might add to a better start and a more optimistic outlook to the future life of the HMV user. Table 18.1 depicts an example generic matrix.

The whole arrangement can include a multitude of players such as the funding agency, centre for HMV, agencies delivering the equipment (special bed, modified wheelchair, oxygen, lift, equipment for communication, disposals), the physiotherapist, the occupational therapist, the social worker, the nurse and the physician. Specific points that should be clarified and settled before discharge are presented in Box 18.1.

If the ventilator-assisted individual will be taken care of by a professional agency whose employees are not trained at the centre for HMV, it is recommended to specify in detail the required qualifications of the hired staff, and also to arrange a signed contract with the agency, and if possible also with the individual employee, to ensure that they possess the claimed knowledge, skills and experience.

No HMV programme is complete without a well-structured follow-up programme. In fact this is the lifelong 'companion' that is supposed to ensure survival, safety and quality of life. Without this, the initiation of HMV carries the risk of being the beginning of the end.

**Table 18.1** Overview of a generic matrix showing the roles of actors involved in training and discharge of the home mechanical ventilation (HMV) user and attendants

| | Time 1 | Time 2 | Time 3 | Time 4 | Time 5 | Time 6 | Time 7 | Time 8 |
|---|---|---|---|---|---|---|---|---|
| Patient | Symptoms | Hires attendants | Education begins | Education continues | Education completed | | HMV user moves home | Check up |
| Department of Neurology | Refers patient to HMV | | | | | | | Check up |
| Centre for HMV | Validates patient for HMV | Initiates 'global' plan | Education of attendants begins | Education continues | Education completed | HMV user is discharged | | Check up |
| Municipality/ insurance | Asked for funding by HMV | Donates funding | | | | | | |
| Agent responsible for change of home | | Contacted by HMV | Begins change of home | | | Home is ready | | |
| Other relevant parties | | | | | | | | |

**Box 18.1 Specific points that should be clarified and settled before discharge**

- Ventilator-assisted individual and attendants are ready and motivated
- In patients with rapidly progressive conditions end-of-life issues should preferably have been discussed, if not clarified
- Ventilator-assisted individual is stable, or is as stable as possible
- All attendants and, where relevant and possible, the ventilator user have completed the specified education and training programme
- Extra ventilator is available if needed (for instance if use of ventilator for more than 12–14 hours a day and/or if the ventilator-assisted individual lives far from a hospital)
- Modifications of wheelchair (to accommodate the ventilator and humidifier for instance) are in place
- Modifications of the home are completed
- A modified vehicle is or will soon be acquired (if funding allows for that)
- A plan for regular delivery of disposables is ready
- Arrangements for school or other institution if relevant have been completed
- Written and illustrated individualized material to take home, reinforcing what has been learned during the training period, is ready
- Arrangements for risk management[6] and emergencies, including back-up for supply of electricity if in area with repeated breakdown of power supply
- Plans for follow-up, including when (routinely and in the case of an exacerbation), where, and with an outline of what issues should be addressed
- A detailed plan for transfer from hospital to home. A nurse from the HMV facility should ideally accompany the ventilator user and the attendant to the ventilator user's living site and help install the necessary device and ensure that the transition takes place in a safe and confident manner

## FUTURE PLANNING

It is obvious that some scenarios will require intensive follow-up and support. In the case of an individual with advanced amyotrophic lateral sclerosis (ALS) who is invasively ventilated, recording a number of variables and adjusting the ventilator a little will not always be sufficient. Planning for how to handle the next deterioration within weeks to a few months is an ongoing and never-ending process, which will require not only medical and logistic skills, but also guidance and help to accept, or at least to some extent cope with, life. End-of-life issues will surface, and in countries where termination of treatment is allowed, the ventilator-assisted individual should be strongly urged to express a decision before a state of lock-in occurs. End-of-life decisions have in some countries been shown commonly to be shared between the involved caregiver and the patient.[7] In our experience, this is often easier the earlier the issue is raised, i.e. even before invasive ventilation is initiated.

In parallel with these problems, the continuously changing and increasing needs of this type of patient will optimally require advanced planning months ahead, comprising a series of practical matters including funding, as expenses may increase over time, and funding agencies may work at a different speed from that of the disease progression.

Although it may seem to be beyond the scope of a follow-up programme for HMV users, it seems reasonable, at least to mention, that after a dramatic deteriorating and sometimes tremendously resource consuming – at a human, emotional and financial level – treatment with a (predictable) fatal outcome, the relatives of the diseased and the attendants can sometimes benefit from a talk, not only with a psychologist or a priest but also with staff at the centre for HMV. The centre may have been one of the main supports in the terminal phase.

## ALTERNATIVES TO THE HOME IN HOME MECHANICAL VENTILATION

In some cases the choice is not between remaining in the acute-care hospital or transfer to the patient's home. In most countries the transfer home is almost impossible for patients who live alone or for whom the caregiver cannot take over the care needed by the patient. Patients with tracheostomy, even without requiring round the clock ventilation, are the most problematic patients at home.

The first consequence of this situation is the increase in hospital stays[8] followed by the financial problems this causes institutions and patients.[9] Some countries have weaning centres where it is easier to make this transition. More than half of patients admitted to centres reach weaning off the ventilator, but 20 per cent require long-term ventilation.[10] Weaning centres play a transitional role in the discharge plan for patients requiring HMV, but in general, they should not be considered as the long-term solution for most of the patients.

Some countries have centres that, while not specifically prepared to receive patients with HMV, can take charge of certain types of these patients. The nomenclature may differ – hospices, nursing homes or long-stay facilities, etc. – but they are all characterized by assurance of basic care in an environment with minimal medical supervision or nursing. The transfer of patients to such centres often requires monitoring by experts, since the caring professionals are not familiar with the use of ventilators. The transfer from hospital to these facilities is not easy in patients with ALS and tracheostomy.

The success of the discharge plan depends largely on the availability of a skilled team that can support the patient and caregivers, both at home and in other healthcare facilities. A good example of this teamwork is in the French non-profit associations that have been working in this field for over 50 years. The ALLP (*Association Lyonnaise de Logistique Posthospitalière,* formerly *Association Lyonnais de Lutte Contre la Poliomyélite*) was established over 50 years ago to facilitate the return home of polio patients requiring long-term ventilatory support.[11] This kind of organization allows support at home, support for ventilated patients who cannot return to their homes and must live in apartments supervised by nurses, as well as the education of both the formal and informal caregivers.

Training and coaching are very important. In general, family caregivers perform properly even more complex procedures. However, in some countries there are regulations that do not allow tracheal suctioning by unlicensed personal care attendants.[12] The organizations that support these restrictive arguments claim that this technique can only be done by specialized professionals (primarily nurses). This point of view, strictly applied, would prevent the return home of many patients, especially children. This extreme position also would hinder the school attendance of patients with HMV. A good strategy for overcoming these legal barriers is the stipulation of formal caregivers (non-graduate) or informal caregivers, as stated by the ALLP. With HMV, as in most chronic conditions, the care plan cannot be finalized without the active participation of the patient (and caregiver) in their own treatment.[13] It is very important to note that the number of potential caregivers involved may be very high. In designing the training, the wide range of those involved in care should be taken into account.

## Team working and coordination of care

The care of patients with chronic diseases is an example of a complex system involving several actors. Decisions are made at different levels of the healthcare system and it is very difficult to control all the details. A decision taken at a point in the health system (for example in the emergency department) can have an enormous impact on the overall treatment plan. The global response to the needs of a patient requires teamwork and a very significant effort to coordinate care.

Wagner defines very well the characteristics of the care team: 'A patient care team is a group of diverse clinicians who communicate with each other regularly about the care of a defined group of patients and participate in that care'.[14] In patients with HMV we can distinguish the 'core team' and a group of professionals involved in patient care. The 'core team' is usually made of a mix of individuals from the hospital expert team (doctors, nurses and physiotherapists) and the community care team (family physician and nurses). Physicians from different specialties may be involved in HMV: chest physicians, paediatricians, anaesthetists or specialists in intensive care. But around this 'core team' we must consider the participation of many other professionals: hospital specialists (speech therapist, nutritionist, ENT, neurologists) and both the hospital and the community can develop rapport with the patient's social workers, occupational therapists, psychologists, technicians supply companies, etc.

The general characteristics that define a team are shown in Box 18.2[15] and the team skills to care for patients with HMV are shown in Box 18.3.[16]

## Care coordinator

The organization of complex care cannot be achieved by the sum of the individual actions of each professional. Spontaneous coordination is impossible. Specialists, particularly physicians, have difficulty getting an overview of the problems of patients. The role of nurses is crucial because they are more holistic in outlook and they are

**Box 18.2 General characteristics that define a team**

- Heterogeneous group of individuals who contribute in different ways
- Clear goals for the group and for each member
- Everyone understands the tasks they have to do
- Clear coordinator role
- There is a supportive, informal atmosphere
- Comfortable with disagreement and feel free to criticise
- A lot of discussion (group members listen to each other)
- Learns from experience

Adapted from: www.kent.ac.uk/careers/sk/teamwork.htm.[13]

**Box 18.3 Team skills to care for patients with HMV**

- Skills related to home mechanical ventilation (HMV) technology and home care
- Ability to assess the adequacy of caregivers
- Knowledge of community resources
- Capacity to integrate home, outpatient, and hospital care
- Designing of guideline-based care plans that integrate the clinical needs and preferences of the patient
- Behavioural counselling and teaching of self-management
- Expertise in group consultations

Adapted from Escarrabill and Goldberg.[14]

more focused on care coordination by training.[17] Moreover, patients clearly value this nursing role and it is obvious that coordination has a direct impact on perceived quality of care.[18]

The role of 'care manager'[19] makes sense from several perspectives. From the perspective of the patient and caregiver it builds confidence and provides competence assurance (it also identifies a single contact in case of problems); from the perspective of other team members it helps to identify the targets; from the perspective of the physician who prescribes the HMV it ensures that all patient needs are covered; and from the perspective of the financier it ensures efficient use of resources. To achieve effective care coordination is essential, in that the professional in charge has the highest decision-making capacity in terms of care organization, planning of visits and the establishment of priorities. The care manager should have the knowledge and skills to organize the care of patients with different diseases but with common problems (in this case the common denominator would be the ventilation) and he/she focuses its critical role in coordinating the different health resources. The care manager must be very accessible to the patient.

Finally, evaluation of healthcare should specifically include an assessment of this coordination.[20]

## Strong and weak relationships

From a practical standpoint, the relationship between HMV prescribing centres and local hospitals or primary care teams is not always easy and clear-cut. In some countries the physician who prescribes does not follow the patient and, therefore, once decisions are made, health professionals who sometimes are not familiar with this complex treatment must assume the long-term follow-up. In other cases, the prescribing team establishes hierarchical relationships with health professionals in the community; this attitude is not the best strategy to promote collaboration. Neither of these two extreme positions is a guarantee of good patient care. There is no health organization (from the high-tech centre to the primary care team) that can single-handedly deal with all the patient's needs in all the possible circumstances.

In addition, although greater centralization improves knowledge, it possibly makes access harder for the patient. Several studies have shown that the best results are achieved by hospitals working as referral centres for the diagnosis and treatment of patients with serious diseases such as ALS. Farrero *et al.*[21] showed that early respiratory evaluation of patients with ALS, performed immediately after diagnosis, improves survival. The care provided by multidisciplinary teams is associated with a better quality of life and increased survival.[22] Traynor *et al.*[23] note that multidisciplinary intervention reduced mortality by 29.7 per cent and, even in patients with bulbar involvement, survival improved by almost 10 months. However, there are some controversial issues. In some studies, benefits are not seen in connection with a multidisciplinary team. This lack of benefit has been attributed to a 'weak' intervention (although the percentage of patients with non-invasive ventilation or percutaneous endoscopic gastrostomy [PEG] was very low in these studies with negative findings).[24]

Hutchinson *et al.*[25] observe that many studies showing benefit of a multidisciplinary approach to ALS have significant selection bias. Certainly patients attending a specialist clinic have a better prognosis; but patients who do not benefit from this kind of attention as they live far from the referral centre have more disabilities, are older, with disease that has been developing for less time or with bulbar onset. In one study, patients referred to a referral centre lived 11 months more than those cared for in the community, which may suggest selection bias rather than more efficacious treatment.[26] Chiò *et al.*[27] also observed improvement in survival in ALS patients treated in tertiary centres. But these patients were younger, they had PEG and non-invasive ventilation (NIV) more frequently, and they were admitted to hospital fewer times than the patients in the control group.

This discussion about the benefits of a referral centre (with a lot of experience and a large number of patients) versus the benefits of a smaller centre (with greater accessibility to the patient but with more limited skills and knowledge) was discussed in the Eurovent survey.[28] This survey revealed a great diversity of strategies in Europe: some countries have fewer facilities with many patients in each (in Denmark there are only two centres that coordinate HMV) whereas others have multiple centres with fewer patients. Moreover, the number of patients do not necessarily reflect the centre's experience in treating critically ill patients. Key skills in HMV are more related to the experience in the care of patients with neuromuscular diseases with or without tracheostomy. The technique of HMV, especially NIV, is not particularly difficult. More and more professionals are becoming familiar with the use of NIV in acute patients and this experience can be transferred in part to the care of chronic patients. The difficulties in HMV are related to the decision making process: choosing the best treatment (which in many cases is not necessarily related to the correction of gas exchange), solving problems and making complex decisions (such as performing tracheostomy in a patient with ALS). The balance between the efficiency of ventilation (measured from the perspective of physiology) and its acceptance by and the comfort of the patient is based more on the caring professionals' deliberation rather than rigid formulas.

The reality, in many cases, is that between the multidisciplinary team and 'nothing' there are many alternatives. As Bonisteel correctly pointed out,[29] the multidisciplinary team is an urban construct that works from a geographically fixed site. At 100 km away from the city, the team has to use existing resources in the community. Moreover, referral organizations have an element of instability. In many cases, the added value offered by these centres is directly related to the characteristics of professionals (the doctors, nurses or physiotherapists) who work in it, and not necessarily the organization itself or the systematic workflow. When people move, the value of the organization also changes. Referral centres cannot grow indefinitely, or in many cases, it is not advisable to grow only in one direction. Furthermore, the concept of referral centre can be useful for part of the care process, but other important aspects of the care process can be performed in centres located closer to the patient's home. The case of ALS may be a good example. The benefits of a referral centre (or very few referral centres) could be for diagnosis and initial assessment of patients with ALS. But for ventilatory support, it is not unreasonable to propose any solution that would allow easy accessibility, especially in regard to proximity of the centre when acute problems occur.

An alternative to the referral centre is networking. But networks should be cooperative rather than hierarchical, and replacing the referral centre by centralized networks is very limited progress. In this sense the so-called 'distributed networks' are more stable[30] and help to identify the roles of each of the components. Table 18.2 summarizes the benefits of networking in the care of patients with HMV.

## Patients like me

Patients have created networks, like 'patientslikeme.com',[31] before the professionals. Patientslikeme aims to promote networking between communities of patients, who share information and experiences about the disease and offer each other support and advice. These communities are also open to health professionals. Currently communities are active on neuromuscular diseases, ALS, Parkinson's, fibromyalgia, multiple sclerosis, diseases related to mood (anxiety, depression, bipolar disorder) and acquired immune deficiency syndrome (AIDS).

Since the introduction of riluzole in 1996, many studies investigated the drugs that delay the progressions of ALS, one of which was published by Fornai *et al.*[32] in February 2008. Fornai *et al.* suggested that daily doses of lithium might slow the progression of ALS in humans during the 15 months of the follow-up. The paper immediately earned the praise of some of the scientific community.[33] However Bedlack *et al.*[34] raised methodological concerns relating to the work of Fornai *et al.*: How were the participants selected? What criteria of inclusion/exclusion were used? How many patients were visited in order to select the 44 participants in the study? Why was the chosen randomization ratio 16:28, rather than 1:1? Was placebo used for patients not receiving lithium? Was the use of ventilatory support or PEG similar in both groups, how were the patients followed up, and what side effects occurred with lithium? Moreover, Vanacore and Galeotti[35] point out that Fornai did not specify the type of intervention in the eight patients in the group not receiving lithium who died.

Through Patientslikeme, Humberto Macedo (ALS patient) and Karen Felzer (daughter of a patient with ALS) analysed in depth the work of Fornai to verify the real impact of lithium in ALS patients. Sceptical about the results, they designed a study to verify the effects of lithium and recruited patients through the network. In less than 6 months they enrolled 217 patients who took lithium regularly (27 per cent with bulbar involvement). Although this was not a randomized study, the group of patients taking lithium was similar to the patients participating in the ALS forum on Patientslikeme (2090 patients; 21 per cent with bulbar involvement). Seven per cent of the lithium participants died during the year, 41 per cent discontinued treatment and for 24 per cent of patients the plasma level of lithium was available. Initial results (of 191 patients followed for 6 months) showed no changes in the rate of disease progression and the rate of progression was not related to levels of lithium. Among the 'collateral effects' they note that low doses of lithium (150 mg/day) might be tried initially for the relief of painful cramps. This study had many limitations from a methodological point of view, but not much more than the Italian study. It was a prospective, observational, patient-led study.[36] But nevertheless, we must recognize that this patient-led study managed to include in a short time a high number of participants that is unthinkable in the conventional academic context. Negative results can neutralize the 'enthusiasm' of the participants to find an immediate remedy to their problems and also evidence obtained for other clinical applications of lithium. However, it is a challenge to conventional clinical research and the study

**Table 18.2** Benefits of networking for patients on home mechanical ventilation

| Network elements | Benefits |
|---|---|
| Sharing data on indication criteria and results | Allows comparison about data rather than opinion |
| Maintaining the skills and knowledge of professionals | Professional development and continuing education |
| Increasing the robustness of healthcare services | Overcome resistance to change or support in cases of both organizational and structural changes |
| Balance between accessibility and excellence | Giving patients quality care close to home |
| Maintaining a portfolio of services including infrequent procedures or highly specialized techniques | The different hospitals in the network can provide specific services to the other centres |
| Ensuring a critical mass (knowledge and experience) | Suggests studies with a large population |

can be either outrightly rejected or be analysed in a thoughtful way. One cannot say that this represents mainstream clinical research in the future, but it is clear that patient networks are an emerging force.

## PATIENT SAFETY

The negative health effects of medical interventions have been known since ancient times. The term 'iatrogenic' refers precisely to this effect: 'produced by the doctor'. Hippocrates (460–360 BC) dictated '*primum non nocere*'. However, the concern about clinical safety developed only recently, after the publication of the report *To Err is Human*, by the Institute of Medicine in the USA.[37]

Worrying about clinical safety makes sense for several reasons. Errors can cause much inconvenience to the patient and are associated with inappropriate stays in hospital, injury, suffering (and death). Whether or not they have impact on the patient, they satisfy no one and are difficult to explain to an increasingly demanding society.

An important aspect related to clinical safety is that there has been a significant qualitative change in the interpretation: the avoidance of blaming individuals for past mistakes and focusing on the organization as the source of the error. Errors do not occur because of 'bad people' but because of bad organization that ignores the formation or the establishment of a protective barrier for the patient. Learnings from safety as developed in industrial activities should be applied to healthcare. A clear example is the safety in all matters relating to air travel.[38]

From a non-health organizational perspective, Spear[39] indicates that hospitals are usually organized by functions. This type of organization tends to lead to fragmentation and, therefore, to creation of ambiguities. To ensure their proper functioning requires a high degree of coordination. Therefore, concerns about clinical safety require the redesign of health systems. The issues around clinical safety are especially relevant in the case of HMV. This is a complex treatment (use of equipment, adaptation of the ventilator, changes in settings in relation to the evolution of the disease, etc.) delivered by various professionals with different degrees of involvement. It is a treatment that takes place beyond the direct control of clinicians and most of the time is supervised by informal caregivers.

During patient care in hospital and when we prepare the discharge plan we can identify hotspots that could compromise safety.[40] Box 18.4 identifies some of these points.

A very important element for patient safety is the transfer of information or the changes to the care team. A patient with a chronic process can see up to 16 different medical specialists in a year.[41] The method of transferring information is crucial when it involves many professionals. Visits to the emergency services are another source of risk. Some patient associations have made recommendations for ventilation users when in the emergency department,[42] and these are summarized in Box 18.5.

### Box 18.4 Risks associated with patients on HMV

- Unplanned admission as a result of poor healthcare management
- Transfer from another acute care hospital
- Transfer from the intensive care unit to general ward
- Transfer from ward to the intensive care unit or another monitored setting
- Any nocturnal transfer behind the hospital
- The weekend in the hospital
- Discharge at the weekend
- Hospital complications developed during admission
- Hospital-acquired infection
- Adverse drug reaction indicated in the chart
- Dissatisfaction with the care received
- Care in emergency departments

### Box 18.5 Recommendations for patients on HMV while attending the emergency department

- Provide all available information (clinical reports, ventilator settings, etc.) and identify the care team
- Remember that oxygen can be dangerous for unventilated patients with neuromuscular diseases
- Anaesthesia may have added risks for patients with neuromuscular diseases
- Insist on being placed in the best position for their stay in the emergency department (in some cases patients are better off in the wheelchair than in the trolley).
- The patient should be autonomous with regard to the equipment (ventilator, assisted cough devices, masks, etc.) until he or she is assured that the health centre can look after their specific needs. It is advisable to avoid hospital admission whenever possible.
- Collect all the data related to the care in the emergency department (or be assured that this information will be sent to the care team).

Fatalities have been reported in patients with HMV in relation to electricity supply problems.[43,44] It is also well documented that patients, when possible, change the settings of the ventilator. Farré *et al.*[45] showed that the percentage of patients with a discrepancy between the prescribed and actual measured main ventilator variable (minute ventilation or inspiratory pressure) was higher than 20 per cent in 13 per cent of the cases and higher than 30 per cent in 4 per cent. Clearly, the HMV carries a certain risk, but zero risk does not exist even in intensive care units. The risk exists, but as Simonds said,[46] the risk can be minimized by sharing clinical information, properly training patients and families and ensuring technical support at home.

In this context, it is easy to overlook some critical points in patient safety. The discharge process is one of these points. Neale *et al.*[47] reported that 10.8 per cent of patients admitted to two large hospitals in Greater London experienced one or more adverse events (most of them preventable) and 18 per cent of adverse events were related to the care at the time of discharge. These figures suggest that the discharge should not be regarded as a bureaucratic procedure but should involve bringing together the patient's condition and care planning outside the hospital. The pressure for short stays (reasonable from the viewpoint of preventing risks to the patient and also to avoid unnecessary costs) generates another source of risk. Sometimes, when discharging the patient, clinicians do not have all the information of the procedures performed in hospital and some of these results can be crucial. Roy *et al.*[6] observed that 41 per cent of patients will receive results after discharge and that 9 per cent of these results will require immediate action. This fact highlights the need for improved communication between hospital and health community resources.[48] Complaints, especially if they relate to the organization, are a good way to improve clinical safety.[49]

Finally, it should be noted that in many cases, the deterioration of the patient with HMV can be very subtle. Chatwin *et al.*[50] analysed home visits due to a suspected malfunction of the ventilator. In 13 per cent of visits no abnormality was detected, but in half the cases the patients did not feel well and were admitted to hospital and two patients died in the course of a month. Perhaps this shows the difficulties faced by patients (and health professionals) in identifying early, subtle changes that suggest a deterioration in lung function or in the general condition. In short, to improve clinical safety, organized care is required to operate unambiguously, as is the continued reinforcement of the training given to patients and caregivers and a high index of suspicion for potential problems.

## DISCHARGE PLANNING IN AGEING PATIENTS OR IN PALLIATIVE CARE

In some circumstances, the discharge plan is designed without a long-term view. This can happen when prescribing HMV in elderly patients or in patients in the advanced stage of their disease.

### Older patients and home mechanical ventilation

It is increasingly common to consider HMV in patients with advanced age. Farrero *et al.*[51] show the benefits of HMV in patients over 75 years. The authors analysed the results of HMV in 43 patients with a mean age of 77.1 ± 1.9 years; 11 per cent of patients stopped treatment (in patients under 75 years cared by the same team the drop-out rate was 2 per cent). In those who continued with HMV there was an improvement in gas exchange, a reduction in hospital admissions and fifty per cent of patients were still alive at 6 years. As Midgren[52] noted, age alone is not a contraindication to HMV. Moreover, Crespo *et al.*[53] found no significant differences in gas exchange or the adverse effects related to the age of patients with HMV.

### Palliative care and home mechanical ventilation

In the patient on long-term HMV, it is sometimes difficult to identify the final stage of the disease, especially in patients with neuromuscular diseases that progress slowly or restrictive respiratory diseases. Despite these difficulties, recognition of the end-of-life stages has a major impact on patients and caregivers,[54] from the emotional, workload and economic viewpoints. In ALS the problems associated with the end-of-life stage are more severe and occur more rapidly than in other patients on HMV.[55] There are situations in which clinical management is especially difficult, as in ALS, patients with diaphragmatic paralysis are intubated before knowing the neurological diagnosis. Decisions may need to be revisited within a few weeks of ventilation, regarding application of invasive ventilation, perhaps without ventilator-free time, because before the acute process it was not possible to make decisions.

In some cases, HMV also could be the only strategy to allow the return home of critically ill patients who cannot be disconnected from the ventilator. In these cases we talk more about 'rescue ventilation' than HMV itself. Rady and Johnson showed that 15 per cent of patients admitted to the ICU were more than 85 years old[56] and 35 per cent of survivors could not return to their homes, requiring admission to a care facility at discharge (the percentage of patients is twice that in the younger patient group).

It can be difficult to provide an individualized prognosis for a COPD patient. Discharge plans for more severe COPD patients require careful identification of suitable candidates, a precise definition of the care needed and a realistic plan to ensure provision of that care.[57] In COPD there is no accepted definition of 'final stage of the disease' so it is difficult to compare different studies.[58] Moreover the use of a cancer model to predict the need for palliative care of COPD patients is unhelpful.[59] In addition, there are no clear criteria for identifying patients with COPD who might benefit from long-term HMV. In some cases, it is clear that HMV is 'rescue ventilation' rather than a formal indication of HMV.

Admission to a hospice (or a centre for chronic patients) is also an alternative in the final stages of life. It is very important to identify the limits of treatment,[60] especially in regard to artificial nutrition, readmission to hospital and resuscitation. These decisions should be written into the medical record. Discharge planning of older patients or patients on palliative care and HMV poses challenges different from those in patients with classic indications. In these cases, the comfort and return to the home are as important as survival. Moreover, in many cases the return home can be very difficult and the patient may require temporary or permanent stay in an institution such as a hospice.

## REFERENCES


1. Luján M, Moreno A, Veigas C *et al.* Non-invasive home mechanical ventilation: effectiveness and efficiency of an outpatient initiation protocol compared with the standard in-hospital model. *Respir Med* 2007; **101**: 1177–82.
2. Chatwin M, Nickol AH, Morrell MJ *et al.* Randomised trial of inpatient versus outpatient initiation of home mechanical ventilation in patients with nocturnal hypoventilation. *Respir Med* 2008; **102**: 1528–35.
3. Bertoye MMA, Garin JP, Vincent P *et al.* Le retour à domicile des insuffisants respiratoires chroniques appareillés. *Lyon Méd* 1965; **38**: 389–410.
4. Fiorenza D, Vitacca M, Clini E. Home hospital monitoring, setting and training for home non invasive ventilation. *Monaldi Arch Chest Dis* 2003; **59**: 119–22.
5. American Association for Respiratory Care. Clinical practice guideline: discharge planning of the respiratory care patient. *Respir Care* 1995; **40**: 1308–12.
6. Roy CL, Poon EG, Karson AS *et al.* Patient safety concerns arising from test results that return after hospital discharge. *Ann Intern Med* 2005; **143**: 121–8.
7. Visser A, van Leeuwen AF, Voogt E *et al.* Clinical decision-making at the end of life: the role of the patient's wish. *Patient Educ Couns* 2003; **50**: 263–4.
8. MacIntyre NR, Epstein SK, Scheinhorn D *et al.* Management of patients requiring prolonged mechanical ventilation: Report of a NAMDRC consensus conference. *Chest* 2005; **128**: 3937–54.
9. White AC, O'Connor HH, Kirby K. Prolonged mechanical ventilation: review of care settings and an update on professional reimbursement. *Chest* 2008; **133**: 539–45.
10. Scheinhorn DJ, Hassenpflug MS, Votto JJ *et al.* Ventilation Outcomes Study Group. Post-ICU mechanical ventilation at 23 long-term care hospitals: a multicenter outcomes study. *Chest* 2007; **131**: 85–93.
11. Association Lyonnaise de Logistique Posthospitalière. Available at: www.allp-sante.com/ (accessed 29 September 2009).
12. Bach JR. *Pulmonary rehabilitation.* Philadelphia: Hanley & Belfus, 1996.
13. Ballangrud R, Bogsti WB, Johansson IS. Clients' experiences of living at home with a mechanical ventilator. *J Adv Nurs* 2009; **65**: 425–34.
14. Wagner EH. The role of patient care teams in chronic disease management. *BMJ* 2000; **320**: 569–72.
15. University of Kent. Teamworking skills. Available at: www.kent.ac.uk/careers/sk/teamwork.htm (accessed 28 September 2009).
16. Escarrabill J. Goldberg A. Training the home health team. In: Ambrosino N, Goldstein R. *Ventilatory support for chronic respiratory failure.* Oxford: Informa Health Care, 2008.
17. Aiken LH. Achieving an interdisciplinary workforce in health care. *N Engl J Med* 2003; **348**: 164–6.
18. Kutney-Lee A, McHugh MD, Sloane DM *et al.* Nursing: a key to patient satisfaction. *Health Aff (Millwood)* 2009; **28**: w669–77.
19. Warren ML, Jarrett C, Senegal R *et al.* An interdisciplinary approach to transitioning ventilator-dependent patients to home. *J Nurs Care Qual* 2004; **19**: 67–73.
20. Tearl DK, Cox TJ, Hertzog JH. Hospital discharge of respiratory-technology-dependent children: role of a dedicated respiratory care discharge coordinator. *Respir Care* 2006; **51**: 744–9.
21. Farrero E, Prats E, Povedano M *et al.* Survival in amyotrophic lateral sclerosis with home mechanical ventilation: the impact of systematic respiratory assessment and bulbar involvement. *Chest* 2007; **127**: 2132–8.
22. Mitsumoto H, Rabkin JG. Palliative care for patients with amyotrophic lateral sclerosis: 'prepare for the worst and hope for the best'. *JAMA* 2007; **298**: 207–16.
23. Traynor BJ, Alexander M, Corr B *et al.* Effect of a multidisciplinary amyotrophic lateral sclerosis (ALS) clinic on ALS survival: a population based study, 1996–2000. *J Neurol Neurosurg Psychiatry* 2003; **74**: 1258–61.
24. Zoccolella S, Beghi E, Palagano G *et al.* ALS multidisciplinary clinic and survival. Results from a population-based study in Southern Italy. *J Neurol* 2007; **254**: 1107–12.
25. Hutchinson M, Galvin R, Sweeney B *et al.* Effect of a multidisciplinary clinic on survival in amyotrophic lateral sclerosis. *J Neurol Neurosurg Psychiatry* 2004; **75**: 1208–9.
26. Sorenson EJ, Mandrekar J, Crum B *et al.* Effect of referral bias on assessing survival in ALS. *Neurology* 2007; **68**: 600–2.
27. Chiò A, Bottacchi E, Buffa C *et al.* PARALS. Positive effects of tertiary centres for amyotrophic lateral sclerosis on outcome and use of hospital facilities. *Neurol Neurosurg Psychiatry* 2006; **77**: 948–50.
28. Lloyd-Owen SJ, Donaldson GC, Ambrosino N *et al.* Patterns of home mechanical ventilation use in Europe: results from the Eurovent survey. *Eur Respir J* 2005; **25**: 1025–31.
29. Bonisteel P. Teamwork. *Can Fam Physician* 2007; **53**: 402.
30. Escarrabill J. Health care support for home mechanical ventilation: networking versus centralization. *Arch Bronconeumol* 2007; **43**: 527–9.
31. Patientslikeme. www.patientslikeme.com/home; requires login (accessed 28 December 2008).
32. Fornai F, Longone P, Cafaro L *et al.* Lithium delays progression of amyotrophic lateral sclerosis. *Proc Natl Acad Sci U S A* 2008; **105**: 2052–7.

33. Talan J. Small doses of lithium slow ALS progression: more trials are planned. *Neurology Today* 2008; **8**: 12.
34. Bedlack RS, Maragakis N, Heiman-Patterson T. Lithium may slow progression of amyotrophic lateral sclerosis, but further study is needed. *Proc Natl Acad Sci U S A* 2008; **105**: E17.
35. Vanacore N, Galeotti F. A clinical specification for a randomized clinical trial on lithium in amyotrophic lateral sclerosis. *Proc Natl Acad Sci U S A* 2008; **105**: E35.
36. Frost JH, Massagli MP, Wicks P *et al.* How the social web supports patient experimentation with a new therapy: the demand for patient-controlled and patient-centered informatics. *AMIA Annu Symp Proc* 2008; **6**: 217–21.
37. Institute of Medicine. *To err is human. Building a safer health system.* Washington: National Academy Press, 2000.
38. Pronovost PJ, Goeschel CA, Olsen KL *et al.* Reducing health care hazards: lessons from the commercial aviation safety team. *Health Aff (Millwood)* 2009; **28**: w479–89.
39. Spear SJ. Fixing health care from the inside, today. HBR, September 2005.
40. Forster AJ, Asmis TR, Clark HD *et al.* Ottawa Hospital Patient Safety Study: incidence and timing of adverse events in patients admitted to a Canadian teaching hospital. *CMAJ* 2004; **170**: 1235–40.
41. Pham HH, Schrag D, O'Malley AS *et al.* Care patterns in Medicare and their implications for pay for performance. *N Engl J Med* 2007; **356**: 1130–9.
42. International Ventilation Users Network. Home ventilator user's emergency preparation checklist. Available at: www.ventusers.org/vume/HomeVentuserChecklist.pdf (accessed 29 September 2009).
43. Lechtzin N, Weiner CM, Clawson L. A fatal complication of noninvasive ventilation. *N Engl J Med* 2001; **344**: 533.
44. Towlson S. *Power cut kills man on home ventilator. The Times*, 14 August 2000.
45. Farré R, Navajas D, Prats E *et al.* Performance of mechanical ventilators at the patient's home: a multicentre quality control study. *Thorax* 2006; **61**: 400–4.
46. Simonds AK. Risk management of the home ventilator dependent patient. *Thorax* 2006; **61**: 369–71.
47. Neale G, Woloshynowych M, Vincent C. Exploring the causes of adverse events in NHS hospital practice. *J R Soc Med* 2001; **94**: 322–30.
48. Kripalani S, LeFevre F, Phillips CO *et al.* Deficits in communication and information transfer between hospital-based and primary care physicians: implications for patient safety and continuity of care. *JAMA* 2007; **297**: 831–41.
49. Vincent C, Davy C, Esmail A *et al.* Learning from litigation. The role of claims analysis in patient safety. *J Eval Clin Pract* 2006; **12**: 665–74.
50. Chatwin M, Heather S, Hanak A *et al.* Analysis of home support and ventilator malfunction in 1211 ventilator dependent patients. *Eur Respir J* 2009 [epub ahead of print].
51. Farrero E, Prats E, Manresa F *et al.* Outcome of non-invasive domiciliary ventilation in elderly patients. *Respir Med* 2007; **101**: 1068–73.
52. Midgren B. Home mechanical ventilation. A growing challenge in an aging society. *Respir Med* 2007; **101**: 1066–7.
53. Crespo A, Muñoz X, Torres F *et al.* Noninvasive home mechanical ventilation in elderly patients. Gerontology 2009 [epub ahead of print].
54. Vitacca M, Grassi M, Barbano L *et al.* Last 3 months of life in home-ventilated patients: the family perception. *Eur Respir J* 2009 [epub ahead of print].
55. Laub M, Midgren B. Survival of patients on home mechanical ventilation: a nationwide prospective study. *Respir Med* 2007; **101**: 1074–8.
56. Rady MY, Johnson DJ. Hospital discharge to care facility: a patient-centered outcome for the evaluation of intensive care for octogenarians. *Chest* 2004; **126**: 1583–91.
57. Escarrabill J. Discharge planning and home care for end-stage COPD patients. *Eur Respir J* 2009; **34**: 507–12.
58. Habraken JM, Willems DL, de Kort SJ *et al.* Health care needs in end-stage COPD: a structured literature review. *Patient Educ Couns* 2007; **68**: 121–30.
59. Simonds AK. Living and dying with respiratory failure: facilitating decision making. *Chron Respir Dis* 2004; **1**: 56–9.
60. Creechan T. Combining mechanical ventilation with hospice care in the home: death with dignity. *Crit Care Nurs* 2000; **20**: 49–53.

# SECTION D

# COPD

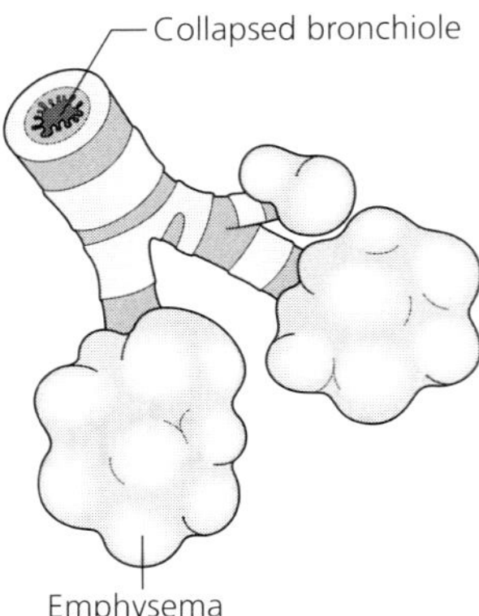


**Figure 20.1** Emphysematous destruction of the alveoli and collapse/closure of the respiratory bronchioles seen in respiratory bronchiolitis.

Hence, in most patients there occur a number of mechanisms by which respiratory failure develops.

In health, gas exchange can be maintained over a wide range of metabolic requirements from basal levels of oxygen consumption during stage III sleep to heavy exercise. Even under conditions when the inspired oxygen falls, as in ascent to high altitude, compensatory mechanisms still defend safe levels of arterial oxygenation (and hence tissue oxygen delivery) with hypoxic vasoconstriction within the lung and an increased total alveolar ventilation tending to mitigate the initial effects of hypoxaemia. In disease the same range of physiological mechanisms come into play but their effectiveness is often compromised. This is particularly true for COPD where the primary problems it produces in lung mechanics not only directly impair the effectiveness of gas exchange but also makes the system more sensitive to changes in carbon dioxide production, mixed venous oxygen tension and cardiac output.

Conventionally gas exchange has been analysed using the three-compartment model developed almost 50 years ago by Riley and colleagues[1] and which is discussed in some detail below. This approach has the virtue of clarity and can be applied relatively easily to clinical situations. However, it is an oversimplification and this is particularly the case in COPD where the wide heterogeneity in pulmonary pathology within an individual can produce quite complex gas exchange abnormalities. The degree of airflow limitation broadly tracks the gas exchange problem with patients in Global Initiative for Chronic Obstructive Lung Disease (GOLD) stages 1 and 2 showing variable widening of the alveolar-arterial oxygen gradient while those in stage 4 may develop severe hypercapnic respiratory failure.

Considerable insights into these complex problems have come from applying the multiple inert gas elimination (MIGET) method to analyse gas exchange in COPD patients in a wide range of settings. This is a mathematically complex and intellectually rigorous approach that involves the analysis of the uptake and excretion of six different gases of variable solubility. Although this has helped our understanding of gas exchange in COPD, and especially the complex causes of hypoxaemia, we will devote most of this chapter to illustrating the general principles of gas exchange using the older approach with some comments on one area in which the MIGET data have changed our understanding of disease.

## DEFINITION OF RESPIRATORY FAILURE

Conventionally respiratory failure is split into two types depending on whether hypercapnia is present.[2] This division is more than simply arbitrary, as it potentially provides important information about the pathophysiological mechanisms leading to respiratory failure. Combined with knowledge of the clinical situation this may help the clinician determine the most appropriate treatment strategy.

Type I or hypoxaemic respiratory failure occurs where there is an abnormally low arterial oxygen tension ($PaO_2$) of <8 kPa (<60 mm Hg) with a normal or low arterial carbon dioxide tension ($PaCO_2$) of <6 kPa (<45 mm Hg) (Table 20.1). This can be considered to be a failure of gas exchange sometimes described as 'lung failure' (Fig. 20.2). Type I respiratory failure is most often caused by abnormalities of the lung parenchyma, the pulmonary vasculature or a

**Table 20.1** Definition of respiratory failure based on level of $PaO_2$ and $PaCO_2$

| | Type of respiratory failure | |
|---|---|---|
| | **Type I** | **Type II** |
| $PaO_2$ level | <8 kPa = <60 mm Hg | <8 kPa = <60 mm Hg |
| $PaCO_2$ level | <6 kPa = <45 mm Hg | >6 kPa = >45 mm Hg |

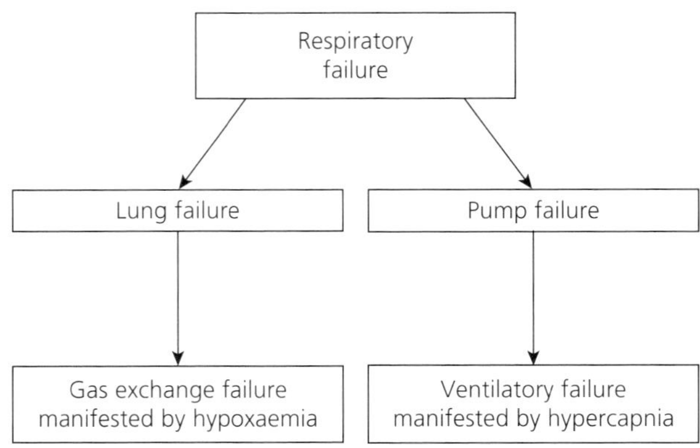


**Figure 20.2** Types of respiratory failure described by Roussos and Koutsoukou.[3]

combination of both. In COPD, several pathophysiological mechanisms might be contributing including:

- ventilation–perfusion ($\dot{V}/Q$) mismatch
- intrapulmonary (right to left) shunt
- impaired alveolar–capillary diffusion

In patients with COPD, alveolar hypoventilation normally exists alongside one or more of the other mechanisms and can accentuate the degree of hypoxaemia. In contrast with hypoventilation in individuals without lung disease, where hypoventilation leads to hypoxaemia with a normal alveolar-arterial gradient ($D_{A-a}O_2$), this combination of mechanisms normally results in widening of the $D_{A-a}O_2$ gradient.

Type II or hypercapnic (hypercarbic) respiratory failure occurs where there is an abnormally low arterial oxygen tension ($PaO_2$) of <8 kPa (<60 mm Hg) with an abnormally raised arterial carbon dioxide tension ($PaCO_2$) of >6 kPa (>45 mm Hg) (Table 20.1). Hence, there is a failure of ventilation which has been described as 'pump failure' – see Figure 20.2. In COPD patients this may be due to fatigue of the respiratory muscles, although the evidence for this outside of the intensive care unit is scant. More commonly the respiratory muscles cannot maintain sufficient alveolar ventilation to prevent hypercapnia in the face of a significantly increased dead space to tidal volume ratio. There is no evidence for a reduced central drive to breathing, although data normalizing this relative to the prevailing mechanical load are lacking.

## PATHOPHYSIOLOGICAL MECHANISMS CAUSING HYPOXAEMIA IN COPD PATIENTS

### Ventilation–perfusion mismatch

This is the most important cause of hypoxaemia and can also contribute to hypercapnia. Ventilation–perfusion mismatching is both physiological and pathological. Mismatch occurs in the normal lung due to gravity/posture, cardiac output and pulmonary artery pressure. Despite this, matching is fairly good as the lung bases receive both more ventilation and greater blood flow than the lung apices as shown in Figure 20.3.

Ventilation–perfusion mismatch is most easily explained using the three-compartment model of dead space ventilation, ideal matching and shunting, but it should be remembered that mismatch is a continuum where each alveolus will have a different relationship. Hence, descriptions of $\dot{V}/Q$ mismatch in the overall lung are a summation of all individual units and the partial pressure of oxygen and carbon dioxide in arterial blood reflect this. Any pathological process that affects the airways, lung parenchyma or pulmonary vasculature will affect the $\dot{V}/Q$ relationship of the lungs and these all exist to different degrees in individuals with COPD.

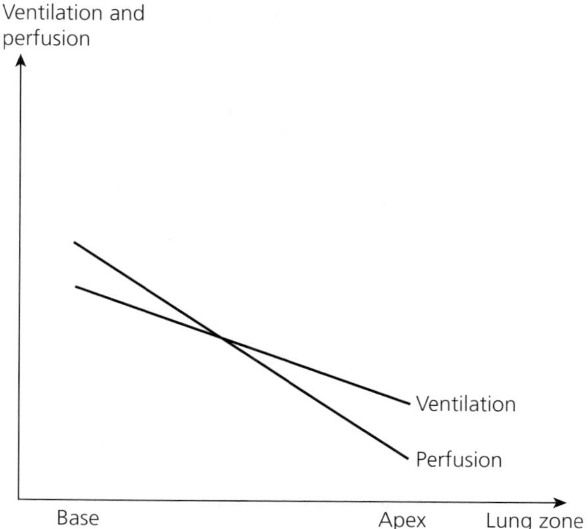


**Figure 20.3** Illustration of the difference in ventilation and perfusion between the lung apex and lung base.

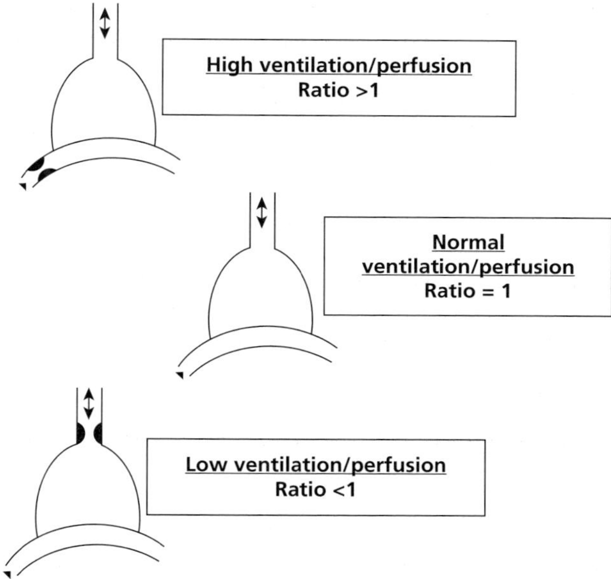


**Figure 20.4** The three-compartment model of ventilation and perfusion illustrating ventilation–perfusion mismatch, physiological dead space and shunting.

The three-compartment model is illustrated in Figure 20.4. In a normal lung, ventilation and perfusion are equally matched and the $\dot{V}/Q$ ratio is 1. In some disease states there is normal ventilation but reduced perfusion and the $\dot{V}/Q$ ratio is high (greater than 1) and at the extreme it is infinity (where blood flow is absent), known as physiological dead space. In another situation there is reduced ventilation but normal perfusion and the $\dot{V}/Q$ ratio is low (less than 1) and at the other extreme it is zero (where ventilation is absent), called physiological shunting. It might be supposed that where ventilation–perfusion mismatch is patchy then areas of normal lung and well-perfused lung would compensate for underperfused areas. However, the oxygen–haemoglobin dissociation curve can be seen to be sigmoid shaped (Fig. 20.5), and this means that well-perfused areas cannot increase blood oxygen saturation above 100 per cent. Hence, $PaO_2$ will fall in the presence of $\dot{V}/Q$ mismatch.

Predominantly emphysematous patients have been shown to ventilate large areas with a high $\dot{V}/Q$ ratio and hardly any areas with a very low $\dot{V}/Q$ ratio or shunt areas. This probably involves both reduction in blood flow to areas of lung due to emphysematous destruction of alveoli in addition to inequality of ventilation. Where low $\dot{V}/Q$ patterns are seen the likely causes are a reduction in ventilation due to mechanical bronchial obstruction due to airway oedema, mucus and airway narrowing, closure and/or collapse. However, perfusion to these areas is also likely to be reduced due to chronic hypoxic vasoconstriction in these areas.[4]

It is very difficult to directly measure ventilation–perfusion mismatching in the lung, and consequently we tend to measure indices of gas exchange which are representative. Gas exchange in the 'ideal' lung (a lung where there was no $\dot{V}/Q$ mismatch) can be represented by the alveolar gas equation:

$$P_AO_2 = P_IO_2 - P_ACO_2/R + F$$

where $P_AO_2$ = partial pressure of oxygen in the alveolus, $P_IO_2$ = partial pressure of inspired oxygen, $P_ACO_2$ = partial pressure of carbon dioxide in the alveolus, R = the respiratory quotient (moles of $CO_2$ produced per mole of $O_2$ consumed) and F is a small correction factor.

The respiratory quotient is also called the respiratory exchange ratio and is determined by tissue metabolism. A commonly used index of gas exchange is the alveolar–arterial oxygen difference where the measured arterial $PO_2$ is subtracted from the 'ideal' alveolar $PO_2$. An increased alveolar–arterial oxygen difference is normally caused by abnormally low ventilation–perfusion ratios within the lung but can be caused by high ratios. It is possible to separate these two situations by calculating the physiological shunt (for low ratios) and the physiological dead space (for high ratios) though in many patients with COPD both exist to a varying degree.

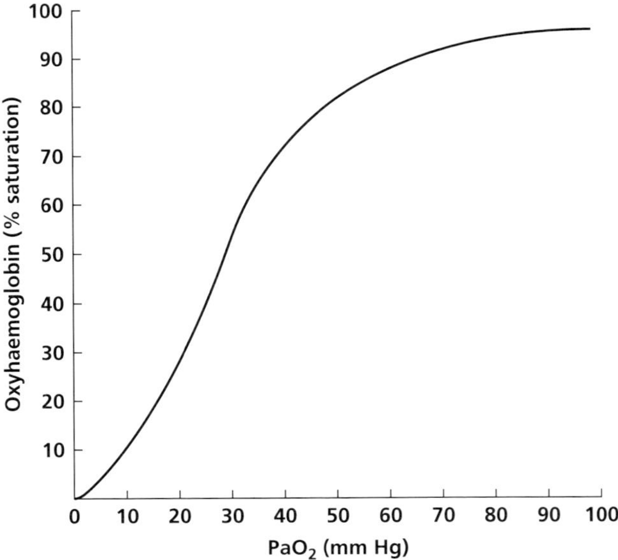


**Figure 20.5** The sigmoid shaped oxygen–haemoglobin dissociation curve illustrating the relationship between oxygen saturation and arterial oxygenation.

## Intrapulmonary shunting

Shunting is one end of the spectrum of ventilation–perfusion mismatch, a situation where deoxygenated blood passes through the pulmonary vascular bed without exposure to ventilation and therefore reduces the $PaO_2$ of arterial blood. A small shunt exists in the normal lung due to blood from the bronchial arteries, and the coronary circulation entering the arterial circulation without passing through ventilated lung.

As considered above, in COPD patients the majority of pathological shunting relates to mechanical bronchial obstruction and closure and/or collapse of alveoli – alveolar collapse contrasting with airways filled with fluid or exudates as seen in conditions such as pulmonary oedema. An important feature of a shunt is that it cannot be completely abolished by administering 100 per cent oxygen as shunted blood will never be exposed to oxygen – albeit the $PaO_2$ will rise because of the higher fraction of inspired oxygen ($FiO_2$) delivered to functioning alveoli. In practice this is not seen in COPD unless there is some coexisting problem such as an undetected atrial septal defect, something which only becomes a problem when gas exchange is disturbed for some other reason, e.g. during an exacerbation.

## Impaired alveolar–capillary diffusion

Emphysema is associated with alveolar destruction (see Fig. 20.1) which can greatly reduce the surface area available for gas diffusion. In theory, during exercise, cardiac output increases and the speed with which blood passes through the capillaries is increased. In these circumstances diffusion impairment could reduce the rate of rise of partial pressure of oxygen in the capillary and contribute to hypoxaemia. However, detailed experiments have shown that ventilation–perfusion inequality and shunt account for all of the hypoxaemia at rest and during exercise and there is no evidence for hypoxaemia caused by diffusion impairment.[4]

## PATHOPHYSIOLOGICAL MECHANISMS CAUSING HYPERCAPNIA IN COPD PATIENTS

The predominant mechanism that produces hypercapnia in COPD patients is alveolar hypoventilation.

### Alveolar hypoventilation

The amount of carbon dioxide eliminated per minute ($VCO_2$) is a function of the concentration of $CO_2$ in the alveoli multiplied by alveolar ventilation ($V_A$); hence:

$$\text{Alveolar } CO_2 \text{ concentration} = VCO_2/V_A$$

By converting the equation to pressures and using factor k (the constant of proportionality) the respiratory equation is obtained which relates arterial $PaCO_2$ to alveolar ventilation:

$$PaCO_2 = k \times (VCO_2/V_A)$$

Since alveolar ventilation ($V_A$) is equivalent to minute ventilation ($V_E$) minus dead space ventilation ($V_D$) then:

$$PaCO_2 = k \times [VCO_2/(V_E - V_D)]$$

Physiological dead space includes anatomical dead space and a component due to dilution of resident gas in the airways. This can then be expressed as:

$$PaCO_2 = k \times VCO_2/V_T \times f \times [1 - (V_D - V_T)]$$

where $V_T$ is tidal volume and f is breathing frequency.

Type II respiratory failure is reflected by hypercapnia and it is clear from these equations that at a constant $VCO_2$, as alveolar ventilation ($V_A$) is reduced the partial pressure of carbon dioxide in the arterial circulation ($PaCO_2$) increases. Hence, alveolar ventilation is a significant cause of type II respiratory failure. Reduced alveolar ventilation also results in a fall in $PaO_2$ but this can be overcome by increasing the concentration of oxygen inspired. The equation also illustrates that decrease in alveolar ventilation can result from a rise in $V_D - V_T$ (by an increase in $V_D$, a reduction in $V_T$ or both), a decrease in $V_E$ or a combination of these factors (seen in many patients with COPD).

An increase in carbon dioxide production will also result in a rise in $PaCO_2$. This can occur during hyperthermia but is most commonly seen during exercise where $VCO_2$ can increase multifold. In normal lungs this would be compensated by a proportional rise in minute ventilation; however, in patients with COPD increase in minute ventilation may be significantly limited as $V_E$ will represent a much higher proportion of maximum voluntary ventilation. This is seen in some patients with severe COPD where $PaCO_2$ increases during exercise and has been shown to relate to dynamic hyperinflation.[5]

### Ventilation–perfusion mismatch

Ventilation–perfusion mismatch is a cause of hypercapnia although this mechanism is less common than hypoventilation. Ventilation–perfusion mismatch delivers carbon dioxide rich blood to the arterial circulation but in the normal lung it does not increase $PaCO_2$ as any increase in $PaCO_2$ is sensed by the chemoreceptors which increase ventilation until the $PaCO_2$ is again normal. This occurs because the transport of carbon dioxide from the blood to the alveoli is linear; hence, when minute ventilation is increased areas where ventilation–perfusion ratio is normal can increase $CO_2$ removal and compensate for mismatching regions. Hence, $\dot{V}/Q$ mismatch is far more important as a cause of hypoxaemia than hypercapnia.

As is evident from the above equations, the situation where it does contribute to hypercapnia is in patients who have an increase in physiological dead space, and consequently increased dead space ventilation, which is seen commonly in COPD patients, particularly those with predominant emphysema.

### Acid–base balance

The concentration of hydrogen ions ($H^+$) is extremely important to cellular metabolism and in particular an increased level impairs normal cell function. The concentration of hydrogen ions is normally expressed as the pH which represents the negative logarithm of $H^+$. It should be remembered that with a logarithmic scale relatively small changes in pH represent large changes in the concentration. In light of the importance to the body pH is normally very tightly controlled.

The main source of hydrogen ions is tissue metabolism as a molecule of carbon dioxide produced combined with water is equivalent to a hydrogen ion and bicarbonate. The body has an effective buffering system to maintain homeostasis. Haemoglobin, proteins and phosphate can all act as buffers but the most important component of the buffering system is the bicarbonate–carbonic acid system expressed as the Henderson–Hasselbalch equation:

$$CO_2 + H_2O \rightleftharpoons H_2CO_3 \rightleftharpoons H^+ + HCO_3^-$$

Balance is maintained by excretion of carbon dioxide through the lungs and excretion of fixed acid by the kidney. Over 100 times more carbon dioxide is excreted by the lungs each day compared with the amount of fixed acids excreted by the kidney; hence, mechanical ventilatory abnormalities seen in patients with COPD significantly affect acid–base balance.

The relationship between pH, $PaCO_2$ and $HCO_3^-$ can be seen in Figure 20.6. If hypercapnia continues but acidosis does not progress then renal buffering will normalize the pH by excreting hydrogen ions through the kidney (compensation) resulting in chronic type II respiratory failure.

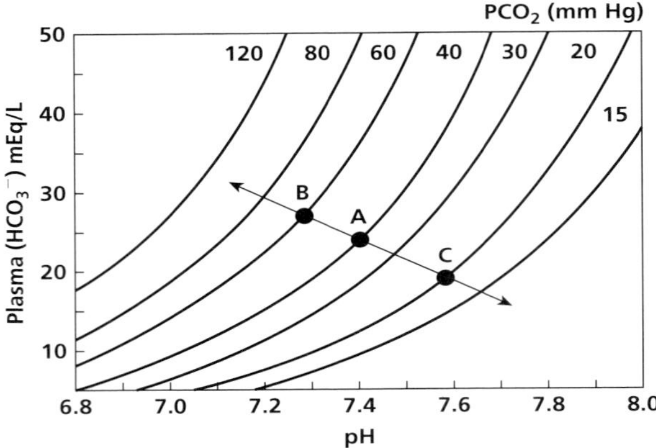


**Figure 20.6** The relationship between pH, $PaCO_2$ and $HCO_3^-$, where A represents the buffer line, B represents respiratory acidosis and C represents respiratory alkalosis.[6]

In COPD, hypercapnia is the principal cause of any acidosis. In stable disease this is compensated as described above but it will usually worsen during exacerbations, where it is a marker of a worse prognosis (although not necessarily the most sensitive one).[7]

## PATHOPHYSIOLOGY OF VENTILATORY FAILURE

As discussed earlier, ventilatory failure is primarily failure of the respiratory pump. Type II respiratory failure results when the respiratory muscles are unable to provide sufficient ventilation to meet metabolic demands. In stable COPD patients this does not usually relate either to abnormalities of central respiratory muscle control/drive, to nerve signalling of the respiratory muscles or to intrinsic defects in respiratory muscle function. On the contrary, current evidence supports a marked increase in respiratory drive consistent with the structural and functional mechanical disadvantage seen in COPD patients which increase ventilatory requirements and relate to disease severity.[8] The combination of airflow obstruction and static and dynamic hyperinflation and presence of intrinsic positive end-expiratory pressure (PEEPi) increase the load on the respiratory muscles. Respiratory muscles operate at a mechanical disadvantage due to geometrical changes in the chest wall and diaphragm in addition to reduced compliance and elastic recoil of the respiratory system, and are less able to produce the negative intrathoracic pressure necessary for respiration.[9] In addition acute changes such as at the time of an exacerbation[10] and during exercise[11] accentuate these mechanical disadvantages by further worsening hyperinflation, airflow obstruction and increasing PEEPi.

Fatigue occurs when the respiratory muscles are unable to generate sufficient pressure to maintain ventilation. The respiratory muscles are relatively resistant to fatigue[12] at rest and at high intensity exercise,[13,14] but changes seen at the time of an exacerbation may lead to fatigue and inadequate pleural pressure generation despite this increased drive. The mechanical changes that occur at the time of an exacerbation are accentuated by a decrease in cardiac output, a worsening of oxygenation and a reduction in nutritional intake at a time of increased energy requirement leading to an acute imbalance of energy supply and demand.

Fundamentally there are a number of pathophysiological processes that contribute to ventilatory failure in COPD patients and these will be examined in turn.

### Increased load on the respiratory system in COPD

#### INCREASED INSPIRATORY RESISTANCE

Inspiratory resistance consists of both airway resistance and the resistance of the lung tissue. In patients with COPD the causes of increased inspiratory resistance have been elegantly described by Hogg *et al.*[15] The causes include airway wall thickening due to inflammation (inflammatory cell infiltration) and oedema, enlargement of mucous glands and airway wall smooth muscle (in the larger airways) and the existence of mucus within the airway (in particular the small, sub 2 mm, airways). In addition, emphysema reduces the number of airway wall to parenchymal attachments, which are important in keeping small airways open. Combined with destruction and fibrosis of the respiratory bronchioles and hyperinflation, this predisposes to dynamic airway collapse and closure, further increasing resistance. Increases in inspiratory resistance of an extent seen in COPD patients can markedly increase work of breathing, contributing to fatigue and ventilatory failure.

#### INCREASED STATIC COMPLIANCE AND REDUCED ELASTIC RECOIL

Lung elastance reflects the recoil of the lung and is defined by a change in pressure over a particular change in lung volume. It is the sum of the elastances of the lung and chest wall and the reciprocal of compliance. Emphysema leads to hyperinflation, destroys parenchymal tissue and reduces airway to parenchymal connections, consequently decreasing static lung elastance and increasing compliance. This results in reduced radial traction applied to the airways, airway collapse and closure and increased inspiratory resistance. In addition it leads to a reduction in maximum expiratory flow, flow limitation and dynamic hyperinflation.

#### INCREASED EXPIRATORY RESISTANCE AND EXPIRATORY FLOW LIMITATION

Ventilatory limitation in COPD patients primarily relates to expiratory flow limitation. Conductance through an airway, at a set lung volume, is a function of alveolar pressure and flow, with increases in alveolar pressure (without forced expiration) increasing flow until maximum expiratory flow is reached. It occurs when, at a specific lung volume, an increase in pressure either does not increase or leads to a reduction in expiratory flow. Individuals with COPD, in particular emphysema, have static hyperinflation and reduced elastic recoil pressures from the lung. With unchanged chest wall recoil pressures acting outwards, the functional residual capacity (FRC) is increased and individuals breathe at a higher lung volume, which reduces airway distensibility and affects the driving force from the alveoli.[16] Compared with normal subjects, equal pressure points are now seen in the more peripheral airways,[17] reducing maximal expiratory flow. Such an individual is only able to increase expiratory flow by breathing at a lower lung volume resulting in dynamic hyperinflation, evidenced by an increase in FRC during exercise. Flow limitation can occur during resting tidal breathing in some patients whereas in others it only occurs during exercise[18] and exacerbations.[10] The impact of worsening hyperinflation on respiratory muscle function and consequently respiratory failure is discussed below.

### MECHANICAL DISADVANTAGE DUE TO CHEST WALL AND DIAPHRAGM POSITION

Pulmonary hyperinflation has significant geometrical effects on the main muscles of respiration, the diaphragm and intercostal muscles. The diaphragm is shortened and flattened and the thoracic cage is expanded, and consequently both diaphragm and intercostal muscles are shortened and operate at a mechanical disadvantage. Maximum force generation is achieved at lower lung volume, usually close to FRC, but shortened muscles[19] have a less favourable length–tension relationship and are able to produce less force for a specific degree of muscle activation.[20] In addition the change in diaphragm shape reduces the number of muscle fibres that are arranged parallel to the chest wall as more are arranged perpendicularly or in series. A result of this is some muscles work isometrically, i.e. they consume energy but do not contribute to force generation.

The change in the shape of the diaphragm reduces potential force generation (Fig. 20.7). The zone of apposition, the area of the costal diaphragm that is in contact with the lateral chest wall, is reduced which in turn reduces the impact of abdominal pressure generation on the thoracic cage thereby limiting thoracic cage expansion.[21] At rest the changes described have relatively little impact on the tidal volume generated but they significantly reduce capacity to increase $V_T$, which is important at the time of an exacerbation or during exercise in particular because a majority of COPD patients dynamically inflate during exercise.[22]

### HYPERINFLATION AND INTRINSIC PEEP

When end-expiratory lung volume exceeds FRC this leads to an elevation of recoil pressure and results in a positive recoil pressure being applied to the alveoli at

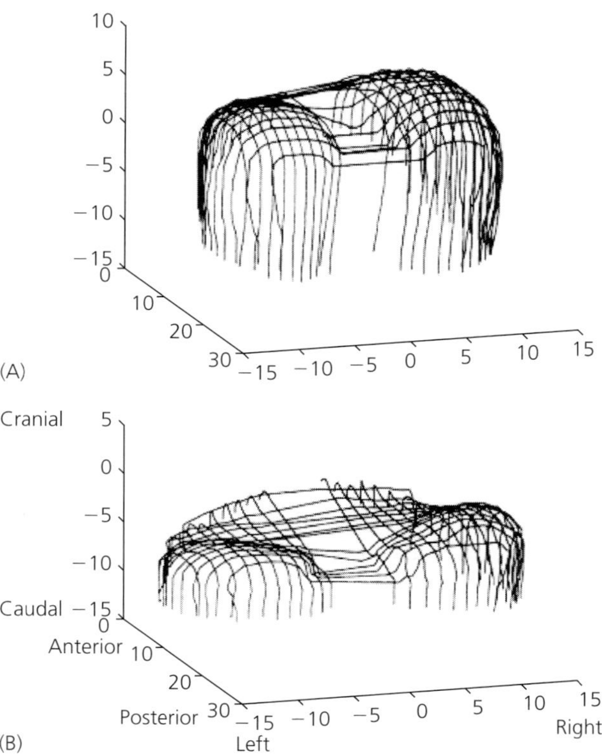


**Figure 20.7** Changes in diaphragm shape due to pulmonary hyperinflation comparing a normal subject (A) with a subject with chronic obstructive pulmonary disease and significant hyperinflation (B). A marked reduction in muscle surface area is seen. Reproduced with permission from Cassart *et al.*[21]

end-expiration. This is seen in COPD patients with hyperinflation, particularly when exercising, and is called PEEPi. It is usually caused by airway compression and reduced expiratory time (discussed further below). When this is present the inspiratory muscles have to overcome this applied pressure before expiratory airflow can commence, which requires increased effort, increases the work of breathing and can contribute to respiratory muscle fatigue.

## Development of hypercapnic respiratory failure

The effect of the above different and interacting pathophysiological abnormalities seen in isolation, or usually in combination, contribute to the development of ventilatory (hypercapnic) respiratory failure. The mean tidal pressure ($P_I$), which needs to be developed for each breath by the inspiratory muscles, is increased and relates to the increased inspiratory load; however, the ability to generate pressure is compromised by impaired diaphragm and intercostal muscle position and function, and both static and dynamic hyperinflation. Furthermore it also decreases as the duty cycle ($T_i/T_{tot}$) increases. In essence expiratory time ($T_e$) is decreased, which has the effect of increasing end-expiratory lung volume and promoting dynamic hyperinflation. This situation is worsened by an increase in breathing frequency (f) which reduces $T_{tot}$ and $T_e$, further promoting dynamic hyperinflation. The decrease in duty cycle also reduces maximum power generated by the respiratory muscles.

The changes all lead to muscle dysfunction and an inability to maintain $V_T$ while weak muscles have greater energy requirements to perform a defined level of work and are more susceptible to fatigue. In addition, the combination of muscular inefficiency and increased energy requirements leads to an increase in oxygen requirements,[23] and this in turn necessitates increased blood flow to the muscle. Blood supply is influenced by cardiac output, the vascular supply to the muscle and the vascular resistance of the muscle, the latter being determined by the intensity and duration of muscle contraction. Hence, in COPD patients the load and inefficiency of the muscles may in turn decrease muscle blood flow, further impairing function and leading to fatigue. The result is that decreased muscle force generation and development of fatigue lead to reductions in tidal volume and minute ventilation, which produces alveolar hypoventilation and leads to hypercapnia and type II respiratory failure by the mechanisms discussed earlier.

## Development of chronic hypercapnic respiratory failure

Development of chronic, compensated type II respiratory failure is a poor prognostic factor for COPD patients.[24] Why this occurs remains unclear. The earlier description of distinct patterns of $\dot{V}/Q$ abnormalities in hypercapnic disease with a bimodal distribution of low and high $\dot{V}/Q$ units[4] has not been consistently supported by subsequent papers using the same methodology. The most consistent abnormality has been the 'rapid shallow' breathing pattern described above but why this should be adopted to different degrees in subjects with apparently similar degrees of mechanical impairment is unknown. It is tempting to speculate that these differences arise from inherent differences in the neural response to mechanical loading, but until more specific imaging methods like functional magnetic resonance imaging are applied to these problems, such explanations must remain a simple conjecture.

## Acute or acute-on-chronic respiratory failure

The development of acidosis due to either the development of hypercapnic respiratory failure or worsening of pre-existing compensated hypercapnic respiratory failure is a poor prognostic sign at the time of a COPD exacerbation and is associated with a worse mortality.[25] At the time of an exacerbation, inspiratory resistance is increased due to bronchospasm and airway inflammation leading to airway narrowing plus frequently a marked increase in airway mucus when a lower respiratory tract infection is present (which is commonly the case). Hyperinflation worsens, which increases expiratory flow resistance, promotes or increases PEEPi and disadvantages diaphragm, intercostal and even accessory muscle function. Increase in breathing frequency to maintain $V_E$ reduces expiratory time and further promotes hyperinflation. Tidal breathing occurs at a steeper part of the pressure–volume curve, which is disadvantageous. In addition the increased energy requirements needed to maintain ventilatory function often correspond with a time of relative anorexia and reduced cardiac output, which potentiates muscle fatigue and promotes acute hypercapnic respiratory failure.

These extrapulmonary factors are important during exacerbations, with 50 per cent of the abnormal gas exchange assessed using the MIGET methodology being explained by increases in metabolic demand, reductions in mixed venous oxygen tension secondary to reduced cardiac output and a fall in minute ventilation relative to these metabolic needs.[26] Instituting non-invasive ventilation improves gas exchange mainly by changing the breathing pattern to a slower deeper one and does not affect the overall $\dot{V}/Q$ distribution within the lung. Although some treatments such as increasing the inspired oxygen concentration can actually worsen intrapulmonary $\dot{V}/Q$ matching, commonly used therapies such as an inhaled β-agonist bronchodilator drug seem to have much less negative impact on $\dot{V}/Q$ matching than similar drugs given intravenously. Indeed treatment with combinations of inhaled β-agonists and anticholinergics can improve operating lung volume and tidal lung mechanics soon after admission, with a shift to a more favourable breathing pattern to improve gas exchange.[10]

# CONCLUSIONS

COPD has many complex effects on gas exchange, which affect patients both acutely during exacerbations and in some cases chronically when persistent hypoxaemia produces secondary pulmonary hypertension and polycythaemia. In mild disease gas exchange, abnormalities are relatively subtle and unlikely to influence the patient's symptoms or require therapy. However, as the disease progresses, abnormalities in blood gas tensions become more frequent and identify patients at greater risk of death or complications. Successfully managing respiratory failure, whether chronically with supplementary oxygen or acutely with non-invasive ventilation, is among the most successful treatment options for COPD and one of the few that reduce the risk of the patient dying, thereby providing a further reason to understand the important and potentially modifiable effects of gas exchange abnormality in this condition.

## REFERENCES


1. Riley RL, Cournard A. Ideal alveolar air and the analysis of ventilation-perfusion relationships in the lungs. *J Appl Physiol* 1949; **1**: 825–47.
2. Campbell EJ. Respiratory failure. *Br Med J* 1965; **i**: 1451–60.
3. Roussos C, Koutsoukou A. Respiratory failure. *Eur Respir J Suppl* 2003; **47**: 3s–14s.
4. Wagner PD, Dantzker DR, Dueck R *et al.* Ventilation-perfusion inequality in chronic obstructive pulmonary disease. *J Clin Invest* 1977; **59**: 203–16.
5. O'Donnell DE, D'Arsigny C, Fitzpatrick M *et al.* Exercise hypercapnia in advanced chronic obstructive pulmonary disease: the role of lung hyperinflation. *Am J Respir Crit Care Med* 2002; **166**: 663–8.
6. West JB. *Respiratory physiology: the essentials*, 8th edn. Lippincott Williams & Wilkins, 2008.
7. Chakrabarti B, Angus RM, Agarwal S *et al.* Hyperglycaemia as a predictor of outcome during non-invasive ventilation in decompensated COPD. *Thorax* 2009; **64**: 857–62.
8. Jolley CJ, Luo YM, Steier J *et al.* Neural respiratory drive in healthy subjects and in COPD. *Eur Respir J* 2009; **33**: 289–97.
9. Polkey MI, Kyroussis D, Hamnegard CH *et al.* Diaphragm strength in chronic obstructive pulmonary disease. *Am J Respir Crit Care Med* 1996; **154**: 1310–17.
10. Stevenson NJ, Walker PP, Costello RW *et al.* Lung mechanics and dyspnea during exacerbations of chronic obstructive pulmonary disease. *Am J Respir Crit Care Med* 2005; **172**: 1510–16.
11. Sinderby C, Spahija J, Beck J *et al.* Diaphragm activation during exercise in chronic obstructive pulmonary disease. *Am J Respir Crit Care Med* 2001; **163**: 1637–41.
12. McKenzie DK, Gandevia SC. Recovery from fatigue of human diaphragm and limb muscles. *Respir Physiol* 1991; **84**: 49–60.
13. Polkey MI, Kyroussis D, Keilty SEJ *et al.* Exhaustive treadmill exercise does not reduce twitch transdiaphragmatic pressure in patients with COPD. *Am J Respir Crit Care Med* 1995; **152**: 959–64.
14. Mador MJ, Kufel TJ, Pineda LA *et al.* Diaphragmatic fatigue and high-intensity exercise in patients with chronic obstructive pulmonary disease. *Am J Crit Care Med* 2000; **161**: 118–23.
15. Hogg JC, Chu F, Utokaparch S *et al.* The nature of small-airway obstruction in chronic obstructive pulmonary disease. *N Engl J Med* 2004; **350**: 2645–53.
16. Leaver DG, Tattersfield AE, Pride NB. Contributions of loss of lung recoil and of enhanced airways collapsibility to the airflow obstruction of chronic bronchitis and emphysema. *J Clin Invest* 1973; **52**: 2117–28.
17. Hogg JC, Macklem PT, Thurlbeck WM. Site and nature of airways obstruction in chronic obstructive lung disease. *N Engl J Med* 1968; **278**: 1355–60.
18. Koulouris NG, Dimopoulou I, Valta P *et al.* Detection of expiratory flow limitation during exercise in COPD patients. *J Appl Physiol* 1997; **82**: 723–31.
19. Gorman RB, McKenzie DK, Pride NB *et al.* Diaphragm length during tidal breathing in patients with chronic obstructive pulmonary disease. *Am J Respir Crit Care Med* 2002; **166**: 1461–9.
20. Roussos C, Macklem PT. The respiratory muscles. *N Engl J Med* 1982; **307**: 786–97.
21. Cassart M, Pettiaux N, Gevenois PA *et al.* Effect of chronic hyperinflation on diaphragm length and surface area. *Am J Respir Crit Care Med* 1997; **156**: 504–8.
22. O'Donnell DE, Revill SM, Webb KA. Dynamic hyperinflation and exercise intolerance in chronic obstructive pulmonary disease. *Am J Respir Crit Care Med* 2001; **164**: 770–7.
23. McGregor M, Becklake MR. The relationship of oxygen cost of breathing to respiratory mechanical work and respiratory force. *J Clin Invest* 1961; **40**: 971–80.
24. Burrows B, Earle RH. Course and prognosis of chronic obstructive lung disease: a prospective study of 200 patients. *N Engl J Med* 1969; **280**: 397–404.
25. Seneff MG, Wagner DP, Wagner RP *et al.* Hospital and 1-year survival of patients admitted to intensive care units with acute exacerbation of chronic obstructive pulmonary disease. *JAMA* 1995; **274**: 1852–7.
26. Barberà JA, Roca J, Ferrer A *et al.* Mechanisms of worsening gas exchange during acute exacerbations of chronic obstructive pulmonary disease. *Eur Respir J* 1997; **10**: 1285–91.

# 21

# Treatment of chronic obstructive pulmonary disease: acute and chronic

BORJA G COSIO, ROBERTO RODRÍGUEZ-ROISIN

ABSTRACT

Chronic obstructive pulmonary disease (COPD) is a preventable and treatable disease characterized by chronic obstruction and inflammation of the airway that flares up during exacerbations. Treatment of the exacerbations follows an 'ABC approach', namely **A**ntibiotics, **B**ronchodilators and **C**orticosteroids. Inhaled bronchodilators, mainly short-acting β-agonists and short-acting antimuscarinic agents, and systemic glucocorticosteroids are the most effective treatments for COPD exacerbations. Antibiotics should be given mainly to patients with increased sputum purulence. Stable disease should be treated based on symptoms and functional impairment. Long-acting bronchodilators and oral theophylline can be used gradually from mild to very severe disease depending upon symptoms. A combination of long-acting β-agonist and inhaled corticosteroid is recommended for severe disease or for patients with frequent exacerbations, due to their beneficial effect on lung function and quality of life, and in reducing exacerbations. Long-term oxygen therapy has been shown to improve survival in selected patients when used properly. Influenza vaccination is effective in all patients with COPD.

## ACUTE EXACERBATIONS OF CHRONIC OBSTRUCTIVE PULMONARY DISEASE

### Background

Exacerbations are periods of acute worsening of chronic obstructive pulmonary disease (COPD) usually defined on the basis of the presenting symptoms, i.e. increased breathlessness, change in cough or sputum volume or purulence. However, patients may also present with other symptoms such as malaise, worsening exercise tolerance, fluid retention, increased fatigue or confusion. During exacerbations, there is a fall in peak expiratory flow (PEF), forced expiratory flow in 1 second ($FEV_1$) and forced vital capacity (FVC), along with increase in residual volume and decrease in inspiratory capacity, indicating airway narrowing, air trapping and lung hyperinflation. Arterial blood gases may also worsen leading to acute or acute-on-chronic respiratory failure in the most severe cases.[1]

A consensual operational definition of COPD exacerbation is a worsening of the patient's condition, from the stable state and beyond day-to-day variations, that is acute in onset and necessitating a change in regular medication in a patient with underlying COPD.[2]

### Pathophysiology

Pathologically, exacerbations of COPD are characterized by enhanced airway inflammation and oedema[3,4] and systemic effects that may be linked to inflammation,[5,6] resulting in more airflow limitation and gas exchange defects due to further mechanical abnormalities in the lung and worsening of ventilation–perfusion matching, along with increased oxygen consumption, altered hypoxic vasoconstriction, and systemic (increased cardiac output) and pulmonary (increased pulmonary artery pressure) haemodynamic abnormalities.[7,8] Interestingly, each of these pathophysiological factors that govern gas exchange can be modulated, at least in part, by the currently available pharmacological and non-pharmacological treatments (Fig. 21.1).[7,9]

Exacerbations of COPD have a negative effect on patients in terms of mortality,[10] health-related quality of life, and

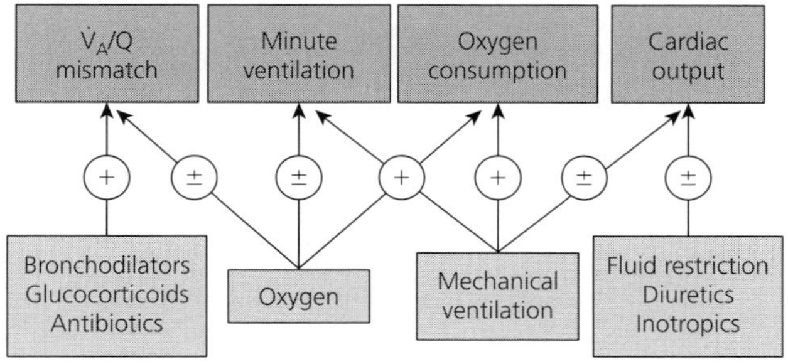


**Figure 21.1** Effect of currently available pharmacological and non-pharmacological options on the pathophysiological factors that govern gas exchange. With permission from Rodriguez-Roisin.[9]

decline in lung function. Hospital mortality of patients admitted for a hypercarbic COPD exacerbation is approximately 10 per cent, reaching 40 per cent at 1 year in those needing mechanical support; the all-cause mortality is even higher (approximately 49 per cent) 3 years after hospitalization for a COPD exacerbation.[11,12] Exacerbations also add a huge socioeconomic burden to healthcare resources.[13] In the UK, exacerbations of COPD account for up to 10 per cent of all medical admissions, equating to more than 100 000 admissions a year. Also, patients with chronic bronchitis exacerbations experience 4.5 times more primary care consultations than the general population.[14]

At the community level, hospital admissions for acute COPD have an impact beyond the emergency department and create seasonally major disruptions in hospital management. Exacerbations of COPD are a major contributor to the clinical load of physicians who, in addition, have access to only limited therapeutic armamentarium.

The poor recognition of COPD exacerbations and insufficient treatment reflects its multidisciplinary nature. Also, the lack of a clearly identified mechanism for exacerbations promotes a non-specific approach to the management and care of many patients with exacerbations, with all available treatments being used.

## Evidence-based treatment

The therapeutic interventions for exacerbations are based on the current evidence,[2,15] which is as follows:

- The most common causes of an exacerbation are infection of the tracheobronchial tree and air pollution, but the cause of about a third of severe exacerbations cannot be identified (evidence level B).
- Inhaled short-acting bronchodilators (particularly inhaled $\beta_2$-agonists with or without anticholinergics) and oral glucocorticosteroids are effective treatments for exacerbations of COPD (evidence level A).
- Patients experiencing COPD exacerbations with clinical signs of airway infection (i.e. increased sputum purulence) may benefit from antibiotic treatment (evidence level B).
- Non-invasive mechanical ventilation in exacerbations improves respiratory acidosis, increases pH, decreases the need for endotracheal intubation, and reduces $PaCO_2$, respiratory rate, severity of breathlessness, the length of hospital stay, and mortality (evidence level A).

## Therapeutic interventions

### PHARMACOLOGICAL INTERVENTIONS

The pharmacological management for COPD exacerbations is summarized by the 'ABC approach', an acronym that reflects the three classes of drugs (**A**ntibiotics, **B**ronchodilators and **C**orticosteroids) commonly used for this condition. However, if we consider only the highest levels of evidence,[2,15] this is only valid for bronchodilators and systemic steroids.

#### Short-acting bronchodilators (SABDs)

*Beta-agonists: short-acting*

Short-acting inhaled $\beta_2$-agonists (SABAs) are the preferred bronchodilators for treatment of exacerbations of COPD (evidence level A). Together with anticholinergic agents, SABAs remain the main treatment modality for exacerbations as they reduce symptoms and improve airflow obstruction. Short-acting $\beta_2$-agonists, such as salbutamol and terbutaline, act by increasing the concentration of cyclic adenosine monophosphate (cAMP),[16] thus they induce rapid bronchodilation by relaxing airway smooth muscle.

*Anti-cholinergics: short-acting*

Anticholinergics, such as ipratropium and oxitropium bromide, are non-selective short-acting muscarinic antagonists (SAMAs), which block the effect of acetylcholine on $M_3$ receptors. If a prompt response to SABAs does not occur, the addition of an anticholinergic is recommended, even though evidence on the effectiveness of this combination is controversial.

There are three relevant issues related to the use of SABDs during exacerbations: efficacy of the drugs, drug combinations, and the delivery system for inhaled treatment. There is no evidence of a difference between the classes of SABDs in terms of bronchodilatation (increased $FEV_1$ range, 150–250 mL) at 90 minutes.[9] When inhaled, the effects of SABAs begin within 5 minutes with maximum peak at 30 minutes; ipratropium begins to take effect after 10–15 minutes with a peak at 30–60 minutes. The effects of the two classes of SABDs decline after 2–3 hours but can last as long as 4–6 hours, depending on their individual properties. Inspiratory capacity also increased significantly at 30 and 90 minutes after nebulized salbutamol 5.0 mg (approximately by 10 per cent each) in inpatients, suggesting a complementary benefit for acute-on-chronic air trapping and lung hyperinflation.[9,17]

By contrast, the efficacy of combinations of SABDs remains debated. Unlike stable COPD, where the simultaneous administration of SABDs is more efficacious than either agent given alone,[18] a combination of SABDs given sequentially in exacerbations does not provide additional benefit. However, increasing the dose and/or the frequency of an existing SABD treatment with SABAs is the strategy recommended by the American Thoracic Society (ATS)/European Respiratory Society (ERS)[19] and the Global Initiative for Chronic Obstructive Lung Disease (GOLD)[2,15] guidelines. In this context, if the clinical response is not immediately favourable the addition of a SAMA is also recommended, despite the uncertainties about combinations of SABDs in this setting. The ATS/ERS guideline[19] and the UK's National Institute for Health and Clinical Excellence (NICE) report[20] recommend the use of SABAs and/or SAMAs. It is most likely, however, that the correct strategy for the physician remains, at least in part, empirical.

Regarding the delivery system, a systematic review of the route of delivery of SABDs found no significant differences in $FEV_1$ between the use of hand-held metered dose inhalers (MDIs) with a good inhaler technique (with or without a spacer device) and nebulizers.[21]

There is accumulating evidence that SABAs may increase the risk of adverse cardiovascular events in patients with obstructive airway disease, a finding of special concern for those patients with underlying cardiovascular comorbidities.[22] However, SABAs did not in any form or at first time use increase the risk of acute myocardial infarction in a cohort of more than 10 000 patients newly diagnosed with COPD, with or without pre-existing concomitant cardiovascular disease.[22,23] Troublesome muscular tremor, hypokalaemia, and increased oxygen consumption also occur. Mild subclinical deterioration in gas exchange within 30–90 minutes of nebulization with further hypoxaemia and/or increased alveolar-to-arterial oxygen difference rarely occurs.[17] The main adverse effect of SAMAs is dry mouth, sometimes associated with a bitter taste. Occasional prostatic symptoms and more rarely glaucoma may also appear.

Although the ATS/ERS guidelines[19] recommend adding long-acting bronchodilators (LABDs) and inhaled steroids as an adjunct to the treatment if patients were not using them, there is no evidence for such a recommendation. Currently, the maintenance or addition of salmeterol during an exacerbation needs to be considered on an individual basis since, when taken in the recommended dosage, it can result in a small but significant decline in $SaO_2$ in stable COPD.[24] There is no evidence whether there are additive side effects when LABAs are used in combination with high doses of SABAs. Alternatively, some non-bronchodilator effects of LABAs,[16] namely inflammatory mediator release inhibition, mucociliary transport stimulation, and neutrophil recruitment attenuation and activation, could be of potential benefit for the pathobiology of exacerbations. The lung hyperinflation observed in patients with exacerbations of COPD[25] may be important as LABDs reduce the impact of hyperinflation both at rest[26] and during exercise.[27]

Of note, recently, it is has been found that high-dose budesonide/formoterol is as effective as prednisolone plus formoterol for the outpatient treatment of non-hospitalized COPD exacerbations, indicating that an early increase of the dose of combination inhalers may be attempted before systemic glucocorticosteroids are used.[28]

### Methylxanthines

Methylxanthines (theophylline or aminophylline) are currently considered second-line intravenous therapy, and are used when there is inadequate or insufficient response to SABDs[2,15] (evidence level B). Possible beneficial effects in terms of lung function and clinical endpoints are modest and inconsistent, whereas adverse effects are significantly increased.[29]

Despite the bronchodilating effects of methylxanthines through directly relaxing the smooth muscle cells in the human airways, possibly by phosphodiesterase inhibition, there is increasing evidence of anti-inflammatory effects at low serum concentrations.[30,31] The recent finding that theophylline activates histone deacetylases – nuclear enzymes involved in the switching off of activated inflammatory genes – is of further pathophysiological and therapeutic interest, and it could be harnessed to reduce the need for glucocorticoids during exacerbations.[31]

When used in the clinical setting, physicians have to be aware of the many unwanted effects of theophylline and interactions with other metabolic factors.

### Systemic and inhaled glucocorticosteroids

Oral or intravenous glucocorticosteroids are recommended as an addition to other therapies in the hospital management of exacerbations of COPD (evidence level A). The exact dose that should be recommended is unknown, but high doses are associated with a significant risk of side effects; 30–40 mg of oral prednisolone daily for 7–10 days can be effective and safe (evidence level C).[2] Prolonged treatment does not result in greater efficacy and increases the risk of side effects (e.g. hyperglycaemia, muscle atrophy). Moreover, therapy with oral prednisolone is not inferior to intravenous treatment within the first 90 days after starting therapy, indicating that the oral route is preferable in the treatment of COPD exacerbations.[32]

The role of systemic corticosteroids in treating patients with exacerbations has remained controversial for almost 20 years. The recommendation is based on relevant randomized controlled trials (RCTs)[33] in outpatients and inpatients with moderate to severe exacerbations of COPD. In addition, conclusive systematic reviews[34] have led to the evidence-based systemic use of corticosteroids for exacerbations of COPD.[9] Compared with placebo, systemic steroids improved symptoms and $PaO_2$ in moderate to severe exacerbations, and reduced treatment failure, relapse and length of hospital stay. Adverse events, however, were more noticeable in the steroid-treated group, hyperglycaemia being the most common and requiring treatment, and also a higher proportion of secondary infections.

Nebulized glucocorticosteroids (budesonide) have shown similar improvement in post-bronchodilator $FEV_1$ within the first 3 days of treatment, to oral prednisolone in patients with severe COPD hospitalized for moderate to severe non-acidotic exacerbations,[35] although other outcomes were not significantly different than placebo. A similar study has reinforced the view that nebulized budesonide may be an effective and safe alternative to systemic glucocorticosteroids in the treatment of exacerbations.[36]

The mechanisms for improving lung function and other outcomes and the patients most likely to benefit from steroid treatment during exacerbations remain contentious. No clinical, biochemical or functional markers can clearly identify which patients will respond better to steroid treatment. Although no effects on airway cytokines have been found in patients with stable COPD,[37] two studies have reported reductions in airway eosinophilic inflammatory markers[38] and in serum C-reactive protein (CRP) after 2 weeks of treatment with oral steroids.[4] The beneficial response to steroids during exacerbations suggests that enhanced airway inflammation and oedema and systemic inflammation are reduced or that the inflammatory pattern is sensitive to corticosteroids. An increased number of eosinophils has been found in patients with mild to moderate COPD exacerbations,[39] possibly related to predominant viral airway infections.

### Antibiotics

The use of antibiotics in exacerbations of COPD remains disputed despite their extensive use. It is unlikely that the majority of patients will benefit from a short course of antibiotics during exacerbations. The most frequent aetiology of an exacerbation is infection of the lower airways and/or air pollution, even though the cause of a third of exacerbations is still unknown. The infectious agents in COPD exacerbations can be viral or bacterial or a combination of both. The predominant bacterial microorganisms recovered from the airways of patients with mild exacerbations are *Haemophilus influenzae*, *Streptococcus pneumoniae* and *Moraxella catarrhalis* whereas, in patients with severe COPD episodes, enteric Gram-negative bacilli and *Pseudomonas aeruginosa* may be more important. The risk factors for *P. aeruginosa* infection are recent hospitalization, frequent administration of antibiotics (four courses in the last year), severe COPD exacerbations, and isolation of *P. aeruginosa* during a previous exacerbation or colonization during a stable period. Viral infections (picornaviruses, influenza A and respiratory syncytial virus) are also likely to play a part in severe exacerbations.

Anthonisen *et al.*[40] provided strong evidence that antibiotics have a significant effect on peak expiratory flow rate (PEFR) and lead to an earlier resolution of all three of the cardinal symptoms defining exacerbations (increased dyspnoea, increased sputum volume and increased sputum purulence). Stockley *et al.*[41] showed a relationship between sputum purulence and the presence of bacteria, suggesting that these patients should be treated with antibiotics if they also have at least one of the other two symptoms (dyspnoea or increased sputum volume). Using a meta-analysis approach, it was concluded that the use of antibiotic treatment in the presence of purulent sputum was associated with a reduction in the risk of mortality, treatment failure and sputum purulence.[42]

Based on the current available evidence antibiotics should be given to:

- patients with exacerbations of COPD with the following three cardinal symptoms: increased dyspnoea, increased sputum volume, and increased sputum purulence (evidence level B)
- patients with exacerbations of COPD with two of the cardinal symptoms, if increased purulence of sputum is one of the two symptoms (evidence level C)
- patients with severe exacerbations of COPD who require mechanical ventilation (invasive or non-invasive) (evidence level B).

The oral route is preferred and is cheaper. The administration should be based on the patterns of local bacterial resistance and they should be used for a period of 3–10 days. If an exacerbation responds poorly to empirical antibiotic treatment, the patient should be re-evaluated for complications with microbiological reassessment if necessary.

## NON-PHARMACOLOGICAL INTERVENTIONS

### Oxygen therapy and mechanical ventilation

Oxygen therapy and mechanical ventilation are of great benefit in acute respiratory failure during exacerbations (see Chapters 22 and 26).

### Pulmonary rehabilitation (physiotherapy)

Pulmonary rehabilitation is a multidisciplinary programme particularly suited to all patients with COPD, except those with stable stage I disease. However, other than manual chest percussion and physiotherapy using positive expiratory pressure masks for selected patients to help in clearing sputum, pulmonary rehabilitation has no indication during the nadir of exacerbations of COPD.[4]

## OTHER MEASURES

Further treatments that can be used in the hospital include: fluid administration (accurate monitoring of fluid balance is essential); nutrition (supplementary when needed); deep venous thrombosis prophylaxis (mechanical devices, heparins, etc.) in immobilized, polycythaemic, or dehydrated

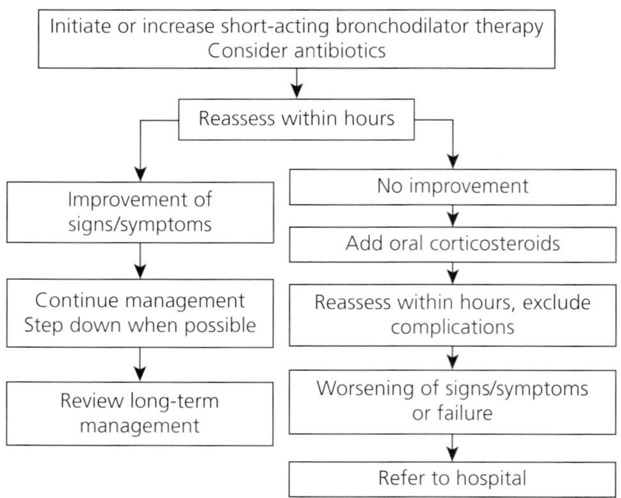


**Figure 21.2** Management of mild to moderate exacerbation of chronic obstructive pulmonary disease. With permission from Rodriguez-Roisin.[9]

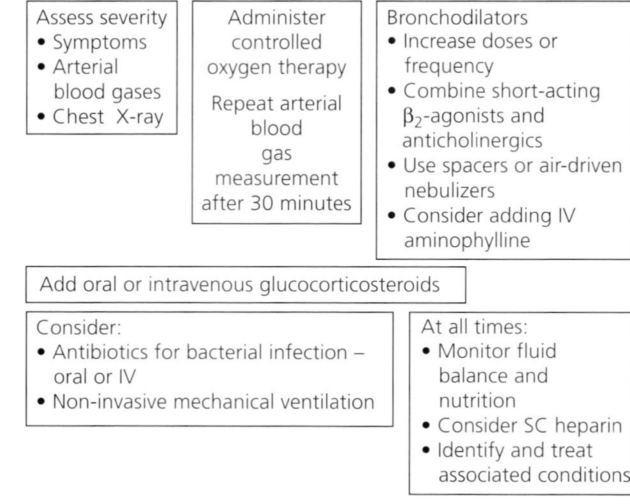


**Figure 21.3** Management of moderate to severe exacerbation of chronic obstructive pulmonary disease. With permission from Rodriguez-Roisin.[9]

patients with or without a history of thromboembolic disease; and sputum clearance (by stimulating coughing and low-volume forced expirations as in home management).

## Therapeutic strategies

### MILD TO MODERATE EPISODES

A management scheme for mild to moderate episodes of COPD exacerbation is shown in Figure 21.2.

### MODERATE TO SEVERE EPISODES

A management scheme for moderate to severe episodes of COPD exacerbation is shown in Figure 21.3.

# STABLE CHRONIC OBSTRUCTIVE PULMONARY DISEASE

## Background

As stated in international guidelines,[2,15] an effective COPD management plan includes four components: assessment of and monitoring disease; reduction of risk factors; management of stable COPD; and management of exacerbations. Although disease prevention is the ultimate goal, once COPD has been diagnosed, effective management should be aimed at: relief of symptoms, prevention of disease progression, improvement in exercise tolerance, improvement in health status, prevention and treatment of complications, prevention and treatment of exacerbations and reduction in mortality. These goals should be reached with minimal side effects from treatment, a particular challenge in COPD patients because they commonly have comorbidities. However, it should be taken into consideration that none of the existing medications for COPD has been shown to modify the long-term decline in lung function that is the hallmark of this disease (evidence level A). Therefore, pharmacotherapy for COPD is used to alleviate symptoms and/or complications.

Likewise, the complex pathophysiology of COPD means that to achieve optimal treatment, it may be important to address more than one component of the disease.[7] This second part of the chapter aims to evaluate and summarize the pharmacological approaches currently available for the treatment of COPD, and to assess their ability to address the underlying multifactorial nature of COPD (Fig. 21.4), with a focus on long-acting $\beta_2$-agonists (LABAs) and their combination with inhaled corticosteroids (ICSs).

## Therapeutic interventions

Pharmacological and non-pharmacological interventions are based on symptoms and the level of severity, measured by $FEV_1$. A management scheme at each stage of severity is shown in Figure 21.5.

### PHARMACOLOGICAL INTERVENTIONS

Since COPD is usually progressive, recommendations for the pharmacological treatment of COPD reflect the following general principles:

- Treatment tends to be cumulative with more medications being required as the disease state worsens.
- Regular treatment needs to be maintained at the same level for long periods of time unless significant side effects occur or the disease worsens.

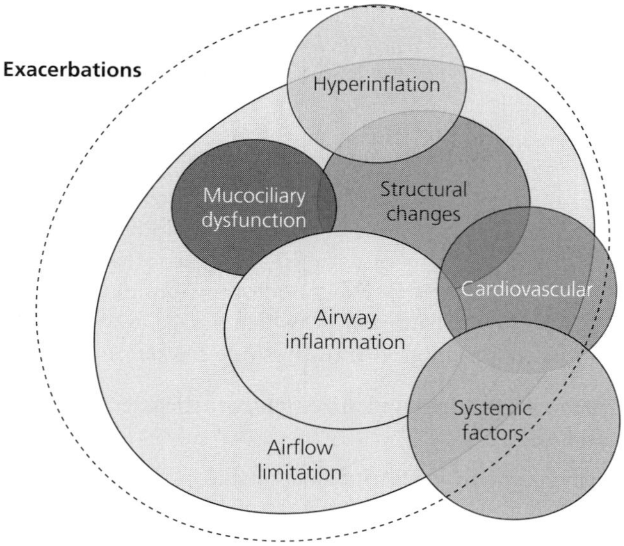

**Figure 21.4** The multifactorial nature of chronic obstructive pulmonary disease. With permission from Rodriguez-Roisin.[7]

- Individuals differ in their response to treatment and in the side effects they report during therapy. Careful monitoring is needed over an appropriate period to ensure that the specific aim of introducing a therapy has been met without an unacceptable cost to the patient.

### Bronchodilators

Regular bronchodilation with drugs that act primarily on airway smooth muscle does not modify the decline of function in stage I (mild) COPD or, by inference, the prognosis of the disease (evidence level B). However, bronchodilator medications are central to the symptomatic management of COPD (evidence level A). They are given either on an as-needed basis for relief of persistent or worsening symptoms, or on a regular basis to prevent or reduce symptoms.

#### *Beta-agonists: short- and long-acting*

$\beta_2$-Agonists stimulate relaxation of the smooth muscle of the airways via $\beta_2$-adrenoceptor-mediated activation of adenylate cyclase and promote bronchodilation. A number of SABAs are available for the treatment of COPD, including salbutamol and terbutaline. These drugs allow brief symptom relief,[43] making them ideal for rescue therapy. However, the short duration of action (4–6 hours) and need for multiple daily dosing means that they are often considered as inconvenient to use as maintenance therapy.

Effects of LABAs such as salmeterol and formoterol last for 12 hours or more, with no loss of effectiveness overnight or with regular use in COPD patients (evidence level A). Both agents have been shown to improve lung function and reduce symptoms and dyspnoea in patients with COPD.[44–46]

#### *Anti-cholinergics: short- and long-acting*

Anticholinergic drugs, such as ipratropium bromide, oxitropium bromide and tiotropium bromide, are muscarinic antagonists and reduce the effects of cholinergic tone and provide effective bronchodilation. Ipratropium

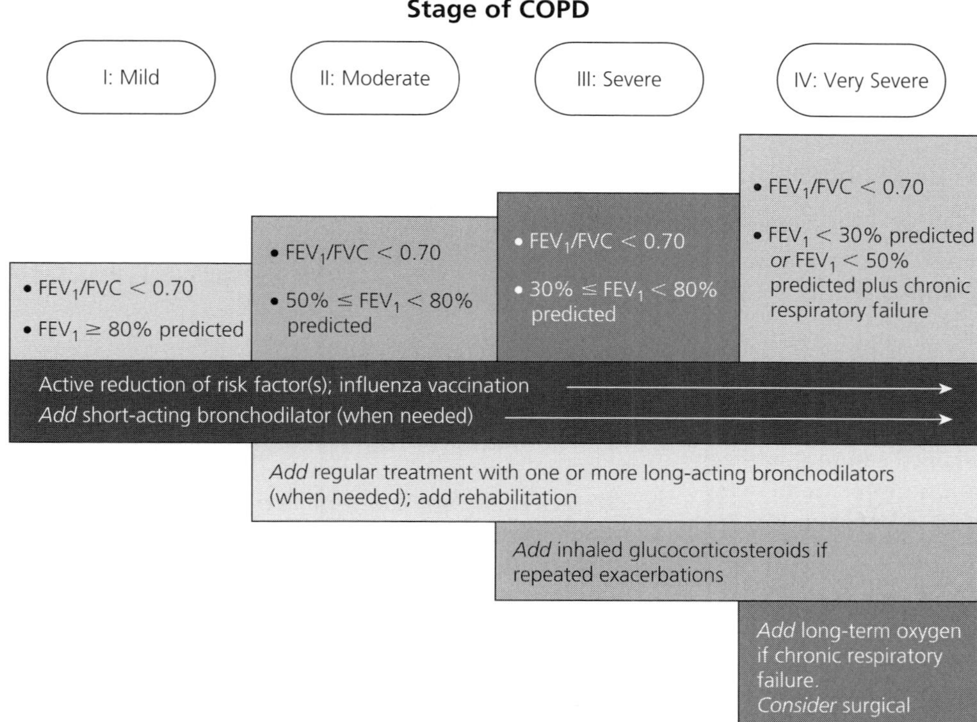


**Figure 21.5** Treatment at each stage of chronic obstructive pulmonary disease. With permission from Rabe *et al.*[2]

bromide and oxitropium at their usually prescribed doses have a short duration of action, which is often inconvenient, although the bronchodilating effect of short-acting inhaled anticholinergics lasts longer than that of SABAs, with some bronchodilator effect generally apparent up to 8 hours after administration (evidence level A). However, long-acting anticholinergics such as tiotropium can be considered to be as effective and convenient as LABAs for the treatment of moderate to very severe COPD. A single dose of tiotropium has been shown to provide effective bronchodilation for more than 24 hours in patients with COPD.[47] In fact, a recent large clinical trial has shown that therapy with tiotropium was associated with improvements in lung function, quality of life and reduction in exacerbations during a 4-year period but did not significantly reduce the rate of decline in $FEV_1$ in patients with COPD treated with other freely prescribed respiratory medications (i.e. inhaled LABAs, inhaled corticosteroids and theophyllines).[48] A sub-analysis of GOLD II patients within this trial showed favourable effects on the rate of decline of lung function as well as the other mentioned outcomes, which suggests a role for these drugs in early intervention.[49]

### Methylxanthines: theophylline (slow release)

Theophyllines produce modest bronchodilatory effects and have been used in the treatment of COPD. The molecular mechanism of bronchodilation is not completely understood. Although theophylline has proven efficacy in COPD, the use of this class of drug is limited by a low risk–benefit ratio, a consequence of widespread side effects due to a non-selective action and pharmacological interaction with other therapies. There is evidence in both asthma and COPD that theophylline has anti-inflammatory properties.[50] However, the molecular mechanisms of this anti-inflammatory action remain uncertain. Proposed mechanisms include adenosine receptor antagonism, interleukin (IL)-10 release, and effects on transcription control and apoptosis.[51] More importantly, theophylline has been shown to activate histone deacetylases, which have a role in suppressing the expression of inflammatory genes.[52]

### Combination bronchodilator therapy

Combining bronchodilators with different mechanisms and durations of action may increase the degree of bronchodilation with equivalent or fewer side effects. For example, a combination of a SABA and an anticholinergic produces greater and more sustained improvements in $FEV_1$ than either drug alone with no evidence of tachyphylaxis over 90 days of treatment.[53] Unfortunately, this combination of bronchodilators has been withdrawn from the market in several western European countries.

### Inhaled glucocorticosteroids

Regular treatment with inhaled glucocorticosteroids does not modify the long-term decline of $FEV_1$ in patients with COPD. However, regular treatment with inhaled glucocorticosteroids is appropriate for symptomatic COPD patients with an $FEV_1$ <50 per cent predicted (stage III [severe] and stage IV [very severe] COPD) and repeated exacerbations (evidence level A). This treatment has been shown to reduce the frequency of exacerbations and thus improve health status (evidence level A), and withdrawal from treatment with inhaled glucocorticosteroids can lead to exacerbations in some patients. It should be taken into account that treatment with inhaled glucocorticosteroids in COPD increases the likelihood of pneumonia and does not reduce overall mortality,[54] which has led to withdrawal of its licence as monotherapy in some countries.

### Combination therapy: inhaled glucocorticosteroids and LABAs

There are two LABA/inhaled glucocorticosteroid combination therapies currently available: salmeterol/fluticasone propionate and formoterol/budesonide. Due to their complementary mechanisms of action, the combination of a LABA and an inhaled glucocorticosteroid can potentially address the underlying multicomponent nature of COPD, and recent data indicate that LABA/inhaled glucocorticosteroid combinations produce wide-ranging effects that are greater than with either agent alone.

An inhaled glucocorticosteroid combined with a LABA is more effective than the individual components in reducing exacerbations and improving lung function and health status (evidence level A). However, combination therapy increases the likelihood of pneumonia, and a large prospective clinical trial has failed to demonstrate a significant effect on mortality.[54]

A large RCT in severe and very severe COPD patients found no difference in exacerbation rate for a combination of inhaled glucocorticosteroid/LABA and tiotropium, although the patients receiving the combination were less likely to withdraw, had better health status and had better survival.[55]

### Oral glucocorticosteroids

Based on the lack of evidence of benefit, and the large body of evidence on side effects, long-term treatment with oral glucocorticosteroids is not recommended in COPD (evidence level A).[2,15]

### Other pharmacological therapies

#### *Vaccines*

Influenza vaccination can reduce serious illness and death in COPD patients by about 50 per cent (evidence level A). Vaccines containing killed or live inactivated viruses are recommended as they are more effective in elderly patients with COPD. Pneumococcal polysaccharide vaccine is recommended for COPD patients 65 years and older.[4]

#### *Mucolytic agents*

The regular use of mucolytics in COPD has been evaluated in a number of long-term studies with controversial results. Although a few patients with viscous sputum may benefit from mucolytics, the overall benefits seem to be very small, and the widespread use of these agents cannot be recommended at present (evidence level D). There is some evidence, however, that in patients who have not been treated with ICS, treatment with mucolytics, such as carbocisteine, may reduce exacerbations.[56]

*Antioxidant agents*

Antioxidants, in particular *N*-acetylcysteine, have been reported, in small studies, to reduce the frequency of exacerbations, leading to speculation that these medications could have a role in the treatment of patients with recurrent exacerbations (evidence level B). However, a large RCT found no effect of *N*-acetylcysteine on the frequency of exacerbations, except in patients not treated with inhaled glucocorticosteroids.[57]

*Antibiotics*

Continuous prophylactic use of antibiotics has been shown to have no effect on the frequency of exacerbations in COPD, and a study that examined the efficacy of winter chemoprophylaxis over a period of 5 years concluded that there was no benefit.[4] There is no current evidence that the use of antibiotics, other than for treating infectious exacerbations of COPD and other bacterial infections, is helpful (evidence level A). A recent trial using macrolides (more specifically, erythromycin) reported a significant reduction in exacerbations of COPD compared with placebo, so that this antibiotic therapy may be effective in decreasing the overburden of this disease in patients with exacerbations.[58]

#### NON-PHARMACOLOGICAL INTERVENTIONS

These include pulmonary rehabilitation, oxygen therapy and domiciliary ventilation. See Chapters 62, 26 and 14, respectively.

**Lung volume reduction surgery**

Lung volume reduction surgery is a surgical procedure that aims to reduce hyperinflation in order to improve respiratory muscle mechanical efficiency. Patients more likely to benefit from this surgical approach are those with upper lobe emphysema and low exercise capacity, as it was shown in a large multicentre study of 1200 patients comparing lung volume reduction surgery with medical treatment after 4.3 years.[59] Patients who received the surgery had a greater survival rate than similar patients who received medical therapy (54 per cent vs 39.7 per cent). Therefore, it should be taken into account that lung volume reduction surgery is an expensive palliative surgical procedure and can be recommended only in carefully selected patients.

**Lung transplantation**

Patients with very severe COPD may benefit from lung transplantation considering they fulfil very restrictive criteria: $FEV_1$ 35 per cent predicted, $PaO_2$ 7.3–8.0 kPa (55–60 mmHg), $PaCO_2$ 6.7 kPa (50 mmHg), and secondary pulmonary hypertension.[60] In this selected group of patients, lung transplantation has been shown to improve quality of life and functional capacity although it does not seem to confer a survival benefit after two years.[61]

### Therapeutic strategies

#### MILD STAGE

For patients with few or intermittent symptoms (stage I COPD), use of a short-acting inhaled bronchodilator as needed to control dyspnoea is sufficient. If inhaled bronchodilators are not available, regular treatment with slow-release theophylline should be considered.

#### MODERATE STAGE

In patients with stage II–IV COPD, in whom dyspnoea during daily activities is not relieved despite treatment with as-needed short-acting bronchodilators, adding regular treatment with a long-acting inhaled bronchodilator is recommended (evidence level A). Regular treatment with long-acting bronchodilators is more effective and convenient than treatment with short-acting bronchodilators (evidence level A). There is insufficient evidence to favour one long-acting bronchodilator over others. For patients on regular long-acting bronchodilator therapy in need of additional symptom control, adding theophylline may produce additional benefits (evidence level B). Pulmonary rehabilitation also needs to be considered due to its evidence proven beneficial effects.

#### SEVERE AND VERY SEVERE STAGES

In patients with a post-bronchodilator $FEV_1$ <50 per cent predicted (stage III and IV COPD) and a history of repeated exacerbations (for example, three in the past 3 years), regular treatment with inhaled glucocorticosteroids should be added to long-acting inhaled bronchodilators, given as a combination inhaler. Chronic treatment with oral glucocorticosteroids should be avoided. Long-term oxygen therapy should be added if chronic respiratory failure is present.

## NEW DIRECTIONS FOR COPD THERAPY

A major phosphodiesterase (PDE) type found in airway inflammatory cells is $PDE_4$; selective inhibition of $PDE_4$ could potentially provide important anti-inflammatory effects in the treatment of COPD. In fact, preclinical studies with two such agents, cilomilast and roflumilast, have demonstrated a range of effects on inflammatory cells and cytokine production. Cilomilast has been shown to reduce key inflammatory cells in bronchial biopsies of patients with COPD; reductions in $CD_{8+}$ cells, $CD_{68+}$ cells, $CD_{4+}$ cells, and neutrophils were indicated compared with placebo.[62] In addition to anti-inflammatory effects, selective $PDE_4$ inhibitors have been shown to improve lung function compared with placebo. A preliminary randomized, dose-ranging trial in patients with COPD demonstrated significantly improved $FEV_1$, FVC and PEF with cilomilast compared with placebo after 6 weeks of therapy.[62] Another study revealed that 24 weeks of roflumilast treatment provided significant improvements in lung function and reduction in exacerbations compared with placebo in patients with COPD.[63,64] This new class of drugs has potential, but more data are needed to establish how they fit into current management strategies.

## REFERENCES


1. O'Donnell DE, Parker CM. COPD exacerbations. 3: Pathophysiology. *Thorax* 2006; **61**: 354–61.
2. Rabe KF, Hurd S, Anzueto A *et al.* Global strategy for the diagnosis, management, and prevention of chronic obstructive pulmonary disease: GOLD executive summary. *Am J Respir Crit Care Med* 2007; **176**: 532–55.
3. Bhowmik A, Seemungal TA, Sapsford RJ *et al.* Relation of sputum inflammatory markers to symptoms and lung function changes in COPD exacerbations. *Thorax* 2000; **55**: 114–20.
4. Sin DD, Lacy P, York E *et al.* Effects of fluticasone on systemic markers of inflammation in chronic obstructive pulmonary disease. *Am J Respir Crit Care Med* 2004; **170**: 760–5.
5. Hurst JR, Wilkinson TM, Perera WR *et al.* Relationships among bacteria, upper airway, lower airway, and systemic inflammation in COPD. *Chest* 2005; **127**: 1219–26.
6. Pinto-Plata VM, Livnat G, Girish M *et al.* Systemic cytokines, clinical and physiological changes in patients hospitalized for exacerbation of COPD. *Chest* 2007; **131**: 37–43.
7. Rodriguez-Roisin R. The airway pathophysiology of COPD: implications for treatment. *COPD* 2005; **2**: 253–62.
8. Barbera JA, Roca J, Ferrer A *et al.* Mechanisms of worsening gas exchange during acute exacerbations of chronic obstructive pulmonary disease. *Eur Respir J* 1997; **10**: 1285–91.
9. Rodriguez-Roisin R. COPD exacerbations. 5: Management. *Thorax* 2006; **61**: 535–44.
10. Soler-Cataluna JJ, Martinez-Garcia MA, Roman SP *et al.* Severe acute exacerbations and mortality in patients with chronic obstructive pulmonary disease. *Thorax* 2005; **60**: 925–31.
11. Donaldson GC, Wedzicha JA. COPD exacerbations.1: Epidemiology. *Thorax* 2006; **61**: 164–8.
12. Patil SP, Krishnan JA, Lechtzin N *et al.* In-hospital mortality following acute exacerbations of chronic obstructive pulmonary disease. *Arch Intern Med* 2003; **163**: 1180–6.
13. Mannino DM, Braman S. The epidemiology and economics of chronic obstructive pulmonary disease. *Proc Am Thorac Soc* 2007; **4**: 502–6.
14. Price LC, Lowe D, Hosker HS *et al.* UK National COPD Audit 2003: Impact of hospital resources and organisation of care on patient outcome following admission for acute COPD exacerbation. *Thorax* 2006; **61**: 837–42.
15. Global initiative for chronic obstructive lung disease. Global strategy for the diagnosis, management, and prevention of chronic obstructive pulmonary disease. Update 2008. Available at: www.goldcopd.com.
16. Johnson M, Rennard S. Alternative mechanisms for long-acting beta-adrenergic agonists in COPD. *Chest* 2001; **120**: 258–70.
17. Polverino E, Gomez FP, Manrique H *et al.* Gas exchange response to short-acting beta2-agonists in chronic obstructive pulmonary disease severe exacerbations. *Am J Respir Crit Care Med* 2007; **176**: 350–5.
18. In chronic obstructive pulmonary disease, a combination of ipratropium and albuterol is more effective than either agent alone. An 85-day multicenter trial. COMBIVENT Inhalation Aerosol Study Group. *Chest* 1994; **105**: 1411–19.
19. Celli BR, MacNee W, Committee members. Standards for the diagnosis and treatment of patients with COPD: a summary of the ATS/ERS position paper. *Eur Respir J* 2004; **23**: 932–46.
20. National Institute for Clinical Excellence (NICE). Chronic obstructive pulmonary disease: national clinical guideline for management of chronic obstructive pulmonary disease in adults in primary and secondary care. *Thorax* 2004; **59** Suppl I: 1–232.
21. Turner MO, Patel A, Ginsburg S *et al.* Bronchodilator delivery in acute airflow obstruction. A meta-analysis. *Arch Intern Med* 1997; **157**: 1736–44.
22. Salpeter SR, Ormiston TM, Salpeter EE. Cardiovascular effects of beta-agonists in patients with asthma and COPD: a meta-analysis. *Chest* 2004; **125**: 2309–21.
23. Suissa S, Assimes T, Ernst P. Inhaled short acting beta agonist use in COPD and the risk of acute myocardial infarction. *Thorax* 2003; **58**: 43–6.
24. Khoukaz G, Gross NJ. Effects of salmeterol on arterial blood gases in patients with stable chronic obstructive pulmonary disease. Comparison with albuterol and ipratropium. *Am J Respir Crit Care Med* 1999; **160**: 1028–30.
25. Parker CM, Voduc N, Aaron SD *et al.* Physiological changes during symptom recovery from moderate exacerbations of COPD. *Eur Respir J* 2005; **26**: 420–8.
26. Celli B, ZuWallack R, Wang S *et al.* Improvement in resting inspiratory capacity and hyperinflation with tiotropium in COPD patients with increased static lung volumes. *Chest* 2003; **124**: 1743–8.
27. O'Donnell DE, Voduc N, Fitzpatrick M *et al.* Effect of salmeterol on the ventilatory response to exercise in

chronic obstructive pulmonary disease. *Eur Respir J* 2004; **24**: 86–94.

28. Stallberg B, Selroos O, Vogelmeier C *et al.* Budesonide/formoterol as effective as prednisolone plus formoterol in acute exacerbations of COPD. A double-blind, randomised, non-inferiority, parallel-group, multicentre study. *Respir Res* 2009; **10**: 11.
29. Barr RG, Rowe BH, Camargo CA Jr. Methylxanthines for exacerbations of chronic obstructive pulmonary disease: meta-analysis of randomised trials. *BMJ* 2003; **327**: 643.
30. Ito K, Lim S, Caramori G *et al.* A molecular mechanism of action of theophylline: Induction of histone deacetylase activity to decrease inflammatory gene expression. *Proc Natl Acad Sci U S A* 2002; **99**: 8921–6.
31. Cosio BG, Iglesias A, Rios A *et al.* Low-dose theophylline enhances the anti-inflammatory effects of steroids during exacerbations of COPD. *Thorax* 2009; **64**: 424–9.
32. de Jong YP, Uil SM, Grotjohan HP *et al.* Oral or IV prednisolone in the treatment of COPD exacerbations: a randomized, controlled, double-blind study. *Chest* 2007; **132**: 1741–7.
33. Niewoehner DE, Erbland ML, Deupree RH *et al.* Effect of systemic glucocorticoids on exacerbations of chronic obstructive pulmonary disease. Department of Veterans Affairs Cooperative Study Group. *N Engl J Med* 1999; **340**: 1941–7.
34. Singh JM, Palda VA, Stanbrook MB *et al.* Corticosteroid therapy for patients with acute exacerbations of chronic obstructive pulmonary disease: a systematic review. *Arch Intern Med* 2002; **162**: 2527–36.
35. Maltais F, Ostinelli J, Bourbeau J *et al.* Comparison of nebulized budesonide and oral prednisolone with placebo in the treatment of acute exacerbations of chronic obstructive pulmonary disease: a randomized controlled trial. *Am J Respir Crit Care Med* 2002; **165**: 698–703.
36. Gunen H, Hacievliyagil SS, Yetkin O *et al.* The role of nebulised budesonide in the treatment of exacerbations of COPD. *Eur Respir J* 2007; **29**: 660–7.
37. Keatings VM, Jatakanon A, Worsdell YM *et al.* Effects of inhaled and oral glucocorticoids on inflammatory indices in asthma and COPD. *Am J Respir Crit Care Med* 1997; **155**: 542–8.
38. Brightling CE, Monteiro W, Ward R *et al.* Sputum eosinophilia and short-term response to prednisolone in chronic obstructive pulmonary disease: a randomised controlled trial. *Lancet* 2000; **356**: 1480–5.
39. Saetta M, Di Stefano A, Maestrelli P *et al.* Airway eosinophilia in chronic bronchitis during exacerbations. *Am J Respir Crit Care Med* 1994; **150**: 1646–52.
40. Anthonisen NR, Manfreda J, Warren CP *et al.* Antibiotic therapy in exacerbations of chronic obstructive pulmonary disease. *Ann Intern Med* 1987; **106**: 196–204.
41. Stockley RA, O'Brien C, Pye A *et al.* Relationship of sputum color to nature and outpatient management of acute exacerbations of COPD. *Chest* 2000; **117**: 1638–45.
42. Ram FS, Rodriguez-Roisin R, Granados-Navarrete A *et al.* Antibiotics for exacerbations of chronic obstructive pulmonary disease. *Cochrane Database Syst Rev* 2006; CD004403.
43. Ram FS, Sestini P. Regular inhaled short acting beta2 agonists for the management of stable chronic obstructive pulmonary disease: Cochrane systematic review and meta-analysis. *Thorax* 2003; **58**: 580–4.
44. Boyd G, Morice AH, Pounsford JC *et al.* An evaluation of salmeterol in the treatment of chronic obstructive pulmonary disease (COPD). *Eur Respir J* 1997; **10**: 815–21.
45. Jones PW, Bosh TK. Quality of life changes in COPD patients treated with salmeterol. *Am J Respir Crit Care Med* 1997; **155**: 1283–9.
46. Mahler DA, Donohue JF, Barbee RA *et al.* Efficacy of salmeterol xinafoate in the treatment of COPD. *Chest* 1999; **115**: 957–65.
47. O'Donnell DE, Fluge T, Gerken F *et al.* Effects of tiotropium on lung hyperinflation, dyspnoea and exercise tolerance in COPD. *Eur Respir J* 2004; **23**: 832–40.
48. Tashkin DP, Celli B, Senn S *et al.* A 4-year trial of tiotropium in chronic obstructive pulmonary disease. *N Engl J Med* 2008; **359**: 1543–54.
49. Decramer M, Celli B, Kesten S *et al.* Effect of tiotropium on outcomes in patients with moderate chronic obstructive pulmonary disease (UPLIFT): a prespecified subgroup analysis of a randomised controlled trial. *Lancet* 2009; **374**: 1171–8.
50. Barnes PJ. Theophylline: new perspectives for an old drug. *Am J Respir Crit Care Med* 2003; **167**: 813–18.
51. Barnes PJ. Theophylline for COPD. *Thorax* 2006; **61**: 742–4.
52. Cosio BG, Tsaprouni L, Ito K *et al.* Theophylline restores histone deacetylase activity and steroid responses in COPD macrophages. *J Exp Med* 2004; **200**: 689–95.
53. Routine nebulized ipratropium and albuterol together are better than either alone in COPD. The COMBIVENT Inhalation Solution Study Group. *Chest* 1997; **112**: 1514–21.
54. Calverley PM, Anderson JA, Celli B *et al.* Salmeterol and fluticasone propionate and survival in chronic obstructive pulmonary disease. *N Engl J Med* 2007; **356**: 775–89.
55. Wedzicha JA, Calverley PM, Seemungal TA *et al.* The prevention of chronic obstructive pulmonary disease exacerbations by salmeterol/fluticasone propionate or tiotropium bromide. *Am J Respir Crit Care Med* 2008; **177**: 19–26.
56. Zheng JP, Kang J, Huang SG *et al.* Effect of carbocisteine on acute exacerbation of chronic obstructive pulmonary disease (PEACE Study): a randomised placebo-controlled study. *Lancet* 2008; **371**: 2013–18.
57. Decramer M, Rutten-van MM, Dekhuijzen PN *et al.* Effects of N-acetylcysteine on outcomes in chronic obstructive pulmonary disease (Bronchitis Randomized on NAC Cost-Utility Study, BRONCUS): a randomised placebo-controlled trial. *Lancet* 2005; **365**: 1552–60.

acidosis ensues (i.e. pH <7.35). A relevant clinical aspect of note is that in this setting (exacerbated COPD) NIV failure and subsequent delivery of invasive ventilation via an endotracheal tube does not carry an increased mortality risk as compared with invasive mechanical ventilation without previous use of NIV. Moreover, some data suggest that NIV can be used even in extremely hypercapnic and acidotic patients who would otherwise need to be intubated. In an adequate environment this 'rescue' strategy is feasible. Although the intubation rate is obviously higher as compared with the usual scenario,[10] even a failed NIV trial in this situation is not harmful as it does not result in additional or attributable mortality.

In experienced centres, changes in practice have been observed: Carlucci *et al.*[11] reported better results in a later period compared with an earlier period – patients with pH <7.2 were three times more likely to be ventilated successfully with NIV after 1997. They were also able to treat more patients outside the ICU.[11] However, patients with multiple comorbidities and higher severity scores are more likely to fail.

The use of NIV for COPD exacerbations has been a revolution in the field of mechanical ventilation and the end result of collaboration between several different fields, mainly respiratory physiology, engineering and clinical science. The numerous and progressive steps taken by investigators, starting with an understanding of the problem at hand (the early physiological and clinical studies), the technical advances facilitating the use of NIV and improving the tolerance of a new technique at the bedside, the initial single-centre studies followed by multicentre randomized studies, all have contributed to the success. Finally, the systematic reproducibility of the beneficial results of NIV in patients with an acute exacerbation of a COPD has been the definitive step to achieve a widespread and routine clinical use.

In the following sections of this chapter we will review the pathophysiology, clinical applications and technical aspects of NIV in COPD, and finally we will offer some comments regarding future avenues of research in this field.

## PHYSIOLOGICAL EFFECTS OF NON-INVASIVE VENTILATION (CONTINUOUS POSITIVE AIRWAY PRESSURE AND PRESSURE SUPPORT VENTILATION/POSITIVE END-EXPIRATORY PRESSURE) IN CHRONIC OBSTRUCTIVE PULMONARY DISEASE

The pathophysiology of respiratory failure is dealt with in detail in Chapter 20. In summary, respiratory drive is increased leading to a decreased inspiratory time (and an increased mean inspiratory flow resulting in a higher burden on the inspiratory muscles) associated with reduced tidal volumes and increased respiratory rate ('rapid-shallow breathing pattern'). In spite of high respiratory drive and increased transdiaphragmatic pressure, tidal volumes remain low and respiratory rate high with reduced alveolar ventilation; as a result $PaCO_2$ increases[3] (Fig. 22.1). In nine patients with COPD in acute respiratory failure, Brochard *et al.*[3] recorded transdiaphragmatic pressures of 19 ± 2 cm $H_2O$ at baseline before NIV initiation. Despite the considerable inspiratory effort, tidal volume was only 289 ± 35 mL in these patients. These values contrast with a transdiaphragmatic pressure of 9 ± 1 cm $H_2O$ and a tidal volume of 699 ± 54 mL that were recorded in 15 clinically stable patients with severe COPD who were scheduled for lung volume reduction surgery.[14] The patient's respiratory pattern of rapid shallow breathing (high frequency and small tidal volumes) is responsible for the two main issues during COPD exacerbation: increased work of breathing (WOB) related to high respiratory rate and increased intrinsic positive end-expiratory pressure (PEEPi); and reduced alveolar ventilation related to low tidal volumes and increased dead space effect (Fig. 22.1).

This vicious circle that is responsible for progressive respiratory muscle exhaustion, increased carbon dioxide with decreased level of consciousness and hypoxaemia may lead to death, unless therapeutic interventions interrupt the cycle. The first-line treatments frequently include bronchodilators, oxygen supplementation, diuretics, anticoagulant agents or antibiotics based on the suspected cause of COPD decompensation. Also, the application of NIV is now part of the first-line recommended treatment with the objective to reverse this cycle:[15,16] to reduce the WOB and restore adequate alveolar ventilation by increasing tidal volumes and reducing the respiratory rate. Brochard *et al.* showed that NIV could achieve these different goals during COPD exacerbation.[3]

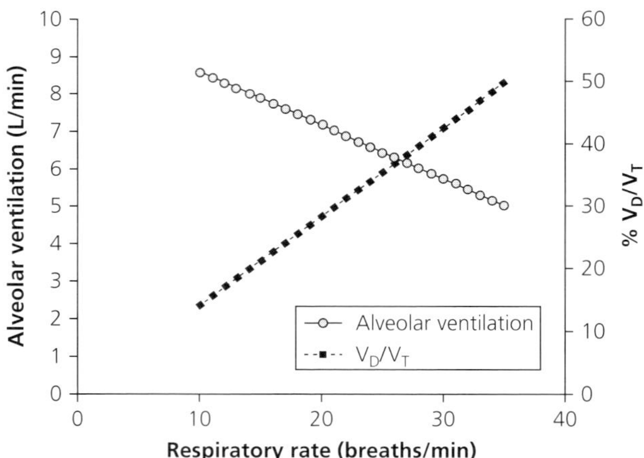


**Figure 22.1** Estimated impact of the respiratory rate (from 10 to 35 breaths/min) on alveolar ventilation for a constant minute ventilation. In this example, minute ventilation is stable at 10 L/min in a male patient, measuring 175 cm, the estimated physiological dead space is 142 mL, based on reference values.[13] The alveolar ventilation decreases when the respiratory rate increases and the impact of dead space is proportional to the respiratory rate.

## Reduction of the work of breathing with non-invasive ventilation

Many studies have demonstrated the impact of NIV on WOB during COPD exacerbation.[12,17–25] In most of the studies, baseline WOB before NIV application was very high, with negative deflections in oesophageal pressure ($\Delta P_{oes}$) or transdiaphragmatic pressure ($\Delta P_{di}$), frequently above 10 cm $H_2O$ with values up to 30 cm $H_2O$.[3,20–22,24–28] Also WOB is frequently above 1 J/L (expressed per litre of ventilation), or 10 J/min (expressed as power). Similarly, a marker of effort to breathe, the pressure–time product (PTP) of the inspiratory muscles ($PTP_{es}$), is frequently above 200 cm $H_2O^*$s/min in this specific population (a normal value would be below 100 cm $H_2O^*$s/min). Mean values for dynamic PEEPi (the lowest alveolar pressure that must be overcome by the inspiratory muscles to initiate inspiratory gas flow) typically exceeded 3 cm $H_2O$ and sometimes 5 cm $H_2O$ in critically ill patients.[3,20] However, when PEEPi is corrected with gastric pressure as described by Lessard *et al.*,[29] values are frequently below 3 cm $H_2O$.[24,26,27] By comparison, in healthy subjects, $\Delta P_{oes}$ is <5 cm $H_2O$, WOB <0.5 J/L, and PEEPi is absent at baseline.[30–32]

With NIV, all indices of effort are reduced in comparison with baseline. WOB is reduced by 30–70 per cent, $\Delta P_{oes}$ and $\Delta P_{di}$ are reduced by 50–75 per cent. In Brochard's study, WOB assessed by transdiaphragmatic pressure was reduced from 19.1 ± 5.4 cm $H_2O$ before NIV to 10.1 ± 5.5 cm $H_2O$ after 45 minutes of NIV.[3] Non-invasive ventilation also reduces diaphragmatic electromyography ($EMG_{di}$) by 20–90 per cent.[17,19,21] Of note, the maximal reduction in $EMG_{di}$ was obtained with values of pressure support of 13 cm $H_2O$ and 17 cm $H_2O$, respectively.[17] The impact of NIV on respiratory effort already appears after a few cycles. Finally, in studies assessing this parameter, the dyspnoea score was reduced by approximately 30–65 per cent.[33–36]

## Impact of pressure support level on indices of effort

During NIV, pressure support is the most frequently used mode of ventilation, most often in association with PEEP. In the most recent multicentre French survey on NIV in ICUs, pressure support was used in 83 per cent of the patients and continuous positive airway pressure (CPAP) alone in 8 per cent of the patients.[1]

The effect of the inspiratory support (pressure support level) and expiratory support (PEEP) must be differentiated.

### INSPIRATORY PRESSURE SUPPORT

Inspiratory pressure support reduces the WOB by supplying a greater proportion of transpulmonary pressure during inspiration and leading to greater tidal volumes.[20] The application of PEEP reduces the WOB by two mechanisms: first, by counterbalancing PEEPi and thereby reducing the threshold load to inspiration;[20] and, second, by increasing respiratory system compliance and thereby reducing the elastic load to inspiration.[37]

Several studies have evaluated the effects of the pressure support level and/or the addition of PEEP during NIV on WOB[19,20,23,38] or dyspnoea.[34] Studying patients with COPD, Vanpee *et al.* found that stepwise application of pressure support in 5 cm $H_2O$ increments between 5 cm $H_2O$ and 20 cm $H_2O$ progressively reduced the indices of effort.[23] Pressure support of 5 cm $H_2O$ had minor impact on $PTP_{di}$ and WOB reduction, while further incremental steps of 5 cm $H_2O$ were associated with substantial reductions of approximately 15–20 per cent at each step.[23]

Carrey *et al.* showed a progressive reduction of $EMG_{di}$ activity from 100 per cent to less than 25 per cent when increasing the level of pressure support from zero to 15 cm $H_2O$ by incremental steps of 5 cm $H_2O$.[17] As previously shown in invasively ventilated patients, the rate of pressurization has an impact both on reduction of patient's effort and on comfort. Prinianakis *et al.* found that PSV with a rapid pressurization rate of 200 cm $H_2O$/s produced the greatest reduction in $PTP_{di}$ (62 per cent) and $\Delta P_{di}$ (54 per cent), but was also associated with the poorest patient tolerance and largest mask leaks.[25]

### EXPIRATORY PRESSURE

In COPD patients with acute exacerbation, CPAP of 5 cm $H_2O$ alone can reduce the WOB in comparison with baseline before NIV application.[20] However, the addition of 10 cm $H_2O$ of inspiratory pressure support is more efficient than CPAP alone or PSV alone[20] (Fig. 22.2). Nava *et al.* also showed that the patient's efforts (assessed by $EMG_{di}$ activity) were reduced in comparison with baseline with PSV of 10 cm $H_2O$ and 20 cm $H_2O$ and further decreased with application of an external PEEP of 5 cm $H_2O$.[19]

Similarly, Vanpee *et al.* showed that adding PEEP of 5 cm $H_2O$ and 10 cm $H_2O$ generally caused a greater decrease in $PTP_{di}$ than did the same level of peak inspiratory pressure without PEEP.[23] Vitacca *et al.*[39] partitioned the inspiratory workload to assess the fraction required to overcome dynamic PEEPi, and then assessed the effects of applied PEEP set to patient comfort versus maximal physiological effect (defined as a 40–90 per cent reduction in $PTP_{di}$). During unassisted spontaneous breathing, dynamic PEEPi accounted for 38 per cent of $PTP_{di}$ (6.7 cm $H_2O$/s per breath). The mean PEEP set to achieve patient comfort and physiological improvement were similar (3.6 cm $H_2O$ vs 3.1 cm $H_2O$, respectively) which resulted in 29 per cent and 20 per cent reductions in the inspiratory work associated with overcoming dynamic PEEPi. Mehta *et al.*[34] reported that NIV with 15 cm $H_2O$ inspiratory support and 5 cm $H_2O$ PEEP improved dyspnoea scores more than CPAP of 10 cm $H_2O$ (62 per cent vs 46 per cent, respectively).

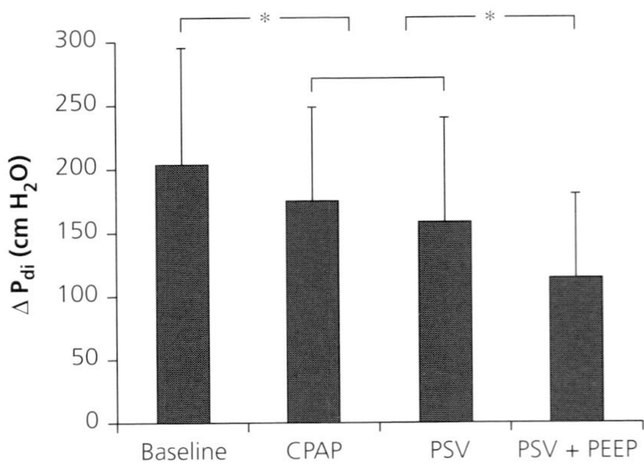


**Figure 22.2** Reduction of the transdiaphragmatic pressure ($\Delta P_{di}$) with different non-invasive ventilatory support in comparison with baseline. Continuous positive airway pressure (CPAP) alone, pressure support ventilation (PSV) and PSV + positive end-expiratory pressure (PEEP) all significantly reduced transdiaphragmatic pressure in comparison with baseline. PSV + PEEP was the most efficient ventilatory support and reduced the $\Delta P_{di}$ significantly more than PSV alone. Reproduced from Appendini *et al.*[20] with permission.

## Impact of NIV on arterial blood gases

The short-term effects of NIV on arterial blood gases in patients with acute exacerbation of COPD are well documented.[3,18–21,24,26,27,34–36,40–45] Across all the studies there has been a consistent finding of either significant improvement or a trend toward improvement in arterial blood gases. In several studies, the reduction of $PaCO_2$ during NIV in comparison with baseline values was predictive of success of the technique, in contrast with patients in whom $PaCO_2$ was stable or deteriorated while on NIV.[41–45]

The improvement in arterial blood gases is related to the inspiratory pressure support more than the expiratory pressure. Appendini *et al.*[20] demonstrated that CPAP alone did not reduce $PaCO_2$ in comparison with baseline, while PSV decreased the $PaCO_2$ in comparison with baseline, but addition of PEEP did not further improve alveolar ventilation. The increase in alveolar ventilation with inspiratory pressure support is related to increased tidal volumes due to increased transpulmonary pressure and to the decrease of the dead space effect with respiratory rate reduction (see Fig. 22.1).

# CLINICAL APPLICATIONS

In 1965, Sadoul *et al.*[46] reported that administering positive pressure ventilation through a face mask instead of a tracheal prosthesis was an efficient way to manage hypercapnic respiratory failure in patients with chronic respiratory disorders, and had little, if any, untoward effects. This was rediscovered during the second half of the 1980s, and in less than 15 years NIV has become a major therapy of acute-on-chronic respiratory failure. The present discussion will focus on the evidence supporting the use of NIV in acute exacerbation of COPD, which includes the prevention of intubation, but also the facilitation of extubation and the prevention of reintubation. Future challenges will be highlighted.

## NIV to prevent intubation in acute-on-chronic respiratory failure

### STRONG EVIDENCE SUPPORTING THE BENEFIT OF NIV IN COPD EXACERBATIONS

The positive results of the first randomized trials that evidenced the benefit of NIV on the risk of endotracheal intubation in the early 1990s[5,47] were confirmed later (Table 22.1).[6,33,48,49,52] In addition, because NIV bypasses weaning issues, which contribute to increased duration of mechanical ventilation, NIV decreases ICU and hospital length of stay in COPD exacerbation.[5,49,50] Finally, a matched controlled study showed that compared with endotracheal intubation, NIV is associated with a lower risk of nosocomial infections (pneumonia, urinary tract infections and bacteraemia).[9] As a consequence of these multiple benefits, NIV reduces the mortality rate of patients admitted for acute COPD exacerbation (Table 22.1).[5,6,47]

The results of these trials have been confirmed by three meta-analyses, which have clearly shown that in acute exacerbation of COPD NIV reduces intubation rate, hospital length of stay and hospital mortality.[7,8,53] However, these meta-analyses also have pointed out that the benefit of NIV with regard to intubation and mortality applies only to severe exacerbations (pH <7.35) and not to mild exacerbations without respiratory acidosis.[51,54]

### THE BENEFIT OF NIV TRANSLATED FROM RANDOMIZED CONTROLLED TRIALS TO THE REAL WORLD

The multiple benefits of NIV in COPD exacerbations are not limited to randomized controlled trials, and have been translated into daily practice. This actual translation is suggested by the results of various single-centre and multicentre studies. As an example, between 1994 and 2001, in a 26-bed ICU, a significant increase in NIV use and a concomitant decrease in mortality and ICU-acquired infection rates were observed.[55] NIV was the only independent factor linked with a reduced risk of death. More recently, a multicentre French survey conducted in 70 ICUs has shown that, in patients with acute-on-chronic respiratory failure, NIV success was an independent predictor of survival while NIV failure was not associated with a higher mortality.[1]

As a consequence of the multiple benefit of NIV, its use has increased over years. Perceived NIV efficacy, which is obvious in many patients, might be a major reason for this large and rapid adoption by physicians.[1,56] A French survey observed that, between 1997 and 2002, NIV use increased

**Table 22.1** Benefit of non-invasive mechanical ventilation (NIV) in respiratory failure related to COPD exacerbation

| Study | Intubation (%) | | | Hospital mortality (%) | | |
|---|---|---|---|---|---|---|
| | Standard therapy | NIV | *p* | Standard therapy | NIV | *p* |
| Bott *et al.* 1993[47] | 7 | 0 | NS | 30 | 10 | NS |
| Brochard *et al.* 1996[5] | 74 | 26 | 0.001 | 29 | 9 | <0.05 |
| Barbe *et al.* 1996[51] | 0 | 0 | NS | 0 | 0 | NS |
| Avdeev *et al.* 1998[50] | 26 | 17 | NS | 31 | 10 | <0.05 |
| Celikel *et al.* 1998[48*] | 13 | 7 | NA | 7 | 0 | NS |
| Plant *et al.* 2000[6] | 27 | 15 | <0.05 | 20 | 10 | 0.05 |
| Dikensoy *et al.* 2002[49] | 41 | 12 | <0.05 | 12 | 6 | NS |
| Conti *et al.* 2002[10†] | 100 | 52 | <0.01 | 19 | 26 | NS |

*Patients in the control group could crossover and receive NIV after failure of the standard medical therapy.
†Intubation was the standard therapy.
NA, not applicable; NS, not significant.

from 50 per cent to 65 per cent in patients with acute-on-chronic respiratory failure who received ventilatory assistance, making this therapy the first-line treatment.[1] More recently, an international survey has shown that, between 1998 and 2004, the use of NIV in acute COPD exacerbation of COPD rose from 17 per cent to 44 per cent.[2] In a survey performed in 2003 among 383 physicians in Ontario, 91 per cent considered NIV 'probably or definitely beneficial' and 95 per cent had used NIV at least once in this indication.[56]

## New challenges for NIV in acute exacerbation of COPD

The benefit of NIV in acute COPD exacerbation is now well established. However, many questions remain, and physicians now not only have to solve various issues regarding NIV practice but they also face new challenges.

### To further improve the proportion of patients who receive NIV

During the past decade, NIV use has increased in France and in international studies.[1,2] However, this improvement is not sufficient as compared with the very well demonstrated benefit of NIV. In a survey performed in 81 acute care hospitals in the states of Massachusetts and Rhode Island in 2002–3, only a third of patients with severe COPD exacerbation were administered NIV.[57] Lack of physician knowledge and inadequate equipment were the top two reasons for the low rate of NIV. In the 2003 Ontario survey, awareness of the literature was predictive of NIV use in COPD exacerbation.[56] Altogether, these data underlie the necessity to develop and implement strategies aimed at increasing appropriate use of NIV in COPD exacerbations. Among these strategies are educational programmes and guidelines. In this direction, a consensus conference on NIV was organized in France in 2006 and gave a grade 2+ (highly recommended) to NIV in acute COPD exacerbation. Recent guidelines now recommend NIV in this indication.

### To improve the NIV success rate

For the past 10 years, the NIV success rate seems to have been stable. Indeed, the various studies devoted to NIV in acute COPD exacerbations found a steady 65–80 per cent success rate.[1,58,59] One might find that the absence of increase of this success rate is disappointing. However, it seems that during the same period, the severity of disease in patients receiving NIV has increased. As an example, in a respiratory ICU, the review of 208 episodes of acute COPD exacerbation showed that the failure rate (17.2 per cent) was constant over years, but that compared with the 1992–6 period, the average pH of patients receiving NIV decreased significantly in the 1997–9 period (7.25 ± 0.07 vs 7.20 ± 0.08, respectively).[11] In this latter period the risk of failure for a patient with a pH <7.25 was threefold lower than in 1992–6. Such data suggest that, with a steady success rate, physicians are able to manage more severe patients, which is clearly a form of improvement.

Late failure is another but still ongoing issue. In a multicentre study, conducted in 137 patients who responded initially to NIV, 23 per cent experienced a new episode of respiratory failure. These patients were more likely to have a poor functional status as well as medical complications. Their prognosis was poor.[60] Here is clearly a major challenge for the forthcoming years.

### To use NIV as an alternative to intubation

In the 1990s, trials that demonstrated the benefit of NIV actually compared NIV to conventional treatment and not to intubation. More recently, two randomized controlled trials showed that NIV administered after failure of standard medical therapy to patients with intubation criteria could reduce the rate of intubation.[10,61] Moreover, a recent case–control study strongly suggested that these results can also apply to patients with moderate to severe encephalopathy (Kelly score of 3 or higher).[62] Altogether, these data suggest that NIV is beneficial as an alternative to intubation. Alteration of consciousness is no longer a contraindication of NIV in acute exacerbation of COPD. In these patients, NIV should be attempted, and pursued when there is rapid improvement of the level of consciousness. Future studies are needed to better determine criteria of selecting these patients.

#### To continue NIV after the acute phase in some patients

Approximately 80 per cent of COPD patients who survive after an NIV treatment are readmitted in the year following discharge, and 63 per cent experience a life-threatening event.[63] Preventing such a relapse is a major therapeutic goal. Obviously, prevention involves optimization of the global treatment of COPD, including medical and physical therapy. However, preliminary results suggest that pursuing NIV during the months following the acute phase may contribute to preventing such relapses.[64] Definitive results are expected.

#### To define more precisely the role of NIV in palliative care settings

The role of NIV when patients and families have decided to forgo intubation remains controversial. In the 2004 European Respiratory Survey, NIV was the ceiling of ventilatory care in 31 per cent of patients with an end-of-life decision.[65] COPD is a predictor of favourable outcome in this context[66] and survival in patients with acute exacerbation of COPD who declined intubation but accepted NIV was about 50–60 per cent.[66,67] However, the 1-year survival is 30 per cent, which is two times less than COPD patients with no care limitation.[68] Although it is even more controversial, NIV may also be administered as a palliative measure when patients and families have chosen to forego all life support, receiving comfort measures only.[69] According to the conclusions of a Society of Critical Care task force, NIV 'should be applied after careful discussion of the goals of care, with explicit parameters for success and failure, by experienced personnel, and in appropriate healthcare settings'.[70]

#### To better define the environment that is required to safely and efficiently administer NIV out of the ICU

For safety reasons, as well as to improve the chances of success, NIV requires an appropriate environment. Elliott *et al.* defined this environment as follows: availability of staff with training and expertise in NIV, adequate staff available throughout the 24-hour period, facilities for monitoring, rapid access to endotracheal intubation and invasive ventilation.[71] Obviously, the ICU setting fulfils all these criteria. Unfortunately, there is clearly an imbalance between ICU beds and the number of patients who need NIV. According to predictions, this imbalance will increase in the future. Indeed, the number of patients requiring mechanical ventilation will grow continuously,[72] while staff shortages currently force ICU bed closures. The strong pressure on ICU beds combined with their high cost has made NIV outside the ICU an attractive option.

Two different 'NIV outside the ICU' settings have been most widely studied: the emergency department and the respiratory diseases ward. Many patients with acute respiratory failure enter the hospital via the emergency department where care is initiated. It seemed therefore logical to evaluate the benefit of NIV in the emergency department. Such benefit remains controversial in acute exacerbations of COPD.[73] Achieving safe and successful NIV in the ward is another challenge. Of course, this is more feasible if the respiratory ward is close to a respiratory ICU. Carlucci *et al*[11] reported that while the severity of disease in patients treated in their respiratory ICU for acute exacerbations of COPD was increasing, more and more less severely ill patients were treated in the nearby ward. Without the vicinity of a respiratory ICU, it is suggested that with adequate staff training NIV can be applied with benefit in the general respiratory ward with the usual ward staff.[6] Furthermore, recent Canadian surveys showed that although NIV was primarily used in monitored areas, initiation or continuation of NIV in general medical or surgical wards was not uncommon.[56,57,74] This observation raises the questions of staffing and training. Finally, a preliminary report stated that NIV might be successfully and safely administered in the ward under the supervision of a medical emergency team.[75] Further studies are needed in this field.

### Non-invasive ventilation to facilitate extubation

Non-invasive ventilation can be used to facilitate extubation and shorten the duration of intubation in COPD patients intubated for an episode of acute respiratory failure. These issues are explored in detail in Chapters 21 and 23. It can also be used to prevent or to treat post-extubation respiratory failure.

## PRACTICAL ASPECTS OF NIV DELIVERY IN COPD PATIENTS

The tolerance of mask ventilation is an important determinant of the success of the technique. Patients with acute exacerbation of COPD often present with some degree of encephalopathy and are not always easily willing to accept a tightly adjusted mask on their face. The time taken by the personnel at the bedside and the quality of explanations given to the patient may have an important part in maximizing tolerance. The comfort of the interface is important; selecting the cheapest mask for purely economic reasons may be cost-ineffective because failures will be higher with a poorly tolerated mask. Fortunately, many different kinds of interface are available, offering similar physiological efficacy.[5]

Pressure support and PEEP (also referred to as bi-level ventilation) is the preferred mode, delivered either with an ICU ventilator offering an 'NIV mode' or by a turbine based NIV dedicated ventilator. The first may offer better monitoring whereas the latter may be better adapted to compensating for leaks. Usually, PEEP does not need to be high and values lower than 5 cm $H_2O$ may be sufficient to offset dynamic intrinsic PEEP. Ventilators designed for NIV usually do not allow setting PEEP below two or three cm $H_2O$, but this may be sufficient. One reason to increase PEEP above 5 cm $H_2O$ is the presence, or the suspicion, of obstructive sleep apnoea syndrome associated with COPD. The coexistence of left heart failure (again proven or suspected) may also be a reason to set PEEP at a minimum of 5 cm $H_2O$. Pressure support usually needs to be between 8 cm $H_2O$ and 15 cm $H_2O$ above PEEP. Too much pressure will generate leaks and may be less comfortable for the patient, but too little pressure will not be sufficient to augment alveolar ventilation. Ideally, bedside monitoring of (exhaled) tidal volume can help this titration, but this possibility will depend on the type of ventilator used. Pressure support breaths are cycled on flow decay, which is usually working reasonably well. For some COPD patients, because of excessive end-inspiratory leaks or because of very poor mechanics, this can generate excessively long insufflation times (longer than 1 second). This may be a reason to limit inspiratory time by using a time cycled mode (an inspiratory time of 1 second is usually sufficient, shorter if the patient is very tachypnoeic) or setting an inspiratory time limit. Another possibility is to set the expiratory threshold (flow threshold) to a value at 50 per cent of peak inspiratory flow or higher. Lastly, expiratory leaks may also generate auto-cycling, which may be uncomfortable for the patient. When this occurs the leak should be minimized or trigger sensitivity can be reduced.

## PERSPECTIVES ON REDUCING FAILURES AND IMPROVING OUTCOMES

### Use of helium

The use of a helium–oxygen mixture is a theoretically attractive approach to improving outcomes from NIV. Helium–oxygen ($HeO_2$) is a gas mixture with a lower density than standard air–oxygen (Air-$O_2$ mixture), and its use is associated with decreased resistance to gas flow.[76] $HeO_2$ reduces inspiratory muscle load when airway resistance is high, thus reducing dyspnoea and improving gas exchange in patients with severe COPD[77] or with severe asthma.[78] The use of $HeO_2$ enhances the unloading effects of NIV. In patients with acute exacerbations of COPD, using $HeO_2$ during NIV reduces dyspnoea, improves carbon dioxide elimination, and decreases the WOB more than conventional NIV with Air-$O_2$.[27,79] Positive results from physiological studies have generated the hypothesis that NIV with $HeO_2$ might improve clinical outcome in patients with acute exacerbation of COPD. This hypothesis has been assessed in two randomized controlled trials that compared the effects of NIV with $HeO_2$ or Air-$O_2$ on intubation rate and other clinical outcomes.[80,81] The two trials failed to show a significant beneficial effect of $HeO_2$ possibly because of a low intubation rate in the control group and, consequently, an insufficient statistical power. Intubation rate tended to be lower, albeit non-significantly, while length of stay in the hospital after the ICU in one study or adverse events in the other were significantly better in the $HeO_2$ group than in the Air-$O_2$ group. The results suggested that $HeO_2$ may have beneficial effects but not as much as hypothesized. These randomized controlled trials suggest that the success of NIV could be improved by using this gas mixture, but more work is needed to prove this; in particular, the cost-effectiveness of this approach needs to be confirmed.

### Late failures

In patients with acute exacerbation of COPD it seems there is no identified risk of trying NIV even at a late stage.[60] In a recent study, a strong association was found between sleep disturbances and late NIV failure.[82] Specifically, late NIV failure (defined as death or endotracheal intubation >48 hours after admission or need for at least 4 hours of NIV per day on day 6 of NIV) in elderly patients with acute hypercapnic respiratory failure was associated with early sleep disturbances including an abnormal electroencephalographic pattern, decreased rapid eye movement (REM) sleep and disruption of the circadian sleep cycle. Paying more attention to sleep quality of COPD patients treated by NIV may therefore be important for their outcome. The data do not show, however, whether sleep disturbances pre-existed and represent a marker of severity or whether the patient's management in the ICU was responsible for part of these abnormalities.

## CONCLUSIONS

NIV has become the gold standard for mild or severe forms of acute exacerbation of COPD, as a means of improving alveolar ventilation, reducing the patient's WOB and avoiding the need for endotracheal intubation and its related complications. Severe forms of exacerbations associated with hypercapnic coma can also be treated with this technique under careful monitoring.[10,83,84] A possible risk of adverse outcome associated with delayed endotracheal intubation in patients who fail a trial of NIV has not been identified in COPD, by contrast to patients with *de novo* acute respiratory failure.[85] In patients who fail NIV, there may be a risk of a longer time on mechanical ventilation[85] but no adverse effect on outcome.[84] Future avenues should consider improvements in patient–ventilator interfaces, reduction in asynchronies through more efficient algorithms for dealing with leaks, use of $HeO_2$ mixtures, and better understanding of late failures. Last, an unresolved but important question concerns the possibility of continuing NIV outside the hospital for patients who benefit from acute treatment with NIV.

## REFERENCES


1. Demoule A, Girou E, Richard JC *et al.* Increased use of noninvasive ventilation in French intensive care units. *Intensive Care Med* 2006; **32**: 1747–55.
2. Esteban A, Ferguson ND, Meade MO *et al.* Evolution of mechanical ventilation in response to clinical research. *Am J Respir Crit Care Med* 2008; **177**: 170–7.
3. Brochard L, Isabey D, Piquet J *et al.* Reversal of acute exacerbations of chronic obstructive lung disease by inspiratory assistance with a face mask. *N Engl J Med* 1990; **323**: 1523–30.
4. Meduri GU, Conoscenti CC, Menashe P *et al.* Noninvasive face mask ventilation in patients with acute respiratory failure. *Chest* 1989; **95**: 865–70.
5. Brochard L, Mancebo J, Wysocki M *et al.* Noninvasive ventilation for acute exacerbations of chronic obstructive pulmonary disease. *N Engl J Med* 1995; **333**: 817–22.
6. Plant PK, Owen JL, Elliott MW. Early use of non-invasive ventilation for acute exacerbations of chronic obstructive pulmonary disease on general respiratory wards: a multicentre randomised controlled trial. *Lancet* 2000; **355**: 1931–5.
7. Keenan SP, Sinuff T, Cook DJ *et al.* Which patients with acute exacerbation of chronic obstructive pulmonary disease benefit from noninvasive positive-pressure ventilation? A systematic review of the literature. *Ann Intern Med* 2003; **138**: 861–70.
8. Lightowler JV, Wedzicha JA, Elliott MW *et al.* Non-invasive positive pressure ventilation to treat respiratory failure resulting from exacerbations of chronic obstructive pulmonary disease: Cochrane systematic review and meta-analysis. *BMJ* 2003; **326**: 185.
9. Girou E, Schortgen F, Delclaux C *et al.* Association of noninvasive ventilation with nosocomial infections and survival in critically ill patients. *JAMA* 2000; **284**: 2361–7.
10. Conti G, Antonelli M, Navalesi P *et al.* Noninvasive vs. conventional mechanical ventilation in patients with chronic obstructive pulmonary disease after failure of medical treatment in the ward: a randomized trial. *Intensive Care Med* 2002; **28**: 1701–7.
11. Carlucci A, Delmastro M, Rubini F *et al.* Changes in the practice of non-invasive ventilation in treating COPD patients over 8 years. *Intensive Care Med* 2003; **29**: 419–25.
12. Azoulay E, Alberti C, Bornstain C *et al.* Improved survival in cancer patients requiring mechanical ventilatory support: impact of noninvasive mechanical ventilatory support. *Crit Care Med* 2001; **29**: 519–25.
13. Radford EP Jr, Ferris BG Jr, Kriete BC. Clinical use of a nomogram to estimate proper ventilation during artificial respiration. *N Engl J Med* 1954; **251**: 877–84.
14. Laghi F, Jubran A, Topeli A *et al.* Effect of lung volume reduction surgery on diaphragmatic neuromechanical coupling at 2 years. *Chest* 2004; **125**: 2188–95.
15. Evans TW. International Consensus Conferences in intensive care medicine: non-invasive positive pressure ventilation in acute respiratory failure. Organised jointly by the American Thoracic Society, the European Respiratory Society, the European Society of Intensive Care Medicine, and the Societe de Reanimation de Langue Francaise, and approved by the ATS Board of Directors, December 2000. *Intensive Care Med* 2001; **27**: 166–78.
16. Keenan SP, Sinuff T, Cook DJ *et al.* Does noninvasive positive pressure ventilation improve outcome in acute hypoxemic respiratory failure? A systematic review. *Crit Care Med* 2004; **32**: 2516–23.
17. Carrey Z, Gottfried SB, Levy RD. Ventilatory muscle support in respiratory failure with nasal positive pressure ventilation. *Chest* 1990; **97**: 150–8.
18. Ambrosino N, Nava S, Bertone P *et al.* Physiologic evaluation of pressure support ventilation by nasal mask in patients with stable COPD. *Chest* 1992; **101**: 385–91.
19. Nava S, Ambrosino N, Rubini F *et al.* Effect of nasal pressure support ventilation and external PEEP on diaphragmatic activity in patients with severe stable COPD. *Chest* 1993; **103**: 143–50.
20. Appendini L, Patessio A, Zanaboni S *et al.* Physiologic effects of positive end-expiratory pressure and mask pressure support during exacerbations of chronic obstructive pulmonary disease. *Am J Respir Crit Care Med* 1994; **149**: 1069–76.
21. Girault C, Richard JC, Chevron V *et al.* Comparative physiologic effects of noninvasive assist-control and pressure support ventilation in acute hypercapnic respiratory failure. *Chest* 1997; **111**: 1639–48.
22. Vitacca M, Clini E, Pagani M *et al.* Physiologic effects of early administered mask proportional assist ventilation in patients with chronic obstructive pulmonary disease and acute respiratory failure. *Crit Care Med* 2000; **28**: 1791–7.
23. Vanpee D, El Khawand C, Rousseau L *et al.* Effects of nasal pressure support on ventilation and inspiratory work in normocapnic and hypercapnic patients with stable COPD. *Chest* 2002; **122**: 75–83.
24. Lellouche F, Maggiore SM, Deye N *et al.* Effect of the humidification device on the work of breathing during noninvasive ventilation. *Intensive Care Med* 2002; **28**: 1582–9.
25. Prinianakis G, Delmastro M, Carlucci A *et al.* Effect of varying the pressurisation rate during noninvasive pressure support ventilation. *Eur Respir J* 2004; **23**: 314–20.

26. Tarabini Fraticelli A, Lellouche F, L'Her E *et al.* Physiological effects of different interfaces during noninvasive ventilation for acute respiratory failure. *Crit Care Med* 2009; **37**: 939–45.
27. Jaber S, Fodil R, Carlucci A *et al.* Noninvasive ventilation with helium-oxygen in acute exacerbations of chronic obstructive pulmonary disease. *Am J Respir Crit Care Med* 2000; **161**: 1191–200.
28. O'Donoghue FJ, Catcheside PG, Jordan AS *et al.* Effect of CPAP on intrinsic PEEP, inspiratory effort, and lung volume in severe stable COPD. *Thorax* 2002; **57**: 533–9.
29. Lessard MR, Lofaso F, Brochard L. Expiratory muscle activity increases intrinsic positive end-expiratory pressure independently of dynamic hyperinflation in mechanically ventilated patients. *Am J Respir Crit Care Med* 1995; **151**: 562–9.
30. Chiumello D, Pelosi P, Taccone P *et al.* Effect of different inspiratory rise time and cycling off criteria during pressure support ventilation in patients recovering from acute lung injury. *Crit Care Med* 2003; **31**: 2604–10.
31. Wysocki M, Meshaka P, Richard JC *et al.* Proportional-assist ventilation compared with pressure-support ventilation during exercise in volunteers with external thoracic restriction. *Crit Care Med* 2004; **32**: 409–14.
32. Racca F, Appendini L, Gregoretti C *et al.* Effectiveness of mask and helmet interfaces to deliver noninvasive ventilation in a human model of resistive breathing. *J Appl Physiol* 2005; **99**: 1262–71.
33. Kramer N, Meyer TJ, Meharg J *et al.* Randomized, prospective trial of noninvasive positive pressure ventilation in acute respiratory failure. *Am J Respir Crit Care Med* 1995; **151**: 1799–806.
34. Mehta S, Jay GD, Woolard RH *et al.* Randomized, prospective trial of bilevel versus continuous positive airway pressure in acute pulmonary edema. *Crit Care Med* 1997; **25**: 620–8.
35. Ambrosino N, Vitacca M, Polese G *et al.* Short-term effects of nasal proportional assist ventilation in patients with chronic hypercapnic respiratory insufficiency. *Eur Respir J* 1997; **10**: 2829–34.
36. Thys F, Roeseler J, Reynaert M *et al.* Noninvasive ventilation for acute respiratory failure: a prospective randomised placebo-controlled trial. *Eur Respir J* 2002; **20**: 545–55.
37. Katz JA, Marks JD. Inspiratory work with and without continuous positive airway pressure in patients with acute respiratory failure. *Anesthesiology* 1985; **63**: 598–607.
38. L'Her E, Deye N, Lellouche F *et al.* Physiologic effects of noninvasive ventilation during acute lung injury. *Am J Respir Crit Care Med* 2005; **172**: 1112–18.
39. Vitacca M, Bianchi L, Zanotti E *et al.* Assessment of physiologic variables and subjective comfort under different levels of pressure support ventilation. *Chest* 2004; **126**: 851–9.
40. Navalesi P, Fanfulla F, Frigerio P *et al.* Physiologic evaluation of noninvasive mechanical ventilation delivered with three types of masks in patients with chronic hypercapnic respiratory failure. *Crit Care Med* 2000; **28**: 1785–90.
41. Ambrosino N, Foglio K, Rubini F *et al.* Non-invasive mechanical ventilation in acute respiratory failure due to chronic obstructive pulmonary disease: correlates for success. *Thorax* 1995; **50**: 755–7.
42. Anton A, Guell R, Gomez J *et al.* Predicting the result of noninvasive ventilation in severe acute exacerbations of patients with chronic airflow limitation. *Chest* 2000; **117**: 828–33.
43. Poponick JM, Renston JP, Bennett RP *et al.* Use of a ventilatory support system (BiPAP) for acute respiratory failure in the emergency department. *Chest* 1999; **116**: 166–71.
44. Putinati S, Ballerin L, Piattella M *et al.* Is it possible to predict the success of non-invasive positive pressure ventilation in acute respiratory failure due to COPD? *Respir Med* 2000; **94**: 997–1001.
45. Soo Hoo GW, Santiago S, Williams AJ. Nasal mechanical ventilation for hypercapnic respiratory failure in chronic obstructive pulmonary disease: determinants of success and failure. *Crit Care Med* 1994; **22**: 1253–61.
46. Sadoul P, Aug M, Gay R. Traitement par ventilation instrumentale de 100 cas d'insuffisants respiratoires chroniques. *Bull Eur Physiopathol Respir Care* 1965; **1**: 549.
47. Bott J, Carroll MP, Conway JH *et al.* Randomised controlled trial of nasal ventilation in acute ventilatory failure due to chronic obstructive airways disease. *Lancet* 1993; **341**: 1555–7.
48. Celikel T, Sungur M, Ceyhan B *et al.* Comparison of noninvasive positive pressure ventilation with standard medical therapy in hypercapnic acute respiratory failure. *Chest* 1998; **114**: 1636–42.
49. Dikensoy O, Ikidag B, Filiz A *et al.* Comparison of non-invasive ventilation and standard medical therapy in acute hypercapnic respiratory failure: a randomised controlled study at a tertiary health centre in SE Turkey. *Int J Clin Pract* 2002; **56**: 85–8.
50. Avdeev SN, Tret'iakov AV, Grigor'iants RA *et al.* Study of the use of noninvasive ventilation of the lungs in acute respiratory insufficiency due exacerbation of chronic obstructive pulmonary disease. *Anesteziol Reanimatol* 1998; **3**: 45–51.
51. Barbe F, Togores B, Rubi M *et al.* Noninvasive ventilatory support does not facilitate recovery from acute respiratory failure in chronic obstructive pulmonary disease. *Eur Respir J* 1996; **9**: 1240–5.
52. Confalonieri M, Potena A, Carbone G *et al.* Acute respiratory failure in patients with severe community-acquired pneumonia. A prospective randomized evaluation of noninvasive ventilation. *Am J Respir Crit Care Med* 1999; **160**: 1585–91.
53. Ram FS, Picot J, Lightowler J *et al.* Non-invasive positive pressure ventilation for treatment of respiratory failure due to exacerbations of chronic obstructive pulmonary disease. *Cochrane Database Syst Rev* 2004; CD004104.

54. Keenan SP, Powers CE, McCormack DG. Noninvasive positive-pressure ventilation in patients with milder chronic obstructive pulmonary disease exacerbations: a randomized controlled trial. *Respir Care* 2005; **50**: 610–16.
55. Girou E, Brun-Buisson C, Taille S *et al.* Secular trends in nosocomial infections and mortality associated with noninvasive ventilation in patients with exacerbation of COPD and pulmonary edema. *JAMA* 2003; **290**: 2985–91.
56. Burns KE, Sinuff T, Adhikari NK *et al.* Bilevel noninvasive positive pressure ventilation for acute respiratory failure: survey of Ontario practice. *Crit Care Med* 2005; **33**: 1477–83.
57. Maheshwari V, Paioli D, Rothaar R *et al.* Utilization of noninvasive ventilation in acute care hospitals: a regional survey. *Chest* 2006; **129**: 1226–33.
58. Carlucci A, Richard JC, Wysocki M *et al.* Noninvasive versus conventional mechanical ventilation. An epidemiologic survey. *Am J Respir Crit Care Med* 2001; **163**: 874–80.
59. Schettino G, Altobelli N, Kacmarek RM. Noninvasive positive-pressure ventilation in acute respiratory failure outside clinical trials: experience at the Massachusetts General Hospital. *Crit Care Med* 2008; **36**: 441–7.
60. Moretti M, Cilione C, Tampieri A *et al.* Incidence and causes of non-invasive mechanical ventilation failure after initial success. *Thorax* 2000; **55**: 819–25.
61. Honrubia T, Garcia Lopez FJ, Franco N *et al.* Noninvasive vs conventional mechanical ventilation in acute respiratory failure: a multicenter, randomized controlled trial. *Chest* 2005; **128**: 3916–24.
62. Scala R, Nava S, Conti G *et al.* Noninvasive versus conventional ventilation to treat hypercapnic encephalopathy in chronic obstructive pulmonary disease. *Intensive Care Med* 2007; **33**: 2101–8.
63. Chu CM, Chan VL, Lin AW *et al.* Readmission rates and life threatening events in COPD survivors treated with non-invasive ventilation for acute hypercapnic respiratory failure. *Thorax* 2004; **59**: 1020–5.
64. Chu CM, Cheung AP, Chan VL *et al.* A randomized trial of home non-invasive ventilation vs. sham ventilation in survivors of acute respiratory failure in COPD. *Am J Respir Crit Care Med* 2008; **177**: A767.
65. Nava S, Sturani C, Hartl S *et al.* End-of-life decision-making in respiratory intermediate care units: a European survey. *Eur Respir J* 2007; **30**: 156–64.
66. Schettino G, Altobelli N, Kacmarek RM. Noninvasive positive pressure ventilation reverses acute respiratory failure in select 'do-not-intubate' patients. *Crit Care Med* 2005; **33**: 1976–82.
67. Levy M, Tanios MA, Nelson D *et al.* Outcomes of patients with do-not-intubate orders treated with noninvasive ventilation. *Crit Care Med* 2004; **32**: 2002–7.
68. Chu CM, Chan VL, Wong IW *et al.* Noninvasive ventilation in patients with acute hypercapnic exacerbation of chronic obstructive pulmonary disease who refused endotracheal intubation. *Crit Care Med* 2004; **32**: 372–7.
69. Shee CD, Green M. Non-invasive ventilation and palliation: experience in a district general hospital and a review. *Palliat Med* 2003; **17**: 21–6.
70. Curtis JR, Cook DJ, Sinuff T *et al.* Noninvasive positive pressure ventilation in critical and palliative care settings: understanding the goals of therapy. *Crit Care Med* 2007; **35**: 932–9.
71. Elliott MW, Confalonieri M, Nava S. Where to perform noninvasive ventilation? *Eur Respir J* 2002; **19**: 1159–66.
72. Needham DM, Bronskill SE, Calinawan JR *et al.* Projected incidence of mechanical ventilation in Ontario to 2026: Preparing for the aging baby boomers. *Crit Care Med* 2005; **33**: 574–9.
73. Wood KA, Lewis L, Von Harz B *et al.* The use of noninvasive positive pressure ventilation in the emergency department: results of a randomized clinical trial. *Chest* 1998; **113**: 1339–46.
74. Paus-Jenssen ES, Reid JK, Cockcroft DW *et al.* The use of noninvasive ventilation in acute respiratory failure at a tertiary care center. *Chest* 2004; **126**: 165–72.
75. Cabrini L, Idone C, Colombo S *et al.* Medical emergency team and non-invasive ventilation outside ICU for acute respiratory failure. *Intensive Care Med* 2009; **35**: 339–43.
76. Pedley TJ, Drazen JM. Aerodynamic theory. In: Macklem PT, Mead J, eds. *Handbook of physiology: the respiratory system III*, vol 3. Bethesda, MD: American Physiological Society; 1986: 41–54.
77. Swidwa DM, Montenegro HD, Goldman MD *et al.* Helium-oxygen breathing in severe chronic obstructive pulmonary disease. *Chest* 1985; **87**: 790–5.
78. Manthous CA, Hall JB, Caputo MA *et al.* Heliox improves pulsus paradoxus and peak expiratory flow in nonintubated patients with severe asthma. *Am J Respir Crit Care Med* 1995; **151**: 310–14.
79. Jolliet P, Tassaux D, Thouret JM *et al.* Beneficial effects of helium:oxygen versus air: oxygen noninvasive pressure support in patients with decompensated chronic obstructive pulmonary disease. *Crit Care Med* 1999; **27**: 2422–9.
80. Jolliet P, Tassaux D, Roeseler J *et al.* Helium-oxygen versus air-oxygen noninvasive pressure support in decompensated chronic obstructive disease: a prospective, multicenter study. *Crit Care Med* 2003; **31**: 878–84.
81. Maggiore SM, Richard JC, Abroug F *et al.* A multicenter, randomized trial of noninvasive ventilation with helium-oxygen mixture in exacerbations of chronic obstructive lung disease. *Crit Care Med* 2010 ; **38**: 145–51.
82. Campo FR, Drouot X, Thille AW *et al.* Poor sleep quality is associated with late noninvasive ventilation failure in patients with acute hypercapnic respiratory failure. *Crit Care Med* 2010; **38**: 477–85.

83. Diaz GG, Alcaraz AC, Talavera JC *et al.* Noninvasive positive-pressure ventilation to treat hypercapnic coma secondary to respiratory failure. *Chest* 2005; **127**: 952–60.
84. Squadrone E, Frigerio P, Fogliati C *et al.* Noninvasive vs invasive ventilation in COPD patients with severe acute respiratory failure deemed to require ventilatory assistance. *Intensive Care Med* 2004; **30**: 1303–10.
85. Demoule A, Girou E, Richard JC *et al.* Benefits and risks of success or failure of noninvasive ventilation. *Intensive Care Med* 2006; **32**: 1756–65.

23

# Non-invasive ventilation in chronic obstructive pulmonary disease

ENRICO M CLINI, ERNESTO CRISAFULLI, NICOLINO AMBROSINO

## ABSTRACT

Advanced chronic obstructive pulmonary disease (COPD) is associated with peripheral and respiratory muscular weakness with nocturnal and daytime arterial blood gas abnormalities (including hypercapnia) leading to chronic respiratory failure (CRF). At present, long-term oxygen therapy (LTOT) is the only recognized long-term treatment that has been shown to significantly improve survival in these patients. An alternative therapeutic approach proposed, especially in patients with worsening hypercapnia, is nocturnal non-invasive ventilation (NIV). The three main theories that explain the efficacy of NIV, as applied by positive pressure (NIPPV), in these patients are: opportunity for resting of fatigued respiratory muscles, improvement in thoracic-pulmonary mechanics, and the 'resetting' of the central respiratory drive. In contrast with the strong evidence favouring the use of NIV in acute exacerbation of COPD, many studies performed in severe but stable patients have shown inconsistent and conflicting results. In the short term, NIV has been shown to reduce the rate of hospitalization, as well as to improve both the patient's quality of life and their functional status. However, long-term assessments did not find any effect on survival and the strongest outcomes were not affected by the use of NIPPV even when added to LTOT. Recommendations of an international consensus conference published in 1999 provided the basis for NIV prescription in stable advanced COPD patients – nocturnal hypoventilation, sleep fragmentation and daytime arterial hypercapnia – which are still considered the optimal indications for domiciliary NIV, in particular in the presence of severe-progressive deterioration of the clinical condition and instability of respiratory function.

## INTRODUCTION

Chronic obstructive pulmonary disease (COPD) is a slowly progressive respiratory disorder characterized by inflammatory and irreversible airway obstruction, associated with muscle deterioration and dysfunction in the advanced stage. Also when stable, COPD patients often have nocturnal and daytime arterial blood gas abnormalities (hypoxaemia and/or hypercapnia) leading to chronic respiratory failure (CRF); this is mainly linked to impaired alveolar ventilation, sleep disorders and increased work of breathing, which in turn cause symptoms. At present, no medication has been shown to change the natural history of COPD. Long-term oxygen therapy (LTOT), when used ≥15 hours/day, is the only therapy that has been shown to significantly improve survival of patients with severe COPD.[1,2]

Non-invasive ventilation (NIV), while specifically providing ventilatory support by means of a mask interface, has been proposed for use in CRF patients with progressive worsening of general and respiratory status. In contrast to the strong evidence for the use of NIV (especially if performed by means of intermittent positive pressure ventilation [IPPV]) to treat acute exacerbations of COPD,[3] several short- and long-term studies provided inconsistent and controversial results in severe but stable patients.[4] Notwithstanding, domiciliary NIV represents the most common indication in COPD across Europe.[5]

In this chapter we describe the pathophysiological basis and available clinical evidence to support the use of long-term NIV in the stable COPD population.

## PATHOPHYSIOLOGY AND EFFECT OF NON-INVASIVE VENTILATION

Chronic obstructive pulmonary disease is a complex disease caused by physiological abnormalities mainly affecting airways and lung parenchyma with alteration of gas exchange. The bronchial alterations are typically related to chronic inflammation that progressively leads to increased airway resistance, decreased expiratory flow and pulmonary hyperinflation.[6] These features contribute to a remarkable compromise of thoracic mechanics including respiratory muscle dysfunction.[7] The latter probably contributes to muscle fatigue (the diaphragm in particular), which in turn may lead to reduced alveolar ventilation and chronic respiratory acidosis.[8] Hypercapnia is, therefore, the hallmark of chronic thoracic pump failure. The flattened diaphragm (with shortened muscle length and diminished maximal force) and the recruitment of additional inspiratory muscles (parasternal and accessory muscles, in particular) is thought to lead to an imbalance between energy supply and demand, thus resulting in a vicious circle of maintaining and then worsening CRF. The load on the respiratory muscles is also increased by the presence of intrinsic positive end-expiratory pressure (PEEPi).[9]

A study by Díaz and colleagues[10] suggests that in severe but stable COPD patients with hypercapnia and dynamic lung hyperinflation the main benefit from NIV is improved gas exchange (reduction in arterial carbon dioxide tension, $CO_2$). These effects during NIV could be explained by a reduction in PEEPi and a reduction of inspiratory load following adoption of a slow/deep pattern of breathing. The intermittent respite for chronically fatigued muscles in COPD patients is, therefore, a logical basis for application of external ventilation (NIV), which may compensate the individual's chronic hypoventilation even if applied at night-time,[11,12] which, at least theoretically, will allow the respiratory muscles to rest and thus improve gas exchange when the individual is awake.

The improvement of chest wall and lung compliance,[13] together with the improvement of respiratory muscle function, could also allow sparing the 'work of breathing'. The underlying mechanism may include both the improved efficiency of the respiratory muscles and the reduction of chronic muscle fatigue with lower oxygen uptake (Fig. 23.1).[15–17] Evidence of respiratory muscle rest and efficiency during non-invasive intermittent positive pressure support ventilation (NIPPV)[18] is provided by the significant reductions that have been seen in diaphragmatic electromyogram activity and the work of breathing.[16,19] Nonetheless, it is still difficult to prove whether changes in respiratory muscle function are the cause rather than consequence of arterial blood gas change under NIPPV.[18,20]

The theory of chronic muscle fatigue is not the only one proposed so far to explain the effectiveness of NIV in COPD.[21] During the night, COPD patients have shorter total sleep time with poorer quality sleep (sleep disruption with a shorter rapid eye movement [REM] period) than normal individuals;[22] thus, NIPPV use is indicated at night to compensate for this high number of episodes of sleep-disordered breathing with associated arterial oxygen desaturation.[23] Although nocturnal hypoxaemia can be easily normalized by means of supplemental oxygen, this may lead to an increase in carbon dioxide levels, especially early in the morning.[24] During REM sleep, respiratory

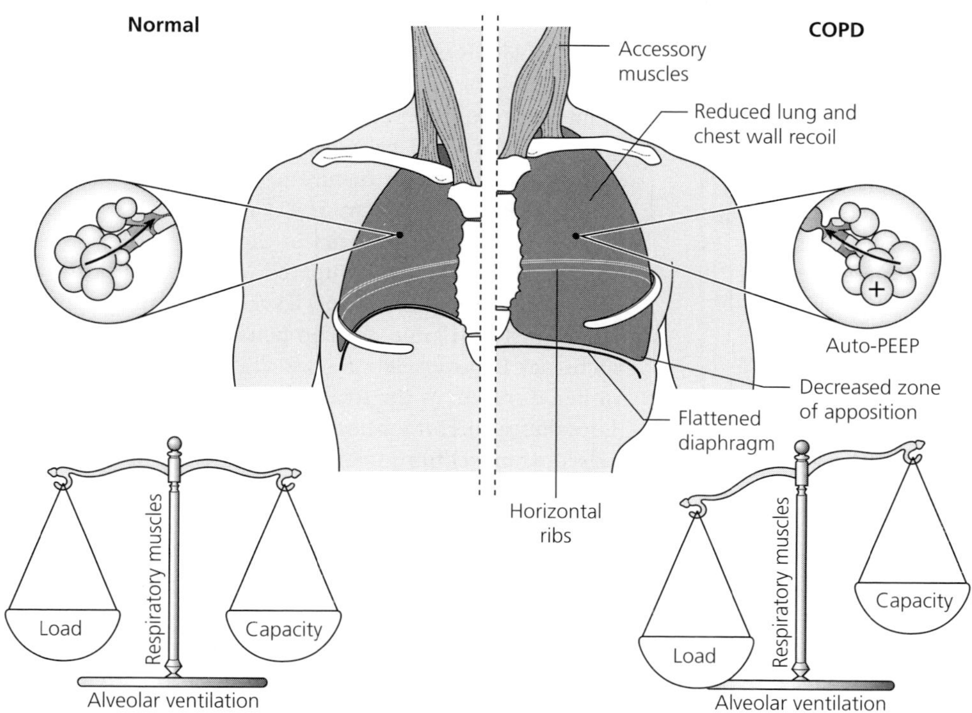


**Figure 23.1** Pathophysiological representation of lung hyperinflation and respiratory muscles dysfunction in chronic obstructive pulmonary disease (COPD) patients (right) as compared with normal individuals (left). Adapted from Sivasothy *et al.*[14] PEEP, positive end-expiratory pressure.

muscle tone and the activity of non-diaphragmatic inspiratory muscles normally diminish in healthy subjects:[25] in patients with CRF due to ventilatory impairment, this reflex activity is further enhanced, thus leading to progressive nocturnal hypoventilation.[26]

Hypoventilation during sleep and the consequent night-to-morning change in carbon dioxide,[27] which may also partly be due to reduced carbon dioxide responsiveness,[28] may be additional factors in the development of chronic 'pulmonary damage' as manifested by pulmonary hypertension.[26,29] Moreover, chronic hypercapnia may further impair diaphragmatic function[30] and also have a deleterious effect on central respiratory drive. Nocturnal NIV prevents sleep-related hypoventilation and improves both quantity and quality (less arousals) of sleep.[31]

Another, and perhaps still unexplored, mechanism behind the success of NIV in these patients is linked to the resetting (lower sensitivity) of the respiratory centre to carbon dioxide levels. In patients with CRF this centre is thought to adjust its output so that the work of the respiratory muscles will not exceed the level that would precipitate muscle fatigue.[7,32,33] In addition, the improvement in oxygenation observed with nocturnal NIV could also have a positive effect when awake. In a study of nocturnal nasal NIPPV applied to COPD patients, Elliott *et al.*[34] found the improvement of blood gases levels to be associated with an increased central chemosensitivity to carbon dioxide. This effect can be related to the correction of the carbon dioxide alveolar–arterial gradient following the improvement in the spontaneous breathing pattern during NIV.

In conclusion, several, not mutually exclusive, pathophysiological theories have been proposed to explain the effect of NIV in stable COPD patients. Overall, the main actions for the efficacy of NIV are 'resetting' of central respiratory drive, improvement of thoracic–pulmonary mechanics with reduced loading of the respiratory muscles, and rest for chronically fatigued respiratory muscles. Finally evidence of stability of pulmonary function after withdrawal of NIV[35] indicates that respiratory muscle fatigue is probably not the most important factor when evaluating patients in a stable state and it seems a less important mechanism than the central resetting of the carbon dioxide drive.

## CLINICAL EVIDENCE

Many trials in patients with severe COPD have reported notable results (reduction of orotracheal intubation and mortality rate) showing efficacy with NIPPV when used in the acute decompensation of the disease.[3] By contrast, (few) controlled trials, and two systematic meta-analyses, of NIV in chronic stable COPD have not reported any consistent benefit of NIPPV in stable COPD with CRF.[4,36,37] So far, studies with similar design have provided conflicting results.

In a 3-month crossover study, Meecham-Jones *et al.*[38] compared the effect of NIPPV added to usual oxygen versus oxygen therapy alone in 18 severe stable patients. In the NIV group, as compared with the conventional oxygen group, the authors demonstrated significant change in diurnal and nocturnal arterial blood gases, improvement of sleep architecture (total time and efficiency), and quality of life. In addition, a good compliance rate with NIV was reported in up to 70 per cent of patients completing the trial. In a similar study in 23 severe COPD patients, Strumpf *et al.*[39] did not find support for any advantage of using NIV as compared with control therapy. Moreover, these authors reported a significantly high dropout rate with NIV (only 30 per cent of patients completed the trial). A similar period of domiciliary treatment with intermittent negative pressure ventilation (INPV) by means of a poncho-wrap was not able to improve inspiratory muscle strength in less severe COPD patients in the study by Shapiro *et al.*[40] Some explanations for these different results may be gained by comparing the baseline characteristics of COPD patients in the two studies. Despite similar degree of severity in airway obstruction, the mean baseline level of carbon dioxide retention in the Strumpf trial was moderate (47 mm Hg) and consistently lower than that (57 mm Hg) recorded by Meecham-Jones *et al.* Notably, patients in these two trials also had differences in impairment of sleep-related disturbances (hypopnoea and oxygen desaturation events). This would suggest that certain subgroups of COPD with more appropriate pathophysiological features might benefit differently from nocturnal domiciliary NIPPV: unfortunately this hypothesis has failed to be proved by two other controlled trials[41,42] in subjects with remarkable hypercapnia.

In a 8-week crossover trial, Lin[41] compared benefits of both long-term oxygen therapy (LTOT) and nasal NIV, alone or as combined treatment. There was no benefit of using NIPPV over and above LTOT with regard to arterial blood gases or pulmonary function, with worse sleep quality when using NIV. Gay and colleagues[42] also found similar results in 13 patients followed for 3 months and receiving active (with inspiratory positive airway pressure [IPAP] set at 10 cm $H_2O$) or sham NIPPV. Less than 50 per cent of patients in the active NIPPV group completed the study as compared with the nearly 100 per cent in the sham group. A low level of ventilatory support, which was not able to compensate for the alveolar nocturnal hypoventilation (see also Fig. 23.1), and the limited duration of the treatment period are advocated as the main reasons for the negative results of these studies.[41,42] Indeed, a longer duration of NIV treatment in observational trials has been associated with better survival when compared with usual LTOT.[1,2]

Casanova *et al.*[43] also studied 20 severe COPD patients under LTOT in a 1-year randomized controlled study (RCT) receiving nocturnal NIPPV plus standard care or standard care alone. Survival as well as the number of acute exacerbations did not differ between groups. The number of admissions to hospital fell significantly at

3 months in the NIPPV group (5 versus 15 per cent) but remained unchanged thereafter. The only benefits observed at 6 months in the NIPPV group were reduction of symptoms (dyspnoea, as measured by the Borg scale) and improvement in neuropsychological tests (psychomotor coordination). Again, it was concluded that there was a marginal benefit of NIPPV in the severe COPD population over a 1-year follow-up.

Other studies designed to show gain in survival with NIV[44,45] have only reported a global reduction of hospital admissions due to acute respiratory failure and unplanned visits at the general practitioner's level. One trial (published as an abstract) indicated that there was no overall survival benefit from NPPV plus LTOT, despite a slight improvement in survival for patients over 65 years.[46]

A multicentre RCT conducted in Italy with 2-year follow-up and including a larger sample ($n = 122$) of patients with severe CRF due to COPD, compared the use of nocturnal NIV (in pressure support modality) plus oxygen versus oxygen alone.[47] This trial aimed at assessing the long-term effect of NIV treatment on severity of hypercapnia, use of healthcare resources and health-related quality of life (HRQoL), measured both by the specific Maugeri Foundation Respiratory Failure Questionnaire (MRF-28) and the St George's Respiratory Questionnaire (SGRQ). There was no advantage with NIV with regard to the mortality rate (18 per cent and 17 per cent in NIV and control groups, respectively). However, a marked trend towards a reduction in hospital admissions (when comparing the follow-up with the follow-back periods) was recorded in favour of NIV, whereas the MRF-28 scores (but not SGRQ) significantly improved in the NIV group only. Positive effects on HRQoL scores (both SGRQ and Nottingham Health Profile) with domiciliary NIPPV were also reported by Perrin *et al.*[48] in 14 patients followed up to 6 months; physical mobility, emotional reactions and energy component scores were the areas showing the best improvement over time.

Finally, a recent Australian prospective trial in 144 stable COPD patients by McEvoy *et al.*[49] is the first to report an effect on survival (mean follow-up 2.21 years) with an adjusted mortality risk reduction of 27 per cent when compared to usual LTOT. Unfortunately, this effect appears to be at the cost of worsening HRQoL, suggesting that patients under NIV had poorer general and mental health status, and reported less vigour with more confusion.

Other, uncontrolled, studies have shown little difference in survival when compared with LTOT. A retrospective over 5-year follow-up analysis in 180 patients with CRF from the UK showed that COPD ($n = 33$) patients were less likely to continue domiciliary NIV in the long term when compared with restrictive disease patients (43 per cent vs 80 per cent, respectively).[50] Comparison of COPD survival rate in this study population was virtually identical to that reported using LTOT.[1,2] Similar results were seen in a study from France.[14] Taken together, these results do not suggest a major effect of NIPPV on survival, as compared with LTOT, and the quality of life data are conflicting.

Another aspect that has been investigated is the effect of NIV when a high inspiratory pressure level is adopted. A study by Windisch *et al.*,[51] albeit uncontrolled, provides some important insights into how NIV might be best used in patients with COPD. NIV was initiated in hospital and the level of inspiratory pressure support was gradually increased, aiming for normocapnia. Previous and preliminary observations of the same authors showed that high inflation pressures can be tolerated, resulting in improved $PaCO_2$ during spontaneous breathing[52] and in better quality of life.[53] Using this strategy, the authors showed that $PaCO_2$ fell during spontaneous breathing by a mean of 7 mm Hg, $PaO_2$ increased by a mean of 6 mm Hg and $FEV_1$ improved by a mean of 140 mL. The 2-year survival rate was 86 per cent. Taken together, these studies suggest that benefit is seen in daytime parameters (physiological and quality of life) when there is a substantial reduction in carbon dioxide during NIV.

Both Díaz *et al.*[10] and Windisch *et al.*[51] reported comparable increases in forced expiratory volume in 1 second ($FEV_1$) after NIV. This raises the possibility that NIV has an effect on the airways themselves; possible mechanisms include a reduction in airway oedema or even stretching open of chronically fibrosed airways. If this is correct, it will probably require a level of pressure to be delivered to the airways for a period of time. If this is an important mechanism, logic would suggest that the higher the pressure and the longer it is applied to the airways, the better. This is entirely speculative, but the improvements in $FEV_1$ were only seen in these trials[10,51] using higher level of inspiratory pressures. Notwithstanding, further evidence is needed before NIV can be considered as standard therapy.

## CLINICAL APPLICATION AND SELECTION OF CANDIDATES

Even if the role of long-term application of NIPPV is not yet clearly established, COPD patients with nocturnal hypoventilation, sleep fragmentation and daytime arterial hypercapnia appear to be the best candidates for home chronic ventilatory support. In the selection of the ideal candidate, repeated hospital admissions for acute hypercapnic respiratory failure (three or more in a year) seems to be a possible guiding factor indicating disease progression and instability.[44] Use of this factor in the selection is also possibly an advantage from the economic point of view in applying domiciliary NIV. Indeed, Tuggey *et al.*,[54] in a trial designed as economic analysis of a selected population of COPD patients with recurrent acidotic exacerbations requiring admission to hospital and acute NIV, have shown that since the adoption of domiciliary NIV the prospective costs from hospitalization and intensive care have greatly reduced. This finding has been further demonstrated in a *post hoc* analysis from the Italian multicentre study on domiciliary NIV,[55] which showed that, given similar charges for drug therapy and oxygen in the follow-up, the cost of acute care in hospital was lower in patients under domiciliary NIV when compared with the LTOT arm (€8.25 ± 10.29/patient/day vs €12.50 ± 20.28/patient/day; $p < 0.05$).

The only guidelines about the use of NIV in stable COPD were published in 1999, the result of a consensus conference rather than the much more rigorous evidence review and development process that would be expected today.[56] The authors recommended that chronic ventilatory support should not be systematically prescribed in all CRF-COPD patients and this remains true today. They did consider that NIPPV may produce some benefits in selected COPD patients with clinical symptoms, signs and functional characteristics as reported in Table 23.1. Although this consensus conference considered the presence of chronic hypercapnia (≥55 mmHg) as the mandatory parameter for indication of NIV (the common opinion is that patients with carbon dioxide ≤55 mm Hg or no carbon dioxide retention appear to gain little or no benefit from NIPPV), the presence of hypercapnia by itself, especially if stable and well tolerated by patients, is not an indication for long-term ventilatory support.

Symptoms linked to nocturnal hypoventilation (frequently underestimated and difficult to screen) are more likely to appear in respiratory patients, with no chance of correction with nocturnal oxygen therapy.[26] Therefore, a recommendation has been made that sleep monitoring should be performed during oxygen supplementation and that the failure to reverse nocturnal desaturation (at a level ≥90 per cent) is a key point in deciding to apply NIPPV during the night.[56] However, although with supplemental oxygen patients may be adequately oxygenated, they develop symptomatic hypercapnia. If adequate oxygenation cannot be maintained with a lower level of oxygen supplementation, NIPPV should be considered. Further data and properly formulated guidelines are required.

## TECHNICAL CONSIDERATIONS

The preset pressure mode of ventilation is the technique of choice for domiciliary NIV applied to COPD patients. Indeed, in hypercapnic COPD, the negative pressure mode of ventilation may cause, especially during the night, upper airway obstruction, which can precipitate rather than improve the nocturnal hypoventilation.

Although a preset pressure mode allows the patient to retain considerable control of breathing pattern and tidal volume, both volume and pressure-limited modes are considered as clinically equivalent and effective in CRF.[57] The usual advice, in COPD patients with increased levels of carbon dioxide, is to utilize pressure support ventilators as the first-line treatment, especially in the pressure-assist mode (such as pressure support ventilation [PSV]) that delivers a preset inspiratory positive airway pressure level (IPAP) to help every spontaneous breathing effort. With this modality, the patient's capacity to vary inspiratory time breath by breath is then warranted, and this allows a close matching with the patient's breathing pattern. Sometimes, these ventilators are commonly referred to as 'bi-level' devices because they cycle between two different positive pressure levels (IPAP and expiratory positive airway pressures [EPAP]).

When setting the ventilator, the level of support is progressively raised in the range 12–20 cm $H_2O$ depending on patient tolerance, with a minimum level of EPAP around 4 cm $H_2O$ in order to improve carbon dioxide removal and counterbalance the PEEPi (physiological value around 4–5 cm $H_2O$, in stable patients).[58,59] Oxygen supplementation, usually needed, is adjusted to correct nocturnal hypoxaemia and maintain oxygen saturation at ≥90 per cent.

During delivery of assist-control NIV, a patient-initiated and adjustable trigger signal is able to synchronize the inspiratory phase, while a threshold reduction of inspira-tory flow is, most commonly, the cause for the ventilator to cycle into expiration. It is possible, moreover, to select many other ventilator parameters such as 'rise time' (time required to reach peak pressure), inspiratory time, inspiratory to expiratory (I:E) ratio, and back-up respiratory rate in order to best suit the patient's breathing pattern and characteristics. All these features may enhance the so-called 'patient–ventilator synchrony' and the overall comfort under NIV.

Portable ventilators including all these setting options are usually prescribed for domiciliary purpose, thanks to their characteristics: easy to use, light (5–10 kg) with

**Table 23.1** Suggested clinical and functional indications for domiciliary non-invasive intermittent positive pressure support ventilation (NIPPV) in patients with severe chronic obstructive pulmonary disease

| Symptoms | Physiological criteria (one of the following) |
|---|---|
| Fatigue | $PaCO_2$ ≥55 mm Hg |
| Dyspnoea | $PaCO_2$ <50 and <54 mmHg and nocturnal desaturation ($O_2$ saturation by pulse oximeter ≤88 per cent for 5 continuous minutes while receiving oxygen therapy with ≥2 L/min) |
| Morning headache, etc. | $PaCO_2$ >50 and <54 mm Hg and hospitalization related to recurrent episodes of hypercapnic respiratory failure (≥2 in a 12-month period) |

Adapted from Windisch *et al.*[51]

compact design, and (relatively) low expense. Since severe COPD patients on NIPPV are generally partially dependent on their machine, the presence of a long-life battery operated ventilator is mandatory only when patients need to be assisted more than 12 hours/day. Sophisticated alarms (high and low pressure) together with monitoring displays are less likely to be required for monitoring the ventilation capacity for these patients when at home.

Given that NIV is usually applied during sleep, overnight monitoring is mandatory. Ventilators without a timed back-up are significantly cheaper and, in the absence of any data confirming that a timed back-up is needed, these should be the machine of choice for domiciliary NIV in COPD. Finally, higher inflation pressures appear to be necessary to influence physiological parameters.[51–53]

More recently, new versions of portable ventilators providing either PSV or volume preset ventilation have opened the marked to novel, powerful turbine pressure support ventilators that can deliver real volume ventilation by means of the so-called average volume assured pressure support ventilation (AVAPS) mode, which seems feasible and effective.[60] More data are needed as to whether this provides benefits that are important to patients.

## FUTURE RESEARCH AND CONCLUSIONS

Despite several trials consistently reporting the true effectiveness of NIV therapy in acute care of COPD patients, the use of domiciliary NIV is still far from being considered the treatment of choice in stable, although hypercapnic, individuals.

Most trials on severe stable COPD have found NIPPV (especially when used overnight) to be effective with regard to short-term outcomes such as exercise tolerance, dyspnoea, and work of breathing. In those severe COPD patients with maximal medical treatment regimens, the use of domiciliary NIPPV may have an adjunctive role in the long-term management of CRF through attenuation of gas exchange alteration, reduction in hospital admission, improvement in the self-perceived HRQoL and functional status. However, there is still no convincing evidence that domiciliary NIV may have an adjunctive role in prolonging survival of the COPD population when compared with usual LTOT. This particular aspect clearly suggests the need to design and conduct studies that can finally answer this open question. Moreover, future trials should include more clear therapeutic endpoints and should consider technical aspects (such as the choice of ventilator mode and settings) according to the severity of the COPD. Finally, it is likely that more specific questionnaires and tools that describe the individual's HRQoL and have been specifically validated in the NIV population would help highlight the outcomes sensitive to changes with this therapy.

## REFERENCES


1. Nocturnal Oxygen Therapy Trial Group. Continuous or nocturnal oxygen therapy in hypoxemic chronic obstructive lung disease: a clinical trial. *Ann Intern Med* 1980; **93**: 391–8.
2. Medical Research Council Working Party. Long-term domiciliary oxygen therapy in chronic hypoxia and cor pulmonale complicating chronic bronchitis and emphysema. *Lancet* 1981; **1**: 681–6.
3. Brochard L, Mancebo J, Wysocki M *et al.* Non invasive ventilation for acute exacerbations of chronic obstructive pulmonary disease. *N Engl J Med* 1995; **333**: 817–22.
4. Rossi A. Non invasive ventilation has not been shown to be ineffective in stable COPD. *Am J Respir Crit Care Med* 2000; **161**: 688–9.
5. Lloyd-Owen SJ, Donaldson GC, Ambrosino N *et al.* Patterns of home mechanical ventilation use in Europe: results from the Eurovent survey. *Eur Respir J* 2005; **25**: 1025–31.
6. Broseghini C, Brandolese R, Poggi R *et al.* Respiratory mechanics during the first day of mechanical ventilation in patients with pulmonary edema and chronic airway obstruction. *Am Rev Respir Dis* 1988; **138**: 355–61.
7. Roussos C. Function and fatigue of respiratory muscles. *Chest* 1985; **88**: 124S–32S.
8. Jeffrey AA, Warren PM, Flenley DC. Acute hypercapnic respiratory failure in patients with chronic obstructive lung disease: risk factors and use of guidelines for management. *Thorax* 1992; **47**: 34–40.
9. Smith TC, Marini JJ. Impact of PEEP on lung mechanics and work of breathing in severe airflow obstruction. *J Appl Physiol* 1988; **65**: 1488–99.
10. Díaz O, Bégin P, Torrealba B *et al.* Effects of non invasive ventilation on lung hyperinflation in stable hypercapnic COPD. *Eur Respir J* 2002; **20**: 1490–8.
11. Rochester DF, Braun NMT, Arora NS. Respiratory muscle strength in chronic obstructive pulmonary disease. *Am Rev Respir Dis* 1979; **119**: 151–4.
12. Braun NM, Marino WD. Effect of daily intermittent rest of respiratory muscles in patients with severe chronic airflow limitation (CAL). *Chest* 1984; **85**: 59S–60S.
13. Grassino AE, Lewinsohn GE, Tyler JM. Effects of hyperinflation of the thorax on the mechanics of breathing. *J Appl Physiol* 1973; **35**: 336–42.
14. Sivasothy P, Smith IE, Shneerson JM. Mask intermittent positive pressure ventilation in chronic hypercapnic respiratory failure due to chronic obstructive pulmonary disease. *Eur Respir J* 1998; **11**: 34–40.
15. Ambrosino N, Nava S, Bertone P. Physiologic evaluation of pressure support ventilation by nasal mask in patients with stable COPD. *Chest* 1992; **101**: 385–91.
16. Nava S, Ambrosino N, Rubini F *et al.* Effect of nasal pressure support ventilation and external PEEP on diaphragmatic activity in patients with severe stable COPD. *Chest* 1993; **103**: 143–50.

17. Macklem PT. The clinical relevance of respiratory muscle research: J Burns Amberson Lecture. *Am Rev Respir Dis* 1986; **134**: 812–15.
18. Goldstein RS, DeRosie JA, Avendano MA *et al.* Influence of non invasive positive pressure ventilation on inspiratory muscles. *Chest* 1991; **99**: 408–15.
19. Renston JP, DiMarco AF, Supinski GS. Respiratory muscle rest using nasal BiPAP ventilation in patients with stable severe COPD. *Chest* 1994; **105**: 1053–60.
20. Elliott MW, Mulvey D, Moxham J *et al.* NIPPV reduces respiratory muscle activity. *Am Rev Respir Dis* 1990; **141**: A722.
21. Shneerson JM. The changing role of mechanical ventilation in COPD. *Eur Respir J* 1996; **9**: 393–8.
22. Catterall JR, Douglas NJ, Calverley PM *et al.* Transient hypoxemia during sleep in chronic obstructive pulmonary disease is not a sleep apnea syndrome. *Am Rev Respir Dis* 1983; **128**: 24–9.
23. Fleetham J, West P, Mezon B *et al.* Sleep, arousals, and oxygen desaturation in chronic obstructive pulmonary disease. The effect of oxygen therapy. *Am Rev Respir Dis* 1982; **126**: 429–33.
24. Goldstein RS, Ramcharan V, Bowes G *et al.* Effect of supplemental nocturnal oxygen on gas exchange in patients with severe obstructive lung disease. *N Engl J Med* 1984; **310**: 425–9.
25. McNicholas WT. Impact of sleep in respiratory failure. *Eur Respir J* 1997; **10**: 920–33.
26. Douglas NJ, Calverley PMA, Leggett RJE *et al.* Transient hypoxemia during sleep in chronic bronchitis and emphysema. *Lancet* 1979; **i**: 1–4.
27. O' Donoghue FJ, Catcheside PG, Ellis EE *et al.* For the Australian trial of Non invasive Ventilation in Chronic Airflow Limitation (AVCAL) investigators. Sleep hypoventilation in hypercapnic chronic obstructive pulmonary disease: prevalence and associated factors. *Eur Respir J* 2003; **21**: 977–84.
28. Ingrassia RS, Nelson SB, Harris CD *et al.* Influence of sleep state on $CO_2$ responsiveness. *Am Rev Respir Dis* 1991; **144**: 1125–9.
29. Wynne JW, Block AJ, Hemenway J *et al.* Disordered breathing and oxygen desaturation during sleep in patients with chronic obstructive lung disease (COLD). *Am J Med* 1979; **66**: 573–9.
30. Juan G, Calverley P, Talamo C *et al.* Effect of carbon dioxide on diaphragmatic function in human beings. *N Engl J Med* 1984; **310**: 874–9.
31. Bach JR, Dominique R, Leger P *et al.* Sleep fragmentation in kyphoscoliotic individuals with alveolar hypoventilation treated by NPPV. *Chest* 1995; **107**: 1552–8.
32. Rochester DF. Does respiratory muscle rest relieve fatigue or incipient fatigue? *Am Rev Respir Dis* 1988; **138**: 516–17.
33. Fleetham JA, Mezon B, West P *et al.* Chemical control of ventilation and sleep arterial oxygen desaturation in patients with COPD. *Am Rev Respir Dis* 1980; **122**: 583–9.
34. Elliott MW, Mulvey DA, Moxham J *et al.* Domiciliary nocturnal nasal intermittent positive pressure ventilation in COPD: mechanisms and underlying changes in arterial blood gas tensions. *Eur Respir J* 1991; **4**: 1044–52.
35. Masa Jiménez JF, Sánchez de Cos Escuin J, Disdier Vicente C *et al.* Nasal intermittent positive pressure ventilation: analysis of its withdrawal. *Chest* 1995; **107**: 382–8.
36. Wijkstra PJ, Lacasse Y, Guyatt GH *et al.* A metaanalysis of nocturnal noninvasive positive pressure ventilation in patients with stable COPD. *Chest* 2003; **124**: 337–43.
37. Kolodziej MA, Jensen L, Rowe B *et al.* Systematic review of non invasive positive pressure ventilation in severe stable COPD. *Eur Respir J* 2007; **30**: 293–306.
38. Meecham-Jones DJ, Paul EA, Jones PW *et al.* Nasal pressure support ventilation plus oxygen compared to oxygen therapy alone in hypercapnic COPD. *Am J Respir Crit Care Med* 1995; **152**: 538–44.
39. Strumpf DA, Millman RP, Carlisle CC *et al.* Nocturnal positive-pressure ventilation via nasal mask in patients with severe chronic obstructive pulmonary disease. *Am Rev Respir Dis* 1991; **144**: 1234–9.
40. Shapiro SH, Ernst P, Gray-Donald K *et al.* Effect of negative pressure ventilation in severe chronic obstructive pulmonary disease. *Lancet* 1992; **340**: 1425–9.
41. Lin CC. Comparison between nocturnal nasal positive pressure ventilation combined with oxygen therapy and oxygen monotherapy in patients with severe COPD. *Am J Respir Crit Care Med* 1996; **154**: 353–8.
42. Gay PC, Hubmayr RD, Stroetz RW. Efficacy of nocturnal nasal ventilation in stable, severe chronic obstructive pulmonary disease during a 3-month controlled trial. *Mayo Clin Proc* 1996; **71**: 533–42.
43. Casanova C, Celli BR, Tost L *et al.* Long-term controlled trial of nocturnal nasal positive pressure ventilation in patients with severe COPD. *Chest* 2000; **118**: 1582–90.
44. Leger P, Bedicam JM, Cornette A *et al.* Nasal intermittent positive pressure ventilation. Long term follow-up in patients with severe chronic respiratory insufficiency. *Chest* 1994; **105**: 100–5.
45. Jones SE, Packham S, Hebden M *et al.* Domiciliary nocturnal intermittent positive pressure ventilation in patients with respiratory failure due to severe COPD: long-term follow up and effect on survival. *Thorax* 1998; **53**: 495–8.
46. Muir JF, Cuvelier A, Tenang B. European task force on mechanical ventilation COPD. Long-term home nasal intermittent positive pressure ventilation (NIPPV) plus oxygen therapy (LTOT) versus LTOT alone in severe hypercapnic COPD. Preliminary results of a European multicentre trial. *Am J Respir Crit Care Med* 1997; **155**: A408.
47. Clini E, Sturani C, Rossi A *et al.* Rehabilitation and Chronic Care Study Group, Italian Association of Hospital Pulmonologists (AIPO). The Italian multicentre study on non invasive ventilation in chronic obstructive pulmonary disease patients. *Eur Respir J* 2002; **20**: 529–38.

48. Perrin C, El Far Y, Vandenbos F *et al.* Domiciliary nasal intermittent positive pressure ventilation in severe COPD: effects on lung function and quality of life. *Eur Respir J* 1997; **10**: 2835–9.
49. McEvoy RD, Pierce R J, Hillman D *et al.* on behalf of the Australian trial of non-invasive Ventilation in Chronic Airflow Limitation (AVCAL) Study Group. Nocturnal non-invasive nasal ventilation in stable hypercapnic COPD: a randomised controlled trial *Thorax* 2009; **64**: 561–6.
50. Simonds AK, Elliott MW. Outcome of domiciliary nasal intermittent positive pressure ventilation in restrictive and obstructive disorders. *Thorax* 1995; **50**: 604–9.
51. Windisch W, Kostic S, Dreher M *et al.* Outcome of patients with stable COPD receiving controlled noninvasive positive pressure ventilation aimed at a maximal reduction of $PaCO_2$. *Chest* 2005; **128**: 657–62.
52. Windisch W, Vogel M, Sorichter S *et al.* Normocapnia during nIPPV in chronic hypercapnic COPD reduces subsequent spontaneous $PaCO_2$. *Respir Med* 2002; **96**: 572–9.
53. Windisch W, Budweiser S, Heinemann F *et al.* The severe respiratory insufficiency questionnaire was valid for COPD patients with severe chronic respiratory failure. *J Clin Epidemiol* 2008; **61**: 848–53.
54. Tuggey JM, Plant PK, Elliott MW. Domiciliary non-invasive ventilation for recurrent acidotic exacerbations of COPD: an economic analysis. *Thorax* 2003; **58**: 867–71.
55. Clini EM, Magni G, Crisafulli E *et al.* Home non-invasive mechanical ventilation and long-term oxygen therapy in stable hypercapnic chronic obstructive pulmonary disease patients: comparison of costs. *Respiration* 2009; **77**: 44–50.
56. ACCP Consensus report. Clinical indications for non invasive positive pressure ventilation in chronic respiratory failure due to restrictive lung disease, COPD, and nocturnal hypoventilation. *Chest* 1999; **116**: 521–34.
57. Windisch W, Storre JH, Sorichter S *et al.* Comparison of volume- and pressure-limited NPPV at night: a prospective randomized cross-over trial. *Respir Med* 2005; **99**: 52–9.
58. Simonds A, ed. *Non invasive respiratory support. A practical handbook*, vol. 1, 3rd edn. London: Hodder Arnold, 2007: 370.
59. Vitacca M, Nava S, Confalonieri M *et al.* The appropriate setting of non invasive pressure support ventilation in stable COPD patients. *Chest* 2000; **118**: 1286–93.
60. Crisafulli E, Manni G, Kidonias M *et al.* Subjective sleep quality during Average Volume Assured Pressure Support (AVAPS) ventilation in patients with hypercapnic COPD. A Physiological Pilot Study. *Lung* 2009; **187**: 299–305.

# SECTION E

# Hypoxaemic respiratory failure

# 24

# Pathophysiology of hypoxaemic respiratory failure

LUKE HOWARD

## ABSTRACT

Hypoxaemic respiratory failure is commonly defined as a partial pressure of oxygen in the arterial blood stream of less than 8 kPa and can be associated with normal, low or high partial pressures of carbon dioxide. It may result from a number of processes in the lung: ventilation–perfusion inequality, hypoventilation, shunt and diffusion limitation, where ventilation–perfusion inequality is usually the greatest contributing factor. Oxygen or positive pressure ventilation administered to treat respiratory failure will affect these processes, in some instances adversely, thus their impact needs to be understood by those attending hypoxaemic patients. In addition, it is not often appreciated that cardiac output and anaemia may interact with gas exchange. In this chapter, these aspects of pathophysiology are explored and applied to examples of common conditions which are often associated with hypoxaemia.

## INTRODUCTION

'Hypoxia' is a broad term, meaning 'low oxygen' and can arise in a number of different situations, for example in the alveolus at high altitude – alveolar hypoxia due to hypobaric hypoxia – or at the cellular level – tissue hypoxia. It is quantified by partial pressure (commonly mm Hg or kPa) and what defines normal levels depends on the tissue compartment in which it is being measured. Levels of partial pressure of oxygen ($PO_2$) decrease from the atmosphere to the mitochondrion where oxygen is utilized: this is known as the oxygen cascade and the integrated response of the lungs, heart and circulation aims to ensure that tissue $PO_2$ at the bottom of this cascade is maintained for aerobic respiration. The $PO_2$ in the arterial blood stream represents the middle portion of this cascade and in the context of acute hypox*aemia* – low $PO_2$ in the blood – other mechanisms such as an increase in cardiac output and recruitment of peripheral vasculature serve to correct for this and maintain oxygen delivery; when chronic, increased erythropoiesis further compensates for hypoxaemia by increasing oxygen content. Lastly, even when compensatory mechanisms fail to maintain oxygen delivery, tissues themselves extract more oxygen from capillary blood, with a lower resultant venous $PO_2$ returning to the heart and lungs.

Despite the multiple mechanisms involved in trying to maintain oxygen transport to the tissues, $PO_2$ is not tightly regulated. This is illustrated by the finding that the normal range for arterial $PO_2$ ($PaO_2$) is wide (10–13 kPa) and that ventilation is not stimulated much below a $PaO_2$ of 8 kPa. During the normal fluctuations of everyday life, it is carbon dioxide production which is most coupled to ventilation. It is perhaps for this reason that hypoxaemic respiratory failure is defined not as a $PaO_2$ below the normal range, but as a $PaO_2$ of less than 8 kPa (type I respiratory failure).[1] By contrast, as soon as $PaCO_2$ is above the normal range (>6 kPa) then type I respiratory failure becomes type II respiratory failure.[1]

## PATHOPHYSIOLOGICAL MECHANISMS OF RESPIRATORY FAILURE

Gas exchange in the lung takes place in the alveolar–capillary unit. Alterations in ventilation and blood flow or perfusion to these building blocks of the lung and changes in how oxygen diffuses across the alveolar–capillary membrane can produce four distinct pathophysiological patterns responsible for development of hypoxaemia: these are ventilation–perfusion inequality, hypoventilation, shunt and diffusion impairment (Fig. 24.1).[2]

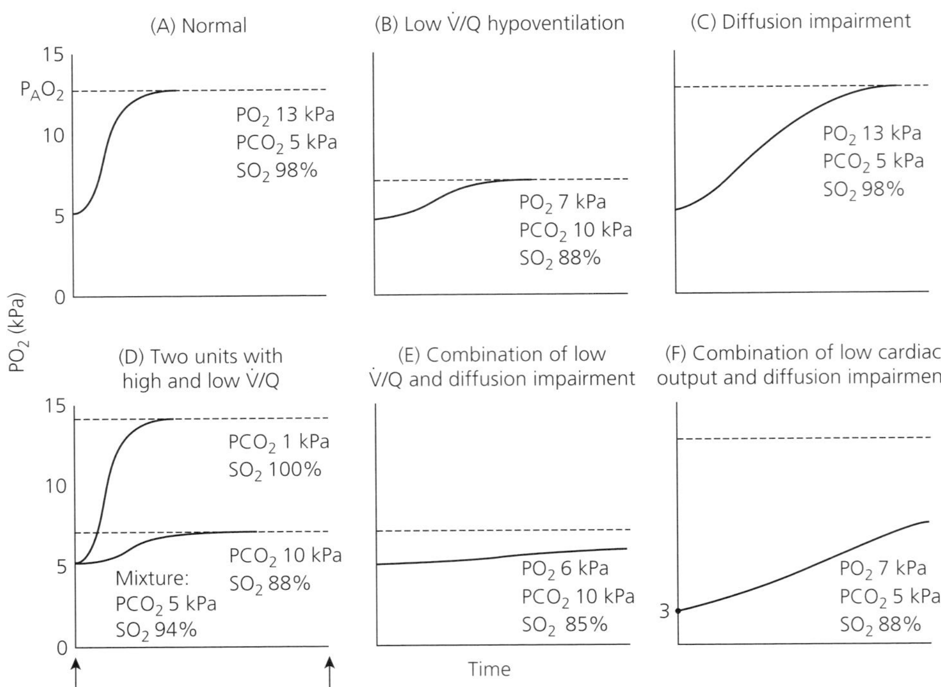


**Figure 24.1** Partial pressure of oxygen ($PO_2$) in the red cell as it passes through the alveolar capillary under different circumstances. On the charts the end-capillary parameters $P_{EC}O_2$, $P_{EC}CO_2$ and $S_{EC}O_2$ have been abbreviated for clarity. $P_AO_2$, alveolar partial pressure of oxygen; V̇/Q, ventilation–perfusion.

## Ventilation–perfusion inequality in health

In health, ventilation and perfusion are not perfectly matched, with the ratio of ventilation to perfusion increasing from the base of the lungs to the apex in the upright position.[3] This occurs due to the lower pressure in the pulmonary artery at the apex of the lung reducing the perfusion pressure, thus blood flow is greatest at the bases. Ventilation also increases from apex to base, but the difference is not as marked as for perfusion. The reason for the regional differences in ventilation relate to the weight of the lung forcing it to operate at lower volume at the base and at less negative intrapleural pressure. This results in more favourable compliance and therefore greater expansion on inspiration.

These physiological principles apply in any position such as lying supine or on one side, which is why patients with unilateral pathology are better oxygenated with the healthy lung in the dependent position. The overall impact of the ventilation–perfusion inequality which exists in the healthy lung however is small.

## Ventilation–perfusion inequality in disease

The ventilation–perfusion relationship may be disturbed in two ways – either increasing or decreasing. By definition higher ratios, such as in underperfused lung due to embolic disease or low cardiac output states, do not have much effect on overall gas exchange as they are receiving relatively little blood flow. It is the increase in the proportion of low ratio units which has the greatest impact. This will classically occur in conditions such as chronic bronchitis, emphysema and asthma, but any lung disease resulting in significant architectural disruption, such as interstitial lung disease, will have marked ventilation–perfusion inequality. Pulmonary venous blood leaving low ratio areas of lung will be hypoxaemic and hypercapnic (Fig. 24.1B). By mixing with blood from areas with normal ventilation–perfusion ratios the venous admixture will tend towards normal depending on the relative proportion of blood from low and normal ventilation–perfusion areas.

The resultant increase in ventilation due to chemoreceptor stimulation[4] will decrease alveolar $PCO_2$ in healthy lung and therefore pulmonary venous $PCO_2$, so that when mixed with the venous return from low ventilation–perfusion areas, $PaCO_2$ will normalize. This can take place as the relationship between $PCO_2$ and carbon dioxide content in the blood is almost linear in the physiological range. This is not the case for oxygen, however, due to the shape of the oxyhaemoglobin dissociation curve. Above a $PO_2$ of 10 kPa, further increases in $PO_2$ will not significantly increase oxygen content, and therefore upon mixing, blood from normal ventilation–perfusion areas cannot compensate low ventilation–perfusion areas in the same way (Fig. 24.1D). For this reason ventilation–perfusion inequality is responsible for hypoxaemia, but not usually hypercapnia; except when circumstances, such as impaired respiratory mechanisms or impaired respiratory drive, limit the ventilatory response.

Given that increases in overall ventilation to the lung are not able to compensate for low ventilation–perfusion units, the respiratory system adopts a different strategy to diminish their impact: hypoxic vasoconstriction.[5,6] This phenomenon is unique to the pulmonary circulation and acts in response to *alveolar* hypoxia to reduce perfusion to low ventilation–perfusion units. Other mechanisms in the lung act in a similar fashion to restore ventilation–perfusion matching and these include hypercapnic vasoconstriction[6] and hypoxic bronchodilation;[7] but these are less well characterized and weaker.

## Hypoventilation

It is reasonable to think of hypoventilation as a form of ventilation–perfusion inequality, with each alveolar–capillary unit receiving reduced ventilation (Fig. 24.1B). The alveolar gas equation:

$$P_AO_2 = P_IO_2 - \left(\frac{P_ACO_2}{RER}\right) + F$$

where $P_AO_2$ is alveolar $PO_2$, $P_IO_2$ is inspired $PO_2$, $P_ACO_2$ is alveolar $PCO_2$, RER is the respiratory exchange ratio and F is a correction factor (~0.3 kPa), describes how oxygen and carbon dioxide behave in a reciprocal fashion, such that for a given increase in $P_ACO_2$, $P_AO_2$, and thus $PaO_2$, will fall. Conceptually, this is perhaps better understood by considering that nitrogen enters and leaves the lung unaltered and the remaining partial pressure in the alveolus is made up of oxygen and carbon dioxide. Any increase in carbon dioxide through hypoventilation will therefore result in alveolar hypoxia. This physiological relationship is crucial when understanding the phenomenon of *rebound hypoxaemia*, which will be discussed later in the chapter.[8]

## Shunt

As with hypoventilation, shunt may also be thought of as a type of ventilation–perfusion inequality; albeit an extreme form of low ventilation–perfusion disturbance. It falls into its own category for a number of reasons. First, it results from underlying acquired or congenital anatomical defects, such as arteriovenous malformations or congenital heart disease. Second, it cannot be regulated by the same physiological mechanisms as the alveolar–capillary unit such as hypoxic vasoconstriction. Third, it takes no part in gas exchange and the consequent severity of hypoxaemia depends on the size of the shunt fraction. A strong clue to the presence of shunt is hypoxaemia which does not correct with administration of 100 per cent oxygen.

## Diffusion impairment

In this situation, ventilation and perfusion may theoretically be matched, but abnormality of the alveolar–capillary interface, such as inflammation or fibrosis, results in impaired diffusion of oxygen. In the normal alveolar–capillary unit at rest, oxygen has equilibrated across the alveolar–capillary membrane one third of the way along the capillary (Fig. 24.1A). When diffusion impairment is present this process may take longer, but rarely will it not equilibrate by the end of the capillary (Fig. 24.1C).[9] Upon exercise, however, less time for equilibration is available due to decreased capillary transit time and desaturation may occur. The other situation in which diffusion impairment may become a significant factor in gas exchange occurs when alveolar $PO_2$ is reduced such as at altitude, hypoventilation or low ventilation–perfusion (Fig. 24.1E). This results in a lower alveolar–capillary gradient down which oxygen can diffuse, making the quality of the alveolar–capillary interface more important.

Diffusion impairment has much less impact on carbon dioxide exchange given its high solubility in the alveolar–capillary membrane, and as a consequence, diffusion impairment is usually associated with type I and not type II respiratory failure.

## Interaction with cardiac output

Reducing cardiac output in the context of constant oxygen consumption necessitates greater oxygen extraction at the tissue level and consequently low mixed venous oxygen saturation returning to the lungs. In the presence of normal gas exchange this will not usually result in any significant arterial hypoxaemia; however, where gas exchange is suboptimal, for any of the reasons described above, then hypoxaemia will be exaggerated by low cardiac states (Fig. 24.1F). Where cardiac output is impaired, if the patient is also anaemic, mixed venous oxygen saturation will fall even further.

# EFFECT OF OXYGEN ADMINISTRATION

Enriching inspired air with oxygen can correct hypoxaemia associated with all of the above physiological abnormalities, apart from shunt where pulmonary arterial blood does not come into contact with alveolar gas. However, it will have the detrimental effect of releasing hypoxic vasoconstriction from low ventilation–perfusion units, thus recruiting more of these units to the pulmonary circulation and hypercapnia may develop in the absence of an adequate ventilatory response. This is one of the major determinants of the rise in carbon dioxide in patients with chronic obstructive pulmonary disease whose respiratory mechanics limit compensatory hyperventilation, but the extent of its contribution is still debated.[10–17]

If oxygen is administered for more than a few minutes to a patient developing type II respiratory failure then carbon dioxide will accumulate not only in the lungs but also in the patient's tissues. Consequently, if oxygen is suddenly removed, profound rebound hypoxaemia[8] may develop as the lungs are flooded with nitrogen again; the remaining partial pressure being exerted by the increased alveolar $PCO_2$ and resultant lower alveolar $PO_2$. This situation may be particularly dangerous and prolonged if carbon dioxide has built up significantly in tissue stores.

## EFFECT OF POSITIVE PRESSURE VENTILATION

Applying positive pressure either by non-invasive ventilation or by endotracheal tube can be associated with a significant improvement in oxygenation through a decrease in shunt and absorption atelectasis. In conditions such as acute lung injury, acute respiratory distress syndrome or pulmonary oedema, recruitment of alveoli through redistribution of oedema and re-expansion of collapsed lung increases ventilation to low ventilation–perfusion areas and opens up areas previously shunting pulmonary arterial blood. By the same token however it may increase dead space fraction by increasing ventilation to high ventilation–perfusion areas. In some cases, usually lung apices, high alveolar pressures may compress alveolar capillaries entirely, shutting down perfusion altogether, although this is rare.[2] Increased lung expansion will also increase anatomical dead space due to airway expansion. Consequently, despite decreased shunt and improved alveolar–arterial gradient for $PO_2$, alveolar dead space may increase, reducing effective alveolar ventilation.

The final important effect of positive pressure ventilation is the effect of increased intrathoracic pressure diminishing venous return to the heart and thus cardiac output. The resultant reduction in mixed venous oxygen saturation may worsen hypoxaemia if gas exchange in the lung is significantly impaired. If the reduction in cardiac output is significant, this may overshadow any benefit gained from increased arterial $PO_2$ with an overall reduction in oxygen delivery.

## CAUSES OF HYPOXAEMIA IN SPECIFIC CONDITIONS (TABLE 24.1)

### Chronic obstructive pulmonary disease

Chronic obstructive pulmonary disease (COPD) is a heterogeneous condition and classically the two 'extremes' of pathology within this broad diagnosis are emphysema and chronic bronchitis. Emphysema is typically associated with type I respiratory failure and less severe hypoxaemia than chronic bronchitis. Some of this difference in presentation may be explained by respiratory drive, and also by architectural differences between these two phenotypes.[18] In emphysema, parenchymal loss due to alveolar destruction will lead to significant increases in dead space ventilation and high ventilation–perfusion units. Hypoxaemia will result both from a combination of decreased capillary transit time (leading to diffusion impairment) due to decreased

**Table 24.1** Contribution of pathophysiological mechanisms to hypoxaemia in common respiratory conditions

| | Ventilation–perfusion inequality | Hypoventilation | Shunt | Diffusion impairment | Low cardiac output |
|---|---|---|---|---|---|
| Obstructive lung disease | | | | | |
| • Emphysema | + | – | +/– | + | – (+ in PH) |
| • Chronic bronchitis | +++ | ++ | +/– | +/– | – (+ in PH) |
| • Asthma | +++ | – | – | – | – |
| Restrictive lung disease | | | | | |
| • Interstitial lung disease | +++ | – | +/– | ++ | – (+ in PH) |
| • Extrapulmonary causes | +/– | +++ | +/– | – | – (+ in PH) |
| Central hypoventilation disorders | +/– | +++ | – | – | – (+ in PH) |
| Vascular disorders | | | | | |
| • Acute PE | ++ | – | +++ | +/– | + |
| • Pulmonary hypertension | ++ | – | + | + | ++ |
| • With PFO | ++ | – | +++ | + | ++ |
| • Pulmonary oedema | ++ | – | ++ | + | +/– |
| • PAVM/HPS | – | – | +++ | + | – |

HPS, hepatopulmonary syndrome; PAVM, pulmonary arteriovenous malformation; PE, pulmonary embolism; PFO, patent foramen ovale; PH, pulmonary hypertension.

capillary cross-sectional area and some low ventilation–perfusion units produced by collapsed airways. In the case of chronic bronchitis, gas exchange is dominated by high numbers of low ventilation–perfusion units due to airway narrowing and obstruction. With a blunted ventilatory response, this sets the scene for type II respiratory failure.

## Asthma

The abnormalities of ventilation–perfusion inequality seen in asthma are similar to those in chronic bronchitis with an increase in low ventilation–perfusion units, resulting in hypoxaemia.[2] Hypoxaemia may be exacerbated in asthma following bronchodilation due to the non-specific relief of vasoconstriction to low ventilation–perfusion areas.[2] Although mucus plugging of airways is a common feature of both asthma and chronic bronchitis, pure shunt is not a major feature and this is presumably due to collateral ventilation.

## Interstitial lung disease

Although the striking histopathological abnormality in interstitial lung diseases is thickening and fibrosis of the alveolar–capillary barrier, ventilation–perfusion inequalities account for most of the impairment of gas exchange leading to hypoxaemia.[9] Diffusion impairment becomes more important on exercise as red cell capillary transit time reduces and mixed venous saturation falls.

## Extrapulmonary restriction

The hypoxaemia associated with extrapulmonary restriction due to neuromuscular or skeletal abnormalities results from hypoventilation to all alveolar–capillary units. The same applies for patients with reduced ventilatory drive such as obesity hypoventilation. Some ventilation–perfusion inequality or shunt may develop due to atelectasis.

## Pulmonary vascular diseases

The mechanisms underlying hypoxaemia resulting from acute pulmonary embolism remain incompletely understood, but several have been proposed.[2] Not surprisingly, studies of ventilation–perfusion relationships demonstrate increases in high ventilation–perfusion units due to embolic occlusion of vessels. This results in significant dead space ventilation. Blood flow is diverted both to normal lung (reducing ventilation–perfusion) and may also pass through haemorrhagic areas of lung or indeed through latent arteriovenous anastomoses. Diverted blood passing through normal lung may suffer from diffusion impairment because of decreased transit time particularly on exercise, causing exertional hypoxaemia. In massive pulmonary embolism, cardiac output may fall, thus reducing mixed venous saturations and further exacerbating hypoxaemia.

Pulmonary oedema results in hypoxaemia due to shunt and ventilation–perfusion inequality.[2] Shunt will develop only by the stage where alveolar–capillary units become cut off because of either direct alveolar filling or airway obstruction due to oedema from adjacent alveoli. Low ventilation–perfusion units develop when this effect is partial or airways become congested. In the earlier stages of pulmonary venous hypertension, when only interstitial oedema is present, some impairment of diffusion may be present, but this is minor as evidenced by relative preservation of gas diffusion and lack of exercise desaturation in heart failure.

Cardiac output can often be elevated in pulmonary oedema, but where it is associated with a low flow state, reduction of mixed venous saturation due to increased peripheral oxygen extraction further worsens arterial $PO_2$ in the face of shunt and ventilation–perfusion inequality.

When the pulmonary arterial system becomes directly affected, as in pulmonary arterial hypertension or chronic thromboembolic pulmonary hypertension, the impact of cardiac output due to right ventricular impairment becomes a key factor. Mixed venous saturations at rest (normally >75 per cent) may often drop below 60 per cent and even much lower, to below 50 per cent in severe disease. When combined with significant ventilation–perfusion inequality, this may lead to significant hypoxaemia. Diffusion impairment may also contribute to desaturation and conceptually this is easiest to comprehend in the setting of chronic thromboembolic disease where blood may be passing rapidly through non-obstructed capillary beds due to a decrease in overall capillary surface area, but this principle will also apply to other forms of pulmonary arterial hypertension.

In patients with pulmonary hypertension and patent foramen ovale, right-to-left intracardiac shunting may develop at rest or on exercise when right atrial pressure exceeds that in the left atrium. Other vascular anomalies in the lung produce shunt, such as pulmonary arteriovenous malformations and capillary dilatation in hepatopulmonary syndrome (HPS). In HPS, oxygen cannot diffuse to blood at the core of the dilated capillary lumen. Since this occurs predominantly at the bases, desaturation is more pronounced in the erect position – a phenomenon termed orthodeoxia.

## Mixed pathologies

Many conditions coexist, either through coincidence, common risk factors or in sequence. Examples would typically include COPD and interstitial lung disease or pulmonary vascular remodelling as a consequence of hypoxic lung disease. This often leads to significantly worse gas exchange. The presence for example of COPD and interstitial lung disease would bring together significant ventilation–perfusion inequality and diffusion impairment (Fig. 24.1E) resulting in pseudonormalization of lung volumes and markedly reduced transfer coefficient and $PaO_2$.

## CONCLUSION

Hypoxaemic respiratory failure can be explained by any combination of ventilation–perfusion inequality, hypoventilation, shunt and diffusion limitation, but by far the commonest and most important factor is ventilation–perfusion inequality. Changes in cardiac output and haemoglobin concentration can interact significantly with these mechanisms, highlighting the crucial role of circulatory resuscitation in the hypoxaemic patient. Administered oxygen and positive pressure ventilation are not passive partners in gas exchange and can alter ventilation–perfusion inequality and cardiac output; thus healthcare professionals treating patients in critical care situations should also understand the physiological consequences of these on gas exchange.

## REFERENCES


1. British Thoracic Society Standards of Care Committee. Non-invasive ventilation in acute respiratory failure. *Thorax* 2002; **57**: 192–211.
2. West JB. *Pulmonary pathophysiology: the essentials*, 7th edn. Baltimore: Lippincott Williams & Wilkins, 2008.
3. West JB. *Respiratory physiology: the essentials*, 8th edn. Baltimore: Lippincott Williams & Wilkins, 2008.
4. Fidone SJ, Gonzalez C. Initiation and control of chemoreceptor activity in the carotid body. In: Cherniack NS, Widdicombe JG, eds. *Handbook of Physiology Section 3: The Respiratory System*. Bethesda, MD: American Physiology Society, 1986: 247–312.
5. Cutaia M, Rounds S. Hypoxic pulmonary vasoconstriction. Physiologic significance, mechanism, and clinical relevance. *Chest* 1990; **97**: 706–18.
6. Dorrington KL, Talbot NP. Human pulmonary vascular responses to hypoxia and hypercapnia. *Pflugers Arch* 2004; **449**: 1–15.
7. Wetzel RC, Herold CJ, Zerhouni EA *et al.* Hypoxic bronchodilation. *J Appl Physiol* 1992; **73**: 1202–6.
8. O'Driscoll BR, Howard LS, Davison AG. BTS guideline for emergency oxygen use in adult patients. *Thorax* 2008; **63** Suppl 6: vi1–68.
9. West JB. State of the art: ventilation-perfusion relationships. *Am Rev Respir Dis* 1977; **116**: 919–43.
10. Berry RB, Mahutte CK, Kirsch JL *et al.* Does the hypoxic ventilatory response predict the oxygen-induced falls in ventilation in COPD? *Chest* 1993; **103**: 820–4.
11. Castaing Y, Manier G, Guenard H. Effect of 26 per cent oxygen breathing on ventilation and perfusion distribution in patients with cold. *Bull Eur Physiopathol Respir* 1985; **21**: 17–23.
12. Dick CR, Liu Z, Sassoon CS *et al.* O2-induced change in ventilation and ventilatory drive in COPD. *Am J Respir Crit Care Med* 1997; **155**: 609–14.
13. Erbland ML, Ebert RV, Snow SL. Interaction of hypoxia and hypercapnia on respiratory drive in patients with COPD. *Chest* 1990; **97**: 1289–94.
14. Aubier M, Murciano D, Fournier M *et al.* Central respiratory drive in acute respiratory failure of patients with chronic obstructive pulmonary disease. *Am Rev Respir Dis* 1980; **122**: 191–9.
15. Feller-Kopman D, Schwartzstein R. The role of hypoventilation and ventilation-perfusion redistribution in oxygen-induced hypercapnia during acute exacerbations of chronic obstructive pulmonary disease. *A J Respir Crit Care Med* 2001; **163**: 1755 (comment).
16. Pain MC, Read DJ, Read J. Changes of arterial carbondioxide tension in patients with chronic lung disease breathing oxygen. *Aust Ann Med* 1965; **14**: 195–204.
17. Robinson TD, Freiberg DB, Regnis JA *et al.* The role of hypoventilation and ventilation-perfusion redistribution in oxygen-induced hypercapnia during acute exacerbations of chronic obstructive pulmonary disease. *Am J Respir Crit Care Med* 2000; **161**: 1524–9.
18. Wagner PD, Dantzker DR, Dueck R *et al.* Ventilation-perfusion inequality in chronic obstructive pulmonary disease. *J Clin Invest* 1977; **59**: 203–16.

# 25

# Home oxygen therapy in chronic respiratory failure

JADWIGA A WEDZICHA, CHRISTINE MIKELSONS

## ABSTRACT

Long-term oxygen therapy corrects chronic hypoxaemia and is associated with reduction in mortality and a number of important physiological benefits if used for at least 15 hours daily. Ambulatory oxygen therapy may prolong the usage of home oxygen though the evidence for longer term benefit on other outcomes is not strong. Short-burst oxygen therapy should not be prescribed for the relief of dyspnoea and other therapies for dyspnoea are more appropriate. Effective home oxygen therapy requires comprehensive assessment of the underlying condition causing respiratory failure and the therapy provided, together with determining oxygen flow rates, appropriate oxygen equipment to match the patient's lifestyle and long-term follow-up.

## INTRODUCTION

Long-term oxygen therapy (LTOT) is an important therapy in patients with chronic respiratory failure as to date it is one of the few interventions that can improve survival in patients with chronic obstructive pulmonary disease (COPD) complicated by chronic respiratory failure. In the early 1980s, two important clinical trials of LTOT were reported,[1,2] which considerably advanced our understanding, prescription and provision of home oxygen therapy. The purpose of home oxygen therapy is to correct hypoxaemia and not primarily as a therapy for breathlessness for which other pharmacological and non-pharmacological interventions will be more appropriate.

There are three main types of oxygen therapy that can be prescribed for home use and these will be discussed in this chapter.[3,4] Home oxygen therapy may also be used in infants and children but paediatric prescription is relatively small and has been covered in detailed elsewhere.[5] This chapter will concentrate on home oxygen therapy for chronic respiratory failure in adults.

### Long-term oxygen therapy

Long-term oxygen therapy is prescribed for patients for continuous use at home usually through an oxygen concentrator with chronic hypoxaemia ($PaO_2$ at or below 7.3 kPa, or 55 mm Hg). In some circumstances, LTOT may also be indicated in patients with a $PaO_2$ between 7.3 and 8 kPa (55–60 mm Hg), if they have evidence of pulmonary hypertension, secondary hypoxaemia, oedema or significant nocturnal arterial oxygen desaturation. There is no benefit in the use of LTOT in COPD patients with a $PaO_2$ above 8 kPa.[6] Once started, this therapy is likely to be lifelong. LTOT is usually given for at least 15 hours daily, to include the overnight period, as arterial hypoxaemia worsens during sleep.

### Ambulatory oxygen therapy

Ambulatory oxygen therapy refers to the provision of oxygen therapy with a portable device during exercise and daily activities. It is usually prescribed in conjunction with LTOT, although a small group of normoxaemic patients may benefit from ambulatory oxygen if they have significant arterial oxygen desaturation on exercise.

### Short-burst oxygen therapy

Short-burst oxygen therapy (SBOT) refers to the intermittent use of supplemental oxygen at home usually provided by static cylinders and normally for periods of about 10–20 minutes at a time to relieve dyspnoea. Although a considerable amount of SBOT is used in the UK, the evidence for benefit of SBOT is weak[7,8] and other treatments for dyspnoea should be used. However, some patients on rare occasions may develop 'intermittent hypoxaemia', e.g. during a COPD exacerbation, and then use of short-term or intermittent oxygen may be appropriate.

## INDICATIONS FOR LONG-TERM OXYGEN THERAPY

There are three main indications for the prescription of LTOT: chronic hypoxaemia, nocturnal hypoventilation and palliative use (Box 25.1).

**Box 25.1 Indications for long-term oxygen therapy**

- Chronic COPD
- Severe chronic asthma
- Interstitial lung disease
- Cystic fibrosis
- Bronchiectasis
- Pulmonary vascular disease
- Primary pulmonary hypertension
- Pulmonary malignancy
- Chronic heart failure

### Chronic hypoxaemia

Identification of patients with chronic hypoxaemia is important, as LTOT is one of the few treatments that can improve prognosis in patients with COPD. Chronic hypoxaemia, with or without carbon dioxide retention, can occur in several respiratory and cardiac disorders, including COPD, chronic severe asthma, interstitial lung disease such as fibrosing alveolitis and asbestosis, cystic fibrosis and pulmonary hypertension. Approximately 60 per cent of prescriptions for home oxygen therapy are for chronic respiratory failure due to COPD. Chronic hypoxaemia leads to an increase in pulmonary arterial pressure, secondary polycythaemia and neuropsychological changes and these complications can be improved with LTOT.

Although two randomized controlled trials showed survival benefit of LTOT in patients with COPD, when used for at least 15 hours daily,[1,2] the precise mechanism of the improvement in survival with oxygen therapy is unknown (Fig. 25.1). Recent epidemiological data have suggested that lack of home oxygen prescription in hypoxaemic patients may predispose to hospital admissions.[10] The two large home oxygen trials did not evaluate

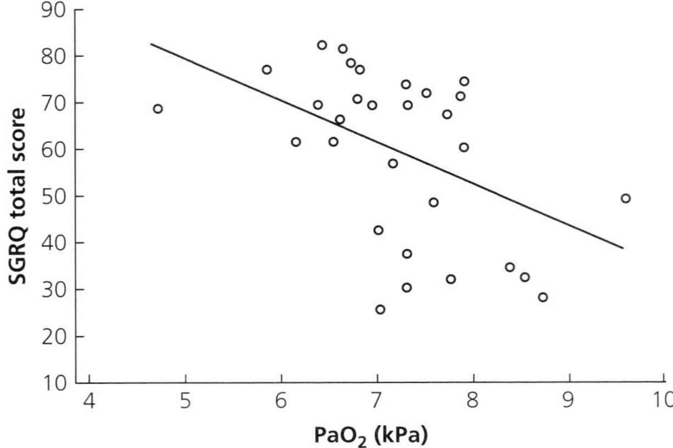


**Figure 25.1** Relation between quality of life and arterial hypoxaemia in chronic obstructive pulmonary disease (COPD). Reproduced from Okubadejo *et al.*[9]

systematically the effects of LTOT on exacerbations, though it is possible that the mortality reduction with LTOT may be due to correction of increasing hypoxaemia at exacerbation.

Previous studies have shown that effects of LTOT on pulmonary artery pressure (PAP) have been small, though PAP may be more useful prognostically and reflect disease severity. Both randomized controlled trials evaluated changes in PAP with LTOT. In the Nocturnal Oxygen Therapy Trial (NOTT) survival was related to the decrease in mean PAP during the first six months of treatment.[11] In the UK Medical Research Council (MRC) trial, LTOT prevented a rise of PAP of 3 mm Hg, seen in the control group, though a fall in PAP was not found.[2] Patients who have daytime hypoxaemia may develop further arterial oxygen desaturation at night during nocturnal hypoventilation and this will contribute to the observed rise in pulmonary artery pressure.[3] Thus LTOT is always prescribed to include the night time as it will reduce the nocturnal hypoxia episodes and thus reduce the peaks of pulmonary hypertension.

The MRC trial showed that only patients who were hypercapnic and who had had a previous documented episode of oedema (cor pulmonale) had benefits after LTOT.[2] On the contrary, the NOTT trial showed that the benefits of LTOT were present in relatively normocapnic patients.[1] It is thus a reasonable assumption that improvements in survival are likely in the presence of chronic hypoxaemia, irrespective of chronic hypercapnia or previous episodes of oedema. This assumption is reflected in the advice of all current international guidelines on the prescription of LTOT. Patients should be prescribed LTOT for at least 15 hours daily, although survival improves when LTOT is used for more than 20 hours daily.[2] Thus the hours of LTOT use should not be restricted especially in severe COPD.

Another complication of chronic hypoxaemia is the development of secondary polycythaemia, though elevation in haematocrit is not consistent in patients in that some develop polycythaemia and others do not. This variability in haematocrit levels may be reflected by the variable erythropoietin levels found in these patients.[12] LTOT as shown in the MRC trial reduces polycythaemia with reductions in haematocrit and red cell mass.[2] Cigarette smoking predisposes to secondary polycythaemia and the variable haematocrit levels may be due to an interaction with smoking. The effect of LTOT on reducing haematocrit may be offset by raised carboxyhaemoglobin levels from cigarette smoking.[13] Patients on home oxygen should stop smoking as the use of oxygen in the presence of smoking can cause burns and is a fire hazard. Any patient who persists in smoking despite using any form of home oxygen must be warned of the potential risks. However there is no objective evidence available that patients who continue smoking have worse outcome on LTOT.

Important relationships have been found between chronic hypoxaemia and health related quality of life. In moderate and severe hypoxaemia, the quality of life score is related to the degree of hypoxaemia, when measured using the St George's Respiratory Questionnaire (SGRQ), a disease specific questionnaire[9] (Fig. 25.1). Anxiety and depression are also related to hypoxaemia and this accounts for psychological comorbidity seen in these patients. Improvements have been found in both anxiety and health status after LTOT. COPD patients have impaired sleep quality with frequent arousals.[14] LTOT corrects nocturnal $SaO_2$, decreases sleep latency and improves sleep quality.[15,16]

Patients with chest wall or neuromuscular diseases who develop hypercapnic respiratory failure usually require ventilatory support with non-invasive ventilation (NIV) rather than LTOT alone. Use of LTOT in these patients may lead to a potentially dangerous rise in hypercapnia overnight with morning headaches. However if chronic hypoxaemia persists while the patient is on ventilatory support, then LTOT should be prescribed but to start at a low oxygen flow rate, e.g. 1 L/min, and titrated with monitoring of overnight hypercapnia. If overnight monitoring is not available, measuring early morning arterial blood gases for the presence of hypercapnia may be useful.

Benefits of LTOT are listed in Box 25.2.

**Box 25.2 Benefits of long-term oxygen therapy**

- Increased survival and quality of life
- Prevention of deterioration of pulmonary haemodynamics
- Reduction of secondary polycythaemia
- Neuropsychological benefit with reduction in symptoms of anxiety and depression
- Improved sleep quality
- Reduction in cardiac arrhythmias
- Increase in renal blood flow

## Nocturnal hypoventilation

Long-term oxygen therapy may also be used in patients with $PaO_2$ above 7.3 kPa but having evidence of nocturnal hypoventilation.[17] This patient group will include those with chest wall disease caused by obesity, chest wall or neuromuscular disease. It may also be used in conjunction with continuous positive airway pressure (CPAP) for obstructive sleep apnoea, though LTOT is not first-line therapy for sleep apnoea. Prescription of LTOT in these situations will require referral to a physician with a specialist interest in these disorders as specialist investigation is required. Although LTOT is usually given lifelong for patients with COPD, in the case of some chest wall disorders and sleep apnoea LTOT may be prescribed for a temporary period, perhaps until the respiratory failure improves with ventilatory support, or weight reduction in the case of sleep apnoea patients has been successful.

## Palliative use

Long-term oxygen therapy may also be prescribed for palliation of severe dyspnoea in patients with lung cancer[18,19] and other causes of disabling dyspnoea such as is found in patients with severe end-stage COPD or neuromuscular disease. However, evidence shows that LTOT is beneficial in a palliative setting when there is also evidence of chronic hypoxaemia. A recent systematic review concluded that oxygen is not beneficial to non-hypoxaemic patients with cancer.[19]

## ASSESSMENT FOR LONG-TERM OXYGEN THERAPY

It essential that all patients as candidates for LTOT undergo a full assessment in a specialist centre with experience in assessing patients for home oxygen therapy. The purpose of assessment is to confirm the presence of hypoxaemia and to ensure that the correct oxygen flow rate is provided to adequately correct the hypoxaemia. Assessment for LTOT depends on measurement of arterial blood gases. Either blood gases from a radial or femoral artery or arterialized ear lobe capillary blood gases can be used for assessments. The advantage of ear lobe gases is that samples can be obtained by various healthcare professionals.[20] Prior to LTOT assessment and prescription, it is essential that there has been optimum medical management of the particular condition and clinical stability. Patients should not be assessed for LTOT during an acute exacerbation of their disease. As exacerbation recovery may be prolonged,[21] hypoxaemia can persist after exacerbation and thus assessment should occur no sooner than at around 5–6 weeks after the patient has recovered from an exacerbation. It is usual to start with a supplemental oxygen flow rate of 2 L/min via nasal cannulas, or from a 24 per cent controlled oxygen face mask, and to aim for a $PaO_2$ value of at least 8 kPa.[4]

Blood gases must be measured, rather than $SpO_2$ with a pulse oximeter, as assessment of hypercapnia and its response to oxygen therapy is required for safe prescription of LTOT. Pulse oximetry has also poor specificity in the crucial $PaO_2$ range for LTOT prescription and thus is unsuitable when used alone for assessment.[22] However, oximetry may prove valuable in screening or case-finding patients with chronic respiratory disease and selecting those patients who require further blood gas analysis.

Patients on LTOT require follow-up after prescription to ensure that there is adequate correction of hypoxaemia and that they are adherent to their oxygen treatment.[23]

## INDICATIONS FOR AMBULATORY OXYGEN THERAPY

Patients with COPD who have chronic hypoxaemia frequently develop worsening arterial oxygen desaturation on exercise, considered significant when the $SpO_2$ falls at least 4 per cent to be below 90 per cent with exercise. A small group of patients without resting hypoxaemia can also develop significant desaturation during exercise and may benefit from ambulatory oxygen. Patients with interstitial fibrosis may develop more severe exercise desaturation for a given level of $PaO_2$. Administration of supplemental oxygen therapy on exercise to patients with hypoxaemia reduces ventilatory demand and may improve operational lung volumes, and alleviates dyspnoea. Although ambulatory oxygen can correct exercise hypoxaemia, reduce breathlessness and increase exercise capacity, short-term responses to ambulatory oxygen are variable amongst patients.[24] As for LTOT, the purpose of ambulatory oxygen is to correct exercise hypoxaemia and not as a therapy with the sole aim of reduction in dyspnoea. However, most of the studies of the effects of ambulatory oxygen are relatively short-term studies and there is less evidence that ambulatory oxygen improves quality of life over the longer term.[25] Indeed short-term responses to ambulatory oxygen with respect to dyspnoea and exercise capacity do not relate to longer-term benefits.[26]

Ambulatory oxygen can be prescribed in three broad groups of patients:[4]

- **Grade 1** – Some patients on LTOT are already housebound and unable to leave the home unaided. In this group ambulatory oxygen will be used for short periods only and intermittently. These patients will generally use ambulatory oxygen at the same flow rate as with their LTOT.
- **Grade 2** – Some patients on LTOT are mobile and need to or can leave the home on a regular basis. In this patient group assessment will need to include a review of activity and oxygen flow rate required to correct hypoxaemia.
- **Grade 3** – These are patients without chronic hypoxaemia ($PaO_2 > 7.3$ kPa), who are not on LTOT, but who show evidence of arterial oxygen desaturation on exercise, with a fall of $SpO_2$ of at least 4 per cent to below 90 per cent. Ambulatory oxygen should only be prescribed if there is evidence of exercise desaturation that is corrected by the proposed ambulatory device.

Ambulatory oxygen therapy is indicated in a number of respiratory conditions, with COPD being the most common. Ambulatory oxygen is not indicated in patients with no evidence of arterial hypoxaemia and is not indicated in patients with chronic heart failure.[27] The other indications are listed in Box 25.3.

**Box 25.3 Indications for ambulatory oxygen**

- Chronic COPD
- Severe chronic asthma
- Interstitial lung disease
- Cystic fibrosis
- Pulmonary vascular disease
- Primary pulmonary hypertension
- Chest wall disease, e.g. kyphoscoliosis

A major issue with ambulatory oxygen is usage of the oxygen outside the home. There is little information on compliance with ambulatory oxygen therapy, though when assessed, compliance has been found to be generally poor, with most patients only using it occasionally to go out of the house or into their gardens and much less than instructed by their healthcare professionals.[28] Lock *et al.* in an early crossover study of oxygen cylinders and liquid systems showed that patients preferred the liquid systems and use them more but did not increase the time outside the home.[29] A number of other studies have reported poor adherence to therapy with ambulatory oxygen therapy.[25,30] Sandland and colleagues have recently shown that in the short term, ambulatory oxygen therapy is not associated with improvements in physical activity, or time spent away from home.[31] However, the use of cylinder oxygen increased over the 8 weeks compared to cylinder air. The authors conclude that patients need time to learn how to use the ambulatory oxygen and thus may then enhance activity.

## ASSESSMENT FOR AMBULATORY OXYGEN

The type of ambulatory oxygen assessment will depend on the patient's grade and thus on the patient's activity and ability to leave the home (Box 25.4). Traditionally assessments for ambulatory oxygen therapy use short-term response to supplemental oxygen therapy during an exercise test (e.g. 6-minute walking test). However, it is now recognized that short-term responses do not predict benefit over a longer period of time and thus the short-term response cannot be used to select patients for ambulatory oxygen. In some cases the weight of the ambulatory device has been shown to negate the benefit of the therapy on the short-term response. Thus the ambulatory oxygen assessment should be used as an opportunity to assess the patient's activity, to set the optimal oxygen flow rate and introduce the patient to the ambulatory device. The assessment should ideally be performed after a course of exercise training as part of a pulmonary rehabilitation programme. The initial assessment should be followed by a review after approximately 2 months of oxygen usage and ambulatory oxygen withdrawn if unhelpful.

**Box 25.4 Ambulatory oxygen therapy: patient assessment based on the British Thoracic Society (BTS) Working Group on Home Oxygen Services[4]**

- Grade 1 oxygen requirements – same flow rate as for static source
- Grade 2 oxygen requirements – evaluate oxygen flow rate to correct exercise $SaO_2$ above 90 per cent using exercise test, e.g. 6-minute walk
- Grade I oxygen requirements – exercise test required, performed on air and oxygen; require evidence of exercise desaturation and improvement with oxygen

Before prescription of ambulatory oxygen, it is important to determine the level of outside activity that the patient is likely to perform, so that the most effective and economic device is provided. Most ambulatory oxygen is provided with lightweight portable cylinders, though small cylinders provide oxygen for a short duration and oxygen conserving devices may be useful in prolonging oxygen availability. However, patient responses to these conserving devices vary owing to varying inspiratory flow rates, and patients should be assessed on the same equipment that they will eventually use when at home. Liquid oxygen systems can provide a longer period of ambulatory oxygen usage but are generally more expensive to provide and not so widely available.

## SHORT-BURST OXYGEN THERAPY

Despite extensive prescription of short-burst therapy, there is no evidence available for benefit of this oxygen modality and other interventions should be used for control of dyspnoea.[7,8] Short-burst oxygen therapy has traditionally been used for pre-oxygenation before exercise, recovery from exercise and control of breathlessness at rest.[32,33] It has also been used after a COPD exacerbation when a patient has not yet recovered from hypoxaemia, though in that case, intermittent (temporary) LTOT would be more appropriate.

## FUTURE RESEARCH

Despite widespread use of home oxygen therapy, there are a number of issues that require further study. More information is required on the mechanisms of long-term benefit with LTOT, especially if LTOT reduces the severity of exacerbations. However further randomized controlled studies of LTOT in hypoxaemic patients are not appropriate, in view of the beneficial effects seen on mortality. Attention is needed to the problem of poor adherence to ambulatory oxygen therapy and how much support and education is required in order that patients use the therapy on a daily basis. Withdrawal of home oxygen in patients with inappropriate short-burst prescriptions also requires evaluation. The goal of a comprehensive home oxygen service for patients with chronic respiratory failure is to ensure that the right person is treated with home oxygen for the correct indications and thus optimal benefits will be obtained with this important but costly therapy.

## REFERENCES


1. Nocturnal Oxygen Therapy Trial Group. Continuous or nocturnal oxygen therapy in hypoxaemic chronic obstructive lung disease. *Ann Intern Med* 1980; **93**: 391–98.
2. Medical Research Council Working Party. Long term domiciliary oxygen therapy in chronic hypoxic cor pulmonale complicating chronic bronchitis and emphysema. *Lancet* 1981; **i**: 681–6.
3. Royal College of Physicians. *Domiciliary Oxygen Therapy Services. Clinical guidelines and advice for prescribers.* London: Royal College of Physicians, 1999.
4. British Thoracic Society (BTS) Working Group on Home Oxygen Services. *Clinical component for the home oxygen service in England and Wales.* London: BTS, 2006.
5. Balfour-Lynn M, Field DJ, Gringras P *et al.* On behalf of the paediatric section of the Home Oxygen Guideline Development Group of the BTS Standards of Care Committee. BTS Guidelines for home oxygen in children. *Thorax* 2009; **64** Suppl 2: ii1–ii26.
6. Gorecka D, Gorzelak K, Sliwinski P *et al.* Effect of long term oxygen therapy on survival in chronic obstructive pulmonary disease with moderate hypoxaemia. *Thorax* 1997; **52**: 674–9.

7. Stevenson NJ, Calverley PMA. Effect of oxygen on recovery from maximal exercise in patients with chronic obstructive pulmonary disease. *Thorax* 2004; **59**: 668–72.
8. Eaton W, Fergusson J, Kolbe CA *et al.* WestShort-burst oxygen therapy for COPD patients: a 6-month randomised, controlled study. *Eur Respir J* 2006; **27**: 697–704.
9. Okubadejo AA, Paul EA, Jones PW *et al.* Quality of life in patients with chronic obstructive pulmonary disease and severe hypoxaemia. *Thorax* 1996; **51**: 44–7.
10. Garcia-Aymerich E, Farrero MA, Félez J *et al.* Risk factors of readmission to hospital for a COPD exacerbation: a prospective study. *Thorax* 2003; **58**: 100–5.
11. Timms RM, Khaja FU, Williams GW *et al.* Hemodynamic response to oxygen therapy in chronic obstructive pulmonary disease. *Ann Intern Med* 1985; **102**: 29–36.
12. Wedzicha JA, Cotes PM, Empey DW *et al.* Serum immunoreactive erythropoietin in hypoxic lung disease with and without polycythaemia. *Clin Sci* 1985; **69**: 413–22.
13. Calverley PMA, Leggett RJ, McElderry L *et al.* Cigarette smoking and secondary polycythaemia in hypoxic cor pulmonale. *Am Rev Respir Dis* 1982; **125**: 507–10.
14. Brezinova V, Catterall JR, Douglas NJ *et al.* Night sleep of patients with chronic ventilatory failure and age matched controls: number and duration of the EEG episodes of intervening wakefulness and drowsiness. *Sleep* 1982; **5**: 123–30.
15. Calverley PMA, Brezinova V, Douglas NJ *et al.* The effect of oxygenation on sleep quality in chronic bronchitis and emphysema. *Am Rev Respir Dis* 1982; **126**: 206–10.
16. Goldstein RS, Ramcharan V, Bowes G *et al.* Effect of supplemental nocturnal oxygen on gas exchange in patients with severe obstructive lung disease. *N Engl J Med* 1984; **310**: 425–29.
17. Douglas NJ, Calverley PMA, Leggett RJ *et al.* Transient hypoxaemia during sleep in chronic bronchitis and emphysema. *Lancet* 1979; **i**: 1–4.
18. Bruera E, de Stoutz N, Valsco-Leiva A *et al.* Effects of oxygen on dyspnoea in hypoxaemic terminal-cancer patients. *Lancet* 1993; **342**: 13–14.
19. Uronis HE, Currow DC, McCrory DC *et al.* Oxygen for the relief of dyspnoea in mildly or non hypoxaemic patients with cancer: a systematic review and meta-analysis. *Br J Cancer* 2008; **98**: 294–9.
20. Pitkin AD, Roberts CM, Wedzicha JA. Arterialised ear lobe blood gas analysis: an underused technique. *Thorax* 1994; **49**: 364–66.
21. Seemungal TAR, Donaldson GC, Bhowmik A *et al.* Time course and recovery of exacerbations in patients with chronic obstructive pulmonary disease. *Am J Respir Crit Care Med* 2000; **161**: 1608–13.
22. Roberts CM, Bugler JR, Melchor R *et al.* Value of pulse oximetry in screening for long-term oxygen requirement. *Eur Respir J* 1993; **6**: 559–62.
23. Restrick LJ, Paul EA, Braid GM *et al.* Assessment and follow-up of patients prescribed long term oxygen treatment. *Thorax* 1993; **48**: 708–13.
24. Bradley JM, Lasserson T, Elborn S *et al.* A systematic review of randomized controlled trials examining the short-term benefit of ambulatory oxygen in COPD. *Chest* 2007; **131**: 278–85.
25. Eaton T, Garrett JE, Young P *et al.* Ambulatory oxygen improves quality of life of COPD patients: a randomised controlled study. *Eur Respir J* 2002; **20**: 306–12.
26. Garrod R, Paul EA, Wedzicha JA. Supplemental oxygen during pulmonary rehabilitation in patients with COPD with exercise hypoxaemia. *Thorax* 2000; **55**: 539–44.
27. Restrick LJ, Davies SW, Noone L *et al.* Ambulatory oxygen in chronic heart failure. *Lancet* 1992; **340**: 1192–3.
28. Lock AH, Paul EA, Rudd RM *et al.* Portable oxygen therapy: assessment and usage. *Respir Med* 1991; **85**: 407–12.
29. Lock SH, Blower G, Prynne M *et al.* Comparison of liquid and gaseous oxygen for domiciliary portable use. *Thorax* 1992; **47**: 98–100.
30. Lacasse Y, Lecours R, Pelletier C *et al.* Randomised trial of ambulatory oxygen in oxygen-dependent COPD. *Eur Respir J* 2005; **25**: 1032–8.
31. Sandland CJ, Morgan MDL, Singh SJ. Patterns of domestic activity and ambulatory oxygen usage in COPD. *Chest* 2008; **134**: 753–60.
32. Woodcock AA, Gross ER, Geddes DM. Oxygen relieves breathlessness in 'pink puffers'. *Lancet* 1981; **i**: 907–9.
33. Evans TW, Waterhouse JC, Carter A *et al.* Short burst oxygen treatment for breathlessness in chronic obstructive airways disease. *Thorax* 1986; **41**: 611–15.

26

# Acute oxygen therapy

MARK ELLIOTT


## ABSTRACT

Oxygen is a drug and like any drug can cause harm as well as benefit. Accepted dogma is that a high $FiO_2$ is protective and gives a margin of safety and therefore that practitioners should err on the side of generous oxygen supplementation. However, patients may be placed at risk by such a strategy. These include patients with chronic stable hypercapnia, those who have received bleomycin even in the distant past and patients with Paraquat poisoning. There is no evidence that giving oxygen in the absence of hypoxia is beneficial. Indeed, in patients with stroke and acute myocardial infarction there is some evidence to suggest that oxygen may actually be harmful. Clinical assessment of the hypoxic patient is unreliable and although pulse oximetry is extremely useful, it does not provide information on pH and $PaCO_2$, vital in the effective management of these patients. A blood gas sample should be obtained in all patients with suspected hypoxaemia. The mitochondrion is the final destination of oxygen, where it is required for aerobic adenosine triphosphate synthesis. Increasing the inspired oxygen concentration is just one part of the strategy for improving tissue oxygen delivery. In particular this must include maintenance of an adequate circulation. When faced with a hypoxic patient it is mandatory to ascertain the cause of the hypoxia, whether the cause is sufficient to explain the degree of hypoxia and to correct what can be reversed. Oxygen should be prescribed and it should be appreciated that oxygen requirements may change over time. It should be targeted to a specific oxygen saturation – 94 per cent to 98 per cent – except in those at risk of hypercapnic respiratory failure, in whom 88 per cent to 92 per cent is the chosen range. It is important to note that an upper as well as a lower limit should be specified. These ranges are appropriate for most patients but may need to be adjusted on a case-by-case basis. (In patients with severe chronic hypoxia, it may be reasonable to accept a lower target range.) These patients will be acclimatized to hypoxia. It is particularly important to appreciate that the need to increase the $FiO_2$ to maintain a target saturation indicates worsening gas exchange and the need for a re-evaluation of the patient's clinical condition. As the patient improves the $FiO_2$ can be reduced, and clear guidance needs to be given about the way in which oxygen can be safely discontinued. The delivery device, initial flow rate and target range should always be prescribed.


## INTRODUCTION

Oxygen is one of the commonest drugs used in medical emergencies. Most breathless patients and a large number of patients with other acute conditions are given supplementary oxygen. Any apparent significant injury at a sporting event is usually accompanied by the immediate administration of oxygen. However, oxygen supplementation is not without risk and there are occasional deaths due to under- or over-use of oxygen. Audits of oxygen use have consistently shown poor performance.[1–6] Unfortunately, there are few randomized controlled trials to guide practice, which is largely guided by precedent.

Tissue hypoxia and cell death can occur, especially in the brain, after just a few minutes of profound hypoxaemia, such as occurs during cardiac arrest. Sudden exposure to low arterial oxygen saturations below about 80 per cent can cause altered consciousness even in healthy subjects. However, the degree of hypoxia that will cause cellular damage is not well established. Patients with chronic lung diseases may tolerate low levels of blood oxygen chronically when in a clinically stable condition, but these levels may not be adequate during acute illness, when the tissue oxygen demand may increase.

Dogma is that a high fraction of inspired oxygen ($FiO_2$) is protective and gives a margin of safety, and therefore

19. Sieker HO, Hickam JB. Carbon dioxide intoxication: the clinical syndrome, its etiology and management with particular reference to the use of mechanical respirators. *Medicine* 1956; **35**: 389–423.
20. Murphy R, Driscoll P, O'Driscoll R. Emergency oxygen therapy for the COPD patient. *Emerg Med J* 2001; **18**: 333–9.
21. Thrush D, Hodges MR. Accuracy of pulse oximetry during hypoxemia. *South Med J* 1994; **87**: 518–21.
22. Aughey K, Hess D, Eitel D *et al.* An evaluation of pulse oximetry in prehospital care. *Ann Emerg Med* 1991; **20**: 887–91.
23. Modica R, Rizzo A. Accuracy and response time of a portable pulse oximeter. The Pulsox-7 with a finger probe. *Respiration* 1991; **58**: 155–7.
24. Severinghaus JW, Naifeh KH. Accuracy of response of six pulse oximeters to profound hypoxia. *Anesthesiology* 1987; **67**: 551–8.
25. Severinghaus JW, Naifeh KH, Koh SO. Errors in 14 pulse oximeters during profound hypoxia. *J Clin Monit* 1989; **5**: 72–81.
26. Kelly AM, McAlpine R, Kyle E. How accurate are pulse oximeters in patients with acute exacerbations of chronic obstructive airways disease? *Respir Med* 2001; **95**: 336–40.
27. Jubran A, Tobin MJ. Reliability of pulse oximetry in titrating supplemental oxygen therapy in ventilator-dependent patients. *Chest* 1990; **97**: 1420–5.
28. Lee WW, Mayberry K, Crapo R *et al.* The accuracy of pulse oximetry in the emergency department. *Am J Emerg Med* 2000; **18**: 427–31.
29. Raffin TA. Indications for arterial blood gas analysis. *Ann Intern Med* 1986; **105**: 390–8.
30. British Thoracic Society. British Guideline on the Management of Asthma. *Thorax* 2008; **63** Suppl 4: iv1–121.
31. Eaton T, Rudkin S, Garrett JE. The clinical utility of arterialized earlobe capillary blood in the assessment of patients for long-term oxygen therapy. *Respir Med* 2001; **95**: 655–60.
32. Murphy R, Thethy S, Raby S *et al.* Capillary blood gases in acute exacerbations of COPD. *Respir Med* 2006; **100**: 682–6.
33. Zavorsky GS, Cao J, Mayo NE *et al.* Arterial versus capillary blood gases: a meta-analysis. *Respir Physiol Neurobiol* 2007; **155**: 268–79.
34. Lightowler JVJ, Elliott MW. Local anaesthetic infiltration prior to arterial puncture: a survey of current practice and a randomised double blind placebo controlled trial. *J R Coll Phys London* 1997; **31**: 645–6.
35. Sado DM, Deakin CD. Local anaesthesia for venous cannulation and arterial blood gas sampling: are doctors using it? *J R Soc Med* 2005; **98**: 158–60.
36. Wimpress S, Vara DD, Brightling CE. Improving the sampling technique of arterialized capillary samples to obtain more accurate $PaO_2$ measurements. *Chronic Respir Dis* 2005; **2**: 47–50.
37. Pitkin AD, Roberts CM, Wedzicha JA. Arterialised earlobe blood gas analysis: an underused technique. *Thorax* 1994; **49**: 364–6.
38. Kelly AM, Kyle E, McAlpine R. Venous pCO and pH can be used to screen for significant hypercarbia in emergency patients with acute respiratory disease. *J Emerg Med* 2002; **22**: 15–19.
39. McVicar J, Eager R. Validation study of a transcutaneous carbon dioxide monitor in patients in the emergency department. *Emerg Med J* 2009; **26**: 344–6.
40. Hebert PC, Wells G, Blajchman MA *et al.* A multicenter, randomized, controlled clinical trial of transfusion requirements in critical care. Transfusion requirements in critical care investigators, Canadian Critical Care Trials Group. *N Engl J Med* 1999; **340**: 409–17.
41. Wilson AT, Channer KS. Hypoxaemia and supplemental oxygen therapy in the first 24 hours after myocardial infarction: the role of pulse oximetry. *J R Coll Phys London* 1997; **31**: 657–61.
42. Agusti AG, Carrera M, Barbe F *et al.* Oxygen therapy during exacerbations of chronic obstructive pulmonary disease. *Eur Respir J* 1999; **14**: 934–9.
43. Nicholson C. A systematic review of the effectiveness of oxygen in reducing acute myocardial ischaemia. *J Clin Nurs* 2004; **13**: 996–1007.
44. Beasley R, Aldington S, Weatherall M *et al.* Oxygen therapy in myocardial infarction: an historical perspective. *J R Soc Med* 2007; **100**: 130–3.
45. Harten JM, Anderson KJ, Kinsella J *et al.* Normobaric hyperoxia reduces cardiac index in patients after coronary artery bypass surgery. *J Cardiothor Vasc Anesth* 2005; **19**: 173–5.
46. Frobert O, Moesgaard J, Toft E *et al.* Influence of oxygen tension on myocardial performance. Evaluation by tissue Doppler imaging. *Cardiovasc Ultrasound* 2004; **2**: 22.
47. Maroko PR, Radvany P, Braunwald E *et al.* Reduction of infarct size by oxygen inhalation following acute coronary occlusion. *Circulation* 1975; **52**: 360–8.
48. Madias JE, Hood WB Jr, Madias JE *et al.* Reduction of precordial ST-segment elevation in patients with anterior myocardial infarction by oxygen breathing. *Circulation* 1976; **53** Suppl 3: 1198–200.
49. Fillmore SJ, Shapiro M, Killip T *et al.* Arterial oxygen tension in acute myocardial infarction. Serial analysis of clinical state and blood gas changes. *Am Heart J* 1970; **79**: 620–9.
50. Waring WS, Thomson AJ, Adwani SH *et al.* Cardiovascular effects of acute oxygen administration in healthy adults. *J Cardiovasc Pharmacol* 2003; **42**: 245–50.
51. Kaneda T, Ku K, Inoue T *et al.* Postischemic reperfusion injury can be attenuated by oxygen tension control. *Jpn Circ J* 2001; **65**: 213–18.
52. Haque WA, Boehmer J, Clemson BS *et al.* Hemodynamic effects of supplemental oxygen administration in congestive heart failure. *J Am Coll Cardiol* 1996; **27**: 353–7.

53. McNulty PH, King N, Scott S *et al.* Effects of supplemental oxygen administration on coronary blood flow in patients undergoing cardiac catheterization. *Am J Physiol Heart Circ Physiol* 2005; **288**: H1057–62.
54. Neill WA, Neill WA. Effects of arterial hypoxemia and hyperoxia on oxygen availability for myocardial metabolism. Patients with and without coronary heart disease. *Am J Cardiol* 1969; **24**: 166–71.
55. Ronning OM, Guldvog B, Ronning OM *et al.* Should stroke victims routinely receive supplemental oxygen? A quasi-randomized controlled trial. *Stroke* 1999; **30**: 2033–7.
56. O'Driscoll BR, Howard LS, Davison AG, on behalf of the British Thoracic Society. BTS guideline for emergency oxygen use in adult patients. *Thorax* 2008; **63** Suppl 6: vi1–68.
57. Gallagher R, Roberts D. A systematic review of oxygen and airflow effect on relief of dyspnea at rest in patients with advanced disease of any cause. *J Pain Palliat Care Pharmacother* 2004; **18**: 3–15.
58. Plant PK, Owen JL, Elliott MW. One year period prevalence study of respiratory acidosis in acute exacerbations of COPD: implications for the provision of non-invasive ventilation and oxygen administration. *Thorax* 2000; **55**: 550–4.
59. Joosten SA, Koh MS, Bu X *et al.* The effects of oxygen therapy in patients presenting to an emergency department with exacerbation of chronic obstructive pulmonary disease. *Med J Aust* 2007; **186**: 235–8.
60. Shahrizaila T, Kinnear W. Recommendations for respiratory care of adults with muscle disorders. *Neuromusc Dis* 2007; **17**: 13–15.
61. Jeffrey AA, Warren PM, Flenley DC *et al.* Acute hypercapnic respiratory failure in patients with chronic obstructive lung disease: risk factors and use of guidelines for management. *Thorax* 1992; **47**: 34–40.
62. Warren PM, Flenley DC, Millar JS *et al.* Respiratory failure revisited: acute exacerbations of chronic bronchitis between 1961–68 and 1970–76. *Lancet* 1980; **1**: 467–70.
63. Comis RL. Bleomycin pulmonary toxicity: current status and future directions. *Semin Oncol* 1992; **19**: 64–70.
64. Demeere JL. Paraquat toxicity. The use of hypoxic ventilation. *Acta Anaesthesiol Belg* 1984; **35**: 219–30.
65. Wedzicha JA. Domiciliary oxygen therapy services: clinical guidelines and advice for prescribers. Summary of a report of the Royal College of Physicians. *J R Coll Phys London* 1999; **33**: 445–7.

27

# Equipment for oxygen therapy

DANIEL SCHUERMANS, LIES VERFAILLIE

ABSTRACT

Two systems are needed to ensure oxygen therapy for a patient: firstly, an oxygen providing system and secondly, an oxygen delivery system. The oxygen providing system delivers generally an oxygen concentration of approximately 99.5 per cent of oxygen. This comes either from a centralized storing system inside the hospital or from more mobile systems like canisters, oxygen concentrators or liquid oxygen systems. The latter three are mostly used for long-term oxygen therapy in home settings. Which one of these systems is preferred depends on the personal context of each patient. The oxygen delivery systems can be divided into two major types: nasal catheter systems and face mask systems. Nasal systems are very comfortable, cheap, effective and user friendly. Therefore they are to be used as primary choice. To prevent side effects, a flow limitation of 4 L/min of oxygen is recommended. One litre of oxygen flow increases the oxygen concentration by 4 per cent. Nasal systems can deliver oxygen concentrations up to 40 per cent of oxygen. However, if you need a higher oxygen concentration, you need to switch to a face mask system. The simple face mask delivers oxygen concentrations up to 60 per cent of oxygen and if a face mask with reservoir is used, oxygen concentrations up to 95 per cent can be achieved. These systems are less user friendly than nasal systems and the oxygen concentration depends on the breathing pattern, the correct positioning and correct use of these masks. Carbon dioxide retention is one of the major problems of incorrectly used face masks. The Venturi mask system can sometimes be a solution to avoid variability of the oxygen concentration. In conclusion, correct oxygen therapy is a challenge and must be tailored to the patient, to achieve satisfactory oxygenation and to optimize personal comfort and compliance.

## INTRODUCTION

An oxygen delivery system is used to normalize or increase arterial oxygen pressure by regulating the oxygen supply to a patient. The oxygen supply depends on a combination of delivery equipment, oxygen flow, breathing pattern, tidal volume and breathing frequency. It has to be correlated with the patient's oxygenation and blood gas values.

Oxygen is given not only to relieve dyspnoea and to maintain oxygenation, but also to improve normal daily activity, to increase endurance exercise capacity and to decrease exacerbations and thus hospitalizations. A fine balance between device comfort, ability to continue normal daily activity and therapeutic effect will determine the choice of a specific oxygen delivery device. If one of these conditions is not fulfilled, lack of compliance will be the consequence.

The choice of a device also depends on many individual factors: quality of life, age, comorbidity, next of kin, social history, etc. Good education of the patient and/or their family is essential for good compliance. In this chapter we present an overview of the different available systems, to enable the reader to make appropriate choices with regard to correct equipment for oxygen delivery, leading to therapeutic success.

## OXYGEN PROVIDING SYSTEMS

There are several oxygen delivery systems: canisters, concentrators and liquid oxygen. The choice of the system depends on the following factors:[1,2]

- expected duration of the therapy
- type of pathology
- breathing pattern of the patient
- need for humidification of the delivered oxygen

- cooperation of the patient
- the needs, restrictions and mobility of the patient
- reliability of the manufacturer and provider
- new developments and research in the field.[3,4]

## Supply of oxygen in the hospital

In most hospitals a centralized storing system is used to supply oxygen. This system is cheap, safe and user friendly. The oxygen has a concentration of at least 99.5 per cent and can be used at all times. When a patient has to be transported in the hospital, a small canister of oxygen is usually used.[3,4]

The correct flow meters and connections must be used and the equipment of the different systems should not be mixed.[1,3]

## Supply of oxygen at home

### CANISTERS

Canisters are cylinders with double metal walls, which contain compressed gaseous oxygen, stored at 200 bar. The oxygen cylinders are colour coded: either a black or dark blue cylinder with a white shoulder or a completely white cylinder.[3] They can contain 5–4400 L of water equivalent which represents 1000–880 000 L of gaseous oxygen, at an oxygen concentration of 99.6 per cent. Before using, the content and the gas concentration of the cylinder should always be checked.[1,3–7]

All oxygen cylinders are provided with a pressure regulator. The construction of the canisters and gas decompression systems has to be of such a quality that the security of patients and staff is ensured during all manipulations. Large canisters must always be secured to the wall with a chain. Portable cylinders are also available but they only last for a few hours.[3,4]

Cylinders can be used at home only for minimum use, e.g. to relieve occasional dyspnoea.[6,8] If a patient needs ≥2 L of oxygen per minute for more than 8 hours a day, other systems are more suitable.[3,4,9] Besides the limited capacity, large canisters are also unwieldy and expensive. However, canisters are always ready to use, and therefore very useful as back-up in case of emergencies.[3,4,6,8]

### OXYGEN CONCENTRATORS

An oxygen concentrator is an electric apparatus that filters ambient air through a molecular sieve, thus absorbing nitrogen and carbon dioxide and delivering high oxygen concentrations.[1,3] It generates an average oxygen concentration between 90 per cent and 95 per cent for flow rates between 0.5 L/min and 5 L/min.[4,7,8,10] The apparatus is comparable with a large vacuum cleaner on wheels (Fig. 27.1). It should be stored in a well-ventilated, clean and dry environment, and should be kept away from open fire and cooking areas.[6,8,9]

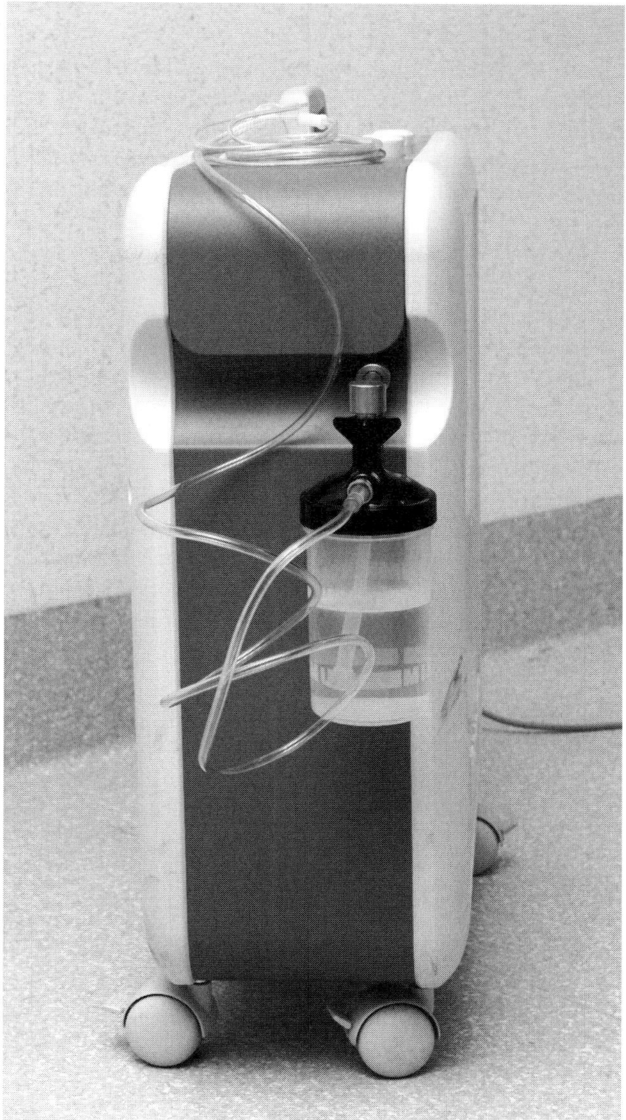

**Figure 27.1** Oxygen concentrator.

As always, thorough maintenance is essential to ensure the correct functioning of the equipment: all inlets and outlets have to be free of dust and obstruction. Oxygen concentrators are compact, reliable, stable and cheap. They need less maintenance than other systems, they make noise at an acceptable level and delivery is necessary only once. Oxygen concentrators need an external energy supply and are therefore usually not portable. Nevertheless it is the most economic way to provide long-term oxygen therapy at home.[4,6]

Recently portable oxygen concentrators on batteries have become available; their weight is approximately 4.5 kg and they are therefore easy to carry. They provide oxygen for several hours depending on the flow and battery capacity. A fully charged battery works for at least 6 hours at a flow of 3 L/min of oxygen.[4,6,7]

## LIQUID OXYGEN

Liquid oxygen systems provide the most flexible oxygen delivery equipment at home. A system consists of two different units: a 'mother unit', which is a big metal tank containing a large amount of liquid oxygen, and a smaller, portable and refillable unit, which gives the patient more mobility.[1,6,11] The mother unit contains 20–40 L of liquid oxygen that evaporates via a valve system as gaseous oxygen. It lasts for 8–10 days at a flow of 2–4 L/min. The liquid oxygen is stored at −183 °C. One litre of liquid oxygen provides 860–900 L of gaseous oxygen.[6,7]

The portable unit is small. When completely filled, it contains between 0.5 L and 1.2 L of liquid oxygen, weighs approximately 4 kg and lasts, depending on the flow, for 4–8 hours (Fig. 27.2).[1,4,6,11]

Liquid oxygen systems have two main advantages when compared with gas cylinders and oxygen concentrators. First, they provide a relatively large oxygen reservoir at home; and second, they offer the possibility to refill the lightweight portable system.[3,7,11] The flow rate needs to be calibrated once a year as inaccurate oxygen delivery can lead to dangerous situations for home care patients without medical supervision. Another danger is the extreme cold, which can give accidental burns when the equipment is wrongly manipulated.

At every delivery the company technician has to inspect all connections and tubes of the system with great precision.[4,6]

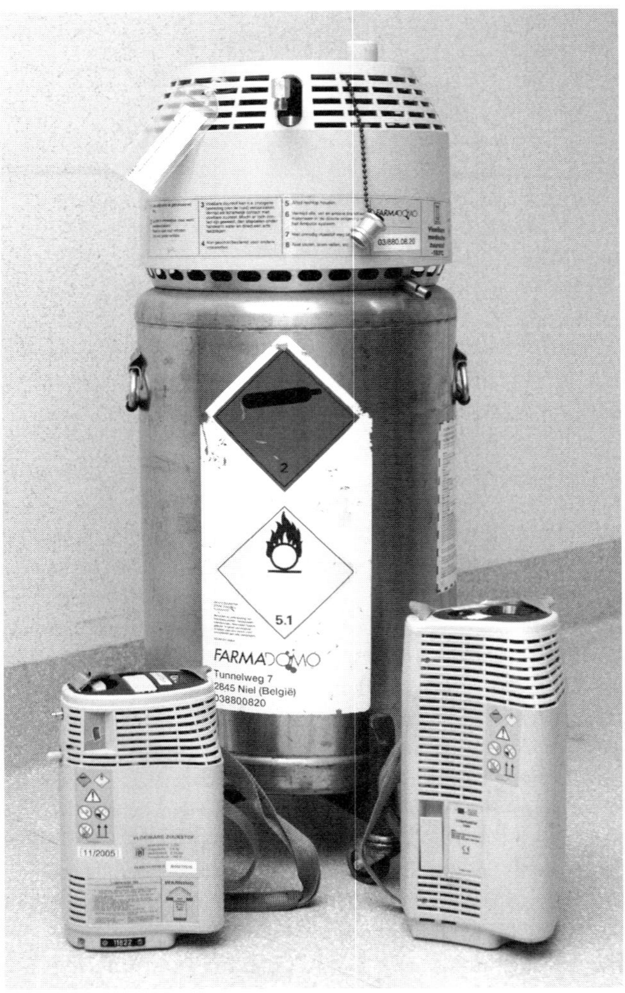


**Figure 27.2** Liquid oxygen.

## OTHER EQUIPMENT FOR OXYGEN DELIVERY

### Flow meter

Minimum marking per 1 L on the flow meter is necessary to deliver the correct flow per minute.[3,4] The delivered flow has to be accurate and calibrated from 0.5 L to 15 L/min.[3,4,11,12] The indicator (mostly a floating metal ball) is correct if the centre of the ball is at the indication level of the litres of oxygen.[3] The limited studies available reveal that most flow meters have unacceptable deviation and must be recalibrated more often than just once a year.[11,12]

### Pressure regulator

The compressed oxygen (up to 200 bar in cylinders) has to be decompressed to atmospheric pressure before being administered to a patient. Each connection has to be airtight and free of lubricant or dust. Each pressure regulator is calibrated during manufacturing, and usually no further calibration is necessary.[1,4,11]

### Tubing and outlet connections

In some situations, there can be more than only one gas supply system, e.g. oxygen, nitrogen, compressed air. The correct connections and tubing must be used without mixing up the different systems. All connections must be made with the greatest caution and checked on a regular basis.[3,4]

The oxygen tubing should not exceed 12 m in length; preferably not more than 5 m. A long tube or a large internal diameter cause a decrease in oxygen flow and thus in oxygen concentration.[1,3,4,11]

## SUMMARY

Table 27.1 compares the features of the various systems described above.

# OXYGEN DELIVERY SYSTEMS

In general three different delivery systems are used to supply oxygen to a patient, depending on the needed oxygen concentration, the patient and the pathology.[3,4] These are nasal prongs or a nasal catheter, a face mask and a transtracheal catheter.[1–4,6,8,13]

The terms low-flow and high-flow systems are not well defined. Sometimes low flow is defined as a flow of

**Table 27.1** Positive (+;+ +;+ + +) and negative (−;− −;− − −) features of each system for oxygen delivery

| | Cylinder | Concentrator | Liquid oxygen |
|---|---|---|---|
| Reliability | + + + | + | + + + |
| Easy maintenance | + + | + + + | + |
| User friendly | + | + + | + + + |
| Pure oxygen | + + + | + | + + + |
| Portable | + + | + | + + + |
| Mobility for the patient | + | + | + + + |
| Noisy | + | + + + | + |
| Delivery frequency | − − − | − | − − |
| Costs | − − | − | − − − |
| Weight | − − | − − − | − |
| Extra energy supply | − | − − − | − |

less than 5 L/min of oxygen where others define it as a flow lower than the tidal breathing flow of the patient. The same ambiguity exists for the definition of the high-flow systems. Therefore we prefer not to use these terms.[4,14–16]

If an oxygen flow lower than tidal breathing flow is used, it is obvious that during inhalation ambient air is inhaled as well, leading to variable oxygen concentrations. The oxygen concentration depends on the dilution with ambient air, breathing frequency and velocity. Using an oxygen flow higher than tidal breathing flow results in a more stable inhaled oxygen concentration.[4,14,15]

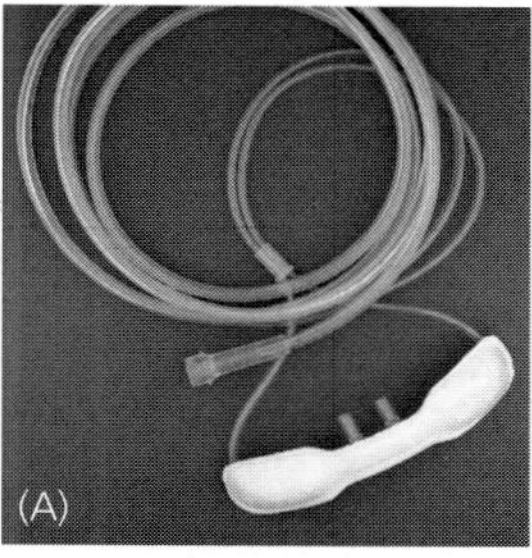

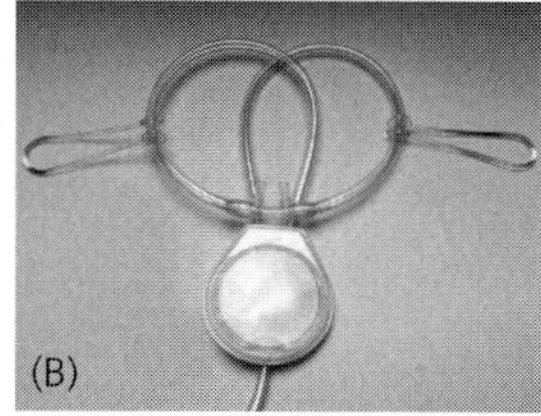

**Figure 27.3** (A) Moustache. (B) Chest reservoir.

## Nasal systems

### NASAL CATHETER

The nasal catheter is a small tube, inserted via the nose until the tip of the tube is visible behind the uvula in the oropharynx. The distance between the tip of the nose and the ear correlates well with the length needed to insert the catheter.[1,3,4,13,15,17] Correct positioning of the catheter is essential for successful oxygenation, since wrong positioning of the catheter can lead to oxygen delivery into the oesophagus. Symptoms of incorrect positioning are nausea, bloating, vomiting and burping.[1,3,4,15,18,19]

### NASAL PRONGS

The nasal prongs consist of a tube with two extensions, placed under the nose with the two soft pronged plastic tubes in the nostrils for about 1 cm.[3,4,13,15] When the prongs are placed into the nostrils, it gives an unpleasant and uncomfortable feeling but after a while the nasal prongs are well tolerated by most patients.[4,13,15] To fix the prongs under the nose, the tubing has to be fitted tightly underneath the chin after positioning it behind the ears. If the tube is fixed too tight it is not well tolerated and after a while it can lead to open wounds. Nasal prongs are useless in cases with nasal obstruction.[3,4,15]

### NASAL SYSTEM WITH A RESERVOIR

There are two nasal systems with an oxygen reservoir. The first system is the so-called 'moustache', consisting of nasal prongs with an enlargement of the diameter of the tubing between the two prongs, thus creating a small reservoir for approximately 20 mL of oxygen (Fig. 27.3A).[4,6,7,18] The second system is the 'pendant', which is an enlargement of the tubing a few centimetres below the nasal prongs and which hangs near the chest of the patient as a reservoir for approximately 30 mL of oxygen (Fig. 27.3B).[4,18]

Both systems are filled during exhalation and provide an extra boost of oxygen at the beginning of the following inhalation. This can reduce oxygen consumption by 25–75 per cent, depending on the used flow when compared to a nasal system without reservoir. They are suitable for the supply of oxygen with a flow of 2–4 L/min, providing an oxygen concentration of 24–50 per cent, respectively.[4,6,7,18]

### THE USE OF NASAL SYSTEMS

For the majority of patients, adequate oxygenation is achieved with 2–3 L/min of oxygen delivered by nasal systems. The inhaled oxygen concentration increases with approximately 4 per cent for each L/min of delivered oxygen, starting at 24 per cent for a flow of 1 L/min. Oxygen flows above 4 L/min often give an uncomfortable feeling with headache and dryness of the nose, especially if the oxygen therapy exceeds 24 hours.[1,3,4,8,15]

Although patients with dyspnoea tend to breathe more by mouth, the inhaled oxygen concentration does not vary much between nasal and mouth breathing. However, the oxygen concentration strongly depends on the breathing frequency and the flow rate.[3,8,17,20]

The big advantages of the nasal systems are that patients are able to continue normal daily activities and they can eat, drink and speak as needed.[3,4,6,8,17] In general, patients prefer nasal devices over masks. Nasal catheters and prongs are simple, cheap and comfortable systems. They are well tolerated by most patients and can be used in home oxygen therapy. Occasionally a patient needs to switch to a face mask, if the nose is too irritated. Furthermore, because patients feel less claustrophobic than with mask systems, nasal systems are removed less frequently.[1,3,4,8,13–15,17] The nasal system is the most commonly used device worldwide, not only for respiratory failure, but also for a variety of other conditions, e.g. cardiac failure, fainting and post surgery.[1,3,4,21]

## Mask systems

### SIMPLE FACE MASKS

This type of face mask must provide at least 5–6 L/min of oxygen to avoid rebreathing of the exhaled carbon dioxide remaining in the mask. The mask fills with oxygen during inhalation while during exhalation the exhaled air is forced out of the mask through side valves.[1,3,4,6,13,17,22,23]

Target flow rate is between 8 L/min and 10 L/min resulting in an oxygen concentration of 40–60 per cent. For flow rates lower than 5 L/min, the oxygen concentration strongly depends on the breathing pattern of the patient. This mask should therefore not be used for patients with low oxygen need.[3,4,13,15,22–24]

### FACE MASKS WITH RESERVOIR BAG

These masks provide an oxygen concentration of 65–95 per cent at a flow rate of 10–15 L/min. This high oxygen concentration is made possible by the use of several one-way valves. A large reservoir bag is attached at the inhalation port of the mask, out of which the patient is breathing directly. Therefore the volume of the reservoir bag needs to be larger than the tidal volume of the patient.[3,4,6,13,15,17,25]

The non-rebreathing mask has a one-way valve at the entrance of the bag and two on the side of the mask. The coordination of these valves avoids mixing inhaled and exhaled air and delivers an oxygen concentration up to 90 per cent.[1,3,13,24,25] The partial rebreathing mask enables the patient to exhale into the bag so that the following inhalation will be a mixture of the exhaled air diluted with pure oxygen.[1,3,4,13,23]

### VENTURI MASKS

This mask has a so called 'Venturi system' at the inhalation port. The Venturi system gives an accurate oxygen concentration regardless of the respiratory flow rate.[3,4,26] Oxygen is delivered at high velocity as a jet flow through a narrow orifice, thus creating a negative pressure. The negative pressure sucks in ambient air via the Venturi adaptor into the system thus diluting the gas flow (Fig. 27.4A). The degree of dilution depends on the flow of the delivered oxygen and the diameter of the Venturi system and therefore provides a fixed oxygen concentration for each Venturi mask.[1,3,4,26] The main advantage of this mask, when compared to traditional masks, is a higher oxygen concentration for the same oxygen flow rate.[1,3,26]

Venturi masks are available for different $O_2$ concentrations (e.g. 24 per cent, 28 per cent, 35 per cent and 40 per cent) (Fig. 27.4B). Another advantage of the Venturi mask, besides the fixed oxygen concentration, is that the flow delivered by the system is usually higher than the inhalation flow of the patient. Only if the respiratory rate exceeds 30 times per minute, the minimum oxygen flow indicated on the mask, has to be adjusted according to blood gas values.[1,3,4,26]

There are two major disadvantages of the Venturi mask. First, inhaled oxygen concentration decreases quickly if the mask is not well adjusted to nose and mouth. Second, the constant blowing of air into the face is considered as very unpleasant by patients. These disadvantages may lead to failure in compliance by some patients.[3,4,15,26]

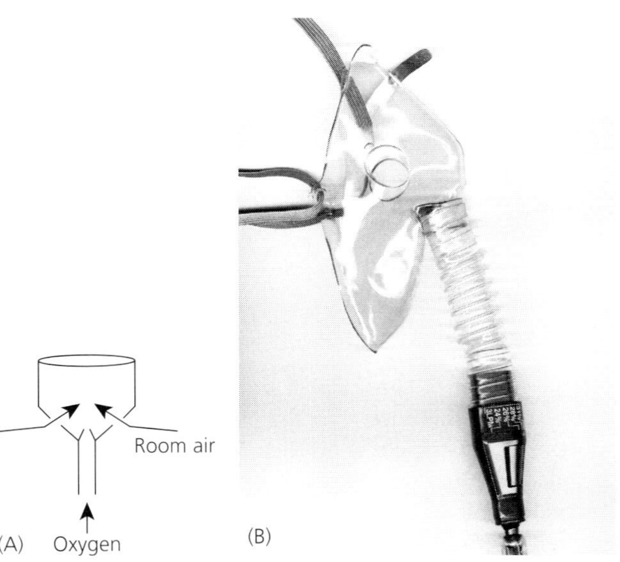


**Figure 27.4** (A) Mechanism of action of the Venturi system. (B) Venturi mask.

### TRACHEOSTOMY MASK

This is a small mask especially designed to place over a tracheostomy and fixed with a rubber ribbon around the neck. Because natural humidification via the nose is bypassed, the oxygen supply has to be humidified.[3,4]

### NASAL MASK

This is a small mask placed over the nose and fixed with a rubber ribbon behind the head of the patient. These masks are not often used, except if the nostrils of the patient are too irritated by the nasal prongs or if a large face mask is not well tolerated.[4]

### THE USE OF MASK SYSTEMS

The mask is placed over mouth and nose and fixed with a rubber ribbon behind the head of the patient. The mask is often provided with a metal strip on top of the nose. Use of the mask may lead to irritation and open wounds on the nose and/or behind the ears.[1,3,15,25,27] The face mask is considered as less user friendly, because of poor fitting to the face and the inability to eat, drink and speak while in use. Furthermore it impedes vision during reading, smells, is noisy and irritates the eyes.[1,4,13,15,23] The mask gives a fixed oxygen concentration, which is not altered by normal variations in respiration. It is a so-called enlargement of the natural anatomic oxygen reservoir.

The use of a simple face mask or rebreathing mask may lead to carbon dioxide retention. Therefore they should be used with caution.[1,3,4,13,15,27] This system is not suited for disoriented, confused or agitated patients. Compliance of the patient regarding a mask system is influenced by understanding its necessity and by its comfort, since uncomfortable devices are usually abandoned after a while.[1,3,4,27]

## Tracheal systems

### TRANSTRACHEAL CATHETER

The transtracheal catheter is a small plastic tube placed between the first and second tracheal ring. It is inserted through a narrow incision, thus bypassing the dead space of the upper airway (Fig. 27.5).[1,6,28,29] It creates an oxygen reservoir in the mouth, larynx and trachea, which leads to a saving of 50 per cent of oxygen at rest and 30 per cent during exercise. A supply of 0.5 L/min of oxygen by the catheter is equivalent to 4 L/min of oxygen given by nasal prongs.[1,6,28] There is no irritation or discomfort at nose, mouth and throat and it is less visible than nasal systems. The transtracheal catheter is often preferred over the nasal systems for long-term use, leading to a better therapy compliance of home care patients.[4,28,30]

The procedure to place this catheter takes several weeks. First, a stent is placed into the trachea. After 1 week it is replaced by the catheter. At 6–8 weeks later, when the fistula is mature and the wound is fully healed, the patient is able to remove the catheter and to clean the fistula. For safety reasons, it is better to hospitalize the patient for at least 24 hours to ensure the correct position of the catheter. This procedure is well tolerated by most patients.[4,28,29]

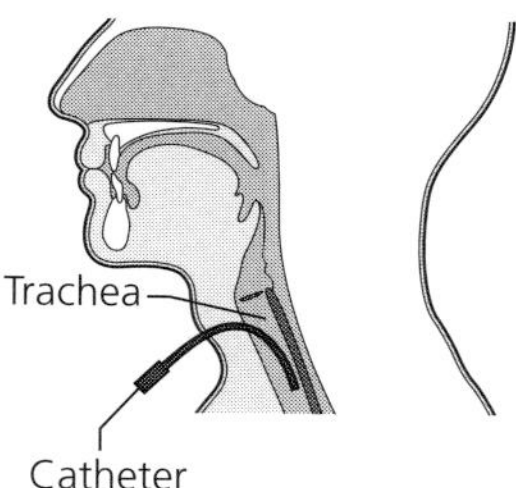


**Figure 27.5** A transtracheal system.

However, this catheter is only an option in long-term oxygen therapy since it is accompanied by a higher incidence of complications. Possible complications are cough, subcutaneous oedema, closure of the fistula, loss of a broken catheter and clotting of mucus around the catheter.[1,28–30] Frequent manipulation of the catheter may cause granulation tissue formation. Other complications mostly involve catheter position and problems reinserting the catheter. Nevertheless most of these complications are temporary and can be solved relatively easy.[1,4,6,28,29] The patient's ability to receive training and education remains the restricting factor in the use of this system.[1,8,15,28–30]

## Enclosures

### OXYGEN TENT

This is a large tent which is placed over the bed of a patient. It is seldom used nowadays due to high cost and substantial loss of oxygen.[2,31–33]

### OXYGEN HAT OR HOOD

This is a system which covers the head of a patient to create an enriched oxygen environment.[31,33] It is often used in neonatal and/or paediatric wards because there is no immediate body contact with the infant.[32]

## The OxyArm

The OxyArm is a minimal contact oxygen delivery device, consisting of a headset and a semi-rigid, in-position adjustable boom, with an oxygen diffuser placed approximately 2 cm in front of both nose and mouth (Fig. 27.6).[34–36] It generates a so-called 'oxygen cloud' with

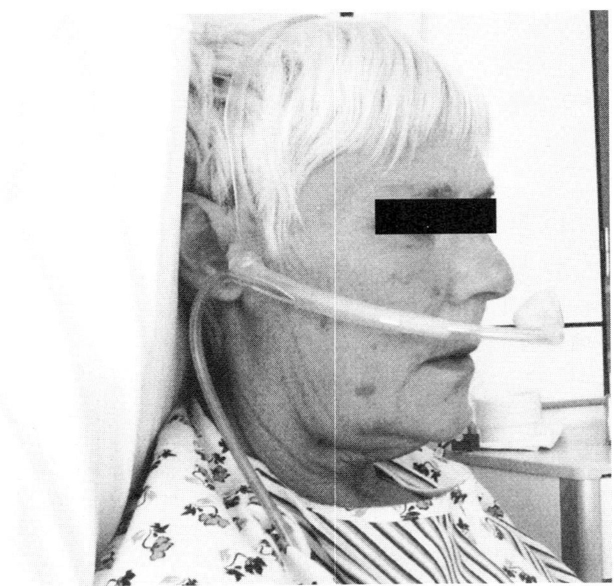

**Figure 27.6** OxyArm.

an oxygen concentration of 28–35 per cent, depending on the flow. In comparison with other systems such as face masks or nasal systems, it is more comfortable for the patient, i.e. there is no claustrophobic feeling and especially there is almost no direct contact between device and face.[4,34–36] This avoids pressure lesions and is therefore better tolerated than other systems.[4,34,36]

## ON-DEMAND OXYGEN DELIVERY SYSTEM

Oxygen saving devices have been developed because the inhalation occupies only a small part of the respiration cycle. During exhalation oxygen delivery is mostly wasted. On-demand oxygen delivery systems (DODS) only supply oxygen during the inhalation phase of the breathing cycle, while storing oxygen in a receptacle during exhalation.[10,37,38] The inhalation starts with an oxygen bolus and during the entire inhalation oxygen delivery is maintained.[6,10,38] There are several different on-demand systems, all triggered by inhalation. Depending on the manufacturer, the period of oxygen delivery is limited by inhalation flow, preset breathing rate, breathing pause or a combination of these factors. Most of these parameters can be partly tailored to the needs of the patient.[37,38]

With this system, oxygen consumption can be decreased by 50 per cent, as the actual oxygen flow time decreases. Total cost of oxygen therapy can be reduced this way.[4,37,38]

The problem with these systems is the short delay between the beginning of inhalation and the actual oxygen delivery.[7,10,38] This can lead to insufficient oxygen delivery even during small exercises.

In summary, DODS is recommended for stable patients at rest. If patients are (very) mobile the DODS could lead to desaturation because of inefficient oxygen delivery.[6,37,38]

## OXYGEN DELIVERY AND NON-INVASIVE VENTILATION SYSTEMS

In patients in respiratory distress, non-invasive ventilation (NIV) should be preferred, as long as possible for postponing intubation, in order to avoid all complications of invasive mechanical ventilation, weaning problems and infection.[39–41]

The success rate of NIV depends not only on the knowledge of the healthcare professionals and how to use the different ventilation modes, but also on the patient's compliance and acceptance. These key factors are strongly influenced by training and experience of the clinical team.[40–43] The oxygen supply during NIV is not well validated and has to be clarified more in detail.[44] The updated guidelines are: oxygen should be given, in whatever amount necessary, to ensure a blood oxygen saturation of at least 85–90 per cent.[39]

Several NIV ventilators do not have a blender to deliver a precise inspired oxygen fraction, but it is always possible to add oxygen supply in the circuit or directly at the mask.[45] Be aware that some determinants can cause oxygen concentration fluctuations during NIV.[39,44,45] First the position of the oxygen injection in the respiration circuit is an important factor of the oxygen concentration. The best place to connect the oxygen is directly before the exhalation valve and not near to the ventilator or close to the mask.[39,44]

The mixing of the exhaled air with the inhaled air during respiration in the semi-closed system is the cause of decrease in the fraction of inspired oxygen ($FiO_2$).[39,44] Oxygen concentrations below 21 per cent are to be expected when no oxygen supply is connected, due to rebreathing into the dead space tubing circuit of the ventilator.[44] Furthermore, the oxygen concentration changes by using different respiration modes and, more specifically, by changing the level of the inspiratory positive airway pressure.[44] Finally, different oxygen flow rates can influence the oxygen concentration without changing other ventilation parameters or settings.[44]

## REFERENCES


1. Lammers J-W, ten Berge E, Duyverman-Slagter C *et al.* Teirlinck richtlijn zuurstofbehandeling thuis kwaliteitsinstituut voor gezondheidzorg. *CBO* 2000; **1**: 23–39.
2. Pruitt W, Jacobs M. Breathing lessons: basics of oxygen therapy. *Nursing* 2003; **33**: 43–5.
3. O'Driscoll B, Howard L, Davison A. On behalf of the British Thoracic Society. BTS guideline for emergency oxygen use in adult patients. *Thorax* 2008; **63** Suppl VI: vi1–vi68.
4. Lodewijckx C, De Bent J, Schuermans D. *Zuurstoftherapie praktische gids voor zorgverstrekkers*, 1st edn. Leuven: ACCO, 2008:41–70.
5. Strickland L, Hogan M, Hogan R *et al.* A randomized multi-arm repeated-measures prospective study of

several modalities of portable oxygen delivery during assessment of functional exercise capacity. *Respir Care* 2009; **54**: 344–9.

6. Rees P, Dudely F. Provision of oxygen at home. *BMJ* 1998; **317**: 935–8.
7. Kampelmacher M, Rooyackers JM, Lammers J. Oxygen therapy at home. *Ned Tijdschr Geneeskd* 2001; **145**: 1975–80.
8. Stretton T. Provision of long term oxygen therapy. *Thorax* 1985; **40**: 801–5.
9. Pfister S. Home oxygen therapy: indications, administration, recertification and patient education. *Nurse Pract* 1995; **20**: 44–7.
10. Nasilowski J, Przybylowski T, Zielinski J *et al.* Comparing supplementary oxygen benefits from a portable oxygen concentrator and a liquid oxygen portable device during a walk test in COPD patients on long term oxygen therapy. *J Respir Med* 2008; **102**: 1021–5.
11. Kampelmacher M, Cornelisse P, Alsbach G *et al.* Accuracy of oxygen delivery by liquid oxygen canisters. *Eur Respir J* 1998; **12**: 204–7.
12. Peters C, Poulima P, Pearson D *et al.* The accuracy of oxygen flow meters in clinical use. *Respir Care* 2002; open forum abstracts.
13. Goldmann, K. Oxygenation and airway management. *Nursecom Educ Technol* 2004; **3**: 54–76.
14. Naresh A, Dewan M D, William C. Effect of low flow and high flow oxygen delivery on exercise tolerance and sensation of dyspnoea. A study comparing the transtracheal catheter and nasal prong. *Chest* 1994; **105**: 1061–5.
15. Eastwood G, O'Connell B, Gardner A *et al.* Patients' and nurses' perspectives on oxygen therapy: a qualitative study. *J Adv Nurs* 2009; **65**: 634–41.
16. Agarwal R, Singhal A, Gupta D. What are high-flow and low-flow oxygen delivery systems? *Stroke* 2005; **36**: 2066–7.
17. Singh C, Singh N, Singh J *et al.* Emergency medicine: oxygen therapy. *J Indian Acad Clin Med* 2001; **3**: 181–3.
18. Hagarty E, Skorodin M, Stiers W *et al.* Performance of a reservoir nasal cannulae (Oxymizer®) during sleep in hypoxemic patients with COPD. *Chest* 1993; **103**: 1129–34.
19. Cigada M, Gavazzi A, Assi E *et al.* Gastric rupture after nasopharyngeal oxygen administration. *Intensive Care Med* 2001; **27**: 939.
20. McConnell EA. Administrating oxygen by nasal cannulae. *Nursing* 1996; **26**: 14–15.
21. American Thoracic Society. Patient information series. Oxygen therapy. *Am J Respir Crit Care Med* 2005; **171**: 2.
22. O'Donohue W. Home oxygen therapy. *Clin Chest Med* 1997; **18**: 535–45.
23. McConnell E. Administering oxygen by masks. *Nursing* 1997; **27**: 26.
24. Sim M, Dean P, Kinsella J *et al.* Performance of oxygen delivery devices when the breathing pattern of respiratory failure is simulated. *Anaesthesia* 2008; **63**: 938–40.
25. Higgings D. Oxygen therapy. *Nurs Time* 2005; **101**: 30–1.
26. Adock CJ, Dawson JS. The Venturi® mask: more than moulded plastic. *Br J Hosp Med (Lond)* 2007; **68**: 28–9.
27. Nerlich S. Oxygen therapy. *Aust Nurs J* 1997; **5**: 23–4.
28. Kampelmacher M, Deenstra M, van Kesteren R *et al.* Transtracheal oxygen therapy: an effective and safe alternative to nasal oxygen administration. *Eur Respir J* 1997; **10**: 828–33.
29. Walsh D, Govan J. Long term continuous domiciliary oxygen therapy by transtracheal catheter. *Thorax* 1990; **45**: 478–81.
30. Magnussen H, Kirsten A, Koehler D *et al.* Lietlinien zur langzeit sauerstofftherapie. *Pneumologie* 2008; **62**: 748–56.
31. Amirav I, Balanov I, Gorenberg M *et al.* Nebulizer hood compared to mask in wheezy infants: aerosol therapy without tears. *Arch Dis Child* 2003; **88**: 719–23.
32. Sherwood B, Indyk L, Indyk LN. Danger of plexiglass oxygen hood: query and clarification. *Pediatrics* 1971; **48**: 333–5.
33. Ambalavanan N, St. John E, Carlo W *et al.* Feasibility of nitric oxide administration by oxygen hood in neonatal pulmonary hypertension. *J Perinatol* 2002; **22**: 50–6.
34. Ling E, McDonald L, Dinesen T *et al.* The OxyArm®: a new minimal contact oxygen delivery system for mouth or nose breathing. *Can J Anesth* 2002; **49**: 297–301.
35. Futrell J, Moore J. The OxyArm®: a supplemental oxygen delivery system. *Anesth Analg* 2006; **102**: 491–4.
36. Dinesen T, McDonnald L, McDonnald S *et al.* A comparison of the OxyArm® oxygen delivery device and standard nasal cannulae in chronic obstructive pulmonary disease patients. *Respir Care* 2003; **48**: 120–3.
37. Roberts C, Bell J, Wedzicha J. Comparison of the efficacy of a demand oxygen delivery system with continuous low flow oxygen in subjects with stable COPD and severe oxygen desaturation on walking. *Thorax* 1996; **51**: 831–4.
38. Braun S, Spratt G, Scott G *et al.* Comparison of six oxygen delivery systems for COPD patients at rest and during exercise. *Chest* 1992; **3**: 694–8.
39. Schönhofer B, Kuhlen R, Neumann P *et al.* Clinical practice guideline: Non-invasive mechanical ventilation as treatment of acute respiratory failure. *Deutsches Ärzteblatt Int* 2008; **105**: 424–33.
40. Nava S, Navalesi P, Conti G. Time of noninvasive ventilation. *Intensive Care Med* 2006; **32**: 361–70.
41. Nava S, Ceriana P. Cause of failure of noninvasive mechanical ventilation. *Respir Care* 2004; **49**: 295–303.
42. Plant P, Eliott M. Chronic obstructive pulmonary disease: management of ventilatory failure in COPD. *Thorax* 2003; **58**: 537–42.
43. Ambrosino N, Vagheggini G. Noninvasive ventilation in exacerbations of COPD. *Int J COPD* 2007; **2**: 471–6.
44. Thys F, Liistro G, Dozin O *et al.* Determinants of $FiO_2$ with oxygen supplementation during noninvasive two-level positive pressure ventilation. *Eur Respir J* 2002: **19**; 653–7.
45. Eliott MW, Ambrosino N, Schönhofer B *et al.* Equipment needs for noninvasive mechanical ventilation. *Eur Respir J* 2002; **20**: 1029–36.

# 28

# Non-invasive ventilation for hypoxaemic respiratory failure

MASSIMO ANTONELLI, GIUSEPPE BELLO

## ABSTRACT

Hypoxaemic acute respiratory failure (ARF) may be caused by several different clinical conditions including pneumonia, acute pulmonary oedema, acute lung injury, acute respiratory distress syndrome, and trauma. The pathophysiological mechanisms that underlie hypoxaemic ARF include shunt, ventilation–perfusion abnormalities and impairment of alveolar–capillary diffusion. The application of positive airway pressure in hypoxaemic ARF patients is proven to open under-ventilated alveoli and increase functional residual capacity, thus decreasing right-to-left intrapulmonary shunt and improving lung mechanics. In these patients, it has been shown that non-invasive ventilation (NIV) can increase oxygenation, reduce dyspnoea and unload respiratory muscles. Also, by lowering left ventricular transmural pressure in patients with left congestive heart failure, positive airway pressure may reduce left ventricular afterload without compromising cardiac index. Current data in the literature are, for the most part, supportive of the use of NIV to treat hypoxaemic patients without hypercapnia. However, an extremely prudent approach is needed, limiting the application of NIV to haemodynamically stable patients who can be closely monitored in the intensive care unit where endotracheal intubation (ETI) is promptly available. Patients at high risk of failure should be closely managed only by experienced personnel and with a low threshold for ETI. Identification of predictors of success or failure may help in recognizing patients who are likely to benefit from NIV and exclude those for whom NIV would be unsafe or ineffective. The risk of NIV failure seems to be higher when patients have a higher severity score, are older or fail to improve after 1 hour of treatment. Controlled studies on the use of NIV in hypoxaemic ARF patients, in which the patient subgroups are differentiated and analysed separately by diagnostic category, would be useful in clarifying the role of NIV.

## INTRODUCTION

Patients with hypoxaemic acute respiratory failure (ARF) are defined as those with a partial pressure of arterial oxygen ($PaO_2$) to inspired oxygen fraction ratio ($FiO_2$) of <200, respiratory rate greater than 35 breaths per minute, and a non-chronic obstructive pulmonary disease (non-COPD) diagnosis, including pneumonia, cardiogenic pulmonary oedema, acute lung injury (ALI), acute respiratory distress syndrome (ARDS), and trauma. In contrast with COPD, the efficacy of non-invasive ventilation (NIV) in patients with hypoxaemic ARF is less clear.

This chapter describes the use of NIV in the heterogeneous group of hypoxaemic ARF patients. The use of NIV in patients with cardiogenic pulmonary oedema and trauma, and the role of NIV in the ventilator weaning process or in post-operative patients, and the accompanying technical aspects, are reported in other chapters of this book.

In the following sections, constant continuous positive airway pressure delivered non-invasively is referred to as CPAP, and non-invasive intermittent positive pressure ventilation with or without positive end-expiratory pressure (PEEP) is referred to as NIPPV (non-invasive positive pressure ventilation). The term NIV is considered to include either CPAP or NIPPV.

## RATIONALE

The pathophysiological mechanisms that underlie hypoxaemic ARF include shunt, ventilation–perfusion abnormalities, and impairment of alveolar–capillary diffusion. The application of positive airway pressure opens under-ventilated alveoli and increases functional residual capacity, thus decreasing right-to-left intrapulmonary shunt, and improving lung mechanics.[1] In patients with ALI, NIPPV is proven to increase oxygenation, reduce dyspnoea and unload respiratory muscles.[2] In these patients, it has been shown that CPAP alone improves gas exchange but fails to unload the respiratory muscles, whereas NIPPV provides a better response, unloading muscles and relieving dyspnoea when compared with CPAP.[2]

By lowering left ventricular transmural pressure in patients with left congestive heart failure, positive airway pressure may reduce left ventricular afterload without compromising cardiac index.[3,4]

## EVIDENCE BASE

Trials of NIPPV in patients with hypoxaemic respiratory failure have yielded conflicting results. In 1989, Meduri *et al.*[5] described one of the first clinical applications of NIPPV in patients with hypoxaemic ARF. Subsequently, in 1994, Pennock *et al.*[6] reported a 50 per cent success rate in a large group of patients with ARF of different aetiologies, and similar good results were achieved by Lapinsky *et al.*,[7] using nasal mask NIPPV. In randomized controlled trials (RCTs), NIPPV has been compared with either usual medical treatment or conventional mechanical ventilation through an endotracheal tube (Table 28.1).

The first RCT on NIPPV in hypoxaemic ARF was reported by Wysocki *et al.*[8] who randomized 41 non-COPD patients with ARF to NIPPV delivered by face mask versus conventional medical therapy. NIPPV reduced the need for endotracheal intubation (ETI), the duration of intensive care unit (ICU) stay, and mortality rate only in those patients with hypercapnia ($PaCO_2$ >45 mm Hg). In a large study[17] on the use of NIPPV to treat respiratory failure of varied origins, 41 of 158 patients were hypoxaemic. These patients required ETI in only 34 per cent of cases, and showed a mortality rate of 22 per cent.

In another RCT,[9] NIPPV was compared to invasive mechanical ventilation in 64 patients with hypoxaemic ARF. After 1 hour of mechanical ventilation, both groups had a significant improvement in oxygenation. Ten (31 per cent) patients treated with NIPPV required ETI. Patients randomized to conventional ventilation more frequently developed septic complications including pneumonia or sinusitis ($p = 0.003$). Among survivors, NIPPV patients had a lower duration of mechanical ventilation ($p = 0.006$) and a shorter ICU stay ($p = 0.002$). Substantially negative results were found in an RCT[10] of 27 patients admitted to the emergency department with hypoxaemic respiratory failure and who received NIPPV or conventional medical therapy. The 16 patients in the NIPPV group had an ETI rate and duration of ICU stay similar to the 11 patients who received medical treatment alone, with a trend towards a greater rate of hospital mortality.

Delclaux *et al.*[14] randomly assigned 123 patients with hypoxaemic ARF ($n = 102$ with ALI and $n = 21$ with cardiac disease) to receive standard medical therapy or CPAP. CPAP provided rapid but transient improvements in oxygenation and dyspnoea but failed to reduce ETI rate, hospital mortality or ICU stay compared with standard therapy.

A subset analysis of 29 patients with non-COPD-related ARF[13] showed that patients treated by non-invasive bi-level positive airway pressure ventilation had a lower ETI rate per 100 ICU days compared with a usual care group (8.5 vs 30.3; $p = 0.01$), although no difference in ICU mortality rates was observed between the groups.

Ferrer *et al.*[16] prospectively randomized 105 patients with severe hypoxaemic ARF to receive NIPPV or high concentration oxygen. Compared with oxygen therapy, NIPPV decreased the need for ETI (25 per cent vs 52 per cent), the incidence of septic shock (12 per cent vs 31 per cent), and the ICU mortality (18 per cent vs 39 per cent), and increased the cumulative 90-day survival ($p < 0.05$ for all the variables).

In ALI/ARDS,[18] transient loss of positive pressure during mechanical ventilation may seriously compromise lung recruitment and gas exchange. For this reason, most NIPPV studies have excluded patients with ALI/ARDS, and limited data are currently available. The first application of NIV (via face mask CPAP) in patients with ARDS was reported by Barach *et al.* in 1938.[19] In a group of 35 patients with ARDS of varied aetiologies, face mask CPAP improved oxygenation within the first hour of therapy.[20] Five patients were ultimately intubated, due to mask discomfort and lack of cooperation. Two RCTs[9,12] reported that in patients with ARDS ($n = 31$), NIPPV avoided ETI in 60 per cent of the cases. In another study on 10 haemodynamically stable patients with severe ALI or ARDS,[21] NIPPV successfully avoided ETI in 6 of 12 episodes of ARF in 10 patients whose mean baseline $PaO_2/FiO_2$ was 102. By contrast, seven ARDS patients included in a larger population with heterogeneous hypoxaemic ARF had an 86 per cent ETI rate.[16] Antonelli *et al.*[22] prospectively investigated the application of NIPPV as first-line intervention in 147 ICU patients with early ARDS. NIPPV improved gas exchange and avoided ETI in 54 per cent of treated patients. NIPPV success was associated with less pneumonia (2 per cent vs 20 per cent, $p < 0.001$) and a lower ICU mortality rate (6 per cent vs 53 per cent, $p < 0.001$) than failures.

Complications associated with ETI in immunosuppressed patients have been widely described.[23–25] In these patients, the use of NIV has provided positive results. In a pilot study[26] on 16 patients with haematological malignancies and ARF, 15 individuals showed a significant improvement in blood gases and respiratory rate within the first 24 hours of nasal mask NIPPV treatment. Five patients died in the ICU following complications independent of the respiratory failure, while 11 were discharged from the ICU in stable condition. Forty recipients of solid organ

**Table 28.1** Randomized controlled studies using non-invasive ventilation in hypoxaemic respiratory failure

| Authors | Year of study | Population | Intervention | | Sample size | Need for ETI | ICU LOS | ICU mortality | Hospital mortality |
|---|---|---|---|---|---|---|---|---|---|
| | | | NIV | Control | (NIV/ Control) | (NIV/ Control, %) | (NIV/ Control, days) | (NIV/ Control, %) | (NIV/Control, %) |
| Wysocki[8] | 1995 | Varied | PSV | UMC | 21/20 | 62/70 | 17 ± 19 / 25 ± 23 | 33/50 | |
| Antonelli[9] | 1998 | Varied | PSV | Invasive MV | 32/32 | 31.3/NA | 9 ± 7 / 16 ± 17* | 28/47 | |
| Wood[10] | 1998 | Varied, emergency dept. | Bi PAP | UMC | 16/11 | 45.5/43.8 | 5.8 ± 5.5 / 4.9 ± 3.2 | | 25/0 |
| Confalonieri *et al.*[11] | †1999 | CAP | PSV | UMC | 16/17 | 37.5/47.1 | 2.9 ± 1.8 / 4.8 ± 1.7 | | 37.5/23.5* |
| Antonelli *et al.*[12] | 2000 | IC | PSV | UMC | 20/20 | 20/70* | 5.5 ± 3 / 9 ± 4* | 20/50* | 35/55 |
| Martin *et al.*[13] | 2000 | Varied | Bi PAP | UMC | 16/13 | 37.5/77* | | 25/54 | |
| Delclaux *et al.*[14] | 2000 | ALI or cardiac disease | CPAP | UMC | 62/61 | 34/39 | 6.5 (1–57) / 6 (1–36) | 21/25 | 31/30 |
| Hilbert *et al.*[15] | 2001 | IC | PSV | UMC | 26/26 | 46/77* | 7 ± 3 / 9 ± 4 | 38/69* | 50/81* |
| Ferrer *et al.*[16] | 2003 | Varied | Bi PAP | UCM | 51/54 | 25/52* | 9.6 ± 12.6 / 11.3 ± 12.6 | 9.2/21.4* | |

BiPAP, bi-level positive airway pressure; CAP, community-acquired pneumonia; ETI, endotracheal intubation; IC, immunocompromised; ICU, intensive care unit; LOS, length of stay; MV, mechanical ventilation; NA, not applicable; NIV, non-invasive ventilation; PSV, pressure support ventilation; UMC, usual medical care.

*Significant difference.

†Subset analysis.

transplantation with ARF were randomized to receive NIPPV versus conventional therapy.[12] Patients treated with NIPPV more often achieved a better oxygenation (60 per cent vs 25 per cent, $p=0.03$) with lower ETI (20 per cent vs 70 per cent, $p=0.002$) and ICU mortality rates (20 per cent vs 50 per cent, $p=0.05$). In an RCT of 52 ARF patients with pneumonia and immunocompromise of varied origin, Hilbert *et al.*[15] showed reductions of ETIs (46 per cent vs 77 per cent, $p=0.03$), and lower mortality rate (50 per cent vs 81 per cent, $p=0.02$) when NIPPV treated patients were compared to controls. NIPPV represents a useful tool to avoid ETI and related complications in selected immunocompromised patients.

The application of NIV to treat pneumonia has yielded no definitive conclusions. In a large RCT[16] on patients with severe hypoxaemic failure, NIPPV prevented ETI and improved ICU survival in a subgroup of 34 patients with pneumonia compared with high-concentration oxygen treatment. NIPPV was associated with a significant reduction in the ETI rate and duration of ICU stay in an RCT including 56 patients with severe community-acquired pneumonia (CAP), in comparison with standard treatment.[11] Post-hoc analysis showed that the benefits occurred only in patients with associated COPD. Jolliet *et al.*[27] used face mask NIPPV in patients with severe (CAP). Despite initial improvements in arterial oxygenation and respiratory rate in 22 of 24 patients, the ETI rate was high (66 per cent). Evaluating the acute effects of NIPPV in a group of non-COPD patients with cardiogenic pulmonary oedema ($n$ = 15) or CAP ($n$ = 18), NIPPV rapidly induced an improvement in arterial oxygenation, but the final outcome was worse in CAP patients, with a higher ETI rate and a longer time spent on ventilation.[28] NIPPV might be indicated in patients with CAP, but great caution should be applied.

## PRACTICAL CONSIDERATIONS

The criteria for selecting appropriate candidates to receive NIV in the ARF setting include clinical indicators such as dyspnoea, tachypnoea, accessory muscle use, paradoxical abdominal breathing and gas exchange deterioration. NIV should be avoided in some clinical conditions as when shock is present (Box 28.1), and criteria for ETI and NIV discontinuation must be thoroughly considered to prevent dangerous delays of invasive ventilation (Box 28.2). Collaboration among physicians, respiratory therapists and nurses is critical to successful application of NIV. During the early phases of milder respiratory failure and after an initial period of continuous administration, NIV can be intermittently applied, with periods of 10–20 minutes interruption. For more severe patients, NIV application has to be continuous for at least 12–24 hours. Aggressive physiotherapy is crucial during the periods of NIV discontinuation.

Identification of predictors of success or failure may help in recognizing patients who are likely to benefit from NIV and exclude those for whom NIV would be unsafe or ineffective. In a multicentre cohort study on patients with hypoxaemic ARF,[29] the risk of NIPPV failure was higher when patients had a higher severity score, were older or failed to improve after 1 hour of treatment. The presence of ARDS or CAP was independently associated with failure of NIPPV, whereas the lowest ETI rate was observed in patients with cardiogenic pulmonary oedema and pulmonary contusion.[29] In a more recent analysis on the use of NIPPV in ARDS,[22] a Simplified Acute Physiology Score II >34 and a $PaO_2/FiO_2 \leq 175$ after 1 hour of therapy were independently associated with NIPPV failure and need for ETI.

### Box 28.1 Criteria for discontinuation of non-invasive ventilation and endotracheal intubation

- Technique intolerance (pain, discomfort or claustrophobia)
- Inability to improve gas exchanges and/or dyspnoea in the first hours (best predictor of success is a good response within 1 hour)
- Haemodynamic instability or evidence of shock, cardiac ischaemia or ventricular arrhythmia
- Inability to improve mental status in agitated patients within 30 minutes after the application of NIV

### Box 28.2 Contraindications to non-invasive ventilation

- Coma, seizures or severe central neurological disturbances
- Inability to protect the airway or clear respiratory secretions
- Unstable haemodynamic conditions (blood pressure or rhythm instability)
- Severe upper gastrointestinal bleeding
- Recent facial surgery, trauma, or burns or inability to fit mask
- Recent gastro-oesophageal surgery
- Undrained pneumothorax
- Vomiting

## CONCLUSIONS AND FUTURE PERSPECTIVES

NIPPV can be used to treat hypoxaemic patients without hypercapnia. However, an extremely prudent approach is needed, limiting the application of NIPPV to haemodynamically stable patients who can be closely monitored in the ICU, where ETI is promptly available. Patients at high risk of failure should be closely managed only by experienced personnel and with a low threshold for ETI.

Controlled studies of NIV in non-hypercapnic respiratory failure, in which the patient subgroups are differentiated and analysed separately by diagnostic category, would be useful in clarifying the role of NIV in the very heterogeneous category of hypoxaemic patients.

## REFERENCES


1. Katz JA, Marks JD. Inspiratory work with and without continuous positive airway pressure in patients with acute respiratory failure. *Anesthesiology* 1985; **63**: 598–607.
2. L'Her E, Deye N, Lellouche F *et al.* Physiologic effects of noninvasive ventilation during acute lung injury. *Am J Respir Crit Care Med* 2005; **172**: 1112–18.
3. Räsänen J, Heikkilä J, Downs J *et al.* Continuous positive airway pressure by face mask in acute cardiogenic pulmonary edema. *Am J Cardiol* 1985; **55**: 296–300.
4. Naughton MT, Rahman MA, Hara K *et al.* Effect of continuous positive airway pressure on intrathoracic and left ventricular transmural pressures in patients with congestive heart failure. *Circulation* 1995; **91**: 1725–31.
5. Meduri GU, Conoscenti CC, Menashe P *et al.* Noninvasive face mask ventilation in patients with acute respiratory failure. *Chest* 1989; **95**: 865–70.
6. Pennock BE, Crawshaw L, Kaplan PD. Noninvasive nasal mask ventilation for acute respiratory failure. Institution of a new therapeutic technology for routine use. *Chest* 1994; **105**: 441–4.
7. Lapinsky SE, Mount DB, Mackey D *et al.* Management of acute respiratory failure due to pulmonary edema with nasal positive pressure support. *Chest* 1994; **105**: 229–31.
8. Wysocki M, Tric L, Wolff MA *et al.* Noninvasive pressure support ventilation in patients with acute respiratory failure: a randomized comparison with conventional therapy. *Chest* 1995; **107**: 761–8.
9. Antonelli M, Conti G, Rocco M *et al.* A comparison of noninvasive positive-pressure ventilation and conventional mechanical ventilation in patients with acute respiratory failure. *N Engl J Med* 1998; **339**: 429–35.
10. Wood KA, Lewis L, Von Harz B *et al.* The use of noninvasive positive pressure ventilation in the emergency department. *Chest* 1998; **113**: 1339–46.
11. Confalonieri M, Potena A, Carbone G *et al.* Acute respiratory failure in patients with severe community-acquired pneumonia. A prospective randomized evaluation of noninvasive ventilation. *Am J Respir Crit Care Med* 1999; **160**: 1585–91.
12. Antonelli M, Conti C, Bufi M *et al.* Noninvasive ventilation for treatment of acute respiratory failure in patients undergoing solid organ transplantation. *JAMA* 2000; **283**: 235–41.
13. Martin TJ, Hovis JD, Costantino JP *et al.* A randomized prospective evaluation of noninvasive ventilation for acute respiratory failure. *Am J Respir Crit Care Med* 2000; **161**: 807–13.
14. Delclaux C, L'Her E, Alberti C *et al.* Treatment of acute hypoxemic nonhypercapnic respiratory insufficiency with continuous positive airway pressure delivered by a face mask: A randomized controlled trial. *JAMA* 2000; **284**: 2352–60.
15. Hilbert G, Gruson D, Vargas F *et al.* Noninvasive ventilation in immunosuppressed patients with pulmonary infiltrates, fever, and acute respiratory failure. *N Engl J Med* 2001; **344**: 481–7.
16. Ferrer M, Esquinas A, Leon M *et al.* Noninvasive ventilation in severe hypoxemic respiratory failure: a randomized clinical trial. *Am J Respir Crit Care Med* 2003; **168**: 1438–44.
17. Meduri GU, Turner RE, Abou-Shala N *et al.* Noninvasive positive pressure ventilation via face mask. *Chest* 1996; **109**: 179–93.
18. Bernard GR, Artigas A, Brigham KL *et al.* The American-European Consensus Conference on ARDS. Definitions, mechanisms, relevant outcomes, and clinical trial coordination. *Am J Respir Crit Care Med* 1994; **149**: 818–24.
19. Barach AL, Martin J, Eckman M. Positive-pressure respiration and its application to the treatment of acute pulmonary edema. *Ann Intern Med* 1938; **12**: 754–95.
20. Covelli HD, Weled BJ, Beekman JF. Efficacy of continuous positive airway pressure administered by face mask. *Chest* 1982; **81**: 147–50.
21. Rocker GM, Mackensie M-G, Willilams B *et al.* Noninvasive positive pressure ventilation: successful outcome in patients with acute lung injury/ARDS. *Chest* 1999; **115**: 173–7.
22. Antonelli M, Conti G, Esquinas A *et al.* A multiple-center survey on the use in clinical practice of noninvasive ventilation as a first-line intervention for acute respiratory distress sindrome. *Crit Care Med* 2007; **35**: 18–25.
23. Estopa R, Torres Marti A, Kastanos N *et al.* Acute respiratory failure in severe hematologic disorders. *Crit Care Med* 1984; **12**: 26–8.
24. Blot F, Guignet M, Nitenberg G *et al.* Prognostic factors for neutropenic patients in an intensive care unit: respective roles of underlying malignancies and acute organ failures. *Eur J Cancer* 1997; **33**: 1031–7.
25. Ewig S, Torres A, Riquelme R *et al.* Pulmonary complications in patients with haematological malignancies treated at a respiratory ICU. *Eur Respir J* 1998; **12**: 116–22.
26. Conti G, Marino P, Cogliati A *et al.* Noninvasive ventilation for the treatment of acute respiratory failure in patients with hematologic malignancies: a pilot study. *Intensive Care Med* 1998; **24**: 1283–8.

27. Jolliet P, Abajo B, Pasquina P *et al.* Non-invasive pressure support ventilation in severe community-acquired pneumonia. *Intensive Care Med* 2001; **27**: 812–21.
28. Domenighetti G, Gayer R, Gentilini R. Noninvasive pressure support ventilation in non-COPD patients with acute cardiogenic pulmonary edema and severe community-acquired pneumonia: acute effects and outcome. *Intensive Care Med* 2002; **28**: 1226–32.
29. Antonelli M, Conti G, Moro ML *et al.* Predictors of failure of noninvasive positive pressure ventilation in patients with acute hypoxemic respiratory failure: a multi-center study. *Intensive Care Med* 2001; **27**: 1718–28.

# SECTION F

# Cardiac failure

# 29

# Pathophysiology and modern management of cardiac failure

MARTIN R COWIE, PAUL M HAYDOCK


## ABSTRACT

Cardiac failure is a clinical syndrome comprising a triad of breathlessness, fatigue and fluid retention. These symptoms can be the result of any disorder, genetic or acquired, affecting the structure or function of the heart in a manner that impairs its ability to act as an efficient pump. Heart failure is not a stand-alone diagnosis – identification of the aetiology and how the body has responded to the cardiac dysfunction is key to providing optimal management of the individual patient. The syndrome can develop relatively suddenly (acute de-novo heart failure), or can be present for many months or years (chronic heart failure). Acute decompensation of the chronic syndrome is not infrequent, particularly where compliance with treatment is poor, monitoring is sub-standard, or with intercurrent illness. The syndrome is characterized by cardiac dysfunction, consequent haemodynamic changes attempting to maintain circulatory homeostasis, changes in breathing pattern, sodium and fluid retention through renal and neurohormonal mechanisms, changes in muscle blood flow, and immune activation. In suspected heart failure, the physician should remember that identification of the syndrome is based on history and examination combined with appropriate investigations; a normal resting electrocardiogram should raise doubt regarding the validity of the diagnosis; plasma natriuretic peptide levels can help to establish the diagnosis; and echocardiography should be used to image the heart for quantifiable determination of cardiac structure and function. Where heart failure is confirmed, management consists of lifestyle measures and the introduction and optimization of medications such as diuretics, inhibitors of the renin–angiotensin–aldosterone axis, and selected β-blockers. For patients fulfilling certain criteria, implantable defibrillators or cardiac resynchronization therapy can also decrease mortality and, in the latter case, improve symptoms. Despite improvements in our understanding of the pathophysiology, and a wider range of therapeutic options, heart failure remains a serious condition, with considerable morbidity and mortality. A condition largely of the elderly, its prevalence is set to rise as the population ages. Optimal management requires close monitoring of the syndrome, multiple medications and increasingly some form of implantable electrical device therapy. Communication between the patient and all professionals involved in their care is essential in optimizing the outcome.


## INTRODUCTION

Heart failure is a clinical syndrome arising as a consequence of the body's response to a heart that is unable to provide a physiologically appropriate output under normal loading conditions. It can occur as the result of any abnormality of the structure or function of the heart.[1] Until the 1980s, understanding of heart failure was based on a haemodynamic model, exemplified by Paul Wood's 1950 definition: 'A state in which the heart fails to maintain an adequate circulation for the needs of the body despite a satisfactory filling pressure.'[2] Recognition that many cases involved increased peripheral vasoconstriction and reduced cardiac contractility resulted in treatment strategies targeted towards improving these haemodynamic parameters by the use of peripheral vasodilators and inotropic agents.

However, work done in the past two decades has greatly increased our understanding of the pathophysiology of heart failure, and it is now accepted that the key to improving symptoms and prognosis is by incremental inhibition of the marked neurohormonal activation that is triggered by the cardiac dysfunction.[3]

Heart failure may occur relatively suddenly – acute *de novo* heart failure – or may be present for months to years – chronic heart failure. The latter may decompensate acutely and lead to hospital admission, similarly to *de novo* heart failure. Acute heart failure syndromes can be classified into several clinical presentations:[4]

- worsening chronic heart failure
- pulmonary oedema
- hypertensive heart failure (high blood pressure and usually relatively preserved left ventricular [LV] systolic function)
- cardiogenic shock
- isolated right heart failure (low output syndrome with no pulmonary congestion but increased jugular venous pressure and low LV filling pressures)
- acute coronary syndrome with heart failure.

Unless the precipitant is completely reversible and there is no lasting damage to the heart, most patients with acute heart failure will enter the chronic phase of the syndrome. Mortality in this group is typically 10 per cent per annum with evidence-based practice,[5] but considerably higher where there is suboptimal treatment or monitoring.

Most patients with heart failure are elderly – the average age at first presentation being 75 in developed countries.[6] Consequently, many patients have considerable comorbidity, such as renal or cognitive dysfunction. Coronary artery disease is the main aetiology in European populations, with hypertension, diabetes, atrial fibrillation (AF) and chronic airways disease frequently also present (Table 29.1). Such comorbidity often limits the amount of therapy that can be safely applied, and necessitates more frequent monitoring.

## HOW DOES HEART FAILURE START?

In a minority of cases, there is a clear insult that can acutely affect overall pump function. This could be acute myocardial infarction, with regional myocardial necrosis leading to a substantial and potentially permanent reduction in ventricular function. Another example is the sudden onset of AF in an elderly hypertensive heart leading to heart failure. In many patients, however, there is no clear single precipitant, and the syndrome is triggered by a number of factors such as chest infection in addition to chronic coronary artery disease, diabetes and hypertension (Fig. 29.1). In chronic valve disease the development of progressive cardiac dysfunction and symptoms is often insidious and the valvular dysfunction may be unsuspected for many years until the full blown heart failure syndrome is diagnosed. It is worth remembering that heritable myopathies and dystrophinopathies (including, but not limited to, Becker and Duchenne) are responsible not only for abnormalities of skeletal muscle, but also have effects on the structure of the myocardium. Respiratory physicians, and others who work with NIV, will encounter these patients more frequently than others in clinical practice and should be attuned to the likely benefits of involving a cardiologist at an early stage of their management, as cardiac dysfunction may not manifest clinically in patients with limited mobility until advanced heart failure has developed. Indeed, there is evidence that developments in respiratory care in such patients have increased the importance of cardiomyopathy, with 10–15 per cent dying from progressive cardiac failure. It is particularly important to note that the prognostically beneficial drug therapies described later in this chapter have also demonstrated improvements in outcome when administered to such patients.[11]

The degree of cardiac dysfunction can be described in a number of ways but typically by using some measure of LV function or dimensions (most often ejection fraction [EF]).

**Table 29.1** Prevalence of comorbidity in heart failure recorded in several multicentre, 'real world' trials (aggregate data from CHARM, 3-CPO and EuroHeart Failure studies)[7–9]

| Comorbidity | Percentage of patients |
|---|---|
| Coronary artery disease | 62 |
| Hypertension | 55 |
| Diabetes mellitus | 28 |
| Hypercholesterolaemia | 41 |
| Atrial fibrillation | 35 |
| Chronic airways disease | 26 |
| Renal dysfunction | 17 |
| Cerebrovascular disease | 15 |
| Peripheral vascular disease | 10 |
| Cognitive impairment/dementia | 12 |

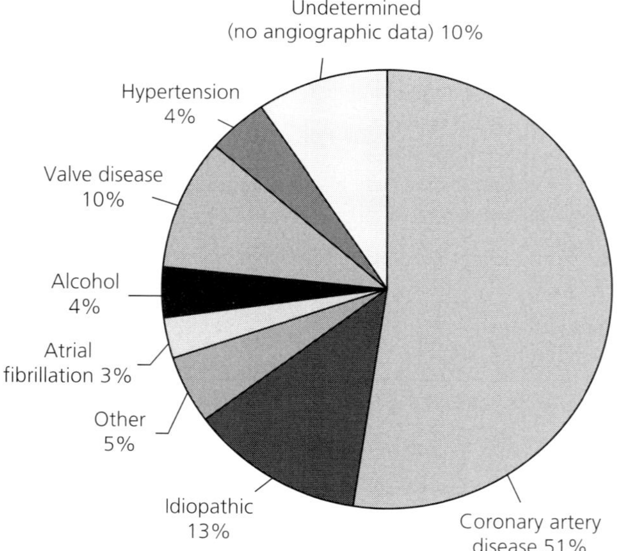


**Figure 29.1** Aetiology of heart failure assessed in 136 under-75s with a new diagnosis of heart failure, using coronary angiography and myocardial perfusion scanning to determine presence of aetiologically important coronary artery disease (author's own data from the Bromley Heart Failure Study).[10]

Such measurements can be made by echocardiography, magnetic resonance imaging or radionuclide angiography. Most of the early drug trials in chronic heart failure recruited patients with severe systolic dysfunction of the LV, e.g. EF <40 per cent. More recently, however, it has been recognized that heart failure can occur even with a relatively normal EF ('diastolic heart failure', 'heart failure with preserved EF'). The clinical presentation with both reduced and preserved EF can be identical[12,13] but the dysfunction in the latter is typically an LV which contracts relatively normally during systole but appears 'stiff' and relaxes slowly in diastole. The classical patient with heart failure with preserved EF has a history of hypertension, with some evidence of LV hypertrophy and at least mild left atrial dilatation.[14,15]

Valve dysfunction is also not uncommon as a cause of HF – with aortic stenosis an increasingly important cause of heart failure in the very elderly. A trigger such as the onset of AF, increase in systemic blood pressure or the development of a chest infection, can also precipitate sudden increases in left atrial pressure and the onset of pulmonary oedema. Such acute decompensation often resolves rapidly with normalization of cardiac rhythm or blood pressure.

## The whole body response to cardiac dysfunction

Cardiac dysfunction results in the activation of mechanical and biochemical homeostatic mechanisms designed to compensate for the potential reduction in cardiac output. While these mechanisms initially produce the desired effect of maintaining organ perfusion, they are ultimately maladaptive and result in the development of progressive heart failure, as the failing heart has to pump against increased peripheral resistance, and reduced muscle perfusion leads to increasing exercise intolerance and fatigue.

The progression of heart failure is usually characterized by a process of LV remodelling, whereby the main pumping chamber becomes increasingly globular and dilated. Such changes can be easily detected by echocardiography or other imaging tests. However, the severity of the syndrome is often only poorly correlated with the size of the ventricle.

Recently, it has been recognized that venous congestion is an important cause of worsening of the heart failure syndrome, with renal perfusion being decreased markedly by high venous pressure in addition to the effects of low cardiac output.[16] Liver congestion is a common feature of advanced heart failure and can cause abdominal discomfort, particularly on exertion. Gut congestion may also play a role in increasing circulating levels of cytokines.

### NEUROHORMONAL ACTIVATION

Key to the severity of the syndrome is the degree of neurohormonal activation that occurs. This affects a large number of homeostatic systems, the most important of which are outlined below.

#### Renin–angiotensin–aldosterone system (RAAS)

Decreased renal perfusion results in the secretion of renin from the juxtaglomerular apparatus. Concurrently, production of angiotensinogen is increased by the liver and there is a consequent increase in circulating angiotensin I. The action of the angiotensin-converting enzyme (ACE) in the lungs converts angiotensin I into the effector hormone angiotensin II. This molecule is a highly potent vasoconstrictor acting on the efferent renal arterioles and the systemic arteriolar bed via both activation of the sympathetic nervous system and stimulation of endothelin release.

Angiotensin II also stimulates aldosterone secretion from the adrenal cortex, promoting salt and water retention (and potassium loss). High levels of antidiuretic hormone (ADH/vasopressin) are also seen in heart failure and some of this increased secretion is due to direct effects of angiotensin II on the pituitary. Both angiotensin II and aldosterone have direct effects on cardiac myocytes, accelerating ventricular remodelling. Angiotensin II causes myocyte hypertrophy and fibrosis, whereas aldosterone results in apoptosis of myocytes and fibrosis.

#### Sympathetic nervous system (SNS)

Angiotensin II stimulates release of noradrenaline (norepinephrine) from sympathetic nerve terminals and inhibits vagal tone. The SNS is also directly stimulated by baroreceptors in response to a fall in perfusion pressure. Increased circulating adrenaline (epinephrine) and noradrenaline act to increase blood pressure and heart rate, with concomitant increased myocardial oxygen demand. Prolonged exposure to high circulating levels of these hormones is toxic to the myocardium. To compound the situation, sympathetic activity itself stimulates the RAAS yet further.

#### Natriuretic peptides

Stretching of the atrial and ventricular walls results in the secretion of ANP (atrial natriuretic peptide) and BNP (B-type natriuretic peptide), respectively. These hormones act to ameliorate the effects of the SNS and RAAS, promoting vasodilatation and natriuresis. Assays are available for the detection of BNP and its inactive N-terminal cleavage fragment (NT-proBNP), which can be helpful in ruling out heart failure – especially in cases where the EF is preserved – as a normal plasma level makes heart failure most unlikely.

### CYTOKINES

It is now recognized that heart failure is an inflammatory state.[17] Levels of tumour necrosis factor (TNF)-$\alpha$, interleukin 1 (IL-1) and IL-6 are elevated and can result in myocyte hypertrophy and apoptosis. These circulating cytokines not only affect the heart but are also at least partially responsible for the cachexia associated with advanced heart failure.[18]

### ARRHYTHMIA

Occasionally, prolonged tachyarrhythmia can lead to a reversible cardiomyopathy.[19] More usually, raised intracardiac pressures and myocardial stretch increase the risk of AF and malignant ventricular dysrrhythmia (sustained tachycardia [VT] or fibrillation [VF]).[7] This risk is compounded by neurohormonal activation, electrolyte abnormalities, and drug toxicities.

The onset of AF can precipitate a sudden worsening of the heart failure syndrome and VT or VF can be life-threatening if they do not terminate speedily. Sudden death as a result of such events is the cause of up to 50 per cent of deaths in heart failure, the others being usually due to progressive heart failure or other cardiovascular events.[20,21]

### CONTROL OF BREATHING

Up to 50 per cent of patients with heart failure show evidence of marked sleep-disordered breathing, with central sleep apnoea or hypopnoea being found in the majority.[22] For further information on this and the potential role of therapy using non-invasive assisted ventilation, see Chapter 31 of this volume.

## MANAGEMENT OF HEART FAILURE

Good diagnosis is the key to good management. Heart failure is not a complete diagnosis in itself, and the nature and cause of the cardiac dysfunction must be determined. Significant comorbidity should also be identified, along with exacerbating or precipitating factors. The aim of treatment is twofold: to improve life-expectancy, and to improve symptoms. Recent international guidelines have been published[4,23–25] and are frequently updated as the evidence base increases.

An emphasis on patient education as well as timely recognition and communication of symptoms heralding decompensation should form the cornerstone of any heart failure management plan, and multidisciplinary input from a range of health professionals is required to ensure that patients achieve the full benefit of their therapies. The risk of emergency hospitalization can be reduced substantially by specialist nurse home visits, telephone support, or remote monitoring.[26]

### DIAGNOSIS

Symptoms of dyspnoea, fatigue or fluid retention should alert the physician to potential heart failure, though symptoms may be non-typical and include dizziness, confusion, anorexia, abdominal bloating or nocturia. Often, a careful history and examination will uncover the more typical signs and symptoms of heart failure. Where such symptoms and signs are present the following tests are recommended to either rule out common masquerading conditions (Box 29.1) or to confirm heart failure and identify the aetiology:

- 12-lead surface electrocardiogram (ECG)
  - where the ECG is normal, heart failure due to systolic dysfunction is unlikely
  - where the ECG is abnormal it may provide clues to the underlying aetiology, e.g. evidence of previous myocardial infarction or LV hypertrophy. Arrhythmia may also be identified which might necessitate medication, electrical cardioversion or permanent pacemaker
- chest radiograph taken in the postero-anterior projection – this may demonstrate cardiomegaly or pulmonary venous congestion, but it is most useful to exclude significant lung pathology
- blood analyses:
  - serum electrolytes, urea and creatinine
  - full blood count
  - thyroid function tests
  - liver function tests including albumin
  - fasting glucose and lipid profile
  - assay of plasma BNP or NT-proBNP concentration
  - in the emergency setting, arterial blood gases. Acidosis and/or carbon dioxide retention is associated with a poor prognosis
- urinalysis for proteinuria and glycosuria
- cardiac imaging by echocardiography – information should be provided on the structure and function of all four cardiac chambers, all valves and the pericardium. If such information cannot be provided then alternative methods of cardiac imaging are required (most usually cardiac magnetic resonance imaging [cMRI]). Such alternative techniques are often required where thoracic abnormalities are present, e.g. radionuclide ventriculography has been demonstrated to be useful in determining LVEF in cases of Duchenne muscular dystrophy.[27]

**Box 29.1 Other conditions that may present with symptoms similar to heart failure**

- Obesity
- Chest disease – including lung, diaphragm or chest wall disease
- Venous insufficiency in lower limbs
- Drug-induced ankle swelling (e.g. amlodipine, nifedipine, felodipine)
- Drug-induced fluid retention (e.g. steroids, non-steroidal anti-inflammatory drugs [NSAIDs])
- Hypoalbuminaemia
- Intrinsic renal or hepatic disease
- Pulmonary embolic disease
- Depression and/or anxiety
- Severe anaemia
- Severe thyroid disease
- Bilateral renal artery stenosis

Occasionally, objective evidence of cardiac dysfunction will be identified in the absence of heart failure symptoms during investigation of other disorders. In such cases, medical therapy is indicated to limit the progression of disease and a full work-up should be done to identify the underlying cause.[28]

### PROGNOSTICATION

It is important that healthcare professionals discuss the diagnosis and prognosis in a sensitive, yet realistic, manner. Life-expectancy is markedly reduced in heart failure and mortality is especially high in the first year following diagnosis – estimated at 20–30 per cent.[29] Overall in-hospital mortality for patients presenting with an acute heart failure syndrome is around 10 per cent, but cardiogenic shock has a considerably poorer outlook.[30] Of all heart failure patients who do survive to discharge one in four will be readmitted within 12 weeks,[31] unless they are entered into a good chronic disease management programme.[32]

Many clinical factors have been shown to affect prognosis, the most important being:[33,34]

- age at first presentation
- extent of comorbidity
- severity of symptoms as expressed by New York Heart Association (NYHA) grade (Table 29.2)
- severity of LV systolic dysfunction (LVSD)
- plasma BNP or NT-proBNP concentration
- renal function and plasma sodium
- blood pressure at presentation
- peak oxygen consumption on cardiopulmonary exercise testing.[35]

Risk stratification is rarely done formally in clinical practice, except for patients who are being considered for transplantation.[36] The involvement of those with palliative care skills can be particularly beneficial towards the end of life, and should be considered for all those with progressive heart failure despite optimal medical therapy.

### ADDRESSING LIFESTYLE ISSUES

Patient education regarding the adoption of beneficial lifestyle measures (and the avoidance of those likely to be harmful) has an important role in the management of chronic heart failure. Few recommendations are based on high level evidence but the following are widely accepted as good practice.

- Fluid restriction is useful in patients with resistant oedema or hyponatraemia. It is not usually required of patients with mild, stable symptoms.
- Restriction of salt intake to a maximum of 6 g per day.
- Alcohol consumption within recommended limits is probably safe, though the fluid load may be excessive. If alcoholic cardiomyopathy is suspected, abstinence should be encouraged as it can lead to marked improvements in ventricular function.
- In all but those patients in NYHA class IV, physical activity should be encouraged to improve symptoms related to deconditioning.[37] Swimming, however, is best avoided as submersion may have undesirable effects on central haemodynamics.

## Disease-modifying drug therapies

Trials in patients with HF due to LV systolic dysfunction have repeatedly confirmed the benefits of drugs that antagonize the maladaptive neurohormonal mechanisms described above. These drugs affect disease progression and improve prognosis. They should be prescribed to all patients with heart failure and LV systolic dysfunction who are able to tolerate them, but need to be introduced at low dose and titrated upwards to target doses with appropriate clinical supervision of symptoms, renal function, blood pressure and side effects.

A role for the use of these agents in heart failure with preserved EF is less clear-cut, with large randomized trials of ACE inhibitors and angiotensin-receptor blockers being

**Table 29.2** New York Heart Association (NYHA) classification of heart failure severity by symptoms

| NYHA class | Description | Category |
|---|---|---|
| I | No limitation: ordinary physical activity does not cause fatigue, breathlessness or palpitations | Asymptomatic |
| II | Slight limitation in physical activity: comfortable at rest but ordinary activity results in fatigue, breathlessness or palpitations | Mild |
| III | Marked limitation of physical activity: comfortable at rest but less than ordinary activity results in fatigue, breathlessness or palpitations | Moderate |
| IV | Unable to carry out any physical activity without discomfort: symptoms of cardiac failure at rest with increased discomfort with any physical activity | Severe |

neutral. Further large-scale trials are awaited to inform better management of these patients in the future.

## ACE INHIBITORS

Angiotensin-converting enzyme inhibitors reduce the relative risk of death by 23 per cent and the relative risk of worsening heart failure by 35 per cent.[38,39] Their beneficial effects have also been seen in asymptomatic left ventricular systolic dysfunction and heart failure post myocardial infarction.[40,41] Angiotensin-converting enzyme inhibitors work by reducing the production of angiotensin II, therefore reducing direct myocyte toxicity and deleterious peripheral and renal vasoconstriction. Several preparations are licensed for use in heart failure (Table 29.3).

When commencing ACE inhibitors, the lowest starting dose should be used and the dose subsequently doubled at fortnightly intervals as blood pressure and renal function allow.[42] The aim should be to stabilize the patient on the target (maximum) dose. Blood pressure or renal dysfunction may limit up-titration.

Important side effects of ACE inhibitors are listed below.

- Troublesome cough – occurs in about 10 per cent of patients. Typically non-productive and clearly related to the commencement of the ACE inhibitors, it is the result of increased circulating bradykinin levels. Care should be taken to exclude lung disease or the onset of pulmonary oedema as an alternative explanation.
- Hypotension – this particularly manifests as orthostatic (postural) hypotension. It can be initially problematic but is often tolerated in the long term.
- Renal dysfunction – incremental rises in urea, creatinine and potassium are to be expected and accepted when using and up-titrating ACE inhibitors. Most physicians would accept a rise in creatinine of 50 μmol/L or to an absolute level of 250 μmol/L (any exaggerated deterioration in renal function following ACE inhibitor introduction should prompt the physician to consider the possibility of renal artery stenosis). Coadministration of nephrotoxic agents such as NSAIDs should be avoided if at all possible.
- Hyperkalaemia – increases to a serum potassium of 5.5 mmol/L are acceptable but these patients require closer monitoring.
- Angio-oedema – this is rare but can happen as an idiosyncratic reaction at any time. ACE inhibitors should be immediately withdrawn if any swelling of the face or tongue is noted.

## ANGIOTENSIN II RECEPTOR ANTAGONISTS

These drugs block angiotensin II at its receptor and consequently reduce the effect of the RAAS. Their clinical effect can be thought of as analogous to ACE inhibitors and they share the same side effect profile, except that they do not produce rises in bradykinin and so do not result in cough.

Again, several different agents are available. However, the evidence base is strongest for the use of candesartan in chronic heart failure[8] and valsartan for use in post myocardial infarction LVSD.[43] These drugs are not considered first-line therapy, but are reserved for use in patients who cannot tolerate ACE inhibitors due to cough.

## β-BLOCKERS

β-Blockers shown to have beneficial effects in heart failure, together with their dosing schedules, are listed in Table 29.4. Well-designed clinical trials have demonstrated β-blockers reduce the risk of all-cause mortality and death due to heart failure by 25 per cent and 35 per cent, respectively.[44–46] Although these long-term benefits are unquestionable, introduction of β-blockers can result in acute deterioration in the control of the heart failure syndrome due to abrupt changes in haemodynamic compensatory mechanisms. These agents should, therefore, be introduced and up-titrated cautiously, paying close attention to heart rate, blood pressure, fluid status and renal function.[42] If decompensation occurs with the introduction of β-blockade then temporary increases in diuretic dosing may improve the situation. These drugs are generally avoided in the acute setting of decompensation, particularly if the patient is fluid overloaded.

**Table 29.3** Angiotensin-converting enzyme (ACE) inhibitors used in the treatment of heart failure (based on recommendations from UK National Institute for Health and Clinical Excellence)[25]

| ACE inhibitor | Starting dose | Target dose |
|---|---|---|
| Captopril | 6.25 mg three times daily | 50 mg three times daily |
| Enalapril | 2.5 mg twice daily | 10–20 mg twice daily |
| Lisinopril | 2.5–5 mg once daily | 20 mg once daily |
| Ramipril | 2.5 mg once daily | 5 mg twice daily or 10 mg once daily |
| Trandolapril | 0.5 mg once daily | 4 mg once daily |

**Table 29.4** β-Blockers used in the treatment of heart failure (based on recommendations from UK National Institute for Health and Clinical Excellence)[25]

| BB | Starting dose | Target dose |
|---|---|---|
| Bisoprolol | 1.25 mg once daily | 10 mg once daily |
| Carvedilol | 3.125 mg twice daily | 25–50 mg twice daily |
| Nebivolol | 1.25 mg once daily | 10 mg once daily |

Side effects of β-blockers are well known, and include bradycardia, heart block and hypotension. Care is needed when considering the use of β-blockers in patients with peripheral vascular disease and chronic airways disease. However, cardioselective agents are considered safe except in cases of definite asthma.[47]

#### ALDOSTERONE ANTAGONISTS

Blockade of the aldosterone receptor is achieved by the use of either spironolactone or eplerenone. Experience with spironolactone in patients with moderate to severe chronic heart failure (NYHA III–IV) has revealed that use of a dose of 25 mg–50 mg is associated with a 30 per cent reduction in the relative risk of death.[48] A trial in mild chronic heart failure is ongoing. Eplerenone is a more selective aldosterone antagonist, of proven benefit in patients with low ejection fraction and either diabetes or heart failure when used in the post myocardial infarction setting.[49] Both drugs may cause hyperkalaemia and renal dysfunction and changes in fluid status can markedly increase this effect. Care should be taken to monitor electrolytes, urea and creatinine when introducing these drugs and when using them in periods of physiological instability. Eplerenone is much less likely to cause endocrine side effects, such as gynaecomastia, than spironolactone.

### Diuretics

Most patients with chronic heart failure will require some oral diuretic therapy. These drugs improve symptoms by easing fluid retention. However, their use may exacerbate neurohormonal activation by decreasing circulating blood volume. It is therefore of paramount importance that diuretics are used at the minimum required dose and in conjunction with the disease-modifying drugs described above. Periods of increased tendency to fluid retention may require higher dosage of diuretic, but this should be reduced again once control has been re-established. Many expert patients adjust their daily dose depending on their weight.

Commonly used diuretics are shown in Table 29.5. Loop diuretics are considered first-line treatment as they are most effective in causing efficient diuresis. A thiazide may be added in cases of resistant fluid retention. Potassium sparing diuretics can be useful in stimulating additional fluid loss, without excessive kaliuresis. (Note: Careful attention should be given to electrolytes and renal function, especially if using these agents with ACE inhibitors, angiotensin II receptor antagonists or aldosterone antagonists.)

In cases of severe decompensated heart failure, mucosal oedema of the gut wall limits the effectiveness of oral preparations and intravenous loop diuretics may be required to stimulate diuresis. In such cases, furosemide infusion can have a more powerful effect than bolus dosing.

### Other drugs used in heart failure

Several other medications are commonly prescribed as adjuncts in the management of heart failure. These are not considered standard therapy, and their use should be reviewed frequently.

#### DIGOXIN

Digitalis has been used for centuries for the treatment of congestive syndromes. There is little evidence to support its modern day use in patients with sinus rhythm but it is often added to conventional treatment in patients who have failed to respond to other therapies.[50] It can be useful in controlling ventricular rates in AF, but β-blockade is preferable and digoxin should be thought of as an 'add in' agent rather than first-line therapy.[51] Toxicity can arise easily in the elderly, particularly with changes in renal function or electrolytes as a result of intercurrent illness.

#### AMIODARONE

Well known as an effective treatment for atrial and ventricular tachyarrhythmia, amiodarone has numerous side effects of which the prescribing physician should be aware. It is vital that liver and thyroid function are routinely monitored in patients taking amiodarone and that these patients and their physicians are attendant to the potential for skin, eye and pulmonary complications. It is often used to suppress ventricular arrhythmia in patients with implantable cardiac defibrillators and thus prevent

**Table 29.5** Diuretics used in the treatment of heart failure (based on recommendations from UK National Institute for Health and Clinical Excellence)[25]

| Drug | Initial dose (mg) | Maximum recommended daily dose (mg) |
|---|---|---|
| Loop diuretics | | |
| – Bumetanide | 0.5–1.0 | 5–10 |
| – Furosemide | 20–40 | 250–500 |
| – Torasemide | 5–10 | 100–200 |
| Thiazides | | |
| – Bendroflumethiazide | 2.5 | 5 |
| – Metolazone | 2.5 | 10 |
| Potassium-sparing diuretics | | |
| – Amiloride | 2.5–5* | 20–40* |
| – Triamterene | 25–50* | 100–200* |

*Lower range appropriate for patient on angiotensin-converting enzyme inhibitor or an angiotensin-receptor blocker.

recurrent shocks. However, there is no evidence for a reduction in sudden cardiac death if it is used in the absence of such devices.[52]

Where AF complicates chronic heart failure, amiodarone may be used in an attempt to restore or maintain sinus rhythm.

#### ANTICOAGULANTS

Vitamin K antagonists are vital in heart failure complicated by AF to reduce thromboembolic risk. Such anticoagulants are also used where intracardiac thrombus has been observed on imaging, where there is evidence of left ventricular aneurysm, or in dilated cardiomyopathy with a history of thromboembolism.[53] Monitoring of anticoagulant control is essential.

#### NITRATE AND HYDRALAZINE COMBINATIONS

This previously widely used combination oral therapy has been superseded by ACE inhibitors. However, benefit has been demonstrated when this combination is added to ACE inhibitors/angiotensin II receptor antagonist and β-blocker in African American populations – probably due to their relative low renin phenotype.[54]

## Surgery and revascularization

Valve repair or replacement is potentially curative in heart failure due to valve dysfunction. Liaison with an experienced cardiac surgeon is necessary to decide on the optimum timing of any procedure. Valve disease should be identified early and monitored closely by a specialist and any acute deterioration should prompt urgent reassessment. Novel percutaneous techniques continue to be assessed for both valve repair and replacement.

Coronary artery bypass grafting and percutaneous revascularization methods have a place in treating ischaemic symptoms in patients with coronary artery disease and heart failure. However, there is only limited evidence for the benefits of revascularization in the absence of ischaemic symptoms, and heart failure patients are typically high-risk operative candidates. Trials to assess the value of revascularization in patients with hibernating myocardium (viable but non-contractile myocardium subtended by a stenosed coronary artery) and no symptoms of angina are ongoing.

## Device therapy

Several large randomized trials of implantable devices have demonstrated improvements in both mortality and morbidity in selected patients with chronic heart failure.[55,56] Their use should be considered as an addition to optimal (or best tolerated) medical therapy.

The benefits to patients are the result of one or both of the following:

- termination of malignant ventricular tachyarrhythmia by implantable cardioverter defibrillator (ICD) technology reduces sudden death
- correction of electromechanical asynchrony by atrio-biventricular pacing – 'cardiac resynchronization therapy' – improves pump efficiency and reduces risk of sudden death.

It has been demonstrated that ICD therapy is of benefit in patients with ischaemic heart disease, LVSD and documented evidence of ventricular arrhythmia or previous cardiac arrest.[52] In patients with no documented arrhythmia, ICD implantation is still recommended for those with LVEF ≤35 per cent in NHYA class II or III (not within 40 days of an acute myocardial infarction). Current guidelines from the UK National Institute for Health and Clinical Excellence (NICE) state that patients should have a reasonable expectation of survival with good functional status for at least 1 year.[57] NHYA class IV patients are not considered eligible as mortality is more likely to be the result of progressive heart failure than sudden cardiac death. International guidelines suggest that the indications for ICD therapy in patients with non-ischaemic causes of heart failure should be similar.[4,24]

Cardiac resynchronization therapy can exist as a pacing system alone (CRT-P) or be combined with ICD technology (CRT-D) for those at particularly high risk of sudden death. Implantation is as for a standard dual-chamber (atrio-right ventricular) pacemaker but with a lead to pace the left ventricle introduced via the coronary sinus. By adjusting the timing of pacing by the atrial and ventricular leads, existing electromechanical asynchrony can be corrected. Asynchrony is very likely in a patient with a QRS duration prolonged beyond 120 ms (bundle branch block) and a low EF.

Currently, CRT-P insertion is recommended in patients with LVEF ≤35 per cent and QRS duration ≥120 ms, who have NYHA class III–IV symptoms, despite optimal medical therapy. This is supported by robust trial data demonstrating the effectiveness of such devices in reducing mortality and repeat hospitalizations.[56,58]

### Heart failure with preserved ejection fraction

The management of chronic heart failure with normal EF is much less clear-cut than that for low EF. Recent randomized trials have been disappointing, and control of background comorbidities, such as hypertension, diabetes or AF remain the mainstay of management, with appropriate use of diuretics to control the degree of fluid retention.

### Acute decompensation and de-novo heart failure

For critically ill patients admitted with heart failure, monitoring of temperature, respiratory rate, heart rate, blood pressure, oxygenation, urine output and electrocardiogram is mandatory. Invasive monitoring with an arterial line should be considered and central venous lines may be used to provide good access to the central circulation as well as monitoring of central venous pressure and oxygen saturation. Pulmonary artery catheterization is now used infrequently, but should be considered in complex cases.

There is a lack of robust data for the management of acute heart failure, and most guidelines are based on expert consensus rather than results of randomized trials. The immediate aim of treatment is to improve symptoms, restore oxygenation, improve organ perfusion and haemodynamics, and limit any cardiac or renal damage, according to the algorithm in Figure 29.2.[4] For further information on this aspect of heart failure management, please refer to Chapters 30 and 31.

Once transferred out of the critical care setting, the aim of management is to optimize the treatment strategy along the lines of chronic heart failure management. The patient should then, ideally, be discharged to a chronic heart failure management programme, with attention to education, rehabilitation and appropriate adjustment and monitoring of drug therapy.[59]

## MANAGEMENT OF ADVANCED HEART FAILURE

Patients with resistant fluid overload can be considered for ultrafiltration in appropriate units. If euvolaemia can be achieved and disease-modifying drugs optimized this may improve prognosis by re-establishing control of the syndrome and reducing organ congestion.[60]

The only definitive treatment currently available for advanced (end stage) heart failure is cardiac transplantation. A shortage of organs, the physical and psychological demands of such a procedure and the sequelae of lifelong immunosuppression are all factors which limit the application of this therapy. Nevertheless, it remains a viable option for individuals with end-stage heart failure, severe symptoms and no serious comorbidity.

For patients awaiting transplants the option of supporting the circulation with an LV assist device is available. Such devices are inserted surgically and can help to optimize the patient prior to transplantation. They can also be used in

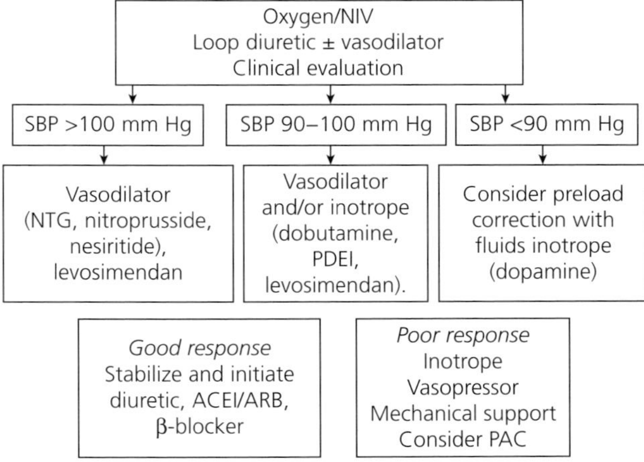


**Figure 29.2** A strategy for treating acute heart failure syndromes according to systolic blood pressure. ACEI, angiotensin-converting enzyme inhibitor; ARB, angiotensin-receptor blocker; NTG, nitroglycerin; PAC, pulmonary artery catheter; PDEI, phosphodiesterase inhibitor. Reproduced from Authors/Task Force Members, Dickstein *et al.*[4] with permission from Oxford Journals.

specialist centres to support patients with potentially reversible acute heart failure, e.g. due to myocarditis or post-partum cardiomyopathy. Newer percutaneous devices are emerging but experience of their use is limited.

For the vast majority of patients with end-stage heart failure, early consideration of palliative and end-of-life care is essential. Expert input, both in hospital and in the community, is desirable.

## CONCLUSIONS

Heart failure is a complex clinical syndrome that can arise from a range of pathologies affecting the heart. The whole body's response to the cardiac dysfunction is variable, and determines prognosis. Therapy is based on a firm diagnosis, full characterization of the syndrome, and introduction of a range of neurohormonal antagonists in addition to diuretic therapy. Increasingly, implantable devices are used to further improve prognosis and symptoms in selected patients. The management of acute decompensation of the chronic syndrome is much less evidence based, but relies on stabilizing haemodynamics and gradually returning the physiology towards the chronic stabilized state. The prognosis of heart failure remains relatively poor, but can be improved markedly by the use of appropriate therapies and the avoidance or early detection and treatment of decompensation.

## REFERENCES


1. Poole-Wilson PA. Chronic heart failure: cause, pathophysiology, prognosis, clinical manifestations, investigations. In: Julian DG, Carom AJ, Fox KF *et al.*, eds. *Diseases of the heart.* London: Ballière-Tindall, 1989: 24–36.
2. Wood P. *Diseases of the heart and circulation.* London: Eyre and Spottiswoode, 1950.
3. Eichhorn EJ, Bristow MR. Medical therapy can improve the biological properties of the chronically failing heart: a new era in the treatment of heart failure. *Circulation* 1996; **94**: 2285–96.
4. Authors/Task Force Members, Dickstein K, Cohen-Solal A *et al.* ESC guidelines for the diagnosis and treatment of acute and chronic heart failure 2008: The task force for the diagnosis and treatment of acute and chronic heart failure 2008 of the European Society of Cardiology. Developed in collaboration with the Heart Failure association of the ESC (HFA) and endorsed by the European Society of Intensive Care Medicine (ESICM). *Eur Heart J* 2008; **29**: 2388–442.
5. Hobbs FDR, Roalfe AK, Davis RC *et al.* Prognosis of all-cause heart failure and borderline left ventricular systolic dysfunction: 5 year mortality follow-up of the Echocardiographic Heart of England Screening Study (ECHOES). *Eur Heart J* 2007; **28**: 1128–34.
6. Cowie MR. Annotated references in epidemiology. *Eur J Heart Fail* 1999; **1**: 101–7.
7. Cleland JGF, Swedberg K, Follath F *et al.* The EuroHeart Failure survey programme: a survey on the quality of care among patients with heart failure in Europe: Part 1: patient characteristics and diagnosis. *Eur Heart J* 2003; **24**: 442–63.
8. Pfeffer MA, Swedberg K, Granger CB *et al.* Effects of candesartan on mortality and morbidity in patients with chronic heart failure: the CHARM-Overall programme. *Lancet* 2003; **362**: 759–66.
9. Gray A, Goodacre S, Newby DE *et al.* Noninvasive ventilation in acute cardiogenic pulmonary edema. *N Engl J Med* 2008; **359**: 142–51
10. Fox KF, Cowie MR, Wood DA *et al.* Coronary artery disease as the cause of incident heart failure in the population. *Eur Heart J* 2001; **22**: 228–36.
11. Ogata H, Ishikawa Y, Ishikawa Y *et al.* Beneficial effects of beta-blockers and angiotensin-converting enzyme inhibitors in Duchenne muscular dystrophy. *J Cardiol* 2009; **53**: 72–8.
12. Sanderson JE. Heart failure with a normal ejection fraction. *Heart* 2007; **93**: 155–8.
13. Paulus WJ, Tschope C, Sanderson JE *et al.* How to diagnose diastolic heart failure: a consensus statement on the diagnosis of heart failure with normal left ventricular ejection fraction by the Heart Failure and Echocardiography Associations of the European Society of Cardiology. *Eur Heart J* 2007; **28**: 2539–50.
14. McMurray JJV, Carson PE, Komajda M *et al.* Heart failure with preserved ejection fraction: clinical characteristics of 4133 patients enrolled in the I-PRESERVE trial. *Eur J Heart Fail* 2008; **10**: 149–56.
15. Cleland JGF, Tendera M, Adamus J *et al.* The Perindopril in Elderly People with Chronic Heart Failure (PEP-CHF) study. *Eur Heart J* 2006; **27**: 2338–45.
16. Damman K, Navis G, Smilde TDJ *et al.* Decreased cardiac output, venous congestion and the association with renal impairment in patients with cardiac dysfunction. *Eur J Heart Fail* 2007; **9**: 872–8.
17. Celis R, Torre-Martinez G, Torre-Amione G. Evidence for activation of immune system in heart failure. Is there a role for anti-inflammatory therapy? *Curr Opin Cardiol* 2008; **23**: 254–60.
18. von Haehling S, Lainscak M, Springer J *et al.* Cardiac cachexia: a systematic overview. *Pharmacol Ther* 2009; **121**: 227–52.
19. Umana E, Solares CA, Alpert MA. Tachycardia-induced cardiomyopathy. *Am J Med* 2003; **114**: 51–5.
20. Mehta PA, Dubrey SW, McIntyre HF *et al.* Mode of death in patients with newly diagnosed heart failure in the general population. *Eur J Heart Fail* 2008; **10**: 1108–16.
21. Orn S. How do heart failure patients die? *Eur Heart J* 2002; **4**: 59.
22. Vazir A, Hastings PC, Dayer M *et al.* A high prevalence of sleep disordered breathing in men with mild

symptomatic chronic heart failure due to left ventricular systolic dysfunction. *Eur J Heart Fail* 2007; **9**: 243–50.

23. Executive Summary: HFSA 2006 Comprehensive heart failure practice guideline. *J Card Fail* 2006; **12**: 10–38.
24. Jessup M, Abraham WT, Casey DE *et al.* 2009 Focused update: ACCF/AHA guidelines for the diagnosis and management of heart failure in adults: a report of the American College of Cardiology Foundation/American Heart Association Task Force on practice guidelines, developed in collaboration with the international society for heart and lung transplantation. *Circulation* 2009; **119**: 1977–2016.
25. National Institute for Clinical Excellence. Guideline 5: *Management of chronic heart failure in adults in primary and secondary care.* London: NICE, 2003.
26. McAlister FA, Stewart S, Ferrua S *et al.* Multidisciplinary strategies for the management of heart failure patients at high risk for admission: a systematic review of randomized trials. *J Am Coll Cardiol* 2004; **44**: 810–19.
27. van Bockel EAP, Lind JS, Zijlstra JG *et al.* Cardiac assessment of patients with late stage Duchenne muscular dystrophy. *Neth Heart J* 2009; **17**: 232–7.
28. McDonagh TA, Morrison CE, Lawrence A *et al.* Symptomatic and asymptomatic left-ventricular systolic dysfunction in an urban population. *Lancet* 1997; **350**: 829–33.
29. Mehta PA, Dubrey SW, McIntyre HF *et al.* Improving survival in heart failure: population-based data from the UK. *Heart* 2009.
30. Dar O, Cowie MR. Acute heart failure in the intensive care unit: epidemiology. *Crit Care Med* 2008; **36**: S3–S8.
31. Rich MW, Freedland KE. Effect of DRGs on three-month readmission rate of geriatric patients with congestive heart failure. *Am J Public Health* 1988; **78**: 680–2.
32. Rich MW, Beckham V, Wittenberg C *et al.* A multidisciplinary intervention to prevent the readmission of elderly patients with congestive heart failure. *N Engl J Med* 1995; **333**: 1190–5.
33. Pocock SJ, Wang D, Pfeffer MA *et al.* Predictors of mortality and morbidity in patients with chronic heart failure. *Eur Heart J* 2006; **27**: 65–75.
34. Levy WC, Mozaffarian D, Linker DT *et al.* The Seattle heart failure model: prediction of survival in heart failure. *Circulation* 2006; **113**: 1424–33.
35. Mancini D, Eisen H, Kussmaul W *et al.* Value of peak exercise oxygen consumption for optimal timing of cardiac transplantation in ambulatory patients with heart failure. *Circulation* 1991; **83**: 778–86.
36. Aaronson KD, Schwartz JS, Chen T-M *et al.* Development and prospective validation of a clinical index to predict survival in ambulatory patients referred for cardiac transplant evaluation. *Circulation* 1997; **95**: 2660–7.
37. O'Connor CM, Whellan DJ, Lee KL *et al.* Efficacy and safety of exercise training in patients with chronic heart failure: HF-ACTION randomized controlled trial. *JAMA* 2009; **301**: 1439–50.
38. Effects of enalapril on mortality in severe congestive heart failure. Results of the Cooperative North Scandinavian Enalapril Survival Study (CONSENSUS). The CONSENSUS Trial Study Group. *N Engl J Med* 1987; **316**: 1429–35.
39. Effect of enalapril on survival in patients with reduced left ventricular ejection fractions and congestive heart failure. The SOLVD Investigators. *N Engl J Med* 1991; **325**: 293–302.
40. Pfeffer M, Braunwald E, Moye L *et al.* Effect of captopril on mortality and morbidity in patients with left ventricular dysfunction after myocardial infarction. Results of the survival and ventricular enlargement trial. The SAVE Investigators. *N Engl J Med* 1992; **327**: 669–77.
41. The Acute Infarction Ramipril Efficacy Study I. Effect of ramipril on mortality and morbidity of survivors of acute myocardial infarction with clinical evidence of heart failure. *Lancet* 1993; **342**: 821–8.
42. McMurray J, Cohen-Solal A, Dietz R *et al.* Practical recommendations for the use of ACE inhibitors, beta-blockers, aldosterone antagonists and angiotensin receptor blockers in heart failure. Putting guidelines into practice. *Eur J Heart Fail* 2005; **7**: 710–21.
43. Pfeffer MA, McMurray JJV, Velazquez EJ *et al.* Valsartan, captopril, or both in myocardial infarction complicated by heart failure, left ventricular dysfunction, or both. *N Engl J Med* 2003; **349**: 1893–906.
44. The Cardiac Insufficiency Bisoprolol Study II (CIBIS-II): a randomised trial. *Lancet* 1999; **353**: 9–13.
45. Effect of metoprolol CR/XL in chronic heart failure: Metoprolol CR/XL Randomised Intervention Trial in-Congestive Heart Failure (MERIT-HF). *Lancet* 1999; **353**: 2001–7.
46. Packer M, Coats AJS, Fowler MB *et al.* Effect of carvedilol on survival in severe chronic heart failure *N Engl J Med* 2001; **344**: 1651–8.
47. Salpeter SR, Ormiston TM, Salpeter EE *et al.* Cardioselective beta-blockers for chronic obstructive pulmonary disease: a meta-analysis. *Respir Med* 2003; **97**: 1094–101.
48. Pitt B, Zannad F, Remme WJ *et al.* The effect of spironolactone on morbidity and mortality in patients with severe heart failure. *N Engl J Med* 1999; **341**: 709–17.
49. Pitt B, Remme W, Zannad F *et al.* Eplerenone, a selective aldosterone blocker, in patients with left ventricular dysfunction after myocardial infarction. *N Engl J Med* 2003; **348**: 1309–21.
50. Ahmed A, Rich MW, Love TE *et al.* Digoxin and reduction in mortality and hospitalization in heart failure: a comprehensive post hoc analysis of the DIG trial. *Eur Heart J* 2006; **27**: 178–86.
51. Gheorghiade M, Adams KF Jr, Colucci WS. Digoxin in the management of cardiovascular disorders. *Circulation* 2004; **109**: 2959–64.
52. Bardy GH, Lee KL, Mark DB *et al.* Amiodarone or an implantable cardioverter-defibrillator for congestive heart failure. *N Engl J Med* 2005; **352**: 225–37.

53. Nair A, Sealove B, Halperin JL *et al.* Anticoagulation in patients with heart failure: who, when, and why? *Eur Heart J Suppl* 2006; **8**: E32–8.
54. Taylor AL, Ziesche S, Yancy C *et al.* Combination of isosorbide dinitrate and hydralazine in blacks with heart failure. *N Engl J Med* 2004; **351**: 2049–57.
55. Bristow MR, Saxon LA, Boehmer J *et al.* Cardiac-resynchronization therapy with or without an implantable defibrillator in advanced chronic heart failure. *N Engl J Med* 2004; **350**: 2140–50.
56. Cleland JGF, Daubert J-C, Erdmann E *et al.* The effect of cardiac resynchronization on morbidity and mortality in heart failure. *N Engl J Med* 2005; **352**: 1539–49.
57. Technology Appraisal 95 – Implantable cardioverter defibrillators for arrhythmias. London: National Institute for Health and Clinical Excellence, 2006.
58. Cleland JGF, Daubert J-C, Erdmann E *et al.* Longer-term effects of cardiac resynchronization therapy on mortality in heart failure (the CArdiac REsynchronization-Heart Failure (CARE-HF) trial extension phase). *Eur Heart J* 2006; **27**: 1928–32.
59. Gheorghiade M, Pang PS. Acute heart failure syndromes. *J Am Coll Cardiol* 2009; **53**: 557–73.
60. Costanzo MR, Guglin ME, Saltzberg MT *et al.* Ultrafiltration versus intravenous diuretics for patients hospitalized for acute decompensated heart failure. *J Am Coll Cardiol* 2007; **49**: 675–83.

# 30

# Acute cardiogenic pulmonary oedema

ALASDAIR J GRAY

## ABSTRACT

A number of high-quality systematic reviews have examined the effectiveness of non-invasive ventilation (CPAP and NIPPV) in patients with cardiogenic pulmonary oedema (CPO) with the following results: NIV significantly reduced endotracheal intubation rate and in-hospital mortality (results remained significant if CPAP was analysed independently); NIPPV was shown to reduce mortality, but not to a statistically significant level ($p = 0.07$), but remained significant for intubation (this probably reflects numbers of patients studied); there was no difference in outcomes between CPAP and NIPPV; there was no difference in myocardial infarction rates between arms. A recent large randomized controlled trial (3CPO) which recruited more patients than the total number included in the meta-analyses did not confirm these findings: there was no difference between 7-day mortality for standard oxygen therapy (9.8%) and NIV (CPAP or NIPPV) (9.5%; $p = 0.87$); NIV was associated with greater reductions in breathlessness, heart rate, acidosis and hypercapnia at one hour; there were no treatment-related adverse events, in particular no increase in myocardial infarction rate; there was no difference in any outcome when CPAP and NIPPV were compared; the breathlessness exhibited by the recruited patients was marked at entrance to the trial. (It seems reasonable for this reason alone to consider NIV to palliate these distressing symptoms. This short-term benefit needs to be balanced, however, with possible intolerance of the mask.) Possible reasons why the large trial gave different results to meta-analyses include: possible differences in patients included; influence of co-treatments; differing thresholds for endotracheal intubation and critical care admission; trial design and interpretation of previous data. In conclusion – in the majority of patients medical therapy, in particular, nitrate therapy, should be instigated as the primary treatment of severe acute CPO and NIV reserved for those patients who have significant respiratory distress and failure or those not improving with standard medical therapy.

## INTRODUCTION

Acute heart failure syndrome[1] (AHFS) is a clinical condition in which the patient with known or *de novo* heart failure has deterioration in their symptoms. These patients primarily present to hospital with signs and symptoms that relate to congestion occurring as a result of elevated left ventricular filling pressures with the accompanying symptoms of dyspnoea and fatigue.[2] Cardiac output, left ventricular ejection fraction, may be impaired or preserved. Patients with preserved left ventricular function, diastolic heart failure, are older and predominantly female.[3,4] Approximately 25–50 per cent of patients will present with acute pulmonary oedema as, at least, part of the clinical syndrome. This may occur with or without systemic congestion and fluid overload.[5–9]

The common clinical classifications of AHFS are detailed in Table 30.1.[10] A number of factors have been identified as common precipitants of hospital admission with AHFS.[11] These include poorly controlled hypertension, acute coronary syndrome, arrhythmias, exacerbation of chronic obstructive pulmonary disease, pneumonia and non-compliance of diet or medication.

Management of AHFS has changed little with the majority of patients receiving diuretic therapy. Increasingly, vasodilator therapies, and in patients with pulmonary oedema and respiratory failure, non-invasive ventilation (NIV) are being used.

## ASSESSMENT AND DIAGNOSIS

Clinical evaluation, including a clear history and examination supported by a 12-lead electrocardiogram (ECG) and plain radiograph of the chest, remains central to making the

**Table 30.1** Common clinical classifications of acute heart failure syndrome

| Clinical status | Heart rate | SBP (mm Hg) | CI (L/min/m²) | PCWP (mm Hg) | Congestion Killip/ Forrester | Diuresis | Hypoperfusion | End-organ hypoperfusion |
|---|---|---|---|---|---|---|---|---|
| I Acute decompensated congestive heart failure | +/- | Low normal/ High | Low normal/High | Mild elevation | K II/F II | + | +/- | - |
| II Acute heart failure with hypertension/ hypertensive crisis | Usually increased | High | +/- | >18 | K II-IV/FII-III | +/- | +/- | +, with CNS symptoms |
| III Acute heart failure with pulmonary oedema | + | Low normal | Low | Elevated | KIII/FII | + | +/- | - |
| IVa Cardiogenic shock*/low output syndrome | + | Low normal | Low, <2.2 | >16 | K III-IV/F I-III | Low | + | + |
| IVb Severe cardiogenic shock | >90 | <90 | <1.8 | >18 | K IV/F IV | Very low | ++ | + |
| V High output failure | + | +/- | + | +/- | KII/FI-II | + | - | - |
| VI Right-sided acute heart failure | Usually low | Low | Low | Low | F I | +/- | +/-, acute onset | +/- |

*The differentiation from low cardiac output syndrome is subjective and the clinical presentation may overlap these classifications.

CI, cardiac index; CNS, central nervous system, PCWP, pulmonary capillary wedge pressure; SBP, systolic blood pressure.

There are exceptions; the above values are general rules.

Modified with permission from Task Force on Acute Heart Failure of the European Society of Cardiology.[10]

Table 30.2 Radiographic and ECG characteristics in acute heart failure syndrome

| Finding | Pooled | | Summary LR (95% CI)* | |
|---|---|---|---|---|
| | Sensitivity | Specificity | Positive | Negative |
| Chest radiography | | | | |
| Pulmonary venous congestion | 0.54 | 0.96 | 12.0 (6.8 to 21.0) | 0.48 (0.28 to 0.83) |
| Interstitial oedema | 0.34 | 0.97 | 12.0 (5.2 to 27.0) | 0.68 (0.54 to 0.85) |
| Alveolar oedema | 0.06 | 0.99 | 6.0 (2.2 to 16.0) | 0.95 (0.93 to 0.97) |
| Cardiomegaly | 0.74 | 0.78 | 3.3 (2.4 to 4.7) | 0.33 (0.23 to 0.48) |
| Pleural effusions(s) | 0.26 | 0.92 | 3.2 (2.4 to 4.3) | 0.81 (0.77 to 0.85) |
| Any oedema | 0.70 | 0.77 | 3.1 (0.60 to 16.0) | 0.38 (0.11 to 1.3) |
| Pneumonia | 0.04 | 0.92 | 0.50 (0.29 to 0.87) | 1.0 (1.0 to 1.1) |
| Hyperinflation | 0.03 | 0.92 | 0.38 (0.20 to 0.69) | 1.1 (1.0 to 1.1) |
| Electrocardiogram | | | | |
| Atrial fibrillation | 0.26 | 0.93 | 3.8 (1.7 to 8.8) | 0.79 (0.65 to 0.96) |
| New T-wave changes | 0.24 | 0.92 | 3.0 (1.7 to 5.3) | 0.83 (0.74 to 0.92) |
| Any abnormal finding | 0.50 | 0.78 | 2.2 (1.6 to 3.1) | 0.64 (0.47 to 0.88) |
| ST elevation | 0.05 | 0.97 | 1.8 (0.80 to 4.0) | 0.98 (0.94 to 1.0) |
| ST depression | 0.11 | 0.94 | 1.7 (0.97 to 2.9) | 0.95 (0.90 to 1.0) |

*LRs are not independent of each other and should not be multiplied in series when multiple findings are considered.
†Pulmonary venous congestion, manifest as distension of pulmonary veins and redistribution to the apices.
CI, confidence interval; LR, likelihood ratio.
Modified with permission from Wang *et al.*[12]

diagnosis of AHFS with pulmonary oedema[12] in emergency care settings. In general, the diagnosis is obvious – a past history of heart failure or ischaemic heart disease, symptoms including orthopnoea, paroxysmal nocturnal dyspnoea or dyspnoea on exercise, clinical findings of a third heart sound, pulmonary crackles, raised jugular venous pressure and leg oedema, all increase the likelihood of acute heart failure in patients presenting with breathlessness.[12] Table 30.2[12] details the radiographic and ECG characteristics that support or refute the diagnosis of an acute heart failure syndrome.

Brain natriuretic peptide (BNP) and proBNP are increasingly used to support the diagnosis of AHFS in emergency patients.[13–16] The results are most helpful in the intermediate clinical risk group of patients, in whom a very low result effectively rules out and a high result effectively rules in the diagnosis of AHFS.[17] Other conditions that result in right heart strain in which BNP-like troponin can rise include chronic obstructive pulmonary disease (COPD) and pulmonary embolism. The results should also be interpreted with caution in older patients and those with renal insufficiency.

A number of factors have been identified as having prognostic implication for AHFS patients. These include age, blood pressure, BNP rise, troponin rise, hyponatraemia, renal dysfunction, previous ischaemic heart disease, ejection fraction and function at discharge,[11,18–22] and some have been evaluated together in clinical prediction rules.[23] The majority of these factors have been identified using registry data encompassing the complete spectrum of AHFS.[11,19] Table 30.3, from a review by Collins *et al.*,[7] provides a concise summary of these risk variables. Moreover, most relate to longer-term outcomes and have not been used to identify those patients at immediate risk of death or need for intervention on presentation. Recently the 3CPO trialists have used data from the 3CPO trial in an attempt to address this in patients with severe cardiogenic pulmonary oedema. Age, systolic blood pressure and the patient's ability to obey commands were factors clearly associated with 7-day mortality.[24]

## CLINICAL MANAGEMENT

The principal treatments for patients with cardiogenic pulmonary oedema have changed little in the past two to three decades. The mainstays of medical management include oxygen, nitrates, diuretics and opioid, although recently some have questioned the benefit of these long-standing agents.[25–27] In the recently published 3CPO trial of 1069 patients with severe cardiogenic pulmonary oedema, 90 per cent, 89 per cent and 51 per cent of patients received nitrates, loop diuretics and opioids, respectively.[28] There is a complete lack of high-quality research to support the effectiveness of any of these agents and some recent observational data suggest an association with worsening outcomes.[29–32] Novel drugs have failed to show clear therapeutic benefit when scrutinized in the setting of large randomized controlled trials. Traditionally, when these therapeutic options have failed or if the patient has presented critically ill, then endotracheal intubation and invasive ventilation has been the only option. Non-invasive ventilation is increasingly used in many emergency care settings for patients with severe acute pulmonary oedema.[33,34]

In contrast, nitrates are more effective at causing venodilatation, vasodilatation and reductions in blood pressure while maintaining cardiac output. In head-to-head comparisons, nitrates have a more favourable haemodynamic profile than furosemide.[49]

### Registry and observational data

Recent observational data from the ADHERE registry suggest an adverse outcome (length of hospital stay and mortality) associated with loop diuretic therapy in patients admitted with AHFS even after controlling for potential confounding factors.[33] Post-hoc analysis of patients with chronic heart failure in the Digoxin Intervention Group study showed that patients receiving diuretics had increased all-cause and cardiovascular mortality, and heart failure related hospitalization independent of severity of illness.[50] This effect is likely to be related to volume depletion activating the renin–angiotensin–aldosterone system in conjunction with electrolyte imbalance despite concomitant use of angiotensin-converting enzyme (ACE) inhibitor therapy.[51] Recent data from the 3CPO trial show no clear benefit in those patients receiving early low-dose loop diuretic, although the majority received the agent.[52]

### Clinical trials

The majority of patients with acute CPO improve rapidly following initiation of therapy. The time course of this recovery and its dissociation from therapy-induced diuresis strongly suggests that intravenous loop diuretic therapy cannot account for clinical improvement. There have been few randomized controlled trials of furosemide therapy, and a literature review[53] reveals only four small-scale studies ($n$ = 28–110). In comparison to furosemide, all report better[48,49] or comparable[54,55] haemodynamic responses with nitrates. In the largest study by Cotter and colleagues,[54] high-dose nitrate and low-dose furosemide was compared to low-dose nitrate and high-dose furosemide. Patients treated with high-dose furosemide had a higher intubation and myocardial infarction rate, and this was mirrored by a slower improvement in pulse rate, respiratory rate and oxygen saturation.

## OPIOIDS

Opioids are commonly used in the initial management of patients with AHFS.[26,27] There is a paucity of evidence of clinical effect although pragmatically it would seem appropriate to use them to relieve pain and distress especially in the context of pulmonary oedema secondary to acute coronary syndrome.[11] This has to be balanced with its central respiratory and central nervous system depressant effects especially in those patients with coexistent respiratory disease such as COPD.

### Theoretical considerations and experimental evidence

There are some data to demonstrate a venodilatory effect of opioids as a result of venous pooling,[56,57] which is postulated to occur due to either histamine release or an alternative action on opioid receptors in vascular smooth muscle. No central effect on pulmonary capillary wedge pressures has been elicited. Indeed, there is some evidence to suggest an increase in heart filling pressures and a reduction in cardiac index due to a direct myocardial depressant effect.[58,59] In addition, opioids may exert an indirect benefit on patients' symptoms and physiology by reducing anxiety and pain, and therefore ameliorating the adverse effects of excess catecholamine drive. However, given the potential detrimental effects of these agents it may be preferable to use alternative agents such as benzodiazepines if anxiolysis is desired.[27]

### Registry and observational data

A number of observational studies have reported poorer outcomes for patients receiving opioids.[30–32] Sachetti and colleagues showed a significant increase in endotracheal intubation (odds ratio [OR] 5.04; $p = 0.001$) and intensive care unit (ICU) (OR 3.08; $p = 0.002$) admission in patients with pulmonary oedema receiving morphine.[31] Clearly, this may be related to underlying severity of disease rather than the direct effect of the drug. A further pre-hospital study investigating different treatment regimens in presumed pulmonary oedema identified an increase in both breathlessness and respiratory rate in those patients administered morphine.[30] More recently, data from the ADHERE registry[32] and unpublished data from the 3CPO trial both demonstrate an association between adverse clinical outcomes and opioid administration.

## VASODILATORS: NITRATES AND SODIUM NITROPRUSSIDE

Glyceryl trinitrate is commonly administered to patients with severe cardiogenic pulmonary oedema and AHFS. In the 3CPO trial, 90 per cent of the recruited 1069 patients received nitrate therapy during initial management in the emergency department.[29] Nitrate is a predominantly a venodilator. At higher doses it provides both coronary and systemic artery dilatation.[60,61] Nitroprusside is an alternative, potent, combined venous and arterial dilator, which is not widely used in clinical practice due to its side effect profile.

### Theoretical considerations and experimental evidence

Nitrates act directly on the vascular smooth muscle with the nitroglycerin transformed into nitrogen oxides, which result in an elevation of cyclic guanosine monophosphate (cGMP). In acute heart failure this results in a reduction in right and left heart filling pressures, systemic vascular resistance and usually an increase in cardiac output. At higher doses there is also the beneficial action of coronary vasodilatation.

### Administration

Vascular and haemodynamic responses are dependent on the route of administration. It can be administered sublingually, transdermally or by intravenous bolus or infusion. There is evidence that a single sublingual dose pre-hospital is associated with improved clinical outcomes.[62] In the majority of instances, glyceryl trinitrate is delivered by bolus or continuous infusion as this allows titration against response and blood pressure. Both are tolerated well if the presentation blood pressure is normal or high and, due to the short length of action, hypotension resolves quickly once the infusion is stopped. Other side effects include headache and rarely methaemoglobinaemia.

#### Registry and observational data

A retrospective analysis from 65 180 patients with AHFS in the ADHERE database reporting on 6549 patients receiving intravenous glyceryl trinitrate showed a lower rate of mortality in these patients than in patients receiving either milrinone or dobutamine. There was no difference in outcomes between glyceryl trinitrate and nesiritide.[63] Unpublished retrospective analysis of nitrate administration in the 3CPO trial showed greater improvement in arterial acidosis (pH) at 1 hour in patients receiving nitrates.

#### Clinical trials

There are no placebo-controlled trials of nitrates in patients with AHFS and pulmonary oedema, but there have been a number of head-to-head comparisons with furosemide (see Diuretics, p. 293). Nitrates were shown to be superior or equivalent in all these small trials.[52] A recent comparative study between glyceryl trinitrate, nesiritide and placebo in addition to 'standard care' is described later.[64]

### VASODILATORS: NESIRITIDE

Nesiritide, a recombinant form of BNP, is a potent arterial and venous dilator with a natriuretic effect[65] licensed in North America for use in patients with AHFS. Approximately 8 per cent of patients in the ADHERE registry received nesitiride.[63]

#### Theoretical considerations and experimental evidence

Early studies demonstrated dose-related reductions in pulmonary capillary wedge pressure (PCWP) and an increase in stroke volume and cardiac index as well as improvement in symptoms.[66,67] There was no significant tolerance, and side effects, principally hypotension, were minimal.

#### Clinical trials

The VMAC investigators compared glyceryl trinitrate with nesiritide and placebo in 489 patients with AHFS and dyspnoea at rest.[64] The primary endpoint was improvement in PCWP and patient dyspnoea at 3 hours after treatment allocation. The trial demonstrated greater reductions in PCWP at 3 and 24 hours in patients receiving nesiritide than in those receiving glyceryl trinitrate. In addition, patients were also reported to have a greater improvement in 'global clinical status' at 24 hours. This trial has been criticized for a number of reasons. All patients received standard management, which invariably included morphine and furosemide prior to randomization. Concomitant therapies were not controlled for despite this being an efficacy trial, e.g. dobutamine, NIV, glyceryl trinitrate regimens were at the discretion of the treating clinician and were relatively low dosage (30–40 μg/min). The 'global clinical status' at 24 hours was poorly described and unvalidated. The differences in PCWP were small and were not shown to be clinically significant or relevant. There was no mortality difference between the two agents. Two recent reviews[68,69] have raised concerns regarding the safety of nesiritide. In three trials reporting data on 862 patients (485 receiving nesiritide) the 30-day mortality was 7.2 per cent compared to 4 per cent in the control group. In the other pooled analysis of five trials and 1269 patients renal dysfunction was significantly higher in the nesiritide treated groups (11.1 per cent compared to 4.2 per cent).

### Other agents

A number of other agents have been evaluated or are used in the management of AHFS. In general, they are used in specialist settings in small subgroups of patients with AHFS, which are resistant to standard therapies or where blood pressure is low. These groups tend not to have pulmonary oedema as the principal clinical finding. Recent novel agents studied include phosphodiesterase inhibitors (milrinone), dobutamine, endothelin antagonists, relaxin, levosimendan and ACE inhibitors.[70–76] A review of all these agents is beyond the scope of this chapter.

## NON-INVASIVE VENTILATION

Non-invasive ventilation is regularly used in patients presenting with cardiogenic pulmonary oedema in the pre-hospital, emergency department and critical care settings. The potential clinical benefit was first described in the 1930s by Barach and Poulton.[77,78] However, it was only with the publication of a number of experimental studies and small randomized controlled trials in the 1980s and subsequent reporting of pooled clinical data that NIV has increasingly been employed in the clinical care of AHFS patients with pulmonary oedema.[79–83] Two principal NIV modalities have been used: continuous positive airway pressure (CPAP) and non-invasive positive pressure ventilation (NIPPV) (sometimes described as BiPAP). Although CPAP is not a true ventilatory modality, given its similar mechanisms of action and use in clinical practice it is included in this chapter. It provides additional positive airway pressure delivered to the patient via a mask interface, which remains consistent in its level throughout the respiratory cycle. NIPPV provides additional pressure applied during inspiration. The potential additional benefit of this modality compared with CPAP is described below. Previously, there had been concern regarding an increase in myocardial infarction rates in patients administered NIPPV,[84] but this was subsequently shown to be unfounded.[28,52,85] A number of recently published meta-analyses[81–83,86–89] suggest a mortality benefit for those patients treated with NIV although this was not supported by results from a large multicentre emergency department trial from the UK, the 3CPO trial,[28,52] published in 2008. Despite theoretical physiological benefits of NIPPV over CPAP, no difference has been found to date in head-to-head comparisons.[28,52,84,90–92] Despite the lack of definitive mortality benefit, NIV is increasingly used in clinical practice and advocated by many specialty organizations.[9,10,93,94]

## Theoretical considerations and experimental evidence

The presumed mechanistic benefits of NIV in cardiogenic pulmonary oedema have been largely extrapolated from research into the effect of NIV in chronic heart failure. This is covered in detail in Chapter 31. Non-invasive ventilation has a number of potentially beneficial effects, including: a dose-dependent afterload lowering effect that improves cardiac function in the failing heart;[95–100] unloading respiratory muscles, with a resultant reduction in the work of breathing that is likely to be due to increased lung compliance secondary to extra-thoracic redistribution of lung water;[101,102] and increasing functional residual capacity and opening collapsed or underventilated alveoli, thus decreasing right to left intrapulmonary shunting, improving lung compliance and oxygenation and decreasing the work of breathing by moving the patient on to a more compliant part of the pressure–volume curve.[103–105]

## Clinical trials

### EFFICACY, EFFECTIVENESS AND OUTCOMES

A number of randomized trials have investigated the efficacy and effectiveness of NIV in the management of acute cardiogenic pulmonary oedema.[84,90–92,106–116] Most of these trials have been small and none has, in isolation, shown mortality benefit. These studies used a variety of endpoints, such as physiological parameters, intubation or predefined treatment failure. They investigated the comparative effectiveness of CPAP and standard oxygen therapy,[106–110] NIPPV and standard oxygen therapy;[111,112] NIPPV and CPAP,[84,85,90,113,114] or either intervention (CPAP and NIPPV) compared with standard oxygen therapy alone.[92,115,116] The majority of these trials showed improvement in physiology or a reduction in endotracheal intubation rate or other surrogate markers of treatment failure in the NIV arm. Two recent larger primary trials will be discussed in greater detail later.[28,52,91]

One of the first trials comparing CPAP with NIPPV in cardiogenic pulmonary oedema was prematurely terminated because of an increase in myocardial infarction rate in the NIPPV arm.[84] Subsequent reanalysis of data suggested that this finding was due to confounding rather than a direct effect of the intervention. A subsequent study by Bellone *et al.* demonstrated no effect of NIPPV on myocardial infarction rate[85] when patients with ischaemic ECGs or raised cardiac biomarkers were excluded before randomization. A systematic review by Peter and colleagues reported a weak relationship between the delivery of NIPPV and an increase in myocardial infarction rate.[82] This finding was largely the result of the weighting of Mehta's study in the pooled data. The 3CPO trial has shown that there is no relationship between myocardial infarction rate and the application of either CPAP or NIPPV.[28]

In an attempt to determine whether a true mortality benefit exists a number of authors have recently reviewed, assimilated and published systematic reviews with meta-analyses.[81–83,86–89] The following section reviews two important meta-analyses and two recent published primary trials.[28,52,81,82,91]

### POOLED DATA

Masip *et al.* conducted a detailed and high-quality systematic review of 15 eligible randomized controlled trials from 10 countries comparing NIV (CPAP or NIPPV) to standard oxygen or CPAP with NIPPV.[81] The details of the different comparative groupings are described in Table 30.5.[81] The primary outcomes for the systematic review were in-hospital mortality and treatment failure. Treatment failure was inconsistently categorized and the authors defined this arbitrarily as the 'need to intubate'. Data on myocardial infarction rate during hospital admission was collected and analysed. All other parameters such as physiology, length of stay, co-treatments and critical care admission were variably reported across the trials. The majority of trials were small and single centre (sample size 26–130) and based in either the ICU or the emergency department. The majority used full face masks and CPAP (2.5–16.0 cm $H_2O$) or NIPPV (8/3–20/5 cm $H_2O$). The complexity of the ventilator used varied considerably. Pooled data included 727 patients for the comparison of NIV (CPAP or NIPPV) to standard oxygen. Patients receiving NIV had a significant reduction in in-hospital mortality ($p$ <0.01; risk ratio 0.55; 95 per cent CI 0.40 to 0.78) and endotracheal intubation ($p$ <0.01; risk ratio 0.48; 95 per cent CI 0.32 to 0.57). Results remained significant if CPAP was analysed independently for both in-hospital mortality and 'need for intubation'. NIPPV was shown to reduce mortality but not to a statistically significant level ($p$ = 0.07), which possibly reflects the numbers of patients included in these trials (total number of patients was 315) but remained significant for intubation ($p$ = 0.02). There was no difference in outcomes between CPAP and NIPPV but these comparisons only included a total of 219 patients. There was no

**Table 30.5** Systematic review of 15 randomized controlled trials comparing non-invasive ventilation (NIV) to standard oxygen or continuous positive airway pressure (CPAP) with non-invasive positive pressure ventilation (NIPPV)

| Source | Location | Sample size* | Mask | CPAP, (cm $H_2O$) | IPAP/EPAP, (cm $H_2O$) | Primary outcomes | Other considerations |
|---|---|---|---|---|---|---|---|
| **Continuous positive airway pressure vs oxygen therapy** | | | | | | | |
| Räsänen *et al.* 1985[107] | 1 ICU in Finland | 40 | Full face | 10 | | Clinical outcomes | |
| Bersten *et al.* 1991[106] | 1 ICU in Australia | 40 (39) | Full face | 10 | | Intubation | |
| Lin *et al.* 1995[108] | 1 ICU in Taiwan | 100 | Full face | 2.5–12.5 | | Intubation In-hospital mortality | Swan-Ganz catheterization |
| Takeda *et al.* 1997[109] | 1 ICU in Japan | 30 (39) | Full face or nasal | 4–10 | | Laboratory parameters | Measurement of plasma endothelin 1 |
| Kelly *et al.* 2002[110] | 1 ED and ICU in the UK | 58 | Full face | 7.5 | | Clinical outcomes Laboratory parameters | Measurement of plasma neurohormonal concentrations |
| L'Her *et al.* 2004[111] | 4 EDs in France | 89 | Full face | 7.5 | | 48-h mortality | Elderly patients (>75 y) |
| **Non-invasive pressure support ventilation vs conventional oxygen therapy** | | | | | | | |
| Masip *et al.* 2000[112] | 1 ICU in Spain | 40 (37) | Full face | | 20/5, Mean | Intubation Resolution time | IPAP was adjusted to tidal volume |
| Levitt, 2001[114] | 1 ED in the United States | 38 | Full face or nasal | | 8/3 Initial | Intubation | Prematurely interrupted when the study by Mehta *et al*[35] was published |
| Nava *et al.* 2003[90] | 5 EDs in Italy | 130 | Full face | | 14.5/6.1, Mean | Intubation | Post hoc analysis in hypercapnic patients |
| **Trials with three study groups** | | | | | | | |
| Park *et al.* 2001[115] | 1 ED in Brazil | 26 | Full face and nasal | 5–12.5 | 8/3 Initial | Intubation | Full face mask for CPAP and nasal for NIPSV |
| Crane *et al.* 2004[92] | 2 EDs in the UK | 60 | Full face | 10 | 15/5 Fixed | Success in ED (2 h) In-hospital mortality | Pre-hospital nitrates therapy evaluated |
| Park *et al.* 2004[116] | 1 ED in Brazil | 83 (80) | Full face | 10 Initial up to 16 | 15/10 Initial | Intubation | |
| **Continuous positive airway pressure vs non-invasive pressure support ventilation** | | | | | | | |
| Mehta *et al.* 1997[84] | 1 ED in the United States | 27 | Nasal and full face | 10 | 15/5 Fixed | Intubation Physiological Improvement | Prematurely stopped for higher rate of AMI in NIPSV group |
| Bellone *et al.* 2004[85] | 1 ED in Italy | 36 | Full face | 10 | 15/5 Initial | AMI | Study restricted to patients with hypercapnia |
| Bellone *et al.* 2005[113] | 1 ED in Italy | 46 | Full face | 10 | 15/5 Initial | Resolution time | Primary endpoint was AMI rate Only non-ischaemic APE |

*Numbers in parentheses denote the number of patients finally included after withdrawals.

AMI, acute myocardial infarction; APE, acute pulmonary oedema; CPAP, continuous positive airway pressure; ED, emergency department; EPAP, positive expiratory airway pressure (equivalent to CPAP); ICU, intensive care unit; IPAP, inspiratory positive airway pressure; NIPSV, bi-level non-invasive pressure support ventilation.

Modified with permission from Masip *et al.*[10]

difference in myocardial infarction rates between arms. The review concluded that NIV should be considered as a first-line treatment for patients presenting with acute cardiogenic pulmonary oedema.

Peter and co-investigators[82] identified 23 eligible studies from 14 countries over an 18-year period. The primary outcomes chosen were in-hospital mortality and the need for intubation and mechanical ventilation. Secondary outcomes included treatment failure, length of hospital stay, length of time of NIV and myocardial infarction rate. Figure 30.1 details the principal data for the review's primary outcomes. There was a mortality reduction for those patients treated with CPAP (relative risk [RR] 0.59, 95 per cent CI 0.28 to 0.90, $p = 0.015$, number needed to treat [NNT] 5). There was a trend towards improved survival with NIPPV. Both CPAP (RR 0.44, 95 per cent CI 0.29 to 0.66, $p = 0.0003$, NNT 6) and NIV (RR 0.50, 95 per cent CI 0.27 to 0.90, $p = 0.02$, NNT 7) showed a reduction in need for endotracheal intubation when compared with standard oxygen therapy. There was no difference in any outcome when CPAP was compared with NIPPV. Finally, there was a trend towards an increase in myocardial infarction rate with NIPPV but this was related to the weighting of a single study.[84]

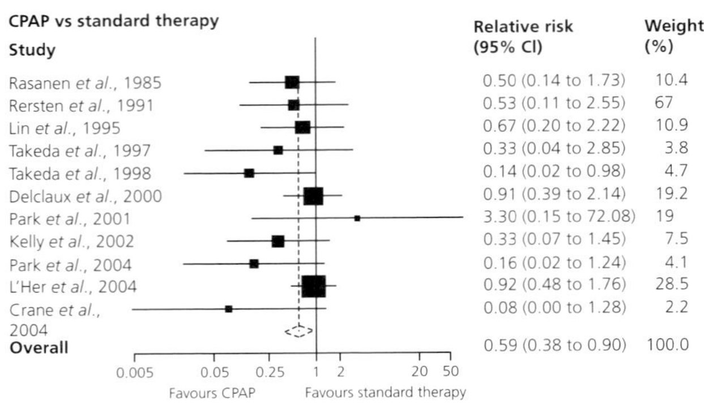


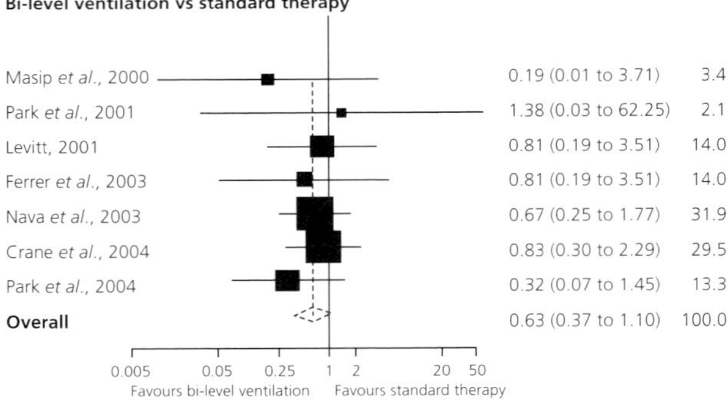


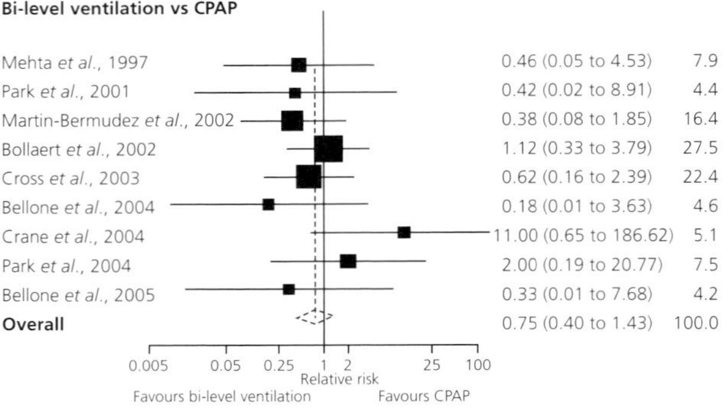


**Figure 30.1** The effect of CPAP, bi-level ventilation and NIPPV on mortality. CPAP, continuous positive airway pressure. Redrawn with permission from Peter *et al.*[82]

## RECENT LARGE PRIMARY TRIALS

The 3CPO trial recruited 1069 patients from 26 UK emergency departments.[28,52] In this multicentre open prospective randomized controlled trial patients with cardiogenic pulmonary oedema were randomized to one of three arms: standard oxygen therapy delivered by variable delivery oxygen mask with resevoir bag, CPAP (5–15 cm $H_2O$) or NIPPV (inspiratory pressure 8–20 cm $H_2O$, expiratory pressure 4–10 cm $H_2O$). Non-invasive ventilation (both CPAP and NIPPV) was delivered through a midrange portable ventilator (Respironics Synchrony). The primary endpoint for the comparison between NIV (CPAP or NIPPV) and standard oxygen was 7-day mortality. The primary endpoint for the comparison between CPAP and NIPPV was 7-day mortality or intubation. Patients with a clinical and radiological diagnosis of cardiogenic pulmonary oedema were included if they were tachypnoeic (respiratory rate >20 breaths/min) and acidotic (pH <7.35) at presentation. Other managment was at the discretion of the treating clinician. As this was a pragmatic trial, there was no predefined treatment failure and patients could, if necessary, cross over between treatment arms. A total of 1069 patients ($78 \pm 10$ years; 43 per cent male) were recruited to standard oxygen therapy ($n = 367$), CPAP ($n = 346$; $10 \pm 4$ cm $H_2O$) or NIPPV ($n = 356$; $14 \pm 5/7 \pm 2$ cm $H_2O$). The mean $\pm$ SD duration of CPAP therapy was $2.2 \pm 1.5$ hours and NIV $2.0 \pm 1.3$ hours. There was no difference between 7-day mortality for standard oxygen therapy (9.8 per cent) and NIV (9.5 per cent; $p = 0.87$). The combined endpoint of 7-day death or intubation rate was similar irrespective of NIV modality (11.7 per cent versus 11.1 per cent, CPAP versus NIV respectively; $p = 0.81$). In comparison with standard oxygen therapy, NIV was associated with greater reductions (treatment difference, 95 per cent confidence intervals) in breathlessness (visual analogue score 0.7, 0.2 to 1.3; $p = 0.008$), heart rate (3 beats per minute, 1 to 6; $p = 0.004$), acidosis (pH 0.03, 0.02 to 0.04; $p < 0.001$) and hypercapnia (0.7 kPa, 0.4 to 0.9; $p < 0.001$) at 1 hour. There were no treatment-related adverse events. There were no differences in other secondary outcomes such as myocardial infraction rate, intubation, length of hospital stay or critical care admission rate.

Moritz and colleagues[91] recruited 120 patients from three French emergency departments to either CPAP or NIPPV. There was no standard oxygen therapy arm.

Patients had either a clinical or radiological diagnosis of pulmonary oedema and two from three of the following criteria: respiratory rate >30 breaths per minute, oxygen saturations of <90 per cent with standard oxygen delivered at least 5 L/min by a variable delivery mask with reservoir or, lastly, use of accessory musculature. CPAP and NIPPV were delivered via a Boussignac system, a simple portable device. CPAP was increased to 10 cm $H_2O$ and NIPPV to obtain a tidal volume of 8–10 mL/kg and expiratory pressure support was set at 5 cm $H_2O$. A combined primary endpoint of death, myocardial infarction or intubation in the first 24 hours of hospital admission, was used. Secondary outcomes included physiology, arterial blood gas analysis, length of hospital stay, in-hospital mortality and work of breathing. During the intervention, mean CPAP levels were 7.7 cm $H_2O$ and for NIPPV 12/4.9 cm $H_2O$. There was no difference between interventions for any outcome. Respiratory distress and physiology improved in both arms. Only 3 per cent of patients required intubation and only one person died within the first 24 hours. Exploratory analysis of patients with and without hypercapnia did not change the rate of improvement or the difference between interventions. Approximately 50 per cent were hypercapnic at presentation. It is of interest that 68 potentially eligible, but non-recruited, patients had non-invasive support applied pre-hospital and another 11 were intubated.

## Interpretation of the evidence

There is unequivocal data to support early symptomatic and physiological benefit in patients with cardiogenic pulmonary oedema receiving either CPAP or NIPPV. This is evident both in large primary trials[28] and pooled data.[79–83,86–89] Previous pooled data[79,80] and recent systematic reviews[81–83,86–89] have concluded that NIV (CPAP or NIPPV) delivers mortality benefit and reduces endotracheal intubation when compared to standard oxygen therapy. Indeed, they have reported up to a 47 per cent reduction in mortality.[82] This is at odds with the results of the 3CPO trial, a large recent pragmatic multicentre trial recruiting more patients than those previously assimilated in published systematic reviews. The 3CPO trial reported no difference in 7-day or 30-day mortality between standard oxygen therapy and NIV in emergency department patients with severe acute cardiogenic pulmonary oedema and acidosis. This was despite early improvements in symptoms and patient physiological parameters. There was no difference found for any primary or secondary outcome for the comparison between NIV and standard oxygen therapy other than breathlessness measured by a visual analogue scale, physiology at 1 hour (pulse rate) and arterial gas exchange parameters at 1 hour (pH and $PCO_2$). It should be noted that the breathlessness exhibited by the recrutied patients was marked with a mean score of 8.9 out of 10 at entrance to the trial. It therefore seems reasonable for this reason alone to consider NIV for palliation of these distressing symptoms. This short-term benefit needs to be balanced, however, with the possible intolerance of the mask.

No data, to date, support the additional benefit of NIPPV over CPAP despite the likely mechanistic advantages,[82] even when a primary trial has been adequately powered,[28] although there are potential reasons why a true benefit may not have been detected.[106] Lastly, despite continuing concerns[9,82,84] regarding the potential for an increase in myocardial infarction rates in patients treated with NIPPV, the 3CPO trial[28] and another trial by Bellone *et al.*[85] have confirmed the safety of the intervention.

It is unclear why the differences in findings between recent pooled data and the 3CPO trial have occurred but there are a number of potential reasons that need to be considered.

### PATIENT POPULATIONS

There may be differences in age, severity of illness and comorbidities in the 3CPO trial patients when compared with those recruited to other previous smaller trials. There may be temporal changes and geographical differences in the underlying aetiology of AHFS patients presenting with cardiogenic pulmonary oedema. This is unlikely for the following reasons. Based on and similar to previous studies, strict criteria were applied for inclusion of patients to the 3CPO trial enabling recruitment of the group of patients most likely to benefit from NIV, i.e. those with respiratory distress and acidosis. Indeed, the recent trial by Nava and colleagues showed a reduction in intubation rates only in a hypercapnic subgroup.[90] The baseline characteristics and event rates in the NIV arms were comparable with previous studies, and demonstrate that the recruited patients had severe disease. There was no evidence of patient selection bias with identical 7-day mortality in non-recruited patients (9.2 per cent).[53] This is further supported by the excellent recruitment rates of eligible patients when compared with those previously reported. There was also no obvious interaction between treatment intervention and disease severity, suggesting that those with milder disease did not obscure potential benefits in the sickest patients.

The 3CPO trial mortality rate has been challenged by some, suggesting that the population may have been less sick than in previous studies.[117,118] However, systematic reviews have used the ill-defined criteria of in-hospital mortality rate. This is likely to be much closer to the 3CPO trial 30-day mortality rate. Moreover, the 3CPO trial patients had significantly higher mortality than registry data (6.7 per cent, EURO HF survey;[119,120] 4 per cent, ADHERE registry).[5] These discrepancies in mortality and patient characteristics betweens studies are likely to reflect differing populations. Acute heart failure registries include all patients with AHFS rather than only those with severe acute pulmonary oedema. Indeed, in the EURO HF registry, only 16 per cent of patients had a qualifying diagnosis of acute pulmonary oedema. Lastly, patient age, male to female ratio and comorbidities are also similar to previous primary trials with mean age between 75 and 80 years, a female preponderance and highly comparable comorbidities such as hypertension, ischaemic heart disease, diabetes, chronic heart failure and COPD.

It is likely that a significant number of patients, given the physiological, age and sex characteristics of recruited patients, had relatively preserved systolic function, so called, diastolic heart failure[3,4] presenting with hypertension,[5,124] although echocardiography was not routine. These patients are likely to be more amenable to rapid pharmacological vasodilatation. Against this is the unequivocal finding, even using the more traditional World Health Organization (WHO) criteria for myocardial infarction definition, that index rates for myocardial infarction are considerably higher than the recent large trial undertaken by Moritz and colleagues[91] from France. Despite this, in-hospital mortality is identical between the two trials.[91]

## INFLUENCE OF CO-TREATMENTS

Although not mandated, the 3CPO trial recommended a set of co-treatments for recruited patients. This specifically included buccal and intravenous nitrates. Approximately 90 per cent of patients received this intervention. It is possible that the cardiovascular beneficial effects of NIV in acute cardiogenic pulmonary oedema have been masked by another treatment working, in particular nitrates, by the same mechanism, i.e. a reduction in preload and afterload.[54] Indeed, Crane identified pre-hospital nitrate as being the only factor associated with improved mortality in a UK observational study of patients with cardiogenic pulmonary oedema.[125] Co-treatments in previous small trials have often been incompletely characterized and documented and nitrate use in registry data is lower and likely to be related to cardiogenic pulmonary oedema only making up a proportion of study patients. It is therefore unclear whether there is consistency in these treatments across trials.

## INCONSISTENCY IN THE DELIVERY OF NIV

The 3CPO trial may have failed to reveal a difference in mortality between NIV and standard oxygen therapy because the intervention was ineffectively delivered. Over 80 per cent of sites had previous experience of NIV prior to the trial starting. There was a comprehensive training programme for all centres to ensure operator competence and consistency throughout the trial. Plant *et al.* have previous reported the safe application of NIV with ward-based staff after similar levels of training and less pre-trial experience and exposure to the intervention.[126] A readily applied portable ventilator that allowed both modalities of ventilation to be delivered as well as a tolerance for leaks around the face mask of up to 50 L/min was used in the 3CPO trial. Although unable to measure the inspired oxygen concentration, the circuit delivered an oxygen concentration up to 60 per cent. This ventilator system is not as sophisticated as some systems used in previous trials but more than others including the recent trial by Moritz *et al.*[91]

Mean pressures for both CPAP (10 cm $H_2O$) and NIPPV (14/7 cm $H_2O$) are highly comparable with previous studies[81,82] and higher than other recent studies.[91] Mean times of delivery of the intervention were a little over 2 hours, suggesting that the patients were physiologically and symptomatically significantly better within this short timeframe and again are similar to recent data from France.[91] There was crossover between interventions in all three arms of the 3CPO trial and these were analysed on an intention-to-treat basis. There were differing reasons with respiratory distress and hypoxia being more likely in the control arm and lack of patient tolerance in the two intervention arms. After these patients were removed from the primary outcome analysis, there remained no significant difference between groups although mortality rates were lower.

## DIFFERING THRESHOLDS FOR ENDOTRACHEAL INTUBATION AND CRITICAL CARE ADMISSION

Previous trials have indicated that the physiological improvement seen with NIV is translated into a reduction in tracheal intubation rates.[81,82] Pooled data from the meta-analysis by Peter *et al.* suggest that 6 patients need to be treated with CPAP and 7 with NIPPV to avoid 1 patient being intubated and mechanically ventilated.[82] The 3CPO trial, however, found no benefit in reducing intubation rates by NIV. This may reflect the relatively low intubation rates. Reasons for this are unclear but may reflect the differing patient populations, concomitant therapies and thresholds for intubation and mechanical ventilation across different countries, clinical environments and time periods. Again some have challenged these low rates, suggesting this reflects withdrawal or ceilings of clinical care rather than a true reflection on severity of illness.[117,118] Intubation rates in the standard therapy arms of previous studies vary from 35–65 per cent in initial trials[106,107] to 5–7 per cent for recent trials in emergency department settings,[92,110] despite similar severity of illness, in-hospital mortality and length of hospital stay. Intubation rate in the intervention arms has also fallen considerably over time with some initial trials reporting an intubation rate of up to 35 per cent whereas recent reports have consistently suggested rates of around 5 per cent. Indeed, the recent French trial by Moritz[91] reported a 3 per cent intubation rate almost identical to that in the 3CPO trial. Given that the present and previous trials were by necessity 'open', there is concern of treatment bias with a differing threshold for intervention according to treatment allocation. For example, patients on standard oxygen may be more likely to undergo intubation than those already gaining the apparent benefit of NIV. Additionally, clinicians may persevere with patients slow to improve with NIV if they believe in its efficacy. It is important to note that intubation did not correlate with mortality in the 3CPO trial.

### Trial design and interpretation of previous data

Recent reviews have included numerous randomized clinical trials. However, the individual trials were composed of small treatment group sizes that varied between 9 and 65 patients with recruitment rates of only 10–30 per cent (*cf.* 62 per cent randomized in the 3CPO trial). In the meta-analyses, the small total number of outcome events was well below the recommended threshold of 200[127] and this limits the generalizability of their findings. There is real concern about reporting, publication and recruitment bias in individual published studies, which will be compounded by pooled analysis. The discrepancy between the 3CPO trial results in the setting of a large multicentre randomized controlled trial and previous pooled data is not unique and the limitations of meta-analysis are well reported.[128]

## TECHNICAL CONSIDERATIONS

There are a number of considerations for services or specialties that want to introduce NIV into clinical practice. Solutions will depend on a number of factors including the size of the hospital, co-location of specialties, numbers of eligible patients and local and national policies and practice. Choices of equipment will also depend on these factors as well as the types of machine in other parts of the hospital and local procurement policies. The majority of patients with cardiogenic pulmonary oedema requiring NIV do not need a complex ventilator. The main factors are a well-fitting, full face mask, the ability to deliver up to a maximum of 100 per cent oxygen, as simple functionality as possible and, ideally, consistency between services to support training and transfer of patients. In addition, NIV should be delivered in a well monitored (minimum of oxygen saturations, heart rate, ECG, respiratory rate, blood pressure) area with resuscitation facilities and adequate levels of appropriately trained nursing staff. There should also be adequate access to blood gas analysis. All services that use NIV for patients with cardiogenic pulmonary oedema and other conditions should audit practice, have clear clinical guidelines and established training programmes.

## Management of pulmonary oedema related to acute heart failure syndromes

As previously stated, pulmonary oedema is one manifestation of patients presenting with AHFS with a number of aetiological factors and spectrums of disease. Increasingly, hypertensive heart failure, so-called vascular failure, is the predominant group.[7,129] Management should be tailored to a number of aspects of the patient's care: relief of symptoms, treatment of the precipitant, e.g. acute coronary syndromes or atrial fibrillation, physiological improvement, respiratory support, and finally prevention of secondary insult to the kidney or heart.[11] Figure 30.2 illustrates a simple algorithm for the early management of AHFS including those with cardiogenic pulmonary oedema based largely on the initial blood pressure. Patient care should be delivered in a clinical area, as detailed in the previous section, with adequate monitoring, staff levels and resuscitation facilities.

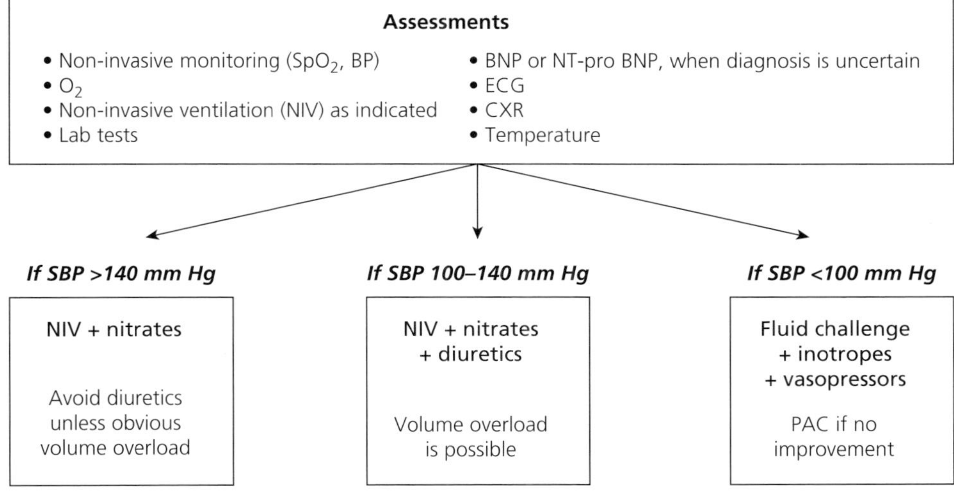


**Figure 30.2** Early management of acute heart failure syndrome. BNP, brain natriuretic peptide; BP, blood pressure; CXR, chest radiograph; ECG, electrocardiogram; PAC, pulmonary artery catheter. Modified with permission from Chatti *et al.*[37]

## CONCLUSIONS

Non-invasive ventilation is widely used in North America, Europe and Australasia for patients with severe acute cardiogenic pulmonary oedema. There are clear mechanistic reasons why these interventions work in acute pulmonary oedema. Indeed multiple small trials revealed that physiological parameters improve quickly with the use of NIV and this reduces endotracheal intubation and potentially in-hospital mortality. These findings have not been supported by the findings of a recent large multicentre clinical effectiveness trial, the 3CPO trial, which has failed to show any clear benefit of NIV for patients with severe acute cardiogenic pulmonary oedema in UK emergency departments, other than early improvement in some physiological characteristics and, importantly, patient symptoms. Despite theoretical advantages for NIPPV over CPAP, no trial data support additional benefit of this modality. The 3CPO trial has unequivocally demonstrated the safety of both NIPPV and CPAP and clearly shows there is no increased risk of myocardial infarction with NIPPV.

In the majority of patients, medical therapy, in particular, nitrate therapy, should be instigated as the primary treatment of severe acute cardiogenic pulmonary oedema, and NIV reserved for those patients who have significant respiratory distress and failure or those not improving with standard medical therapy. Further research is required to investigate whether certain subgroups of patients will gain particular benefit from NIV. These may include patients with normal or low blood pressure, valvular heart disease or patients with coexistent chronic respiratory disease such as COPD. Non-invasive ventilation (CPAP or NIPPV) provides significant early improvement in patient symptoms and markers of disease severity but perhaps unsurprisingly this does not translate into a reduction in subsequent mortality.

## REFERENCES


1. Adams KF Jr, Fonarow GC, Emerman CL *et al.* Characteristics and outcomes of patients hospitalized for heart failure in the United States: rationale, design, and preliminary observations from the first 100,000 cases in the Acute Decompensated Heart Failure National Registry (ADHERE). *Am Heart J* 2005; **149**: 209–16.
2. De Luca L, Fonarow GC, Adams KF Jr *et al.* Acute heart failure syndromes: clinical scenarios and pathophysiologic targets for therapy. *Heart Fail Rev* 2007; **12**: 97–104.
3. Owan TE, Hodge DO, Herges RM *et al.* Trends in prevalence and outcome of heart failure with preserved ejection fraction. *N Engl J Med* 2006; **355**: 251–9.
4. Aurigemma GP, Gaasch WH, Aurigemma GP *et al.* Clinical practice. Diastolic heart failure. *N Engl J Med* 2004; **351**:1097–105.
5. Gheorghiade M, Zannad F, Sopko G *et al.* Acute heart failure syndromes: current state and framework for future research. *Circulation* 2005; **112**: 3958–68.
6. Developed in collaboration with the American College of Chest Physicians and the International Society for Heart and Lung Transplantation, endorsed by the Heart Rhythm Society, Hunt SA, Abraham WT, Chin MH *et al.* ACC/AHA 2005 guideline update for the diagnosis and management of chronic heart failure in the adult – summary article: a report of the American College of Cardiology/American Heart Association Task Force on practice guidelines (writing committee to update the 2001 guidelines for the evaluation and management of heart failure). *J Am Coll Cardiol* 2005; **46**: 1116–43.
7. Collins S, Storrow AB, Kirk JD *et al.* Beyond pulmonary edema: diagnostic, risk stratification, and treatment challenges of acute heart failure management in the emergency department. *Ann Emerg Med* 2008; **51**: 45–57.
8. Nieminen MS, Bohm M, Cowie MR *et al.* Executive summary of the guidelines on the diagnosis and treatment of acute heart failure: the Task Force on Acute Heart Failure of the European Society of Cardiology. *Eur Heart J* 2005; **26**: 384–416.
9. American College of Emergency Physicians Clinical Policies Subcommittee (Writing Committee) on acute heart failure syndromes, Silvers SM, Howell JM *et al.* Clinical policy: critical issues in the evaluation and management of adult patients presenting to the emergency department with acute heart failure syndromes. *Ann Emerg Med* 2007; **49**: 627–69.
10. Task Force on Acute Heart Failure of the European Society of Cardiology. Executive summary of the guidelines on the diagnosis and treatment of acute heart failure. *Eur Heart J* 2005; **26**: 384–416.
11. Gheorghiade M, Pang PS. Acute heart failure syndromes. *J Am Coll Cardiol* 2009; **53**: 557–73.
12. Wang CS, Fitzgerald JM, Schulzer M *et al.* Does this dyspneic patient in the Emergency Department have congestive heart failure. *JAMA.* 2005; **294**: 1944–56.
13. Schwann E. B-type natriuretic peptide for diagnosis of heart failure in emergency department patients: a critical appraisal. *Acad Emerg Med* 2004; **11**: 681–91.
14. Knudsen CW, Omland T, Clopton P *et al.* Diagnostic value of B-type natriuretic peptide and chest radiographic finings in patients with acute dyspnea. *Am J Med* 2004; **116**: 363–8.
15. Harrison A, Morrison LK, Krishnaswamy P *et al.* B-type natriuretic peptide predicts future events in patients presenting to the Emergency Department with dyspnea. *Ann Emerg Med* 2002; **39**: 131–8.
16. McCullough PA, Nowak RM, McCord J *et al.* B-Type natriuretic peptide and clinical judgement in emergency diagnosis of heart failure. *Circulation* 2002; **106**: 416–22.
17. Maisel AS, Krishnaswamy P, Nowak RM *et al.* Rapid measurement of B-type natriuretic peptide in the emergency diagnosis of heart failure. *N Engl J Med* 2002; **347**: 161–7.

18. Gheorghiade M, Abraham WT, Albert NM *et al.* For the OPTIMIZE-HF investigators. Systolic blood pressure at admission, clinical characteristics, and outcomes in patients hospitalized with acute heart failure. *JAMA* 2006; **296**: 2217–26.
19. Mueller C, Scholer A, Laule-Kilian K *et al.* Use of B-type natriuretic peptide in the evaluation and management of acute dyspnea. *N Engl J Med* 2004; **350**: 647–54.
20. Lee DS, Austin PC, Rouleau JL *et al.* Predicting mortality among patients hospitalized for heart failure. *JAMA* 2003; **290**: 2581–7.
21. Fonarow GC, Abraham TW, Nancy MA *et al.* for the OPTIMIZE-HF investigators. Factors Identified as precipitating hospital admissions for heart failure and clinical outcomes. *Arch Int Med* 2008; **168**: 847–54.
22. Fonarow GC, Adams KF, Abraham TW *et al.* for the ADHERE scientific advisory committee, study group and investigators. Risk stratification for in-hospital mortality in acutely decompensated heart failure. Classification and regression tree analysis. *JAMA* 2005; **293**: 572–80.
23. Auble TE, Hsleh M, McCausland JB *et al.* Comparison of four clinical prediction rules for estimating risk in heart failure. *Ann Emerg Med* 2007; **50**: 127–35.
24. Gray A, Goodacre S, Masson M *et al.* A simple risk score to predict early outcome in acute cardiogenic pulmonary oedema. *Circulation*: Heart Failure; published on line ahead of print 30 October 2009.
25. Graham CA. Pharmacological therapy of acute cardiogenic pulmonary oedema in the emergency department. *Emerg Med Australas* 2004; **16**: 47–54.
26. Mattu A, Martinez JP, Kelly BS. Modern management of cardiogenic pulmonary oedema. *Emerg Med Clin North Am* 2005; **23**: 1105–25.
27. Northridge D. Frusemide or nitrates for acute heart failure. *Lancet* 1996; **247**: 667–8.
28. Gray A, Goodacre S, Newby D *et al.* on behalf of the 3CPO trialists. Noninvasive ventilation in acute cardiogenic pulmonary edema. *N Engl J Med* 2008; **359**: 24–33.
29. Hoffman JR, Reynolds S. Comparison of nitroglycerin, morphine and furosemide in the treatment of presumed pre-hospital pulmonary edema. *Chest* 1987; **92**: 923–7.
30. Sacchetti A, Ramoska E, Moakes ME *et al.* Effect of ED management on ICU use in acute pulmonary edema. *Am J Emerg Med* 1999; **17**: 571–4.
31. Peacock WF, Hollander JE, Diercks DB *et al.* Morphine and outcomes in acute decompensated heat failure: an ADHERE analysis. *Emerg Med J* 2008; **25**: 205–9.
32. Peacock WF, Costanzo MR, De Marco T *et al.* for the ADHERE Scientific Advisory Committee and Investigators. Impact of intravenous loop diuretics on outcomes of patients hospitalized with acute decompensated heart failure: insights from the ADHERE registry. *Cardiology* 2009; **13**: 12–19.
33. Browning J, Atwood B, Gray A. CPO trial group. Use of non-invasive ventilation in UK emergency departments. *Emerg Med J* 2006; **23**: 920–1.
34. Tallman TA, Peacock WF, Emerman CL *et al.* Noninvasive ventilation outcomes in 2430 acute decompensated heart failure patients: An ADHERE Registry analysis. *Acad Emerg Med* 2008; **15**: 355–62.
35. Fonarow GC, Heywood JT, Heidenreich PA *et al.* Temporal trends in clinical characteristics, treatments, and outcomes for heart failure hospitalizations, 2002 to 2004: findings from Acute Decompensated Heart Failure National Registry (ADHERE). *Am Heart J* 2007; **153**: 1021–8.
36. Silvers SM, Howell JM, Kosowsky JM *et al.* from the American College of Emergency Physicians clinical policies subcommittee. Clinical policy: critical issues in the evaluation and management of adult patients presenting to the emergency department with acute heart failure syndromes. *Ann Emerg Med* 2007; **49**: 627–69.
37. Chatti R, Fradj NB, Trabelsi W *et al.* Algorithm for therapeutic management of acute heart failure syndromes. *Heart Fail Rev* 2007; **12**: 113–17.
38. Figueras J, Weil MH. Blood volume prior to and following treatment of acute cardiogenic pulmonary edema. *Circulation* 1978; **57**: 349–55.
39. Figueras J, Weil MH. Hypovolaemia and hypotension complicating management of acute cardiogenic pulmonary edema. *Am J Cardiol* 1979; **44**: 1349–55.
40. Henning RJ, Weil MH. Effect of afterload reduction on plasma volume during acute heart failure. *Am J Cardiol* 1978; **42**: 823–7.
41. Francis GS, Siegel RM, Goldsnmith SR *et al.* Acute vasoconstrictor response to intravenous frusemide in patients with chronic congestive heart failure. *Ann Intern Med* 1985; **103**: 106.
42. Ikram H, Chan W, Espiner EA *et al.* Haemodynamic and hormone responses to acute and chronic frusemide therapy in congestive heart failure. *Clin Sci* 1980; **59**: 443–9.
43. Nelson GI, Ahuja RC, Silke B *et al.* Haemodynamic effects of frusemide and its influence in the repetitive rapid volume loading in acute myocardial infarction. *Eur Heart J* 1983; **4**: 706–11.
44. Dormans TPJ, Pickkers P, Russel FGM *et al.* Vascular effects of loop diuretics. *Cardiovasc Res* 1996; **32**: 988–97.
45. Pickkers P, Dormans TPJ, Smits P. Direct vasoactivity of frusemide. *Lancet* 1996; **347**: 1338–9.
46. Kraus PA, Lipman J, Becker PJ. Acute preload effects of furosemide. *Chest* 1990; **98**: 586–93.
47. Kubo SH, Clark M, Laragh JH *et al.* Identification of normal neurohormonal activity in mild congestive heart failure and stimulating effect of upright posture and diuretics. *Am J Cardiol* 1987; **60**: 1322–8.
48. Verma SP, Silke B, Hussain M *et al.* First-line treatment of left ventricular failure complicating acute myocardial infarction: a randomised evaluation of immediate effects of diuretic, venodilator, arteriodilator, and positive inotropic drugs on left ventricular function. *J Cardiovasc Pharmacol* 1987; **10**: 38–46.

49. Nelson GI, Silke B, Ahuja RC *et al.* Haemodynamic advantages of isosorbide dinitrate over frusemide in acute heart failure following myocardial infarction. *Lancet* 1983; **1**: 730–3.
50. Domanski M, Tian X, Haigney M *et al.* Diuretic use, progressive heart failure, and death in patients in the DIG study. *J Card Fail* 2006; **12**: 327–32.
51. Krum H, Cameron P. Diuretics in the treatment of heart failure: mainstay of therapy or potential hazard. *J Card Fail* 2006; **12**: 333–5.
52. Gray A, Goodacre S, Newby D *et al.* on behalf of the 3CPO trialists. Noninvasive ventilation in acute cardiogenic pulmonary edema. *Health Technol Assess* 2009; **13**.
53. Johnson A, Mackway-Jones K. Frusemide or nitrates in acute left ventricular failure. *Emerg Med J* 2001; **18**: 59–60.
54. Cotter G, Metzkor E, Kaluski E *et al.* Randomised trial of high-dose isosorbide dinitrate plus low-dose furosemide versus high-dose furosemide plus low-dose isosorbide dinitrate in severe pulmonary oedema. *Lancet* 1998; **355**: 389–93.
55. Beltrame JF, Zeitz CJ, Unger SA *et al.* Nitrate therapy is an alternative to furosemide/morphine therapy in the management of acute cardiogenic pulmonary edema. *J Card Fail* 1998; **4**: 271–9.
56. Vismara LA, Leaman DM, Zelis R. The effects of morphine on venous tone in patients with acute pulmonary edema. *Circulation* 1976; **18**: 455–60.
57. The cardiovascular effects of morphine. The peripheral capacitance and resistance vessels in human subjects. *J Clin Invest* 1974; **18**: 455–60.
58. Timmis AD, Rothman MT, Henderson MA *et al.* Haemodynamic effect of intravenous orphine on patients with acute myocardial infarction complicated by severe left ventricular failure. *BMJ* 1980; **280**: 980–2.
59. Amsterdam EA, Zelis R, Kohfeld DB *et al.* Effect of morphine on myocardial contractility negative inotropic action during hypoxia ad reversal by isoprterenol. *Circulation* 1971; **135** Suppl II: 43–4.
60. Haber HL, Siek CL, Bergin JD *et al.* Bolus intravenous nitroglycerin predominantly reduces afterload in patients with severe congestive heart failure. *J Am Coll Cardiol* 1993; **22**: 251–7.
61. Imhof PR, Ott B, Frankhauser P *et al.* Differences in nitroglycerin dose response in the venous and arterial beds. *Eur J Clin Pharamacol* 1980; **18**: 455–60.
62. Crane SD, Elliott MW, Gilligan P *et al.* Randomised controlled comparison of continuous positive airways pressure, bilevel non-invasive ventilation, and standard treatment in emergency department patients with acute cardiogenic pulmonary oedema. *Emerg Med J* 2004; **21**: 155–61.
63. Abraham WT, Adams KF, Fonarow GC *et al.* In-hospital mortality in patients with decompensated heart failure requiring vasoactive medications: an analysis of the Acute Decompensated Heart Failure National Registry (ADHERE). *J Am Coll Cardiol* 2005; **46**: 57–64.
64. Publication committee for the VMAC investigators. Intravenous nesiritide vs nitrogylcerin for treatment of decompensated congestive heart failure: a randomized controlled trial. *JAMA* 2002; **287**: 1531–40.
65. Hollenberg SM. Vasodilators in acute heart failure. *Heart Fail Rev* 2007; **12**: 143–7.
66. Colucci WS, Elkayam U, Horton DP *et al.* Intravenous nesiritide, a natiuretic peptide, in the treatment of decompensated congestive heart failure. *N Engl J Med* 2000; **343**: 246–53.
67. Moazemi K, Chana J, Willard AM *et al.* Intravenous vasodilator therapy in congestive heart failure. *Drugs Aging* 2003; **20**: 485–508.
68. Sacker-Bernstein JD, Skopocki HA, Aaronson K. Risk of worsening renal function with Nesiritide in patients with acutely decompensated heart failure. *Circulation* 2005; **111**: 1487–91.
69. Sacker-Bernstein JD, Kowalski M, Fox M *et al.* short-term risk of death after treatment with Nesiritide for decompensated heart failure: a pooled analysis of randomized controlled trials. *JAMA* 2005; **293**: 1900–5.
70. Teerlink JR. Overview of randomised clinical trials in acute heart failure syndromes. *Am J Cardiol* 2005; **96**: 59G–67G.
71. Cuffe MS, Califf RM, Adams KF Jr *et al.* Short-term intravenous milrinone for acute exacerbation of chronic heart failure. *JAMA* 2002; **287**: 1541–7.
72. Teerlink JR, Metra M, Felker GM *et al.* Relaxin for the treatment of patients with acute heart failure (Pre-RELAX-AHF): a multicentre, randomised, placebo-controlled, parallel-group, dose finding phase IIb study. *Lancet* 2009; **373**: 1429–39.
73. Dschietzig T, Teichman SL, Unemori E *et al.* Intravenous recombinant human relaxin in compensated heart failure: a safety, tolerability and pharmacodynamic trial. *J Card Fail* 2009; **15**: 182–90.
74. Follath F, Cleland JG, Just H, *et al.* Efficacy and safety of intravenous levosimendan compared with dobutamine in severe low-output heart failure (the LIDO study): a randomised double-blind trial. *Lancet.* 2002; **360**: 196–202.
75. McMurray JJ, Teerlink JR, Cotter G *et al.* Effects of tezosentan on symptoms and clinical outcomes in patients with acute heart failure: the VERITAS randomised controlled trials. *JAMA* 2007; **298**: 2009–19.
76. Hamilton RJ, Carter WA, Gallagher EJ. Rapid improvement of acute pulmonary edema with sublingual captopril. *Acad Emerg Med* 1996; **3**: 205–12.
77. Barach AL, Martin J, Eckman M. Positive pressure respiration and its application to the treatment of acute pulmonary edema. *Ann Intern Med* 1938; **12**: 754–95.
78. Poulton EP, Oxon DM. Left-sided heart failure with pulmonary oedema its treatment with the 'pulmonary plus pressure machine'. *Lancet* 1936; **228**: 981–3.
79. Pang D, Keenan SP, Cook DJ *et al.* The effect of positive pressure airway support on mortality and the need for intubation in cardiogenic pulmonary edema: a systematic review. *Chest* 1998; **114**: 1185–92.

80. Kelly C, Newby DE, Boon NA *et al.* Support ventilation versus conventional oxygen. *Lancet* 2001; **357**: 1126.
81. Masip J, Roque M, Sanchez B *et al.* Noninvasive ventilation in acute cardiogenic pulmonary edema: systematic review and meta-analysis. *JAMA* 2005; **294**: 3124–30.
82. Peter JV, Moran JL, Phillips-Hughes J *et al.* Effect of non-invasive positive pressure ventilation (NIPPV) on mortality in patients with acute cardiogenic pulmonary oedema: a meta-analysis. *Lancet* 2006; **367**: 1155–63.
83. Collins SP, Mielniczuk LM, Whittingham HA *et al.* The use of noninvasive ventilation in emergency department patients with acute cardiogenic pulmonary edema: a systematic review. *Ann Emerg Med* 269; **48**: 260–9.
84. Mehta S, Jay GD, Woolard RH *et al.* Randomized, prospective trial of bilevel versus continuous positive airway pressure in acute pulmonary oedema. *Crit Care Med* 1997; **25**: 620–8.
85. Bellone A, Monari A, Cortellaro F *et al.* Myocardial infarction rate in acute pulmonary edema: noninvasive pressure support ventilation versus continuous positive airway pressure. *Crit Care Med* 2004; **32**: 1860–5.
86. Ho KM, Wong K. A comparison of continuous and bi-level positive airway pressure non-invasive ventilation in patients with acute cardiogenic pulmonary oedema: a meta-analysis. *Crit Care* 2006; **10**: R49.
87. Winck JC, Azevedo LF, Costa-Pereira A *et al.* Efficacy and safety of non-invasive ventilation in the treatment of acute cardiogenic pulmonary edema – a systematic review and meta-analysis. *Crit Care* 2006; **10**: R69.
88. Agarwal R, Aggarwal AN, Gupta D *et al.* Non-invasive ventilation in acute cardiogenic pulmonary oedema. *Postgrad Med J* 2005; **81**: 637–43.
89. Nadar S, Prasad N, Taylor RS *et al.* Positive pressure ventilation in the management of acute and chronic cardiac failure: a systematic review and meta-analysis. *Int J Cardiol* 2005; **99**: 171–85.
90. Nava S, Carbone G, DiBattista N *et al.* Noninvasive ventilation in cardiogenic pulmonary edema: a multicenter randomized trial. *Am J Respir Crit Care Med* 2003; **168**: 1432–7.
91. Moritz F, Brousse B, Gellee B *et al.* Continuous positive airway pressure versus bilevel noninvasive ventilation in acute cardiogenic pulmonary edema: a randomized multicenter trial. *Ann Emerg Med* 2007; **50**: 666–75.
92. Crane SD, Elliott MW, Gilligan P *et al.* Randomised controlled comparison of continuous positive airways pressure, bilevel non-invasive ventilation, and standard treatment in emergency department patients with acute cardiogenic pulmonary oedema. *Emerg Med J* 2004; **21**: 155–61.
93. British Thoracic Society. Guidelines on non-invasive ventilation in acute respiratory failure. *Thorax* 2002; **57**: 192–211.
94. Evans TW. International consensus conferences in intensive care medicine: non-invasive positive pressure ventilation in acute respiratory failure. Organised jointly by the American Thoracic Society, the European Respiratory Society, the European Society of Intensive Care Medicine, and the Societe de Reanimation de Langue Francaise, and approved by the ATS Board of Directors, December 2000. *Intensive Care Med* 2001; **27**: 166–78.
95. Pinsky MR, Summer WR, Wise RA *et al.* Augmentation of cardiac function by elevation of intrathoracic pressure. *J Appl Physiol* 1983; **54**: 950–5.
96. Pinsky MR, Summer WR. Cardiac augmentation by phasic high intrathoracic pressure support in man. *Chest* 1983; **84**: 370–5.
97. Pinsky MR, Marquez J, Martin D *et al.* Ventricular assist by cardiac cycle-specific increases in intrathoracic pressure. *Chest* 1987; **91**: 709–15.
98. Grace MP, Greenbaum DM. Cardiac performance in response to PEEP in patients with cardiac dysfunction. *Crit Care Med* 1982; **10**: 358–60.
99. De Hoyos A, Liu PP, Benard DC *et al.* Haemodynamic effects of continuous positive airway pressure in humans with normal and impaired left ventricular function. *Clin Sci* 1995; **88**: 173–8.
100. Acosta B, DiBenedetto R, Rahimi A *et al.* Hemodynamic effects of noninvasive bilevel positive airway pressure on patients with chronic congestive heart failure with systolic dysfunction. *Chest* 2000; **118**: 1004–9.
101. Naughton MT, Rahman MA, Hara K *et al.* Effect of continuous positive airway pressure on intrathoracic and left ventricular transmural pressures in patients with congestive heart failure. *Circulation* 1995; **91**: 1725–31.
102. Lenique F, Habis M, Lofaso F *et al.* Ventilatory and hemodynamic effects of continuous positive airway pressure in left heart failure. *Am J Respir Crit Care Med* 1997; **155**: 500–5.
103. Katz JA. PEEP and CPAP in perioperative respiratory care. *Respir Care* 1984; **29**: 614–29.
104. Katz JA, Marks JD. Inspiratory work with and without continuous positive airway pressure in patients with acute respiratory failure. *Anesthesiology* 1985; **63**: 598–607.
105. Branson RD, Hurst JM, DeHaven CB Jr. Mask CPAP: state of the art. *Respir Care* 1985; **30**: 846–57.
106. Bersten AD, Holt AW, Vedig AE *et al.* Treatment of severe cardiogenic pulmonary edema with continuous positive airway pressure delivered by face mask. *N Engl J Med* 1991; **325**: 1825–30.
107. Rasanen J, Heikkila J, Downs J *et al.* Continuous positive airway pressure by face mask in acute cardiogenic pulmonary edema. *Am J Cardiol* 1985; **55**: 296–300.
108. Lin M, Yang YF, Chiang HT *et al.* Reappraisal of continuous positive airway pressure therapy in acute cardiogenic pulmonary edema. Short-term results and long-term follow-up. *Chest* 1995; **107**: 1379–86.

109. Takeda S, Nejima J, Takano T *et al.* Effect of nasal continuous positive airway pressure on pulmonary edema complicating acute myocardial infarction. *Jap Circ J* 1998; **62**: 553–8.
110. Kelly CA, Newby DE, McDonagh TA *et al.* Randomised controlled trial of continuous positive airway pressure and standard oxygen therapy in acute pulmonary oedema; effects on plasma brain natriuretic peptide concentrations. *Eur Heart J* 2002; **23**: 1379–86.
111. L'Her E, Duquesne F, Girou E *et al.* Noninvasive continuous positive airway pressure in elderly cardiogenic pulmonary edema patients. *Intensive Care Med* 2004; **30**: 882–8.
112. Masip J, Betbese AJ, Paez J *et al.* Non-invasive pressure support ventilation versus conventional oxygen therapy in acute cardiogenic pulmonary oedema: a randomised trial. *Lancet* 2000; **356**: 2126–32.
113. Bellone A, Vettorello M, Monari A *et al.* Noninvasive pressure support ventilation vs. continuous positive airway pressure in acute hypercapnic pulmonary edema. *Intensive Care Med* 2005; **31**: 807–11.
114. Levitt MA. A prospective, randomized trial of BiPAP in severe acute congestive heart failure. *J Emerg Med* 2001; **21**: 363–9.
115. Park M, Lorenzi-Filho G, Feltrim MI *et al.* Oxygen therapy, continuous positive airway pressure, or noninvasive bilevel positive pressure ventilation in the treatment of acute cardiogenic pulmonary edema. *Arq Bras Cardiol* 2001; **76**: 221–30.
116. Park M, Sangean MC, Volpe MS *et al.* Randomized, prospective trial of oxygen, continuous positive airway pressure, and bilevel positive airway pressure by face mask in acute cardiogenic pulmonary edema. *Crit Care Med* 2004; **32**: 2407–15.
117. McDermid RC, Bagshaw S. Noninvasive ventilation in cardiogenic pulmonary edema. *N Engl J Med* 2008; **359**: 2068–9.
118. Masip J, Mebazaa A, Filippatos G. Noninvasive ventilation in cardiogenic pulmonary edema. *N Engl J Med* 2008; **359**: 2068–9.
119. Cleland JG, Swedberg K, Follath F *et al.* The EuroHeart Failure survey programme – a survey on the quality of care among patients with heart failure in Europe. Part 1: patient characteristics and diagnosis. *Eur Heart J* 2003; **24**: 442–63.
120. Nieminen MS, Brutsaert D, Dickstein K *et al.* EuroHeart Failure Survey II (EHFS II): a survey on hospitalized acute heart failure patients: description of population. *Eur Heart J* 2006; **27**: 2725–36.
121. Bhatia RS, Tu JV, Lee DS *et al.* Outcome of heart failure with preserved ejection fraction in a population-based study. *N Engl J Med* 2006; **355**: 260–9.
122. Alla F, Zannad F, Filippatos G. Epidemiology of acute heart failure syndromes. *Heart Fail Rev* 2007; **12**: 91–5.
123. Crane SD. Epidemiology, treatment and outcome of acidotic, acute, cardiogenic pulmonary oedema presenting to an emergency department. European *J Emerg Med* 2002; **9**: 320–4.
124. Plant PK, Owen JL, Elliott MW. Early use of non-invasive ventilation for acute exacerbations of chronic obstructive pulmonary disease on general respiratory wards: a multicentre randomised controlled trial. *Lancet* 2000; **335**: 1931–5.
125. Flather MD, Farkouh ME, Pogue JM *et al.* Strengths and limitations of metanalysis: larger studies may be more reliable. *Control Clin Trials* 1997; **18**: 568–79.
126. Le Lorier J, Gregoire G, Benhaddad A *et al.* Discrepancies between meta-analyses and subsequent large randomised controlled trials. *N Engl J Med* 1997; **337**: 536–42.
127. Fillippatos G and Zannad F. An introduction to acute heart failure syndromes: definition and classification. *Heart Fail Rev* 2007; **12**: 87–90.

# 31

# Assisted ventilation in chronic congestive cardiac failure

MATTHEW T NAUGHTON

## ABSTRACT

Congestive heart failure is a costly and debilitating condition associated with high mortality and morbidity. Fortunately, it is highly responsive to non-invasive positive airway pressure ventilation (NIV) in many cases. For the purposes of this chapter, NIV will refer mainly to continuous positive airway pressure (CPAP), bi-level positive airway pressure (BiPAP), auto-titrating positive airway pressure (APAP) and adaptive servo-controlled ventilation (ASV). By virtue of the simultaneous pulmonary, cardiac and upper airway pneumatic actions, both cardiac and respiratory work can be alleviated with NIV by approximately 10 and 40 per cent, respectively. With time, cardiac remodelling may also occur and thereby reduce the frequency of acute deteriorations. In patients with heart failure and obstructive sleep apnoea (OSA), CPAP and BiPAP have been shown to improve systolic function, quality of life and neurohumoral activity. In patients with heart failure and central sleep apnoea (CSA), CPAP has been shown to improve systolic function, neurohormonal activity and exercise capacity. In stable heart failure, with either OSA or CSA, an improvement in survival with NIV is yet to be confirmed.

## INTRODUCTION

Congestive heart failure is a common and costly condition.[1] Acute cardiogenic pulmonary oedema (APO) is responsible for the majority of acute hospital admissions in people aged above 65 years, of whom ~50 per cent are readmitted for the same reason within a year. Both incidence and prevalence of chronic heart failure are increasing, due to an ageing population and improved management of most medical conditions (including ischaemic heart disease), such that >10 per cent of people now aged 80 years have heart failure. The 5-year mortality, from the time of heart failure diagnosis, is 50 per cent, which rivals many malignancies. Thus new and imaginative heart failure management strategies are required.

One such strategy, namely non-invasive positive airway pressure 'assisted' ventilation (NIV), has been gaining momentum over the past 80 years.[2] In this review, the term NIV will encompass positive airway pressure (PAP) delivered via a mask to a spontaneously breathing patient. These include 'pressure' (as opposed to 'volume') set devices in either continuous (i.e. fixed) (continuous positive airway pressure [CPAP]), bi-level (bi-level positive airway pressure [BiPAP]), auto-titrating positive airway pressure (APAP) or adaptive servo-controlled ventilation (ASV) modes.

## PATHOPHYSIOLOGY

### Heart failure

Circulatory failure occurs when the heart is unable to pump sufficient blood to meet the metabolic needs of the body, caused by cardiac (i.e. heart failure) and non-cardiac causes (Box 31.1). The causes and classifications of heart failure are important to appreciate when one considers the role of NIV as some types of heart failure will be more responsive to NIV than others. For example, disorders of cardiac pump function are more likely to be responsive to positive airway pressure than would heart failure secondary to disorders of cardiac rhythm or rate.

Systolic heart failure is defined by impaired left ventricular contractility and measured by a left ventricular ejection

**Box 31.1 Causes of circulatory failure**

Heart failure

- Myocardial (systolic and diastolic)
  - coronary artery disease (large and small vessel)
  - hypertension
- Infiltrative (e.g. sarcoid)
  - inflammatory
  - congenital
  - associated with neuromuscular (Duchenne)
  - toxic (e.g. alcohol)
  - post-partum (i.e. pregnancy associated)
- Pericardial
- Valvular
  - rhythm and conduction
  - fibrillation
  - extreme tachycardia or bradycardia
  - asynchrony

Non-cardiac causes

- Thyroid (hypo- or hyperthyroid)
- Anaemia
- Blood volume loss (e.g. haemorrhage)
- Inadequate oxyhaemoglobin (e.g. high altitude)
- Increased capacity of vascular bed (e.g. septic shock, anaphylaxis)
- Increased venous return (e.g. excessive intravenous fluids)
- Decreased peripheral resistance (e.g. arteriovenous fistula, cirrhosis)

fraction (LVEF) estimated by nuclear angiography or echocardiography of <55 per cent or left ventricular fractional shortening (LVFS) measured by echocardiography of <28 per cent. Diastolic heart failure or heart failure with normal systolic function is defined by symptoms of heart failure[3] with elevated left ventricular filling pressures in the setting of impaired left ventricular relaxation and normal systolic contraction. It is commonly due to 'stiff' ventricular walls which can result from hypoxia, tachycardia[4] and hypertension. Objectively, diastolic heart failure is defined by an elevated left ventricular filling pressure measured during a right heart catheter study (i.e. pulmonary capillary wedge pressure [PCWP] of >12 mm Hg) in the setting of normal systolic function (i.e. LVEF >55 per cent). Unfortunately heart failure symptoms do not parallel reliably the main objective marker of systolic and diastolic heart failure, namely PCWP.[5]

## Sleep-disordered breathing

As with exercise, sleep can place adverse stresses upon the cardiovascular system. The stress of sleep is due to body posture (horizontal vs upright) and state change (sleep vs wake). During sleep, heart rate, systemic blood pressure, minute ventilation, airway calibre and lung volumes are reduced by ~20 per cent. In non-rapid eye movement (REM) sleep, sympathetic activity is usually withdrawn and parasympathetic activity increased. In REM sleep, both sympathetic and parasympathetic activity become active, although regional blood flow differs from wakefulness (e.g. blood is directed away from skeletal muscles which are actively inhibited during REM sleep). In normal circumstances, the above changes have no adverse effects as metabolic rate also is diminished.

In obstructive sleep apnoea (OSA), sleep-related loss of upper airway muscle tone and upper airway collapse contributes to hypopnoea and apnoea (partial and complete obstruction for >10 seconds, respectively) in concert with strong diaphragmatic contractions, large negative intrathoracic pressure (ITP) swings accompanied by hypoxaemia and hypercapnia, terminated by an arousal from sleep, an acute rise in systemic and pulmonary blood pressure and sympathetic activity. Usually OSA is associated with greatest hypoxaemia in REM sleep. The combined negative ITP and elevated systemic blood pressure result in elevated transmural pressure to which the cardiac chambers are exposed.[6] Recurring hypoxia and hypercapnia result in endothelial cell damage and oxygen radical formation which may lead to premature or accelerated atherosclerosis.[7] Left untreated, OSA may contribute to the development of heart failure through systemic hypertension, premature atherosclerosis and coronary artery disease and increased left ventricular transmural pressure.

In patients with established systolic heart failure, elevated PCWP[1,8] and catecholamines,[1,9] hyperventilation and hypocapnia[10] may occur. When combined with lung to brain circulatory delay, advanced heart failure results in a waxing and waning pattern of ventilation known as Cheyne–Stokes respiration or central sleep apnoea (CSA) (Fig. 31.1). Typically, CSA occurs in non-REM sleep, and arousals occur at the peak of ventilation, with mild hypoxaemia and symptoms of orthopnoea and paroxysmal nocturnal dyspnoea. Some patients with heart failure have an overlap of CSA and OSA.[11] In one study of single-night analyses of heart failure patients, the frequency of OSA dropped from 69 to 23 per cent and CSA increased from 32 to 78 per cent associated with a ~2 mm Hg fall in mean transcutaneous $PCO_2$ from the first to last quarter of the night in 12 patients with heart failure.[12] It is important to note that CSA is alleviated by more than 50 per cent when in the lateral[13] and similarly by the elevated head position[14] compared with the horizontal supine position.

## Pulmonary effects of heart failure

With heart failure, PCWP increases, fluid extravasates into the interstitium, then along the interlobular septa, towards the peribronchovascular space and thereafter towards

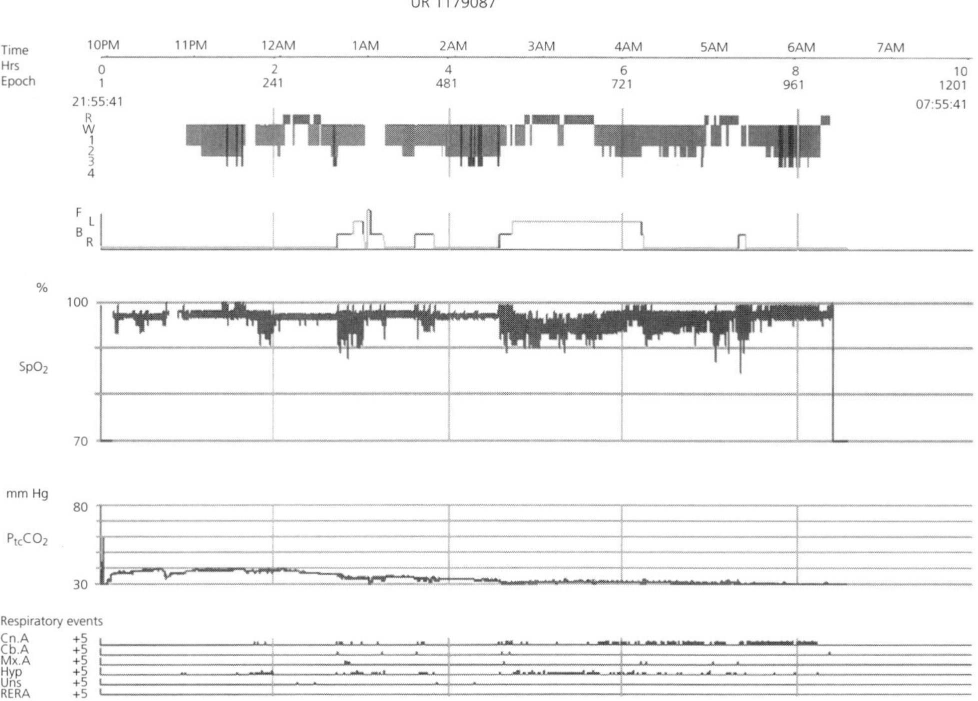


**Figure 31.1** Typical polysomnogram illustrating hyperventilation during sleep in a HF patient with central sleep apnoea (CSA). Note from top: time, sleep stages (non-REM and REM), body position (front, left, back, right), $SpO_2$, transcutaneous $PCO_2$ and respiratory events (central and obstructive apnoeas and hypopnoeas). Note the episodic fall in $SpO_2$ to values generally about 90 per cent, peak values to 100 per cent, and corresponding gradual reduction in $P_{tc}CO_2$ to 30 mm Hg. This indicates the presence of hyperventilation associated with central sleep apnoea.

the hila.[15] In addition, fluid accumulates in the pleural spaces, where ~25 per cent of the total body fluid accumulated in heart failure is deposited. In heart failure, the lymphatic drainage is estimated to increase 10-fold allowing drainage of fluid from the pleural space and interlobar septa.

Pulmonary complications related to heart failure (Box 31.2) include a reduced total lung capacity (TLC) and functional residual capacity (FRC), bronchial wall oedema with associated airflow obstruction. Pulmonary restriction correlates inversely with cardiac size.[16] Respiratory muscle weakness occurs with heart failure, which in APO may lead to hypercapnia (~20–45 per cent of APO). Usually <1 per cent of cardiac output is needed by respiratory muscles, however this increases disproportionately with increased work of breathing at a time of reduced cardiac output.[17] In APO, the carbon monoxide diffusing capacity is usually elevated, related to increased pulmonary blood volume, but falls with medical management of APO.[15] Chronic heart failure with long-standing interstitial oedema and interstitial haemosidereosis may lead to ossific nodules.[18] The pulmonary effects of heart failure may depend on age of onset and duration; for example heart failure effects related to mitral stenosis of rheumatic origin in youth may differ from hypertensive heart failure in the elderly.[15] This may be due to the rate of deterioration and compensatory processes. Therefore, knowing the severity and temporal change in symptoms (hours vs decades), the cause of heart failure, the age of symptom onset (youth vs elderly), the response to treatment and the presence or absence of coexisting pulmonary conditions are all important. Also, given the commonality of cigarette smoking in heart and lung disease plus the pulmonary side effects of cardiac treatment (e.g. amiodarone, β-blockers, pacemakers, thoracotomy) interpretation of lung function testing (including cardiopulmonary testing [Fig. 31.2] and sleep studies) and the understanding of mechanisms of dyspnoea in heart failure can be challenging.

### Box 31.2 Pulmonary complications of heart failure

- Restrictive ventilatory defect
- Obstructive ventilatory defect
- Diffusing capacity increased (acute heart failure) and reduced (chronic heart failure)
- Respiratory muscle weakness
- Hyperventilation

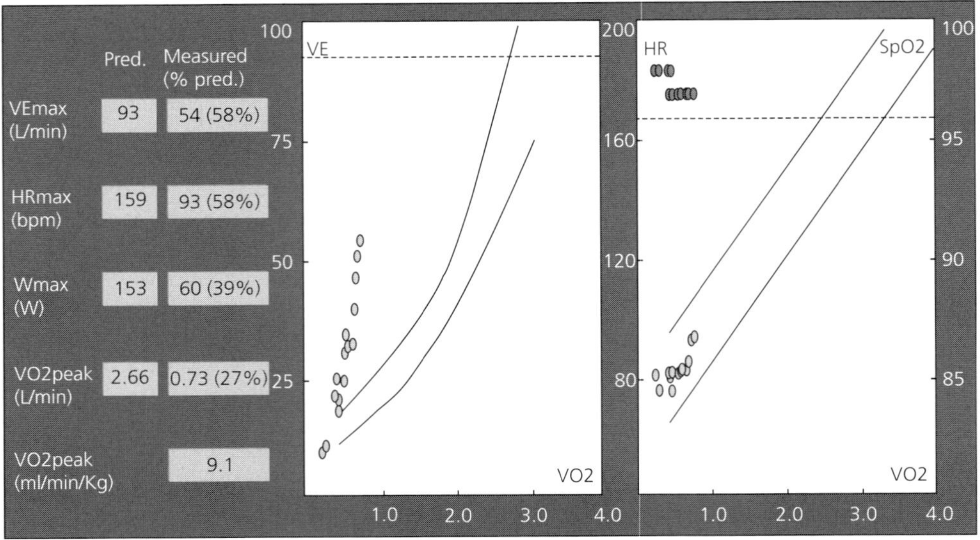


**Figure 31.2** Typical cardiopulmonary exercise test illustrating hyperventilation during exercise in a patient with heart failure. Note in the left graph of minute ventilation (VE) vs oxygen consumption ($VO_2$) the near vertical display of dots (representing 30 second data points) to the left of the expected normal. Patient's VE reaches only 58 per cent of predicted maximum (maximum displayed as dotted horizontal line). The right graph displays heart rate and $SpO_2$ vs $VO_2$. Note little change in heart rate due to negative inotropic drugs with a maximum heart rate achieved of 58 per cent predicted. Note also absence of hypoxaemia (minimum $SpO_2$ 97 per cent).

In normal subjects, acute volume loading results in reductions in TLC and FVC.[19] In stable heart failure, acute volume loading causes small airway obstruction.[20] Recovery from pulmonary oedema in non-smokers with heart failure is associated with a rise in TLC, FVC, forced expiratory volume in 1 second ($FEV_1$) and $FEV_1$/FVC ratio.[21]

With acute heart failure, capillary filtration of water leads to alveolar oedema. Over months to years, compensatory mechanisms may occur and reduce capillary filtration by as much as 50 per cent. Therefore, a reduced pulmonary diffusing capacity in heart failure may indicate a compensatory thickening of the alveolar capillary membrane which may prevent alveolar oedema. In support of this theory, reduced diffusing capacity with increased pulmonary dry weight suggesting an interstitial process made up of insoluble protein, lipid and cellular infiltrate, greater numbers of alveolar type 2 cells (source of surfactant) and an increase in surfactant was observed in a rodent model of heart failure.[22] The increase in alveolar surfactant would reduce surface tension and thereby reduce the work of breathing (WOB).

## MECHANISMS OF NON-INVASIVE VENTILATION IN HEART FAILURE

The proposed mechanisms of NIV in heart failure are listed in Box 31.3 and discussed below.

### UPPER AIRWAY STABILIZATION

The provision of NIV via a mask allows pneumatic splinting of the upper airway while breathing spontaneously. This action is most important during sleep in patients with OSA or when the sleep-deprived APO patient becomes drowsy and their neck flexes forwards.

**Box 31.3 Effects of NIV in heart failure**

- Upper airway splinting
- Pulmonary effects:
  - ↑ lung volume
  - bronchodilatation
  - ↑ ventilation–perfusion ratio
  - assist inspiratory respiratory muscles
  - ↑ dead space
- Cardiac effects:
  - ↓ afterload: ↓ transmural pressure; ↓ cardiac chamber size; ↓ systemic blood pressure
  - ↓ preload
- Autonomic effects:
  - attenuate sympathetic activity
  - accentuate parasympathetic activity

### INCREASE IN LUNG VOLUME

Heart failure, supine position and sleep are associated with a restrictive ventilatory defect. The lungs contain 50 per cent of the oxygen stores – thus a fall in TLC will increase the propensity to tissue hypoxaemia. CPAP of 10 cm $H_2O$ increases lung volume (~0.5–1.0 L) and tidal volume[23] associated with a fall in $dSpO_2/dt$ (from 0.42 to 0.20 per cent/s).[24]

## BRONCHODILATATION

Positive airway pressure has a bronchodilating effect, particularly if the cause of bronchoconstriction is a mechanical factor (obesity) or oedema (heart failure). Bronchogram studies indicate that CPAP is associated with a 30 per cent increase in airway diameter.[25] Lenique *et al.*[26] estimated lung resistance to fall with CPAP in adults with subacute heart failure by 40 per cent.

## RESPIRATORY MUSCLE

Respiratory muscle weakness of heart failure may be overcome with CPAP by assisting inspiratory muscles and reducing increasing pulmonary compliance. Using the tension time index (Fig. 31.3),[27] it is estimated that CPAP reduces $P_i$/MIP and $T_i/T_{tot}$ and thereby WOB and avoiding fatigue. In 3-month studies of CPAP in heart failure and CSA, respiratory muscle strength improves.[28]

## LUNG MECHANICS

In patients with subacute APO, CPAP was shown to be associated with a 45 per cent increase in lung compliance,[26] which is similar effect to that seen with surfactant in the rodent model of heart failure.[22] Work of breathing falls by 40 per cent in stable heart failure patients with CPAP associated with a 35 per cent reduction in pleural pressure amplitude and 7 per cent reduction in respiratory rate.[29] Others have shown similar reductions in WOB following APO with CPAP compared with T-piece breathing.[23]

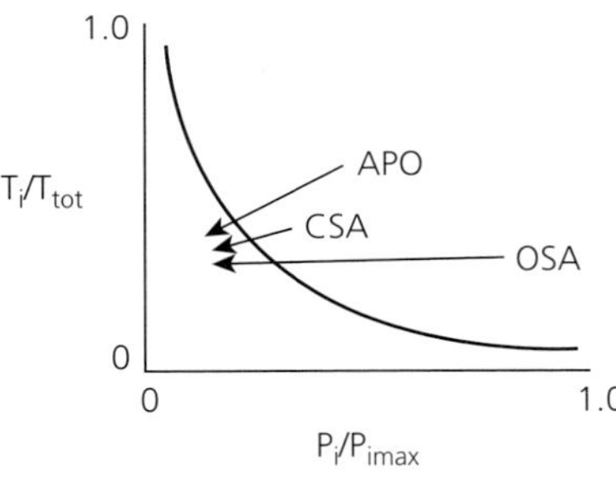


**Figure 31.3** Schematic representation of respiratory muscle fatigue.[27] On the vertical axis is the ratio of inspiratory time to total inspiratory and expiratory time (i.e. $T_i/T_{tot}$). The horizontal axis is the ratio of inspiratory pressure to maximum inspiratory pressure ($P_i$/MIP). The area to the right of the line represents a condition of high predisposition to fatigue, whereas to the left of the line low chance of fatigue. Estimates of the positions of patients with heart failure and obstructive sleep apnoea (OSA), central sleep apnoea (CSA) and acute cardiogenic pulmonary oedema (APO) are marked. Arrows indicate the expected direction when continuous positive airway pressure is applied.

## VENTILATORY DRIVE

Heart failure is associated with an increased respiratory drive during sleep and exercise[7,10,30] and CPAP during sleep causes a reduction in ventilation and a carbon dioxide rise.[31] The fall in ventilation and rise in carbon dioxide with CPAP is due to improved oxygenation (increased lung volume), improved cardiac output and a reduction in sympathetic activity. Increased dead space (due to dilated conducting airways and mask volume) may also contribute to hypercapnia.

Whether BiPAP is more beneficial than CPAP in heart failure has not been shown. Theoretically, it was thought that BiPAP may be more effective than CPAP in correcting the physiological disturbance of heart failure. However, one study suggested more biochemically proven myocardial infarction following admission with APO with BiPAP compared with CPAP.[32] This was not reproduced in later trials. Whether ASV, designed to maintain ventilation in CSA at ~90 per cent of minute ventilation and abolish the periodic breathing of CSA, is more effective that simple CPAP in heart failure remains to be determined.[33]

## CARDIAC AFTERLOAD

In heart failure, cardiac output is critically dependent upon left ventricular afterload, defined by Laplace's Law:

$$\text{Afterload} = \frac{(\text{systolic blood pressure} - \text{intrathoracic pressure}) \times \text{LV radius}}{\text{LV wall thickness}}$$

Thus LV afterload is increased when systolic blood pressure is raised, the ITP is more negative, the radius of the ventricle is increased on the wall of the left ventricle is decreased. These variables will change to differing degrees during APO, OSA and CSA, as illustrated in Figure 31. 4A–E.

In heart failure, the stroke volume is sensitive to changes in afterload: any factors which reduce afterload should increase stroke volume (unless there are conduction defects).[34] CPAP at pressures of 5–10 cm $H_2O$ has been shown to reduce systemic blood pressure acutely and chronically,[35] elevate intrathoracic pressures and reduce LV chamber radius.[36] Due to reductions in LV transmural pressure and heart rate, significant reductions in cardiac work have also been reported.[29,37,38] CPAP in stable heart failure patients has been associated with reductions in myocardial oxygen uptake[37] and cardiac sympathetic activity.[38]

The effects of CPAP directly on cardiac output are variable. Increased stroke volume in stable heart failure patients with elevated filling pressures (PCWP >18 mm Hg) has been shown acutely,[39,40] whereas others could not confirm this if in atrial fibrillation.[41,42] Other studies have shown an increase in LVEF over 1–3 months in OSA[43,44] and

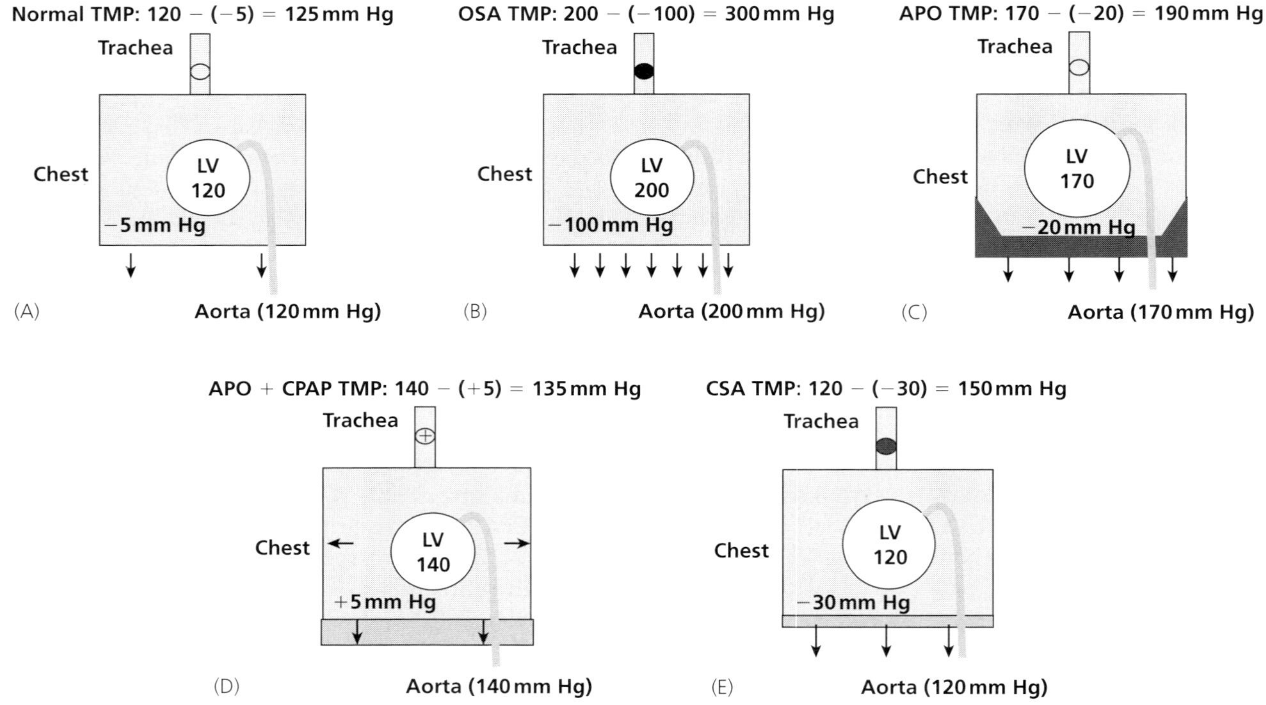


**Figure 31.4** A–E The effects of intrathoracic and systemic blood pressure on left ventricular transmural pressure during systole (TMP). (A) A normal situation during inspiration and systole with systolic blood pressure of 120 mm Hg and normal inspiratory pressures of − 5 mm Hg, accounting for a TMP of 125 mm Hg. (B) A patient with obstructive sleep apnoea (OSA) and heart failure: note very elevated systolic blood pressure and very large negative intrathoracic pressures with corresponding TMP of 300 mm Hg. (C) A patient with acute pulmonary oedema (APO): note elevated systolic BP and large negative intrathoracic pressures with corresponding TMP of 190 mm Hg. Also note development of effusions and further loss of total lung capacity. (D) A patient with APO on 10 mm Hg (~12 cm $H_2O$) continuous positive airway pressure: note fall in systolic blood pressure, positive change in intrathoracic pressures and abolition of pleural effusions and reduction in left ventricular chamber size with overall reduction in TMP to 135 mm Hg. (E) A patient with central sleep apnoea (CSA) and heart failure: note elevated systolic blood pressure and large negative intrathoracic pressures, greater cardiomegaly and elevated TMP of 150 mm Hg. Also note loss of total lung capacity and left ventricular chamber dilatation.

CSA patients[45,46] with LV remodelling plus reductions in mitral regurgitation and cardiac chamber dimensions.[47]

### PRELOAD

The elevation of intrathoracic pressure will impede venous return by up to 40 per cent in canine models given 10 mm Hg CPAP.[48] In normal subjects this may result in elevation of heart rate to maintain cardiac output. In heart failure, a small amount of CPAP (5–10 cm $H_2O$) may independently augment stroke volume (by virtue of ascending the Starling curve). High levels of CPAP may impair venous return and reduce cardiac output (e.g. heart failure with dehydration, sepsis) and in such circumstances BiPAP may be more beneficial.

### AUTONOMIC EFFECTS

Based on heart rate variability analysis (both temporal and power spectral analysis), the acute effects of CPAP in heart failure have been shown to increase vagal and attenuate sympathetic activity.[38,49] Reductions in urinary and blood noradrenaline (norepinephrine) have been observed associated with improvement in cardiac function with CPAP in patients with heart failure and OSA[43,44] and CSA.[45,46] Moreover, other neurohumoral markers of heart failure and LV wall stress (e.g. brain natriuretic peptide [BNP]) have also been shown to fall with ASV.[50] Baroreceptor function and heart rate variability has been shown to improve over 4 weeks with CPAP in heart failure and OSA patients.[51]

## EVIDENCE BASE FOR NON-INVASIVE VENTILATION IN CHRONIC HEART FAILURE

Non-invasive ventilation has been used in various areas of heart failure. In acute heart failure (i.e. APO), NIV (both CPAP and BiPAP) have been shown to be effective in terms of improvement in physiology, reduced intubation risk and survival (CPAP only) in carefully selected patients.[32] In one study, >50 per cent of hospital inpatients recuperating from APO had OSA, which when treated with APAP resulted in significant improvements in

LVEF.[52] In heart failure patients without sleep apnoea, CPAP was found to have no impact upon cardiac function or survival over 5 years.[53] Thus the balance of this section will be confined to chronic heart failure with OSA and CSA (Table 31.1).

### OBSTRUCTIVE SLEEP APNOEA

Obstructive sleep apnoea occurs in ~25 per cent of heart failure patients[11] and CPAP over 1–3 months has been shown to improve LVEF, autonomic control and quality of life[43,44] whereas improvements in long-term mortality are suggested in uncontrolled studies.[54,55]

In the first randomized controlled, parallel design, trial of CPAP in stable heart failure with OSA,[43] 24 patients (~55 yrs) with heart failure (mean LVEF 27 per cent, ~50 per cent on β-blocker therapy) and OSA (apnoea hypopnoea index [AHI] 41 eph, minimum $SpO_2$ 80 per cent) were randomized to CPAP or no CPAP for one month. Optimal medical therapy continued in both groups. Compared with the untreated control group, the CPAP-treated group (9 cm $H_2O \times 6$ h/night) experienced a significant improvement in LVEF (25–34 per cent) associated with falls in heart rate, systolic blood pressure plus left ventricular end systolic and diastolic volumes. Similar changes were noted in the β-blocker and non-β-blocker treated groups.

Sympathetic nerve activity, measured by muscle sympathetic nerve activity (MSNA) recordings, were taken during wakefulness from the common peroneal nerve at baseline and at one-month follow-up in 17 patients:[56] the MSNA fell by ~15 per cent in the CPAP-treated group. In 18 of the 24 patients, the frequency of premature ventricular beats also fell (170 to 70/h) with CPAP over one month whereas there was no significant change in the control group.[57] In another retrospective study from the same investigators, the control group (i.e. stable heart failure with untreated OSA) had a significantly worse 3-year survival than the heart failure group without OSA.[54] Although there was no significant difference in survival between OSA treated and untreated groups, a trend for improved survival with CPAP emerged.

The second randomized controlled, parallel design, trial of CPAP treatment for OSA in stable heart failure by Mansfield *et al.*[44] involved 55 patients (~57 years, LVEF 35 per cent, β-blocker use 78 per cent, AHI 28 eph and minimum $SpO_2$ 78 per cent), of whom 40 completed the 3-month trial. They were randomized to CPAP (8 cm $H_2O \times 6$ h/night) or control. The change in LVEF was significant (38–43 per cent), as was the 42 per cent fall in overnight urinary noradrenaline and improved quality of life (Medical Outcome Survey Short Form 36 and chronic heart failure) with 3 months of nocturnal CPAP compared with the untreated control group. However there was no significant change in maximum oxygen uptake during incremental cycle ergometry exercise. Although survival was not a primary endpoint, two deaths occurred in the CPAP group: one spontaneous and the other a complication of a pacemaker insertion, whereas there were no deaths in the control arm. Thus the call for longer trials with death as an endpoint is warranted.

A third, crossover design, trial assessed APAP in heart failure.[58] It enrolled 26 patients (~61 yrs, 80 per cent on β-blockers, LVEF 29 per cent, AHI 36 eph) for treatment with APAP/sham (6 weeks on each), and 23 patients completed the trial. Mean CPAP was 7 cm $H_2O$ in use for only 3.5 h/night. A significant improvement in sleepiness was observed, but no significant improvements were seen in the other primary or secondary endpoints (exercise capacity, LVEF, quality of life, plasma neurohumoral markers). The negative outcomes may be due to study design (crossover), relatively low levels of CPAP and hours of use and absence of a follow-up sleep study to ensure abolition of OSA.

**Table 31.1** Various actions of positive airway pressure (CPAP, BiPAP, ASV) in different situations of heart failure

| | OSA | CSA | APO |
|---|---|---|---|
| Upper airway stability | + + + | + | – |
| Increases lung volume | + | + + | + + + |
| Increases alveolar pressure | + | + + | + + + |
| Decreases left ventricular transmural pressure: | | | |
| • by alleviating negative ITP | + + + | | |
| • by elevating ITP | – | + + | + |
| Assists inspiratory muscles | – | + + | + + + |
| Bronchodilation | – | + | + + + |
| Prevents expiratory muscle recruitment (e.g. BiPAP) | – | – | + |
| Prevents fluctuation in tidal volume (e.g. ASV) | – | + | – |

APO, acute cardiogenic pulmonary oedema; ASV, adaptive servo-controlled ventilation; BiPAP, bi-level positive airway pressure; CPAP, continuous positive airway pressure; CSA, central sleep apnoea; ITP, intrathoracic pressure; OSA, obstructive sleep apnoea.

### CENTRAL SLEEP APNOEA

CSA occurs in ~25 per cent of heart failure patients.[11] A single-centre randomised trial of CPAP in stable heart failure with CSA before the routine use of BB included 24 patients (~59 yrs, LVEF 20 per cent, AHI 38 eph); those randomised to CPAP (10 cm $H_2O \times 6$ hrs/night) experienced a significant improvement in LVEF (21 to 29 per cent), quality of life and markers of neurohormonal activity[45] compared with a control group. Unlike CPAP for OSA (which responds immediately), CPAP for CSA was slowly titrated with careful inpatient observation for 2–3 nights, from 5 to 13 cm $H_2O$ with the knowledge that CSA may take days-weeks to resolve. Importantly in this group of patients there was a fall in minute ventilation and a rise in transcutaneous $CO_2$ levels.[31] Taken together, these data suggested an improvement in cardiac function, a fall in sympathetic activity, a reduction in hyperventilation (with rise in $PaCO_2$) and resultant stabilization of ventilation during sleep with CPAP over weeks to months.

However, two other groups were unable to confirm these findings. Davies *et al.*[59] reported no significant improvements in LVEF or symptom outcomes in an observational trial of eight patients with heart failure due to a variety of causes (e.g. one elderly patient with aortic stenosis) who were given 7.5 cm $H_2O$ CPAP for 2 weeks. This negative outcome may have been due to a low level and short duration of CPAP and the heterogeneous population studied. Similarly Buckle *et al.*[60] reported no change in AHI in a single night of CPAP (5–7.5 cm $H_2O$) in 8 patients with congestive heart failure (LVEF 24 per cent) and CSA (20 per cent of the night with CSA increasing to 28 per cent on CPAP).

These trials led to the larger CANPAP trial[46] with transplant-free survival as the primary outcome. This trial was conducted in 11 centres with 258 patients recruited (~63 years, LVEF 24 per cent, β-blocker use 77 per cent, AHI 40 eph, minimum $SpO_2$ 82 per cent). Patients continued medical therapy and were randomized to CPAP or no CPAP. The mean follow-up period was 2.2 years and 85 per cent completed the trial (CPAP 9 cm $H_2O$ × 4 h/night). There was no significant improvement in the primary outcome, namely transplant-free survival, nor in two secondary outcomes (hospitalizations and quality of life). However, there were significant improvements in other secondary outcomes (plasma noradrenaline, LVEF, nocturnal oxygenation, AHI and 6-minute walk distance).

A *post-hoc* analysis[61] of transplant-free survival based upon the 'suppressability' of the AHI during a repeat sleep study at 3 months in 210 of the original 258 CANPAP patients indicated that AHI fell to <15 eph in 57 per cent of patients randomized to CPAP. This CSA suppression with CPAP at 3 months was associated with a significant improvement in LVEF (25.6 to 29.2 per cent). Most importantly, the transplant-free survival at 60 months follow-up was greater in the CSA suppressed group compared with the untreated control and non-suppressed CSA groups (~95 vs ~50 per cent, respectively).

Another study compared BiPAP with medical therapy in 21 patients (~51 years) with chronic heart failure (LVEF 33 per cent, β-blocker use 67 per cent), and CSA (AHI >20 eph, mean ~28 eph).[62] Patients who were randomized to BiPAP (inspiratory positive airway pressure [IPAP] 11 cm $H_2O$, expiratory positive airway pressure [EPAP] 8 cm $H_2O$ × 4.8 h/night) or control. Over 3 months, those on BiPAP experienced an increase in LVEF (31 to 51 per cent), a reduction in AHI (28 to 5 eph), arousals, urinary noradrenaline (40 per cent reduction), whereas there were no changes in LVEF (35 to 38 per cent) or other parameters. A crossover study by Kohnlein *et al.*[63] compared 2 weeks of CPAP (8.5 cm $H_2O$) with 2 weeks of BiPAP (IPAP 8.5 and EPAP 3 cm $H_2O$) in random order and observed similar reductions in AHI (27 to ~8 eph), arousal indices (31 to 16/h) and lung to finger circulation times in 16 patients (aged 62 years) with heart failure (LVEF 24 per cent) and CSA. In addition, sleep quality and quality of life improved. Thus the studies of Noda[62] and Kohlein[63] both confirm the benefits of NIV in improving cardiac function.

Recently, ASV was developed for use in CSA.[33] This device detects and maintains a patient's ventilation at 90 per cent of their prior 3-minute moving average by providing a small amount of CPAP (~5 cm $H_2O$) plus a small amount of inspiratory pressure support (~4 cm $H_2O$). During central apnoeas, it provides greater inspiratory support (5–8 cm $H_2O$) at 15 breaths per minute sufficient to maintain ventilation.

In a series of single night studies, Teschler *et al.*[33] compared the effects of a single night of supplemental oxygen (2 L/m), CPAP (mean 9.3 cm $H_2O$), BiPAP (IPAP 13.5 and EPAP 5.2 cm $H_2O$), and ASV (mean 7–9 cm $H_2O$) on consecutive nights, in random order in 14 heart failure patients with CSA. The AHI declined significantly from 45 eph (control) to 28 eph (oxygen) to 27 eph (CPAP) and 15 eph (BiPAP) and 6 eph (ASV). Improvements in sleep quality (combined slow-wave sleep and REM sleep) occurred only in the BiPAP and ASV treatment groups. The effects on cardiovascular function were not assessed. The group mean $PtcCO_2$ and arterialized $PaCO_2$ increased overnight with ASV and CPAP (2.0 mm Hg and 3.6 mm Hg with ASV and 2.5 mm Hg and 4.2 mm Hg with CPAP) compared with baseline control night. The rise in $PCO_2$ with ASV was attributed to a fall in minute volume of ventilation (although not measured) related to greater slow wave and REM sleep and less arousals. Alternatively, it may have been due to dead space provided by ASV. Similar to ASV, night flow-targeted dynamic BiPAP was found to be effective in eliminating CSA, however, cardiac variables were not measured.[64] Thus further acute studies are warranted to determine the precise mechanisms of action of the ASV device.

Several medium duration clinical trials of ASV followed. A 1-month randomized, controlled, single-centre trial of ASV (mean 10 cm $H_2O$) vs sham (2 cm $H_2O$)[50] showed less sleepiness (greater Osler test by 9 minutes) lower plasma BNP levels and 24-hour urinary adrenaline levels with ASV. Mean usage of therapeutic and sham ASV were 5 and 3.6 hours per night. There were no changes on echocardiography or in questionnaires. Unfortunately follow-up polysomnographs were not performed and as such the effect of intervention on AHI and sleep quality were not determined. The lack of an effect on cardiac function may be explained by a lower mean pressure than CPAP with insufficient unloading of the left ventricle or increase in lung volume.

Two studies have assessed ASV over 6 months. The first randomized trial[65] compared ASV (5 cm $H_2O$ CPAP with 3–10 cm $H_2O$ swing) with CPAP (mean 8 cm $H_2O$) in 25 patients (mean age 62 years, LVEF 29 per cent, β-blocker use 72 per cent, AHI 43 eph). Average NIV use was 4.3 hours per night. The study had incomplete data, however, the group mean LVEF improved with ASV (29 to 35 per cent) whereas there was no change with CPAP (30 to 28 per cent).

The other 6-month ASV trial (non-randomized) compared ASV (mean 10 cm $H_2O$) with an untreated control group[66] and reported a marked improvement in LVEF (29 to 37 per cent) with ASV compared with controls (36 to 31 per cent). This study included 19 patients (61 years, BMI 32 kg/m$^2$, β-blocker use >90 per cent, LVEF 32 per cent, AHI 40 eph both central and obstructive in type) who received a ASV pressure range of 6–10 cm $H_2O$ for 4.5 h/night over 6 months.

The only 12-month study of ASV reported comes from Germany,[67] and in 15 patients (LVEF ~30 per cent, NYHA 2+3) randomized to CPAP (10 cm $H_2O$) with ASV (5–15 cm $H_2O$) it indicated similar reductions in AHI (CPAP 48 to 12 eph) and ASV (47 to 9 eph) whereas there were trends of improvements in $VO_2$ max with CPAP (16.6 to 19.8 L/min/kg) whereas no change was noted in the ASV group. Adherence to therapy was slightly better with CPAP (6 vs 4 hours per night). In both groups there were no changes in fractional shortening determined by echocardiography.

Thus ASV is a promising new version of CPAP, which may provide improved sleep quality, yet medium- and long-term trials with cardiac outcomes are lacking. Currently, ASV is the subject of large-scale, long-term randomized trials (e.g. SERVE-heart failure; http://servehf.com) in order to evaluate its effects on cardiovascular outcomes in heart failure with CSA.

### Limitations of studies

The major concerns with much of the published data relate to study design and absence of appropriate endpoints. When dealing with heart failure patients it is important to include a control group and robust markers of cardiac function (e.g. mortality, admissions, LVEF, BNP) in addition to general and disease-specific quality of life (i.e. heart failure and sleep apnoea) – composite endpoints may be used. The level, duration and mode of NIV needs to be adequate and include reporting of leak mask type and efficacy (i.e. follow-up AHI). Accurate descriptions of heart failure are also required and include aetiology, cardiac rhythm, rate and any associated features of heart failure (e.g. anaemia, renal failure, etc). Duration of heart failure should also be included, as the features of mitral stenosis in youth may differ from ischaemic cardiomyopathy in the elderly.

## TECHNICAL ASPECTS

#### SUPPLEMENTAL OXYGEN

The role of oxygen therapy in heart failure with sleep-disordered breathing has been influenced by a number of studies which have shown marginal effects upon markers of CSA and no significant changes in cardiac function.[7] The alleviation of AHI may relate to attenuation of peripheral and central chemosensitivity, although this remains to be proven. Although avoidance of hypoxia is thought to be important, so too is the avoidance of hyperoxia as it can impair pulmonary and cardiac function and cause coronary vasoconstriction.[7]

#### CPAP TITRATION IN CSA

Unlike CPAP for OSA (which usually responds immediately) CPAP for CSA should be slowly titrated with careful observation for 2–3 nights, from 5 cm $H_2O$ to 13 cm $H_2O$ with the knowledge that CSA may take days to weeks to resolve.

## FUTURE DIRECTIONS

Many questions lie ahead to be answered in forthcoming trials of NIV in heart failure and sleep-disordered breathing. Most studies have been marred by viewing sleep-disordered breathing as a static condition, i.e. its presence or absence in a particular patient at a finite time. It appears likely that the severity and presence of either type of sleep-disordered breathing is dependent on several factors including body weight, fluid accumulation, drugs, posture and head elevation. Also, whether NIV remodels the failing heart, acutely or chronically, and for how long is unknown, as is whether the trajectory of the underlying heart failure prognosis and severity can be altered.

The effects of heart failure therapies (from medications, pacemakers to transplantation) on sleep-disordered breathing need further investigation, as it is possible that the treatment of heart failure will attenuate this condition. The optimal mode and duration of the various NIV settings and devices to treat sleep apnoea in heart failure remain unknown. Whether BiPAP or ASV devices are beneficial over commonplace and less expensive CPAP remains speculative.

The best outcome variable in patients with heart failure and sleep-disordered breathing remains to be determined. The AHI may not be best suited for the CSA group as shorter cycle length (indicating better cardiac function) and less hypoxaemia (indicating increased oxygen stores) may be dismissed by a higher AHI. Cycle length, markers of oxygenation and carbon dioxide, sleep quality, patient comfort and quality of life plus markers of autonomic control (e.g. heart rate, heart rate variability, overnight urinary noradrenaline) and BNP may be best.

The use of ASV may negate central apnoeas and hypopnoeas measured in the usual way, i.e. by chest and abdominal plethysmography and oronasal airflow, and thus drop the AHI. However, the underlying pathophysiological periodic breathing may persist and only be detected by measurement of the fluctuating swings in peak inspiratory pressures. Whether persistent underlying periodic breathing is of clinical importance remains to be determined.

A more intricate knowledge of cardiopulmonary interaction in heart failure is required particularly related

59. Davies RJO, Harrington KJ, Ormerod OJ *et al.* Nasal continuous positive airway pressure in chronic heart failure with sleep disordered breathing. *Am Rev Respir Dis* 1993; **147**: 630–4.
60. Buckle P, Millar T, Kryger M. The effect of short term nasal CPAP on Cheyne-Stokes respiration in congestive heart failure. *Chest* 1992; **102**: 31–5.
61. Arzt M, Floras JS, Logan AG *et al.* Suppression of central sleep apnea by continuous positive airway pressure and transplant-free survival in heart failure: a post hoc analysis of the Canadian Continuous Positive Airway Pressure for Patients with Central Sleep Apnea and Heart Failure Trial (CANPAP). *Circulation* 2007; **115**: 3173–80.
62. Noda A, Izawa H, Asano H *et al.* Beneficial effect of bilevel positive airway pressure on left ventricular function in ambulatory patients with idiopathic dilated cardiomyopathy and central sleep apnea-hypopnoea. A preliminary study. *Chest* 2007; **131**: 1694–701.
63. Kohnlein T, Welte T, Tan LB *et al.* Assisted ventilation for heart failure patients with Cheyne Stokes respiration. *Eur Resp J* 2002; **20**: 934–41.
64. Arzt M, Wenzel R, Montalvan S *et al.* Effects of dynamic bilevel positive airway pressure support on central sleep apnea in men with heart failure. *Chest* 2008; **134**: 61–6.
65. Phillipe C, Stoica-Herman M, Drouot X *et al.* Compliance with and effectiveness of adaptive servoventilation versus continuous positive airway pressure in the treatment of Cheyne-Stokes respiration in heart failure over a six month period. *Heart* 2006; **92**: 337–42.
66. Hastings PC, Vazir A, Meadows GE *et al.* Adaptive servo-ventilation in heart failure patients with sleep apnea: a real world study [letter]. *Int J Cardiol* 2009; **139**: 17–24.
67. Randerath WJ, Galetke W, Domanski U *et al.* Efficacy of adaptive servo-ventilation versus constant positive airway pressure therapy in patients with heart failure and Cheyne-Stokes respiration. *Am J Respir Crit Care Med* 2004; **169**: A466.

# SECTION G

# Neuromuscular disease

# 32

# Muscle disorders and ventilatory failure

DAVID HILTON-JONES

## ABSTRACT

Ventilation is dependent upon the normal functioning of the respiratory muscles – the most important being the intercostals and diaphragm. These are skeletal muscles and they can be involved to a greater or lesser extent in those diseases that primarily affect muscles (myopathies) as well as those that cause secondary muscle weakness through denervation (neurogenic disorders). This chapter reviews those myopathies in which ventilatory failure, requiring long-term non-invasive ventilation, is a risk, and distinguishes between those conditions in which such involvement is a late consequence of the disease, when the patient may be profoundly affected by weakness, and those rare conditions in which there is a predilection for involvement of the respiratory muscles and ventilatory failure may ensue when the patient is still ambulant. The classification of the myopathies are discussed and the major clinical features of each condition reviewed.

## INTRODUCTION

Ventilation is ultimately achieved through the contraction and relaxation of the muscles of the chest wall and diaphragm. They are voluntary muscles of the same general composition as the skeletal musculature. It is therefore not surprising that primary muscle disorders may be complicated by the development of ventilatory insufficiency. Given that many such myopathies are progressive in nature and have no specific treatment, it is unarguable that one of the greatest successes of management in the past 20 years has been the introduction of non-invasive ventilatory techniques which have given enormous benefit with respect to quality of life, together with, in some disorders, a very substantial increase in life expectancy.[1]

Much of the rest of this volume is devoted to the basics of clinical and laboratory assessment of ventilatory insufficiency and its subsequent management. Such details will not be repeated here except in so much that there may be specific issues concerning individual disorders. A major aim of this chapter is to educate respiratory specialists about the often individually very rare muscle disorders that they will come across while providing non-invasive ventilation. Their knowledge need not be encyclopaedic, but greater insight must help overall patient management.

Many individual myopathies are extremely rare but as the ventilatory consequences, and their management, are essentially independent of the pathological process causing the myopathy there is no need for the respiratory specialist to have detailed knowledge of all forms of myopathy. This chapter will concentrate on the more common muscle diseases associated with ventilatory insufficiency and the need for ventilatory support, noting the rarer entities in passing.

At the clinical level a fundamentally important distinction is between those conditions in which ventilatory insufficiency is invariably a late feature of the disease (by which time the patient has long been wheelchair dependent), and those conditions in which significant ventilatory insufficiency, requiring intervention, may develop while the patient is still ambulant. Arguably these latter patients are at greatest risk because neither the patient, nor the managing clinician if not specializing in the area, may be aware of the risks or be attuned to the premonitory symptoms until problems ensue. In rare instances ventilatory failure may be the first manifestation of a myopathy.

This chapter is concerned primarily with late-childhood and adult muscle disorders. It deals with conditions in which the pathological process involves some part of muscle fibre, including the neuromuscular junction. Most of the conditions covered will require long-term ventilatory support once insufficiency has developed, although in some instances temporary non-invasive ventilation may be required to cover complications such as pneumonia, or the post-operative period.

The other major part of the motor unit is the anterior horn cell and motor neurone. Brief comment will be made about spinal muscular atrophy as in the clinic it is commonly seen alongside primary muscle disorders and shares similarities of management with muscular dystrophy. Acquired disorders such as poliomyelitis and neuropathies, such as Guillain–Barré syndrome, will not be covered here. Similarly, amyotrophic lateral sclerosis (motor neurone disease) will not be discussed, but is covered in Chapter 35. There are a number of neuromuscular disorders which present in the neonatal period and require invasive ventilation, and often have a poor prognosis (e.g. type 1 spinal muscular atrophy, Pompe's disease) and they will also not be discussed here.

## CLASSIFICATION OF MUSCLE DISORDERS

There is no uniquely applicable or useful system of classification but nevertheless it is valuable to have a framework, particularly for those less familiar with the field of neuromuscular disorders. A fundamental distinction is between acquired and inherited disorders. At the time of writing a fair generalization is that there are no specific treatments for inherited disorders, and that most acquired disorders can either be treated successfully or will remit if the cause is withdrawn. Exceptions may include enzyme replacement therapy for acid maltase deficiency (Pompe's disease), as a treatable inherited disorder,[2] and inclusion body myositis as an untreatable acquired disorder. Not surprisingly, therefore, the main burden with respect to the provision of non-invasive ventilation is for patients with inherited muscle disorders.

The main categories of acquired and inherited muscle disorders, and the more common conditions within each category, are shown in Boxes 32.1 and 32.2, respectively. Those conditions commonly associated with significant ventilatory problems are shown in italics. In other words, those conditions highlighted represent the bulk of the clinical workload.

### Box 32.1 Acquired muscle disorders

(Conditions commonly associated with ventilatory problems are in italics)

Endocrinopathies

- Hypothyroidism
- Hyperthyroidism
- Cushing's syndrome

Drug-induced: numerous but including:

- any drug causing hypokalaemia (e.g. diuretic, liquorice)
- penicillamine (causing myasthenic syndrome)
- statins
- anti-retroviral drugs (mitochondrial myopathy)
- *steroid/neuromuscular blocker acute quadriplegic myopathy*

Idiopathic inflammatory myopathies

- Polymyositis (often with connective tissue disease)
- Dermatomyositis
- Inclusion body myositis

Metabolic myopathies

- Glycogenoses
- Disorders of lipid metabolism (e.g. carnitine palmitoyl-transferase deficiency)

Infection

- Viruses (e.g. myalgia associated with flu)
- Bacteria (abscess formation)
- Numerous helminths and protozoa

## MUSCLE DISORDERS ASSOCIATED WITH LATE VENTILATORY INSUFFICIENCY

In the conditions discussed below, ventilatory insufficiency is inevitable in later stages of the disease. Early manifestations include increased susceptibility to chest infections (compounded by aspiration in those with pharyngeal muscle involvement) and delayed recovery following general anaesthesia. Either may precipitate ventilatory failure, which may be transient or permanent. In myotonic dystrophy sleep-disordered breathing may contribute to excessive daytime sleepiness (although central mechanisms are more important). All boys with Duchenne will eventually develop ventilatory failure, whereas only a small proportion of men with the allelic disorder Becker dystrophy will do so. Similarly, only a small proportion of patients with myotonic dystrophy require, or as will be mentioned will tolerate, long-term assisted ventilation.

### Duchenne muscular dystrophy

That this was the first clearly defined dystrophy simply reflects the facts that it is the most common inherited myopathy presenting in childhood and has a stereotypic clinical presentation. It is an X-linked recessive disorder and thus typically affects males but is transmitted by carrier females. The incidence is 1 in 3500 live male births. Up to

**Box 32.2 Inherited muscle disorders**

(Conditions commonly associated with ventilatory problems are in italics)

Muscular dystrophies

- X-linked recessive:
  - *Duchenne*
  - Becker
  - Emery–Dreifuss syndrome (Emerin deficiency)
- Autosomal dominant:
  - facioscapulohumeral
  - limb-girdle: Type 1B (allelic with autosomal dominant Emery-Dreifuss syndrome), Type 1C
  - Emery–Dreifuss syndrome (lamin A/C deficiency)
  - oculopharyngeal
- Autosomal recessive: limb girdle: numerous types numbered 2A–2O, *Type 2I (FKRP deficiency)*

Congenital muscular dystrophy

- *Numerous subtypes*

Myotonic dystrophy

- *Type 1 (Steinert's disease, DMPK gene CTG repeat)*
- Type 2 (Proximal myotonic myopathy, *ZNF9* gene CCTG repeat)

Myofibrillar myopathies

- *Desminopathy*

Congenital myopathies

- *Collagen VI disorders (Bethlem and Ullrich myopathies)*
- Central core disease
- *Nemaline myopathy*
- *Rigid spine disorders (SEPN1 and RyR1 mutations)*

Metabolic myopathies

- Glycogenoses:
  - *acid maltase deficiency (Pompe's disease)*
  - McArdle's disease (myophosphorylase deficiency)
- Lipidoses: carnitine palmitoyltransferase deficiency)
- Mitochondrial cytopathies: numerous phenotypes

Muscle channelopathies

- Sodium
  - Hyperkalaemic periodic paralysis
  - Normokalemic periodic paralysis
- Calcium
  - Hypokalaemic periodic paralysis
- Potassium
  - Andersen's syndrome
- Chloride
  - Autosomal dominant and recessive myotonia congenita

10 per cent of carrier females manifest muscle features, but they are generally mild and asymptomatic. Features in carriers include elevated serum creatine kinase levels, calf muscle hypertrophy, and proximal limb weakness; such weakness is very rarely severe.

### MOLECULAR ASPECTS

Duchenne muscular dystrophy (DMD) is caused by mutations in the gene coding for the very large structural protein dystrophin,[3] whose main function is supporting the muscle fibre membrane. It is allelic with Becker muscular dystrophy (BMD), discussed below, and these and related conditions are sometimes referred to as the dystrophinopathies. The main consequence of the defect is increased membrane fragility, which leads to abnormal calcium homoeostasis, activation of proteases and muscle fibre necrosis. The commonest mutations are large deletions (about 70 per cent) which are readily detected by relatively simple molecular tests. The remaining mutations include small deletions, duplications and point mutations which, within an extremely large gene, had proved difficult to identify with conventional technology. Previously the approach to diagnosis included testing for larger deletions, and if they were absent to demonstrate absence of dystrophin by immunohistochemistry on a muscle biopsy specimen – when appropriate more detailed, and expensive, mutational analysis could be undertaken. Recent advances have meant that rapid, cost-effective, laboratory testing is increasingly becoming available, with the imminent arrival of 'DNA-chip' diagnosis.

In DMD the mutation is 'out of frame' resulting in disruption of the reading frame and failure of protein production.[4] Thus muscle biopsy immunohistochemistry shows complete lack of dystrophin. In BMD there is a mutation in the same gene, but it is 'in frame' allowing production of a truncated version of dystrophin which is partly functional. Muscle immunohistochemistry typically shows patchiness of dystrophin staining and western blotting shows reduced quantities of dystrophin of reduced molecular weight.

### CLINICAL FEATURES

No clinical features are evident at birth but if the serum creatine kinase is measured it is invariably massively elevated – this has formed the basis of neonatal screening programmes.[5] Typically motor milestones are slightly delayed, but often not by enough to cause any immediate concern. It gradually becomes apparent that the boy is not gaining motor skills. He appears clumsy in his movements, can walk but not run, and cannot hop or jump. Speech delay is common. In some boys learning difficulties are apparent, thought to relate to the fact that dystrophin is expressed in the brain.[6] Behavioural difficulties are common, which may again reflect abnormal dystrophin expression in the brain, but also may be a reaction to the physical consequences of the disorder. Despite the stereotypical nature of the presentation and the relative ease of diagnosis (a massively elevated serum creatine kinase together with such clinical features is essentially diagnostic) delayed diagnosis is common.[7]

The weakness invariably affects the proximal lower limb muscles first. Often there is hypertrophy of the calf muscles – this may initially be due to compensatory muscle fibre hypertrophy but the end-stage process is replacement of muscle by fat and fibrous tissue; hence the commonly used term pseudohypertrophy. Such hypertrophy is particularly common in DMD and BMD, but can be seen in other dystrophies and spinal muscular atrophy.[8] Tongue hypertrophy is often striking. The proximal weakness is reflected in Gower's manoeuvre, in which the boy trying to rise from the floor has to use his hands against his legs in ladder fashion to push himself up. The boys pass through a period of maintaining mobility by the use of aids (in the 8–10-year age range) but become increasingly restricted and all are wheelchair dependent by the age of 12 years.

The weakness spreads to involve the proximal upper limb muscles, the paraspinal muscles, and the respiratory muscles. Hand function is preserved late into the course of the disorder and computer keyboard and joystick control abilities remain vital assets. Paraspinal muscle weakness leads to lumbar lordosis which, combined with the proximal lower limb weakness, gives a characteristic waddling gait. A major consequence of the dorsal kyphoscoliosis is further ventilatory compromise, in addition due to that caused by respiratory muscle weakness, due to mechanical restriction of movement.

The age of onset of significant ventilatory impairment is variable. In the early teens forced vital capacity is substantially reduced. There is increased risk of chest infection. It is at this age that spinal surgery (insertion of rods to straighten the spine) is often considered – the potential benefits include improvement in ventilation due to correction of kyphoscoliosis and improvement of posture (and thus reduction of discomfort) in the wheelchair.[9] But the reduced vital capacity and nature of the surgery carry with them the risk of substantial peri- and post-operative complications requiring detailed pre-operative assessment. A further complicating issue for surgery is the presence, almost inevitably, of cardiomyopathy (see below). The symptomatology and management of hypoventilation is discussed in detail elsewhere in this volume.

Cardiac dystrophin expression is impaired and cardiomyopathy is inevitable. Initial features include electrocardiographic (ECG) changes followed by the development of a dilated cardiomyopathy. Despite the severity of the echocardiographic changes, symptomatic heart involvement is relatively uncommon probably because of the patient's profound immobility and lack of 'stress' on the heart. Given that the introduction of non-invasive ventilation has substantially lengthened life expectancy, cardiac involvement is likely to become a more important issue. Regular cardiac surveillance should start early in the second decade, and despite lack of evidence from specific trials it is accepted practice to treat pre-symptomatic cardiomyopathy, for example with angiotensin-converting enzyme (ACE) inhibitors and β-blockers.[10] Some have advocated even more intensive prophylaxis.[11]

## Becker muscular dystrophy

As discussed above this disorder is allelic to DMD. Becker defined the disorder on the basis of a characteristic presentation with onset in childhood/adolescence, relatively slow progression, and a distribution of weakness paralleling that seen in DMD. The pattern of inheritance was X-linked and there was debate for many years as to whether it was an allelic disorder to DMD or related to involvement of a different gene, the former eventually being proven when the dystrophin gene was identified. In one extensive study of BMD about 10 per cent of patients required a wheelchair by the age of 40 years, reflecting the much milder prognosis compared with DMD.[12]

The phenotypic variability of the dystrophinopathies (Box 32.3) relates to the nature of the underlying mutation. Firstly, the position of the mutation within the gene is a major determinant of whether the phenotype is restricted to cardiomyopathy or also involves skeletal muscle or involves skeletal muscle alone. Secondly, the position of the mutation and the extent that the mutation leads to truncation of the protein product has a major effect on the severity of muscle involvement. This raises issues with respect to nosology. The disorder that Becker recognized is outlined above and discussed in more detail below. But some patients present with the same pattern of muscle involvement at a much earlier age, are wheelchair dependent by early teens, and thus overlap with those patients with milder forms of DMD. Others are so mildly affected that they remain asymptomatic until they present with quadriceps weakness in late-middle age. Others never develop weakness but have a cramp/myalgia syndrome, and a very small number are asymptomatic but have an elevated creatine kinase. To use the eponym Becker for all of these variants, and some even include those with only cardiomyopathy, seems inappropriate and confusing, for doctors and patients. The more general term dystrophinopathy therefore has its merits.

The description below is of the condition that Becker would have recognized, and is indeed the most prevalent form of dystrophinopathy in adult life.

**Box 32.3 Phenotypic expression of the dystrophinopathies**

- Duchenne muscular dystrophy
- Becker muscular dystrophy
- Manifesting female carriers
- Cramp/myalgia syndrome
- Asymptomatic hypercapnia
- Late-onset quadriceps myopathy
- Isolated cardiomyopathy

### MOLECULAR ASPECTS

These were discussed above. From a practical point of view, a patient suspected of having BMD should have DNA analysis as the first approach to diagnosis (noting that as in DMD the serum creatine kinase is invariably elevated). The same issues with respect to deletions and smaller mutations apply. It has recently been recognized that autosomal recessive limb-girdle muscular dystrophy type 2I (due to mutations in the *FKRP* gene) can look exactly like BMD, including raised serum creatine kinase and cardiac involvement, and exclusion of that by DNA testing should be performed prior to considering muscle biopsy.

### CLINICAL ASPECTS

Although the incidence of BMD is lower than DMD, the much longer survival means that its prevalence is higher than DMD. The diagnosis is typically made in adolescence with the history of symptoms dating back to very early teens. A history of calf cramps, often attributed to 'growing pains', and toe-walking is common. Calf hypertrophy may have been noted. The onset of weakness is invariably in the proximal lower limb/pelvic area and examination shows weakness of hip flexion and knee extension (quadriceps). The greater involvement of quadriceps than the hamstrings (knee flexors) is characteristic and distinguishes Becker from many forms of limb-girdle muscular dystrophy. As in DMD a rather characteristic waddling gait develops. An oft repeated history is that the boy was poor at games, coming last in races and being clumsy during sporting activities. Subsequently difficulties climbing stairs are noted, and then difficulty getting up from low chairs.

At a later stage peri-scapular muscle involvement becomes evident with some winging of the shoulder blades. Rather strikingly in some patients weakness of grip can become troublesome. As the proximal lower limb weakness advances rising from a chair becomes extremely difficult and stairs impossible without hand-rails. Falls, due mainly to quadriceps weakness and thus lack of knee support, are inevitable. There is an increasing need for walking aids and then occasional use of a wheelchair. However, the majority of patients retain a degree of independent ambulation into late middle age.

Significant ventilatory insufficiency is very much less common than in DMD and few patients require long-term non-invasive ventilation – and then only in patients who have been wheelchair dependent for a long period (Fig. 32.1). Chest infections and post-operative respiratory depression may require short-term ventilatory support. Many patients retain a normal, or only minimally reduced, forced vital capacity throughout their lives. Life expectancy is reduced in those with more severe muscle involvement, leading to wheelchair dependence, and in those with cardiomyopathy, but in many is normal.

The development of cardiomyopathy is highly variable and unlike in DMD is not inevitable.[13] But some patients may develop severe cardiomyopathy even in the presence of only mild limb muscle involvement, so cardiac surveillance is essential from diagnosis. There have been many reports of patients requiring cardiac transplantation while still fully ambulant.[14]

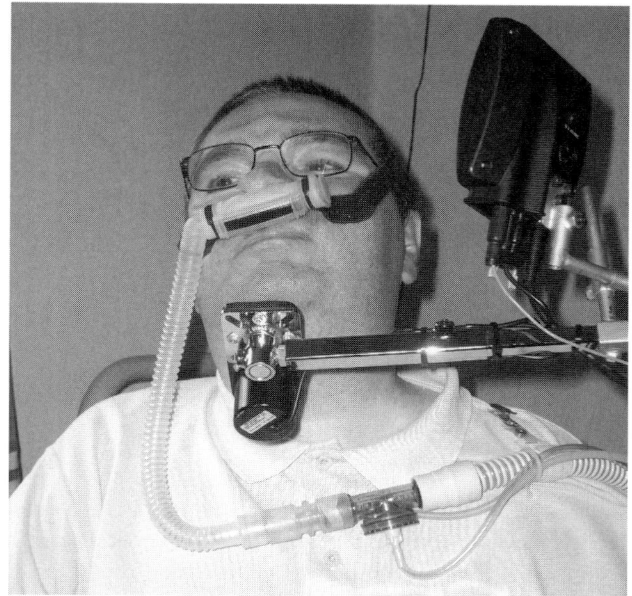

**Figure 32.1** This patient with Becker muscular dystrophy developed ventilatory insufficiency after having been wheelchair dependent for many years. Initially he required nocturnal ventilation only, but subsequently became dependent on daytime ventilation. His degree of immobility is profound and he uses an environmental control system operated by the chin apparatus.

## Myotonic dystrophy

This is the commonest inherited disorder seen in adult muscle clinics and has a prevalence of ~12/100 000 population.[15] It is clinically highly variable and has important systemic manifestations other than skeletal and cardiac muscle involvement.[16] For reasons that will be discussed, despite the almost inevitable involvement of the respiratory muscles the use of long-term non-invasive ventilation is relatively uncommon.

### MOLECULAR ASPECTS

Myotonic dystrophy occurs due to an unstable trinucleotide repeat expansion in a gene (*DMPK*) coding for a protein kinase. It is believed that most of the manifestations of the disorder are a consequence of disturbed RNA metabolism rather than dysfunction of the gene in which the mutation is located.[17] Thus, altered splicing of the chloride channel gene causes the characteristic myotonia, of the insulin receptor gene insulin resistance, and of cardiac and CNS genes the common conduction abnormalities and cognitive features.

The mutation is unstable and an increase in size in mitosis explains some of the progression of the disorder during life. More importantly an increase in size, sometimes dramatic, in meiosis means that the offspring have a tendency to develop the condition at an earlier age (anticipation); earlier-onset cases are inclined to show a rather different pattern of clinical involvement with cognitive and behavioural problems initially predominating over muscle involvement. Although there is significant overlap it is convenient in clinical practice to recognize four major phenotypes:

- asymptomatic/oligosymptomatic
- adult-onset (classical Steinert's disease)
- childhood onset
- congenital onset.

The size of the expansion increases down the group. Thus most normal individuals have ~12 repeats. Up to ~100 repeats may be asymptomatic, typical adult-onset disease is seen with ~100–500 repeats, childhood-onset with somewhat larger repeats, and the most severe congenital form with over 1000 repeats. The figures given are only a rough approximation such that a DNA result alone is of little use for prognostication. A major reason for this is that repeat size is determined from a blood sample (lymphocytes), and as a consequence of instability of the mutation during mitosis different tissues from the same individual may show widely differing numbers of repeats.

## CLINICAL ASPECTS

Those with very small expansions may be asymptomatic but cataracts, often presenting at a relatively young age, are common. Significant skeletal muscle involvement is not seen, cardiac complications are rare, and assisted ventilation is not an issue. Congenital myotonic dystrophy presents as a floppy infant with feeding and respiratory difficulties. Although both may need support in most they settle down within a few days; more severe cases remain ventilator dependent and do not survive. The child then makes progress but milestones are somewhat delayed and learning difficulties are inevitable. Relatively mild skeletal involvement is evident, but the learning difficulties and behavioural problems present the major challenge. The facial appearance is characteristic due to facial muscle weakness and underlying skeletal dysmorphism which in itself relates to the long-standing weakness. In early adulthood the muscular manifestations progress, as in the adult-onset form, and there is a high morbidity and mortality in the third and fourth decades from cardiorespiratory problems.[18] The childhood-onset form presents in the first decade with cognitive and behavioural problems with little or no evidence of skeletal muscle involvement, such that the diagnosis is often missed for some considerable time.

The remainder of this section will deal with the multisystemic features seen in adult-onset myotonic dystrophy – by far and away the most common form encountered in clinical practice. Onset of symptoms is typically in adolescence and early adult life. Most commonly it is limb skeletal muscle features that lead to presentation, more rarely excessive daytime sleepiness or cardiorespiratory problems. In women, the diagnosis may come to light following the birth of a congenitally affected child.

### Skeletal muscle

Myotonia is a hallmark of the disease and describes the phenomenon of delayed muscle relaxation after contraction. The patient complains of stiffness of their hands and difficulty relaxing the hand after gripping something tightly. Myotonia may also affect the muscles in the throat region, causing difficulties swallowing and a feeling of clumsiness of the tongue when speaking.

The pattern of muscle weakness is essentially invariable involving the facial, neck flexor, and distal limb muscles (and respiratory muscles as discussed below). Proximal limb weakness is a late feature and thus strikingly different to most myopathies. Before the patient is aware of symptoms it is possible to show weakness of the facial muscles (incomplete burying of the eyelids), neck flexion and grip. Although the facial weakness may become quite severe, few patients complain of it – however, it may contribute to some of the difficulties in establishing non-invasive ventilation (Fig. 32.2). The facial weakness, combined with ptosis and receding hairline, gives rise to the characteristic facies.

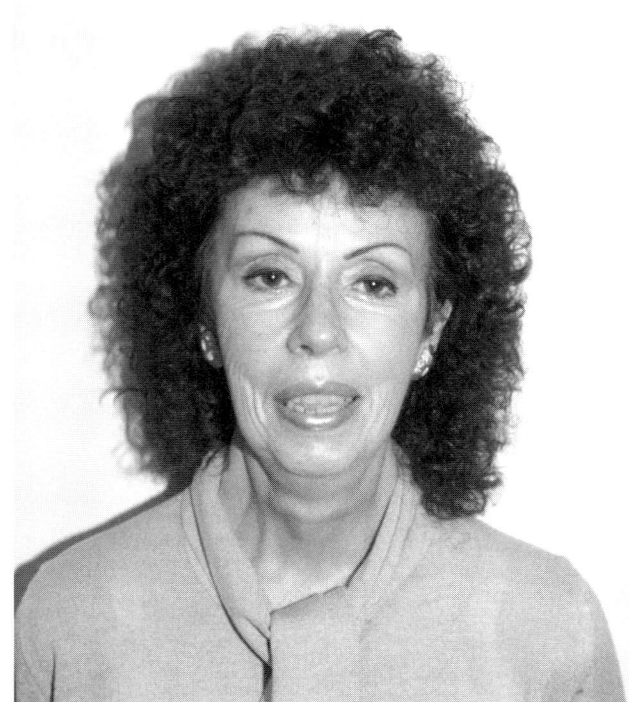

**Figure 32.2** Myotonic dystrophy. Characteristic facial weakness due to atrophy of the facial and masticatory muscles, and ptosis. The facial muscle weakness, and in some patients dysmorphic features, may hinder use of masks for non-invasive ventilation.

The respiratory muscles are involved early and in our experience many patients have a significantly reduced forced vital capacity (less than 50 per cent predicted) even at first presentation when other features of skeletal muscle involvement may be minimal. The forced vital capacity (FVC) falls with time and many adults have values below 2 L. This, combined with swallowing impairment due to pharyngeal muscle weakness, contributes to the high incidence of chest infections which are a major source of morbidity and mortality.[19] Many studies have shown nocturnal compromise of ventilation with associated sleep fragmentation.[20,21] While this might be thought to be a contributing factor to excessive daytime sleepiness (EDS) it is striking that treatment with non-invasive nocturnal ventilation may not help,[22] and that EDS can be a major symptom in those with no evidence of respiratory compromise – all supporting the view that EDS largely relates to central nervous system dysfunction.

Delayed recovery of ventilation following anaesthesia is extremely common and undiagnosed patients may be first identified in this setting. At diagnosis all patients should be advised of the risks of surgery and anaesthesia. The highest morbidity has been associated with gallbladder surgery, presumably because of additional direct effects of the surgery on the adjacent diaphragm.

#### Heart

Cardiac conduction abnormalities are extremely common,[23] whereas symptomatic cardiomyopathy is rare. Typical ECG changes include progressive lengthening of the PR interval, broadening of the QRS complex, and the development of various forms of block including partial and complete bundle branch block and complete heart block. Brady-arrhythmias may be treated by pacemaker insertion but there is increasing evidence that many patients die from tachyarrhythmias which may appropriately be treated by insertion of an implantable defibrillator. Despite numerous publications the best approach to cardiac surveillance and management remains unclear.[24] Annual ECG is a minimum requirement. Changes on the ECG and the development of cardiac symptoms indicates the need for further assessment which will include 24-hour recording and possibly intracardiac electrophysiology.

#### Brain

As a group, these patients have a slightly lower IQ than average. More striking is a characteristic psychological profile which largely reflects frontal lobe dysfunction and practically is associated with apathy and impaired organizational skills.[25] Apathy and related behavioural issues have a profound effect for some individuals with respect to employment, social interactions, and clinical management.[26] It partly explains why patients with myotonic dystrophy have a reputation for being poor attendees in clinic, although it can be argued that some clinics offer little of benefit to the patients who therefore see no reason to attend. These factors are also relevant with respect to non-compliance with non-invasive ventilation.

Excessive daytime sleepiness is extremely common but under-recognized.[27] It can be debilitating for the patient, and seriously compromise employability, and can be particularly irksome for family and friends, who may perceive it as the patient showing boredom and lack of interest. The fact that many patients show sleep-disordered breathing might suggest it would respond to non-invasive ventilation, but it is striking that it rarely does so. On the other hand, stimulant drugs such as modafinil can be highly effective.[28]

#### Additional features

Cataracts develop at a younger age than normal. Fertility can be impaired, particularly in males, who may develop azoospermia. Premature, male pattern, balding is more striking in males than females. Insulin resistance is common, but frank diabetes rare. It is more common in the older obese patient and essentially behaves like, and is managed in the same way as, maturity-onset diabetes. Irritable bowel symptoms are very common. Bladder involvement is probably underestimated.

### Other dystrophies

Ventilatory failure may occur in the limb-girdle dystrophies, but as in BMD this is rare other than in patients who have substantial limb weakness and have long been wheelchair dependent. The same is true for facioscapulohumeral dystrophy, one of the commonest dystrophies in adults, and overall the need for non-invasive ventilation is very rare.

## MUSCLE DISORDERS ASSOCIATED WITH EARLY VENTILATORY INSUFFICIENCY

In these disorders ventilatory failure may occur while the patient is still ambulant. Non-invasive ventilation is life-saving, improves quality of life, and allows long-term survival. Each is rare, and only the major clinical and management features will be described.

### Acid maltase deficiency

This is an autosomal recessive disorder that may present in two major fashions, depending on the level of residual enzyme activity. The most severe form is classical Pompe's disease presenting early in the first decade and associated with ventilatory failure, widespread weakness and organomegaly. Death was inevitable until the recent introduction of enzyme replacement therapy.[29]

A later onset form is associated with proximal muscle weakness and respiratory muscle weakness selectively affecting the diaphragm.[30] Onset is typically in adolescence but can be much later, in to early middle age. The pattern of proximal limb weakness is non-specific and an incorrect initial diagnosis of limb-girdle dystrophy or myositis is often made. A proportion of patients first present in respiratory failure but on closer assessment nearly all have signs, and usually also previously unrecognized symptoms, of proximal limb weakness. In those presenting with limb weakness evidence of diaphragmatic weakness (a significant fall in FVC when the patient is lying compared with standing) may be found and point towards the diagnosis. In those who develop ventilatory failure non-invasive ventilation is highly effective. Most will require, at least initially, nocturnal ventilation only, but as the condition advances daytime ventilation may become necessary. Those who are still ambulant are unlikely to require daytime ventilation.

The diagnosis is often not considered unless there is the additional clue of early respiratory muscle involvement. Once thought of the diagnosis is established or refuted by enzymological studies which can be performed on a blood sample.[31,32] In some patients the diagnosis is suggested by the appearance on muscle biopsy (accumulation of glycogen and increased acid phosphatase activity) but the biopsy can be normal.

### Congenital myopathies

This title is misleading because many of these conditions (Box 32.2) are not truly congenital (evidence of disease at birth) but have their onset in the first few years of life. Although genetically and pathologically very heterogeneous they share many clinical similarities. Perhaps the most striking attribute is that despite early onset they are relatively non-progressive, unlike the dystrophies. Much of the apparent progression in childhood and adolescence is due to enlargement of the skeleton without the musculature keeping pace. Once the individual is fully grown, and throughout adult life, there is very little progression of weakness. What they also share in common is rather diffuse proximal and distal muscle involvement, without the marked proximal predilection seen in most myopathies. The weakness is typically modest with the individual retaining independent ambulation. In many of these conditions ventilatory failure, requiring the introduction of non-invasive ventilation, develops in childhood or adolescence.

### Emery–Dreifuss syndrome

This rare syndrome was first described as an X-linked disorder and was subsequently shown to be due to mutations in a gene (*STA*) producing the nuclear envelope protein emerin. It was subsequently realized that most patients with this phenotype have an autosomal dominant disorder due to mutations in the *LMNA* gene coding for another nuclear envelope protein lamin A/C,[33] and that it is allelic to autosomal dominant limb-girdle muscular dystrophy type 2B.

The phenotype is defined by the triad of early muscle contractures, a humero-pelvic distribution of muscle weakness and cardiac involvement (which carries high mortality). Contractures develop in the advanced stages of most myopathies, when the patient is very immobile, but in Emery–Dreifuss syndrome they are an early feature, when the patient is fully ambulant, and characteristically affect the neck, elbows and ankles. Most patients retain ambulation but it becomes increasingly difficult because of the contractures and abnormal posture. Cardiac arrhythmias carry a high mortality and current evidence supports the implantation of a defibrillator.[34,35] The development of ventilatory failure is relatively common.

### LGMD 2I

As noted, this autosomal recessive limb-girdle dystrophy can mimic BMD, including cardiac involvement.[36] Unlike BMD, ventilatory insufficiency can develop while the patient is still ambulant and requires regular monitoring.

## COMMENTS ON OTHER MYOPATHIES AND RELATED CONDITIONS

For the intensivist the most common neuromuscular disorders that they will see on an intensive care unit (ICU) are Guillain–Barré syndrome and myasthenia gravis. They share in common the need for invasive ventilation during the acute stage (e.g. myasthenic crisis) but both are self-limiting. It is very rare for patients with myasthenia to need long-term non-invasive ventilation, although that need is slightly more common in patients with anti-MuSK antibodies as opposed to anti-acetylcholine receptor antibodies. Ventilatory failure is much less common in Lambert–Eaton myasthenic syndrome than myasthenia gravis.

Another condition that is seen on ICU is acute quadriplegic myopathy due to the combined use of high-dose steroids and a neuromuscular blocking drug – typically in a patient with acute asthma.[37,38] Invasive ventilation is required, and sometimes non-invasive ventilation during the recovery period, but not long-term. Desmin mutations are one cause of so-called myofibrillar myopathies.[39] Slowly progressive proximal weakness develops from early middle age. Diaphragmatic involvement is common and ventilatory failure may develop in an ambulant patient. Although not a myopathy, spinal muscular atrophy is a common condition whose management is typically in the same clinic as those patients with muscular dystrophies. The commonest form, autosomal recessive proximal spinal muscular atrophy, is due to mutations affecting the *SMN* gene and four major categories are recognized:

- type 1 – diagnosed by 6 months of age; ventilator dependence and early death
- type 2 – diagnosed by 2 years of age; can sit but never walk

- type 3 – diagnosed between 18 months and adolescence; can walk
- type 4 – onset in adult life.

As with DMD, patients with type 2 spinal muscular atrophy, and to a lesser extent type 3, have problems with kyphoscoliosis which may, together with respiratory muscle weakness, contribute to ventilatory insufficiency requiring long-term non-invasive ventilation. Despite the early onset in some patients, and substantial early disability, progression throughout life is extremely slow and many with type 3 will have a normal life expectancy. The major cause of morbidity is chest infection.

## RESPIRATORY CARE OF ADULTS WITH MUSCLE DISORDERS

The rest of this book is devoted to this! But it has been recognized that deficiencies exist in current services with the clinicians looking after patients with muscle diseases not being expert respiratory physicians, and respiratory physicians managing non-invasive ventilation not having experience of other aspects of the patient's condition. With this in mind the Muscular Dystrophy Campaign (a UK charity devoted to patients with primary muscle disorders) convened a workshop to develop 'best practice' guidelines, and some of the same authors reviewed the features of respiratory involvement in inherited myopathies.[40,41] These are useful documents to provide a framework for effective management of such patients.

From all of the above it is apparent that there is an urgent need for cooperation between specialist chest physicians, neurologists and paediatricians to optimize the care of this particular population of patients.

## REFERENCES


1. Eagle M, Baudouin SV, Chandler C *et al.* Survival in Duchenne muscular dystrophy: improvements in life expectancy since 1967 and the impact of home nocturnal ventilation. *Neuromuscul Disord* 2002; **12**: 926–9.
2. Katzin LW, Amato AA. Pompe disease: a review of the current diagnosis and treatment recommendations in the era of enzyme replacement therapy. *J Clin Neuromuscul Dis* 2008; **9**: 421–31.
3. Muntoni F, Torelli S, Ferlini A. Dystrophin and mutations: one gene, several proteins, multiple phenotypes. *Lancet Neurol* 2003; **2**: 731–40.
4. Tuffery-Giraud S, Beroud C, Leturcq F *et al.* Genotype-phenotype analysis in 2,405 patients with a dystrophinopathy using the UMD-DMD database: a model of nationwide knowledgebase. *Hum Mutat* 2009; **30**: 934–45.
5. Kemper AR, Wake MA. Duchenne muscular dystrophy: issues in expanding newborn screening. *Curr Opin Pediatr* 2007; **19**: 700–4.
6. Donders J, Taneja C. Neurobehavioral characteristics of children with Duchenne muscular dystrophy. *Child Neuropsychol* 2009; **15**: 295–304.
7. Ciafaloni E, Fox DJ, Pandya S *et al.* Delayed diagnosis in Duchenne muscular dystrophy: data from the muscular dystrophy surveillance, tracking, and research network (MD STARnet). *J Pediatr* 2009; **155**: 380–5.
8. Reimers CD, Schlotter B, Eicke BM *et al.* Calf enlargement in neuromuscular diseases: a quantitative ultrasound study in 350 patients and review of the literature. *J Neurol Sci* 1996; **143**: 46–56.
9. Eagle M, Bourke J, Bullock R *et al.* Managing Duchenne muscular dystrophy – the additive effect of spinal surgery and home nocturnal ventilation in improving survival. *Neuromuscul Disord* 2007; **17**: 470–5.
10. Kaspar RW, Allen HD, Montanaro F. Current understanding and management of dilated cardiomyopathy in Duchenne and Becker muscular dystrophy. *J Am Acad Nurse Pract* 2009; **21**: 241–9.
11. Nigro G, Politano L, Passamano L *et al.* Cardiac treatment in neuro-muscular diseases. *Acta Myol* 2006; **25**: 119–23.
12. Bushby KM, Gardner-Medwin D. The clinical, genetic and dystrophin characteristics of Becker muscular dystrophy. I. Natural history. *J Neurol* 1993; **240**: 98–104.
13. Finsterer J, Stollberger C. Cardiac involvement in Becker muscular dystrophy. *Can J Cardiol* 2008; **24**: 786–92.
14. Finsterer J, Bittner RE, Grimm M. Cardiac involvement in Becker's muscular dystrophy, necessitating heart transplantation, 6 years before apparent skeletal muscle involvement. *Neuromuscul Disord* 1999; **9**: 598–600.
15. Harper PS. *Myotonic dystrophy*, 3rd edn. Major problems in neurology. London: WB Saunders, 2001:436.
16. Harper PS, Van Engelen B, Eymard B *et al. Myotonic dystrophy: present management, future therapy.* Oxford: Oxford University Press, 2004:251.
17. Machuca-Tzili L, Brook D, Hilton-Jones D. Clinical and molecular aspects of the myotonic dystrophies: a review. *Muscle Nerve* 2005; **32**: 1–18.
18. Reardon W, Newcombe R, Fenton I *et al.* The natural history of congenital myotonic dystrophy: mortality and long term clinical aspects. *Arch Dis Child* 1993; **68**: 177–81.
19. de Die-Smulders CE, Howeler CJ, Thijs C *et al.* Age and causes of death in adult-onset myotonic dystrophy. *Brain* 1998; **121**: 1557–63.
20. Kumar SP, Sword D, Petty RK *et al.* Assessment of sleep studies in myotonic dystrophy. *Chron Respir Dis* 2007; **4**: 15–18.
21. Laberge L, Begin P, Dauvilliers Y *et al.* A polysomnographic study of daytime sleepiness in

myotonic dystrophy type 1. *J Neurol Neurosurg Psychiatry* 2009; **80**: 642–6.

22. Guilleminault C, Philip P, Robinson A. Sleep and neuromuscular disease: bilevel positive airway pressure by nasal mask as a treatment for sleep disordered breathing in patients with neuromuscular disease. *J Neurol Neurosurg Psychiatry* 1998; **65**: 225–32.
23. Cudia P, Bernasconi P, Chiodelli R *et al.* Risk of arrhythmia in type I myotonic dystrophy: the role of clinical and genetic variables. *J Neurol Neurosurg Psychiatry* 2009; **80**: 790–3.
24. Dello Russo A, Mangiola F, Della Bella P *et al.* Risk of arrhythmias in myotonic dystrophy: trial design of the RAMYD study. *J Cardiovasc Med (Hagerstown)* 2009; **10**: 51–8.
25. Modoni A, Silvestri G, Vita MG *et al.* Cognitive impairment in myotonic dystrophy type 1 (DM1): a longitudinal follow-up study. *J Neurol* 2008; **255**: 1737–42.
26. Rubinsztein JS, Rubinsztein DC, Goodburn S *et al.* Apathy and hypersomnia are common features of myotonic dystrophy. *J Neurol Neurosurg Psychiatry* 1998; **64**: 510–15.
27. Hilton-Jones D. Myotonic dystrophy – forgotten aspects of an often neglected condition. *Curr Opin Neurol* 1997; **10**: 399–401.
28. Talbot K, Stradling J, Crosby J *et al.* Reduction in excess daytime sleepiness by modafinil in patients with myotonic dystrophy. *Neuromuscul Disord* 2003; **13**: 357–64.
29. Schoser B, Hill V, Raben N. Therapeutic approaches in glycogen storage disease type II/Pompe Disease. *Neurotherapeutics* 2008; **5**: 569–78.
30. Muller-Felber W, Horvath R, Gempel K *et al.* Late onset Pompe disease: clinical and neurophysiological spectrum of 38 patients including long-term follow-up in 18 patients. *Neuromuscul Disord* 2007; **17**: 698–706.
31. Goldstein JL, Young SP, Changela M *et al.* Screening for Pompe disease using a rapid dried blood spot method: experience of a clinical diagnostic laboratory. *Muscle Nerve* 2009; **40**: 32–6.
32. Winchester B, Bali D, Bodamer OA *et al.* Methods for a prompt and reliable laboratory diagnosis of Pompe disease: report from an international consensus meeting. *Mol Genet Metab* 2008; **93**: 275–81.
33. Bonne G, Di Barletta MR, Varnous S *et al.* Mutations in the gene encoding lamin A/C cause autosomal dominant Emery-Dreifuss muscular dystrophy. *Nat Genet* 1999; **21**: 285–8.
34. Sanna T, Dello Russo A, Toniolo D *et al.* Cardiac features of Emery-Dreifuss muscular dystrophy caused by lamin A/C gene mutations. *Eur Heart J* 2003; **24**: 2227–36.
35. Golzio PG, Chiribiri A, Gaita F. 'Unexpected' sudden death avoided by implantable cardioverter defibrillator in Emery Dreifuss patient. *Europace* 2007; **9**: 1158–60.
36. Poppe M, Cree L, Bourke J *et al.* The phenotype of limb-girdle muscular dystrophy type 2I. *Neurology* 2003; **60**: 1246–51.
37. Larsson L. Acute quadriplegic myopathy: an acquired 'myosinopathy'. *Adv Exp Med Biol* 2008; **642**: 92–8.
38. Argov Z. Drug-induced myopathies. *Curr Opin Neurol* 2000; **13**: 541–5.
39. Schroder R, Schoser B. Myofibrillar myopathies: a clinical and myopathological guide. *Brain Pathol* 2009; **19**: 483–92.
40. Shahrizaila T, Kinnear W. Recommendations for respiratory care of adults with muscle disorders. *Neuromuscul Disord* 2007; **17**: 13–15.
41. Shahrizaila N, Kinnear WJ, Wills AJ. Respiratory involvement in inherited primary muscle conditions. *J Neurol Neurosurg Psychiatry* 2006; **77**: 1108–15.

# 33

# Pathophysiology of respiratory failure in neuromuscular diseases

FRANCO LAGHI, HAMEEDA SHAIKH, GOKAY GUNGOR

## ABSTRACT

Respiratory failure is one of the most important causes of increased morbidity and mortality in patients with neuromuscular diseases. The pathophysiology of respiratory failure in these patients is complex and includes alveolar hypoventilation, impaired gas exchange or both. Alveolar hypoventilation can result from impaired control of breathing and increased mechanical load on the respiratory muscles. In most patients, however, respiratory muscle weakness is the main culprit for the development of alveolar hypoventilation. Impaired gas exchange results from ventilation/perfusion inequality or, less often, increased intrapulmonary shunt. These derangements in gas exchange occur when patients affected by neuromuscular diseases develop bulbar and expiratory muscle weakness. Weakness of the bulbar and expiratory muscles increases the risk for pulmonary aspiration, retention of secretions, and pneumonia. In addition, bulbar and expiratory muscle weakness can increase the likelihood of atelectasis in patients with inspiratory muscle weakness. Diagnosis of respiratory impairment frequently goes undetected in patients with neuromuscular diseases until ventilatory failure is precipitated by aspiration pneumonia or cor pulmonale. Diagnosis is delayed because limb muscle weakness prevents patients from exceeding their limited ventilatory capacity. In specific cases the lack of dyspnoea may reflect the difficulty in communicating symptoms because of cognitive impairment. It follows that the diagnosis of respiratory dysfunction resulting from neuromuscular diseases requires a high index of clinical suspicion and, in selected cases, the use of specific tests. In this chapter we discuss the multifaceted pathophysiology of respiratory failure in patients with neuromuscular diseases.

## INTRODUCTION

According to the level of anatomical involvement, neuromuscular diseases (NMDs) can be grouped in those involving upper motor neurones, lower motor neurones, peripheral nerves, neuromuscular junction and peripheral muscles (Box 33.1). In patients affected by NMDs, respiratory failure is one of the most important causes of excess morbidity and premature mortality.[1] Ventilatory support is the only intervention known to extend survival in patients who develop respiratory failure as a result of NMDs.[1]

## PATHOPHYSIOLOGY OF RESPIRATORY FAILURE IN NEUROMUSCULAR DISEASES

Alveolar hypoventilation – defined as alveolar ventilation inappropriately low for the patient's level of carbon dioxide production – is the primary mechanism responsible for respiratory failure in NMDs. The rise in the partial pressure of carbon dioxide in the alveoli that accompanies hypoventilation causes a decrease in the partial pressure of oxygen. This means that hypoventilation can cause hypoxaemia even when the lung parenchyma is normal, i.e. hypercapnia with normal alveolar-to-arterial oxygen gradient (A-a$DO_2$, see Appendix 33.1). When NMDs cause pulmonary complications that impair gas exchange and, thus, increase A-a$DO_2$, hypoxaemia can be out of proportion to the degree of alveolar hypoventilation. In patients with increased A-a$DO_2$ the magnitude of neuromuscular derangement causing hypercapnia can be less than in patients with NMDs and normal gas exchange. When gas exchange is impaired – or when the pattern of breathing is rapid and shallow – alveolar hypoventilation can occur despite normal or increased total minute ventilation.[2] In the sections that follow we will discuss

**Box 33.1 Examples of neuromuscular diseases that can be associated with respiratory failure grouped according to the level of anatomical involvement**

Upper motor neurone

- Amyotrophic lateral sclerosis
- Multiple sclerosis
- Stroke
- Trauma
- Post-polio syndrome

Lower motor neurone

- Spinal cord injury
- Post-polio syndrome
- Amyotrophic lateral sclerosis
- Spinal muscle atrophies

Peripheral nerves

- Guillain–Barré syndrome
- Tick paralysis
- Shellfish poisoning

Neuromuscular junction

- Botulism
- Myasthenia gravis
- Drugs (neuromuscular blocking agents)

Muscle fibres

- Inflammatory/autoimmune myopathies (dermatomyositis, polymyositis)
- Myotonic dystrophies
- Duchenne muscular dystrophy
- Metabolic myopathies (glycogen storage disease, abnormal lipid metabolism)
- Endocrine myopathies (hyperthyroidism)

mechanisms responsible for alveolar hypoventilation and impaired gas exchange in patients with NMDs. In addition we will discuss selected diagnostic tools to identify patients at risk of respiratory failure.

## Alveolar hypoventilation

In patients with NMDs, alveolar hypoventilation can result from decreased respiratory drive, increased mechanical load, diminished respiratory muscle performance, and impaired cardiovascular performance.

### ALVEOLAR HYPOVENTILATION: DECREASED RESPIRATORY DRIVE

Structural lesions of the central nervous system can contribute to, or cause, alveolar hypoventilation and hypercapnic respiratory failure (Box 33.1). These lesions can be the result of trauma, infections, post-polio syndrome, paraneoplastic syndromes (anti-Hu autoantibodies) and cerebrovascular accidents.[1] Patients with cerebrovascular accidents caused by acute hemispheric infarction require mechanical ventilation 25 per cent of the time usually because of impaired consciousness, impaired airway protection or hypoxaemia. More than 80 per cent of intubated patients die, mostly because of midbrain herniation.[1]

When present severe hypercapnia depresses the central nervous system and decreases respiratory motor output. A vicious cycle can arise, whereby hypercapnia causes depressed drive leading to more hypercapnia.[1] Hypercapnia can decrease diaphragmatic contractility, although not consistently.[3] Acidosis may be more important than hypercapnia in causing respiratory muscle impairment (mortality is more closely related to acidosis than to hypercapnia).[3] Even this last possibility is uncertain because diaphragmatic contractility was not affected by acidosis in one study.[4]

### ALVEOLAR HYPOVENTILATION: INCREASED MECHANICAL LOAD

In patients with NMDs, upper airway obstruction and reduced chest wall and lung compliances can limit the ability of the respiratory muscles to generate and sustain adequate alveolar ventilation.

#### Upper airway obstruction

Parkinson's disease, multiple system atrophy (a Parkinson-like syndrome that causes progressive degenerative disease of the central nervous system), amyotrophic lateral sclerosis (ALS) and botulism are some of the NMDs that can cause vocal cord dysfunction and frank vocal cord paralysis.[1] Presence of vocal cord dysfunction or paralysis can predispose the patient to upper airway obstruction and, thus, contribute to ventilatory failure and death.[1]

#### Impaired chest wall and lung mechanics

Severe weakness of the inspiratory muscles produces a restrictive pattern with decreases in vital capacity, total lung capacity and functional residual capacity.[1] When respiratory muscle strength is less than 50 per cent of predicted the loss in vital capacity is greater than expected.[1] The decrease is secondary to decreases in compliance of the chest wall and lungs. Several factors can decrease chest wall compliance:[1]

- thoracic scoliosis – this can be particularly severe in those patients in whom respiratory and vertebral muscle weakness is present before spinal growth is complete

- obesity – a common occurrence in patients with spinal cord injury
- stiffening of tendons and ligaments of the rib cage, and ankylosis of the costosternal and thoracovertebral joints.

Decrease in lung compliance can result from inflammatory and fibrotic changes of the lung parenchyma. The last two processes can be triggered by recurrent aspiration of gastric contents and impaired cough. (Other factors that can decrease lung compliance include diffuse microatelectasis and, in patients with cardiac impairment, pulmonary congestion.[1])

## ALVEOLAR HYPOVENTILATION: DIMINISHED RESPIRATORY MUSCLE PERFORMANCE

Respiratory muscle weakness frequently goes undetected in patients with NMDs until ventilatory failure is precipitated by aspiration pneumonia or cor pulmonale.[1] Diagnosis is delayed because limb muscle weakness prevents patients from exceeding their limited ventilatory capacity.[1] In specific cases such as multiple sclerosis or ALS, the lack of dyspnoea may reflect the difficulty in communicating symptoms because of cognitive impairment.[1] In patients with NMDs, respiratory muscle weakness may be present at birth (type 1 spinal muscular dystrophy), arise later in the course of the disease (myotonic dystrophy, Duchenne muscular dystrophy) or be acquired (spinal cord injury, poliomyelitis, post-polio syndrome, ALS).[1]

Few patients develop severe respiratory muscle weakness despite little or no peripheral muscle weakness[5] and some develop severe diaphragmatic weakness – or even diaphragmatic paralysis – in the absence of a systemic NMD. Severe diaphragmatic weakness or paralysis can occur with disease processes that damage the phrenic nerve such as trauma, mediastinal malignancies, herpes zoster, diphtheria, Lyme disease, malnutrition, alcoholism, diabetes, lead toxicity, vasculitis and porphyria.[1]

In clinical practice it may be impossible to identify the specific cause of diaphragmatic weakness/paralysis. It is likely that many of these cases of 'idiopathic' diaphragm weakness/paralysis are secondary to neuralgic amyotrophy. Neuralgic amyotrophy is an inflammatory condition of unknown aetiology that is usually limited to the brachial plexus. One to five per cent of patients affected by neuralgic amyotrophy develop unilateral or bilateral diaphragmatic paralysis.[1] Dyspnoea occurs after a prodromal flu-like episode, followed by acute severe neck and shoulder pain with or without arm weakness.[1] The first episode of dyspnoea may also be precipitated by surgery. More than 90 per cent of patients recover upper limb function within 3 years after the onset of weakness or paralysis.[6] Recovery of diaphragmatic function is slower and less complete.[1,5] Similar to limb muscles, diaphragmatic paralysis can recur after complete recovery. No specific therapy is available for patients with neuralgic amyotrophy. It has been reported that in patients with persistent bilateral paralysis who develop cor pulmonale, plication of both hemidiaphragms can improve ventilation and gas exchange and can resolve orthopnoea.[1]

Patients with respiratory muscle weakness take rapid shallow breaths, possibly as a result of afferent signals in weakened respiratory muscles, intrapulmonary receptors, or both.[1] $PaCO_2$ may be reduced early in the disease, but hypercapnia is likely when respiratory muscle strength falls to 25 per cent of predicted.[1] Reduction in strength, however, does not consistently predict alveolar hypoventilation,[7] because factors such as elastic load and breathing pattern also contribute.[8] Abnormalities in respiratory muscle performance and in alveolar ventilation may initially be evident only during exercise or sleep.[1] When inspiratory strength and vital capacity are 50 per cent of predicted, hypoventilation can occur with minor upper respiratory tract infections.[9]

Orthopnoea that develops within seconds of lying down is often reported as a classic symptom of bilateral diaphragmatic paralysis and, less often, unilateral diaphragmatic paralysis.[1] This contrasts with the more gradual onset of orthopnoea in patients with congestive heart failure.[10] In general orthopnoea occurs when maximal transdiaphragmatic pressure is less than 30 cm $H_2O$.[10]

The increased hydrostatic pressure surrounding an individual immersed in water decreases chest wall compliance[11,12] and, as a result of movement of blood into the thorax,[13] it decreases lung compliance. These unfavourable changes in lung mechanics cause a rise in the elastic load on the respiratory muscles. Not surprisingly, when immersed in water, patients with severe diaphragmatic weakness or with diaphragmatic paralysis often complain of dyspnoea[1] and experience greater reductions in lung volumes and greater increases in respiratory drive than healthy subjects.[14]

Patients with bilateral paralysis often complain of dyspnoea when bending or lifting – activities that require expiratory muscle recruitment.[1] These symptoms may arise because the paralysed diaphragm cannot prevent the rise in intrathoracic pressure (and the cessation of inhalation) caused by expiratory muscle recruitment. The variability of symptoms, loss of lung volume, and inspiratory strength among reports is probably related to the coexistence of weakness of other inspiratory and expiratory muscles in some patients but not in others.[1] In contrast to the orthopnoea in patients with diaphragmatic paralysis, patients with quadriplegia can report platypnoea (dyspnoea when sitting and relieved in the supine position).[15] In the supine position the area of apposition of the diaphragm with respect to the abdominal wall and its resting length are increased.[15] These two factors enhance the force generation capacity of the muscle.[15]

Irrespective of the primary pathology, patients with NMDs commonly develop abnormalities during sleep: frequent arousals, increased stage 1 sleep, decreased rapid eye movement (REM) sleep, hypoventilation, and hypoxaemia.[1] Patients with diaphragmatic weakness or diaphragmatic paralysis, such as patients affected by ALS, are at particular risk of developing hypoventilation during REM sleep[1] (when the diaphragm is almost the only active muscle).[16] To decrease this likelihood, the central nervous system can adopt two strategies: phasic recruitment of inspiratory muscles other than the diaphragm during REM sleep, or suppression of REM sleep. The failure of some patients to develop these adaptative strategies may explain discrepancies among reports on oxygenation during sleep in patients with isolated diaphragmatic paralysis.[1]

Sleep-disordered breathing usually precedes, and probably contributes to, daytime ventilatory failure.[1] Patients commonly report symptoms of nocturnal hypoventilation and sleep disruption (insomnia, morning headache, daytime somnolence, decreased intellectual performance).[17,18] Sleep-disordered breathing usually develops when vital capacity in the supine position is <60 per cent of the predicted value[19] or maximal inspiratory pressure is less negative than –34 cm $H_2O$.[19] The degree of abnormality parallels the extent of respiratory weakness.[19] Hypopnoeas and apnoeas in NMDs can be central, pseudo-central (inspiratory effort too weak to be identified on polysomnography) or obstructive.[1] The central events result from involvement of the central nervous system. Obstructive events typically result from weakness of the upper airway musculature. Hypoventilation and daytime hypercapnia may be aggravated by resetting of the chemoreceptors during sleep, which is reversible with chronic nocturnal ventilation.[1]

Hypopnoeas predominate in the early stage of an NMD.[19] As the respiratory muscle weakness progresses, clear short-lasting hypopnoeas tend to be replaced by more prolonged episodes of hypoventilation that are not captured by the apnoea–hypopnoea score.[19] Accordingly, apnoea–hypopnoea scores can underestimate the effect of nocturnal hypoventilation on quality of life or functional status.[20] Sleep disruption in patients with NMDs may also result from an inability to change position during sleep, muscle twitches, and leg jerks.[21]

#### ALVEOLAR HYPOVENTILATION: IMPAIRED CARDIOVASCULAR PERFORMANCE

NMDs caused by genetic abnormalities such as myotonic dystrophy, Duchenne muscular dystrophy, type II glycogenosis and mitochondrial syndromes can cause myocardial dysfunction.[1] Myocardial dysfunction, *per se*, can cause respiratory muscle weakness. According to investigations conducted in laboratory animals and in patients with heart failure (without NMDs), respiratory muscle weakness associated with heart failure can result from several mechanisms:[1]

- decreased number of type IIb fibres – these fibres produce 1.5–2 times more force than type I fibres
- reduced cross-sectional area of all types of muscle fibres in the rib cage and diaphragm – potential mechanisms include decreased regional blood flow and activation of the ubiquitin–proteasome proteolytic pathway by tumour necrosis factor
- structural abnormalities of diaphragmatic fibres
- decrease in the voluntary drive to the diaphragm during maximal inspiratory efforts.

As with respiratory muscle strength, endurance too is reduced in heart failure.[1] Two factors may contribute to the decreased endurance: decreased circulatory supply of energy substrates and increased work of breathing caused by decreased static lung compliance (when pulmonary congestion or pleural effusions are present).[1]

### Impaired gas exchange

Ventilation/perfusion inequalities and less often increased intrapulmonary shunt can complicate the clinical course of NMDs. The mechanisms for such impairments in gas exchange include development of diffuse microatelectasis, ineffective cough with retention of secretions/bronchopneumonia and heart failure.

#### IMPAIRED GAS EXCHANGE: DIFFUSE MICROATELECTASIS

In the past investigators considered the presence of diffuse microatelectasis a common occurrence in patients with NMDs. Purported mechanisms for the development of microatelectasis include infrequent (and small) sighs[22] and rapid and shallow breathing.[23] The real impact of diffuse microatelectasis in NMDs has been put into question.[24] On high-resolution computed tomography diffuse microatelectasis was found in only two of 14 patients with NMDs who had a 30 per cent decrease in lung compliance.[24]

#### IMPAIRED GAS EXCHANGE: INEFFECTIVE COUGH/BRONCHOPNEUMONIA

Ineffective cough is a common cause of retention of secretions and bronchopneumonia in patients with NMDs. Ineffective cough can result from inspiratory muscle weakness, expiratory muscle weakness and/or bulbar muscle impairment.[1] Inspiratory muscle weakness decreases the effectiveness of cough because the inhaled volume preceding the expulsive phase of cough is smaller. Smaller inhaled volume limits the increase in length (and thus in force output) of the expiratory muscles during the expulsive phase of cough. Expiratory muscle weakness decreases the effectiveness of cough because of impairment in cough-induced dynamic airway compression, leading to a reduction in the velocity of airflow. Dysfunction of the bulbar muscles – i.e. musculature of the mouth, pharynx, palate, tongue, and larynx – can impair cough through involuntary closure of the vocal cords during rapid exhalation.[1] Moreover, bulbar muscle dysfunction predisposes to aspiration of secretions and foreign material into the airway. Bulbar muscle impairment can occur in several NMDs including ALS, post-polio syndrome, botulism, myasthenia, Parkinson's disease and tick paralysis.[1]

### IMPAIRED GAS EXCHANGE: DECREASED CARDIAC FUNCTION

In patients with NMDs and decreased cardiac function, impaired gas exchange can result from pulmonary congestion/alveolar flooding and pleural effusions. The combination of impaired gas exchange and decreased mixed venous oxygen content – caused by increased oxygen extraction in the peripheral circulation of patients with heart failure – can contribute to worsening of hypoxaemia.[2]

## DIAGNOSIS

Early identification of bulbar, inspiratory and expiratory muscle impairment is of critical importance to reduce excess morbidity and premature mortality in patients affected by NMDs.[1,25] It would seem logical and acceptable to perform respiratory muscle testing less often in patients with slowly progressive NMDs (e.g. myotonic dystrophy, Duchenne muscular dystrophy) and more often in patients with rapidly progressive NMDs (e.g. ALS) and even more often in hospitalized patients who have an evolving NMD (e.g. Guillain–Barré syndrome, botulism). Unfortunately, for most NMDs it remains unclear how often respiratory muscle testing should be performed (and when ventilatory support should be initiated).

### Bulbar muscle impairment

In patients with NMDs, bulbar muscle impairment is commonly unrecognized. A high level of suspicion and clinical observation are the primary means to assess these patients. Signs of incipient bulbar dysfunction may include nasal tonality of the voice, dysarthria, oral accumulation of saliva, impaired gag reflex, dysphagia and weak cough. Early consultation with an experienced speech therapist can give objective quantification of the complex action of swallowing.

### Inspiratory muscle impairment

Signs of respiratory muscle impairment in NMDs may be limited to tachypnoea, inability to finish long sentences (staccato speech) or list numbers from 1 to 20 without pausing to take a breath, increased use of accessory neck muscles, paradoxical breathing. Complaints of non-refreshing sleep and frequent nocturnal awakenings should be considered warning signs of imminent neuromuscular respiratory failure. Unfortunately, all these findings are non-specific. A more objective assessment of inspiratory muscle impairment in NMDs can be obtained by recording maximal inspiratory airway pressure, sniff pressure and, less often, maximal transdiaphragmatic inspiratory pressure and transdiaphragmatic twitch pressure elicited by phrenic nerve stimulation (Table 33.1).

**Table 33.1** Respiratory compromise due to neuromuscular diseases causing respiratory muscle weakness*

| Finding | Compromise |
|---|---|
| Pressures | |
| MIP ≤34 cm $H_2O$ | Sleep-disordered breathing |
| MIP ≤20 cm $H_2O$ | Inability to ventilate adequately |
| MEP <40 cm $H_2O$ | Impaired cough, inability to clear secretions |
| Twitch gastric pressure <7 cm $H_2O$ | Impaired cough, inability to clear secretions |
| Vital capacity | |
| <30 mL/kg | Impaired cough/sleep-disordered breathing |
| <20 mL/kg | Inability to sigh or prevent atelectasis |
| <10 mL/kg | Inability to ventilate adequately |
| Bulbar weakness/paralysis | Inability to protect the airway and to avoid aspiration |

*The large variability of pressures and volumes associated with clinical compromise limit usefulness/generalizability of specific diagnostic thresholds (see text for details).
MEP, maximal expiratory airway pressure; MIP, maximal inspiratory airway pressure.

Measurements of maximal airway pressure (MIP) during forceful inhalation against an occluded airway reflect global inspiratory muscle strength;[10] MIP is usually measured after exhalation to residual volume.[10] This manoeuvre, however, is not easy to perform and MIP values are often larger when recorded at functional residual capacity than at residual volume. Maximal airway pressure can be recorded using a bedside manometer fitted with a mouthpiece. In general, an MIP more negative than –70 cm $H_2O$ for women and –100 cm $H_2O$ for men excludes clinically significant weakness. Poor mouth sealing due to facial muscle weakness may render bedside respiratory function testing less reliable.

Global inspiratory muscle strength can also be quantified by recording nasal pressures during a sniff manoeuvre (SNIP). In general, a SNIP more negative than –50 cm $H_2O$ for women and –60 cm $H_2O$ for men excludes clinically significant weakness.[26]

Maximal transdiaphragmatic inspiratory pressure recordings may be useful in identifying diaphragmatic impairment and – in those patients who are unable or unwilling to make voluntary efforts – transdiaphragmatic twitch pressure elicited by phrenic nerve stimulation can be used to obtain objective assessment of inspiratory muscle impairment. Phrenic nerve stimulation can be achieved with either an electrical stimulator[27] or a magnetic stimulator,[27] though the latter is easier to use in mechanically ventilated patients (Fig. 33.1).[28–30] In healthy volunteers, magnetic stimulation elicits twitch pressures which average 31–39 cm $H_2O$.[10] In patients with severe chronic obstructive

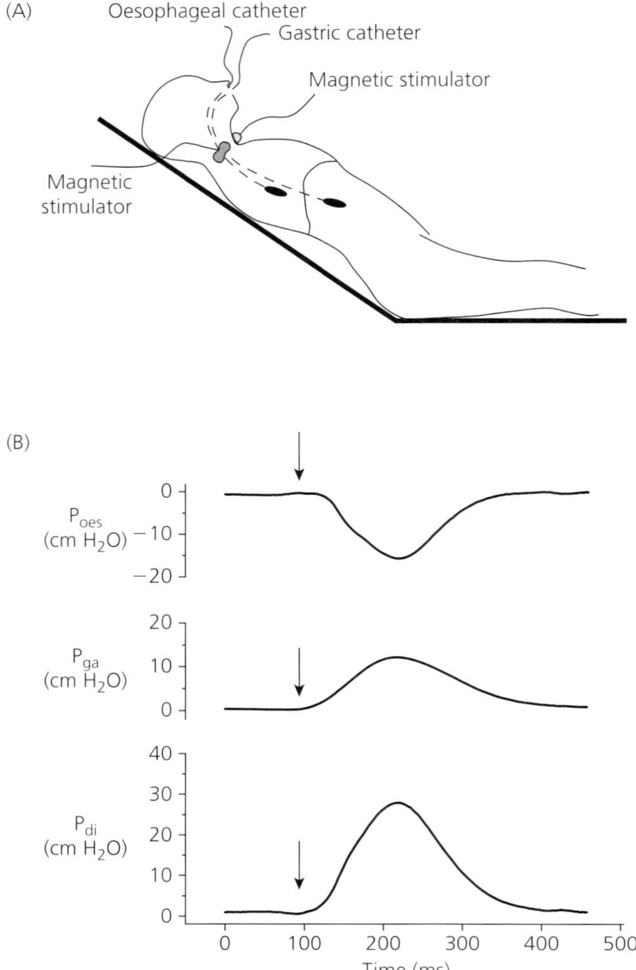


**Figure 33.1** Recording of transdiaphragmatic twitch pressure. (A) An oesophageal and a gastric balloon are passed through the nares. Magnetic stimulation of the phrenic nerves elicits diaphragmatic contraction. (B) Continuous recordings of oesophageal ($P_{oes}$) and gastric pressures ($P_{ga}$) and transdiaphragmatic pressure ($P_{di}$) – calculated by subtracting $P_{oes}$ from $P_{ga}$. Phrenic nerve stimulation (arrows) results in contraction of the diaphragm with consequent fall in intrathoracic pressure (negative defection of $P_{oes}$) and rise in intra-abdominal pressure (positive deflection of $P_{ga}$). These swings in pressure are responsible for the transdiaphragmatic twitch pressure. The smaller the transdiaphragmatic twitch pressure, the smaller the force generation capacity of the diaphragm. Redrawn with permission from Laghi F. Hypoventilation and respiratory muscle dysfunction. In: Parillo JE, Dellinger RP, eds. *Critical care medicine: principles of diagnosis and management in the adult,* 3rd edn. St. Louis: Mosby, 2002.

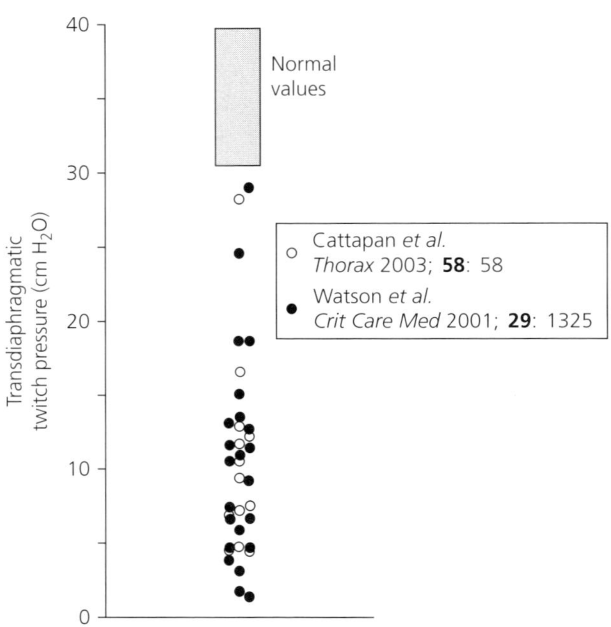


**Figure 33.2** Transdiaphragmatic twitch pressure recorded in mechanically ventilated patients recovering from an episode of acute respiratory failure. Box represents range of transdiaphragmatic twitch pressures recorded in healthy subjects. Most mechanically ventilated patients had evidence of diaphragmatic weakness (data from Cattapan *et al.*[29] (open circles), and from Watson *et al.*[30] (closed circles).) Modified from Laghi F. *Respir Care Clin* 2005; **11**: 173.

pulmonary disease, twitch pressures average 19–20 cm $H_2O$.[31,32] The value of transdiaphragmatic twitch pressure in patients recovering from an episode of acute respiratory failure is about a third of that recorded in healthy subjects (Fig. 33.2).[28–30] This marked reduction in twitch pressure[29,30] indicates the presence of respiratory muscle weakness in most of these patients. Purported mechanisms of respiratory muscle weakness in critical ill patients include critical illness neuropathy and myopathy (Table 33.2).

Diaphragmatic ultrasonography is a new method of assessing diaphragmatic function.[33,34] In 30 patients with suspected diaphragmatic paralysis, diaphragmatic motion was abnormal in 22 patients.[33] Fluoroscopy (with sniff) was technically impossible in four patients and it missed the motion abnormalities in another five patients. Ultrasonography can also be used to measure diaphragmatic thickness in the zone of apposition.[34] Diaphragmatic thickness at functional residual capacity of less than 2 mm combined with a less than 20 per cent increase in thickness during inspiration provided perfect discrimination between a paralysed and normal diaphragm.[34]

## Expiratory muscle impairment

Measurement in gastric pressure following electrical or magnetic stimulation of the abdominal wall muscles (while patients relax at end-exhalation) – or twitch gastric pressure ($P_{gatw}$) – provides a selective and quantitative measure of expiratory muscle function.[35] In healthy subjects, the mean (±SD) value of $P_{gatw}$ is $24 \pm 5$ cm $H_2O$.[36] In patients with ALS, an effective cough is unlikely when $P_{gatw}$ is less than 7 cm $H_2O$.[37]

**Table 33.2** Characteristics of acute and subacute paralysis

| | Guillain-Barré | Critical illness polyneuropathy | Critical illness myopathy | Spinal cord lesion | Poliomyelitis | Tick paralysis | Botulism |
|---|---|---|---|---|---|---|---|
| Progression | Days to weeks | Days to weeks | Days to weeks | Slow or immediate | Days to weeks | Hours to days | Days |
| Evolution of motor deficit | Usually ascending | Generalized | Generalized | Focal | Asymmetrical | Ascending | Descending |
| Fever | Uncommon | Commonly present | Uncommon | Absent | Present | Fever | Uncommon |
| Meningeal signs | Uncommon | Absent | Absent | Absent | Present | Absent | Absent |
| Ataxia | Uncommon | Absent | Absent | Sometimes present | Absent | Present | Absent |
| Tendon reflexes | Absent | Reduced or absent | Reduced or absent | Variable | Absent | Absent | Reduced or absent |
| Babinski sign | Absent | Absent | Absent | Present | Absent | Absent | Absent |
| Sensory deficit | Mild | Mild | Absent | Present | Absent | Absent | Absent |
| CSF: protein | High | – | Normal | Normal or high | High | Normal | – |
| CSF: white cells (per mm$^3$) | <10 | – | – | Variable | >10 | <10 | – |
| Recovery time | Weeks to months or no recovery | Weeks to months or no recovery | Weeks to months or no recovery | Variable according to aetiology | Months to years or no recovery | <24 hours (North America),* >2 weeks (Australia)* | Weeks to months |

*After tick removal.
CSF, cerebrospinal fluid.
From Laghi and Tobin.[1]

## Tests of inspiratory and expiratory muscle impairment

Generation of vital capacity maneouvres, maximal expiratory efforts from total lung capacity (including whistling),[38] require maximal voluntary recruitment of the inspiratory muscles followed by maximal voluntary recruitment of the expiratory muscles. This means that these tests are affected by impairment of the inspiratory and/or of the expiratory muscles. The normal vital capacity in adults is approximately 50 mL/kg, and elimination of secretions with coughing is impaired when the vital capacity declines to <30 mL/kg.[39] Serial vital capacity measurements that decline to <15–20 mL/kg increase the likelihood that ventilator assistance will be necessary. Ventilatory failure occurs at a vital capacity of around 10 mL/kg.[39]

Maximal expiratory pressure (MEP) is the airway pressure recorded during a maximal effort at total lung capacity using a bedside manometer fitted with a mouthpiece. Normal values for MEP are approximately 100 cm $H_2O$ for women and approximately 150 cm $H_2O$ for men. When the MEP is <40 cm $H_2O$ coughing is unlikely to be effective. Due to the voluntary nature of the manoeuvre, great caution has to be taken in interpretation of low MEP values. For instance, Man and co-workers[40] reported that among 171 patients with suspected respiratory muscle dysfunction and MEP values below the lower 95 per cent confidence interval recorded in healthy volunteers, 72 patients (42 per cent) had normal expiratory muscle strength.

## Arterial blood gas and electrolytes

Monitoring arterial blood gas – even in rapidly progressive neuromuscular diseases such as ALS or Guillain–Barré syndrome – can give a false sense of security because gas exchange can be largely maintained despite severe respiratory muscle impairment.[41,42] Of 81 patients with ALS, more than half of those with a vital capacity of 19–50 per cent of predicted were normocapnic.[42] Most patients with a MIP or MEP of less than 25 per cent of predicted were not hypercapnic.[42] These observations indicate that, at least in patients with ALS, measurements of arterial blood gases alone are of little value in monitoring disease progression[42,43] until the last four to five months of life. At that point, patients may show a precipitous fall in serum chloride (an indirect marker of respiratory acidosis), making it a more promising indicator of patient outcome than measurements of respiratory muscle strength during the terminal phase of the disease.[43] (For an additional discussion on the diagnostic approach to NMDs and ventilatory failure please see Chapter 32.)

## FUTURE RESEARCH/CONCLUSION

Respiratory failure occurs with numerous NMDs. Severe impairment of respiratory muscle function may be recognized early in the disease process, as in the case of bilateral diaphragmatic paralysis, or it may go unrecognized until hypercapnic respiratory failure develops, as in the case of Duchenne muscular dystrophy. Neuromuscular diseases involving the respiratory muscles often lead to breathing disturbances during sleep and pulmonary aspiration. Dyspnoea may not develop until respiratory impairment is so far advanced because activity sufficient to induce dyspnoea is limited by associated weakness of the limb muscles. Accordingly, a high level of suspicion is necessary to recognize the presence of respiratory muscle impairment and allow the institution of specific therapies. While the understanding of the pathophysiological mechanisms of respiratory failure in NMDs has greatly improved during the past two decades, the type of diagnostic tests to be employed in the identification of patients at risk of respiratory failure and the frequency with which these tests should be obtained remains elusive. Future research must focus on the development of disease-specific diagnostic strategies that will accurately monitor disease progression and identification of impending respiratory failure in patients with NMDs.

## APPENDIX 33.1

The A-a$DO_2$ is calculated as $P_AO_2 - PaO_2$, where $P_AO_2$ (alveolar $O_2$ tension) can be estimated according to the simplified alveolar gas equation $P_AO_2 = FiO_2 \times (PB - PH_2O) - PaCO_2/R$, where $FiO_2$ = fractional concentration of inspired $O_2$ (about 0.21 when breathing room air), PB = barometric pressure (about 760 mm Hg at sea level), $PH_2O$ = water vapour pressure (usually taken as 47 mm Hg at 37°C) and R = respiratory exchange ratio of the whole lung.

The respiratory exchange ratio (R) = $CO_2$ production/$O_2$ consumption ($VCO_2/VO_2$). R is normally ~0.8. In steady state, R is determined by the relative proportions of free fatty acids, protein and carbohydrate consumed by the tissues. In this equation, it is assumed that alveolar $PCO_2$ and $PaCO_2$ are the same (usually they nearly are). In healthy young subjects (≤30 years old) breathing air at sea level, A-a$DO_2$ is usually <10 mm Hg and increases by ~ 3 mm Hg per decade after 30 years.

## REFERENCES


1. Laghi F, Tobin MJ. Disorders of the respiratory muscles. *Am J Respir Crit Care Med* 2003; **168**: 10–48.
2. Laghi F, Tobin MJ. Indications for mechanical ventilation. In: Tobin MJ, ed. *Principles and practice of mechanical ventilation*, 2nd edn. New York: MacGraw-Hill, 2006:129–62.
3. Laghi F. Weaning from mechanical ventilation. In: Gabrielli A, Layon AJ, Yu M, eds. *Civetta, Taylor and Kirby's critical care*, 4th edn. Lippincott Williams & Wilkins, 2008.
4. Sassoon CS, Gruer SE, Sieck GC. Temporal relationships of ventilatory failure, pump failure, and diaphragm fatigue. *J Appl Physiol* 1996; **81**: 238–45.
5. Hughes PD, Polkey MI, Moxham J *et al.* Long-term recovery of diaphragm strength in neuralgic amyotrophy. *Eur Respir J* 1999; **13**: 379–84.
6. Tsairis P, Dyck PJ, Mulder DW. Natural history of brachial plexus neuropathy. Report on 99 patients. *Arch Neurol* 1972; **27**: 109–17.
7. Gibson GJ, Gilmartin JJ, Veale D *et al.* Respiratory muscle function in neuromuscular disease. In: Jones NL, Killian KJ, eds. *Breathlessness. The Campbell symposium.* Hamilton, Ontario: Boehringer-Ingelheim, 1992:66–73.
8. Misuri G, Lanini B, Gigliotti F *et al.* Mechanism of CO2 retention in patients with neuromuscular disease. *Chest* 2000; **117**: 447–53.
9. Poponick JM, Jacobs I, Supinski G *et al.* Effect of upper respiratory tract infection in patients with neuromuscular disease. *Am J Respir Crit Care Med* 1997; **156**: 659–64.
10. Tobin MJ, Laghi F. Monitoring respiratory muscle function. In: Tobin MJ, ed. *Principles and practice of intensive care monitoring.* New York: McGraw-Hill, 1998: 497–544.
11. Sharp JT, Henry JP, Sweaney SK *et al.* Effects of mass loading the respiratory system in man. *J Appl Physiol* 1964; **19**: 959–66.
12. Hong SK, Cerretelli P, Cruz JC *et al.* Mechanics of respiration during submersion in water. *J Appl Physiol* 1969; **27**: 535–8.
13. Dahlback GO, Jonsson E, Liner MH. Influence of hydrostatic compression of the chest and intrathoracic blood pooling on static lung mechanics during head-out immersion. *Undersea Biomed Res* 1978; **5**: 71–85.
14. Schoenhofer B, Koehler D, Polkey MI. Influence of immersion in water on muscle function and breathing pattern in patients with severe diaphragm weakness. *Chest* 2004; **125**: 2069–74.
15. Baydur A. Mechanical ventilation in neuromuscular disease. In: Tobin MJ, ed. *Principles and practice of mechanical ventilation*, 2nd edn. New York: MacGraw-Hill, 2006: 679–89.
16. Tusiewicz K, Moldofsky H, Bryan AC *et al.* Mechanics of the rib cage and diaphragm during sleep. *J Appl Physiol* 1977; **43**: 600–2.

17. Nugent AM, Smith IE, Shneerson JM. Domiciliary-assisted ventilation in patients with myotonic dystrophy. *Chest* 2002; **121**: 459–64.
18. Midgren B. Lung function and clinical outcome in postpolio patients: a prospective cohort study during 11 years. *Eur Respir J* 1997; **10**: 146–9.
19. Ragette R, Mellies U, Schwake C *et al.* Patterns and predictors of sleep disordered breathing in primary myopathies. *Thorax* 2002; **57**: 724–8.
20. Bourke SC, Shaw PJ, Gibson GJ. Respiratory function vs sleep-disordered breathing as predictors of QOL in ALS. *Neurology* 2001; **57**: 2040–4.
21. Labanowski M, Schmidt-Nowara W, Guilleminault C. Sleep and neuromuscular disease: frequency of sleep-disordered breathing in a neuromuscular disease clinic population. *Neurology* 1996; **47**: 1173–80.
22. McKinley AC, Auchincloss JH Jr, Gilbert R *et al.* Pulmonary function, ventilatory control, and respiratory complications in quadriplegic subjects. *Am Rev Respir Dis* 1969; **100**: 526–32.
23. Lotano R. Nonpulmonary causes of respiratory failure. In: Parrillo JE, Dellinger PR, eds. *Critical care medicine: Principles of diagnosis and management in the adult*, 3rd edn. Philadelphia: Mosby, 2008: 853–65.
24. Estenne M, Gevenois PA, Kinnear W *et al.* Lung volume restriction in patients with chronic respiratory muscle weakness: the role of microatelectasis. *Thorax* 1993; **48**: 698–701.
25. Bourke SC, Tomlinson M, Williams TL *et al.* Effects of non-invasive ventilation on survival and quality of life in patients with amyotrophic lateral sclerosis: a randomised controlled trial. *Lancet Neurol* 2006; **5**: 140–7.
26. Uldry C, Fitting JW. Maximal values of sniff nasal inspiratory pressure in healthy subjects. *Thorax* 1995; **50**: 371–5.
27. Laghi F, Harrison MJ, Tobin MJ. Comparison of magnetic and electrical phrenic nerve stimulation in assessment of diaphragmatic contractility. *J Appl Physiol* 1996; **80**: 1731–42.
28. Laghi F, Cattapan SE, Jubran A *et al.* Is weaning failure caused by low-frequency fatigue of the diaphragm? *Am J Respir Crit Care Med* 2003; **167**: 120–7.
29. Cattapan SE, Laghi F, Tobin MJ. Can diaphragmatic contractility be assessed by airway twitch pressure in mechanically ventilated patients? *Thorax* 2003; **58**: 58–62.
30. Watson AC, Hughes PD, Louise HM *et al.* Measurement of twitch transdiaphragmatic, esophageal, and endotracheal tube pressure with bilateral anterolateral magnetic phrenic nerve stimulation in patients in the intensive care unit. *Crit Care Med* 2001; **29**: 1325–31.
31. Polkey MI, Kyroussis D, Hamnegard CH *et al.* Diaphragm strength in chronic obstructive pulmonary disease. *Am J Respir Crit Care Med* 1996; **154**: 1310–17.
32. Laghi F, Jubran A, Topeli A *et al.* Effect of lung volume reduction surgery on diaphragmatic neuromechanical coupling at 2 years. *Chest* 2004; **125**: 2188–95.
33. Houston JG, Fleet M, Cowan MD *et al.* Comparison of ultrasound with fluoroscopy in the assessment of suspected hemidiaphragmatic movement abnormality. *Clin Radiol* 1995; **50**: 95–8.
34. Gottesman E, McCool FD. Ultrasound evaluation of the paralyzed diaphragm. *Am J Respir Crit Care Med* 1997; **155**: 1570–4.
35. Man WD, Moxham J, Polkey MI. Magnetic stimulation for the measurement of respiratory and skeletal muscle function. *Eur Respir J* 2004; **24**: 846–60.
36. Kyroussis D, Mills GH, Polkey MI *et al.* Abdominal muscle fatigue after maximal ventilation in humans. *J Appl Physiol* 1996; **81**: 1477–83.
37. Polkey MI, Lyall RA, Green M *et al.* Expiratory muscle function in amyotrophic lateral sclerosis. *Am J Respir Crit Care Med* 1998; **158**: 734–41.
38. Chetta A, Harris ML, Lyall RA *et al.* Whistle mouth pressure as test of expiratory muscle strength. *Eur Respir J* 2001; **17**: 688–95.
39. O'Donohue WJ Jr, Baker JP, Bell GM *et al.* Respiratory failure in neuromuscular disease. Management in a respiratory intensive care unit. *JAMA* 1976; **235**: 733–5.
40. Man WD, Kyroussis D, Fleming TA *et al.* Cough gastric pressure and maximum expiratory mouth pressure in humans. *Am J Respir Crit Care Med* 2003; **168**: 714–17.
41. Vitacca M, Clini E, Facchetti D *et al.* Breathing pattern and respiratory mechanics in patients with amyotrophic lateral sclerosis. *Eur Respir J* 1997; **10**: 1614–21.
42. Lyall RA, Donaldson N, Polkey MI *et al.* Respiratory muscle strength and ventilatory failure in amyotrophic lateral sclerosis. *Brain* 2001; **124**: 2000–13.
43. Stambler N, Charatan M, Cedarbaum JM. Prognostic indicators of survival in ALS. ALS CNTF Treatment Study Group. *Neurology* 1998; **50**: 66–72.

# 34

# Slowly progressive neuromuscular diseases

JOSHUA O BENDITT, LOUIS BOITANO

## ABSTRACT

A large number of neuromuscular disorders result in a slow progression of respiratory muscle weakness. The rate of progression may be quite rapid in the case of spinal muscular atrophy type 1 or very slow as in cases showing late effects of polio (post-polio syndrome). Different portions of the respiratory system may be involved including inspiratory muscles, expiratory muscles and glottic musculature. It is therefore important for the clinician who cares for these patients to have a logical and consistent approach, evaluating each portion of the respiratory system at each visit.

## INTRODUCTION

A wide variety of progressive neuromuscular disorders can result in dysfunction of the ventilatory muscles that in turn can lead to respiratory failure, pneumonia and even death. Breathing disorders are recognized as the leading cause of mortality in neuromuscular disease.[1] Neuromuscular disease can affect almost any part of the neurological system leading to changes in the respiratory system. In this chapter we will focus on a number of different conditions that affect the respiratory system in a progressive manner and review the pathophysiology and data pertinent to respiratory function where available.

Since respiratory impairment is a leading cause of morbidity and death in this population and because appropriate respiratory interventions can be instituted that prevent complications and prolong life in individuals with neuromuscular disease,[2,3] we have found it very useful to take a 'respiratory care' approach to the patient with respiratory muscle weakness from any cause.[4] We and others[4–6] have divided the respiratory system into three main areas of dysfunction (Fig. 34.1):[7]

- ventilatory function determined predominantly by the inspiratory muscles
- swallowing and airway protection determined by glottic muscles
- cough function which is determined by inspiratory, expiratory and glottic function.

Relatively simple testing can be performed at each clinic visit that can ensure that no potential problems are missed (Box 34.1). Specific therapies for ventilatory failure, cough insufficiency and swallowing issues can be employed. These techniques are detailed in other chapters.

## SPECIFIC DISEASES COVERED

Although there are a large number of neurological diseases that can affect the respiratory system, we will focus on the following disease processes during the rest of the chapter, in large part because not a great deal of data are available on respiratory issues pertaining to many of the disorders:

- spinal muscular atrophy (SMA)
- myasthenia gravis
- post-polio syndrome
- myotonic dystrophy
- glycogen storage disease
- congenital myopathies
- mitochondrial myopathy.

## SPINAL MUSCULAR ATROPHY

### DEFINITION AND PATHOPHYSIOLOGY

Spinal muscular atrophy is an autosomal recessive disease that is the leading genetic cause of infant death. It results from a

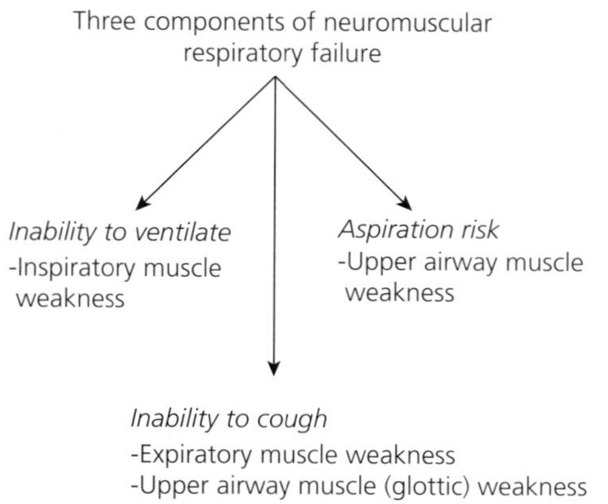


**Figure 34.1** The three components of neuromuscular respiratory failure.

**Box 34.1 Potential clinical measures for respiratory system function**

Ventilatory function

- Vital capacity
- Maximal inspiratory pressure
- Carbon dioxide:
  - end-tidal
  - arterial
  - transcutaneous

Cough function

- Peak cough expiratory flow
- Maximal expiratory pressure

Swallowing function

- Historical data
- Observed barium study
- Endoscopic evaluation

defect in a gene called survival motor neurone 1 (*SMN1*) and occurs in about 1 in 6000 to 1 in 10 000 live births[8] and has a carrier frequency of 1 in 50.[9] Although previously EMG and muscle biopsy were required for the diagnosis of the disease, genetic testing can now diagnose 95 per cent of the patients.[10] The defective gene results in degeneration of motor neurones in the spinal cord, which leads to hypotonia and muscle weakness in individuals affected. Clinical manifestations include hypotonia and muscle weakness and wasting of voluntary muscles. The lower extremities are weaker and proximal muscles are weaker than distal muscles. Tongue fasciculations and bulbar muscle involvement can occur particularly in SMA type 1. Sensation is intact and intellectual function is normal. SMA has classically been divided into three categories depending on the severity of disease and age of presentation.

SMA type 1 (Werdnig–Hoffman) is the most common (50 per cent) and severe presentation of the disease.[11] It is diagnosed within the first 6 months of life and individuals have profound hypotonia with flaccidity. They are unable to sit upright or hold their head erect without assistance. Death occurs within 2 years due to respiratory failure if respiratory interventions are not employed.[10] SMA type 2 is diagnosed between ages 6 and 18 months of age. It is sometimes referred to as the intermediate form. Individuals have less hypotonia and are able to sit but not stand unsupported. The phenotypic presentation is less severe and individuals can survive into the third decade of life even without respiratory intervention.[10] SMA type 3 (Kugelberg–Welander disease) is the least severe form of the disease and presents at or after 18 months of age. Individuals have an abnormal gait but a normal life expectancy. Recently, SMA type 4 (adult onset) has been added to include very mild disease.[12,13]

## RESPIRATORY CLINICAL ISSUES

In this discussion, we will focus on SMA types 1 and 2 as the most severe respiratory impairment occurs there. Intercostal muscles are more significantly affected and the diaphragm is relatively spared, which results in paradoxical movement of the chest wall during respiration with inward movement of the rib cage and outward movement of the diaphragm. The chest wall in the first year of life is particularly compliant and this results in distortion of the chest wall and development of a bell-shaped configuration of the chest wall with pectus excavatum that results from this muscular imbalance.

The physiological result of this chest wall and muscle problem is:[13]

- chest wall and lung underdevelopment
- impaired cough resulting in poor clearance of lower airway secretions
- recurrent infections that exacerbate muscle weakness
- hypoventilation during sleep.

Left untreated, there is a progression of respiratory failure beginning with anatomic changes that lead to repeat respiratory infections, progressive respiratory failure initially at night but later during the day[14,15] and ultimately full-time respiratory failure and death if untreated. A consensus statement for standard of care in SMA has been developed to aid in standardizing clinical care and also to make uniform study protocols.[13]

## RESPIRATORY MANAGEMENT

Respiratory assessment for SMA was recommended according to the severity of the disease, starting with SMA type 1 ('non-sitters'). Evaluation should include observation of breathing, observation of cough function and evaluation of gas exchange that includes measurement of pulse oximetry, and carbon dioxide evaluation via end-tidal or transcutaneous methods. Formal measurement of pulmonary function including vital capacity, maximal inspiratory and maximal expiratory pressures may be impossible, particularly in infants with SMA type 1 and even type 2. Therefore the most useful evaluation of overall respiratory function may be that of direct visualization of cough function and airway clearance.[13] It was also suggested that physical examination alone could provide very valuable information as to the requirement for airway clearance, which is the area of greatest weakness in SMA. Elevated respiratory rate, cyanosis or pallor, paradoxical breathing including intercostal muscle retractions may be indicators of airway clearance issues. A pulse oximetry reading of 94 per cent or less suggests that augmentative airway clearance efforts should be under-taken. Overnight chart recording of pulse oximetry can be helpful in identifying sleep-disordered breathing. It was also suggested that end-tidal and transcutaneous carbon dioxide monitoring as well as home sleep monitoring could be helpful in assessing sleep-disordered breathing, but their utility has not been studied and, if doubt exists, a full polysomnogram should be obtained to look for treatable sleep-disordered breathing. If recurrent respiratory infections are noted despite adequate cough therapy then swallowing assessment should be undertaken. A baseline chest radiograph was suggested for comparison during the likely occurrence of an infection. It was suggested that formal clinic evaluation occur every 3–6 months, more frequently warranted by symptoms at home.

For those who are able to sit (SMA type 2) respiratory evaluation should continue to focus on the physical examination, but in this case more formal pulmonary function testing may be possible, especially in older children. In addition, careful observation for kyphoscoliosis was suggested as this is a common occurrence in this form of the disease and is potentially correctable. For those who are able to walk (SMA types 3 and 4) physical examination continues to be important but greater emphasis falls on routine pulmonary function evaluation which can be obtained more easily due to greater cooperation with greater age. Other evaluation should be directed by clinical symptoms and indications.

In both acute and chronic situations, airway clearance is of critical importance. A variety of methodologies are available including chest physiotherapy, postural drainage and mechanically assisted cough devices such as the mechanical insufflator-exsufflator (MIE). This can be required up to every few hours or more during an acute episode and is suggested on a daily basis in more severely affected individuals. A protocol has been devised at the University of Wisconsin that involves a combination of initial applications of the MIE device followed by manual or mechanical chest percussion followed by postural drainage and a repeat of the MIE. In this protocol, which is used at home, those with SMA type 1 perform this twice per day and those with SMA type 2 when the child is well.[10] Those with SMA type 3 and 4 rarely need cough assistance, most often following operative intervention or significant respiratory illness only.

The individual with SMA type 1 may need immediate ventilatory support in the neonatal period. It is now possible with small paediatric interfaces to initiate non-invasive positive pressure ventilation (NIPPV).

The benefits reported for NIPPV for children with SMA type 1 include the potential for ventilatory support without a surgical intervention,[16] amelioration of the chest wall deformity and improvement in lung development[17,18] and potentially lung function. The long-term goals for NIPPV in SMA as in other neuromuscular diseases are amelioration of sleep quality, quality of life and avoidance of surgical interventions.[19] Complications of NIPPV include those related to prolonged use (16–18 hours/day) including skin irritation and breakdown and distortion of the midface (midface hypoplasia).[20] Gastric distention and emesis can also occur and can result in aspiration and pneumonia and possibly death.[10] As NIPPV is not always effective, the options of invasive (tracheostomy) ventilation and palliative care need to be discussed with each family individually and carefully, particularly for those individuals with SMA type 1. These discussions will need to occur early because of rapid progression.

Invasive ventilation is not required chronically for SMA type 2,[21] although for both SMA type 2 and SMA type 1 viral respiratory tract infection can lead to a situation where non-invasive methodologies are unsuccessful. Intubation until improvement in secretion management and oxygenation occurs can provide a bridge to further non-invasive management. Patients with SMA type 3 rarely if ever need non-invasive ventilatory support other than in instances of perioperative care or if they develop sleep apnoea with ageing. This is the same with SMA type 4.[10]

Patients with SMA type 1 and 2 are at risk of respiratory complications during surgery or procedures. It has been strongly suggested that a team including a nutritionist, pulmonologist and anaesthesiologist as well as surgeon should be used as a team in the pre- and post-operative period (Fig. 34.2). Less invasive procedures, if at all possible, should be considered.

## MYASTHENIA GRAVIS

### PATHOPHYSIOLOGY

Although myasthenia gravis is not necessarily a progressive disease, we have included it here because it is the most common disease affecting neuromuscular junction transmission. It is an autoimmune disease characterized by an antibody-mediated immune attack directed at acetylcholine receptors and/or receptor-associated proteins in the postsynaptic membrane of the neuromuscular junction. It causes weakness of many muscle groups including the respiratory muscles. The respiratory muscles are particularly susceptible to fatigue during the severe, potentially life-threatening exacerbations

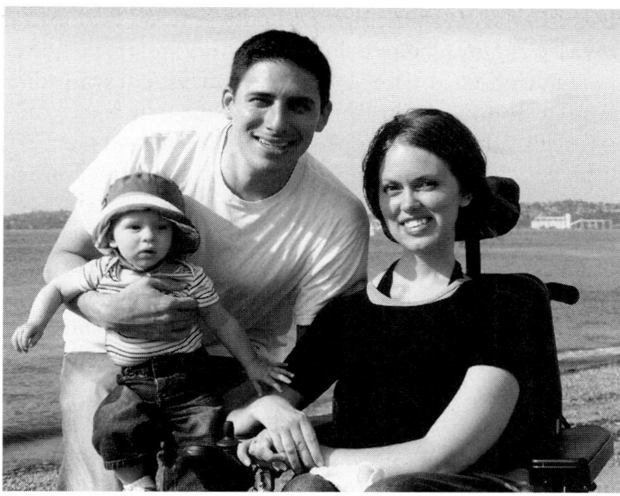

**Figure 34.2** Female patient with spinal muscular atrophy type 2, who successfully completed a pregnancy and delivered a healthy infant with non-invasive ventilatory support.

known as myasthenic crises. Acute treatment of myasthenic crises focuses on rapid therapies including intravenous immunoglobulin (IVIG) as well as plasmapheresis and corticosteroid therapy.[22,23] Assiduous attention to respiratory care permits support of the patient while allowing time for therapy of the underlying myasthenia to be effective.

Myasthenia gravis can also occur as a paraneoplastic syndrome in association with thymoma. It has been estimated that approximately 15 per cent of all patients with thymoma will exhibit myasthenia gravis. Removal of the thymoma may result in amelioration of the myasthenia symptoms.

### RESPIRATORY CLINICAL ISSUES

There are a number of physiological issues that put the patient with myasthenia gravis at risk for respiratory failure during an exacerbation of the disease. First, upper airway compromise due to weakness can lead to aspiration and difficulty with swallowing. In addition, the same bulbar muscles can lead to obstruction and loss of adequate ventilation. Weakness of inspiratory muscles can lead to frank hypoventilation, atelectasis and hypoxaemia. Lastly, expiratory muscle weakness can lead to poor cough function. Therefore judging when intubation and mechanical ventilation with protection of the upper airway and respiratory system is needed is critical for survival. Absolute indications for intubation in myasthenic crisis have been reported to be cardiac or respiratory arrest, impaired consciousness shock, arrhythmias, blood–gas alterations, and bulbar dysfunction with confirmed aspiration. Much more difficult is the decision to intubate when such strict criteria are not met. Over time a number of objective criteria have been proposed and used although rarely studied in a prospective manner. These objective criteria have included a vital capacity of less than 1 L, one that falls by 50 per cent from baseline or one that is <15 mL/kg ideal body weight. A maximal inspiratory pressure ≥30 cm $H_2O$ and maximal expiratory pressure <40 cm $H_2O$ have also been used. However, a number of subjective assessments have been developed to aid in alerting earlier those myasthenia gravis patients who may be getting into trouble. These have included the presence of rapid shallow breathing, tachycardia, weak cough, staccato speech, accessory muscle use, abdominal muscle paradox, single breath count of <15, and cough after swallowing.[24] A very high index of suspicion must be maintained and early rather than late intervention is certainly preferable.

### RESPIRATORY MANAGEMENT

There is debate as to the role of NIPPV in treatment of myasthenic crisis and there are studies that lend some credence to its use in selected patients. Seneviratne *et al.*[25] in a retrospective manner studied 60 episodes of myasthenic crisis in 52 patients. Bi-level positive airway pressure (BiPAP) was the initial method of ventilatory support in 24 episodes and endotracheal intubation was performed in 36 episodes. In 14 episodes treated using BiPAP, intubation was avoided. The mean duration of BiPAP in these patients was 4.3 days. The only predictor of BiPAP failure (i.e. requirement for intubation) was a $PaCO_2$ level exceeding 45 mm Hg on BiPAP initiation ($p = 0.04$). There were no differences in patient demographics or in baseline respiratory variables and arterial gases between the groups of episodes initially treated using BiPAP versus endotracheal intubation. The mean ventilation duration was 10.4 days. The intensive care unit and hospital lengths of stay statistically significantly increased with ventilation duration ($p < 0.001$ for both). The only variable associated with decreased ventilation was the initial use of BiPAP. However, because bulbar musculature is often involved in myasthenia gravis, air blowing through a mask can lead to aspirated secretions and great care must be taken when using this modality.

## POST-POLIO SYNDROME (PPS)

### DEFINITION AND PATHOPHYSIOLOGY

In the developed world, the major health issue arising from polio currently is the post-polio syndrome, in which new weakness develops in survivors of the polio epidemics of the mid-twentieth century.[26,27] Generally accepted criteria for the post-polio syndrome include:[28]

- confirmed history of polio
- partial or fairly complete recovery after acute episode
- period of 15 or more years of neurological and functional stability
- onset of new neurogenic weakness
- two or more of the following symptoms: fatigue, new muscle or joint pain, muscle atrophy, new weakness in

previously unaffected muscles, functional loss or cold intolerance

- no other medical explanation found.

Estimates of prevalence of post-polio syndrome will vary greatly depending on the criteria used to define the syndrome. If patients are asked whether they have a new symptom related to previous polio prevalence, the syndrome is reported at 50 per cent or higher.[29] If new onset weakness is included as an identifying criterion the prevalence may drop to as low as 20–30 per cent of overall polio survivors. The prevalence of PPS worldwide has been reported to be between 15 per cent and 80 per cent of individuals surveyed.[30]

It has been suggested that electromyography (EMG) may be of assistance in assessing individuals with suspected post-polio syndrome in showing the typical lower motor neurone involvement; to assess the extent of neuronal involvement; to exclude other causes of new weakness such as entrapment syndromes; and to assess other possible concomitant neuromuscular disease.[28] It should be noted that EMG cannot differentiate findings related to the original polio injury from post-polio syndrome but is more useful in assessing extent of involvement and excluding other causes of weakness.

Muscle biopsy is probably not useful in the evaluation of electromyography as the findings are non-specific and can be seen in patients with both the absence and presence of findings of new weakness in a particular muscle group.[31]

### CLINICAL RESPIRATORY ISSUES

Reduced pulmonary function due to weak respiratory muscles and chest wall deformity can occur in patients with electromyography.[32] In one of the earlier and larger studies of pulmonary function in patients with electromyography, Dean *et al.*[33] performed a cross-sectional study of 74 patients with a distant history ofpolio. These were subjects recruited by advertisement and were not using any respiratory aids at the time nor were they being treated for any form of cardiorespiratory disease that they were aware of. There was a fairly wide spread of normal and abnormal pulmonary function with the most striking finding a very significant reduction in maximal expiratory pressure (MEP). Factors associated with a decrease in pulmonary function included ventilator support at the onset of polio, and age of onset of polio after age 10 but not >35 years (previously described by others). In addition, they asked about shortness of breath to their patients. In those individuals with shortness of breath, pulmonary function tended to be lower. The authors suggested all patients with a history of polio, particularly with ventilatory support at the time of initial presentation and onset after age 10, should undergo careful screening for late respiratory effects of polio.

### RESPIRATORY MANAGEMENT

It is well known that individuals with a history of polio and post-polio syndrome have a high incidence of sleep-disordered breathing.[34,35] Findings of low forced vital capacity, chest wall restriction, ventilatory support requirement during the initial bout of polio and current symptoms of sleep-disordered breathing such as daytime hypersomnolence are predictors for likely sleep-disordered breathing. A high index of suspicion should be maintained when evaluating these individuals.

Diurnal ventilatory insufficiency will be present in some individuals with polio (either from the time of the original polio infection or due to late effects of polio) such that full-time ventilation is required. Sometimes frank ventilatory failure will be triggered by a respiratory tract infection that results in increased work of breathing and an inability to maintain adequate blood gas homeostasis. A number of methodologies have been employed including tracheostomy ventilation, full-time mask ventilation, and mouthpiece ventilation (see Chapter 6).

In summary, it is quite possible to support individuals with late-onset effects of polio with non-invasive methodologies.

## MYOTONIC DYSTROPHY

### DEFINITION AND PATHOPHYSIOLOGY

Myotonic dystrophy is the most frequently inherited neuromuscular disease with an estimated frequency worldwide of 2.1–14.3 in 100 000 births.[36] Myotonic dystrophy is an autosomal dominant disorder that is genetically heterogeneous with variable phenotypic expression. There are two major classifications including DM1, formerly known as Steinert's disease, and DM2, a more mild disease form. Myotonic dystrophy often has multisystem affects including cardiac conduction abnormalities, cataracts, infertility and insulin resistance. In addition, DM1 patients may have severe developmental delay. Based upon the age of clinical onset DM1 can be classified congenital, classical or minimal. Congenital DM1 presents at birth or within the first year of life as a severe form. In the classical form symptoms develop between the second and fourth decade with slow progression over time. Minimal DM1 is characterized by the development of mild symptoms after 50 years of age. Only the adult onset form has been found in DM2.

The genetic basis for the multisystemic effect in DM1 is the expansion of a CTG trinucleotide repeat in the 3'-untranslated region of the dystrophia myotonic protein kinase gene on chromosome 19q 13.3 and an expanded CCTG tetranucleotide repeat expansion located on intron 1 of the zinc finger protein 9 gene on chromosome 3q 21.3 in DM2.[37] The cause of muscle weakness and wasting is not yet known. A characteristic phenotypic feature of skeletal muscle weakness is facial muscle weakness in DM1, which is mild and occurs later in DM2. Oropharyngeal muscle weakness can result in dysphagia and dysarthria. Limb weakness is associated with the weakness of thigh, hip flexor and extensor muscles. Myotonia, a slowed relaxation following a normal muscle contraction, can be periodic but is more pronounced and severe in DM1 than in DM2. Cardiac abnormalities include both conduction disturbances and structural defects.

### RESPIRATORY CLINICAL ISSUES

Respiratory muscle weakness is common in DM1 resulting in variable restrictive pulmonary impairment and alveolar hypoventilation. In congenital DM1, infants develop respiratory failure requiring continuous ventilation. Infants that survive the first year can develop improved motor function but are at a higher risk for cardiorespiratory mortality. In the classical form of DM1 restrictive pulmonary impairment can be mild to moderate requiring nocturnal ventilatory support or severe and chronic requiring continuous ventilation. Oropharyngeal muscle weakness can result in dysphagia and the liability of chronic aspiration but is more commonly associated with sleep-disordered breathing. Sleep-disordered breathing and nocturnal hypoxaemia has been shown to be common in myotonic dystrophy. The severity of nocturnal hypoxaemia has been associated with the degree of obesity. Daytime hypercapnia has also been observed and worsens with sleep. While polysomnography studies of myotonic dystrophy patients with daytime hypersomnolence have identified a significant degree of obstructive sleep apnoea other studies have also identified a significant degree of central sleep apnoea. In one study a majority of patients showed periodic breathing patterns indicating a central auto-regulatory dysfunction. The incidence of sudden death in myotonic dystrophy is associated with ventricular arrhythmias, and nocturnal hypoxaemia secondary to sleep-disordered breathing is a significant risk factor for cardiac arrhythmia.

### RESPIRATORY CLINICAL MANAGEMENT

The respiratory management of myotonic dystrophy should include serial pulmonary function testing to assess respiratory muscle strength. Vital capacity testing and static mouth pressure testing has been commonly used to assess neuromuscular respiratory function.[38] The predominance of sleep-disordered breathing in this population should prompt the clinician to screen the patient for symptoms of sleep-disordered breathing.[39,40] Periodic evaluation using nocturnal oximetry studies can identify the need for polysomnography testing to evaluate the degree of sleep-disordered breathing which is often affected by a combination of upper airway obstruction, central breathing dysfunction and respiratory muscle weakness.[41,42] Most patients will have a combined obstructive and central sleep-disordered breathing affected by restrictive pulmonary impairment. These patients will require non-invasive bi-level pressure support ventilation with a spontaneous/timed back-up rate to adequately support nocturnal ventilation. Nocturnal bi-level pressure ventilation has been associated with sustained improved ventilation and with improved survival.[43,44] Bi-level pressure titration with polysomnography monitoring may be necessary to determine the most supportive pressure regimen for nocturnal ventilation. Respiratory muscle aids including cough augmentation therapy may also be required for patients with weak cough strength secondary to restrictive pulmonary impairment. Peak expiratory cough flow, a measure of cough strength, should be done to serially evaluate cough effectiveness, and MIE can be used to support cough clearance in myotonic patients with inadequate cough strength. Myotonic patients with severe oropharyngeal muscle weakness may develop chronic upper airway airflow restriction or aspiration. A tracheostomy may be indicated in order to better support these patients.

While NIPPV has been associated with improved survival there are limitations in the use of this therapy for myotonic dystrophy patients. The characteristic facial muscle weakness in this patient population often limits the ability to successfully apply positive pressure mask ventilation. Cognitive impairment also has been associated with a significant limitation in the patient's compliance to the nightly use of positive pressure mask ventilation.[45]

## GLYCOGEN STORAGE DISEASE

### DEFINITION AND PATHOPHYSIOLOGY

Glycogen is the stored form of glucose reserves that provides an energy substrate during periods of high energy expenditure or when glucose availability is low. Disorders that result in the abnormal storage of glycogen are identified as glycogen storage diseases. There are a number of genetic mutations in the synthesis of proteins involved in glycogen synthesis, degradation and regulation that can result in the abnormal storage of glycogen.[46] The primary effects of glycogen storage disease in muscle tissue are muscle cramps, exercise intolerance, fatigue and progressive muscle weakness. A number of glycogen metabolism defects that result in the abnormal storage of glycogen have been classified. Lysosomal acid maltase deficiency, or Pompe's disease, is the glycogen storage disease type that has been found to most affect respiratory function. The incidence of Pompe's disease is estimated to be between 1 in 40 000 and 1 in 600 000 depending on geographical and ethnic factors. Pompe's disease has been classified as infantile, juvenile and adult forms depending on the age of onset. Infants are severely affected with cardiomegaly, hepatosplenomegaly, mental retardation and severe myopathy and generally do not survive past the age of 2 as a result of hypertrophic cardiomyopathy.[47] The juvenile or childhood and adult forms are milder with slower progression. In these forms skeletal muscle weakness is the primary symptom with progressive proximal weakness in the limb-girdle distribution.[48] Respiratory muscle weakness occurs in both forms and in adults respiratory insufficiency can be the first sign.

Pompe's disease is an autosomal recessive disorder that results from a deficiency of the glycogen degrading lysosomal enzyme acid $\alpha$-glucosidase (GAA). Symptom expression and disease severity are dependent on the amount of residual GAA activity.[49]

### RESPIRATORY ISSUES

Unlike most other neuromuscular diseases where limb weakness usually occurs before respiratory involvement, respiratory insufficiency can be one of the first indications of the disease.[50,51] Diaphragmatic weakness is the predominant contributing factor and weakness in the inspiratory muscles of the chest can also contribute to respiratory insufficiency.[49] Upper airway weakness can also contribute to sleep-disordered breathing and can be either independent of or more affected by inspiratory muscle weakness.[52] Chronic nocturnal hypoventilation can produce symptoms of hypercarbia including restlessness, frequent awakenings, nocturia, vivid nightmares, morning headaches and poor sleep quality.[53] Progressive inspiratory muscle weakness can also affect cough strength by limiting the inspiratory volume necessary to produce an adequate peak expiratory cough flow in order to clear pulmonary secretions. In Pompe's disease, where respiratory involvement is often the primary limitation, mild subclinical outward symptoms may not be apparent to the clinician. Acute respiratory failure, which is a common presentation, is most often precipitated by pulmonary congestion secondary to respiratory infection in the face of cough insufficiency and hypoventilation.[49,52]

### RESPIRATORY CLINICAL MANAGEMENT

Patients who are diagnosed with Pompe's disease before an acute respiratory event should be immediately referred for a neuromuscular respiratory assessment to evaluate their respiratory status and thereafter undergo serial respiratory assessment to monitor their respiratory status.[52,54] Upright and supine FVC spirometry, and maximum inspiratory and expiratory pressure testing should be done to determine the degree of diaphragmatic weakness and global respiratory muscle weakness.[55] Peak cough flow testing should also be done to assess cough strength.[56] Diaphragmatic and upper airway muscle weakness should prompt the clinician to screen for symptoms of sleep-disordered breathing and a referral for diagnostic polysomnography testing should be made for any indication of symptoms.[49] NIPPV has been shown to support nocturnal ventilation and improve the longevity of Pompe's patients.[52,57] A spontaneous/timed mode of bi-level pressure support is necessary to support severe diaphragmatic limited ventilation during REM sleep. Cough insufficiency may be augmented by either manual or mechanical cough augmentation.[58] Manual hyperinflation combined with abdominal thrust has been shown to augment limited cough strength, and MIE has also been shown to augment cough in patients who do not experience significant bulbar symptoms.

# CONGENITAL MYOPATHIES

Congenital myopathies are muscle disorders that are caused by genetic abnormalities of muscle development.[59] These disorders are present at birth though symptoms may not develop until later in infancy or childhood, and in rare cases in adults. The most common disorders with respiratory involvement include nemaline myopathy, centronuclear (myotubular) myopathy and multicore myopathy. Congenital myopathies generally have the same clinical features including hypotonia, primarily proximal muscle weakness, decreased tendon reflexes and skeletal deformities associated with developmental muscle weakness.

## Nemaline myopathy

### DEFINITION AND PATHOPHYSIOLOGY

Nemaline myopathy is characterized by thread-like bodies in the longitudinal sections of muscle tissue. This disease has been classified into three forms based upon the onset of clinical presentation including mild to severe infantile, moderate congenital (classic) and adult onset forms.[60] In the severe infantile form, there is severe generalized weakness and hypotonia of the facial, bulbar and respiratory muscles.[61] In the milder infantile, congenital and adult forms, symptoms are less severe and progressive. Nemaline myopathy results from mutations in genes encoding for several different protein components in the thin filaments of skeletal muscle.[62]

### RESPIRATORY CLINICAL ISSUES

In the severe infantile disease form marked respiratory muscle weakness and bulbar dysfunction generally result in respiratory failure and death within the first year although prolonged survival with improvement has been reported.[63] In the milder congenital and adult forms diaphragmatic weakness appears to be the primary restrictive respiratory limitation. In addition nemaline myopathy has also been associated with impairment of the central respiratory drive during REM sleep.[64] A discrepancy between the rate of deterioration in motor function and the development of respiratory impairment has also been reported.[65,66]

## Centronuclear (myotubular) myopathy

### DEFINITION

Centronuclear myopathy is a clinically and genetically variable disorder with characteristic large nuclei located in the centre of muscle fibres that resemble myotubes, the early foetal muscle fibres. There are two primary clinical presentations. The more common milder form consisting of both autosomal dominant and autosomal recessive subforms consist of relatively mild skeletal muscle weakness and hypotonia that can be present in the newborn or have a later onset and slow progression. The more severe X-linked form presents in males at birth. Infants present with marked skeletal muscle weakness and hypotonia, bulbar dysfunction.[67] Respiratory muscle weakness leads to early respiratory failure.[68] In autosomal dominant and recessive forms the distribution of weakness is predominantly proximal with additional distal involvement. Facial weakness and ocular abnormalities including ophthalmoplegia and ptosis are variable depending on the form.[69]

#### PATHOPHYSIOLOGY

Mutations responsible for the X-linked form are in the gene encoding for myotubularin, a protein required for muscle cell differentiation.[70] In general the autosomal dominant form has been associated with later onset and milder course whereas the autosomal recessive form is generally intermediate in respect to onset and course.[71]

#### RESPIRATORY CLINICAL ISSUES

In the X-linked severe form marked respiratory muscle weakness results in early respiratory failure and only continuous mechanical ventilation can support survival.[72] In the autosomal recessive form respiratory impairment can be mild to severe and associated cardiomyopathy has been reported.[73] While the more mild autosomal dominant form generally does not have cardiorespiratory involvement, earlier-onset cases may develop restrictive respiratory impairment.[74]

### Multicore myopathy

#### DEFINITION

Multicore myopathy is characterized by the multifocal myofibrillar degeneration that is smaller in size and number as compared to larger central core degeneration. Type I fibres are predominantly affected but both type I and type II may be affected.[75] Autosomal dominant and recessive patterns of inheritance as well as sporadic occurrence have been found. Multicore myopathy had previously been recognized as primarily infantile and benign with relatively non-progressive mostly proximal weakness, hypotonia and hyporeflexia.[76] Clinical features include facial and respiratory muscle weakness, joint contractures, chest deformities, and scoliosis. More recent reports have described later adult-onset cases with respiratory involvement and cardiomyopathy.[77,78]

#### PATHOPHYSIOLOGY

The pathophysiology of multicore myopathy is not well understood. Mitochondrial depletion and mitochondrial, myofibrillar function is thought to have a predominant effect on skeletal muscle weakness.

#### RESPIRATORY CLINICAL ISSUES

In multicore myopathy the intercostal muscles have been found to be affected more than the diaphragm in patients with respiratory involvement.[79] Paraspinal muscle contracture with resulting scoliosis induced chest wall restriction has also been reported.[80] Nocturnal hypoventilation progressing to respiratory failure has been reported in adolescent and adult patients.[80]

### Respiratory management of congenital myopathies

The severity of the respective disease form will affect the course of respiratory management. The more severe infantile disease forms will most often require either continuous or nocturnal mechanical ventilation via tracheostomy.[72] In general earlier-onset forms may develop more severe respiratory impairment whereas later-onset forms tend to have lesser cardiorespiratory involvement. Respiratory assessment should include upright and supine vital capacity testing, static mouth pressures to assess inspiratory and expiratory muscle strength[52] and peak cough flow. Arterial blood gas testing, end-tidal carbon dioxide and transcutaneous carbon dioxide testing can be used to monitor for developing hypercapnic respiratory failure.[52,81] A serial assessment for symptoms of sleep-disordered breathing should also be included. Polysomnography testing combined is indicated for any suspicion of sleep-disordered breathing.[66,82] Non-invasive mask ventilation has been shown to successfully support noc-turnal hypoventilation in congenital myopathies with respiratory insufficiency.[83,84] Polysomnography with bi-level pressure titration should be done in order to determine the most effective bi-level pressure support and back-up rate regimen.[82]

## MITOCHONDRIAL MYOPATHY

#### DEFINITION AND PATHOPHYSIOLOGY

Mitochondria are cellular organelles responsible for oxidative phosphorylation, which produces adenosine triphosphate (ATP), the energy substrate for metabolic function. Defects in the process of oxidative phosphorylation that affects skeletal muscle alone or in conjunction with central nervous system disease are identified as mitochondrial myopathy. Myopathy can occur alone or as a part of a multisystem disease. Clinical manifestations of myopathy can include myalgia, exercise intolerance, proximal muscle weakness, external ophthalmoplegia and facioscapulohumeral syndrome. The diagnosis of mitochondrial myopathy is based on muscle biopsy showing morphological abnormalities in muscle mitochondria. Skeletal muscle and brain tissue are selectively affected by mitochondrial dysfunction as a result of the high energy demand of these tissues.

### RESPIRATORY CLINICAL ISSUES

Respiratory failure has been reported in adults with mitochondrial disease either as an acute event sometimes associated with respiratory infection or as a chronic recurrent problem.[85,86] Respiratory muscle weakness has been identified on spirometry testing and diaphragmatic paralysis has been reported. Impaired ventilatory response to hypercapnia and hypoxia has also been reported.[87] There have been case reports of sleep apnoea associated with mitochondrial disease. Muscle weakness and phrenic nerve involvement may also contribute to sleep apnoea. Respiratory arrest during sleep has also been reported.[88]

### RESPIRATORY MANAGEMENT

A neuromuscular respiratory assessment should be included with regular clinical evaluation.[89] The patient should be screened for symptoms of sleep-disordered breathing since sleep apnoea has been associated with a decreased ventilatory drive. Patients with symptoms of sleep-disordered breathing should be evaluated by polysomnography testing and non-invasive ventilation should be applied according to the findings of polysomnography with pressure titration.[82,90]

## SUMMARY

In summary, there are a wide variety of neuromuscular disorders that can affect respiratory function. Almost every facet of the respiratory system can be affected. Careful screening for symptoms, evaluation of respiratory function at clinic visits and a high index of suspicion for respiratory issues is key in providing the best level of care for patients with neuromuscular disease. Non-invasive methodologies for ventilatory and cough support are widely available and should be offered to appropriate patients.

## REFERENCES


1. Bergofsky EH. Respiratory failure in disorders of the thoracic cage. *Am Rev Respir Dis* 1979; **119**: 643–69.
2. Bourke SC, Tomlinson M, Williams TL *et al.* Effects of non-invasive ventilation on survival and quality of life in patients with amyotrophic lateral sclerosis: a randomised controlled trial. *Lancet Neurol* 2006; **5**: 140–7.
3. Simonds AK, Ward S, Heather S *et al.* Impact of nasal ventilation on survival in hypercapnic Duchenne muscular dystrophy. *Thorax* 1998; **53**: 949–52.
4. Benditt JO. The neuromuscular respiratory system: physiology, pathophysiology, and a respiratory care approach to patients. *Respir Care* 2006; **51**: 829–37; discussion 837–9.
5. Bach JR. *Nonivasive mechanical ventilation*, 1st edn. Philadelphia: Hanley and Belfus, 2002:348.
6. Perrin C, Unterborn JN, Ambrosio CD *et al.* Pulmonary complications of chronic neuromuscular diseases and their management. *Muscle Nerve* 2004; **29**: 5–27.
7. Leith DE, Butler JP, Sneddon SL *et al.* Cough, in handbook of physiology: the respiratory system, vol. 3. In: Macklem PT, Mead J, eds. *Mechanics of breathing, Part 2.* Bethesda: American Physiologic Society, 1990: 315–36.
8. Koul R, Al Futaisi A, Chacko A *et al.* Clinical and genetic study of spinal muscular atrophies in Oman. *J Child Neurol* 2007; **22**: 1227–30.
9. Lunn MR, Wang CH. Spinal muscular atrophy. *Lancet* 2008; **371**: 2120–33.
10. Schroth MK. Special considerations in the respiratory management of spinal muscular atrophy. *Pediatrics* 2009; **123** Suppl 4: S245–9.
11. Markowitz JA, Tinkle MB, Fischbeck KH. Spinal muscular atrophy in the neonate. *J Obstet Gynecol Neonatal Nurs* 2004; **33**: 12–20.
12. Russman BS. Spinal muscular atrophy: clinical classification and disease heterogeneity. *J Child Neurol* 2007; **22**: 946–51.
13. Wang CH, Finkel RS, Bertini ES *et al.* Consensus statement for standard of care in spinal muscular atrophy. *J Child Neurol* 2007; **22**: 1027–49.
14. Mellies U, Dohna-Schwake C, Stehling F *et al.* Sleep disordered breathing in spinal muscular atrophy. *Neuromuscul Disord* 2004; **14**: 797–803.
15. Mellies U, Ragette R, Dohna Schwake C *et al.* Long-term noninvasive ventilation in children and adolescents with neuromuscular disorders. *Eur Respir J* 2003; **22**: 631–6.
16. Oskoui M, Levy G, Garland CJ *et al.* The changing natural history of spinal muscular atrophy type 1. *Neurology* 2007; **69**: 1931–6.
17. Bach JR, Bianchi C. Prevention of pectus excavatum for children with spinal muscular atrophy type 1. *Am J Phys Med Rehabil* 2003; **82**: 815–19.
18. Perez A, Mulot R, Vardon G *et al.* Thoracoabdominal pattern of breathing in neuromuscular disorders. *Chest* 1996; **110**: 454–61.
19. Bach JR, Baird JS, Plosky D *et al.* Spinal muscular atrophy type 1: management and outcomes. *Pediatr Pulmonol* 2002; **34**: 16–22.
20. Houston K, Buschang PH, Iannaccone ST *et al.* Craniofacial morphology of spinal muscular atrophy. *Pediatr Res* 1994; **36**: 265–9.
21. Bach JR, Niranjan V, Weaver B. Spinal muscular atrophy type 1: A noninvasive respiratory management approach. *Chest* 2000; **117**: 1100–5.
22. Gajdos P, Chevret S. Toyka K. Intravenous immunoglobulin for myasthenia gravis. *Cochrane Database Syst Rev* 2008: CD002277.
23. Qureshi AI, Choudary MA, Akbar MS *et al.* Plasma exchange versus intravenous immunoglobulin treatment in myasthenic crisis. *Neurology* 1999; **52**: 629–32.

24. Mehta S. Neuromuscular disease causing acute respiratory failure. *Respir Care* 2006; **51**: 1016–21; discussion 1021–3.
25. Seneviratne J, Mandrekar J, Wijdicks EF *et al.* Noninvasive ventilation in myasthenic crisis. *Arch Neurol* 2008; **65**: 54–8.
26. Rekand T, Korv J, Farbu E *et al.* Lifestyle and late effects after poliomyelitis. A risk factor study of two populations. *Acta Neurol Scand* 2004; **109**: 120–5.
27. Willen C, Thoren-Jönsson AL, Grimby G *et al.* Disability in a 4-year follow-up study of people with post-polio syndrome. *J Rehabil Med* 2007; **39**: 175–80.
28. Farbu E, Gilhus NE, Barnes MP *et al.* EFNS guideline on diagnosis and management of post-polio syndrome. Report of an EFNS task force. *Eur J Neurol* 2006; **13**: 795–801.
29. Bruno RL. Post-polio sequelae: research and treatment in the second decade. *Orthopedics* 1991; **14**: 1169–70.
30. Farbu E, Rekand T, Gilhus NE. Post-polio syndrome and total health status in a prospective hospital study. *Eur J Neurol* 2003; **10**: 407–13.
31. Jubelt B, Cashman NR. Neurological manifestations of the post-polio syndrome. *Crit Rev Neurobiol* 1987; **3**: 199–220.
32. Kidd D, Williams AJ, Howard RS *et al.* Late functional deterioration following paralytic poliomyelitis. *Q J Med* 1997; **90**: 189–96.
33. Dean E, Ross J, Road JD *et al.* Pulmonary function in individuals with a history of poliomyelitis. *Chest* 1991; **100**: 118–23.
34. Bergholtz B, Mollestad SO, Refsum H. Post-polio respiratory failure. New manifestations of a forgotten disease. *Tidsskr Nor Laegeforen* 1988; **108**: 2474–5.
35. Howard RS, Wiles CM, Spencer GT. The late sequelae of poliomyelitis. *Q J Med* 1988; **66**: 219–32.
36. Mathieu J, Allard P, Potvin L *et al.* A 10-year study of mortality in a cohort of patients with myotonic dystrophy. *Neurology* 1999; **52**: 1658–62.
37. Brook JD, McCurrach ME, Harley HG *et al.* Molecular basis of myotonic dystrophy: expansion of a trinucleotide (CTG) repeat at the 3' end of a transcript encoding a protein kinase family member. *Cell* 1992; **69**: 385.
38. Griggs RC, Donohoe KM. The recognition and management of respiratory insufficiency in neuromuscular disease. *J Chronic Dis* 1982; **35**: 497–500.
39. Cirignotta F, Mondini S, Zucconi M *et al.* Sleep-related breathing impairment in myotonic dystrophy. *J Neurol* 1987; **235**: 80–5.
40. Gilmartin JJ, Cooper BG, Griffiths CJ *et al.* Breathing during sleep in patients with myotonic dystrophy and non-myotonic respiratory muscle weakness. *Q J Med* 1991; **78**: 21–31.
41. Finnimore AJ, Jackson RV, Morton A *et al.* Sleep hypoxia in myotonic dystrophy and its correlation with awake respiratory function. *Thorax* 1994; **49**: 66–70.
42. Kumar SP, Sword D, Petty RKH *et al.* Assessment of sleep studies in myotonic dystrophy. *Chron Respir Dis* 2007; **4**: 15–18.
43. Nitz J, Burke B. A study of the facilitation of respiration in myotonic dystrophy. *Physiother Res Int* 2002; **7**: 228–38.
44. Nugent AM, Smith IE, Shneerson JM. Domiciliary-assisted ventilation in patients with myotonic dystrophy. *Chest* 2002; **121**: 459–64.
45. Gamez J, Calzada M, Cervera C *et al.* Non-compliance of domiciliary ventilatory treatment in patients with myotonic dystrophy. *Neurologia* 2000; **15**: 371.
46. Nakajima H, Raben N, Hamaguchi T *et al.* Phosphofructokinase deficiency; past, present and future. *Curr Mol Med* 2002; **2**: 197–212.
47. Kishnani PS, Nicolino M, Volt T *et al.* A retrospective, multinational, multicenter study on the natural history of infantile-onset Pompe disease. *J Pediatr* 2006; **148**: 671–6.
48. Engel AG. Acid maltase deficiency in adults: studies in four cases of a syndrome which may mimic muscular dystrophy or other myopathies. *Brain* 1970; **93**: 599–616.
49. Kishnani PS, Steiner RD, Bali D *et al.* Pompe disease diagnosis and management guideline. *Genet Med* 2006; **8**: 267–88.
50. Rosenow EC 3rd, Engel AG. Acid maltase deficiency in adults presenting as respiratory failure. *Am J Med* 1978; **64**: 485–91.
51. Keunen RW, Lambregts PC, Op de Coul AA *et al.* Respiratory failure as initial symptom of acid maltase deficiency. *J Neurol Neurosurg Psychiatry* 1984; **47**: 549–52.
52. Mellies U, Dohna-Schwake C, Voit T. Respiratory function assessment and intervention in neuromuscular disorders. *Curr Opin Neurol* 2005; **18**: 543–7.
53. Mellies U, Ragette R, Schwake C *et al.* Sleep-disordered breathing and respiratory failure in acid maltase deficiency. *Neurology* 2001; **57**: 1290–5.
54. Pellegrini N, Laforet P, Orlikowski D *et al.* Respiratory insufficiency and limb muscle weakness in adults with Pompe's disease. *Eur Respir J* 2005; **26**: 1024–31.
55. Fromageot C, Lofaso F, Annane D *et al.* Supine fall in lung volumes in the assessment of diaphragmatic weakness in neuromuscular disorders. *Arch Phys Med Rehabil* 2001; **82**: 123–8.
56. Dohna-Schwake C, Ragette R, Teschler H *et al.* Predictors of severe chest infections in pediatric neuromuscular disorders. *Neuromuscul Disord* 2006; **16**: 325–8.
57. Mellies U, Stehling F, Dohna-Schwake C *et al.* Respiratory failure in Pompe disease: treatment with noninvasive ventilation. *Neurology* 2005; **64**: 1465–7.
58. Trebbia G, Lacombe M, Fermanian C *et al.* Cough determinants in patients with neuromuscular disease. *Respir Physiol Neurobiol* 2005; **146**: 291–300.
59. Sarnat HB. Myotubular myopathy: arrest of morphogenesis of myofibres associated with persistence of fetal vimentin and desmin. Four cases compared with fetal and neonatal muscle. *Can J Neurol Sci* 1990; **17**: 109–23.

60. Martinez BA, LakeBD. Childhood nemaline myopathy: a review of clinical presentation in relation to prognosis. *Dev Med Child Neurol* 1987; **29**: 815–20.
61. Sarnat HB. New insights into the pathogenesis of congenital myopathies. *J Child Neurol* 1994; **9**: 193–201.
62. Sanoudou D, Beggs AH. Clinical and genetic heterogeneity in nemaline myopathy – a disease of skeletal muscle thin filaments. *Trends Mol Med* 2001; **7**: 362–8.
63. Banwell BL, Singh NC, Ramsay DA. Prolonged survival in neonatal nemaline rod myopathy. *Pediatr Neurol* 1994; **10**: 335–7.
64. Riley DJ, Santiago TV, Daniele RP *et al.* Blunted respiratory drive in congenital myopathy. *Am J Med* 1977; **63**: 459–66.
65. Sasaki M, Yoneyama H, Nonaka I. Respiratory muscle involvement in nemaline myopathy. *Pediatr Neurol* 1990; **6**: 425–7.
66. Kudou M, Kobayashi Y, Yamashita K *et al.* Two cases of nemaline myopathy diagnosed after episodes of respiratory failure. *Nihon Kokyuki Gassai Zasshi* 2006; **44**: 474–8.
67. Oldfors A, Kyllerman M, Wahlstrom J *et al.* X-linked myotubular myopathy: clinical and pathological findings in a family. *Clin Genet* 1989; **36**: 5–14.
68. Braga SE, Gerber A, Meier C *et al.* Severe neonatal asphyxia due to X-linked centronuclear myopathy. *Eur J Pediatr* 1990; **150**: 132–5.
69. Jeannet PY, Bassez G, Eymard B *et al.* Clinical and histologic findings in autosomal centronuclear myopathy. *Neurology* 2004; **62**: 1484–90.
70. Blondeau F, Laporte J, Bodin S et al. Myotubularin, a phosphatase deficient in myotubular myopathy, acts on phosphatidylinositol 3-kinase and phosphatidylinositol 3-phosphate pathway. *Hum Mol Genet* 2000; **9**: 2223–9.
71. Wallgren-Pettersson C, Clarke A, Samson F *et al.* The myotubular myopathies: differential diagnosis of the X-linked recessive, autosomal dominant and autosomal recessive forms and present state of DNA studies. *J Med Genet* 1995; **32**: 673–9.
72. Herman GE, Finegold M, Zhao W *et al.* Medical complications in long-term survivors with X-linked myotubular myopathy. *J Pediatr* 1999; **134**: 206–14.
73. Verhiest W, Brucher JM, Goddeeris P *et al.* Familial centronuclear myopathy associated with 'cardiomyopathy'. *Br Heart J* 1976; **38**: 504–9.
74. Bitoun M, Bevilacqua JA, Prudhon B *et al.* Dynamin 2 mutations cause sporadic centronuclear myopathy with neonatal onset. *Ann Neurol* 2007; **62**: 666–70.
75. Gardner-Medwin D. Neuromuscular disorders in infancy and childhood. In: Walton J, Karpati G, Hilton-Jones D. *Disorders of voluntary muscle*. Edinburgh: Churchill Livingstone, 1994.
76. Penegyres PK, Kakulas BA. The natural history of minicore-multicore myopathy. *Muscle Nerve* 1991; **14**: 411–15.
77. Shuaib A, Martin JM, Mitchell LB *et al.* Multicore myopathy: not always a benign entity. *Can J Neurol Sci* 1988; **15**: 10–14.
78. Magliocco AM, Mitchell LB, Brownell AK *et al.* Dilated cardiomyopathy in multicore myopathy. *Am J Cardiol* 1989; **63**: 150–1.
79. Rimmer KP, Whitelaw WA. The respiratory muscles in multicore myopathy. *Am Rev Respir Dis* 1993; **148**: 227–31.
80. Rowe PW, Eagle M, Pollitt C *et al.* Multicore myopathy: respiratory failure and paraspinal muscle contractures are important complications. *Dev Med Child Neurol* 2000; **42**: 340–3.
81. Kotterba S, Patzold T, Malin JP *et al.* Respiratory monitoring in neuromuscular disease – capnography as an additional tool? *Clin Neurol Neurosurg* 2001; **103**: 87–91.
82. Sasaki M *et al.* Respiratory failure in nemaline myopathy. *Pediatr Neurol* 1997; **16**: 344–6.
83. Bielen P, Sliwiński P, Kamiński D *et al.* Respiratory failure during the course of congenital myopathy effectively treated with nocturnal noninvasive nasal positive pressure ventilation. *Pneumonol Alergol Pol* 2000; **68**: 151–5.
84. Shahrizaila N, Lim WS, Robson DK *et al.* Tubular aggregate myopathy presenting with acute type II respiratory failure and severe orthopnoea. *Thorax* 2006; **61**: 89–90.
85. Barohn RJ, Clanton T, Sahenk J *et al.* Recurrent respiratory insufficiency and depressed ventilatory drive complicating mitochondrial myopathies. *Neurology* 1990; **40**: 103–6.
86. Kim GW, Kim SM, Sunwoo IN *et al.* Two cases of mitochondrial myopathy with predominant respiratory dysfunction. *Yonsei Med J* 1991; **32**: 184–9.
87. Carroll JE, Zwillich C, Weil JV *et al.* Depressed ventilatory response in oculocraniosomatic neuromuscular disease. *Neurology* 1976; **26**: 140–6.
88. Tatsumi C, Takahashi M, Yorifuji S *et al.* Mitochondrial encephalomyopathy, ataxia, and sleep apnea. *Neurology* 1987; **37**: 1429–30.
89. Dandurand RJ, Matthews PM, Arnold DL *et al.* Mitochondrial disease. Pulmonary function, exercise performance, and blood lactate levels. *Chest* 1995; **108**: 182–9.
90. Bye PT, Ellis ER, Issa FG *et al.* Respiratory failure and sleep in neuromuscular disease. *Thorax* 1990; **45**: 241–7.

35

# Amyotrophic lateral sclerosis

STEPHEN C BOURKE, G JOHN GIBSON

## ABSTRACT

Non-invasive ventilation (NIV) has been less widely used in amyotrophic lateral sclerosis (ALS) than in more slowly progressive neuromuscular disease but recent data have confirmed that it improves quality of life and, at least in those without severe bulbar impairment, increases survival. Due to the relatively rapid decline of respiratory muscle function, regular monitoring of vital capacity and respiratory muscle pressures is advised; NIV should be considered in patients with maximum inspiratory pressures <40 per cent of predicted or with milder weakness if severe orthopnoea is present, even in the absence of hypercapnia. In ALS, careful attention to detail is vital for successful treatment with NIV, particularly in relation to adequacy of the interface, control of saliva and assistance with coughing. Further research is required to define the criteria and optimal time for starting NIV and to clarify more precise indications for using NIV in patients with more severe bulbar impairment.

## INTRODUCTION

Amyotrophic lateral sclerosis (ALS) is a progressive neurological disease of unknown cause characterized by degeneration of upper and lower motor neurones. The broader term 'motor neurone disease' (MND) is sometimes used to include conditions limited to either the spinal motor neurones (spinal muscular atrophy) or the upper motor neurones (primary lateral sclerosis) but both variants usually progress to involve upper and lower motor neurones. In effect, the terms ALS and MND are synonymous. In most patients the condition is relentlessly progressive, with median survival from symptom onset of about 3 years and death usually due to respiratory failure secondary to respiratory muscle weakness. Until recently, NIV has been used less frequently in ALS than in patients with more slowly progressive muscle weakness, because of uncertainty about its benefits in this population and concerns over possibly prolonging suffering. Recent evidence, however, has confirmed that, for many patients with ALS, NIV improves both survival and quality of life (QoL).

## EPIDEMIOLOGY

ALS is mainly a disease of late middle age, with median onset around 60 years, a slight male predominance[1,2] and an incidence of ~2.5/100 000.[3,4]

## PATHOPHYSIOLOGY

ALS results in varying combinations of weakness of limb, axial, facial, bulbar and respiratory muscles. Weakness of bulbar muscles impairs phonation, swallowing, and protection of the airway. An effective cough requires adequate force and coordination of inspiratory, expiratory and laryngeal muscles and weakness of any of these impairs clearing of respiratory secretions. In most individuals the severity of diaphragmatic weakness parallels weakness of the other respiratory muscles.[5] Respiratory muscle weakness reduces vital capacity and may increase residual volume, while total lung capacity can remain within the normal range despite fairly severe weakness.[5] The reduction of vital capacity is due to loss of inspiratory and expiratory force and a reduction in pulmonary compliance.[6] A fall in vital capacity in the supine posture is an index of the severity of diaphragmatic weakness.[7]

Respiratory muscle function is assessed more directly by measurements of maximal pressures – either maximum static pressure measured at the mouth (MIP, MEP) or during a forceful sniff (sniff nasal inspiratory pressure – SNIP). With respiratory muscle weakness, pressure measurements are more sensitive in the earlier stages of disease and vital capacity falls significantly only with moderate or severe weakness.[8] Consequently, even if progression of disease were linear with time, a non-linear relation of VC to duration of illness would be predicted with accelerating decline in the later stages, a pattern confirmed by measurements over extended periods.[9] Respiratory and/or bulbar muscle weakness reduces peak flow during coughing (cough peak flow) and 'cough spikes' may be absent on the maximum flow volume curve if the subject is asked to cough forcefully during expiration.[10]

The ventilatory response to $CO_2$ is reduced in proportion to the severity of respiratory muscle weakness.[5] Elevation of $PaCO_2$ in ALS usually implies severe weakness and a poor prognosis. Hypercapnia is related in non-linear fashion to the severity of weakness, with vital capacity and maximum inspiratory pressures severely impaired before chronic hypercapnia supervenes (Fig. 35.1).[11] No such relationship holds in patients with severe bulbar weakness, probably because assessment of respiratory muscle strength by volitional tests is then reliable.[11]

## Abnormalities during sleep

Sleep-disordered breathing and disruption of sleep architecture are both common in ALS.[12,13] Sleep disruption can result from sleep-disordered breathing and orthopnoea, as well as muscle cramps and difficulty dealing with respiratory secretions.

The reported prevalence of sleep-disordered breathing in ALS has varied from 17 per cent to 76 per cent and clearly depends on patient selection. Individuals with more severe weakness are particularly vulnerable during rapid eye movement (REM) sleep, when, normally, ventilation is almost entirely dependent on the diaphragm. Possibly as an adaptation to this vulnerability, individuals with severe diaphragmatic weakness may show reduced or even absent REM sleep.[14]

The common pattern of sleep-disordered breathing is REM sleep-related hypopnoea and oxygen desaturation, together, in patients with more severe weakness, with overall hypoventilation. Otherwise, discrete breathing events are relatively infrequent and consequently the apnoea/hypopnoea index (AHI) is an insensitive index of the severity of sleep-disordered breathing in ALS.[12,14] Obstructive apnoeas have been reported only occasionally and bulbar weakness appears to have little effect on the severity or type of sleep-disordered breathing.[12,13]

## Relation of daytime and nocturnal function

Sleep-disordered breathing is sometimes detectable in the relatively early stages of ALS but, overall, measurements asleep and awake correlate with each other: nocturnal oxygenation declines with vital capacity and maximum inspiratory pressures, though not necessarily in linear fashion.[12,15] Nocturnal transcutaneous $PCO_2$ is elevated before daytime $PaCO_2$ is raised.[11] Inevitably, once daytime hypercapnia and hypoxaemia supervene, nocturnal oxygenation deteriorates further.

# CLINICAL FEATURES

## Patterns of presentation

The clinical picture of ALS varies depending on the muscle groups most affected. Patterns at presentation include predominant involvement of limb, trunk, bulbar or respiratory muscles, but most patients later develop weakness of other muscle groups. Less than 20 per cent are aware of respiratory symptoms at presentation, although respiratory muscle weakness is demonstrable in most if appropriate measurements are made.[16] Patients with severe early respiratory muscle involvement occasionally present with breathlessness[17] and sometimes in respiratory failure. With long-term ventilatory support,[18,19] the prognosis with this presentation may not be as gloomy as previously reported.[20]

## Symptoms and signs

The main symptoms reflect the predominant group of muscles involved at the time of assessment, most commonly limb weakness with variably present bulbar symptoms, in

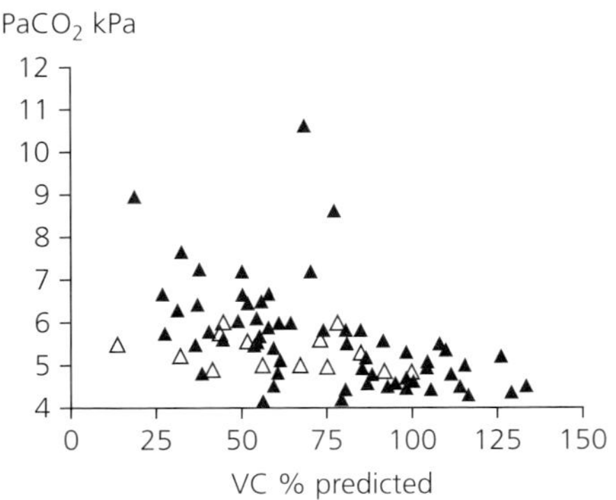


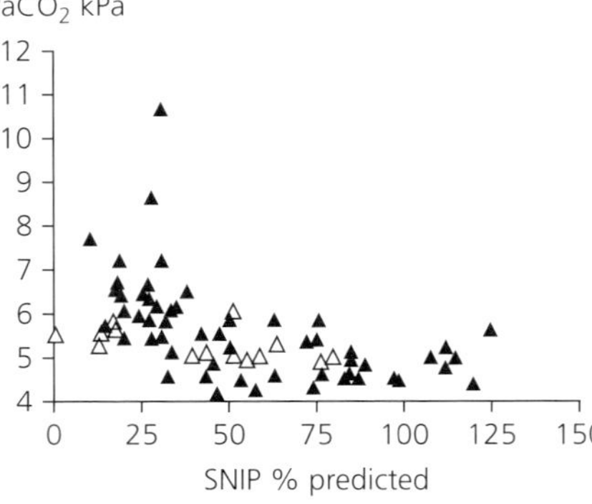


**Figure 35.1** Relations of arterial $PCO_2$ to (left) vital capacity (VC) and (right) sniff nasal inspiratory pressure (SNIP), both expressed as percentage of predicted values. Open symbols represent patients with predominant bulbar features; horizontal lines indicate normal range of $PCO_2$. Modified with permission from Lyall *et al.*[11]

particular dysphagia and dysarthria. Respiratory symptoms include shortness of breath, sometimes with pronounced orthopnoea. Breathlessness on exertion is, however, often a late feature as many patients are too incapacitated to exercise significantly. Bulbar features can be graded using the ALS functional rating scale (ALS-FRS),[21] or a simple six-point bulbar score.[22]

Sleep-related symptoms are often unrecognized unless specifically sought; these include insomnia, restless and unrefreshing sleep, excessive daytime sleepiness, lethargy, fatigue and sometimes headaches.[12,13] Physical examination typically shows widespread weakness, muscle fasciculation and increased reflexes. One important physical sign is an audibly weak voluntary cough; other signs may include use of accessory respiratory muscles during quiet breathing and paradoxical movement of the abdominal wall.[7]

About 5 per cent of patients develop frontotemporal dementia; this is associated with bulbar onset, older age, poor compliance with NIV and percutaneous endoscopic gastrostomy (PEG) feeding and shorter survival.[23] Milder degrees of cognitive dysfunction are more common. Chronic respiratory failure and sleep deprivation may also contribute to cognitive impairment.

## Respiratory and sleep investigations

The most appropriate respiratory function tests for routine clinical use are vital capacity and maximum inspiratory pressure (MIP and SNIP). Vital capacity should be measured both upright and supine. Maximum pressures are often impaired early, even when vital capacity is still within the normal range.[24] Overall, SNIP is the best predictor of daytime $PaCO_2$, but with severe respiratory muscle weakness $P_{Imax}$ may be more reliable.[25] Many patients find reproducible performance of the forceful sniff manoeuvre easier than maximum static pressure, but in others the reverse is the case; therefore, ideally, both should be attempted and the numerically larger used as the 'true' measurement. More invasive measurements such as transdiaphragmatic pressure are impracticable for routine clinical use. The reliability of all volitional measurements is suspect in patients with severe bulbar impairment.

Routine monitoring of daytime oxygen saturation is also recommended, and if $SaO_2$ is $<95$ per cent, arterial blood gases may be indicated. Instruments for measuring transcutaneous (and hence arterial) $PCO_2$ are becoming more reliable and more widely available, such that regular monitoring of $PCO_2$ is likely to become routine clinical practice in the future.

A sleep study (full or limited polysomnography) is appropriate for patients with sleep-related symptoms. Periodic monitoring of overnight saturation by oximetry is recommended by some and may be of value in patients with severe bulbar impairment, but, in those with good bulbar function, it is doubtful whether this adds usefully to simpler daytime monitoring either in terms of predicting prognosis or in determining the optimal time for treatment with NIV (see below).

## Prognosis

In one recent series the median delay from initial symptom to diagnosis was 10 months,[1] with a median survival from diagnosis of only 1.4 years. However, in this series 20 per cent survived more than 5 years and 8 per cent more than 10 years from diagnosis. Calculated from the onset of initial weakness, median survival was 2.5 years, with 5- and 10-year survival of 25 and 15 per cent, respectively.

The rate of decline of respiratory function is variable.[16] Although the initial rate of decline of vital capacity is nonlinear,[9] once weakness is sufficiently severe to cause respiratory symptoms the decline is approximately rectilinear. The average rate of decline in three series ranged from 2.4 to 4.1 per cent of predicted vital capacity per month.[16,24,26] Some authors have estimated the average rate of decline of vital capacity from first symptoms by extrapolation, using a single measurement and assuming that the premorbid value was 100 per cent predicted.[26,27]

Respiratory features are very well established predictors of survival in ALS: respiratory onset of symptoms, vital capacity, actual and estimated decline in vital capacity, maximum pressures and nocturnal hypoxaemia all convey prognostic information.[1,15,27–29] Hypercapnia is generally regarded as an ominous prognostic feature and raised serum bicarbonate and low chloride concentrations (which accompany respiratory acidosis) predict shorter survival. Other adverse predictive variables include poor nutritional status, older age, bulbar onset of disease and the time interval between initial symptoms and diagnosis (the longer the period, the slower the progression).[1,2,29]

# USE OF NON-INVASIVE VENTILATION IN AMYOTROPHIC LATERAL SCLEROSIS

## Current guidelines and practice

Most patients with ALS die in respiratory failure, but only a minority receive ventilatory support.[4,30–33] The American Academy of Neurology ALS Practice Parameter guidelines (1999) recommended 3-monthly assessment, including spirometry, with counselling about NIV when either respiratory symptoms or (forced) vital capacity $<50$ per cent are present.[34] A consensus report on the indications for NIV recommended initiating NIV in progressive neuromuscular conditions if symptoms (fatigue, dyspnoea, morning headache, etc.) were present plus at least one of the following: $PaCO_2 \geq 45$ mm Hg (6.0 kPa); nocturnal oxygen saturation $<88$ per cent for 5 consecutive minutes; maximal inspiratory pressures $<60$ cm $H_2O$; forced vital capacity (FVC) $<50$ per cent of predicted.[35]

These guidelines lack a strong evidence base, are poorly followed and are in need of updating. Surveys of clinical practice in the past 10 years have shown that many neurologists do not routinely monitor spirometry in patients with ALS,[4,31] and even fewer measure respiratory pressures (MIP, MEP, SNIP).[33] Once orthopnoea or symptomatic hypercapnia develops, some patients survive for only a few weeks or months, leaving a narrow 'window of opportunity' to initiate ventilatory support.[22,36] Regular monitoring of respiratory muscle function is therefore essential.

## Non-invasive ventilation and survival

In non-randomized studies of NIV initiated for symptoms or declining respiratory function, intolerance was associated with shorter survival from the onset of respiratory insufficiency.[37–39] The results of these studies are, however, inconclusive, as factors that influence tolerance of NIV, particularly bulbar function, may also independently affect survival, while non-compliance with NIV might also imply non-compliance with other aspects of care. A recent prospective randomized controlled trial has confirmed that NIV improves survival in subjects with normal, or at most moderately impaired, bulbar function.[22] The trial was inclusive; no patients were excluded on the basis of bulbar function, level of disability, social support or views on life-prolonging therapy (Fig. 35.2). Initially, 92 patients were enrolled and assessed every 2 months. Those who developed orthopnoea with $P_{Imax}$ <60 per cent predicted (of whom 20 were normocapnic) or symptomatic hypercapnia within the timeframe of the study were randomized to receive NIV ($n = 22$) or standard care ($n = 19$). In patients with normal or only moderately impaired bulbar function, NIV increased median survival by 205 days ($p < 0.006$), with improvements in, and maintenance of, QoL for most of this period. Although patients with severe bulbar impairment showed no survival benefit, some QoL indices improved.[22]

## Non-invasive ventilation versus tracheostomy ventilation

Long-term ventilatory support via tracheostomy is now rarely used in ALS,[4,30,33] with the notable exception of Japan.[40] This may reflect concern that it may commit the patient to institutional care and lead to ventilator entrapment, potentially with the patient totally unable to communicate. Compared to NIV, patients receiving tracheostomy ventilation survive longer, particularly if bulbar function is poor,[41] but they are less likely to be cared for at home[42] and overall report poorer QoL.[43] Although patients on tracheostomy ventilation cared for at home report similar QoL to those on NIV,[43] this is at the cost of greater caregiver burden,[41,44] while NIV is not accompanied by increased caregiver burden.[39] Other advantages of NIV are that speech and swallowing are better preserved, natural airway defences are not compromised, ventilator entrapment is less of an issue, and there probably are psychological benefits, such as a feeling of better control. Patients who have experienced both NIV and tracheostomy ventilation usually prefer the former.[45] Consequently, tracheostomy ventilation should generally be considered only for patients with severe bulbar impairment or those who are intolerant of, or failing on, NIV.

## Quality of life and cognitive function

In a progressive and debilitating condition such as ALS, it is important that interventions that improve survival do not prolong suffering, but rather extend life with symptom control and quality of life that are acceptable to the patient. Several prospective cohort studies[46–48] and non-randomized controlled trials[39,49,50] have shown sustained improvements in QoL with NIV, but none included a contemporaneous and equivalent control group. The largest improvements were seen in domains assessing sleep-related problems and mental health. Of importance, normocapnic subjects with orthopnoea showed similar improvements to those with hypercapnia or nocturnal

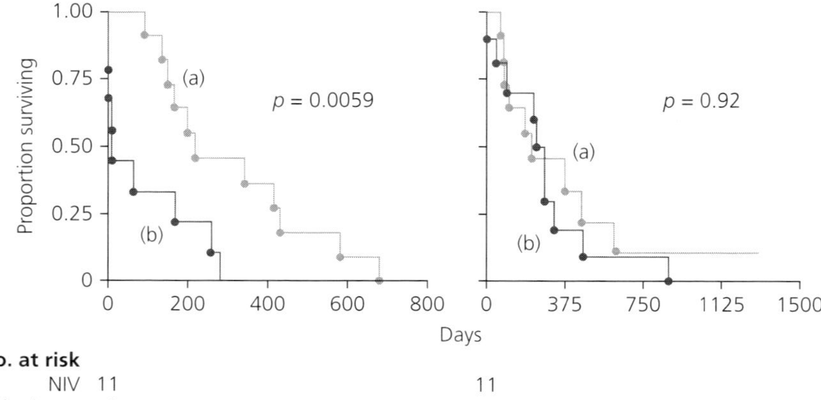


**Figure 35.2** Survival from randomization in randomized controlled trial of non-invasive ventilation (NIV) (a) versus standard care (b). Patients with normal or only moderately impaired bulbar function (left) had significantly longer survival, while those with severe bulbar impairment (right) did not. Modified with permission from Bourke *et al.*[22]

oxygen desaturation and reliance on the latter as essential criteria for initiating NIV may deprive many patients of benefit.[48] The QoL benefits associated with NIV in these studies were confirmed in a randomized controlled trial.[22] Compared to controls, subjects with normal or only moderately impaired bulbar function showed sustained benefit in all domains of the Medical Outcome Survey Short Form 36 (SF-36) (except physical function), Chronic Respiratory Questionnaire (CRQ) and the Sleep Apnea Quality of Life Index (SAQLI). Even in subjects with severe bulbar impairment the CRQ dyspnoea domain and some domains of the SAQLI improved. Following initiation of NIV, improvements in some aspects of cognitive function have been reported,[51] although in a subsequent study only a favourable trend was seen.[39]

Comparison of the strain, anxiety, depression and QoL of caregivers of ALS patients receiving NIV and a control group of caregivers of patients with similar disability but without respiratory muscle weakness showed no differences in caregiver stain, although the SF-36 energy vitality domain was lower at 12 months in the NIV caregivers' group. These results compare favourably with the greater burden experienced by caregivers of patients receiving tracheostomy ventilation.[41,44]

### Respiratory function

Studies comparing subjects who use NIV and those who refuse NIV or are intolerant of it have shown a slower decline of vital capacity in the former.[38,48] In hypercapnic patients receiving nocturnal NIV, pulmonary gas exchange improves during both the period of assisted ventilation and spontaneous breathing. The sustained reduction in $PaCO_2$ probably results mainly from 'unloading' $CO_2$ during the period of assisted ventilation, thus reversing the associated chronic respiratory acidosis and increasing the ventilatory stimulus during daytime spontaneous ventilation.[52] A small increase in lung compliance, possibly due to reversal of atelectasis, has been reported after a session of treatment with NIV,[6] but it is unclear whether this is sustained.

## CLINICAL APPLICATION OF NON-INVASIVE VENTILATION IN AMYOTROPHIC LATERAL SCLEROSIS

### Indications and timing

Non-invasive ventilation should be considered in all patients with ALS and respiratory insufficiency. In the individual case, the decision to initiate treatment should take account of the patient's views on potentially life-prolonging therapy, where he or she wishes to be cared for, the level of caregiver and social support and factors likely to influence adherence to, and benefit from, NIV (including age, nutritional status and upper limb, bulbar and cognitive function).

The optimum time to start treatment is unclear. Most studies have included several criteria for initiation of NIV and few have compared different criteria. One small prospective study compared five different criteria: orthopnoea, sleep-related symptoms, AHI >10, nocturnal oxygen desaturation and daytime hypercapnia. Orthopnoea (even in normocapnic subjects) was associated with a large improvement in QoL and good adherence to NIV. Nocturnal desaturation and daytime hypercapnia were also associated with good results, but reliance on these alone would have excluded several patients with orthopnoea who benefited. Sleep-related symptoms were sensitive, but less specific, predictors of benefit and AHI >10 was unhelpful.[48] The rate of disease progression varies greatly in ALS and survival following the development of orthopnoea or daytime hypercapnia may be short, possibly only a few weeks. This highlights the importance of close monitoring of respiratory muscle function and lends support to earlier initiation of NIV, particularly in patients with rapidly progressive disease. Regular formal assessment of respiratory symptoms and function reduces the likelihood of emergency intubation, increases the proportion of patients treated with NIV and, in patients with preserved bulbar function, improves survival.[53] Measurement of MIP[12] and SNIP[15] should be included in routine monitoring.

On current evidence, the authors recommend routine assessment of relevant symptoms (orthopnoea, breathlessness on mild exertion, restless and unrefreshing sleep, vivid dreams, morning headaches, excessive daytime sleepiness, fatigue and poor appetite) and respiratory muscle function (*good bulbar function*: $SaO_2$, MIP, MEP, SNIP, VC sitting and supine ± peak cough flow; *poor bulbar function*: $SaO_2$ and, if normal but symptomatic, nocturnal oximetry ± $PCO_2$) every 2–3 months. Patients with orthopnoea plus evidence of respiratory muscle weakness can be offered NIV without further investigation. Those with symptoms suggesting hypercapnia or nocturnal hypoventilation should have arterial/capillary blood gases measured and, if these are normal, further investigation should include overnight monitoring (e.g. respiratory polysomnography or nocturnal oximetry, combined with transcutaneous $PCO_2$ if available). Those with evidence of daytime or nocturnal respiratory failure should be offered NIV. NIV is intrusive and adherence to treatment may be poor and later treatment may be compromised if NIV is introduced too early. However, earlier introduction of NIV should be considered in patients showing a rapid decline in respiratory muscle strength based on measurements of SNIP and MIP. In one study the best predictor of daytime hypercapnia was SNIP <32 per cent predicted.[11] To allow time to initiate NIV, we suggest considering NIV once the better of SNIP and MIP <40 per cent predicted, with at least mild respiratory symptoms.

Suggested criteria for introducing non-invasive ventilation are (any one of):

- orthopnoea with evidence of respiratory muscle weakness (SNIP/MIP <60 per cent predicted, fall in vital capacity supine >20 per cent or sitting vital capacity <80 per cent)
- daytime hypercapnia

- nocturnal desaturation ($SaO_2$ <90 per cent for >5 per cent sleep or 5 consecutive minutes)
- nocturnal hypercapnia (transcutaneous $PCO_2$ >6.5 kPa)
- better of SNIP and MIP <40 per cent predicted (particularly if disease progression is rapid).

The role of NIV in patients with early (pre-symptomatic) respiratory muscle weakness is unclear. As NIV appears to reduce the rate of decline of vital capacity,[38] it is plausible that earlier introduction might improve survival. A retrospective cohort study concluded that survival from diagnosis was better in patients starting treatment with NIV early (FVC ≥65 per cent) compared with those in whom it was initiated once respiratory function was more severely compromised (FVC <65 per cent).[54] However, MIP was better preserved in the early intervention arm, despite the interval between diagnosis and initiation of NIV being similar in both groups, suggesting that the rate of progression of respiratory muscle weakness was slower in the early NIV group and possibly explaining the apparent survival advantage. No randomized controlled trial of early (pre-symptomatic) and standard NIV has been reported in ALS, but a trial of this type in Duchenne muscular dystrophy, surprisingly, showed higher mortality with earlier intervention[55] (see Chapter 36) and therefore definitive guidance on this point is not yet possible.

### Effect of bulbar function

Moderate or severe bulbar impairment is associated with poor adherence to NIV,[22,37,48,56] however there is some evidence that patients with bulbar impairment survive longer if they can tolerate NIV.[37] Some authors have suggested early use of NIV in patients with bulbar disease, to improve adherence. However, one cohort study showed that in the bulbar subgroup NIV tolerance was associated with better survival only in hypercapnic subjects.[53]

Some cohort studies have reported good outcomes with bulbar *onset* disease treated with NIV,[38,57] but bulbar function at *initiation of NIV* is more relevant. Further confounding factors in cohort studies are that patients with bulbar impairment perform volitional respiratory function tests poorly[11] and the sensation of choking on lying flat may be confused with orthopnoea due to respiratory muscle weakness. Consequently, in such patients, NIV may be initiated at a time when their true respiratory muscle strength is better than assumed, which may explain the apparent survival advantage. This conclusion is supported by the results of our randomized controlled trial of NIV in ALS: compared with subjects with better bulbar function, those with severe bulbar impairment had apparently similar vital capacity, MIP and SNIP, but lower $PaCO_2$ (5.8 kPa vs 6.6 kPa, $p = 0.019$) at randomization and, in the control arm, survived longer.[22]

### Outcome of acute presentation in respiratory failure

Acute or acute on chronic respiratory failure may be triggered by mucus plugging, upper[58] or lower respiratory tract infections, pneumonia, uncontrolled oxygen therapy[59] or sedative drugs. Virtually all survivors require long-term ventilatory support.[18,19] In patients without severe bulbar impairment, NIV offers significant advantages over invasive ventilation even in the acute setting, including lower mortality, fewer treatment failures, shorter ICU stay and fewer complications.[19,60] Mechanical cough assistance may help clearance of secretions and avoid the need for mini-tracheostomy.[61] Mucolytics, such as *N*-acetylcysteine 1–2 g nebulized 4 hourly, are often a helpful adjunct.

Patients with ALS may present with acute respiratory failure before the diagnosis is clear,[18] but in those with an established diagnosis this should usually be avoidable by regular monitoring. Issues, such as ventilatory support and alternative palliative therapies, should be openly discussed with patients at an early stage. Advance directives should be drawn up and respected and effective palliative therapy offered instead of ventilation when appropriate. Communication is better preserved with NIV than with invasive ventilation, which is of particular importance in the acute setting when patients present *in extremis* and their views on long-term ventilation are unclear. If such patients are invasively ventilated initially (often reflecting the inexperience of the receiving team or in order to facilitate transfer between units) they can usually be extubated and weaned onto NIV subsequently.

## TECHNICAL ASPECTS OF NON-INVASIVE VENTILATION IN AMYOTROPHIC LATERAL SCLEROSIS

The general technical aspects of NIV are covered in Part I of this volume. Certain aspects more specific to ALS warrant particular mention.

### Interface

A suitable and comfortable interface is essential and a wide selection of interfaces from various manufacturers should be available. Custom-made masks may be considered for individual patients if it is difficult to obtain a good seal with standard interfaces. Mouth leak is particularly common with bulbo-facial weakness. In our experience, most prefer an oronasal interface to a nasal mask and chin strap. When using an oronasal mask, it is important to ensure that the patient can remove it in an emergency or, at the very least, raise an alarm quickly. This may entail customizing headgear (e.g. rip cord) and fitting an alarm system which the patient can easily activate. Those needing intermittent ventilatory support during the daytime may prefer to use a mouthpiece; a lip-seal can be added to reduce problems with mouth leak.

### Saliva

Bulbar impairment causes difficulty swallowing, with consequent pooling of saliva, choking episodes and drooling. Education on safe swallowing techniques, frequent swallowing, attention to posture to prevent saliva pooling in the throat and use of suction are helpful. Pooling of watery saliva, combined with impaired airway protection, is particularly problematic when the patient requires NIV as saliva is easily blown into the trachea. This may trigger coughing bouts, contribute to lower respiratory tract infections and reduce tolerance of NIV. Measures to reduce the volume and increase the viscosity of the saliva include drugs (amitriptyline, hyoscine, glycopyrronium, atropine), injection of botulinum toxin into the salivary glands[62] and irradiation of the salivary glands.[63]

In some patients, thick viscous saliva results from dehydration, mouth breathing or over-treatment of excessive thin saliva. Ensuring adequate fluid intake, avoiding dairy products and drinking fruit juice may help. Mucolytics, such as carbocysteine, and artificial saliva should be considered if the problem persists. If the patient is using NIV, an oronasal mask to prevent mouth-leak and the addition of a heated humidifier should be considered. Whether the initial problem is pooling of watery saliva or thick viscous secretions, achieving the optimum balance between volume and viscosity can be difficult.

### Cough

Methods to improve the effectiveness of cough include huffing, active cycle of breathing, breath stacking and thoraco-abdominal thrusts. An Ambu bag or volume cycled ventilator can be used to facilitate breath stacking and the technique may be combined with thoraco-abdominal thrusts. Mechanically assisted cough, using an insufflator-exsufflator, can generate a clinically effective cough in most patients with respiratory muscle weakness, at least when stable,[64–66] and is more effective than physiotherapist-assisted cough and well tolerated.[66] The technique is less effective with severe bulbar impairment, probably due to upper airway collapse during exsufflation.[64] With severe bulbar impairment, a Guedel airway may be used to support the upper airway during mechanically assisted coughing. Cohort studies have suggested that in stable patients with ALS, NIV plus mechanically assisted coughing is associated with prolonged survival[67] and, during acute decompensation, can avoid intubation with low in-hospital mortality, provided bulbar function is not severely impaired.[19]

### Gastrostomy tube placement

In ALS, difficulty swallowing, breathlessness during eating, difficulty feeding and loss of independence may all contribute to nutritional depletion. Placement of a gastrostomy tube should be considered if, despite conservative measures, the patient is failing to maintain adequate intake, has great difficulty swallowing such that eating is tiring, or has an unsafe swallow. In cohort studies, patients fed via gastrostomy survive longer than those who decline[68] or are fed via a nasogastric tube.

The traditional approach of PEG tube placement under conscious sedation is associated a high complication rate in patients with vital capacity <50 per cent.[68,69] Early placement of a PEG tube should be considered in patients with rapidly declining respiratory function, again emphasizing the importance of regular monitoring. In patients with serious respiratory compromise (vital capacity <50 per cent, MIP/SNIP <40 per cent predicted, daytime or nocturnal hypercapnia), radiologically guided insertion of a gastrostomy (RIG) tube may be safer than PEG as sedation is not required, NIV is more easily provided during the procedure and the patient does not have to lie completely supine.[70–72] Although successful PEG insertion with NIV support has been described,[73] there will be a large air leak, so substantial increases in pressure support and $FiO_2$ are likely to be required. Alternatively, the patient may be briefly intubated and ventilated during PEG insertion and then extubated onto NIV. The approach in individual centres will be strongly influenced by local experience and skill. Regardless of the technique employed, the 30-day mortality is higher than the mortality during the procedure.[69,70] Diaphragmatic splinting and post-procedure pneumonia contribute to the complication rate; careful post-procedure care is essential.

## FUTURE RESEARCH

### Optimal timing of initiation of non-invasive ventilation

In ALS, NIV is often commenced following the development of orthopnoea or symptomatic hypercapnia. If such patients do not receive NIV, survival may be very short,[22,39] leaving a very narrow 'window of opportunity' to initiate treatment. Earlier intervention might be more appropriate, perhaps based on the presence of mild respiratory symptoms and evidence of respiratory muscle weakness, although published data in Duchenne muscular dystrophy suggest that this is not necessarily the case. Non-invasive ventilation is also a relatively intrusive therapy and adherence to treatment may be poor in asymptomatic subjects. The optimal criteria for initiation of NIV remain unclear and need to be addressed by large multicentre randomized controlled trials. The results of such trials should be analysed separately for subjects with normal or only moderate bulbar impairment and those with severe impairment.

## Bulbar impairment

In patients with severe bulbar impairment, different cohort studies have shown conflicting results.[37,38,48,53,56] In our RCT, NIV conveyed no survival advantage in those with severe bulbar impairment,[22] but the study was not powered to detect a survival advantage in this subgroup and some indices of QoL did improve. The role of, and indications for, NIV in patients with more severe bulbar involvement therefore remain unclear.

Volitional tests of respiratory muscle function are unreliable in patients with bulbar impairment[11] and interpretation of symptoms is also difficult as such patients may have difficulty distinguishing the sensation of choking on lying flat from orthopnoea. Others may avoid lying supine to prevent pooling of secretions at the back of the throat and thus may not be aware of orthopnoea. Consequently, compared to subjects with better bulbar function, a different approach to routine monitoring of respiratory muscle function is required and the optimal criteria for initiating NIV may be different. Options worthy of further study include nocturnal and daytime oximetry and transcutaneous $PCO_2$.

## Cough

In ALS, impaired cough is an important cause of morbidity and mortality and the ability to generate an effective assisted cough may influence survival, including in patients established on NIV. In addition to ensuring effective airway clearance, several techniques to assist coughing include an active insufflation stage (e.g. breath stacking ± use of an Ambu bag or volume cycled ventilator, mechanical cough assist), which may also help to reverse atelectasis. The effect of routine use of such techniques, especially mechanical cough assistance, on the frequency of acute decompensation due to mucus plugging or respiratory tract infections, lung function, QoL and survival warrants further study.

## REFERENCES


1. Louwerse ES, Visser CE, Bossuyt PM *et al.* Amyotrophic lateral sclerosis: mortality risk during the course of the disease and prognostic factors. The Netherlands ALS Consortium. *J Neurol Sci* 1997; **152** Suppl **1**: S10–17.
2. Tysnes OB, Vollset SE, Larsen JP *et al.* Prognostic factors and survival in amyotrophic lateral sclerosis. *Neuroepidemiology* 1994; **13**: 226–35.
3. PARALS. Incidence of ALS in Italy: evidence for a uniform frequency in Western countries. *Neurology* 2001; **56**: 239–44.
4. Bourke SC, Williams TL, Bullock RE *et al.* Non-invasive ventilation in motor neuron disease: current UK practice. *Amyotroph Lateral Scler Other Motor Neuron Disord* 2002; **3**: 145–9.
5. Serisier DE, Mastaglia FL, Gibson GJ. Respiratory muscle function and ventilatory control. I in patients with motor neurone disease. II in patients with myotonic dystrophy. *Q J Med* 1982; **51**: 205–26.
6. Lechtzin N, Shade D, Clawson L *et al.* Supramaximal inflation improves lung compliance in subjects with amyotrophic lateral sclerosis. *Chest* 2006; **129**: 1322–9.
7. Lechtzin N, Wiener CM, Shade DM *et al.* Spirometry in the supine position improves the detection of diaphragmatic weakness in patients with amyotrophic lateral sclerosis. *Chest* 2002; **121**: 436–42.
8. De Troyer A, Borenstein S, Cordier R. Analysis of lung volume restriction in patients with respiratory muscle weakness. *Thorax* 1980; **35**: 603–10.
9. Fallat RJ, Jewitt B, Bass M *et al.* Spirometry in amyotrophic lateral sclerosis. *Arch Neurol* 1979; **36**: 74–80.
10. Chaudri MB, Liu C, Hubbard R *et al.* Relationship between supramaximal flow during cough and mortality in motor neurone disease. *Eur Respir J* 2002; **19**: 434–8.
11. Lyall RA, Donaldson N, Polkey MI *et al.* Respiratory muscle strength and ventilatory failure in amyotrophic lateral sclerosis. *Brain* 2000; **124**: 2000–13.
12. Gay PC, Westbrook PR, Daube JR *et al.* Effects of alterations in pulmonary function and sleep variables on survival in patients with amyotrophic lateral sclerosis. *Mayo Clin Proc* 1991; **66**: 686–94.
13. David WS, Bundlie SR, Mahdavi Z. Polysomnographic studies in amyotrophic lateral sclerosis. *J Neurol Sci* 1997; 152 Suppl **1**: S29–35.
14. Arnulf I, Similowski T, Salachas F *et al.* Sleep disorders and diaphragmatic function in patients with amyotrophic lateral sclerosis. *Am J Respir Crit Care Med* 2000; **161**: 849–56.
15. Morgan RK, McNally S, Alexander M *et al.* Use of sniff nasal-inspiratory force to predict survival in amyotrophic lateral sclerosis. *Am J Respir Crit Care Med* 2005; **171**: 269–74.
16. Schiffman PL, Belsh JM. Pulmonary function at diagnosis of amyotrophic lateral sclerosis. Rate of deterioration. *Chest* 1993; **103**: 508–13.
17. Nightingale S, Bates D, Bateman DE *et al.* Enigmatic dyspnoea: an unusual presentation of motor neurone disease. *Lancet* 1982; **i**: 933–5.
18. Bradley MD, Orrell RW, Clarke J *et al.* Outcome of ventilatory support for acute respiratory failure in motor neurone disease. *J Neurol Neurosurg Psychiatry* 2002; **72**: 752–6.
19. Servera E, Sancho J, Zafra M *et al.* Alternatives to endotracheal intubation for patients with neuromuscular diseases. *Am J Phys Med Rehabil* 2005; **84**: 851–7.
20. Shoesmith CL, Findlater K, Rowe A *et al.* Prognosis of amyotrophic lateral sclerosis with respiratory onset. *J Neurol Neurosurg Psychiatry* 2007; **78**: 629–31.
21. Cedarbaum JM, Stambler N. Performance of the Amyotrophic Lateral Sclerosis Functional Rating Scale (ALSFRS) in multicenter clinical trials. *J Neurol Sci* 1997; 152 Suppl **1**: S1–9.

22. Bourke SC, Tomlinson M, Williams TL *et al.* Effects of non-invasive ventilation on survival and quality of life in patients with amyotrophic lateral sclerosis: a randomised controlled trial. *Lancet Neurol* 2006; **5**: 140–7.
23. Olney RK, Murphy J, Forshew D *et al.* The effects of executive and behavioral dysfunction on the course of ALS. *Neurology* 2005; **65**: 1774–7.
24. Fitting J-W, Paillex R, Hirt L *et al.* Sniff nasal pressure: A sensitive respiratory test to assess progression of amyotrophic lateral sclerosis. *Ann Neurol* 1999; **46**: 887–93.
25. Hart N, Polkey MI, Sharshar T *et al.* Limitations of sniff nasal pressure in patients with severe neuromuscular weakness. *J Neurol Neurosurg Psychiatry* 2003; **74**: 1685–7.
26. Vender R, Mauger D, Walsh S *et al.* Respiratory systems abnormalities and clinical milestones for patients with amyotrophic lateral sclerosis with emphasis upon survival. *Amyotroph Lateral Scler* 2007; **8**: 36–41.
27. Armon C, Graves MC, Moses D *et al.* Linear estimates of disease progression predict survival in patients with amyotrophic lateral sclerosis. *Muscle Nerve* 2000; **23**: 874–82.
28. Desport JC, Preux PM, Truong TC *et al.* Nutritional status is a prognostic factor for survival in ALS patients. *Neurology* 1999; **53**: 1059–63.
29. Stambler N, Charatan M, Cedarbaum JM. Prognostic indicators of survival in ALS. ALS CNTF Treatment Study Group. *Neurology* 1998; **50**: 66–72.
30. Lechtzin N, Wiener CM, Clawson L *et al.* Use of noninvasive ventilation in patients with amyotrophic lateral sclerosis. *Amyotroph Lateral Scler Other Motor Neuron Disord* 2004; **5**: 9–15.
31. Borasio GD, Shaw PJ, Hardiman O *et al.* Standards of palliative care for patients with amyotrophic lateral sclerosis: results of a European survey. *Amyotroph Lateral Scler Other Motor Neuron Disord* 2001; **2**: 159–64.
32. Bradley WG, Anderson F, Bromberg M *et al.* Current management of ALS: comparison of the ALS CARE Database and the AAN Practice Parameter. The American Academy of Neurology. *Neurology* 2001; **57**: 500–4.
33. Melo J, Homma A, Iturriaga E *et al.* Pulmonary evaluation and prevalence of non-invasive ventilation in patients with amyotrophic lateral sclerosis: a multicenter survey and proposal of a pulmonary protocol. *J Neurol Sci* 1999; **169**: 114–17.
34. Miller RG, Rosenberg JA, Gelinas DF *et al.* Practice parameter: the care of the patient with amyotrophic lateral sclerosis (an evidence-based review): report of the Quality Standards Subcommittee of the American Academy of Neurology: ALS Practice Parameters Task Force. *Neurology* 1999; **52**: 1311–23.
35. Clinical indications for noninvasive positive pressure ventilation in chronic respiratory failure due to restrictive lung disease, COPD, and nocturnal hypoventilation – a consensus conference report. *Chest* 1999; **116**: 521–34.
36. Mustfa N, Walsh E, Bryant V *et al.* The effect of noninvasive ventilation on ALS patients and their caregivers. *Neurology* 2006; **66**: 1211–17.
37. Aboussouan LS, Khan SU, Meeker DP *et al.* Effect of noninvasive positive-pressure ventilation on survival in amyotrophic lateral sclerosis. *Ann Internal Med* 1997; **127**: 450–3.
38. Kleopa KA, Sherman M, Neal B *et al.* BiPAP improves survival and rate of pulmonary function decline in patients with ALS. *J Neurol Sci* 1999; **164**: 82–8.
39. Mustfa N, Walsh E, Bryant V *et al.* The effect of noninvasive ventilation on ALS patients and their caregivers. *Neurology* 2006; **66**: 1211–17.
40. Kawata A, Mizoguchi K, Hayashi H. A nationwide survey of ALS patients on tracheostomy positive pressure ventilation (TPPV) who developed a totally locked-in state (TLS) in Japan. *Rinsho Shinkeigaku* 2008; **48**: 476–80.
41. Marchese S, Lo Coco D, Lo Coco A. Outcome and attitudes toward home tracheostomy ventilation of consecutive patients: A 10-year experience. *Respir Med* 2008; **102**: 430–6.
42. Cazzolli PA, Oppenheimer EA. Home mechanical ventilation for amyotrophic lateral sclerosis: Nasal compared to tracheostomy-intermittent positive pressure ventilation. *J Neurol Sci* 1996; **139** Suppl: 123–8.
43. Moss AH, Oppenheimer EA, Casey P *et al.* Patients with amyotrophic lateral sclerosis receiving long-term mechanical ventilation: advance care planning and outcomes. *Chest* 1996; **110**: 249–55.
44. Gelinas DF, O'Connor P, Miller RG. Quality of life for ventilator-dependent ALS patients and their caregivers. *J Neurol Sci* 1998; 160 Suppl **1**: S134–S6.
45. Bach JR. A comparison of long-term ventilatory support alternatives from the perspective of the patient and care giver. *Chest* 1993; **104**: 1702–6.
46. Hein H, Schucher B, Magnussen H. Intermittent assisted ventilation in neuromuscular diseases: course and quality of life. *Pneumologie* 1999; 53 Suppl **2**: S89–90.
47. Aboussouan LS, Khan SU, Banerjee M *et al.* Objective measures of the efficacy of noninvasive positive-pressure ventilation in amyotrophic lateral sclerosis. *Muscle Nerve* 2001; **24**: 403–9.
48. Bourke SC, Bullock RE, Williams TL *et al.* Noninvasive ventilation in ALS: indications and effect on quality of life. *Neurology* 2003; **61**: 171–7.
49. Pinto AC, Evangelista T, Carvalho M *et al.* Respiratory assistance with a non-invasive ventilator (Bipap) in MND/ALS patients: survival rates in a controlled trial. *Journal of the Neurol Sci* 1995; **129** Suppl: 19–26.
50. Lyall RA, Donaldson N, Fleming T *et al.* A prospective study of quality of life in ALS patients treated with noninvasive ventilation. *Neurology* 2001; **57**: 153–6.
51. Newsom-Davis IC, Lyall RA, Leigh PN *et al.* The effect of non-invasive positive pressure ventilation (NIPPV) on cognitive function in amyotrophic lateral sclerosis (ALS): a prospective study. *J Neurol Neurosurg Psychiatry* 2001; **71**: 482–7.

52. Annane D, Quera-Salva MA, Lofaso F *et al.* Mechanisms underlying effects of nocturnal ventilation on daytime blood gases in neuromuscular diseases. *Eur Respir J* 1999; **13**: 157–62.
53. Farrero E, Prats E, Povedano M *et al.* Survival in amyotrophic lateral sclerosis with home mechanical ventilation. *Chest* 2005; **127**: 2132–8.
54. Lechtzin N, Scott Y, Busse AM *et al.* Early use of non-invasive ventilation prolongs survival in subjects with ALS. *Amyotroph Lateral Scler* 2007; **8**: 185–8.
55. Raphael JC, Chevret S, Chastang C *et al.* Randomised trial of preventive nasal ventilation in Duchenne muscular dystrophy. French Multicentre Cooperative Group on Home Mechanical Ventilation Assistance in Duchenne de Boulogne Muscular Dystrophy. *Lancet* 1994; **343**: 1600–4.
56. Lo Coco D, Marchese S, Pesco MC *et al.* Noninvasive positive-pressure ventilation in ALS: predictors of tolerance and survival. *Neurology* 2006; **67**: 761–5.
57. Peysson S, Vandenberghe N, Philit F *et al.* Factors predicting survival following noninvasive ventilation in amyotrophic lateral sclerosis. *Eur Neurol* 2008; **59**: 164–71.
58. Poponick JM, Jacobs I, Slipinski G *et al.* Effect of upper respiratory tract infection in patients with neuromuscular disease. *Am J Respir Crit Care Med* 1997; **156**: 659–64.
59. Gay PC, Edmonds LC. Severe hypercapnia after low-flow oxygen therapy in patients with neuromuscular disease and diaphragmatic dysfunction. *Mayo Clin Proc* 1995; **70**: 327–30.
60. Vianello A, Bevilacqua M, Arcaro G *et al.* Non-invasive ventilatory approach to treatment of acute respiratory failure in neuromuscular disorders. A comparison with endotracheal intubation. *Intensive Care Med* 2000; **26**: 384–90.
61. Vianello A, Corrado A, Arcaro G *et al.* Mechanical insufflation-exsufflation improves outcomes for neuromuscular disease patients with respiratory tract infections. *Am J Phys Med Rehabil* 2005; **84**: 83–8.
62. Jackson CE, Gronseth G, Rosenfeld J *et al.* Randomized double-blind study of botulinum toxin type B for sialorrhea in ALS patients. *Muscle Nerve* 2009; **39**: 137–43.
63. Neppelberg E, Haugen DF, Thorsen L *et al.* Radiotherapy reduces sialorrhea in amyotrophic lateral sclerosis. *Eur J Neurol* 2007; **14**: 1373–7.
64. Sancho J, Servera E, Diaz J *et al.* Efficacy of mechanical insufflation-exsufflation in medically stable patients with amyotrophic lateral sclerosis. *Chest* 2004; **125**: 1400–5.
65. Mustfa NM, Aiello MM, Lyall RAM *et al.* Cough augmentation in amyotrophic lateral sclerosis. *Neurology* 2003; **61**: 1285–7.
66. Chatwin M, Ross E, Hart N *et al.* Cough augmentation with mechanical insufflation/exsufflation in patients with neuromuscular weakness. *Eur Respir J* 2003; **21**: 502–8.
67. Bach JRMDF. Amyotrophic lateral sclerosis: prolongation of life by noninvasive respiratory aids. *Chest* 2002; **122**: 92–8.
68. Mazzini L, Corra T, Zaccala M *et al.* Percutaneous endoscopic gastrostomy and enteral nutrition in amyotrophic lateral sclerosis. *J Neurol* 1995; **242**: 695–8.
69. Kasarskis EJ, Scarkata D, Hill R *et al.* A retrospective study of percutaneous endoscopic gastrostomy in ALS patients during the BDNF and CNTF trials. *J Neurol Sci* 1999; **169**: 118–25.
70. Lewis D, Ampong MA, Rio A *et al.* Mushroom-cage gastrostomy tube placement in patients with amyotrophic lateral sclerosis: a 5-year experience in 104 patients in a single institution. *Eur Radiol* 2009; **19**: 1763–71.
71. Desport JC, Mabrouk T, Bouillet P *et al.* Complications and survival following radiologically and endoscopically-guided gastrostomy in patients with amyotrophic lateral sclerosis. *Amyotroph Lateral Scler Other Motor Neuron Disord* 2005; **6**: 88–93.
72. Chio A, Galletti R, Finocchiaro C *et al.* Percutaneous radiological gastrostomy: a safe and effective method of nutritional tube placement in advanced ALS. *J Neurol Neurosurg Psychiatry* 2004; **75**: 645–7.
73. Gregory S, Siderowf A, Golaszewski AL *et al.* Gastrostomy insertion in ALS patients with low vital capacity: respiratory support and survival. *Neurology* 2002; **58**: 485–7.

# 36

# Duchenne muscular dystrophy

ANITA K SIMONDS

ABSTRACT

Duchenne muscular dystrophy (DMD) is one of the commonest inherited disorders of childhood and the outlook for young men with this condition has improved markedly over the past 20 years. Non-invasive ventilation has played a major part in changing outcomes, but new problems and challenges have arisen as the prevalence of men with DMD in their late 20s and 30s grows.

## INTRODUCTION

Duchenne muscular dystrophy (DMD) is important to the field of non-invasive ventilation for several notable reasons. Rideau,[1] one of the pioneers of non-invasive ventilation (NIV), first explored nasal delivery in this group in the mid to late 1980s, and DMD has become the paradigm for a progressive neuromuscular condition in which management of the respiratory consequences has a marked effect of survival. This is quite different from NIV use in chest wall disease or post tuberculous lung disease where the precipitating cause is static although the pathophysiological decline has become a vicious circle. Furthermore, use of NIV in DMD has been a stepping stone to its application in older patients with acquired neuromuscular disease, e.g. amyotrophic lateral sclerosis/motor neurone disease and extension into younger paediatric groups with inherited neuromuscular and neurological conditions.

## PATHOPHYSIOLOGY

Duchenne muscular dystrophy is due to deficiency of the sarcolemmal related protein, dystrophin. The dystrophin gene on the X chromosome is huge, being the largest gene described in humans so far. Its genomic sequence makes up about 1.5 per cent of the human genome. The size of the dystrophin gene makes it more liable to mutations, most of which affect the muscle isoform leading to DMD or Becker muscular dystrophy (BMD).[2] There are several other isoforms of the gene which are expressed in the brain or cardiac muscle. Dystrophin is a rod-shaped protein which at a cellular level interacts at the sarcolemma with integral membrane proteins (dystroglycans, syntrophin and dystrobrevin complexes) to form the dystrophin–glycoprotein complex. The key role of this complex is to stabilize the sarcolemma and protect muscle fibres from contraction-related damage. This may explain why, while dystrophin has been shown to be absent by the second trimester in affected foetuses, the cumulative consequences of mechanical damage do not become evident until the child is several years old. As there is no evidence of the disease or muscular weakness at birth, strictly speaking DMD is not a congenital muscular dystrophy.

Deletions in the gene occur in about 60–65 per cent of DMD and BMD patients, duplications are rarer and range from 5 per cent to 15 per cent. Although deletions can arise anywhere in the dystrophin gene the two commonest deletion 'hotspots' are in the central part of the gene and towards the end. Interestingly there is no relationship whatsoever between the size of the deletion and phenotypic impact, for example very large deletions which involve up to 50 per cent of gene may result in mild Becker variants. The phenotype depends instead on whether the deletion or duplication affects the reading frame of the dystrophin gene. As described by Muntoni *et al.*[2] mutations that maintain the reading frame (in-frame) tend to result in abnormal but partly functional dystrophin. If the deletion or duplication disrupts the reading frame (frame-shift) unstable RNA results leading to the production of virtually indetectable levels of abnormal protein. This hypothesis correctly classifies over 90 per cent of DMD and BMD cases.

The brain and retina are also affected by lack of dystrophin. Results are somewhat variable, however, and can range from very occasional severe retardation to less severe effects. The overall IQ in DMD is about 1 standard deviation below the mean and there is some evidence of preferential effect on verbal memory. However, there is no evidence that intellectual impairment is progressive or correlated with the severity or duration of the muscle disease. There are a few rare mutations that cause cardiac muscle involvement alone (X-linked cardiomyopathy). Cardiac involvement in typical DMD is discussed below.

## CLINICAL COURSE

Clinically, the consequences of DMD are first seen in early childhood: 50 per cent of DMD children do not walk until 18 months and 25 per cent are only walking by the age of 2 years.[3] Parents are often alerted by a waddling gait, tendency to fall and pseudohypertrophy of calf muscles. About 20 per cent of cases are diagnosed by the age of 2 years and 75 per cent by 4 years. On average patients required a wheelchair for mobility by the age of 10–12 years, but the introduction of steroid therapy and walking orthoses have extended the period individuals can remain ambulant. This is important as about 50 per cent of DMD cases develop a scoliosis and progression of spinal curvature is associated with increasing muscle weakness and the adolescent growth spurt. If steroid therapy reduces the decline in muscle strength there will be less overlap with growth spurt, and scoliosis (and impact on chest wall restriction) should be less marked. For example, in one non-randomized study[4] of boys matched for age and pulmonary function at baseline, a scoliosis of >20 degrees occurred in 67 per cent of a control group but only 17 per cent of the steroid (deflazocort)-treated group. These factors may feed into better peak lung function and ultimately better survival although there have been no definitive randomized controlled trials of steroid therapy.

The distribution of muscle involvement in DMD is relatively characteristic. Overall, lower limbs are affected more than upper limbs and proximal muscles more than distal groups. Preferential involvement of the sternomastoids, latissimus dorsi, glutei and quadriceps is usually seen. Inspiratory and expiratory muscles are usually similarly affected (unlike spinal muscular atrophy where early expiratory muscle weakness may be seen). Facial, buccal, sphincter and swallowing muscles are only involved late in the course of the disease. Indeed old textbooks report swallowing muscles are 'never affected' but this was the case before ventilatory support had produced long-term survival and late complications (see below). Progression in muscle weakness is not linear, and there may be periods of apparent arrest in the course of the disease. Once individuals are using wheelchairs full-time, contractures of the hips, knees and elbows can occur with a talipes equinovarus, and typical frog-leg posture.

The evolution of lung function changes in DMD falls into three stages.[5] In the first stage during the first decade or so, forced vital capacity (FVC) increases as predicted. In the second phase lung volumes plateau as inspiratory muscle weakness ± scoliosis becomes manifest. In a final phase, FVC initially falls slowly and then may decline by as much as 250 mL/year. Peak vital capacity in the absence of ventilatory support is a prognostic factor in that a peak vital capacity of less than 1.2 L was associated with average age of death at 15.3 years and those with a peak vital capacity in excess of 1.7 L survived to an average of 21 years. With ventilatory support it is now possible to support individuals with an unrecordably low VC for many years, but peak vital capacity is still likely to be a prognostic marker and indicates whether NIV is likely to be needed sooner rather than later.

Assessment with sleep studies is important as the first signs of ventilatory compromise are seen during sleep. Rapid eye movement (REM)-related hypoventilation tends to occur when vital capacity is less than 60 per cent predicted and hypoventilation progresses to non-REM sleep and ultimately daytime ventilatory failure[6] unless that pathophysiological sequence is addressed (see below). The clinical course is frequently punctuated by chest infections due to weakness of inspiratory muscles and reduced cough efficacy due to decreased expiratory muscle strength.

Cardiac involvement takes the form of conduction defects or left ventricular disease. A cardiomyopathy may involve the right ventricle, but since the advent of effective respiratory support, cor pulmonale is unheard of. There is no correlation between extent of cardiomyopathy and limb muscle weakness in young children. Nigro *et al.*[7] found preclinical evidence of cardiac disease in 25 per cent DMD under the age of 6 years and almost 60 per cent between the ages of 6 and 10 years. Clinically apparent cardiac involvement in this series was present in all patients by the age of 18 years and 72 per cent of patients were symptomatic. Although not conclusively demonstrated, NIV may alter the course of cardiomyopathy as fewer patients seem to be symptomatic in current cohorts, although this may reflect early use of angiotensin-converting enzyme (ACE) inhibitor[8] drugs and β-blockers.

## EVIDENCE BASE FOR NON-INVASIVE VENTILATION

The outlook for DMD patients without ventilatory support is very poor. With a FVC of less than 1 L, the 5-year survival is 8 per cent.[9] In the 1970s and 1980s DMD patients were treated with tracheostomy ventilation, although it is difficult to compare results with studies done today. While there has been no randomized controlled study of NIV in DMD, Vianello *et al.*[10] compared the 2-year course in hypercapnic patients who received NIV and those who did not. All NIV recipients survived, whereas 4/5 who did not receive NIV died. In a single centre cohort treated with NIV, once they had become hypercapnic during the day, 1-year and 5-year survival rates were 85 per cent and 73 per cent, respectively.[11] This compares with an earlier trial[12] in which asymptomatic patients with vital capacity between 20 per cent and 50 per cent predicted were randomized to NIV or a control group in order to see whether NIV halted the decline in lung function. The results showed no impact on lung function, moreover there were excess deaths in the NIV group. This trial has been criticized on the grounds that cardiological function was significantly worse in the NIV limb, families were given no advice about use of NIV or other techniques for secretion clearance, and families in the control group were also aware that NIV was available should respiratory problems occur so might have sought help earlier. Furthermore, patients did not undergo sleep studies, so it is unclear whether sleep-disordered breathing was present, although would be expected in at least a proportion with vital capacity in the 20–50 per cent range. Even taking into account these factors, there are no good grounds to recommend NIV as preventive therapy in asymptomatic DMD boys with no evidence of nocturnal hypoventilation.

To clarify this point, another randomized controlled trial[3] explored used of NIV at an intermediate stage, i.e. in patients with nocturnal hypoventilation but daytime normocapnia. Subjects were mixed and did not solely comprise those with DMD. However results in the control (non-NIV) group showed virtually all patients who had nocturnal hypoventilation became hypercapnic within the following 12–24 months. Nocturnal blood gas tensions and quality of life measures improved in the group randomized to NIV, but deteriorated in controls (Fig. 36.1). This provides evidence that the best time to introduce NIV is at the stage of symptomatic nocturnal hypoventilation. Eagle *et al.*[14] have shown the impact of NIV on successive cohorts of DMD patients.

## QUALITY OF LIFE

Kohler *et al.*[15] evaluated health-related quality of life in DMD patients using the Medical Outcome Survey Short Form 36 (SF-36). While physical function was reduced with age as expected, domains representing general and mental health, emotional health, social function and pain were not reduced and were near values in populations without chronic illness. Despite a greater reduction in pulmonary function and activities of daily living, individuals receiving NIV had similar health-related quality of life scores to those who did not need ventilatory support.

In addition Bach and team[16] have shown consistently that life satisfaction in DMD may be underestimated by

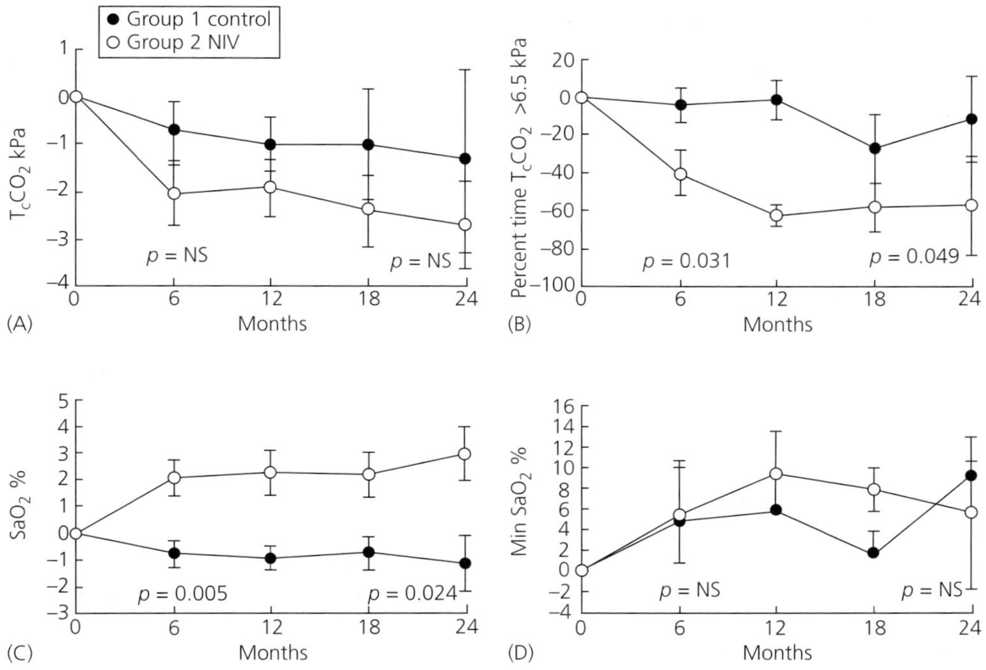


**Figure 36.1** Randomized controlled trial of non-invasive ventilation in patients with nocturnal hypoventilation but normal daytime $PCO_2$. Differences from baseline values and at 6, 13, 18 and 24 months in (A) peak nocturnal transcutaneous carbon dioxide, (B) time transcutaneous carbon dioxide >6.5 kPa, (C) mean nocturnal $SaO_2$ and (D) minimum nocturnal $SaO_2$. *p* values given at 6 and 24 months. Error bars represent standard error (SE). With permission from Eagle *et al.*[14]

health professionals. While most DMD patients rate their quality of life as good, there can be major psychosocial pressures on parents and siblings. These often exacerbated by frustrations over practical issues such as housing, transportation, seating, electric beds and availability of caregivers. It is important always to keep a focus on the family as well as the patient. Getting the ventilator settings right is but a small part of the overall care plan.

### Titration of results

Most teams titrate ventilator settings to overnight monitoring. Oximetry and transcutaneous carbon dioxide monitoring are helpful. Leaks often fragment sleep by causing arousals. More detailed polysomnography studies are only required if problems cannot be solved by simpler monitoring or symptoms persist despite apparent good overnight control of ventilation.

## TECHNICAL CONSIDERATIONS

### Ventilators

Early studies used volume ventilators in the main, but more recently pressure support ventilation has been widely used in neuromuscular groups.[17] In truth neuromuscular patients are relatively easy to ventilate, however, expiratory positive airway pressure (EPAP) in bi-level devices may be helpful in reducing tendency to upper airway collapse, recruiting functional residual capacity and dealing with atelectasis. Increasing EPAP, say, from 5 cm $H_2O$ to 7 cm $H_2O$ may be helpful in these situations especially when atelectasis complicates an acute chest infection.[18] Bi-level NIV use may also improve cardiac function by offloading the left ventricle but this effect is difficult to separate out from improvement in $PaO_2$ and $PCO_2$ that is also likely to occur. Volume ventilators have the advantage in that they can be used to help the patient breath stack but applying serial tidal volume insufflations. However, this function can also be achieved by using an Ambu bag with one-way valve or cough insufflator-exsufflator (see Chapter 35).

Patients with neuromuscular disease can be prone to gastric bloating which can be reduced by adjusting sleeping position or decreasing inspiratory peak airways pressure. Usually bi-level ventilators are less likely to provoke gastric bloating than volume ventilators.

Importantly most Duchenne patients wish to get out and about during the day. Ventilators must be suitable to fit beneath a wheelchair and have long-term battery power. Battery power is also crucial as patients become more dependent on ventilation to manage risks such as power failures/disruptions in power supplies, and practicalities such as the transfer of patients on NIV, e.g. to hospital or between hospital wards.

### Interfaces

There are a number of important considerations when choosing interfaces. Leaks can be problematical because of facial characteristics and the inability to close the mouth due to weakness or jaw contractures. Further, to retain independence where possible, neuromuscular patients wish to place their own mask. This is often not possible in Duchenne patients as upper limb strength is lost. If a full face mask is used and the patient cannot remove it himself there is a theoretical risk of aspiration if the patient vomits, although in practice this seems rare and choices should be made balancing the risk of aspiration against consequences of leaks and inadequate ventilation. Decision making should also be recorded in the patient's notes. Use of a mask may also limit the patient's ability to communicate, so consideration should be given to additional means of communication such as a buzzer at night.

### Daytime non-invasive ventilation

Oral delivery of non-invasive ventilation in neuromuscular disease has a long track record.[19] Toussaint *et al.*[20] have explored the use of mouthpiece NIV during the day having established this in patients already on nocturnal NIV but in whom uncontrolled hypercapnia is occurring during the day due to progression of disease. This is simply assessed by daytime transcutaneous carbon dioxide measurements. Initially $PCO_2$ control and symptom relief can be achieved by short top-ups of NIV in the day, e.g. an hour after lunch or on coming home from college in the evening. If that is not sufficient then NIV via a mouthpiece (supported with a headstand) can be helpful, provided the individual has neck power to turn to access the mouthpiece as needed. The Belgian group[20] showed that mouthpiece ventilation in their cohort was introduced on average $4.1 \pm 2.5$ years after initiation of nocturnal NIV, and 1, 3, 5 and 7-year survival rates from initiation were 88 per cent, 77 per cent, 58 per cent and 51 per cent, respectively. Symptoms resolved, and in six out of seven patients swallowing function also improved. Increasing daytime NIV is often required once vital capacity drops below around 400 mL.

### Tracheostomy ventilation

The proportion of DMD patients receiving non-invasive and invasive ventilation varies considerably from country to country. The main indications for tracheostomy ventilation are listed in Box 36.1. There have been comparisons of pulmonary morbidity in DMD groups on tracheostomy invasive positive pressure support (T-IPPV) and NIV showing less pulmonary morbidity and hospitalizations than in those on NIV.[21] These comparisons are fraught in that groups may not be comparable. However, Soudon *et al.*[22] showed worse morbidity in the

**Box 36.1 Indications for tracheostomy ventilation in DMD**

- Swallowing dysfunction with recurrent aspiration
- Failure to thrive on NIV
- Intractable upper airway or interface problems
- Failure to wean to NIV after acute episode of decompensation
- Patient preference

full-time tracheostomy ventilated group (mucus hypersecretions and tracheal injury) although nutritional supplementation was needed more frequently in the NIV group, who were younger. In many centres now, most DMD patients are on NIV with T-IPPV reserved for those with swallowing issues that cannot be resolved with a combination of NIV, cough assistance and percutaneous endoscopic gastrostomy (PEG) feeding. The care package for those with a tracheostomy is inevitably more complex[23] and there is a relatively high risk of other complications such as tracheal haemorrhage.

## TRANSITIONAL CARE

Transition from paediatric to adult care is an important issue for DMD patients as problems with sleep-disordered breathing are likely to be developing in the mid teenage years. Ideally paediatric and adult care can be carried out in the same institution, but if not a gradual planned handover helps both the boys and their parents and is likely to reduce unplanned admissions. Paediatric care is often more multidisciplinary than adult care and so exact team plans may be difficult to replicate. However cardiology, respiratory, physiotherapy, occupational therapy and nutritional support are vital. Neurological input is helpful and new orthopaedic issues may arise. Psychological support for the family needs to meet individual requirements, with the young Duchenne patient gradually encouraged to assume an increasing role in decision making. Social networking is likely to play an increasing role.

## LONG-TERM FINDINGS AND LATER COMPLICATIONS

With improved survival and reduced respiratory morbidity and mortality, the natural history of DMD has changed with many living into their late 20s and 30s.[14,24] More young men now die of cardiomyopathy (Fig. 36.2). Cardiosurveillance should occur 2 yearly from diagnosis, and then from the age of 10 years once a year with echo and electrocardiography (ECG), together with 24-hour monitoring if required.[25] In many protocols, an ACE

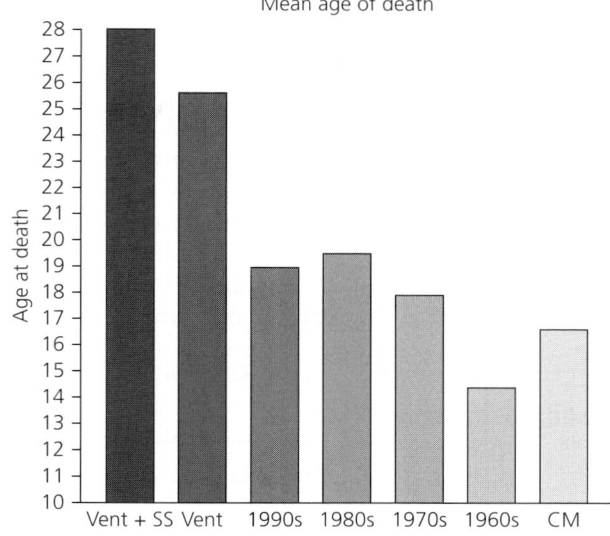


**Figure 36.2** Trends in survival in Duchenne muscular dystrophy. SS, scoliosis surgery; CM, cardiomyopathy; Vent, non-invasive ventilation. With permission from Bushby K *et al.*[25]

inhibitor is added once left ventricular fractional shortening falls below 28 per cent and a β-blocker then added to stabilize the heart rate.

Osteoporosis may add to orthopaedic problems particularly in young men who have received steroid therapy. In young patients in their late 20s and 30s we have seen an increased incidence of bowel pseudo-obstruction exacerbated by weakness of abdominal muscles to expel bowel motions, and renal/urinary calculi and urinary retention. It is not clear in these patients whether there is an additional smooth muscle involvement. Most patients can tolerate surgery with careful specialist management and use of NIV in the peri-operative period. There is a consensus document[26] of peri-operative care which is essential reading for teams managing these patients.

## SUPPORTIVE CARE, PALLIATION OF SYMPTOMS AND PROGRESSIVE CARE PLANS

Although survival has been extended, ultimately most DMD patients become ventilator dependent for most of the day and night by their late 20s or 30s. Orthopaedic and back pain and worsening cardiomyopathy require comprehensive symptom relief, and more frequent chest infections can complicate the course. Symptom palliation is key and of course there is no contraindication to pain relief including opiates for severe discomfort as ventilator settings can be adjusted to control $PCO_2$. Muscle pain and nerve root pain may be helped by a range of drugs including baclofen and pregabalin. In our experience most DMD patients wish to have full supportive measures when resuscitation choices are discussed until a very late stage, but this is of course an individual decision. All young men should be invited to take part in decision making at an age and emotionally appropriate time. When providing information about outcomes and choice it is important to provide written information for patients to take away and digest, as verbal memory problems may limit understanding and recollection of discussions. When individuals with DMD are admitted to a hospital that has few such patients and limited experience with DMD it is vital to liaise with specialist centres and transfer carried out if required to reduce any tendency to nihilism.

## Standards of care

There are consensus documenents[27,28] for the respiratory management of DMD children and adults, but in practice care including respiratory support for DMD patients is variable. Parents and families are not always informed about ventilatory options and often discussion occurs too late,[29] increasing the risk of uncontrolled decompensation. As the natural history is clear it should be possible to plan the timing of initiation of therapy around the patient and family.[13] In selected stable patients outpatient initiation of NIV may be as effective as inpatient initiation and more convenient for families.[30] In one recent UK report,[31] 67 per cent of parents rated their local medical care as poor to really poor, and 68 per cent of parents did not feel well informed – although this varied considerably from region to region, and in some areas patients and families were content with care. This variability probably represents care provision elsewhere in Europe. It is clear that in a complex and evolving condition such as DMD, NIV is one part of the management, and a multidisciplinary, informed approach is vital.[25,32,33]

## REFERENCES


1. Rideau Y, Gatin G, Bach J *et al.* Prolongation of life in Duchenne's muscular dystrophy. *Acta Neurol* 1983; **5**: 118–24.
2. Muntoni F, Torelli S, Ferlini A. Dystrophin and mutations: one gene, several proteins, multiple phenotypes. *Lancet Neurol* 2003; **2**: 731–8.
3. Emery AEH. Duchenne muscular dystrophy or Meryon's disease. In: Emery AEH, ed. *The muscular dystrophies.* Oxford: Oxford University Press, 2001: 55–71.
4. Alman BA, Raza SN, Biggar WDB. Steroid treatment and the development of scoliosis in males with Duchenne Muscular Dystrophy. *J Bone Joint Surg Am* 2004; **86**: 519–24.
5. Baydur A, Gilgoff I, Prentice W *et al.* Decline in respiratory function and experience with long term assisted ventilation in advanced Duchenne's muscular dystrophy. *Chest* 1990; **97**: 884–9.
6. Ragette R, Mellies U, Schwake C *et al.* Patterns and predictors of sleep disordered breathing in primary myopathies. *Thorax* 2002; **57**: 724–8.
7. Nigro G, Coni LI, Politano L *et al.* The incidence and evolution of cardiomyopathy in Duchenne muscular dystrophy. *Int J Cardiol* 1990; **26**: 271–7.
8. Duboc D, Meaune C, Lerebours G *et al.* Effect of perindopril on the onset and progression of left ventricular dysfunction in Duchenne muscular dystrophy. *J Am Coll Cardiol* 2005; **45**: 855–7.
9. Phillips MF, Smith PE, Carroll N *et al.* Nocturnal oxygenation and prognosis in Duchenne muscular dystrophy. *Am J Respir Crit Care Med* 1999; **160**: 198–202.
10. Vianello A, Bevilacqua M, Salvador V *et al.* Long-term nasal intermittent positive pressure ventilation in advanced Duchenne's Muscular Dystrophy. *Chest* 1994; **105**: 445–8.
11. Simonds AK, Muntoni F, Heather S *et al.* Impact of nasal ventilation on survival in hypercapnic Duchenne muscular dystrophy. *Thorax* 1998; **53**: 949–52.
12. Raphael J-C, Chevret S, Chastang C *et al.* Randomised trial of preventive nasal ventilation in Duchenne muscular dystrophy. *Lancet* 1994; **343**: 1600–4.
13. Ward SA, Chatwin M, Heather S *et al.* Randomised controlled trial of non-invasive ventilation (NIV) for nocturnal hypoventilation in neuromuscular and chest wall disease patients with daytime normocapnia. *Thorax* 2005; **60**: 1019–24.
14. Eagle M, Baudouin S, Chandler C *et al.* Survival in Duchenne muscular dystrophy: improvements in life expectancy since 1967 and the impact of home nocturnal ventilation. *Neuromusc Disord* 2002; **12**: 926–9.
15. Kohler M, Clarenbach CF, Boni L *et al.* Quality of life, physical disability, and respiratory impairment in Duchenne muscular dystrophy. *Am J Respir Crit Care Med* 2005; **172**: 1032–6.
16. Bach JR, Campagnolo DI, Hoeman S. Life satisfaction of individuals with Duchenne muscular dystrophy using long-term mechanical ventilatory support. *Am J Phys Med Rehabil* 1991; **70**: 129–35.
17. Lloyd-Owen SJ, Donaldson GC, Ambrosino N *et al.* Patterns of home mechanical use in Europe: results from the Eurovent survey. *Eur Respir J* 2005; **25**: 1025–31.
18. Simonds AK. Acute non-invasive ventilation in neuromuscular disease, chest wall disorders and cystic fibrosis and bronchiectasis. In: Simonds AK, ed. *Non-invasive respiratory support: a practical handbook.* London: Hodder Arnold, 2007: 73–80.
19. Bach JR, Alba AS, Bohatiuk G *et al.* Mouth intermittent positive pressure ventilation in the management of postpolio respiratory insufficiency. *Chest* 1987; **91**: 859–64.
20. Toussaint M, Steens M, Wasteels G *et al.* Diurnal ventilation via mouthpiece: survival in end-stage Duchenne patients. *Eur Respir J* 2006; **28**: 549–55.

21. Bach JR, Ishikawa Y, Kim H. Prevention of pulmonary morbidity for patients with Duchenne muscular dystrophy. *Chest* 1998; **112**: 1024–8.
22. Soudon P, Steens M, Toussaint M. A comparison on invasive versus noninvasive fulltime mechanical ventilation in Duchenne muscular dystrophy. *Chronic Respir Dis* 2008; **5**: 87–93.
23. Simonds AK. Discharging the ventilator-dependent patient and the home ventilatory care network. In: Simonds AK, ed. *Non-invasive respiratory support: a practical handbook.* London: Hodder Arnold, 2007: 229–48.
24. Jeppesen J, Green A, Steffensen BF *et al.* The Duchenne muscular dystrophy population in Denmark, 1977–2001: prevalence, incidence and survival in relation to the introduction of ventilator use. *Neuromusc Disord* 2003; **13**: 804–12.
25. Bushby K, Bourke J, Bullock R *et al.* The multidisciplinary management of Duchenne muscular dystrophy. *Curr Pediatr* 2005; **15**: 292–300.
26. Birnkrant DJ, Panitch HB, Benditt JO *et al.* American college of chest physicians consensus statement on the respiratory and related management of patients with Duchenne muscular dystrophy undergoing anesthesia or sedation. *Chest* 2007; **132**: 1977–86.
27. Finder J, Birnkrant D, Carl J *et al.* ATS Consensus Statement: Respiratory care of the patient with Duchenne muscular dystrophy. *Am J Respir Crit Care Med* 2004; **170**: 456–65.
28. Shahrizaila T, Kinnear W. Recommendations for respiratory care of adults with muscle disorders. *Neuromusc Disord* 2007; **17**: 13–15.
29. Kinali M, Manzur AY, Gibson BE *et al.* UK Physicians' attitudes and practices of long term non-invasive ventilation of children with Duchenne muscular dystrophy. *Pediatr Rehabil* 2006; **9**: 351–64.
30. Chatwin M, Nickol AH, Morrell MJ *et al.* Randomised trial of inpatient versus outpatient initiation of home mechanical ventilation in patients with nocturnal hypoventilation. *Respir Med* 2008; **102**: 1528–35.
31. Action Duchenne. Duchenne families standards of care consultations. Report 2009.
32. Bushby K, Finkel R, Case LE *et al.* Diagnosis and management of Duchenne muscular dystrophy. 1: Diagnosis, and pharmacological and psychosocial management. *Lancet Neurol* 2010; **9**: 1–16.
33. Bushby K, Finkel R, Case LE *et al.* Diagnosis and management of Duchenne muscular dystrophy. 2: Implementation of multidisciplinary care. *Lancet Neurol* 2010; **9**: 177–89.

# 37

# Central sleep apnoea

PATRICK LÉVY, JEAN-CHRISTIAN BOREL, RENAUD TAMISIER, BERNARD WUYAM, JEAN-LOUIS PÉPIN

## ABSTRACT

Central sleep apnoea (CSA) is an heterogeneous group of diseases that can be further divided into two classes depending on the presence or absence of hypercapnia during the day. Pathophysiology depends on the aetiology. Non-hypercapnic CSA including CSA with Cheyne–Stokes respiration (CSA-CSR) is mainly due to hyperventilation and a reduction in the carbon dioxide level, which leads to a lowering of the prevailing $PaCO_2$ near the apnoeic threshold, with the difference defining the carbon dioxide reserve. Conversely, hypercapnic CSA, i.e. congenital central hypoventilation syndrome, narcotic-induced central apnoea, obesity hypoventilation syndrome and impaired respiratory motor control, are related to various mechanisms, resulting in nocturnal loss of ventilatory output to respiratory muscles. Heart failure (CSA-CSR) is the main cause of non-hypercapnic CSA. The prevalence of CSA-CSR remains high despite new treatment modalities in heart failure and CSA-CSR appears to significantly alter survival and morbidity in heart failure. There are at the present time no evidence-based therapeutic options. Large randomized controlled trials are currently being conducted to assess the effects of adaptive servo-ventilation on survival in heart failure presenting with CSA-CSR. Hypercapnic CSA although including many different medical conditions is usually best treated with non-invasive nasal ventilation, but very few large trials have been conducted and thus many therapeutic issues remain unresolved.

## INTRODUCTION

Central sleep apnoea (CSA) is characterized by episodes of apnoea or hypopnoea related to loss of ventilatory output from the central respiratory generator located in the brainstem. However, owing to the complexity of the control of ventilation, many structures may be structurally or functionally involved in the loss of ventilatory drive, including medullary neurones, carotid bodies or feedback from respiratory muscle afferents. The nosology of CSA remains debated although several recommendations/classifications have been published in the past 10 years.[1] The reason is probably the disparity in prevalence between the different clinical entities. Although CSA is very frequent in heart failure and thus commonly seen in clinical practice,[2] idiopathic CSA or tumours and trauma-induced lesions of the brainstem are rare.[3] However, it has been suggested to divide CSA into two classes based on the presence or absence of hypercapnia during daytime.[4] This classification seems to be pertinent with respect to both pathophysiology and different treatment options.[3] In this chapter, we will review the classification and pathophysiology of CSA. We will also discuss CSA in heart failure, specific aetiologies such as complex sleep apnoea or opioid-induced sleep apnoea, and hypercapnic central sleep apnoea with special emphasis on the treatment issues.

## CLASSIFICATION

### Non-hypercapnic central sleep apnoea

#### CSA WITH CHEYNE–STOKES RESPIRATION (CSA-CSR)

This breathing disorder is seen in 30–80 per cent of patients with advanced congestive heart failure (CHF).[5–7] The polysomnographic pattern is characterized by the presence of central apnoeas and hypopnoeas, alternating with periods of crescendo-decrescendo tidal volume (Fig. 37.1). CSA-CSR has been associated, in a severity-dependent

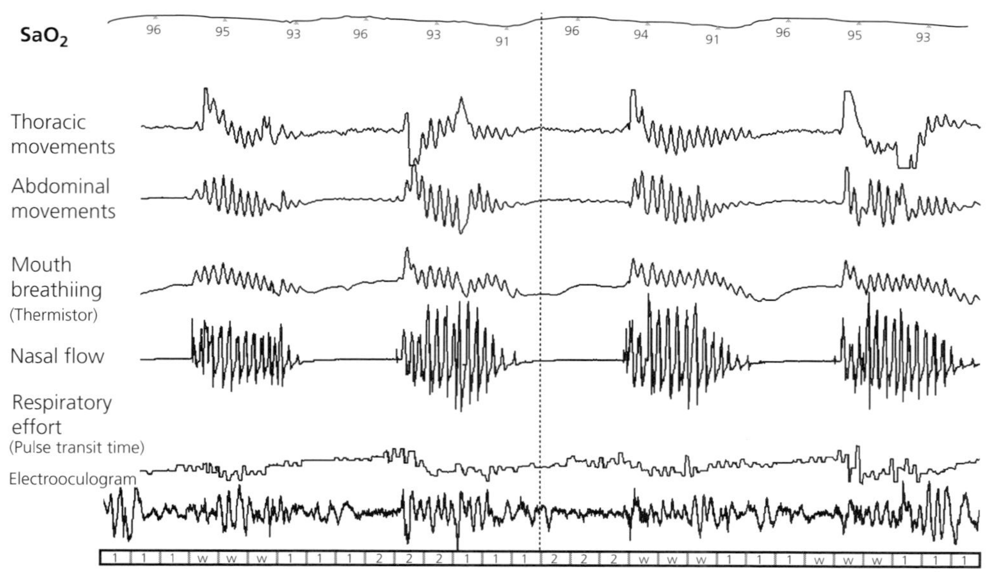


**Figure 37.1** Typical polygraphic tracing in a patient with heart failure presenting with Cheyne-Stokes respiration and central apnoea. This is a 5-minute tracing.

manner, with elevations of sympathetic nervous activity in CHF patients, and is an important predictor of CHF progression,[8] arrhythmias[9] and mortality.[10]

#### IDIOPATHIC CSA

Idiopathic CSA is a relatively rare disorder with poorly understood pathophysiology and natural history. From a clinical standpoint, idiopathic CSA represents an exclusion diagnosis in CSA without a recognized causal factor. Although there is increased ventilatory response to carbon dioxide and a high loop gain predisposing to ventilatory control instability and resulting in low daytime $PaCO_2$, the typical polysomnographic pattern is not waxing and waning as in CSA-CSR but rather abrupt hyperventilation associated with arousals.[11] The arousal typically occurs at the end of the event, the cycling period being usually shorter than in CSA-CSR. Clinically, frequent awakenings during the night, insomnia and daytime somnolence are often reported. Sleep fragmentation may indeed favour ventilatory control instability since wake–sleep transitions tend to reduce the carbon dioxide reserve and to allow crossing the apnoeic threshold (see Pathophysiology below).

### Hypercapnic central sleep apnoea

Patients with hypercapnic CSA present with sleep hypoventilation, which means that there is hypercapnia during the daytime that worsens during sleep.[3] This can be related either to abnormal central pattern generator output or to impairment of respiratory motor output originating below the brainstem.

## PATHOPHYSIOLOGY

### CSA-CSR and other non-hypercapnic central sleep apnoeas

#### APNOEIC THRESHOLD AND CARBON DIOXIDE RESERVE

When $PaCO_2$ falls below a critical threshold called the apnoeic threshold, central respiratory drive ceases. However, over time, when stable sleep is obtained, the reduction in ventilation leads to a gradual rise in $PaCO_2$ ranging from 3 mm Hg to 8 mm Hg and a new sleep-specific carbon dioxide set point (close to 45 mm Hg).[12] Thus, the difference between the carbon dioxide set point and the apnoeic threshold (i.e. the carbon dioxide reserve) is increased, which leads to breathing stability. Breathing instability can arise from a change in the carbon dioxide set point as seen during the transition from sleep to wake, e.g. from 45 mm Hg to 40 mm Hg, or from an increase in the apnoeic threshold, both resulting in reduced carbon dioxide reserve. Conversely, any intervention leading to an increased carbon dioxide reserve will stabilize ventilation (Fig. 37.2). The carbon dioxide reserve is increased when ventilation is augmented with the notable exception of hypoxia[13] and heart failure. In CHF presenting with CSA-CSR, it has been evidenced that eupnoeic $PCO_2$ is not increased, suggesting an additional ventilatory stimulant during sleep while the apnoeic threshold is not reduced despite the additional ventilatory stimulation, thus leading to a reduced carbon dioxide reserve in a similar manner to what has been shown during hypoxia.[14] Hypoxia does not seem to contribute in CSA but both conditions may have a common mechanism.[14]

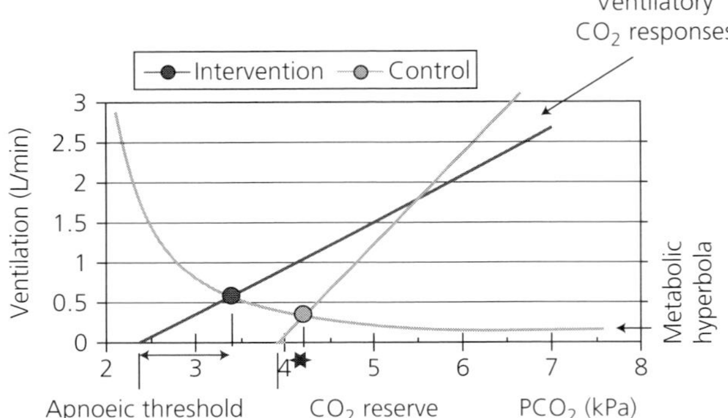


**Figure 37.2** Respiratory and metabolic carbon dioxide ($CO_2$) control. Breathing instability may arise from an increase in carbon dioxide ventilatory response *or* an increase in apnoeic threshold and/or a reduction in the carbon dioxide set point, the difference between the latter defining the carbon dioxide reserve. Any intervention increasing the carbon dioxide reserve will conversely stabilize breathing.

### OTHER MECHANISMS

There is evidence that *hyperventilation* has a role in the genesis of periodic breathing and central apnoeas in heart failure, suggesting permanent hyperventilation in patients with CSA-CSR.[3,12] The role of hyperventilation is also supported by data obtained during manipulation of the carbon dioxide blood level. An increase in $PaCO_2$ during sleep with low levels of inspired carbon dioxide (2–3 per cent) and/or the addition of an external dead space during sleep have been shown to efficiently stabilize ventilation and remove apnoeas, in both CSA-CSR[15] and idiopathic CSA.[16] Stimulation of the vagal pulmonary C-fibres by venous congestion and interstitial oedema has been suggested as a possible cause of hyperventilation in heart failure, as patients with CSA-CSR have a significantly higher pulmonary capillary wedge pressure (PCWP) than those without CSA-CSR, with a significant negative correlation between PCPW and awake $PaCO_2$.[17] Also, increased ventilatory response to carbon dioxide has been reported to occur in CSA-CSR.[18] Finally, elevated sympathoneural activity, an important feature in the pathogenesis of heart failure owing to its detrimental effects on the function of the failing myocardium,[19] has been evidenced in CSA-CSR.[20,21]

The role of *circulation time* has also been discussed. Early observations led to the hypothesis that the delays in the transport of the oxygenated blood to the brain (or possibly to the carotid chemoreceptors) could be responsible for CSR. Circulatory delay, as reflected by lung-to-ear circulation time (LECT), has been shown, however, to influence the total time of the breathing cycle and the length of the hyperpnoeic phase of CSR (the longer the circulation time the longer the total cycle time and the hyperventilatory phase) but not the apnoea length *per se*.[22]

## Hypercapnic central sleep apnoea

Congenital central hypoventilation syndrome (CCHS) is a rare disease with an estimated incidence at 1 per 200 000 live births.[23] It is diagnosed in the absence of primary neuromuscular, lung or cardiac disease or an identifiable brainstem lesion, and is characterized by generally adequate ventilation while the patient is awake but alveolar hypoventilation with typically normal respiratory rates and shallow breathing (diminished tidal volume) during sleep.[24] More severely affected children hypoventilate both while awake and asleep. While asleep, children with CCHS experience progressive hypercapnia and hypoxaemia.[24] They have absent or negligible ventilatory sensitivity to hypercapnia and absent or variable ventilatory sensitivity to hypoxaemia during sleep. Thus these patients need lifelong ventilatory support. The identification of *$PHOX_2B$* as the disease-causing gene in CCHS[25] has been an important step forward. There have been since several reports of adults exhibiting sleep-related hypoventilation or central apnoeas and severe hypoxaemia, with *$PHOX_2B$* mutations.[26] More generally, *$PHOX_2B$* appears pivotal to the development of respiratory networks.[27]

Several diseases may be responsible for hypercapnic CSA, all of them being associated with *anatomical or functional defect of the respiratory controller*.[28] These include the Shy Drager syndromes and dysautonomia, in which impaired control of breathing is associated with autonomic nervous system dysfunction also affecting the cardiovascular system.[29] Similarly, diabetes mellitus and familial dysautonomia, and a series of diseases affecting the central nervous system (CNS, may be associated with CSA: stroke, poliomyelitis, encephalitis, multiple sclerosis and vascular anomalies. Central sleep apnoea has also been reported after trauma, cervical posterior cordotomy, and in Chiari malformations,[30,31] suggesting that lesions in the motor neurones descending from the medulla to the respiratory muscles can lead to similar functional deficits.

*Chronic opioid use* has become an important concern in Western countries.[32] Central sleep apnoea has been found in stable patients treated with methadone, a synthetic opioid commonly used in the treatment of addiction, as well as in patients receiving opioid analgesics. CSA in opioid chronic use is different from CSA-CSR and idiopathic CSA, with no crescendo-decrescendo pattern and a much shorter period. It seems to correspond frequently to an ataxic type of breathing that is dose dependent.[33] The pathophysiology is unclear. However, blunted central chemosensitivity (diminished ventilatory response to carbon dioxide) with enhanced peripheral chemosensitivity (increased hypoxic ventilatory response) seems to be important.[34] One explanation may be the opioid differential effects at the CNS level. There is evidence of novel morphine-induced acetylcholine release at the hypoglossal motor nucleus.[35] As mentioned by Horner,[36] this release of acetylcholine, while a reduction in more rostral regions implicated in arousal or rapid eye movement (REM) control, was dose dependent, and blocked by μ but not κ opioid receptor antagonists.[35] These μ receptors seem to be expressed at the pre-Bötzinger complex level with a similar release of acetylcholine. Since this particular region is critical in the generation of respiratory rhythm and the subsequent expression of this rhythmic activity in other medullary respiratory neurones,[36] it might explain at least partly the ataxic breathing seen in chronic opioid use.

Although *obesity hypoventilation syndrome* is sometimes classified as such,[3] this condition is associated with obesity plus daytime hypercapnia unexplained by another reason and is not CSA. Sleep apnoea may or may not be present and is essentially obstructive in nature.

Hypercapnic patients with intact central respiratory output from respiratory centres may exhibit CSA due to anomalies in the motor neurones to the respiratory muscles. This is the case in a wide range of neuromuscular disorders including myasthenia gravis, amyotrophic lateral sclerosis, post-polio syndrome and myopathies as well as in chest wall syndromes such as kyphoscoliosis.[3]

## CENTRAL SLEEP APNOEA AND HEART FAILURE

### Epidemiology

Reported prevalence rates of CSA-CSR in patients with heart failure vary greatly from 30 per cent to 100 per cent.[2] Javaheri *et al.* recently reported on a prospective study of 100 of 114 consecutive eligible patients with heart failure and left ventricular ejection fraction (LVEF) <45 per cent[6] with 37 per cent with CSA and 12 per cent with obstructive sleep apnoea (OSA).

One critical and highly discussed question is whether with the new treatments of heart failure the incidence of CSA has dropped, as suggested by the CANPAP study published in 2005.[37] Although there are data supportive of a reduction in CSA-CSR prevalence[38] others have found a persistent high prevalence despite a high rate of use of β-blockers.[7,39] In any case, severity of heart failure is critical.

### Diagnosis and management of CSA-CSR

It has been questioned whether CSA-CSR is only a marker of CHF severity. However, CSA-CSR, independently of other risk factors, seems to increase the risk of mortality in CHF by two- to threefold,[10,40,41] although this has not been confirmed in all studies.[42] However, it suggests that diagnosis and treatment of CSA-CSR are mandatory. This is emphasized in the recommendations recently published by the European Society of Cardiology mentioning higher morbidity in heart failure patients presenting with sleep-disordered breathing and recommending specific treatment for sleep-disordered breathing.[43]

#### DIAGNOSIS[44]

The diagnosis should be systematically established in severe cardiac failure patients (stages III–IV of the New York Heart Association classification and LVEF <40 per cent). Typically, patients with idiopathic dilated cardiomyopathy are the best candidates. Several factors have been identified as risks factors for sleep-disordered breathing, namely male gender, age more than 40, daytime hypocapnia and atrial fibrillation.[45]

Overnight monitoring is mandatory after screening in the clinical context, e.g. daytime fatigue, excessive daytime sleepiness and markers of hyperventilation. Although complete polysomnography would be desirable, it has certainly not been adapted to epidemiological needs.[44] Thus simplified techniques are required. Respiratory effort can be determined by oesophageal pressure, which still remains the reference method.[1] The non-invasive alternative techniques include recognition of inspiratory flow limitation using nasal pressure or persistent or augmented respiratory effort using pulse transit time.[44] These techniques should ideally be used together to allow classifying the respiratory events either as central or obstructive. In order to avoid misclassifications and establish the adequate treatment, oximetry alone should not be used.[46]

#### MANAGEMENT

There is a major role for any treatment that may improve cardiac function. As previously discussed, β-blockers are now systematically prescribed in CHF patients. It seems at least in some patients that this treatment may reduce CSA-CSR.[47]

With oxygen therapy, reductions in the severity of CSA-CSR, decrease in overnight urinary noradrenaline (norepinephrine) levels, and increase in peak oxygen consumption during graded exercise with nightly use have been reported.[48,49] However, oxygen has not been shown to improve direct measures of cardiac function.[50] In any case, large randomized controlled trials are lacking in this area.[51]

Long-term nightly use of continuous positive airway pressure (CPAP) over 1–3 months has been shown to alleviate CSA-CSR,[52,53] increase LVEF,[54] inspiratory muscle strength, and reduce mitral regurgitation, atrial natriuretic peptide,[55] and adrenergic tone.[20] It has also been shown to improve quality of life.[54] Regarding survival, the largest study was reported in 2005.[37] As previously mentioned, the study had to be stopped due to the reduced incidence of CSA-CSR.[37] There also was a trend towards an increased mortality in the CPAP arm in the first 18 months while further improvement in the treated group did not reach significance when the study was stopped (Fig. 37.3A).[37] A *post-hoc* analysis of these data showed that these disappointing results were at least partly related to the degree of correction of the respiratory events under CPAP with a much improved survival in the responders than in

eupnea during sleep. *Am J Respir Crit Care Med* 2002; **165**: 1251–60.

14. Dempsey JA, Smith CA, Przybylowski T *et al.* The ventilatory responsiveness to CO(2) below eupnoea as a determinant of ventilatory stability in sleep. *J Physiol* 2004; **560**: 1–11.
15. Steens RD, Millar TW, Su X *et al.* Effect of inhaled 3 per cent $CO_2$ on Cheyne-Stokes respiration in congestive heart failure. *Sleep* 1994; **17**: 61–8.
16. Badr MS, Grossman JE, Weber SA. Treatment of refractory sleep apnea with supplemental carbon dioxide. *Am J Respir Crit Care Med* 1994; **150**: 561–4.
17. Lorenzi-Filho G, Azevedo ER, Parker JD *et al.* Relationship of carbon dioxide tension in arterial blood to pulmonary wedge pressure in heart failure. *Eur Respir J* 2002; **19**: 37–40.
18. Wilcox I, McNamara SG, Dodd MJ *et al.* Ventilatory control in patients with sleep apnoea and left ventricular dysfunction: comparison of obstructive and central sleep apnoea. *Eur Respir J* 1998; **11**: 7–13.
19. Jessup M, Brozena S. Heart failure. *N Engl J Med* 2003; **348**: 2007–18.
20. Naughton MT, Benard DC, Liu PP *et al.* Effects of nasal CPAP on sympathetic activity in patients with heart failure and central sleep apnea. *Am J Respir Crit Care Med* 1995; **152**: 473–9.
21. Spaak J, Egri ZJ, Kubo T *et al.* Muscle sympathetic nerve activity during wakefulness in heart failure patients with and without sleep apnea. *Hypertension* 2005; **46**: 1327–32.
22. Hall MJ, Xie A, Rutherford R *et al.* Cycle length of periodic breathing in patients with and without heart failure. *Am J Respir Crit Care Med* 1996; **154**: 376–81.
23. Trang H, Dehan M, Beaufils F *et al.* The French congenital central hypoventilation syndrome registry: general data, phenotype, and genotype. *Chest* 2005; **127**: 72–9.
24. American Thoracic Society. Idiopathic congenital central hypoventilation syndrome: diagnosis and management. *Am J Respir Crit Care Med* 1999; **160**: 368–73.
25. Amiel J, Laudier B, Attie-Bitach T *et al.* Polyalanine expansion and frameshift mutations of the paired-like homeobox gene PHOX2B in congenital central hypoventilation syndrome. *Nat Genet* 2003; **33**: 459–61.
26. Trang H, Laudier B, Trochet D *et al.* PHOX2B gene mutation in a patient with late-onset central hypoventilation. *Pediatr Pulmonol* 2004; **38**: 349–51.
27. Gallego J, Dauger S. PHOX2B mutations and ventilatory control. *Respir Physiol Neurobiol* 2008; **164**: 49–54.
28. Plum F, Leigh R. Abnormalities of the central mechanisms. In: Hornbein TF, ed. *Regulation of breathing.* New York: Marcel Dekker, 1981:989–1067.
29. Guilleminault C, Briskin JG, Greenfield MS *et al.* The impact of autonomic nervous system dysfunction on breathing during sleep. *Sleep* 1981; **4**: 263–78.
30. Gagnadoux F, Meslier N, Svab I *et al.* Sleep-disordered breathing in patients with Chiari malformation: improvement after surgery. *Neurology* 2006; **66**: 136–8.
31. Dauvilliers Y, Stal V, Abril B *et al.* Chiari malformation and sleep related breathing disorders. *J Neurol Neurosurg Psychiatry* 2007; **78**: 1344–8.
32. Wang D, Teichtahl H. Opioids, sleep architecture and sleep-disordered breathing. *Sleep Med Rev* 2007; **11**: 35–46.
33. Walker JM, Farney RJ, Rhondeau SM *et al.* Chronic opioid use is a risk factor for the development of central sleep apnea and ataxic breathing. *J Clin Sleep Med* 2007; **3**: 455–61.
34. Teichtahl H, Wang D, Cunnington D *et al.* Ventilatory responses to hypoxia and hypercapnia in stable methadone maintenance treatment patients. *Chest* 2005; **128**: 1339–47.
35. Skulsky EM, Osman NI, Baghdoyan HA *et al.* Microdialysis delivery of morphine to the hypoglossal nucleus of Wistar rat increases hypoglossal acetylcholine release. *Sleep* 2007; **30**: 566–73.
36. Horner RL. Morphine-induced acetylcholine release at the hypoglossal motor nucleus: implications for opiate-induced respiratory suppression. *Sleep* 2007; **30**: 551–2.
37. Bradley TD, Logan AG, Kimoff RJ *et al.* Continuous positive airway pressure for central sleep apnea and heart failure. *N Engl J Med* 2005; **353**: 2025–33.
38. Schulz R, Blau A, Borgel J *et al.* Sleep apnoea in heart failure. *Eur Respir J* 2007; **29**: 1201–5.
39. MacDonald M, Fang J, Pittman SD *et al.* The current prevalence of sleep disordered breathing in congestive heart failure patients treated with beta-blockers. *J Clin Sleep Med* 2008; **4**: 38–42.
40. Hanly PJ, Zuberi-Khokhar NS. Increased mortality associated with Cheyne-Stokes respiration in patients with congestive heart failure. *Am J Respir Crit Care Med* 1996; **153**: 272–6.
41. Lanfranchi PA, Braghiroli A, Bosimini E *et al.* Prognostic value of nocturnal Cheyne-Stokes respiration in chronic heart failure. *Circulation* 1999; **99**: 1435–40.
42. Roebuck T, Solin P, Kaye DM *et al.* Increased long-term mortality in heart failure due to sleep apnoea is not yet proven. *Eur Respir J* 2004; **23**: 735–40.
43. Dickstein K, Cohen-Solal A, Filippatos G *et al.* ESC Guidelines for the diagnosis and treatment of acute and chronic heart failure 2008. *Eur Heart J* 2008; **29**: 2388–442.
44. Pepin JL, Chouri-Pontarollo N, Tamisier R *et al.* Cheyne-Stokes respiration with central sleep apnoea in chronic heart failure: proposals for a diagnostic and therapeutic strategy. *Sleep Med Rev* 2006; **10**: 33–47.
45. Sin DD, Fitzgerald F, Parker JD *et al.* Risk factors for central and obstructive sleep apnea in 450 men and women with congestive heart failure. *Am J Respir Crit Care Med* 1999; **160**: 1101–6.
46. Series F, Kimoff RJ, Morrison D *et al.* Prospective evaluation of nocturnal oximetry for detection of sleep-related breathing disturbances in patients with chronic heart failure. *Chest* 2005; **127**: 1507–14.
47. Tamura A, Kawano Y, Naono S *et al.* Relationship between beta-blocker treatment and the severity of central sleep apnea in chronic heart failure. *Chest* 2007; **131**: 130–5.

48. Andreas S, Clemens C, Sandholzer H *et al.* Improvement of exercise capacity with treatment of Cheyne-Stokes respiration in patients with congestive heart failure. *J Am Coll Cardiol* 1996; **27**: 1486–90.
49. Javaheri S, Ahmed M, Parker TJ *et al.* Effects of nasal $O_2$ on sleep-related disordered breathing in ambulatory patients with stable heart failure. *Sleep* 1999; **22**: 1101–6.
50. Krachman SL, Nugent T, Crocetti J *et al.* Effects of oxygen therapy on left ventricular function in patients with Cheyne-Stokes respiration and congestive heart failure. *J Clin Sleep Med* 2005; **1**: 271–6.
51. Javaheri S. Pembrey's dream: the time has come for a long-term trial of nocturnal supplemental nasal oxygen to treat central sleep apnea in congestive heart failure. *Chest* 2003; **123**: 322–5.
52. Takasaki Y, Orr D, Popkin J *et al.* Effect of nasal continuous positive airway pressure on sleep apnea in congestive heart failure. *Am Rev Respir Dis* 1989; **140**: 1578–84.
53. Naughton MT, Benard DC, Rutherford R *et al.* Effect of continuous positive airway pressure on central sleep apnea and nocturnal $PCO_2$ in heart failure. *Am J Respir Crit Care Med* 1994; **150**: 1598–604.
54. Naughton MT, Liu PP, Bernard DC *et al.* Treatment of congestive heart failure and Cheyne-Stokes respiration during sleep by continuous positive airway pressure. *Am J Respir Crit Care Med* 1995; **151**: 92–7.
55. Tkacova R, Liu PP, Naughton MT *et al.* Effect of continuous positive airway pressure on mitral regurgitant fraction and atrial natriuretic peptide in patients with heart failure. *J Am Coll Cardiol* 1997; **30**: 739–45.
56. Arzt M, Floras JS, Logan AG *et al.* Suppression of central sleep apnea by continuous positive airway pressure and transplant-free survival in heart failure: a post hoc analysis of the Canadian Continuous Positive Airway Pressure for Patients with Central Sleep Apnea and Heart Failure Trial (CANPAP). *Circulation* 2007; **115**: 3173–80.
57. Pepin JL, Krieger J, Rodenstein D *et al.* Effective compliance during the first 3 months of continuous positive airway pressure. A European prospective study of 121 patients. *Am J Respir Crit Care Med* 1999; **160**: 1124–9.
58. Teschler H, Dohring J, Wang YM *et al.* Adaptive pressure support servo-ventilation: a novel treatment for Cheyne-Stokes respiration in heart failure. *Am J Respir Crit Care Med* 2001; **164**: 614–19.
59. Kohnlein T, Welte T, Tan LB *et al.* Assisted ventilation for heart failure patients with Cheyne-Stokes respiration. *Eur Respir J* 2002; **20**: 934–41.
60. Arzt M, Schulz M, Schroll S *et al.* Time course of continuous positive airway pressure effects on central sleep apnoea in patients with chronic heart failure. *J Sleep Res* 2009; **18**: 20–5.
61. Noda A, Izawa H, Asano H *et al.* Beneficial effect of bilevel positive airway pressure on left ventricular function in ambulatory patients with idiopathic dilated cardiomyopathy and central sleep apnea-hypopnea: a preliminary study. *Chest* 2007; **131**: 1694–701.
62. Pepperell JC, Maskell NA, Jones DR *et al.* A randomized controlled trial of adaptive ventilation for Cheyne-Stokes breathing in heart failure. *Am J Respir Crit Care Med* 2003; **168**: 1109–14.
63. Philippe C, Stoica-Herman M, Drouot X *et al.* Compliance with and effectiveness of adaptive servoventilation versus continuous positive airway pressure in the treatment of Cheyne-Stokes respiration in heart failure over a six month period. *Heart* 2006; **92**: 337–42.
64. Arzt M, Wensel R, Montalvan S *et al.* Effects of dynamic bilevel positive airway pressure support on central sleep apnea in men with heart failure. *Chest* 2008; **134**: 61–6.
65. Davies RJ, Harrington KJ, Ormerod OJ *et al.* Nasal continuous positive airway pressure in chronic heart failure with sleep-disordered breathing. *Am Rev Respir Dis* 1993; **147**: 630–4.
66. Liston R, Deegan PC, McCreery C *et al.* Haemodynamic effects of nasal continuous positive airway pressure in severe congestive heart failure. *Eur Respir J* 1995; **8**: 430–5.
67. Randerath WJ, Galetke W, Kenter M *et al.* Combined adaptive servo-ventilation and automatic positive airway pressure (anticyclic modulated ventilation) in co-existing obstructive and central sleep apnea syndrome and periodic breathing. *Sleep Med* 2009; **10**: 898–903.
68. Thomas RJ. Effect of added dead space to positive airway pressure for treatment of complex sleep-disordered breathing. *Sleep Med* 2005; **6**: 177–8.
69. Morgenthaler TI, Kagramanov V, Hanak V *et al.* Complex sleep apnea syndrome: is it a unique clinical syndrome? *Sleep* 2006; **29**: 1203–9.
70. Thomas RJ, Terzano MG, Parrino L *et al.* Obstructive sleep-disordered breathing with a dominant cyclic alternating pattern – a recognizable polysomnographic variant with practical clinical implications. *Sleep* 2004; **27**: 229–34.
71. Endo Y, Suzuki M, Inoue Y *et al.* Prevalence of complex sleep apnea among Japanese patients with sleep apnea syndrome. *Tohoku J Exp Med* 2008; **215**: 349–54.
72. Kuzniar TJ, Pusalavidyasagar S, Gay PC *et al.* Natural course of complex sleep apnea – a retrospective study. *Sleep Breath* 2008; **12**: 135–9.
73. Allam JS, Olson EJ, Gay PC *et al.* Efficacy of adaptive servoventilation in treatment of complex and central sleep apnea syndromes. *Chest* 2007; **132**: 1839–46.
74. Issa FG, Sullivan CE. Reversal of central sleep apnea using nasal CPAP. *Chest* 1986; **90**: 165–71.
75. Perez de Llano LA, Golpe R, Ortiz Piquer M *et al.* Short-term and long-term effects of nasal intermittent positive pressure ventilation in patients with obesity-hypoventilation syndrome. *Chest* 2005; **128**: 587–94.
76. Mokhlesi B, Kryger MH, Grunstein RR. Assessment and management of patients with obesity

hypoventilation syndrome. *Proc Am Thorac Soc* 2008; **5**: 218–25.

77. Mokhlesi B. Positive airway pressure titration in obesity hypoventilation syndrome: continuous positive airway pressure or bilevel positive airway pressure. *Chest* 2007; **131**: 1624–6.
78. Banerjee D, Yee BJ, Piper AJ *et al.* Obesity hypoventilation syndrome: hypoxemia during continuous positive airway pressure. *Chest* 2007; **131**: 1678–84.
79. Storre JH, Seuthe B, Fiechter R *et al.* Average volume-assured pressure support in obesity hypoventilation: a randomized crossover trial. *Chest* 2006; **130**: 815–21.
80. Piper AJ, Wang D, Yee BJ *et al.* Randomised trial of CPAP vs bilevel support in the treatment of obesity hypoventilation syndrome without severe nocturnal desaturation. *Thorax* 2008; **63**: 395–401.
81. Redolfi S, Corda L, La Piana G *et al.* Long-term non-invasive ventilation increases chemosensitivity and leptin in obesity-hypoventilation syndrome. *Respir Med* 2007; **101**: 1191–5.
82. Chouri-Pontarollo N, Borel JC, Tamisier R *et al.* Impaired objective daytime vigilance in obesity-hypoventilation syndrome: impact of noninvasive ventilation. *Chest* 2007; **131**: 148–55.

# SECTION H

# Chest wall deformity

# 38

# Scoliosis

WILLIAM J M KINNEAR

## ABSTRACT

Scoliosis is a rotational deformity of the spine. Most cases are either idiopathic or associated with a neuromuscular disorder involving the paraspinal muscles. Congenital cases are rare and related to vertebral abnormalities. Spinal deformity in scoliosis is measured by the Cobb angle. Respiratory problems are unusual if this angle is less than 90°, or if the vital capacity is more than 50 per cent of predicted. Patients with scoliosis have ventilation–perfusion mismatching, reduced lung and chest wall compliance, increased work of breathing, respiratory muscle weakness and reduced respiratory drive. Gas exchange is worst during rapid eye movement (REM) sleep. Nocturnal non-invasive ventilation should be started in any patient with scoliosis who develops daytime hypercapnia. It should also be used in patients with symptomatic nocturnal hypoventilation, bearing in mind that these symptoms may be vague and under-reported by patients. Asymptomatic nocturnal hypoventilation needs to be monitored regularly. Non-invasive ventilation improves gas exchange during sleep, relieves respiratory muscle fatigue and allows recovery of respiratory drive. Pressure control modes should be used, with high inspiratory pressures. Timings should be similar to the patient's spontaneous breathing pattern, the aim being that they should not be triggering the ventilator, which should provide – rather than support – respiration.

## INTRODUCTION

The bony structure of the spinal column reminds us that we are segmental organisms. In our quadripedal ancestors, the spine was suspended between the shoulder and pelvic girdles. Adopting an upright posture has brought us many advantages, but we pay a price in that the spine no longer hangs in the configuration for which it evolved: a column of blocks stacked on-top of each other is inherently unstable.

When we assumed the upright posture, we maintained the spinal curvature of our ancestors. Forward curvature of the spine is called kyphosis. A gentle kyphosis appears to make the spine more stable: loss of this curvature is an important predictor of the likelihood of developing the rotational deformity of scoliosis.[1] Thoracic kyphosis is normally associated with lumbar lordosis (inward curvature).

In quadripeds, the scope for rotational distortion of the spine is limited: since all four limbs touch the ground, the pelvic and shoulder girdles remain in alignment. This corrective mechanism is lost in bipeds, and the spine is vulnerable to rotational deformity. If you look at the spinous processes on the X-ray of a patient with scoliosis, you can see how the vertebrae twist round at the apex of the deformity, emphasizing that this is a rotational problem and not just lateral curvature.

Cervical and lumbar spinal deformities have little effect on the mechanics of respiration. If the thoracic spine is involved, the rib cage is inevitably distorted. In mild cases the effects may only be cosmetic, but more severe disruption of the normal configuration of the ribs constrains their movement. On the concave side of the curve the ribs are crushed together, whereas on the convex side they are splayed apart, although they must still join together anteriorly onto the sternum (Fig. 38.1).

Although scoliosis is a rotational deformity, its severity is often assessed by measuring the angulation in a two-dimensional plane, in this case the coronal (as opposed to the sagittal angulation of kyphosis). To do this we need a frontal X-ray of the spine, on which we calculate the Cobb angle. Draw a line through the middle of the two vertebrae

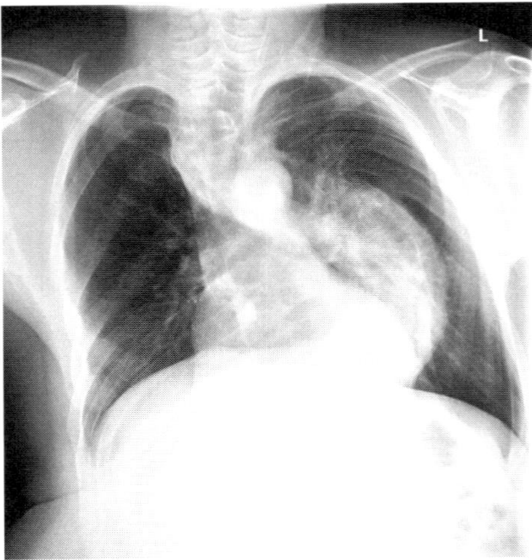


**Figure 38.1** Chest X-ray of a patient with thoracic scoliosis. Note the narrow gaps between the ribs posteriorly in the left upper zone, compared with the wider gaps on the right.

at the top and bottom of the curved segment; Cobb realized that drawing two lines perpendicular to those you drew through the vertebrae allows you to measure the angle of curvature.[2] Respiratory failure is uncommon if the angle of spinal curvature is less than 100° (i.e. approximately a right angle).

If the thoracic spine is curved, the affected person will try to get their head back into vertical alignment by developing a compensatory curve in the unaffected segments. (If you look carefully at a patient with scoliosis, you will notice that their head is not centred over their pelvis.) If the primary abnormality is lumbar, the thoracic curve which develops in compensation is rarely severe enough to compromise gas exchange (Fig. 38.2).

Scoliosis causes loss of vertical height. Another clinical clue to the presence of scoliosis is the length of a patient's arms compared to the height of their trunk. Arm span is similar to vertical height, a trick we use to estimate what the height would be without the spinal curvature when calculating predicted lung function parameters for a patient with scoliosis.[3]

On the convex side of the spinal curvature, the ribs are splayed apart. This may form a 'rib hump' which is a cosmetic issue for the patient, sometimes corrected by the operation of costoplasty. On the concave side, the ribs are crowded together, and there may be discomfort where the lower ribs rub against the iliac crest. The longer the segment of thoracic spine affected, the more severe the effects on respiration.

Most cases of scoliosis are idiopathic (Box 38.1). Rarely, congenital absence of one half of the vertebra or fusion of adjacent vertebrae will lead to a scoliosis. These congenital curves are important in that the full complement of alveoli do not develop in the lung on the concave side of the curve. An echocardiogram should be performed to look for associated cardiac defects.

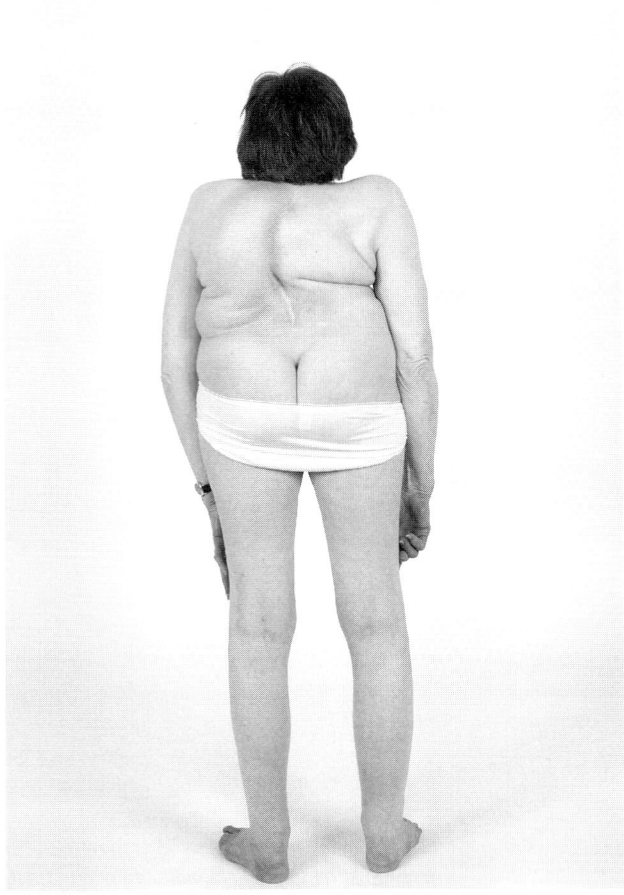

**Figure 38.2** Thoracic scoliosis: note the rib hump, how the person's head is not centred over the pelvis, and how long the arms are compared with the trunk.

**Box 38.1 Classification of scoliosis**

- Congenital (vertebral abnormalities, myelomeningocele)
- Neuromuscular
- Idiopathic
- Connective tissue diseases (Marfan's syndrome, osteogenesis imperfecta)
- Neurofibromatosis
- Vertebral destruction (infection, trauma, tumour, radiation, etc.)
- Thoracoplasty

Familial aggregation of idiopathic scoliosis implies a genetic component to the disease, but other factors affecting bone growth, muscles, nerves, collagen, blood vessels, ligaments etc. are likely to be involved. Much work remains to be done to elucidate the genetics of this disease. For reasons that are not clear, adolescent idiopathic scoliosis is more common in females, with curvature convex to the left. Screening programmes have been put in place to detect asymptomatic scoliosis, with a view to intervening before the curve progresses too far, but their value is much debated. Look carefully for clinical features of an underlying skeletal condition in all patients with scoliosis.

## Scoliosis in neuromuscular disorders

The spine is flanked by two large groups of muscles – the paraspinal muscles. The stabilizing influence of these muscles is illustrated by the fact that patients with diseases such as muscular dystrophy develop scoliosis. When the paraspinal muscles on one side are weak – for example when affected by poliomyelitis – spinal deformity is very common. These curves are sometimes referred to as 'paralytic' scoliosis. The muscle weakness may not become apparent until limb muscles become affected, sometimes many years later. Keep the possibility of an underlying neuromuscular aetiology in mind whenever you review a patient with 'idiopathic' scoliosis.

## Tuberculosis

In the days prior to anti-tuberculous chemotherapy, the operation of thoracoplasty was performed as a means of collapsing upper lobe cavities. Several ribs were removed – sometimes under local anaesthesia. Scoliosis usually developed subsequently, because of loss of the stabilizing effect of the ribs on the spine. These patients always had severe pulmonary tuberculosis (TB), inevitably leaving them with fibrosis and bronchiectasis. They often had other procedures such as phrenic nerve crush or artificial pneumothorax. The aetiology of hypercapnic respiratory failure as a late complication involves many different influences on the work of breathing and capacity of the respiratory muscles. In many published series these patients are referred to as 'sequelae of tuberculosis' rather than 'thoracoplasty'. For simplicity, I will use the term 'post-TB'.

# PATHOPHYSIOLOGY

## Ventilation

As we have noted, scoliosis causes the ribs on the concave side of the curve to be crushed together. Ventilation is reduced on that side. On the convex side, the ribs are splayed apart. If you look carefully at a patient with severe scoliosis, when they breathe in there may well be parts of the rib cage which move in rather than out; this paradoxical motion wastes the inspiratory force generated by the respiratory muscles. Post-TB patients may also have paradoxical motion of the segment of the rib cage where their ribs were removed. We will come back to the mechanics of the rib cage in more detail shortly.

## Perfusion

On the convex side of the spinal curvature, the lungs are over-distended. The pulmonary vascular tree is also stretched, which reduces the size of the vessels. On the concave side, the vessels are less affected, so ventilation–perfusion imbalance is inevitable.[4,5] Ventilation–perfusion matching is worse the more severe the spinal curvature (and the lower the vital capacity) and deteriorates with age.[6] As a result, hypoxia with pulmonary hypertension and right heart failure are common in adults with severe scoliosis.

Right heart failure may be exacerbated by chronic nocturnal hypoxia.[7] Schonhofer *et al.*[8] documented a mean fall in pulmonary artery pressure of 8.5 mm Hg in patients with scoliosis or post-TB after a year of nocturnal non-invasive ventilation (NIV), without any significant change in lung volumes. Mean overnight oxygen saturation increased from 72.5 per cent to 90.5 per cent. It is impossible to work out whether the pulmonary hypertension that persists in many patients despite nocturnal NIV is related to distortion of the pulmonary vascular tree, or reflects irreversible damage from repeated episodes of nocturnal hypoxia over many years (see Sleep below).

## Compliance

Clearly, distorted ribs will be more difficult to expand, so the compliance of the chest wall will be reduced in scoliosis. Compliance is the increase in volume for a set amount of applied inflation pressure. A stiff chest wall will show a smaller increase in size for any given pressure, compared to a more compliant chest wall. The compliance of the whole respiratory system can be measured by observing the increase in volume when positive pressure is applied to the airway (or negative pressure around the outside of the chest, for example in an iron lung), but of course this reflects the compliance of the lungs as well as the rib cage. Alternatively, you could inflate the lungs by a known amount – let us say half a litre – and get the subject to relax onto an occluded mouthpiece; the pressure measured at the mouthpiece is called the elastic recoil pressure, which again includes the pressure from the rib cage and the lungs as they try to deflate back to their normal resting volume. You will gather that it is quite difficult to measure the compliance of the rib cage, because of the need to measure lung compliance as well (which requires an estimate of pleural pressure, such as oesophageal pressure) and to ensure that none of the respiratory muscles are contracting when the pressure measurements are made. Most of the data on rib cage compliance in scoliosis come from patients undergoing spinal surgery under general anaesthesia.

It is less obvious why the compliance of the lung should also be reduced in scoliosis.[9] In congenital scoliosis, the total number of alveoli is less than normal, so the lungs will be less compliant. In addition, chronic under-expansion may lead to changes in the elastic properties of the lung. Inflation to larger lung volumes – as happens with NIV – should help correct these changes. This hypothesis is supported by the observation that 5 minutes of positive pressure breathing in patients with scoliosis resulted in an increase in lung compliance.[10]

## Resistance

Airway calibre is proportional to lung volume. Patients with scoliosis breathe at low lung volumes, so their airway resistance is high[11] and they may be flow-limited towards the end of expiration.[12] Anecdotally, anaesthetists have observed when intubating patients prior to spinal surgery that the trachea is sometimes distorted in severe scoliosis, and that this kinking improves when the spinal curvature is corrected.

The ANTADIR series[13] found that airflow obstruction is an independent predictor for the development of hypercapnic respiratory failure in post-TB and scoliotic patients. Whilst much of this may be post-tuberculous endobronchial scarring or volume-related changes in airway calibre, the possibility of concomitant asthma or chronic obstructive pulmonary disease (COPD) should not be overlooked. Consider a trial of bronchodilator therapy in scoliotic and post-TB patients if they have audible wheeze or obstructive spirometry.

## Work of breathing

The work of breathing in scoliosis at rest is high and related to the extent of restriction.[4,6] Most of this is caused by low compliance rather than increased resistance. In order to keep the work of breathing as low as possible, the person increases their respiratory rate and keep their tidal volumes low.[14] If they need to increase ventilation, for example on exercise or if they become unwell, they are forced to increase their tidal volume. At this point of their compliance curve, it requires much more pressure to produce any change in volume, with the result that the work of breathing increases rapidly.

## Respiratory muscle strength

Contraction of the inspiratory muscles moves the rib cage to produce lung expansion. When the ribs are distorted, the mechanical coupling of the respiratory muscles is disrupted, so the force they exert is less efficient in producing movement of the rib cage. Similarly, the diaphragm is displaced from its normal position and is less effective at displacing the abdominal contents in order to inflate the lungs. Indeed, you may see paradoxical inward motion of some parts of the rib cage during inspiration in patients with scoliosis – another indicator of the mechanical inefficiency of the respiratory muscles, whereby work is wasted on moving the chest wall without producing ventilation.

Many studies have documented low respiratory muscle strength in scoliosis.[9,15–20] After starting NIV, maximum inspiratory pressures are often considerably better. This improvement, in the absence of any significant change in the size or shape of the rib cage, is consistent with the hypothesis that the muscles are weakened by the work they have to do to expand the stiff rib cage. Hypoxia and hypercapnia impair muscle contraction, but there is no consistent relationship between changes in arterial blood gases and the improvement in maximum mouth pressures. The most likely explanation for improvement in these volitional measures of strength after NIV is that the subjects are more awake, feel better and try harder at the tests.

## Respiratory muscle fatigue

So, the respiratory muscles are less effective than normal, but are faced with increased work. Accessory muscles are recruited to help.[9] With each breath, if the force needed to produce an adequate tidal volume starts to approach the maximum available force, then the inspiratory muscles will become fatigued. This may happen insidiously as the chest becomes stiffer and age-related changes weaken the muscles, or acutely when an event such as an infection increases the work of breathing or the ventilation which must be achieved to maintain normal gas exchange.

Some evidence for the existence of respiratory muscle fatigue in scoliosis comes from observations of the effects of NIV. Schonhofer *et al.*[21] documented an improvement in respiratory muscle endurance after three months of nocturnal NIV. The threshold load against which the inspiratory muscles had to work was set at 33 per cent of baseline maximum inspiratory pressure (MIP); this represented only 22 per cent of MIP after NIV, on account of an increase from 43 to 66 cm $H_2O$, so the endurance task was not strictly comparable. Nevertheless, the improvement in endurance time was substantial and likely to represent a real improvement in their resistance to fatigue.

## Respiratory drive

In mild scoliosis, the drive to breathe may be greater than normal in order to maintain normal ventilation, but in more severe cases ventilatory drive is usually reduced.[6] In measuring the ventilatory output in response to elevation of carbon dioxide levels, the drive to breathe might be normal but mechanical factors prevent the patient from increasing tidal volume. This is overcome by looking at the pressure generated when the airway is occluded briefly – one tenth of a second, hence the term P0.1.

Impaired ventilatory drive could be a protective strategy, allowing the arterial carbon dioxide to rise in order to protect the respiratory muscles if they are in danger of becoming fatigued. This implies a reduction in alveolar ventilation to a level which the muscles may be able to sustain. In addition, a rise in arterial carbon dioxide levels increases the back pressure driving carbon dioxide out of the blood stream into the air which is to be exhaled, so overall carbon dioxide elimination from the body is increased.

Bicarbonate accumulates in patients with chronic hypercapnic respiratory failure. This larger pool of buffer blunts any change in pH with any further increases in carbon dioxide, which means that the ventilatory response to carbon dioxide is impaired. Possibly the most likely explanation for the blunted respiratory drive in scoliosis is that it is the consequence of sleep deprivation and repeated periods of hypoventilation at night. Improvement in the ventilatory response to carbon dioxide is a fairly consistent finding after NIV, even in the absence of any change in chest wall mechanics or respiratory muscle strength.[21–23]

## Sleep

Sleep is associated with a reduction in ventilation and ventilatory drive, and elevation of arterial carbon dioxide levels. In scoliosis, rapid eye movement (REM) sleep seems to be the most vulnerable period.[7,24–28] Central hypoventilation and periodic breathing are the most common abnormalities. Apnoeas are usually central, although obstructive episodes have been described.[24]

During REM sleep, breathing is less regular and tidal volumes fall. The intercostal and accessory muscles are inhibited in this phase of sleep, and the diaphragm alone may be incapable of maintaining adequate alveolar ventilation. Loss of intercostal tone will reduce functional residual capacity; since there is less oxygen within the lungs to act as a buffer, any episodes of hypoventilation will have a more profound effect on arterial oxygen saturation.

The vulnerability of this group of patients to problems during sleep is emphasized by studies of NIV withdrawal. Hill *et al.*[29] reported the effects of withdrawing nocturnal NIV from patients with chronic hypercapnic respiratory failure. Of the six patients studied, two had scoliosis and two had a thoracoplasty. The intention was to stop NIV for 2 weeks, but only two patients managed this because of sleep disturbance and recurrence of their daytime symptoms, associated with deterioration in nocturnal gas exchange. Masa Jiménez *et al.*[26] investigated the effect of withdrawing NIV for 15 days in five patients with scoliosis or post-TB. During REM sleep, gas exchange was much worse than it had been when they were on NIV, with disruption of their sleep pattern.

## Respiratory effects of spinal surgery for scoliosis

Surgical correction of spinal curvature may be undertaken for cosmetic appearances. In muscular dystrophy, stabilization of the spine may be necessary for maintenance of posture, but the effect on lung function is often disappointing.[30,31] In idiopathic scoliosis, good quality evidence on the respiratory consequences of spinal surgery is sparse. Overall, it seems that any improvement in the mechanics of respiration is likely to be small, and surgery should not be undertaken for this reason alone. A period of halo traction pre-operatively may help identify those patients whose curvature can be improved, with concomitant increase in vital capacity.[32] Spinal surgery is a major undertaking with a significant mortality,[33] although this may change with refinement of surgical techniques. The post-operative use of NIV will be considered below.

## Scoliosis and the risk of hypercapnic respiratory failure

On the basis of the pathophysiology we have considered and the evidence of large observational studies,[4,34–36] patients with scoliosis who have the following features should be considered at greater risk of developing ventilatory failure:

- the thoracic spine is involved
- the curvature was present before the age of 5 years
- the angle of curvature is greater than 90°
- the vital capacity is less than 50 per cent of predicted
- the spine has never been surgically stabilized
- the scoliosis is secondary to neuromuscular weakness (including poliomyelitis)
- there is additional lung disease such as asthma or COPD.

This may help you identify patients who need to be kept under regular review. In addition to measuring vital capacity, you should have a low threshold for measuring arterial blood gases and assessing gas exchange overnight.

## Post-tuberculosis

These patients are almost invariably hypoxic, on account of their extensive pulmonary scarring.[37,38] The work of breathing is high, and the mechanical efficiency of the chest wall impaired as a consequence of removal of ribs. The capacity of the inspiratory muscles may be impaired by phrenic nerve crush or avulsion. On this basis it seems reasonable to suggest that they might develop respiratory muscle fatigue, which NIV could relieve. Although detailed studies are lacking, REM sleep is likely to be a vulnerable period for this group of patients, for exactly the same reasons as for those with scoliosis.

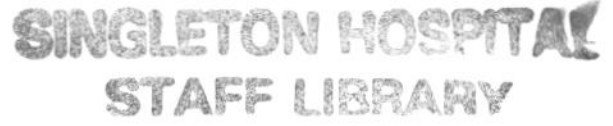

## EVIDENCE BASE

### Early trials

In 1988, Ellis *et al.*[39] reported a study of seven patients with scoliosis who were in hypercapnic respiratory failure. Two improved on CPAP, but the remaining five needed NIV. Traditional volume controlled ventilators designed for home use were fitted to customized nasal masks. Abnormal gas exchange during sleep was corrected, accompanied by improvement in sleep quality. After 3 months of NIV, daytime blood gases and maximum inspiratory pressure were also better. This new technique was soon taken up by centres around the world that historically had provided ventilatory support via a tracheostomy or older non-invasive techniques such as external negative pressure ventilation or rocking beds. Bach and Alba[40] included five patients with scoliosis in a mixed group of 52 patients transferring to NIV from other methods of ventilatory support, in whom it was shown to be effective in maintaining normal gas exchange. In Bach's centre and many others this signalled a rapid drift away from the use of tracheostomy.

Zaccaria *et al.*[41] reported their experience with 17 scoliotic patients. The more severely compromised patients were managed with a tracheostomy, the remainder with NIV. They noted similar improvements in gas exchange in both groups, suggesting that they were equally effective. Leger *et al.*[42] reported reduction in hospitalization and improvement in blood gases in 105 scoliotic and 80 post-TB patients. Three years after starting NIV, survival was 76 per cent for the post-TB and scoliosis groups. The survival of patients with scoliosis secondary to poliomyelitis was noted to be just as good as for idiopathic scoliosis. Pehrsson *et al.*[43] included 13 patients with scoliosis and 5 post-TB in a survey of patients on home mechanical ventilation, in which they found good psychosocial functioning and mental wellbeing, in spite of severe physical limitations.

Jackson *et al.*[44] followed 32 post-TB patients who were treated with different methods of NIV. The 5-year survival was 74 per cent. Arterial blood gases improved in the first few days of NIV, but with little further improvement subsequently. Slowly deteriorating arterial blood gases were associated with worsening right heart failure and a poor prognosis.

### Wider experience

As the size of reported series became larger, confidence grew in NIV as an effective long-term treatment. Simmonds and Elliott[45] reported 5-year survival of 79 per cent for scoliosis ($n = 47$), 100 per cent for polio ($n = 30$) and 94 per cent for post-TB ($n = 20$). As other groups had noted, arterial blood gases improved in the months after starting and NIV and remained stable thereafter.

In 1996, Chailleux *et al.*[13] reported the French ANTADIR experience of over 26 000 patients using oxygen or ventilators at home. NIV was associated with increased survival, particularly for scoliosis compared to post-TB. In 2005, Lloyd-Owen *et al.*[46] reported the results of the Eurovent study, in which approximately a third of patients had thoracic deformity as the aetiology of their ventilatory failure.

### Mechanisms

#### MECHANICS

Once it was clear that NIV was effective, attention turned to how it worked. Some studies showed an increase in vital capacity,[47] but in the majority of reports there was little change. The consistent improvement in gas exchange is unlikely to be explained by changes in the mechanics of the lungs or rib cage.

#### MUSCLES

Respiratory muscle strength often improves with NIV. The study of Schonhofer *et al.*[21] showing improved respiratory muscle endurance is consistent with the hypothesis that NIV rests the respiratory muscles and allows them to recover from respiratory muscle fatigue. Gonzalez *et al.*[48] undertook a prospective study of 16 patients with scoliosis who were treated with NIV for 3 years. Vital capacity and minimal inspiratory pressure increased, with the result that the duty cycle of the inspiratory muscles moved away from the critical fatigue threshold. The possibility remains that the improvement in respiratory drive seen with NIV (see below) is only possible because the respiratory muscles regain the capacity to do the work necessary to maintain normal alveolar ventilation.

#### DRIVE

Non-invasive ventilation leads to an improvement in ventilatory drive. Dellborg *et al.*[22] showed improvement in the ventilator response to hypercapnia after 9 months of NIV in patients with alveolar ventilation from a variety of causes, including four with scoliosis. The magnitude of improvement correlated with changes in daytime and overnight carbon dioxide levels. Nickol *et al.*[23] included eight patients with scoliosis in a study of the mechanism of improvement of respiratory failure with NIV. After 3 months, this subgroup showed similar improvement in $PaCO_2$ and hypercapnic respiratory drive to the patients with neuromuscular problems.

Increased ventilatory drive is likely to be a pivotal mechanism for the longer term changes seen with NIV. The changes in drive seem to correlate well with improved gas exchange, both during NIV and while breathing spontaneously. It is unclear whether the improvement in gas exchange causes the increase in drive, or the other way round.

### SLEEP

Gas exchange is undoubtedly worse during sleep in scoliosis, and is corrected by NIV. Masa *et al.*[27] included seven scoliotic and one post-TB patient in a study of 21 patients with nocturnal hypoventilation. Gas exchange was much worse in REM sleep, and these abnormalities were corrected more effectively by NIV than supplementary oxygen. Schonhofer and Kohler[28] studied 11 patients with scoliosis of which four were post-TB. Polysomnography showed improvement in sleep architecture. On the other hand, Buyse *et al.*[47] failed to show much change in sleep architecture with NIV in their patients, despite improvement in gas exchange. Bach *et al.*[49] studied seven patients with scoliosis (one secondary to pleuroparietal TB) who had been using NIV at night for 3 months or more. Symptoms, hospitalization rates, daytime $PaCO_2$ and overnight oxygenation improved, but again polysomnographic sleep parameters were not significantly different.

Further light on the relevance of sleep comes from a study by Schonhofer *et al.*[50] comparing nocturnal with diurnal NIV. Seventeen patients were included in each group, six with scoliosis and seven post-TB. In both groups, gas exchange during the day and overnight improved and sleep studies showed an improvement in sleep architecture even with daytime NIV.

In summary, improving alveolar ventilation using NIV leads to recovery of respiratory drive. This leads to increased ventilation when breathing spontaneously, which can only be maintained because the respiratory muscles are in better shape than they were before NIV was started. Sleeping better probably helps, but is not pivotal.

## CLINICAL APPLICATIONS

### Hypercapnic respiratory failure

An elevated daytime $PaCO_2$ in a scoliotic or post-TB patient almost always means they have passed a critical point whereby their respiratory muscles are too fatigued to maintain normal alveolar ventilation. Non-invasive ventilation should be started soon, since a small further reduction in alveolar ventilation will result in a disproportionately large – and potentially dangerous – rise in $PaCO_2$. If the daytime $PaCO_2$ has risen during an acute illness and returned to normal, it is usually appropriate to discuss starting NIV anyway: the transient elevation in $PaCO_2$ implies very little reserve, and the likelihood of needing NIV within a year is very high.

### Nocturnal hypoventilation

Patients who hypoventilate during the daytime will always be worse at night. During the progression towards diurnal respiratory failure, there will be a stage where they are normocapnic during the day, but hypoventilate at night. Periods of oxygen desaturation are seen commonly when performing screening sleep studies on patients with scoliosis who have no symptoms of nocturnal hypoventilation. More detailed monitoring will reveal that these periods occur in REM sleep and are associated with a rise in $PaCO_2$. These episodes may be truly asymptomatic, but it is important to question the patient carefully – the classical morning headaches are much less common than vaguer symptoms such as poor appetite, lethargy, tiredness etc. Masa *et al.*[27] noted that their patients considered themselves asymptomatic, but reported that they felt a lot better on NIV.

Ward *et al.*[51] reported a prospective trial of elective NIV versus a wait-and-watch approach in 26 patients with nocturnal hypoventilation but normal daytime arterial blood gases. Most of the patients had neuromuscular problems but small numbers of patients with scoliosis were included in each group. The main conclusion of the study was that patients with asymptomatic nocturnal hypoventilation are likely to need NIV within the following 2 years. It is difficult to know how well this applies to the scoliotic subgroup: the authors of the paper themselves noted that nocturnal hypoventilation may evolve more slowly than in neuromuscular patients.

### Daytime non-invasive ventilation

Schonhofer *et al.*[48] suggested that daytime NIV is as effective as nocturnal use. Clearly it is less intrusive for the patients to use NIV at night, but if they are unable to sleep with the ventilator on – as sometimes happens – then daytime use is an alternative. There will be a time on NIV below which it is ineffective, but even a few hours is probably better than nothing. Highcock *et al.*[52] studied daytime NIV to see if this improved exercise capacity on a treadmill in scoliosis, but it appears to be ineffective in this regard. An hour or two of NIV in the middle of the day may be beneficial for a patient using nocturnal NIV who finds they are struggling to last all day breathing spontaneously. Whether this works by resting the respiratory muscles or altering the mechanics of the lungs and/or chest wall is not known.

### Post-operative (spinal surgery)

It can often be anticipated that a patient with scoliosis undergoing spinal surgery is likely to need ventilatory support for a few days post-operatively. Traditionally, this has involved an elective tracheostomy, but NIV may be an alternative in selected patients. Given that the surgery is almost always planned well in advance, the opportunity should be taken to get the patient accustomed to NIV pre-operatively. This improves the chances of avoiding a tracheostomy post-operatively, since the patient has had time to become accustomed to the mask and ventilator.

## TECHNICAL CONSIDERATIONS

### Mode

Bi-level pressure support ventilators, commonly used to treat hypercapnic respiratory failure in acute exacerbations of COPD, are not ideal for correcting hypoventilation in scoliosis. Given their wide availability, they can be used when patients present acutely,[27,29] but as soon as possible the patient should be transferred onto a ventilator which has a 'control' mode.

The aim of NIV in scoliosis is to provide adequate alveolar ventilation, resting the respiratory muscles and normalizing arterial blood gases. This is achieved by using a control mode of ventilation, whereby the patient is not required to trigger the ventilator on or off. This can be thought of as 'providing' rather than 'supporting' ventilation. Pressure- or volume-targeted modes can be used, although the former are used much more commonly these days. Volume control remains an option for patients in whom normalization of gas exchange is problematical.

Schonhofer *et al.*[53] studied a group of 30 patients with chronic ventilatory failure which included four with scoliosis and eight post-TB. After 1 month of volume controlled NIV, respiratory rate, $PaCO_2$, P0.1, P0.1/MIP, MIP and VT had all improved. When switched to pressure controlled NIV, some patients deteriorated, only to recover when they returned to the volume controlled mode. These patients were slightly more hypoxic and more hypercapnic before treatment, but it was not possible to predict at the outset which mode would suit which patient. In practice, pressure controlled NIV is likely to be the first choice, but the option of changing to volume controlled should be borne in mind if the patient does not improve after a month or so.

Tuggey and Elliott[54] compared pressure- and volume-targeted NIV in 13 patients with chest wall deformity. There was no difference in efficacy between the two modes. The authors noted patients would settle for a low back-up rate, even when this compromised nocturnal ventilation. Leakage was the main cause of persisting hypoventilation in both groups.

### Pressure

We have already noted that the compliance of the chest wall is low in patients with scoliosis, so they need high pressures to inflate their chest. This pressure is likely to be at least 25 cm $H_2O$, and this should be the starting pressure for pressure-targeted modes.

If a bi-level pressure ventilator is used, the expiratory pressure should be kept as low as possible.

### Rate

Patients with scoliosis will allow their respiratory rate to drop during sleep, even if this means that they do not maintain adequate alveolar ventilation. For this reason, the back-up rate should be set fairly high.

It is vital for the patient to coordinate with the ventilator during NIV. Patients with scoliosis may breathe at rates of 30 or more breaths per minute. Start with a rate similar to their spontaneous rate; as they get used to NIV, their rate may slow down a little, and you can reduce the back-up rate accordingly. For most patients with scoliosis the range will be 15–20 breaths per minute, but occasionally you will need to leave them with a higher rate in order to maintain coordination with the ventilator.

### Inspiratory time

In order to minimize the peak pressure which the inspiratory muscles have to develop, patients with scoliosis may prolong their inspiratory time. An inspiratory:expiratory ratio of 1:1 or even higher may be necessary for full inflation of the chest. In the majority of patients, expiration is not a problem, so they tolerate short expiratory times without becoming hyperinflated.

### Rise time

In ventilators with the facility to adjust this parameter, rise time should be set initially to match the patient's own spontaneous breathing pattern. Further adjustments should be guided by how comfortable the patient feels on the ventilator.

### Oxygen

Ventilation–perfusion imbalance can cause persistent hypoxia in scoliosis. Asymptomatic desaturation in REM sleep is quite common in patients with scoliosis on NIV, but if right heart failure does not resolve despite correction of nocturnal hypoventilation, then it seems reasonable to add in supplementary oxygen, aiming for a mean oxygen saturation greater than 90 per cent.

## FUTURE RESEARCH

The aetiology of scoliosis seems likely to be multifactorial, but more research is needed to identify the genetic factors involved and their interaction with environmental influences. As surgical techniques are refined and become less invasive, there will be a need for studies to review the effect of correcting the deformity on lung function. More sophisticated imaging techniques may allow us to study the physiology of respiration in real time, for example how ventilation and perfusion are distributed in the lungs of patients, and whether NIV has an effect on this.

While there seems little doubt that the respiratory muscles develop fatigue, more studies are needed on how they adapt to changes in their operational length – because of distortion of the rib cage – and increased workload. Allowing arterial carbon dioxide levels to rise may be a protective mechanism to prevent irreversible damage in respiratory muscles in the face of a load/capacity ratio that is unsustainable. This hypothesis is supported by the recovery of drive when NIV is started, but serial studies of the hypercapnic ventilatory response as patients with scoliosis approach respiratory failure would be interesting.

## SUMMARY

- Patients with a scoliosis are at risk of hypercapnic respiratory failure if:
  - the thoracic spine is involved
  - the curvature was present before the age of 5 years
  - the angle of curvature is greater than 90°
  - the vital capacity is less than 50 per cent of predicted
  - the spine has never been surgically stabilized
  - the scoliosis is secondary to neuromuscular weakness (including poliomyelitis)
  - there is additional lung disease such as asthma or COPD.
- If the daytime $PaCO_2$ is elevated in a patient with scoliosis, they need to start nocturnal NIV and stay on it indefinitely.
- NIV parameters in a patient with scoliosis should be:
  - pressure control mode (i.e. the patient triggers neither the start nor the end of inspiration)
  - inspiratory positive airway pressure (IPAP) of at least 25 cm $H_2O$
  - lowest expiratory positive airway pressure (EPAP) possible if bi-level circuit used
  - respiratory rate and inspiratory time approximately the same as the patient's spontaneous breathing pattern.

## REFERENCES


1. Kearon C, Viviani GR, Kirkley A. Factors determining pulmonary function in adolescent idiopathic thoracic scoliosis. *Am Rev Respir Dis* 1993; **148**: 288–94.
2. Cobb JR. Outline for the study of scoliosis. *Instr Course Lect* 1948; **5**: 261–75.
3. Hepper NGG, Black LF, Fowler WS. Relationship of lung volume to height and arm span in normal subjects and in patients with spinal deformity. *Am Rev Respir Dis* 1965; **91**: 356–62.
4. Bergofsky EH, Turino GM, Fishman AP. Cardiorespiratory failure in kyphoscoliosis. *Medicine (Baltimore)* 1959; **38**: 263–317.
5. Giordano A, Fuso L, Calcagni ML *et al.* Evaluation of pulmonary ventilation and diaphragmatic movement in idiopathic scoliosis using radioaerosol ventilation scintigraphy. *Nucl Med Commun* 1997; **18**: 105–11.
6. Kafer ER. Idiopathic scoliosis. Gas exchange and the age dependence of arterial blood gases. *J Clin Invest* 1976; **58**: 825–33.
7. Mezon BL, West P, Israels J *et al.* Sleep breathing abnormalities in kyphoscoliosis. *Am Rev Respir Dis* 1980; **122**: 617–21.
8. Schonhofer B, Barchfeld T, Wenzel M *et al.* Long term effects of non-invasive mechanical ventilation on pulmonary haemodynamics in patients with chronic respiratory failure. *Thorax* 2001; **56**: 524–8.
9. Estenne M, Derom E, De Troyer A. Neck and abdominal muscle activity in patients with severe thoracic scoliosis. *Am J Respir Crit Care Med* 1998; **158**: 452–7.
10. Sinha R, Bergovsky EH. Prolonged alteration of lung mechanics in kyphoscoliosis by positive pressure hyperinflation. *Am Rev Respir Dis* 1972; **106**: 47–57.
11. van Noord JA, Cauberghs M, Van de Woestijne KP *et al.* Total respiratory resistance and reactance in ankylosing spondylitis and kyphoscoliosis. *Eur Resp J* 1991; **4**: 945–51.
12. Bjure J, Grimby G, Kasalicky J *et al.* Respiratory impairment and airway closure in patients with untreated idiopathic scoliosis. *Thorax* 1970; **25**: 451–6.
13. Chailleux E, Fauroux B, Binet F *et al.* Predictors of survival in patients receiving domiciliary oxygen therapy or mechanical ventilation. A 10-year analysis of ANTADIR observatory. *Chest* 1996; **109**: 741–9.
14. Ramonatxo M, Milic-Emili J, Prefaut C. Breathing pattern and load compensatory responses in young scoliotic patients. *Eur Resp J* 1988; **1**: 421–7.
15. Jones RS, Kennedy JD, Hasham F *et al.* Mechanical inefficiency of the thoracic cage in scoliosis. *Thorax* 1981; **36**: 456–61.
16. Cook CD, Barrie H, DeForest SA *et al.* Lung volumes, mechanics of respiration and respiratory muscle strength in scoliosis. *Pediatrics* 1960; **25**: 766–74.
17. Smyth RJ, Chapman KR, Wright TA *et al.* Pulmonary function in adolescents with mild idiopathic scoliosis. *Thorax* 1984; **39**: 901–4.
18. Lisboa C, Moreni R, Fava M *et al.* Inspiratory muscle function in patients with severe kyphoscoliosis. *Am Rev Respir Dis* 1985; **132**: 48–52.
19. Szeinberg A, Canny GJ, Rashed N *et al.* Forced vital capacity and maximal respiratory pressures in patients with mild and moderate scoliosis. *Pediatr Pulmonol* 1988; **4**: 8–12.
20. Cooper DM, Rojas JV, Mellins RB *et al.* Respiratory mechanics in adolescents with idiopathic scoliosis. *Am Rev Respir Dis* 1984; **130**: 16–22.
21. Schonhofer B, Wallstein S, Wiese C *et al.* Noninvasive mechanical ventilation improves endurance performance in patients with chronic respiratory failure due to thoracic restriction. *Chest* 2001; **119**: 1371–8.
22. Dellborg C, Olofson J, Hamnegard C-H *et al.* Ventilatory response to CO2 re-breathing before and after nocturnal nasal intermittent positive pressure ventilation in patients with chronic alveolar hypoventilation. *Respir Med* 2000; **94**: 1154–60.

23. Nickol AH, Hart N, Hopkinson NS *et al.* Mechanisms of improvement of respiratory failure in patients with restrictive thoracic disease treated with non-invasive ventilation. *Thorax* 2005; **60**: 754–60.
24. Guilleminault C, Kurland G, Winkle R *et al.* Severe kyphosis, breathing and sleep. *Chest* 1982; **79**: 626–30.
25. Sawicka EH, Branthwaite MA. Respiration during sleep in kyphoscoliosis. *Thorax* 1987; **42**: 801–8.
26. Masa Jiménez JF, Sénchez de Cos Escuin J, Disdier Vicente C *et al.* Nasal intermittent positive pressure ventilation. Analysis of its withdrawal. *Chest* 1995; **107**: 382–8.
27. Masa JF, Celli B, Riesco JA *et al.* Noninvasive positive pressure ventilation and not oxygen may prevent overt ventilatory failure in patients with chest wall diseases. *Chest* 1997; **112**: 207–13.
28. Schonhofer B, Kohler D. Effect of non-invasive mechanical ventilation on sleep and nocturnal ventilation in patients with chronic respiratory failure. *Thorax* 2000; **55**: 308–13.
29. Hill NS, Eveloff SE, Carlisle CC *et al.* Efficacy of nocturnal nasal ventilation in patients with restrictive thoracic disease. *Am Rev Respir Dis* 1992; **145**: 365–71.
30. Larsson E-LC, Aaro SI, Normelli HCM *et al.* Long-term follow-up of functioning after spinal surgery in patients with neuromuscular scoliosis. *Spine* 2005; **30**: 2145–52.
31. Kennedy JD, Staples AJ, Brook PD *et al.* Effect of spinal surgery on lung function in Duchenne muscular dystrophy. *Thorax* 1995; **50**: 1173–8.
32. Swank SM, Winter RB, Moe JH. Scoliosis and cor pulmonale. *Spine* 1982; **7**: 343–54.
33. Rizzi PE, Winter RB, Lonstein JE *et al.* Adult spinal deformity and respiratory failure. Surgical results in 35 patients. *Spine* 1997; **22**: 2517–31.
34. Branthwaite MA. Cardiorespiratory consequences of unfused idiopathic scoliosis. *Chest* 1986; **80**: 360–9.
35. Pehrsson K, Bake B, Larsson S *et al.* Lung function in adult idiopathic scoliosis: a 20 year follow up. *Thorax* 1991; **46**: 474–8.
36. Pehrsson K, Nachemson A, Olofson J *et al.* Respiratory failure in scoliosis and other thoracic deformities. A survey of patients with home oxygen or ventilator therapy in Sweden. *Spine* 1992; **17**: 714–18.
37. Phillips MS, Kinnear WJ, Shneerson JM. Late sequelae of pulmonary tuberculosis treated by thoracoplasty. *Thorax* 1987; **42**: 445–51.
38. Phillips MS, Miller MR, Kinnear WJ *et al.* Importance of airflow obstruction after thoracoplasty. *Thorax* 1987; **42**: 348–52.
39. Ellis ER, Grunstein RR, Chan S *et al.* Noninvasive ventilatory support during sleep improves respiratory failure in kyphoscoliosis. *Chest* 1988; **94**: 811–15.
40. Bach JR, Alba AS. Management of chronic alveolar hypoventilation by nasal ventilation. *Chest* 1990; **97**: 52–7.
41. Zaccaria S, Zaccaria E, Zanaboni S *et al.* Home mechanical ventilation in kyphoscoliosis. *Monaldi Arch Chest Dis* 1993; **48**: 161–4.
42. Leger P, Bedicam JM, Conrnette A *et al.* Nasal intermittent positive pressure ventilation. Long-term follow-up in patients with severe chronic respiratory insufficiency. *Chest* 1994; **105**: 100–5.
43. Pehrsson K, Olofson J, Larsson S *et al.* Quality of life of patients treated by home mechanical ventilation due to restrictive disorders. *Resp Med* 1994; **88**: 21–6.
44. Jackson M, Smith I, King M *et al.* Long term domiciliary assisted ventilation for respiratory failure following thoracoplasty. *Thorax* 1994; **49**: 915–19.
45. Simonds AK, Elliott MW. Outcome of domiciliary nasal intermittent positive pressure ventilation in restrictive and obstructive disorders. *Thorax* 1995; **50**: 604–9.
46. Lloyd-Owen SJ, Donaldson GC, Ambrosino N *et al.* Patterns of home mechanical ventilation use in Europe: results of the Eurovent survey. *Eur Resp J* 2005; **25**: 1025–31.
47. Buyse B, Meersseman W, Demedts M. Treatment of chronic respiratory failure in kyphoscoliosis: oxygen or ventilation? *Eur Resp J* 2003; **22**: 525–8.
48. Gonzalez C, Ferris G, Diaz J *et al.* Kyphoscoliotic ventilatory insufficiency. Effects of long-term intermittent positive-pressure ventilation. *Chest* 2003; **124**: 857–62.
49. Bach JR, Robert D, Leger P *et al.* Sleep fragmentation in kyphoscoliotic individuals with alveolar hypoventilation treated by NIPPV. *Chest* 1995; **107**: 1552–8.
50. Schonhofer B, Geibel M, Sonneborn M *et al.* Daytime mechanical ventilation in chronic respiratory insufficiency. *Eur Resp J* 1997; **10**: 2840–6.
51. Ward S, Chatwin M, Heather S *et al.* Randomised controlled trial of non-invasive ventilation (NIV) for nocturnal hypoventilation in neuromuscular and chest wall disease patients with daytime normocapnia. *Thorax* 2005; **60**: 1019–24.
52. Highcock MP, Smith IE, Shneerson JM. The effect of noninvasive intermittent positive-pressure ventilation during exercise in severe scoliosis. *Chest* 2002; **121**: 1555–60.
53. Schonhofer B, Sonneborn M, Haidl P *et al.* Comparison of two different modes for non-invasive mechanical ventilation in chronic respiratory failure: volume versus pressure controlled device. *Eur Resp J* 1997; **10**: 184–91.
54. Tuggey JM, Elliott MW. Randomised crossover study of pressure and volume non-invasive ventilation in chest wall deformity. *Thorax* 2005; **60**: 859–64.

# SECTION I

# Obesity

# 39

# The endocrinologist and respiratory failure

JOHN P H WILDING

## ABSTRACT

Respiratory failure may be associated with a variety of endocrine disorders, for example muscle weakness due to Cushing's syndrome, and exogenous corticosteroids may contribute to respiratory failure in some conditions; the strongest associations are with obesity, which has several adverse effects on lung function, reducing lung volumes, increasing airways resistance and increasing ventilation–perfusion mismatch. This may contribute to increased risk of respiratory failure in a variety of clinical conditions such as asthma and chronic obstructive pulmonary disease. The most severe manifestations lead to development of obesity-related hypoventilation. Effects of obesity on the upper airways are a major factor in the aetiology of obstructive sleep apnoea, which is independently associated with hypertension, dyslipidaemia, insulin resistance and type 2 diabetes. Interventions to improve nocturnal apnoeas, such as continuous positive airway pressure (CPAP), may have beneficial metabolic effects, and weight loss will benefit both conditions. Patients with obesity-related hypoventilation will require non-invasive ventilation until they successfully lose weight. Interventions to help weight loss include lifestyle change, drugs and surgery. The beneficial effects of weight loss on respiratory conditions and the risk of respiratory failure have not been systematically investigated in prospective clinical trials, although observational studies suggest benefit is likely.

## INTRODUCTION

Specialists in endocrine disease may become involved in the care of patients requiring non-invasive ventilation (NIV) for two main reasons.

- An endocrine or metabolic disorder is the primary reason for ventilation. In most cases this will be because the patient is severely obese or has a multisystem disease (for example myotonic dystrophy) with associated endocrine abnormalities.
- A patient requiring NIV has an underlying endocrine disorder that may complicate or contribute to the requirement for NIV. Common examples here include diabetes, hypercortisolism (Cushing's syndrome or exogenous steroid treatment), hypothalamic–pituitary disease and hypothyroidism.

Much of the associated pathology is associated with or the result of obesity, so this chapter will focus on the relationship between obesity and respiratory function and disease, with reference to other metabolic and endocrine diseases as appropriate.

## PATHOPHYSIOLOGY OF OBESITY

### Definitions and classification

Obesity describes an increase in body fat to the level at which it has adverse effects on health. The degree of obesity is usually defined using the body mass index (BMI), calculated as weight (kg)/height ($m^2$), and this is generally used in clinical practice and epidemiological studies (Table 39.1).[1] Body mass index is only a surrogate measure of adiposity; studies using more accurate measures such as dual emission X-ray absorptiometry (DEXA) or magnetic resonance imaging show that there is a large variance in body fatness and of body fat distribution at any given level of BMI. Measurement of waist circumference or

**Table 39.1** Classification and disease risk associated with obesity, based on body mass index and waist circumference

| | Body mass index | Waist circumference | | |
|---|---|---|---|---|
| | | <80 cm women <94 cm men | >80 cm women >94 cm men | >94 cm women >102 cm men |
| Underweight | <18.5 | | | |
| Healthy weight | 18.6–25.0 | Low | Increased | High |
| Overweight | 25.1–30.0 | Low | Increased | High |
| Obese Class I | 30.1–35.0 | Increased | High | Very high |
| Obese Class 2 | 35.1–40.0 | High | Very high | Very high |
| Obese Class 3 | >40.0 | Very high | Very high | Very high |

Sources: World Health Organization, National Institute for Health and Clinical Excellence Clinical guideline 43 (2007).

waist/hip ratio may provide a better index of total body adiposity than BMI and therefore may better predict the risk of metabolic complications of obesity, such as diabetes and heart disease (Table 39.1).

## Epidemiology

Obesity has become increasingly common in most Western societies over the past 20–30 years and is rapidly spreading to the developing world. For example in the UK, 6 per cent of men and 8 per cent of women were obese in 1980; by 2007 this had risen to 23.6 per cent of men and 24.4 per cent of women.[2] In the USA, prevalence rates of 30 per cent are now common in many states. The International Obesity Task Force (www.iotf.org) provides comprehensive data on obesity prevalence throughout the world.

### SEVERE (MORBID) OBESITY

As obesity has become more common, severe obesity (BMI >40 kg/m$^2$) has also increased rapidly. In the UK, this now affects 1.3 per cent of men and 2.2 per cent of women.[2] Such individuals are at particularly high risk of obesity-related disease, particularly diabetes, respiratory disorders including sleep apnoea and obesity hypoventilation syndrome, cardiac disease, sudden death, arthritis, immobility and psychological problems.

Recently some authors have suggested an alternative classification, with staging of obesity based on the presence of comorbidity and disability;[3] although this is yet to be widely accepted, it may provide a useful framework for use in clinical practice.

## Aetiology

The aetiology of obesity is complex. Fundamentally weight gain results from an imbalance between energy intake and energy expenditure over time. In humans (as opposed to experimental rodents, where metabolic rate is quantitatively more important because of their small body size), this is usually the result of increased food intake. The degree of energy imbalance required to gain substantial amounts of weight over many years is not great: an additional 100 kcal per day could result in 5 kg weight gain over a year. Genetic, psychological, social and environmental factors all play a part in determining an individual's BMI. Although it is clear that genetics cannot explain the recent rise in obesity in the population, genetic studies clearly show that at least 50–70 per cent of the population variance in BMI is due to inheritable factors.[4] The importance of appetite control is demonstrated by a number of rare single gene disorders that result in extreme obesity. All of these are due to defects in pathways that regulate appetite, and include deficiency of the adipose-tissue hormone leptin, which signals body fat content to the central nervous system, and defects in downstream pathways responsive to leptin, including the melanocortin-4 receptor (POMC), and brain-derived neurotrophic factor.[5] Much of the population risk is polygenic, with individual genes only contributing to a small proportion of risk; the most powerful of these, *FTO* (discovered as a result of a genome-wide scan looking for genes for type 2 diabetes), is associated with a 1.5 kg greater weight for heterozygotes, and 3 kg for homozygotes.[6]

The societal and environmental factors causing the current epidemic are complex, but include easy availability of energy dense food of high hedonic value, coupled with an increasingly sedentary lifestyle. Individual psychological factors are also important and may promote or help maintain obesity in susceptible individuals. A more detailed discussion of the aetiology of obesity can be found in the UK government's *Foresight report* (www.foresight.gov.uk/OurWork/ActiveProjects/Obesity/Obesity.asp).

## Medical complications of obesity

Obesity is associated with an increased risk of many diseases. Most focus has been on the metabolic consequences of obesity, including insulin resistance, type 2 diabetes, dyslipidaemia (increased low-density lipoprotein [LDL] and total cholesterol, decreased high-density lipoprotein [HDL] cholesterol and increased triglycerides), hypertension and greater risk of vascular disease, particularly ischaemic heart disease and stroke. Other metabolic consequences of obesity include hyperuricaemia and disorders of sex hormone metabolism, including polycystic ovarian syndrome. Several cancers are more common in the obese; many of these are hormone dependent (such as breast, endometrial and prostate).[7] Mechanical consequences of obesity include joint pain, osteoarthritis, skin problems such as intertrigo and lymphoedema and respiratory problems including breathlessness (often in the absence of overt lung or cardiac disease), increased snoring, obstructive sleep apnoea and obesity hypoventilation syndrome.[8] Many epidemiological studies also report increased rates of asthma in the obese, although this may be confounded by breathlessness in the absence of objective evidence of bronchial hyper-reactivity.[9,10]

### Mechanisms of disease in obesity

The mechanisms by which obesity adversely affects metabolism are not fully understood. Obese individuals are more likely to be resistant to the actions of insulin; increased fat mass may contribute to insulin resistance in a number of ways. These include increased availability of free fatty acids, which may compete with glucose for metabolism within the cell; expanded adipocytes produce increased amounts of some secreted proteins, termed adipokines. For example tumour necrosis factor α, interleukin-6 and resistin may contribute to the development of insulin resistance either by directly interfering with insulin receptor action or by other mechanisms.[11] Adipocytes also produce a protective factor, adiponectin. Circulating adiponectin falls as fat mass rises, which may contribute to insulin resistance.[12] Sympathetic nervous system activity is high in obesity, which also promotes insulin resistance and hypertension.[13]

Fat deposition outside adipocytes (ectopic fat) may also cause insulin resistance and contribute to obesity-related disease. The main sites of ectopic fat deposition are the liver (contributing to insulin resistance in the liver, and to the development of non-alcoholic fatty liver disease, which may progress to cirrhosis), muscles, contributing to insulin resistance, reduced exercise capacity and the islets of Langerhans in the pancreas where it might contribute to islet dysfunction and the development of type 2 diabetes mellitus.[14]

Increased insulin resistance, with greater activity of insulin on insulin-like growth factor 1 receptors, may contribute to increased risk of pancreas, bowel and renal cancers, but other unknown factors may also contribute.

## EFFECTS OF OBESITY ON LUNG FUNCTION

Obesity alters several indices of pulmonary function, including lung volumes, airway resistance and compliance, ventilation–perfusion mismatch, and response to exercise. In general these effects are detrimental, and most prominent in those people with severe obesity.

### Lung volumes

Lung volumes (vital capacity, total lung capacity [TLC] and residual volume) fall in a linear fashion with increasing BMI, with the greatest changes seen in those with a BMI >40 kg/m$^2$. In such individuals the expiratory reserve volume (ERV) is also reduced, which can result in breathing occurring at close to residual volume in the most extreme cases.[15]

There is some evidence that these changes are greater in those with higher degrees of abdominal obesity, as assessed by waist/hip ratio; changes in other adipose tissue compartments, including within the thoracic cavity itself, may also contribute.[16] The most severely obese may also experience greater problems when sitting or supine, probably as a result of increased abdominal fat affecting diaphragmatic function.[17]

### Airway resistance and compliance

Spirometric values are reduced in some but not all studies of obese individuals. One study found that a 10 kg weight increase was associated with a 96 mL fall in forced expiratory volume in 1 second ($FEV_1$) in men and a 51 mL fall in women. This may be partly related to decreased chest wall compliance, but other factors include a reduction in airway calibre, which may be greater than the expected reduction seen with the decreased lung volumes found in obesity.[18]

### Ventilation–perfusion mismatch

Reduced lung volumes resulting in areas of atelectasis may result in some ventilation–perfusion mismatch in obesity; this may be more pronounced in the lower zones. In very severe obesity this may contribute to hypoxia.

## OBESITY AND THE UPPER AIRWAYS

Collapse of the upper airway during sleep leading to snoring and upper airway obstruction is common during sleep in obese subjects, although other factors such as variations in jaw, tongue and soft palate anatomy also contribute. The risk is generally proportional to BMI, although other measures such as neck circumference (which may partly reflect fat deposition in the neck) may be better predictors of the presence of snoring, upper airway resistance syndrome and obstructive sleep apnoea.

### Response to exercise

Energy requirements at rest are generally higher in obese than lean subjects as a result of increased lean body mass as well as increased adipose tissue mass. The work of breathing at rest is also increased as a result of the various mechanical factors described above.[19] When obese subjects exercise, oxygen uptake and carbon dioxide production increase in a linear fashion as would be expected in normal weight subjects, albeit at a higher level, reflecting the increased workload and energy requirements of obesity. Not all studies show decreased exercise capacity or increased perception of dyspnoea in obesity, but this may be confounded by underlying cardiorespiratory fitness. Expiratory flow limitation may also occur during exercise in obese subjects.

### Effects of weight loss

There is limited information about the effects of weight loss on lung mechanics and lung function in obesity, but studies in patients who have lost weight following bariatric surgery generally show improvements in all of the measures of lung volume described above, suggesting that such abnormalities are largely reversible with weight loss.

## OBESITY AND RESPIRATORY DISEASE

A number of respiratory conditions are associated with obesity, many of which respond to treatment with continuous positive airway pressure (CPAP) or NIV; the most prevalent of these is obstructive sleep apnoea (OSA), which is also independently associated with a greater risk of hypertension, diabetes, metabolic syndrome and cardiovascular disease.[20]

### Obstructive sleep apnoea

Obstructive sleep apnoea is part of the spectrum of sleep-related breathing disorders. It affects between 2 per cent and 4 per cent of the population, is more common in men and is strongly associated with obesity.[21] It is characterized by episodic reduction or cessation of breathing during sleep due to collapse of the upper airways. These hypopnoeas or apnoeas are considered to have occurred if there is 50 per cent reduction or cessation of airflow for at least 10 seconds, associated with a reduction in oxyhaemoglobin saturation and arousal from sleep. Obstructive sleep apnoea is diagnosed if more than five such episodes occur per hour slept; more than 15 episodes suggests moderate OSA and more than 30, severe. The gold standard for diagnosis is polysomnography conducted in a sleep laboratory, but limited sleep studies, conducted at home using portable equipment that monitors oxygen saturation, airflow and chest wall movement, are increasingly being used for screening and diagnosis in clinical practice.[22]

The interest to the endocrinologist comes not only from the associated obesity, but also from the associations between OSA and hypertension, diabetes, metabolic syndrome and vascular disease that may be partly independent of obesity.[23–26] Epidemiological studies have consistently shown that individuals with OSA are more likely to have each of these disorders, but it has been more difficult to establish whether this observation is truly independent of obesity, and fully understand the mechanisms involved. Potential mechanisms include the sympathetic nervous system activation that occurs during arousals from sleep, which might directly increase blood pressure and contribute to insulin resistance;[27,28] associated daytime tiredness may also increase stress and increase blood pressure further. Intermittent hypoxaemia may also be an important factor; hypoxia has recently been implicated in altering the synthesis and release of various factors from adipose tissue that may play a role in the pathogenesis of insulin resistance and the metabolic syndrome.[29,30] Adipose tissue is already hypoxic in obesity and the additional intermittent nocturnal hypoxia could further the increased release of adipokines that promote insulin resistance and other metabolic abnormalities.[31]

The most convincing evidence for an independent effect of OSA on metabolic syndrome components is for hypertension. Several epidemiological studies have confirmed associations between OSA and increased blood pressure that are statistically independent of obesity,[32] apnoeic episodes are associated with arousal from sleep, and increased sympathetic activity and CPAP treatment has been shown to reduce daytime blood pressure in both hypertensive and normotensive patients with OSA.[33–35]

Obstructive sleep apnoea is also associated with metabolic syndrome and type 2 diabetes. Up to 80 per cent of obese patients with OSA are likely to have metabolic syndrome (compared to 40 per cent of similarly obese patients without OSA) and 23 per cent type 2 diabetes.[28] There is some support for the suggestion that CPAP treatment might improve these abnormalities, although the evidence is less convincing in relation to dyslipidaemia and raised blood glucose than it is for hypertension.[34,36,37] One retrospective study was able to show that CPAP treatment appeared to reduce cardiovascular mortality in comparison to untreated patients who declined CPAP,[38] but the proposal that CPAP reduces mortality in OSA by decreasing metabolic risk is yet to be established in a prospective study.

### Obesity hypoventilation syndrome (see Chapter 40)

Obesity hypoventilation syndrome is characterized by daytime hypoxia and hypercapnia, usually in association with extreme obesity. It is usually considered to be at the extreme end of the spectrum of sleep-related breathing disorders, although some patients may not have coexisting OSA, and many will benefit from NIV for effective management. Weight loss can also improve the symptoms, and if sufficient can reverse the respiratory failure.

### Asthma/chronic obstructive pulmonary disease

Asthma has been associated with obesity in a number of epidemiological studies, but this observation may well be confounded by misdiagnosis of asthma in obese individuals who are more likely to complain of breathlessness than those who are not obese. Nevertheless, the abnormalities in lung function found in obese individuals, including effects on lung volumes and increased likelihood of airway collapse, might make pre-existing asthma more severe.[39] Finally, obesity is a proinflammatory state, and it is possible that this contributes to increased asthma severity. The same may also be true for chronic obstructive pulmonary disease (COPD), where the presence of obesity may contribute to decreased lung volumes, increase the work of breathing and decrease exercise capacity. In addition, recent work has highlighted hyperglycaemia as a marker of poor outcomes in patients with COPD requiring NIV during acute exacerbations.[40]

### Neuromuscular disorders and obesity

Some neuromuscular disorders, for example myotonic dystrophy, are associated with both obesity and an increased risk of respiratory failure. It is not known whether weight loss will benefit such patients in terms of improved lung function and research is needed in this area.

## OTHER ENDOCRINE DISORDERS AND RESPIRATORY DISEASE

### Cushing's syndrome and exogenous corticosteroid use

Steroid hormones are known to cause weakness of respiratory muscles and there are several reports of steroid treatment for Cushing's syndrome being associated with respiratory muscle weakness, although this is not a usual feature of Cushing's syndrome. Although it would be uncommon for this to be the sole cause of respiratory failure, it may contribute, for example in patients being treated with steroids for conditions such as COPD or asthma, and has been reported during corticosteroid treatment in patients with dermatomyositis.

### Hypothyroidism

Hypothyroidism is often associated with moderate weight gain, but this would rarely result in presentation to an NIV unit. Severe hypothyroidism, 'myxoedema coma', is fortunately rare but should respond to thyroxine treatment.

### Hypothalamic and pituitary disease

Hypopituitarism and treatment of hypothalamic and pituitary tumours are frequently associated with rapid weight gain,[41] and may present with OSA or obesity hypoventilation syndrome. Such patients will usually be known to have the condition and be taking pituitary hormone replacements, but physicians should be alert to the possibility that weight gain and development of OSA or obesity hypoventilation may be the first presentation of hypothalamic–pituitary disease and consider endocrine testing and scanning of the pituitary if symptoms of hypopituitarism or other suggestive features such as headache or visual field loss are present.

## CLINICAL IMPLICATIONS AND EVIDENCE BASE FOR INTERVENTION

### Benefits of weight loss

The benefits of weight loss are best documented from interventional studies in metabolic conditions such as impaired glucose tolerance and diabetes, and for improvements in blood pressure and other risk factors, where modest weight loss (of about 5–10 per cent of starting body weight) has been shown to reduce the risk of diabetes by up to 58 per cent in high-risk patients as well as lower blood pressure and improve circulating lipids.[42,43] The evidence base for benefits of similar degrees of weight loss on respiratory disease is less compelling, and most data come from studies of significant weight loss following bariatric surgery, but even this is very limited in scope and quality.[44] The available data do suggest that weight loss is likely to be of benefit in patients with OSA and possibly in obese patients with asthma, although the latter currently relates to one small study, using very low calorie diets in short-term treatment only, which may not be generalizable to the wider population of obese patients with asthma.[45]

### Interventions to aid weight loss

Energy restriction, increased physical activity and psychological support provide the basis for all interventions aimed at helping people lose weight. Although severe energy restriction can produce more rapid weight loss, modest restriction of 600 kcal below calculated metabolic rate is better tolerated, is more likely to result in sustainable long-term changes in eating habits and has been shown to produce at least equivalent weight loss in the long term compared with fixed, low-energy diets.[46] Some individuals may benefit from the more rigid meal plans offered by meal replacements, and this approach can be helpful when more rapid weight loss is needed, for example prior to surgery and in some cases of obesity hypoventilation. Physical activity is an important component of any weight loss programme, and although it may contribute less to weight loss than reduced energy intake, increased activity has other health benefits, and contributes to weight maintenance after successful weight loss.

Drug therapy should be considered as an adjunct to lifestyle intervention, rather than as a substitute, and can be helpful for some patients. The two drugs currently licensed and recommended for long-term use are the intestinal lipase inhibitor, orlistat, and the centrally acting satiety agent, sibutramine. These drugs both result in weight loss that is greater than placebo (for orlistat mean weight loss is 3.4 kg and for sibutramine 4.5 kg, with 50–60 per cent of patients achieving an overall weight loss of 5 per cent).[47–49] Orlistat and sibutramine both have modest additional lipid lowering effects that are independent of weight loss. Sibutramine may increase blood pressure and pulse rate in some patients, and this should be monitored carefully during the first 3 months of therapy. Sibutramine is contraindicated in patients at high cardiovascular risk (e.g. previous MI), but the licence for sibutramine was withdrawn in Europe in January 2010, as preliminary results of a long-term trail suggested increased cardiovascular events in patients at high cardiovascular risk. Other drugs that result in weight loss, which can be useful in specific clinical conditions (although not licensed for the treatment of obesity), include the glucagon-like peptide 1 analogues exenatide and liraglutide, used for the treatment of type 2 diabetes,[50] and the anticonvulsants topiramate and zonisamide.[51,52]

Bariatric surgery is now well established as an appropriate intervention for the more severely obese patients; current international guidelines suggest that surgery may be appropriate for patients with a BMI >40 kg/m$^2$, or >35 kg/m$^2$ for those with significant comorbidities, such as diabetes. Three main procedures in widespread use are laparoscopic gastric banding, laparoscopic Roux-en-Y gastric bypass and laparoscopic duodenal switch. Long-term weight loss with each of these procedures ranges from 15–20 per cent with gastric banding to 30 per cent with the bypass and 35–40 per cent with the duodenal switch. Surgery (particularly those procedures which bypass the duodenum) can produce dramatic improvements in type 2 diabetes, with up to 70 per cent of patients achieving remission.[53] Long-term follow-up suggests that this can be sustained for over 10 years, with concomitant improvements in other comorbidities, and lower mortality compared with age- and gender-matched patients who did not undergo surgery.[54] Surgery can also reduce requirements for CPAP in patients with sleep apnoea.[44]

### Other interventions

Recognition of the associations between obesity, respiratory disease and metabolic risk is important and there is now consensus that the high co-occurrence of these conditions warrants clinical vigilance in looking for the presence of diabetes, dyslipidaemia and hypertension in patients with OSA, and consideration to the possibility of OSA in patients with diabetes and in those with vascular disease.

## FUTURE RESEARCH

The potential beneficial effects of CPAP treatment on metabolic disease are potentially of considerable clinical significance, and further work is needed to more fully understand the mechanisms involved and investigate fully whether promising uncontrolled data is supported by randomized clinical trials.

Finally, there is a real need to conduct properly controlled clinical trials (of lifestyle, pharmacotherapy and surgery) to assess the potential effects of weight loss in patients with respiratory disease that may be caused or exacerbated by obesity.

## REFERENCES

1. World Health Organization. *Obesity – preventing and managing the global epidemic.* World Health Organization (WHO), Geneva, 1998.
2. Health and Social Care Information Centre. *Health survey for England 2007.* London: Health and Social Care Information Centre, 2008.
3. Sharma AM, Kushner RF. A proposed clinical staging system for obesity. *Int J Obes* 2009; **33**: 289–95.
4. Walley AJ, Asher JE, Froguel P. The genetic contribution to non-syndromic human obesity. *Nat Rev Genet* 2009; **10**: 431–42.
5. Farooqi S, O'Rahilly S. Genetics of obesity in humans. *Endocr Rev* 2006; **27**: 710–18.
6. Frayling TM, Timpson NJ, Weedon MN *et al.* A common variant in the FTO gene is associated with body mass index and predisposes to childhood and adult obesity. *Science* 2007; **316**: 889–94.
7. Calle EE, Rodriguez C, Walker-Thurmond K *et al.* Overweight, obesity, and mortality from cancer in a prospectively studied cohort of US adults. *N Engl J Med* 2003; **348**: 1625–38.
8. Guerra S, Sherrill DL, Bobadilla A *et al.* The relation of body mass index to asthma, chronic bronchitis, and emphysema. *Chest* 2002; **122**: 1256–63.
9. Mokdad AH, Ford ES, Bowman BA *et al.* Prevalence of obesity, diabetes, and obesity-related health risk factors, 2001. *JAMA* 2003; **289**: 76–9.

10. Aaron SD, Vandemheen KL, Boulet LP *et al.* Overdiagnosis of asthma in obese and nonobese adults. *CMAJ* 2008; **179**: 1121–31.
11. Kos K, Wilding JPH. Adipokines as emerging therapeutic targets. *Curr Opin Investig Drugs* 2009; **10**: 1061–8.
12. Arita Y, Kihara S, Ouchi N *et al.* Paradoxical decrease of an adipose-specific protein, adiponectin, in obesity. *Biochem Biophys Res Commun* 1999; **257**: 79–83.
13. Landsberg L. Pathophysiology of obesity-related hypertension: role of insulin and the sympathetic nervous system. *J Cardiovasc Pharmacol* 1994; **23** Suppl 1: S1–8.
14. Szendroedi J, Roden M. Ectopic lipids and organ function. *Curr Opin Lipidol* 2009; **20**: 50–6.
15. Jones RL, Nzekwu MMU. The effects of body mass index on lung volumes. *Chest* 2006; **130**: 827–33.
16. Chen Y, Rennie D, Cormier YF *et al.* Waist circumference is associated with pulmonary function in normal-weight, overweight, and obese subjects. *Am J Clin Nutr* 2007; **85**: 35–9.
17. Benedik PS, Baun MM, Keus L *et al.* Effects of body position on resting lung volume in overweight and mildly to moderately obese subjects. *Respir Care* 2009; **54**: 334–9.
18. Parameswaran K, Todd DC, Soth M. Altered respiratory physiology in obesity. *Can Respir J* 2006; **13**: 203–10.
19. Kress JP, Pohlman AS, Alverdy J *et al.* The impact of morbid obesity on oxygen cost of breathing (Vo(2RESP)) at rest. *Am J Respir Crit Care Med* 1999; **160**: 883–6.
20. Berg S. Obstructive sleep apnoea syndrome: current status. *Clin Respir J* 2008; **2**: 197–201.
21. Davies RJ, Stradling JR. The epidemiology of sleep apnoea. *Thorax* 1996; **51** Suppl 2: S65–S70.
22. Mulgrew AT, Fox N, Ayas NT *et al.* Diagnosis and initial management of obstructive sleep apnea without polysomnography: a randomized validation study. *Ann Intern Med* 2007; **146**: 157–66.
23. Peker Y, Kraiczi H, Hedner J *et al.* An independent association between obstructive sleep apnoea and coronary artery disease. *Eur Respir J* 1999; **14**: 179–84.
24. Carlson JT, Hedner JA, Ejnell H *et al.* High prevalence of hypertension in sleep apnea patients independant of obesity. *Am J Respir Crit Care Med* 1994; **150**: 72–7.
25. Coughlin SR, Mawdsley L, Mugarza JA *et al.* Obstructive sleep apnoea is independently associated with an increased prevalence of metabolic syndrome. *Eur Heart J* 2004; **25**: 735–41.
26. Parish JM, Adam T, Facchiano L. Relationship of metabolic syndrome and obstructive sleep apnea. *J Clin Sleep Med* 2007; **3**: 467–72.
27. Narkiewicz K, van de Borne PJH, Cooley RL *et al.* Sympathetic activity in obese subjects with and without obstructive sleep apnoea. *Circulation* 1998; **98**: 776.
28. West SD, Nicoll DJ, Stradling JR. Prevalence of obstructive sleep apnoea in men with type 2 diabetes. *Thorax* 2006; **61**: 945–50.
29. Somers VK, Mark AL, Abboud FM. Sympathetic activation by hypoxia and hypercapnia: implications for sleep apnea. *Clin Exp Hypertens A* 1988; **10** Suppl 1: 413–22.
30. Hedner JA, Wilcox I, Laks L *et al.* A specific and potent pressor effect of hypoxia in patients with sleep apnea. *Am Rev Respir Dis* 1992; **146**: 1240–5.
31. Trayhurn P, Wood IS. Signalling role of adipose tissue: adipokines and inflammation in obesity. *Biochem Soc Trans* 2005; **33**: 1078–81.
32. Nieto FJ, Young TB, Lind BK *et al.* Association of sleep-disordered breathing, sleep apnea, and hypertension in a large community-based study. *JAMA* 2000; **283**: 1829–36.
33. Minemura H, Akashiba T, Yamamoto H *et al.* Acute effects of nasal continuous positive airway pressure on 24-hour blood pressure and catecholamines in patients with obstructive sleep apnea. *Intern Med* 1998; **37**: 1009–13.
34. Coughlin S, Mawdsley L, Mugarza JA *et al.* Cardiovascular and metabolic effects of CPAP in obese men with OSA. *Eur Respir J* 2007; **29**: 720–7.
35. Pepperell JC, Ramdassingh-Dow S, Crosthwaite N *et al.* Ambulatory blood pressure after therapeutic and subtherapeutic nasal continuous positive airway pressure for obstructive sleep apnoea: a randomised parallel trial. *Lancet* 2002; **359**: 204–10.
36. Harsch IA, Schahin SP, Bruckner K *et al.* The effect of continuous positive airway pressure treatment on insulin sensitivity in patients with obstructive sleep apnoea syndrome and type 2 diabetes. *Respiration* 2004; **71**: 252–9.
37. Harsch IA, Hahn EG, Schahin SP. Effect of CPAP on insulin resistance in patients with obstructive sleep apnoea and type 2 diabetes. *Thorax* 2008; **63**: 384–5.
38. Marin JM, Carrizo SJ, Vicente E *et al.* Long-term cardiovascular outcomes in men with obstructive sleep apnoea-hypopnoea with or without treatment with continuous positive airway pressure: an observational study. *Lancet* 2005; **365**: 1046–53.
39. Shore SA. Obesity and asthma: Possible mechanisms. *J Allerg Clin Immunol* 2008; **121**: 1087–93.
40. Baker EH, Janaway CH, Philips BJ *et al.* Hyperglycaemia is associated with poor outcomes in patients admitted to hospital with acute exacerbations of chronic obstructive pulmonary disease. *Thorax* 2006; **61**: 284–9.
41. Daousi C, Dunn AJ, Foy PM *et al.* Endocrine and neuroanatomic features associated with weight gain and obesity in adult patients with hypothalamic damage. *Am J Med* 2005; **118**: 45–50.
42. Tuomilheto J, Lindstrom J, Erickson JG *et al.* Prevention of type 2 diabetes mellitus by changes in lifestyle anongst subjects with impaired glucose tolerance. *N Engl J Med* 2001; **344**: 1343–50.
43. Avenell A, Broom J, Brown TJ *et al.* Systematic review of the long-term effects and economic consequences of treatments for obesity and implications for health improvement. *Health Technol Assess* 2004; **8**: 1–182.

44. Simard B, Turcotte H, Marceau P *et al.* Asthma and sleep apnea obesity: Outcome after bariatric surgery. *Obes Surg* 2004; **14**: 1381–8.
45. Stenius-Aarniala B, Poussa T, Kvarnstrom J *et al.* Immediate and long term effects of weight reduction in obese people with asthma: randomised controlled study. *BMJ* 2000; **320**: 827–32.
46. Avenell A, Brown TJ, Mcgee MA *et al.* What are the long-term benefits of weight reducing diets in adults? A systematic review of randomized controlled trials. *J Hum Nutr Diet* 2004; **17**: 317–35.
47. James WPT, Astrup A, Finer N *et al.* Effect of sibutramine on weight maintenance after weight loss: a randomised trial. *Lancet* 2000; **356**: 2119–25.
48. Sjostrom L, Rissanen A, Andersen T *et al.* Weight loss and prevention of weight regain in obese patients: a 2-year, European, randomised trial of orlistat. *Lancet* 1998; **352**: 167–72.
49. Padwal RS, Majumdar SR. Drug treatments for obesity: orlistat, sibutramine, and rimonabant. *Lancet* 2007; **369**: 71–7.
50. Ratner RE, Maggs D, Nielsen LL *et al.* Long-term effects of exenatide therapy over 82 weeks on glycaemic control and weight in over-weight metformin-treated patients with type 2 diabetes mellitus. *Diabetes Obes Metab* 2006; **8**: 419–28.
51. Wilding J, Van Gaal L, Rissanen A *et al.* A randomized double-blind placebo-controlled study of the long-term efficacy and safety of topiramate in the treatment of obese subjects. *Int J Obes* 2004; **28**: 1399–410.
52. Gadde KM, Franciscy DM, Wagner HR *et al.* Zonisamide for weight loss in obese adults: a randomized controlled trial. *JAMA* 2003; **289**: 1820–5.
53. Pories WJ, Swanson MS, MacDonald KG *et al.* Who would have thought it – an operation proves to be the most effective therapy for adult-onset diabetes-mellitus. *Ann Surg* 1995; **222**: 339–52.
54. Sjostrom L, Lindroos AK, Peltonen M *et al.* Lifestyle, diabetes, and cardiovascular risk factors 10 years after bariatric surgery. *N Engl J Med* 2004; **351**: 2683–93.

# 40

# Pathophysiology of respiratory failure in obesity

FRANCESCO FANFULLA

## ABSTRACT

The prevalence of obesity is increasing in both the developed and developing worlds, but the respiratory consequences are often underappreciated. Obesity may lead to several alterations in every aspect of respiratory function. The most common problems include elevated work of breathing, respiratory muscle inefficiency and reduced respiratory compliance. Decreased functional residual capacity and expiratory reserve volume, with a high closing volume, are associated with the closure of peripheral lung units, abnormalities in the ventilation-to-perfusion ratio and hypoxaemia. The consequences of these alterations is respiratory impairment, although the severity of this impairment varies greatly between patients. Obesity is a major risk factor for sleep-disordered breathing, usually obstructive sleep apnoea or obesity hypoventilation syndrome, which leads to more severe respiratory impairment. The final result is the development of hypoxaemia, carbon dioxide retention, pulmonary hypertension and chronic cor pulmonale with severe disability. Although this chronic respiratory failure usually develops progressively, most patients receive respiratory care at the time of the first acute episode of respiratory failure. New fields of future research, in particular modification of control of breathing induced by repetitive episodes of hypoxia or hypercapnia, are discussed.

## INTRODUCTION

Obesity is a major public health problem and is now considered a worldwide epidemic. A huge number of subjects, nearly 1.5 billion adults, are estimated to be overweight, whereas 400 million adults are obese.[1] Once considered a problem only in developed countries, excess weight and obesity are now increasing in less developed countries, primarily because of the growing intake of energy-dense ('junk') food and sedentary lifestyles promoted by urbanization. Indeed, the numbers of overweight and obese subjects are rising everywhere, but the average body mass index (BMI) of Europeans (26.5 kg/m$^2$) is now one of the highest of all World Health Organization regions.

Obesity has considerable effects on morbidity and mortality. The term 'metabolic syndrome' is increasingly used to describe the cluster of abdominal obesity with hypertension, dyslipidaemia and impaired insulin resistance; this problem affects 20–30 per cent of the total population in the European region.[2] The burden of disease attributable to a high BMI among adults in the European region amounted to more than 1 million deaths and about 12 million life-years of ill health (disability-adjusted life-years [DALYs]) in 2000.[3] Data from the Framingham study in the USA show that obesity reduces life expectancy: obesity at the age of 40 years led to a reduction in life-expectancy of 7 years in women and 6 years in men.[4]

## THE EFFECTS OF OBESITY ON RESPIRATORY PHYSIOLOGY

Obesity has been demonstrated to lead to alterations in all components of respiratory physiology: mechanical properties of the respiratory system, airway resistance, control of breathing, gas exchange, work of breathing, etc. These effects are summarized in Table 40.1.

The number and severity of the respiratory alterations do, however, vary considerably between patients. Indeed, in clinical practice, there are obese subjects with little or no impairment in lung function as well as patients with severe respiratory failure due to obesity hypoventilation syndrome. The source of this variability is not well understood. Numerous factors may contribute to an individual's

Table 40.1 Main respiratory function alterations in obesity

| Function | Alteration |
|---|---|
| Respiratory physiology | Impairment due to obesity |
| Respiratory mechanics | Decreased total respiratory system compliance |
| | Increased airway resistance |
| Lung volumes | Mild to moderate reduction |
| | Variable changes in residual volume |
| Gas exchange | Reduced $PaO_2$ |
| | Increased A–$aO_2$ gradient |
| | Increased $PaCO_2$ |
| Work of breathing | Increased work of breathing |
| | Increased oxygen cost of breathing |

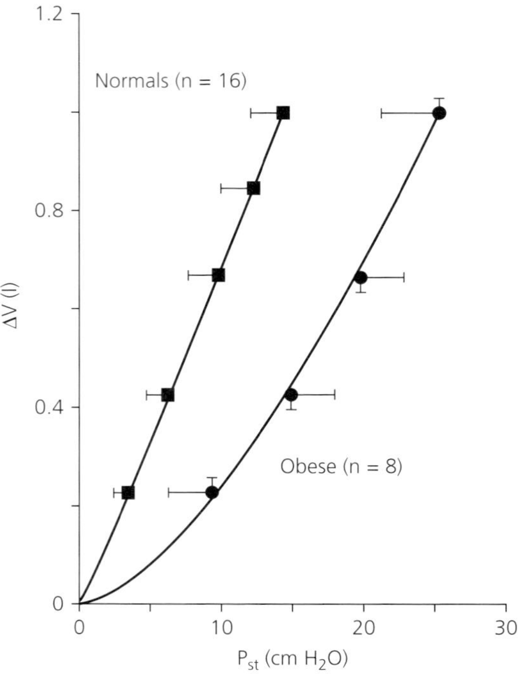


Figure 40.1 Average static volume (ΔV)–pressure ($P_{st}$) curve of the total respiratory system in eight morbidly obese patients and 16 normal anaesthetized subjects. Data are expressed as mean ± SD. Reproduced with permission from Pelosi *et al.*[7]

clinical and physiological status, including age, severity of obesity, distribution of fat, fertility status in females, smoking, physical activity, control of breathing, sleep-disordered breathing, sleep restrictions, medications and comorbid conditions.

Many years ago, Naimark and Cherniak reported a decrease, of as much as two-thirds of normal values in total respiratory system compliance in obese subjects.[5] They attributed this finding to the greater adiposity around the ribs, diaphragm and abdomen, or to limited movements of the ribs caused by thoracic kyphosis and lumbar hyperlordosis as a result of excessive abdominal fat. In a study performed on sedated, paralysed, post-operative, morbidly obese patients, Pelosi *et al.* found that, compared with normal subjects, the obese patients had a lower respiratory system compliance, caused by decreases in both lung and chest wall compliance, higher lung resistance with marked increases in airway and lung resistance, and a smaller functional residual capacity (FRC).[6] In another physiological study, again conducted in sedated, paralysed, morbidly obese patients and normal subjects, Pelosi *et al.* found that the obese patients had marked alterations of the mechanical properties of the respiratory system, largely explained by a reduction in lung volumes due to the excessive unopposed intra-abdominal pressure. The average static volume–pressure curves of the total respiratory system indicated an overall higher elastance in obese subjects and the presence of an 'inflection point' at a pressure between 5 cm $H_2O$ and 15 cm $H_2O$, after which the volume increased linearly with pressure (Fig. 40.1).[7] The pattern of elastance of the total respiratory system was different in normal and in obese subjects: in normal subjects the elastance did not change with increasing volume whereas in obese patients elastance dropped sharply along the inflection point (from 0 L to 0.6 L) and subsequently remained constant (Fig. 40.2).

Several studies investigating the relationship between body weight and various spirometric indices have shown that increased body weight decreases lung volumes.[8–10]

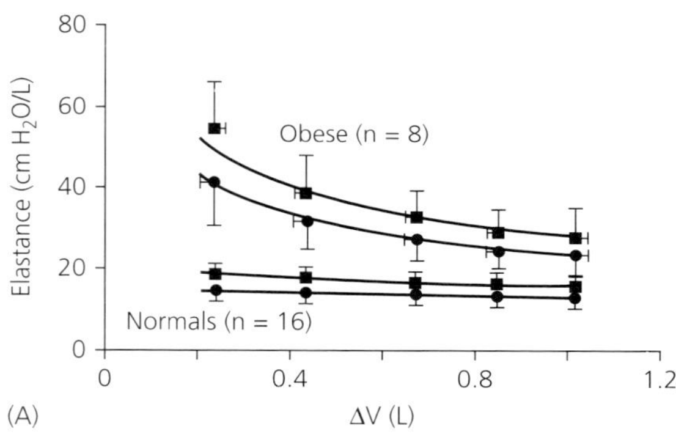


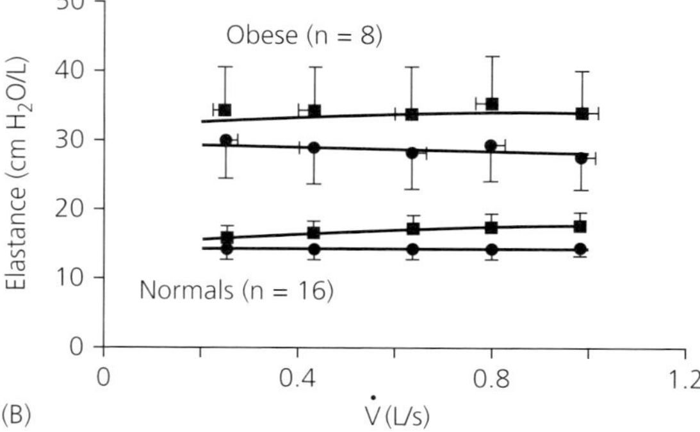


Figure 40.2 Relationship of static (filled dots) and dynamic (filled squares) elastance with (A) average static volume (ΔV) and (B) flow ($\dot{V}$) in eight morbidly obese patients and 16 normal anaesthetized paralysed subjects. Data are expressed as mean ± SD. Reproduced with permission from Pelosi *et al.*[7]

Lung function impairment as well as the metabolic syndrome have been associated with an increased risk of cardiovascular disease and premature death.[11,12] Recently, in a large-scale population-based study a positive relationship was found between lung function impairment and the metabolic syndrome; this was due mainly to abdominal obesity and was independent of major cardiovascular risk factors, including BMI.[13] Since abdominal obesity has been related to a higher risk of respiratory death, respiratory function evaluation should be considered mandatory in all subjects with increased body weight, especially those with an increasing abdominal circumference.[14–16]

Recently, Jones *et al.* collected pulmonary function test data from 373 patients and showed that BMI had a significant effect on all lung volumes.[17] The patients were divided into five groups according to BMI. An inverse linear relationship was observed between BMI and vital capacity and total lung capacity, but the group mean values remained within the normal ranges even for the morbidly obese patients. The most dramatic effects of BMI were seen for FRC and expiratory reserve volume since there were significant differences between the group with a BMI of 20–25 kg/m$^2$ and all other groups with higher BMI. The FRC and expiratory reserve volume decreased exponentially with increasing BMI, such that morbid obesity resulted in patients breathing near their residual volume; the greatest declines in FRC and expiratory reserve volume were found among the overweight patients and those with mild obesity.

Relationships between obesity and respiratory function were investigated in the European Prospective Investigation into Cancer and Nutrition cohort in Norfolk (EPIC-Norfolk), which included 9674 men and 11 876 women aged from 45 to 79 years with no known pre-existing serious illness.[18] In this study, Canoy *et al.* found that forced expiratory volume in one second and forced vital capacity were linearly and inversely related across the entire range of waist-to-hip ratios in both men and women, and that this relation persisted after adjustment for age, BMI, cigarette smoking, social class, physical activity, prevalent bronchitis/emphysema and prevalent asthma.

Postural changes in lung volumes are different in normal and obese subjects. In normal subjects there is a reduction in FRC and an increase in airflow resistance when the supine posture is adopted; most of the reduction in FRC is related to gravitational effects of the abdominal contents, so that the diaphragm takes a more expiratory position. In contrast, in obese subjects there is no supine decrease in FRC or total lung capacity, as recently demonstrated by Watson and Pride.[19] The mechanism of this different pattern of postural changes in lung volumes in obese subjects is not understood. However, the lack of a further decrease in FRC has a favorable effect of restricting increases in inspiratory work of breathing and deterioration in gas exchange during tidal breathing when supine.

The effects of longitudinal changes of BMI on spirometric indices and diffusion capacity of the lung were investigated in the general population by Bottai *et al.* in an 8-year follow-up survey.[20] The authors evaluated the effects of weight changes over time in a group of 1426 adults aged >24 years. They found that lung function loss tended to be greater among those who, at baseline, reported higher BMI values; the loss was greater in males than in females. The detrimental effect of gaining weight might be reversible in many adults since those whose BMI decreased over time had an improvement in lung function.

It was recognized 20 years ago that expiratory flow rate could decrease in non-smoking obese individuals.[21] Maximal expiratory flow rates decrease progressively with decreasing lung volume, so that breathing at a low lung volume is associated with a reduction in expiratory flow reserve, which can further diminish in the presence of airway obstruction. This phenomenon is more likely to occur with the subject in the supine position, during which the relaxation volume of the respiratory system and FRC are lower than in the sitting position because of the gravitational effect of the abdominal contents. Tidal expiratory flow limitation (EFL) promotes dynamic hyperinflation with a concurrent increase in work of breathing due to the presence of intrinsic positive end-expiratory pressure (PEEPi). All these findings were reported by Pankow *et al.* who compared data obtained from a small group of severely obese subjects with those from a normal weight control group.[22] Several mechanisms could induce EFL in obesity. Airflow is dependent on lung volume so that any decrease in FRC determines a decrease in expiratory flow reserve. Breathing at very low lung volumes may promote airway closure and air trapping, as demonstrated in subjects breathing at low lung volumes due to chest strapping.[23] On the other hand, these data revealed that, in severe obesity, inspiratory muscles are loaded not only by decreased compliance of the total respiratory system but also by the presence of PEEPi. Similar features were also found in morbidly obese, post-operative, mechanically ventilated patients. Koutsoukou *et al.* demonstrated the presence of EFL, associated with dynamic hyperinflation and a concurrent risk of low lung volume injury, in 10 of 15 patients.[24] Only the application of a relatively high level of PEEPe abolished all these mechanical abnormalities.

Several studies performed in normal subjects have demonstrated that there is a straight relationship between body weight and arterial oxygen concentration.[25,26] Indeed, in the reference equation for $PaO_2$ in middle-aged and elderly subjects proposed by Cerveri *et al.*, BMI is one of the main factors explaining the variability of arterial oxygen tension in the general population.[26] The physiological basis of this finding is not well understood. Many years ago, Ulmer *et al.* demonstrated a great variation in lung ventilation/perfusion ratio according to BMI.[27] They studied a group of subjects with BMI in the normal range and found that higher BMI is associated with increasing mismatch between ventilation and perfusion, and lower value of $PaO_2$. Holley *et al.* studied lung ventilation and perfusion in a group of obese subjects and found significant ventilation/perfusion ratio abnormalities, consisting of more prevalent perfusion in lower zones of the lung where ventilation was considerably reduced.[28] Recently, Yamane *et al.* demonstrated that hypoxia in obese subjects in the supine position is caused primarily by insufficient gas exchange in the regions of lung linked to the inferior pulmonary veins.[29] They found an inverse relationship between BMI and $PO_2$ in the inferior pulmonary veins suggesting a possible subclinical manifestation of obesity-related respiratory insufficiency. The authors attributed these findings in part to the regional alveolar ventilation–perfusion mismatch caused by the closure of dependent airways within the range of tidal breathing[30] and in part to alveolar hypoventilation.

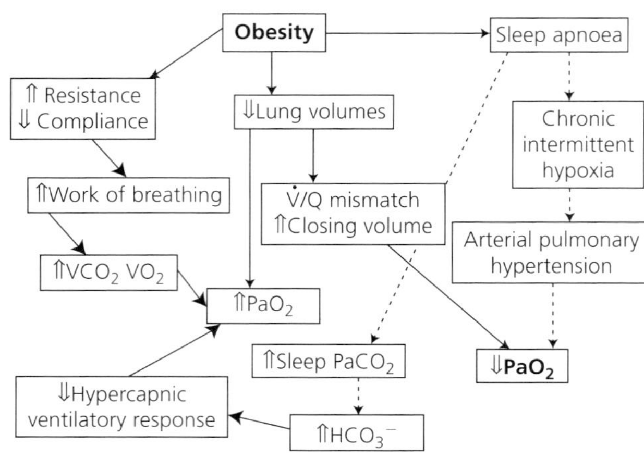


**Figure 40.3** Mechanisms by which obesity may lead to chronic hypoxaemia and hypercapnia. Dashed lines represent modifications induced directly by obstructive sleep apnoea.

## SLEEP-DISORDERED BREATHING: OBSTRUCTIVE SLEEP APNOEA SYNDROME AND OBESITY HYPOVENTILATION SYNDROME

Sleep is associated with normal changes in many physiological functions, including respiration. The relevant differences in comparison with wakefulness affect control of breathing, airflow resistance, ventilatory response to increased load, activity of respiratory muscles and body position. Sleep results in a decrease of about 10–15 per cent in minute ventilation, essentially as a result of a nearly 20 per cent decrease in tidal volume not fully compensated by an increase in respiratory rate. As a consequence, the reduction in ventilation results in an increase of 3–7 mm Hg in $PaCO_2$, and a decrease of 4–9 mm Hg in $PaO_2$, whereas $SaO_2$ decreases by about 2 per cent. The sleep-related decrease in the ventilatory responses to hypercapnia and hypoxia explains the absence of a compensatory increase in ventilation to changes in blood gases.

All these physiological changes in respiration are particularly exaggerated in the presence of increased body weight. Obesity is a condition associated with a high prevalence of sleep-disordered breathing that, untreated, leads to daytime hypoxia and chronic respiratory failure. The two most important diseases associated with obesity, at least from an epidemiological point of view, are obstructive sleep apnoea syndrome (OSAS) and obesity hypoventilation syndrome (OHS). The mechanisms by which obesity may lead to chronic hypoxaemia and hypercapnia are summarized in Figure 40.3.

Obstructive sleep apnoea syndrome is defined as the repetitive collapse of the upper airways during sleep, occurring more than five times per hour of sleep. Intermittent hypoxaemia, hypercapnia, large negative intrathoracic pressure swings associated with arousals and sleep fragmentation are typical findings of this syndrome.[31] Classical symptoms reported by patients or relatives are excessive daytime sleepiness, unrefreshing sleep, nocturia, snoring, witnessed apnoeas and nocturnal choking. Signs include systemic (or difficult to control) hypertension, premature cardiovascular disease, atrial fibrillation and heart failure. Factors contributing to the development of OSAS include increasing age, gender, an anatomically narrow upper airway, a tendency to have a more collapsible upper airway, individual differences in neuromuscular control of upper airway muscles and variations in ventilatory control mechanisms. Obesity seems to explain only 30–50 per cent of the variance in the apnoea hypopnoea index (AHI), with a prevalent effect in patients aged <60 years.[32] Obesity may predispose to OSAS by accumulation of fat around the neck, resulting in increased extraluminal pressure and a propensity to upper airway collapse or in a modification of the geometry of the airways. Abdominal obesity, through its negative effects on lung volumes, determines a reduction in longitudinal traction predisposing to upper airway collapse. Finally, changes in body weight in patients with OSAS are associated with changes in the severity of the syndrome. Data from the Wisconsin sleep cohort suggest that weight gain has a greater effect on OSAS than an equivalent weight loss: a 20 per cent increase in weight was associated with a 70 per cent increase in AHI, whereas a 20 per cent reduction in weight was associated with a 48 per cent decrease in AHI.[33] The development of respiratory failure in patients with OSAS is still a matter of discussion.[34] Generally, the presence of chronic daytime hypoxaemia has been attributed to pre-existing lung disease such as chronic obstructive pulmonary disease, so that airway obstruction and lung hyperinflation have been considered to have major roles in determining the lower values of $PaO_2$.[35–37] However, Fanfulla *et al.* recently demonstrated that patients with OSAS, in the absence of lung comorbidity such as diffuse airway obstruction, had lower values of $PaO_2$ than those expected on the basis of age.[38] The main factor responsible for this reduction in daytime $PaO_2$ was the degree of nocturnal hypoxia. The authors attributed their findings to various factors, including repeated nocturnal desaturation that may lead to recurrent pulmonary hypertension and pulmonary vascular injury that in turn may lead to mild hypoxaemia.

The term OHS, formerly 'Pickwickian syndrome', has been used with different meanings over time in the literature. However, the term is now universally used to define patients with obesity (generally morbid obesity), chronic alveolar hypoventilation leading to daytime hypercapnia ($PaCO_2$ >45 mm Hg) and hypoxaemia ($PaO_2$ <70 mm Hg) associated with sleep-disordered breathing. Generally, the respiratory alteration during sleep consists in a picture of severe OSAS (~90 per cent of patients with OHS), while the remaining cases have severe, prolonged sleep hypoventilation with rare episodes of obstructive apnoea/hypopnoea (<5 events per hour of sleep). In these latter cases, the patients' $PaCO_2$ during sleep may be at least 10 mm Hg higher than that recorded in a supine position during the quiet wakefulness preceding the onset of sleep.[38] Finally, it should be remembered that some individual patients with OSAS may develop daytime chronic hypercapnia in the absence of obesity (BMI <30 kg/m$^2$). Few data are available about the prevalence of OHS in the general population. The prevalence in patients attending sleep laboratories or admitted to hospital ranges from 11 per cent to 38 per cent.[39–42]

The mechanisms leading to chronic carbon dioxide retention in obese patients are not completely understood. It is known that the clinical and functional disorders in patients with OHS are generally more severe than those in patients with the same degree of obesity but with OSAS. At this point, is not clear whether OHS is the final step in the natural clinical history of OSAS, as postulated by Lugaresi *et al.* many years ago, or whether OHS is a separate clinical entity with a specific pathophysiology.[43] Indeed, although the likelihood of developing diurnal hypercapnia increases as BMI rises, weight alone does not explain the presence of hypercapnia.[44] As mentioned above, in patients with OHS, the respiratory function impairment is usually enhanced, causing a two-threefold increase in the work of breathing compared with that in lean subjects.[5,6] Similarly, global oxygen consumption ($VO_2$) is increased in obesity, as reported by Kress *et al.*,[45] who measured $VO_2$ during spontaneous breathing in morbidly obese patients immediately prior to scheduled gastric bypass surgery, and again during mechanical ventilation to determine the effects of morbid obesity on oxygen consumption dedicated to respiratory muscle work. They found that morbid obesity is associated with a substantial increase in $VO_2$ dedicated to respiratory muscle work during quiet breathing when compared with that in normal control patients. This increase in energy expenditure could represent a limited ventilatory reserve which may predispose such patients to respiratory failure during acute pulmonary or systemic illnesses.

The presence of altered control of breathing in patients with OHS is a matter of concern. Several studies have reported abnormalities in ventilatory control of patients with OHS.[46–48] In other studies, the respiratory drive of obese eucapnic patients was increased in order to compensate for the respiratory system changes associated with obesity,[49] whereas obese patients who developed hypoventilation while awake did not show this augmented drive.[46] On the other hand, Leech *et al.* documented that the great majority of a group of patients with OHS were able to normalize $PaCO_2$ during voluntary hyperventilation.[50]

The presence of a reduced ventilatory response to increased mechanical load and/or carbon dioxide level is considered by many authors to be an acquired phenomenon, since most patients show improvements in ventilatory responsiveness after appropriate treatment.[51–53] A mutual relationship between OHS and sleep-induced upper airway obstruction[40,54] has been proposed by several investigators on the basis of various considerations: the great majority of OHS patients still have severe OSAS, the clinical presentation of OHS with and without OSAS is identical, and a high proportion of patients with OHS with pure sleep hypoventilation at presentation go on to develop OSAS once daytime hypercapnia improves with nocturnal ventilation.[55]

The mechanism by which OSAS could cause chronic hypercapnia during wakefulness has been intensively investigated.[56–59] Berger *et al.* demonstrated that minute ventilation during sleep is not reduced (and is, indeed, sometimes increased) in those OSAS patients with daytime hypercapnia because of the marked hyperventilation at the end of each apnoea/hypopnoea event (inter-critical period).[56] Minute ventilation during the inter-critical period is strictly related to carbon dioxide loading during the obstructive event[57] (Fig. 40.4). Berger *et al.* demonstrated the presence of a strong inverse relationship between the post-event ventilatory response slope (the ratio between the ventilatory response and $CO_2$ loading during the event) and chronic awake arterial $PCO_2$ ($r$ = 0.90, $p$ <0.001), suggesting that this mechanism is impaired in patients with chronic hypercapnia (Fig. 40.5). Patients may fail to eliminate carbon dioxide completely during the post-apnoeic period when the ratio between the duration of the obstructive event and the hyperventilation period is higher than 3:1. In this case, the wash-out of carbon dioxide loaded during the apnoea/hypoponea may not be complete, leading to progressive carbon dioxide retention during sleep.[58] Norman *et al.* identified bicarbonate retention compensating for the acute rise in carbon dioxide, as well as the inability to unload the increased carbon dioxide and bicarbonate during wakefulness, as important mechanisms which would further blunt respiratory drive and promote awake hypercapnia. A raised level of serum bicarbonate is a typical clinical finding in patients with OHS.[59]

The role of leptin in the development of chronic hypoventilation is a much debated issue.[60–62] Obese subjects usually have higher circulating levels of leptin than do normal subjects; further increases have been found in patients with OSAS and OHS.[60–63] A possible explanation

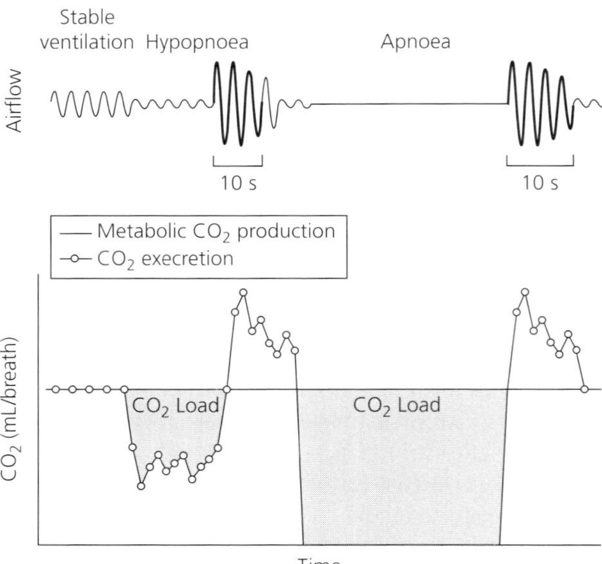


**Figure 40.4** Carbon dioxide ($CO_2$) loading and unloading during respiratory events. Shaded areas represent $CO_2$ loading due to reduced $CO_2$ excretion during obstructive events. Clear areas represent $CO_2$ unloading due to compensatory hyperventilation between events. Reproduced with permission from Berger *et al.*[56]

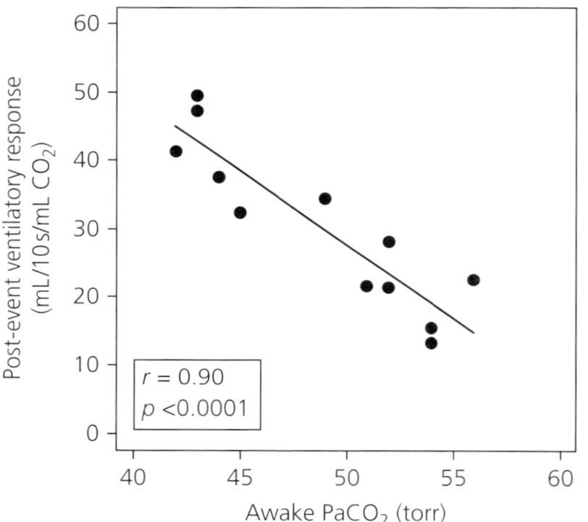


**Figure 40.5** Relationship between post-event ventilatory response slope and awake $PaCO_2$. Reproduced with permission from Berger *et al.*[57]

of the conflicting data from human and animal models is that the increased leptin levels in humans are necessary to maintain adequate minute ventilation as a consequence of the increased ventilatory load.[60] However, in the presence of so-called 'leptin resistance' this compensatory mechanism would be lost and hypercapnia during wakefulness could emerge.[61] Campo *et al.* found an association between higher serum leptin levels and reductions in baseline respiratory drive and chemoresponsiveness to $CO_2$ in obese subjects, but it has still not been established whether this is linked to the development of daytime chronic hypercapnia.[64]

## AREAS FOR FUTURE RESEARCH

In clinical practice there is a great variability in respiratory impairment in individual patients, ranging from small changes in lung volumes to severe acute-on-chronic respiratory failure needing admission to an intensive care unit. The source of this variability is far from having been identified since most of the studies that have generated data were cross-sectional or characterized by small sample sizes.

Other aspects that need thorough investigation are the adaptive behavioural and physiological responses elicited by obesity itself or by the changes in respiratory functions induced by obesity, mechanisms that regulate the ventilatory drive under increased mechanical load, as well as intermittent or chronic alterations in blood gas levels or pH. Recent studies have led to an increasing awareness of the importance of the hypothalamus in maintaining normal breathing by means of the activity of specific neurones that contain peptide transmitters called orexins/hypocretins.[65] Orexins (orexin-A and orexin-B) are hypothalamic neuropeptides that were first discovered to enhance appetite and consciousness;[66] subsequent studies have revealed their involvement in the regulation of circulation, respiration and analgesia.[67] Williams *et al.* demonstrated in mice that acidification increases intrinsic excitability of orexin neurons, whereas alkalinization depresses it, suggesting a new mechanism of controlling breathing comparable to that of the classical chemosensory neurones of the brainstem.[65] Deng *et al.* showed that orexin knock-out mice had a blunted hypercapnic chemoreflex in comparison to that of wild-type animals, and that this reflex was partially restored after supplementation with orexins; similarly, the hypercapnic chemoreflex was reduced in wild-type mice after injection of an orexin antagonist.[68]

Exposure to hypoxia elicits ventilatory acclimatization and different forms of respiratory plasticity through various mechanisms, predominantly related to type of hypoxic stimulus (continuous or intermittent).[69–71] Chronic hypoxia usually induces long-term facilitation or progressive augmentation through mechanisms involving the peripheral carotid body chemoreceptors, whereas intermittent hypoxia acts on the brainstem and spinal cord. Long-term facilitation is a form of neuronal plasticity characterized by a progressive increase in respiratory output during the normoxic periods that separate hypoxic episodes and by a sustained elevation in respiratory activity for up to 90 min after exposure to hypoxia; progressive augmentation is characterized by a gradual increase in the magnitude of the hypoxic ventilatory response from the initial to the final hypoxic episode of a protocol of intermittent hypoxia exposure. How these mechanisms are involved in the pathogenesis of chronic respiratory failure remains to be clarified. Mateika *et al.*

demonstrated a significant inverse correlation between the ventilatory response to hypoxia/hypercapnia and the severity of apnoea in individuals with OSAS. Chronic intermittent hypoxia may have a differential effect on this response, initially causing an enhancement but later leading to depression.[72] Finally, extracellular adenosine triphosphate (ATP) signalling seems to play a role in ventilatory control, mediating both peripheral and central chemosensory transduction in response to changes in arterial levels of oxygen and carbon dioxide, but the exact role of this newly discovered pathway in the control of breathing still needs to be elucidated.[73]

## REFERENCES

1. World Health Organization. *The challenge of obesity in the WHO European Region and strategies of response.* Available at: www.euro.who.int/document/E90711.pdf (accessed 15 February 2010).
2. Branca F, Nikogosian H, Lobstein T. *The challenge of obesity in the WHO European Region and the strategies for response: summary*, 2007.
3. James WPT, Jackson-Leach R, Ni Mhurchu C *et al.* Overweight and obesity (high body mass index). In: Ezzati M, Lopez AD, Rodgers A *et al.*, eds. *Comparative quantification of health risks: global and regional burden of disease attribution to selected major risk factors*, Chapter 8, vol. 1. Geneva: World Health Organization, 2004:497–596.
4. Peeters A, Barendregt JJ, Willekens F *et al.* Obesity in adulthood and its consequences for life expectancy: a life-table analysis. *Ann Intern Med* 2003; **138**: 24–32.
5. Naimark A, Cherniack RM. Compliance of the respiratory system and its components in health and obesity. *J Appl Physiol* 1960; **15**: 377–82.
6. Pelosi P, Croci M, Ravagnan I *et al.* Total respiratory system, lung, and chest wall mechanics in sedated-paralyzed postoperative morbidly obese patients. *Chest* 1996; **109**: 144–51.
7. Pelosi P, Croci I, Ravagnan I *et al.* Respiratory system mechanics in sedated, paralyzed morbidly obese patients. *J Appl Physiol* 1997; **82**: 811–18.
8. Ray CS, Sue DY, Bray G *et al.* Effects of obesity on respiratory function. *Am Rev Respir Dis* 1983; **128**: 501–6.
9. Collins LC, Hoberty PG, Walker JF *et al.* The effect of body fat distributions on pulmonary function tests. *Chest* 1995; **107**: 1298–302.
10. Lazarus R, Sparrow D, Weiss ST. Effects of obesity and fat distribution on ventilatory function. *Chest* 1997; **111**: 891–8.
11. Young RP, Hopkins R, Eaton TE. Forced expiratory volume in one second: not just a lung function test but a marker of premature death from all causes. *Eur Respir J* 2007; **30**: 616–22.
12. Lakka HM, Laaksonen DE, Lakka TA *et al.* The metabolic syndrome and total and cardiovascular disease mortality in middle-aged men. *JAMA* 2002; **288**: 2709–16.
13. Leone N, Courbon D, Thomas F *et al.* Lung function impairment and metabolic syndrome. *Am J Resp Crit Care Med* 2009; **179**: 509–16.
14. Pischon T, Boeing H, Hoffmann K *et al.* General and abdominal adiposity and risk of death in Europe. *N Engl J Med* 2008; **359**: 2105–20.
15. Lee HM, Chung SJ, Lopez VA *et al.* Association of FVC and total mortality in US adults with metabolic syndrome and diabetes. *Chest* 2009; **136**: 171–6.
16. Ochs-Balcom HM, Grant BJB, Muti P *et al.* Pulmonary function and abdominal adiposity in the general population. *Chest* 2006; **129**: 853–62.
17. Jones RL, Nzekwu MMU. The effects of body mass index on lung volumes. *Chest* 2006; **130**: 827–33.
18. Canoy D, Luben R, Welch A *et al.* Abdominal obesity and respiratory function in men and women in the EPIC-Norfolk Study, United Kingdom. *Am J Epidemiol* 2004; **159**: 1140–9.
19. Watson RA, Pride NB. Postural changes in lung volumes and respiratory resistance in subjects with obesity. *J Appl Physiol* 2005; **98**: 512–17.
20. Bottai M, Pistelli F, Di Pede F *et al.* Longitudinal changes of body mass index, spirometry and diffusion in a general population. *Eur Respir J* 2002; **20**: 665–73.
21. Rubinstein I, Zamel N, DuBarry L *et al.* Airflow limitation in morbidly obese, nonsmoking men. *Ann Intern Med* 1990; **112**: 828–32.
22. Pankow W, Podszus T, Gutheil T *et al.* Expiratory flow limitation and intrinsic positive end-expiratory pressure in obesity. *J Appl Physiol* 1998; **85**: 1236–43.
23. Caro CG, Butler J, DuBois AB. Some effects of restriction of chest cage expansion on pulmonary function in man. An experimental study. *J Clin Invest* 1960; **39**: 573–83.
24. Koutsoukou A, Koulouris N, Bekos *et al.* Expiratory flow limitation in morbidly obese postoperative mechanically ventilated patients. *Acta Anaesthesiol Scand* 2004; **48**: 1080–8.
25. Hardie JA, Vollmer WM, Buist AS *et al.* Reference values for arterial blood gases in the elderly. *Chest* 2004; **125**: 2053–60.
26. Cerveri I, Zoia MC, Fanfulla F *et al.* Reference values of arterial oxygen tension in the middle-aged and elderly. *Am J Respir Crit Care Med* 1995; **152**: 934–41.
27. Ulmer WT, Reichel G. Untersuchungen uber die Altersabhangigkeit der aleolaren und arteriellen Sauerstoff-und Kohlensauredrucke. *Klein Wochenschr* 1963; **41**: 1–6.
28. Holley HS, Milic-Emili J, Becklake MR *et al.* Regional distribution of pulmonary ventilation and perfusion in obesity. *J Clin Invest* 1967; **46**: 475–81.
29. Yamane T, Date T, Tokuda M *et al.* Hypoxemia in inferior pulmonary veins in supine position is dependent on obesity. *Am J Respir Crit Care Med* 2008; **178**: 295–8.

30. Farebrother MJB, McHardy GJR, Munro JF. Relationship between pulmonary gas exchange and closing volume before and after substantial weight loss in obese subjects. *Br Med J* 1974; **3**: 391–3.
31. American Academy of Sleep Medicine. *International classification of sleep disorders*, 2nd edn. Diagnostic and coding manual. Westchester, Illinois: American Academy of Sleep medicine, 2005.
32. Young T, Peppard PE, Taheri S. Excess weight and sleep-disordered breathing. *J Appl Physiol* 2005; **99**: 1592–9.
33. Peppard PE, Young T, Palta M *et al.* Longitudinal study of moderate weight change and sleep-disordered breathing. *JAMA* 2000; **284**: 3015–21.
34. Sajkov D, McEvoy RD. Obstructive sleep apnea and pulmonary hypertension. *Prog Cardiovasc Dis* 2009; **51**: 363–70.
35. Krieger J, Sforza E, Apprill M *et al.* Pulmonary hypertension, hypoxemia, and hypercapnia in obstructive sleep apnea patients. *Chest* 1989; **96**: 729–37.
36. Chaouat A, Weitzemblum E, Krieger J *et al.* Association of chronic obstructive pulmonary disease and sleep apnea syndrome. *Am J Respir Crit Care Med* 1995; **151**: 82–6.
37. Weitzenblum E, Krieger J, Appril M *et al.* Daytime pulmonary hypertension in patients with obstructive sleep apnea syndrome. *Am Rev Respir Dis* 1988; **138**: 345–9.
38. Fanfulla F, Grassi M, Taurino AE *et al.* The relationship of daytime hypoxemia and nocturnal hypoxia in obstructive sleep apnea syndrome. Sleep 2008; **31**: 249–55.
39. Resta O, Foschino MP, Carpagnano GE *et al.* Diurnal $PaCO_2$ tension in obese women: relationship with sleep disordered breathing. *Int J Obes Relat Metab Disord* 2003; **27**: 1453–8.
40. Laaban JP, Chailleux E. Daytime hypercapnia in adult patients with obstructive sleep apnea syndrome in France, before initiating nocturnal nasal continuous positive airway pressure therapy. *Chest* 2005; **127**: 710–15.
41. Akashiba T, Kawahara S, Kosaka N *et al.* Determinants of chronic hypercapnia in Japanese men with obstructive sleep apnea syndrome. *Chest* 2002; **121**: 415–21.
42. Nowbar S, Burkart KM, Gonzales R *et al.* Obesity-associated hypoventilation in hospitalized patients: prevalence, effects, and outcome. *Am J Med* 2004; **116**: 1–7.
43. Lugaresi E, Cirignotta F, Gerardi R *et al.* Snoring and sleep apnea: natural history of heavy snorers disease. In: Guilleminault C, Partinen M, eds. *Obstructive sleep apnea syndrome*. New York: Raven Press, 1990: 25–36.
44. Mokhlesi B, Krygher MH, Grunstein RR. Assessment and management of patients with obesity hypoventilation syndrome. *Proc Am Thorac Soc* 2008; **5**: 218–25.
45. Kress JP, Pohlman AS, Alverdy J *et al.* The impact of morbid obesity on oxygen cost of breathing ($O_{2RESP}$) at rest. *Am J Respir Crit Care Med* 1999; **160**: 883–6.
46. Sampson MG, Grassino A. Neuromechanical properties in obese patients during carbon dioxide rebreathing. *Am J Med* 1983; **75**: 81–90.
47. Lopata M, Onal E. Mass loading, sleep apnea, and the pathogenesis of obesity hypoventilation. *Am Rev Respir Dis* 1982; **126**: 640–5.
48. Chouri-Pontarollo N, Borel JC, Tamisier R *et al.* Impaired objective daytime vigilance in obesity-hypoventilation syndrome: impact of noninvasive ventilation. *Chest* 2007; **131**: 148–55.
49. Burki NK, Baker RW. Ventilatory regulation in eucapnic morbid obesity. *Am Rev Respir Dis* 1984; **129**: 538–43.
50. Leech J, Onal E, Aronson R *et al.* Voluntary hyperventilation in obesity hypoventilation. *Chest* 1991; **100**: 1334–8.
51. Jokic R, Zintel T, Sridhar G *et al.* Ventilatory responses to hypercapnia and hypoxia in relatives of patients with the obesity hypoventilation syndrome. *Thorax* 2000; **55**: 940–5.
52. de Lucas-Ramos P, de Miguel-Diez J, Santacruz-Siminiani A *et al.* Benefits at 1 year of nocturnal intermittent positive pressure ventilation in patients with obesity hypoventilation syndrome. *Respir Med* 2004; **98**: 961–7.
53. Redolfi S, Corda L, La Piana G *et al.* Long-term non-invasive ventilation increases chemosensitivity and leptin in obesity-hypoventilation syndrome. *Respir Med* 2007; **101**: 1191–5.
54. Akashiba T, Akahoshi T, Kawahara S *et al.* Clinical characteristics of obesity-hypoventilation syndrome in Japan: a multi-center study. *Intern Med* 2006; **45**: 1121–5.
55. De Miguel Diez J, De Lucas Ramos P, Perez Parra JJ *et al.* Analysis of withdrawal from noninvasive mechanical ventilation in patients with obesity-hypoventilation syndrome. Medium term results. *Arch Bronconeumol* 2003; **39**: 292–7.
56. Berger KI, Ayappa I, Sorkin IB *et al.* $CO_2$ homeostasis during periodic breathing in obstructive sleep apnea. *J Appl Physiol* 2000; **88**: 257–64.
57. Berger KI, Ayappa I, Sorkin IB *et al.* Postevent ventilation as a function of CO2 load during respiratory events in obstructive sleep apnea. *J Appl Physiol* 2002; **93**: 917–24.
58. Ayappa I, Berger KI, Norman RG *et al.* Hypercapnia and ventilatory periodicity in obstructive sleep apnea syndrome. *Am J Respir Crit Care Med* 2002; **166**: 1112–15.
59. Norman RG, Goldring RM, Clain JM *et al.* Transition from acute to chronic hypercapnia in patients with periodic breathing: predictions from a computer model. *J Appl Physiol* 2006; **100**: 1733–41.
60. O'Donnell CP, Tankersley CG, Polotsky VP *et al.* Leptin, obesity, and respiratory function. *Respir Physiol* 2000; **119**: 163–70.
61. O'Donnell CP, Schaub CD, Haines AS *et al.* Leptin prevents respiratory depression in obesity. *Am J Respir Crit Care Med* 1999; **159**: 1477–84.
62. Phipps PR, Starritt E, Caterson I *et al.* Association of serum leptin with hypoventilation in human obesity. *Thorax* 2002; **57**: 75–6.
63. Shimura R, Tatsumi K, Nakamura A *et al.* Fat accumulation, leptin, and hypercapnia in obstructive

sleep apnea-hypopnea syndrome. *Chest* 2005; **127**: 543–9.

64. Campo A, Fuhbeck G, Zulueta JJ *et al.* Hyperleptinaemia, respiratory drive and hypercapnic response in obese patients. *Eur Respir J* 2007; **30**: 223–31.
65. Williams RH, Jensen LT, Verkhratsky A *et al.* Control of hypothalamic orexin neurons by acid and $CO_2$. *PNAS* 2007; **107**: 10685–90.
66. Willie JT, Chemelli RM, Sinton CM *et al.* To eat or to sleep? Orexin in the regulation of feeding and wakefulness. *Ann Rev Neurosci* 2001; **24**: 429–58.
67. Young JK, Wu M, Manaye KF *et al.* Orexin stimulates breathing via medullary and spinal pathways. *J Appl Physiol* 2005; **98**: 1387–95.
68. Deng BS, Nakamura A, Zhang W *et al.* Contribution of orexin in hypercapnic chemoreflex: evidence from genetic and pharmacological disruption and supplementation in mice. *J Appl Physiol* 2007; **103**: 1772–9.
69. Mateika JH, Narwani G. Intermittent hypoxia and respiratory plasticity in humans and other animals: does exposure to intermittent hypoxia promote or mitigate sleep apnoea? *Exp Physiol* 2009; **94**: 279–96.
70. Wilkerson JER, MacFarlane PM, Hoffman MS *et al.* Respiratory plasticity following intermittent hypoxia: roles of protein phosphatases and reactive oxygen species. *Biochem Soc Trans* 2007; **35**: 1269–72.
71. MacFarlane PM, Mitchell GS. Respiratory long-term facilitation following intermittent hypoxia requires reactive oxygen species formation. *Neuroscience* 2008; **152**: 189–97.
72. Mateika JH, Ellythy M. Chemoreflex control of ventilation is altered during wakefulness in humans with OSA. *Respir Physiol Neurobiol* 2003; **138**: 45–57.
73. Ackland GL, Kasymov V, Gourine AV. Physiological and pathophysiological roles of extracellular ATP in chemosensory control of breathing. *Biochem Soc Trans* 2007; **35**: 1264–8.

# 41

# Non-invasive ventilation in acute and chronic respiratory failure due to obesity

JUAN F MASA, ISABEL UTRABO, FRANCISCO JAVIER GÓMEZ DE TERREROS

## ABSTRACT

Obesity is a growing phenomenon associated with increased morbidity and mortality. The mechanisms by which diurnal hypercapnia improves with non-invasive ventilation (NIV) are complex and not entirely understood. Combined action is probably the most reasonable explanation for understanding the effects of NIV on obesity hypoventilation syndrome (OHS). Intermittent positive pressure ventilation and continuous positive airway pressure (CPAP) are used extensively worldwide. Clinical series have reported improvements in symptoms, arterial blood gases and sleep disorders with these treatments. Although CPAP corrects nocturnal obstructive events in patients with OHS, daytime $PaCO_2$ does not return to a normal value in all cases. Response to CPAP can depend on the predominance of nocturnal obstructive events. Non-invasive ventilation can prevent obstructive events and reduce hypoventilation during sleep. Both NIV and CPAP could decrease nocturnal hypercapnia, leading to lower daytime serum bicarbonate and, consequently, less blunting of the central carbon dioxide response. Currently, the most frequent OHS ventilation mode is pressure support, although average volume assured pressure support could decrease daytime $PaCO_2$ more effectively. While 90 per cent of patients with OHS have concurrent sleep apnoea, treatment with NIV has not classically been titrated during sleep. Although there is no standard recommendation, expiratory positive air pressure (EPAP) could be employed as it is used to treat conventional sleep apnoea, together with inspiratory positive airways pressure (IPAP) to improve nocturnal hypoventilation, or EPAP used to prevent apnoeas and IPAP to prevent hypopnoeas and improve nocturnal hypoventilation as well. Given that, there are no randomized controlled trials that demonstrate, in non-selected patients, whether NIV is superior to CPAP and if one (or both) of them is more effective than the historic treatment (weight loss and oxygen). Future research must focus on the comparative value of the above-mentioned treatments in the short-term and long-term settings.

## INTRODUCTION

Non-invasive ventilation (NIV) is a recognized therapy for several diseases that result in nocturnal and daytime hypoventilation, especially neuromuscular diseases and conditions that cause restriction of the chest wall.

Obesity is a growing phenomenon worldwide,[1] associated with increased morbidity and mortality[2,3] (see Chapter 39). Obesity compromises waking respiratory function, primarily in the supine position. This difficulty and the tendency for decreased ventilation in normal sleep physiology, hypotonia of the intercostal muscles and lower lung volume, can lead to nocturnal oxyhaemoglobin desaturation and hypercapnia. Moreover, the accumulation of fat in the lateral parts of the pharynx intensifies extra-luminal pressure and can modify the geometry of the upper airway, facilitating collapse[4] (apnoeas and hypopnoeas). These mechanisms can lead to daytime hypercapnic respiratory failure called obesity hypoventilation syndrome (OHS; see Chapter 40).

The therapeutic mechanisms resulting in nocturnal and daytime gas exchange improvement in patients with restrictive chest wall diseases (e.g. kyphoscoliosis) treated with NIV are not completely understood. Since OHS can generate mechanical difficulties and nocturnal hypoventilation similar to kyphoscoliosis, NIV may be effective in OHS. The first effective treatments for OHS, used in small series of patients, were continuous positive airway pressure (CPAP) in 1982[5] and intermittent positive pressure ventilation in 1992,[6] both used non-invasively.

The aim of this chapter is to review the role of NIV (intermittent positive pressure ventilation [IPPV]) and CPAP in OHS, in particular the mechanisms that produce improvement, the available evidence, clinical applications, technical considerations and future research.

## PATHOPHYSIOLOGY (POTENTIAL MECHANISMS FOR ACHIEVING NON-INVASIVE VENTILATION IMPROVEMENT)

### Chronic failure

The mechanisms by which diurnal hypercapnia improves with NIV are complex and not entirely understood. The principal mechanisms are improvement in: abnormal respiratory mechanics (including respiratory muscle dysfunction); central responses to hypercapnia and/or neurohormonal dysfunction (leptin resistance); and sleep-disordered breathing (see Chapter 40 and Fig. 41.1).

#### RESPIRATORY MECHANICS

Mechanical alterations in the respiratory system produced by the obesity component of OHS can result in respiratory muscle dysfunction[7] and, potentially, daytime hypercapnia. Non-invasive ventilation can reduce inspiratory muscular activity[8] and, consequently, it could decrease mechanical load, favouring greater muscular efficacy after NIV treatment (during the day).

The evidence of improvement in vital capacity and lung volume with long-term NIV is contradictory. Several studies[9–11] have shown no change in lung volumes or forced vital capacity in OHS after effective treatment with NIV therapy. On the other hand, two more recent studies in patients with OHS[12,13] have reported significant improvements in vital capacity and expiratory reserve volume after NIV therapy.

#### BREATHING CONTROL

The altered response to hypercapnia observed in OHS[11] can improve with NIV treatment,[11,13] suggesting that improvement in central chemosensitivity could result in daytime normocapnia. However, this improvement cannot be caused by a direct effect on the neural drive, but can be the consequence of NIV acting to improve other mechanisms (mechanical, neurohormonal dysfunction and sleep-disordered breathing improvements).

The hormone leptin, produced by fat cells, is implicated in appetite reduction and may also act on the nervous system to increase ventilation.[14] Consequently, if leptinaemia

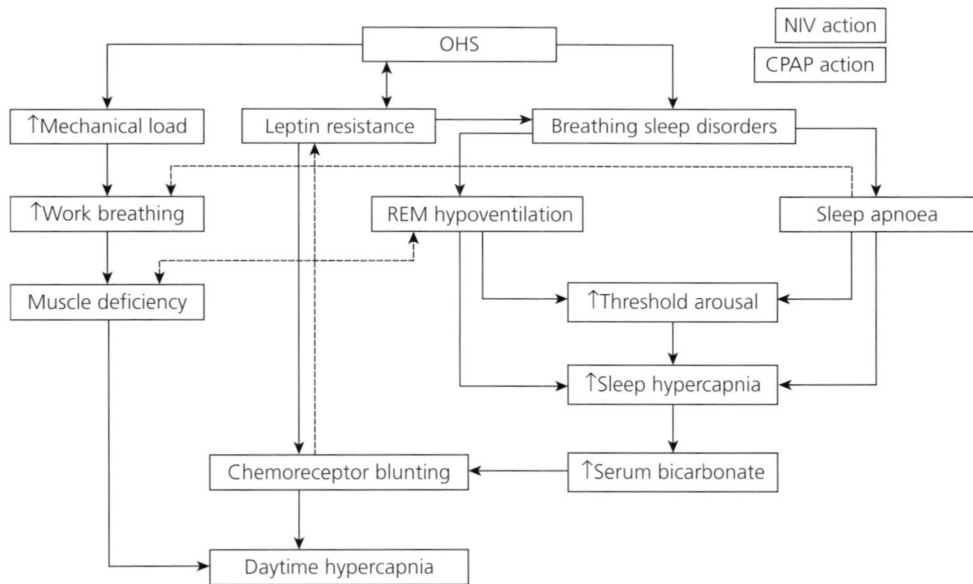


**Figure 41.1** Potential mechanisms for achieving improvement with non-invasive ventilation (NIV). Daytime hypercapnia in obesity hypoventilation syndrome (OHS) can result in increased mechanical respiratory load, central leptin resistance, breathing sleep-disorders or a combination of all of these (see Chapter 40). Continuous positive airway pressure (CPAP) prevents nocturnal obstructive events and consequently decreases sleep hypercapnia, serum bicarbonate and chemoreceptor blunting. It can alleviate breathing effort as well, and NIV can resolve sleep apnoeas and nocturnal hypoventilation caused by non-apnoeic episodes. In addition, NIV decreases breathing effort and may produce improvement in respiratory drive, decreasing central leptin resistance. REM, rapid eye movement. Modified with permission from the figure published in M Kryger, ed., *Principles and practice in sleep medicine*, Masa JF, Kryger M. Restrictive lung disorders, Copyright: Elsevier (in press).

is low or normal, but there is a central resistance to leptin, daytime hypercapnia could develop. The level of serum leptin decreases to normal limits in patients with sleep apnoea hypopnoea syndrome (SAHS) treated with CPAP,[15] but it is assumed that apnoeas and hypopnoeas are the cause of the elevated leptin levels rather than being the result of them.[16] Leptinaemia also decreases with NIV treatment[17] as does daytime hypercapnia, and some studies have shown a correlation between leptinaemia and a reduction in the hypercapnic ventilatory response.[18] Nevertheless, a recent study[19] reported contradictory results – leptin increased with NIV. Therefore, the role of leptin in how NIV treatment achieves improvement is still unclear.

#### SLEEP

Nocturnal hypoventilation is the confluent factor of all sleep-breathing disorders. Although OHS can exist without sleep apnoea, approximately 90 per cent of OHS patients have sleep apnoea.[9,20] Despite correction of nocturnal obstructive events with CPAP in patients with OHS, daytime $PaCO_2$ does not return to normal in all cases. Several studies have emphasized that the CPAP response may depend on the predominance of nocturnal obstructive events.[21,22] Thus, if the time with apnoeas is a high proportion of total sleep time, CPAP can be effective in reverting daytime $PaCO_2$.[23] Non-invasive ventilation can prevent obstructive events and reduces hypoventilation during sleep. Both NIV and CPAP should decrease nocturnal hypercapnia, leading to lower daytime serum bicarbonate and consequently less blunting of the central carbon dioxide response.[24] Because most of the mechanisms that improve with NIV are inter-related, the combined action of all (or the majority) of them is the most reasonable explanation for understanding the action of NIV in OHS (Fig. 41.1).

### Acute failure

Limited information is available about mechanisms by which NIV produces improvement in an acute setting. They are probably not very different from those mentioned above, although decreasing breathing effort by reducing the load on respiratory muscles and opening microatelectasis, as well as improvement of central chemosensitivity, may be the most important factors.[25]

## EVIDENCE BASE

### Chronic failure

Weight loss is the ideal treatment for OHS. It can improve respiratory failure, pulmonary hypertension and sleep disorders.[26] However, it is difficult to achieve and maintain significant weight loss in these patients. Limited long-term data are available about the efficacy of bariatric surgery in OHS[27] and it is not an alternative for most patients because of significant morbidity and mortality.[28] Moderate weight loss can also improve $PaCO_2$, although this outcome has not been confirmed over the long term.[26]

Currently, NIV and CPAP are used extensively worldwide. Clinical series have reported improvements in symptoms, arterial blood gases and sleep disorders with these treatments (Table 41.1). As mentioned above, improvement in spirometry, lung volumes and chemosensitivity to carbon dioxide were reported in some studies but not in others. In non-controlled longitudinal studies, decreases in days of hospital admission have been observed.[10,29,30] There are no controlled trials assessing mortality, and decreased mortality was only observed in series of treated patients when compared with other studies in which they were not treated.[31] Only one clinical series reported higher mortality in treated patients compared with patients who rejected treatment.[9]

Continuous positive airway pressure treatment is able to prevent nocturnal obstructive events in patients with OHS, but nocturnal and daytime $PaCO_2$ do not revert to normal values in all cases. A controlled study[36] compared the impact of overnight CPAP titration in 23 patients with OHS and 23 patients with eucapnic SAHS who were matched for body mass index (BMI), apnoea hypopnoea index (AHI), and lung function. Forty-three per cent of patients with OHS had refractory hypoxaemia during CPAP titration. From this and other studies,[32,37–39] patients unresponsive to CPAP treatment appeared to have more obesity, higher $PaCO_2$, and lower $PaO_2$, and nocturnal oxygen saturation ($SaO_2$), than responsive patients.

At the present time, only one randomized controlled study has ascertained and compared the short-term efficacy of NIV and CPAP treatments in 36 OHS patients, selected for their favourable response to an initial night of CPAP treatment.[15] From 45 eligible patients, nine (20 per cent) did not achieve acceptable improvement with CPAP based in the following criteria: $SaO_2$ remaining below 80 per cent continuously (>10 min) in the absence of apnoeas; acute increase in transcutaneous $PaCO_2$ during REM sleep (>10 mm Hg); or increase in afternoon to morning $PaCO_2$ of >10 mm Hg in patients with an awake $PaCO_2$ >55 mm Hg. Daytime sleepiness, $PaCO_2$ and polysomnographic improvements were similar in both the CPAP and NIV groups. However, there are no randomized controlled trials demonstrating which of these two treatments are more effective in non-selected patients, or whether these treatments are more successful than weight loss. No controlled trials have evaluated whether the repercussions of OHS (arterial and pulmonary hypertension, cardiovascular events, hospital days and mortality) decrease to a similar extent with each type of treatment, or if some are more effective than others.

In one study, obese patients with nocturnal hypoventilation but without daytime hypercapnia were treated first with oxygen and then with NIV. Oxygen increased

**Table 41.1** Efficacy of non-invasive ventilation and continuous positive airway pressure in chronic hypercapnic respiratory failure

| Authors (year) | Patients | Study type | Intervention | Duration | Clinical improvement | Respiratory function improvement | Sleep disorder improvement | Hospitalization and mortality reduction |
|---|---|---|---|---|---|---|---|---|
| Sullivan *et al.*[5] (1983) | 2 | Case reports | CPAP | 1–3 m | Oedema, EDS; mental function | $PaO_2$, $PaCO_2$ | SDB, $SatO_2$ | |
| Berg *et al.*[29] (2001) | 20 | Retrospective | NIV-CPAP | 2 y | | | SDB, $SatO_2$ | Hospital days |
| Janssens *et al.*[30] (2003) | 71 | Retrospective | NIV | 7 y | | $PaO_2$, $PaCO_2$ | | Hospital days, mortality |
| Budweiser *et al.*[31] (2007) | 126 | Retrospective | NIV | 10 y | | $PaO_2$, $PaCO_2$ $FEV_1$, IVC, TLC, RV/TLC | | Mortality |
| Piper *et al.*[32] (1994) | 13 | Retrospective | NIV | 3 m | | $PaO_2$, $PaCO_2$ | $PaCO_2$tc | |
| Piper *et al.*[33] (2008) | 36 | RCT | NIV vs CPAP | 3 m | Similar EDS; NIV: better sleep quality | Similar $PaCO_2$ and $SatO_2$ | | |
| Storre *et al.*[34] (2006) | 10 | RCT | NIV vs AVAPS | 1.5 m | Sleep quality, QoL | $PaCO_2$ with AVAPS | Sleep architecture, SDB, $SatO_2$ with both treatments. $PaCO_2$tc with AVAPS | |
| Hida *et al.*[35] (2003) | 26 | Before/after | CPAP | 3 m | EDS, QoL | | | |
| Chouri-Pontarollo *et al.*[11] (2007) | 15 | Before/after | NIV | 5 n | EDS, objective vigilance | $PaCO_2$ | Sleep architecture, SDB, $SatO_2$ | |
| Masa *et al.*[10] (2001) | 22 | Before/after | NIV | 4 m | EDS, headache, oedema, dyspnoea, mental function | $PaO_2$, $PaCO_2$ | | Hospital days |
| Berger *et al.*[21] (2001) | 23 | Before/after | NIV-CPAP | 4 d–7 y | | $PaCO_2$ | | |
| De Lucas *et al.*[13] (2004) | 13 | Before/after | NIV | 12 m | | $PaO_2$, $PaCO_2$, FVC, $CO_2$ chemosensitivity | | |
| Pérez de Llano *et al.*[9] (2005) | 20 | Retrospective | NIV-CPAP | 7 y | EDS, dyspnoea | $PaO_2$, $PaCO_2$ | | Higher mortality in rejected NIV |
| Redolfi *et al.*[19] (2007) | 6 | Before/after | NIV | 6–20 m | | $PaO_2$, $PaCO_2$, $CO_2$ chemosensitivity | | |
| Heinemann *et al.*[12] (2007) | 35 | Before/after | NIV | 12–24 m | | $PaO_2$, $PaCO_2$, VC, TLC, RV/TLC | | |

AVAPS, average volume assured pressure support; CPAP, continuous positive airway pressure; EDS, excessive daytime sleepiness; m, months; n, nights; NIV, non-invasive ventilation; $PaCO_2$, $PaO_2$, partial arterial carbon dioxide and oxygen pressures; $PaCO_2$tc, transcutaneous $PaCO_2$; QoL, quality of life; RTC, randomized controlled trial; $SatO_2$, oxygen saturation; SDB, sleep-disordered breathing; y, years.

transcutaneous $PaCO_2$ during sleep compared with NIV.[40] However, no randomized studies have been carried out to show the efficacy of long-term oxygen therapy in OHS, or oxygen therapy together with weight loss. In addition, oxygen treatment has not been compared with CPAP or NIV in OHS. While oxygen therapy is commonly combined with NIV in patients with persistent hypoxaemia, there are no available data about the long-term benefits of this procedure.

## Acute failure

Little published information is available about the efficacy of NIV and CPAP in acute hypercapnic respiratory failure in OHS (Table 41.2). Non-controlled and non-randomized trials have been performed, and NIV was used more frequently than CPAP and improvement in pH and $PaCO_2$ was the norm. Apparently, the number of intubations and deaths were low. One study showed lower mortality with NIV than with invasive ventilation (23.5 per cent and 15 per cent, respectively)[41] and the other studies, already mentioned above, reported lower mortality in patients treated with NIV compared with those who refused it (3 per cent with NIV and 57 per cent without).[9]

# CLINICAL APPLICATIONS

## Non-invasive ventilation or continuous positive airway pressure

As mentioned above, NIV (pressure or volume limited) and CPAP have a role in OHS treatment. Nocturnal hypoventilation can be effectively improved with CPAP in between 47 per cent to 80 per cent of the OHS patients[22,33,36] and diurnal $PaCO_2$ reduced or restored (to normal values).[33] However, in clinical practice, the selection of patients for one or the other treatment is not clearly established. According to the only controlled and randomized study[33] the selection of patients should be performed based on their initial response to a night of CPAP treatment. Therefore, if CPAP prevents obstructive events and maintains adequate oxygenation and ventilation, CPAP should be best for long term treatment, and NIV should be used if this is not the case. However, some non-controlled studies have shown that NIV may be more strongly indicated than CPAP in patients with a predominance of hypoventilation over obstructive events during sleep, higher obesity, higher $PaCO_2$ and lower $PaO_2$ while awake.[21,23,32,36–39] Therefore a more refined selection of patients for NIV or CPAP treatment could be also used until more information becomes available. Patients with a large number of apnoeas and, consequently, high sleep time in apnoea can very probably respond to CPAP[23] (see Pathophysiology section). On the other hand, in patients without a significant number of apnoeas, their nocturnal hypoventilation could depend on other mechanisms (i.e. obesity); then NIV should be preferable (Fig. 41.2).

In patients with acute failure, both NIV and CPAP could be used (Table 41.2), but NIV should be the first choice, due to an apparently higher efficacy, the severity of respiratory failure and the difficulty of performing a sleep study to determine the presence of SAHS.

## Length of treatment

Unless drastic weigh loss occurs, NIV or CPAP treatments seem necessary indefinitely. However, some patients treated effectively with NIV can be switched to CPAP or even discontinue treatment for a period of time.

Some clinical series[6,32,39,44] have reported that patients who are non-responsive to CPAP treatment (daytime hypercapnia unresolved), but who are effectively treated with NIV for several weeks, could return to CPAP for long periods of time without the reappearance of daytime hypercapnic respiratory failure (Fig. 41.2). In a prospective study,[22] 24 patients effectively treated with NIV were switched to CPAP. In 13 patients (54 per cent), oxygen desaturation persisted after elimination of apnoeas and hypopnoeas and they were returned to NIV. The remaining patients continued with CPAP, maintaining slightly better daytime $PaCO_2$ and oxygenation (daytime and nocturnal) than the OHS group treated with NIV.

In another prospective study,[45] 12 OHS patients successfully treated with NIV for 1 year were required to cease the treatment for 3 months. They had diurnal and nocturnal $PaO_2 \geq 60$ mm Hg and $PaCO_2 \leq 45$ mm Hg as well

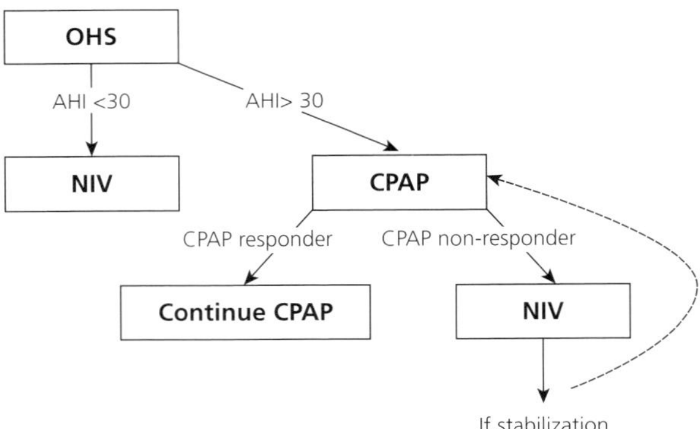


**Figure 41.2** Treatment of choice. Patients with obesity hypoventilation syndrome (OHS) and significant sleep apnoea should initially be treated with continuous positive airway pressure (CPAP). If relevant nocturnal or daytime hypoventilations remain (non-responder patients) non-invasive ventilation (NIV) is the best treatment option. Once appropriate improvement in nocturnal and daytime hypoventilation has been present for a long time, patients can be treated again with CPAP. Patients with OHS but without significant sleep apnoea who have been unsuccessful with dietary therapy should be treated directly with NIV. AHI, apnoea hypopnoea index.

**Table 41.2** Efficacy of non-invasive ventilation and continuous positive airway pressure in acute hypercapnic respiratory failure

| Authors (year) | Patients | Study type | Intervention | Clinical improvement | Respiratory function improvement | Intubations and mortality |
|---|---|---|---|---|---|---|
| Pérez de Llano *et al.*[9] (2005) | 34 | Retrospective | NIV-CPAP | | pH, $PaO_2$, $PaCO_2$ | No intubations, 1 patient died |
| Duarte *et al.*[41] (2007) | 33 | Retrospective | NIV-CPAP | | pH, $PaCO_2$ | 36% intubated, 5 patients died |
| Shivaram *et al.*[42] (1993) | 6 | Before/after | CPAP | Mental function | pH, $PaO_2$, $PaCO_2$ | No intubations, 1 patient died |
| Ortega *et al.*[43] (2006) | 17 | Before/after | NIV | | pH, $PaCO_2$ | No intubations or deaths |

CPAP, continuous positive airway pressure; NIV, non-invasive ventilation.

as nocturnal $SaO_2$ ≥90 per cent for more than 70 per cent of the night. After the withdrawal period, daytime and nocturnal pH, $PaO_2$ and $PaCO_2$ were similar to the previous period. Although these patients would probably show worse blood gas measurements with greater withdrawal time, this study suggests the possibility of discontinuing NIV for short (weekend) or intermediate (vacation) periods in some patients who desire it.

## When to treat

The standard indication is obese patients (BMI >30 kg/m$^2$) with daytime hypercapnia ($PaCO_2$ >45 mm Hg) and without other potential causes of hypercapnia such as severe obstructive or restrictive pulmonary disease (significant kyphoscoliosis or neuromuscular diseases), severe hypothyroidism or other central hypoventilation syndromes.[46]

However, some patients with obesity have relevant nocturnal hypoventilation and secondary clinical symptoms without daytime hypercapnia. This situation could be considered an early phase of OHS, at least in some individuals, resulting in daytime hypercapnia after a progressive increase of bicarbonate (Fig. 41.1). A non-randomized study, mentioned above,[40] compared the efficacy of sequential treatments with oxygen and NIV in a group of 11 patients with obesity who had nocturnal hypoventilation without daytime respiratory failure or relevant apnoeic episodes during sleep. Only NIV improved all clinical symptoms and nocturnal $PCO_2$, maintaining a level of oxygenation similar to oxygen therapy. Early initiation of NIV treatment can improve clinical symptoms and possibly prevent the development of OHS.

## Additional oxygen therapy

As mentioned, supplementing NIV with oxygen is common and the rule in acute failure. Chronic oxygen treatment is used in approximately half of OHS patients,[9,12,47] although the necessity of oxygen therapy can decrease after weeks or months of NIV use.[9,47] The goal should be to maintain the $SaO_2$ >90 per cent during the night when NIV cannot achieve this alone, although no studies have demonstrated that this approach provides additional benefits for patients.

## Follow-up

There are no standard recommendations for carrying out follow-up of OHS patients treated with NIV. However, follow-up is essential to verify the efficacy of treatment and to ensure proper adherence and compliance. A study has shown that improvements in clinical symptoms and blood gases depend on adherence to NIV. Accordingly, daytime $PaCO_2$ decreased 1.84 mm Hg per hour of real daily use.[47]

# TECHNICAL CONSIDERATIONS

There are no guidelines for the technical application of NIV in OHS, and this can lead to the assumption that there are no treatment differences with other restrictive chest wall diseases. However, some considerations must be highlighted, since patients with OHS have high impedance in the respiratory system, especially when extremely obese, and have a significant number of apnoeas and hypopnoeas.

## Setting and titration

### CONTINUOUS POSITIVE AIRWAY PRESSURE

The CPAP level is positively correlated with BMI.[48] Therefore, the pressure used for OHS treatment is usually higher than that used for patients with SAHS (without daytime hypercapnia), at about 14 cm $H_2O$.[33,36]

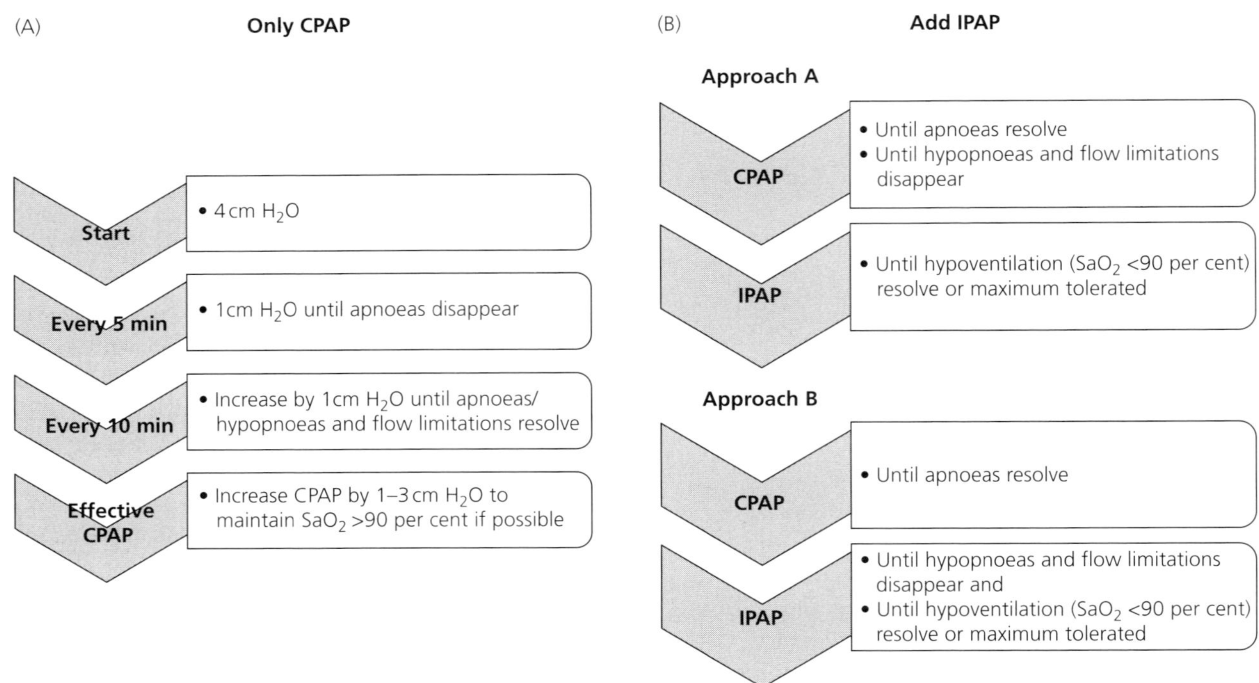


Figure 41.3 Continuous positive airway pressure (CPAP) and non-invasive ventilation (NIV) titration for obesity hypoventilation syndrome (OHS. (A) Only CPAP: starting at 4 cm $H_2O$, the technician increases CPAP by 1 cm $H_2O$ every 5 minutes until the apnoeas resolve, and then increases pressure by 1 cm $H_2O$ every 10 minutes until hypopnoeas and flow limitation resolve. Finally, CPAP is increased by 1–3 cm $H_2O$ to maintain $SaO_2$ >90 per cent or until the limit of tolerance is reached. (B) Add intermittent positive airway pressure (IPAP): approach A – CPAP as it used above to prevent apnoeas, hypopnoeas and flow limitations and then IPAP is increased to maintain $SaO_2$ >90 per cent or until the limit of tolerance is reached; approach B – CPAP as it used above to resolve apnoeas and then IPAP is increased to prevent hypopnoeas, flow limitations and to maintain $SaO_2$ >90 per cent or until the limit of tolerance is reached.

Determining optimal CPAP in SAHS patients is well understood.[49] For OHS, in some studies[33,36] pressure was increased once obstructive events were eliminated to improve nocturnal oxygen desaturation (Fig. 41.3). However, it is not clear if this process has benefits for nocturnal or daytime hypercapnic respiratory failure.

Today, auto-CPAP titration is a common procedure for achieving optimal CPAP in SAHS patients,[50] but most studies of the efficacy of auto-titration excluded patients with OHS. As a result, the efficacy of these devices is unknown. Conventional CPAP titration is required for OHS patients.

## NON-INVASIVE VENTILATION

The first studies testing the efficacy of NIV in OHS mainly used volume limited ventilators[10,32] but more recent studies employed pressure limited ventilators. There are no studies comparing the two types of ventilators in OHS, although a study including patients with chronic respiratory failure showed similar efficacy between the two.[51] At present, the use of pressure limited ventilators (or hybrid ventilators with pressure modes) is the rule in daily clinical practice. Bi-level pressure support is the most frequently employed mode. Inspiratory positive air pressure (IPAP) can be high, although the average is frequently around 16–18 cm $H_2O$.[30,33] The level of expiratory positive air pressure (EPAP) or CPAP can vary depending on the presence and severity of SAHS (see below). Although a fixed respiratory rate is not required in this ventilation mode (pressure support), most studies use a security rate of 12–15 breaths/minute.

Recent designs of non-invasive ventilator have a ventilation mode which guarantees a preset volume, called average volume assured pressure support (AVAPS) or target volume. There are two modes: the respirator analyses the tidal volume within a breath and responds, if the previously set tidal volume cannot be maintained, by volume limited ventilation (intra-breath analysis); or the respirator continuously analyses (breath-to-breath) the tidal volume and the minute volume, adjusting the level of pressure support. Technically this is pressure support ventilation, but with adaptive pressure.

Storre *et al.*[34] compared bi-level pressure support with AVAPS in a randomized crossover trial. Ten patients with OHS who did not respond to CPAP treatment were included. Six weeks of therapy with AVAPS achieved greater improvement in nocturnal and daytime $PaCO_2$ than bi-level pressure support. However, changes in sleep quality and quality of life were similar between the two ventilation modes. The interference of NIV with sleep quality has been insufficiently studied, and a study in patients with OHS[52] observed frequent patient–ventilator asynchronies, which degraded sleep quality. More studies are necessary to confirm and assess the effect of correcting these asynchronies.

Classically, treatment with NIV in OHS has not been nocturnally titrated. However, most patients with OHS have concurrent sleep apnoea, requiring EPAP adjustment. Furthermore, IPAP can prevent hypopnoeas and hypoventilation, depending on the level of pressure used. Therefore, arguments for performing titration during sleep in OHS are similar to those for SAHS. At the moment, there is no standard methodology. However, two approaches are recommended (Fig. 41.3): conventional titration of EPAP (CPAP) as it is used in SAHS, and IPAP used to improve nocturnal desaturation ($SaO_2$ >90 per cent);[33,53] EPAP could be used to prevent apnoeas (static obstruction) and IPAP to prevent hypopnoeas (dynamic obstruction) and improve nocturnal desaturation (hypoventilation).[54] The second method can result in lower EPAP and similar IPAP, which would be more comfortable for the patient, potentially improving adherence and compliance. Future studies need to investigate this possibility.

When acute respiratory failure is present, the main objective is to reverse respiratory acidosis as soon as possible. In this circumstance, no titrated ventilation setting is advisable. High EPAP pressure (12–14 cm $H_2O$) can prevent obstructive events during sleep. If this level of EPAP is poorly tolerated, intermediate pressure (7–9 cm $H_2O$) can prevent apnoeas and additional IPAP completes the treatment of obstructive events (hypopnoeas). Relatively high IPAP pressure (18–20 cm $H_2O$) or even higher is recommended initially, primarily in extreme obesity. Daytime $PaCO_2$ and nocturnal $SaO_2$ (and transcutaneous $PCO_2$) should help adjust EPAP and IPAP. If repetitive, continuing decreases in $SaO_2$ are observed, EPAP should be increased, and if persistent desaturation (or persistent elevations of transcutaneous $PCO_2$) occurs, IPAP should be increased.[25] A pre-set safety respiratory rate could be more recommendable in acute than in chronic respiratory failure. Alternative ventilation modes such as AVAPS, pressure control or volume control ventilation can be considered.

### Treatment time

Most patients with chronic failure only need nocturnal NIV to obtain dramatic improvement. In patients with extreme obesity and residual daytime hypercapnia, one option is to extend treatment to the daytime, although there is no formal evidence for the effectiveness of this regimen in OHS. In acute respiratory failure, ventilation time must be maximized during the first 12–24 hours, with some brief interruptions, because expected pH improvement should occur in the first hours of therapy.[25]

### Interfaces

The most extensive experience in long-term treatment for chronic failure is with the nasal mask. Nevertheless, as with other diseases treated using NIV, switching to another kind of mask or nasal prongs could be beneficial if there is a justifiable cause (e.g. important oral leakage might indicate a switch to an oronasal mask).[55] Masks with an intentional leak could impede efficient IPAP when the intentional leak increases.[56] Therefore, it is advisable to use an expiratory valve (preferably inside a ventilator with a double circuit) in acute respiratory failure. In these patients, oronasal or face masks may be the best choice in the initial setting to guarantee a more hermetic circuit and prevent oral leakage.

## FUTURE RESEARCH

Obesity hypoventilation syndrome is a relatively recent indication for NIV,[57] but today it is probably the illness most frequently requiring long-term treatment in the developed world. Despite extensive use, the level of evidence about its efficacy is intermediate or low, and future research must focus on the following topics.

#### EFFICACY

Randomized controlled studies must demonstrate, in OHS patients who are not pre-selected, whether NIV is superior to CPAP and if either (or both) are more effective than the historic treatment (weight loss and oxygen). This research should analyse both short-term (respiratory function, polysomnographic parameters and quality of life improvements) and long-term (arterial and pulmonary hypertension, incidence of cardiovascular events, days of hospitalization and survival) effects of treatment. In addition, the benefit of adding oxygen to NIV to improve residual desaturation should be clarified.

#### PATHOGENESIS

The treatment effect makes it possible to explore causality. In this way, the role of sleep apnoea or leptin in the genesis of daytime hypercapnia can be investigated in CPAP responders and non-responders.

#### PROPHYLACTIC TREATMENT

Non-invasive ventilation is indicated for symptomatic nocturnal hypoventilation based on clinical series.[57] Nocturnal hypoventilation may be the principal factor leading to daytime hypercapnia. It remains to be demonstrated whether early initiation of NIV (for nocturnal hypoventilation without daytime hypercapnia) can prevent the development of daytime hypercapnia.

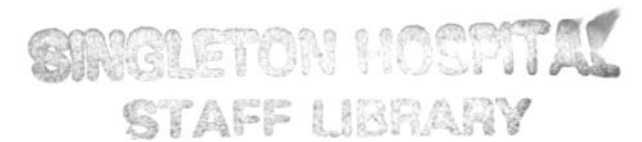

### TECHNICAL CONSIDERATIONS

The optimal NIV settings and modes for OHS are not well established. Future research and consensus should focus on standardizing this procedure. Studies should show whether NIV titration using EPAP for preventing only apnoeas (and IPAP for abolishing hypopneas and hypoventilation) achieves similar efficacy, adherence and compliance as EPAP used for completely preventing obstructive events (apnoeas and hypopnoeas) and IPAP for hypoventilation.

## REFERENCES


1. Wang Y, Beydoun MA. The obesity epidemic in the United States-gender, age, socio-economic, racial/ethnic, and geographic characteristics: a systematic review and meta-regression analysis. *Epidemiol Rev* 2007; **29**: 6–28.
2. World Health Organization. Obesity: *Preventing and managing the global epidemic* – Report of a WHO consultation on obesity. Geneva: World Health Organization, 1998:1–276.
3. Zhang C, Rexrode KM, Van Dam RM *et al.* Abdominal obesity and the risk of all-cause, cardiovascular and cancer mortality: sixteen years of follow-up in US women. *Circulation* 2008; **117**: 1658–67.
4. Crummy F, Piper AJ, Naughton MT. Obesity and the lung: 2. Obesity and sleep-disordered breathing. *Thorax* 2008; **63**: 738–46.
5. Sullivan CE, Berthon-Jones M, Issa FG. Remission of severe obesity-hypoventilation syndrome after short-term treatment during sleep with nasal continuous positive airway pressure. *Am Rev Respir Dis* 1983; **128**: 177–81.
6. Waldhorn RE. Nocturnal nasal intermittent positive pressure ventilation with bi-level positive airway pressure ($B_iPAP$) in respiratory failure. *Chest* 1992; **101**: 516–21.
7. Kress JP, Pohlman AS, Alverdy J *et al.* The impact of morbid obesity on oxygen cost of breathing (VO(2RESP)) at rest. *Am J Respir Crit Care Med* 1999; **160**: 883–6.
8. Pankow W, Hijjeh N, Schüttler F *et al.* Influence of noninvasive positive pressure ventilation on inspiratory muscle activity in obese subjects. *Eur Respir J* 1997; **10**: 2847–52.
9. Pérez de Llano LA, Golpe R, Ortiz Piquer M *et al.* Short-term and long-term effects of nasal intermittent positive pressure ventilation in patients with obesity-hypoventilation syndrome. *Chest* 2005; **128**: 587–94.
10. Masa JF, Celli BR, Riesco JA *et al.* The obesity hypoventilation syndrome can be treated with noninvasive mechanical ventilation. *Chest* 2001; **119**: 1102–7.
11. Chouri-Pontarollo N, Borel JC, Tamisier R *et al.* Impaired objective daytime vigilance in obesity-hypoventilation syndrome: impact of noninvasive ventilation. *Chest* 2007; **131**: 148–55.
12. Heinemann F, Budweiser S, Dobroschke J *et al.* Non-invasive positive pressure ventilation improves lung volumes in the obesity hypoventilation syndrome. *Respir Med* 2007; **101**: 1229–35.
13. De Lucas-Ramos P, de Miguel-Díez J, Santacruz-Siminiani A *et al.* Benefits at 1 year of nocturnal intermittent positive pressure ventilation in patients with obesity-hypoventilation syndrome. *Respir Med* 2004; **98**: 961–7.
14. O'Donnell CP, Schaub CD, Haines AS *et al.* Leptin prevents respiratory depression in obesity. *Am J Respir Crit Care Med* 1999; **159**: 1477–84.
15. Ip MSM, Lam KSL, Ho C *et al.* Serum leptin and vascular risk factors in obstructive sleep apnea. *Chest* 2000; **118**: 580–6.
16. Fitzpatrick M. Leptin and the obesity hypoventilation syndrome: a leap of faith? *Thorax* 2002; **57**: 1–2.
17. Yee, BJ, Cheung J, Phipps P *et al.* Treatment of obesity hypoventilation syndrome and serum leptin. *Respiration* 2006; **73**: 209–12.
18. Campo A, Freihbeck G, Zueta JJ *et al.* Hypercapnic response in obese patients. *Eur Respir J* 2007; **30**: 223–31.
19. Redolfi S, Corda L, La Piana G *et al.* Long-term noninvasive ventilation increases chemosensitivity and leptin in obesity-hypoventilation syndrome. *Respir Med* 2007; **101**: 1191–95.
20. Kessler R, Chaovat A, Schinkewitch P *et al.* The obesity-hypoventilation syndrome revisited: a prospective study of 34 consecutive cases. *Chest* 2001; **120**: 369–76.
21. Berger KI, Ayappa I, Chatramontri B *et al.* Obesity hypoventilation syndrome as a spectrum of respiratory disturbances during sleep. *Chest* 2001; **120**: 1231–38.
22. Pérez de Llano LA, Golpe R, Ortiz Piquer M *et al.* Clinical heterogeneity among patients with obesity hypoventilation syndrome: therapeutic implications. *Respiration* 2008; **75**: 34–9.
23. Ayappa I, Berger KI, Norman RG *et al.* Hypercapnia and ventilatory periodicity in obstructive sleep apnea syndrome. *Am J Respir Crit Care Med* 2002; **166**: 1112–15.
24. Mokhlesi B, Tulaimat A, Faibursowitsch I *et al.* Obesity hypoventilation syndrome: prevalence and predictors in patients with obstructive sleep apnea. *Sleep Breath* 2007; **11**: 117–24.
25. Lee WY, Mokhlesi B. Diagnosis and management of obesity hypoventilation syndrome in the ICU. *Crit Care Clin* 2008; **24**: 533–49.
26. Olson AL, Zwillich C. The obesity hypoventilation syndrome. *Am J Med* 2005; **118**: 948–56.
27. Martí-Valeri C, Sabaté A, Masdevall C *et al.* Improvement of associated respiratory problems in morbidly obese patients after open roux-en-y gastric bypass. *Obes Surg* 2007; **17**: 1102–10.
28. Surgeman HJ, Fairman RP, Sood RK *et al.* Long-term effects of gastric surgery for treating respiratory insufficiency of obesity. *Am J Clin Nutr* 1992; **55**: 5975–6015.
29. Berg G, Delaive K, Manfreda J *et al.* The use of health-care resources in obesity-hypoventilation syndrome. *Chest* 2001; **120**: 377–83.

30. Janssens JP, Derivaz S, Breitenstein E *et al.* Changing patterns in long-term noninvasive ventilation: a 7 year prospective study in the Geneva lake area. *Chest* 2003; **123**: 67–79.
31. Budweiser S, Riedl SG, Jörres RA *et al.* Mortality and prognostic factors in patients with obesity-hypoventilation syndrome undergoing non-invasive ventilation. *J Intern Med* 2007; **261**: 375–83.
32. Piper AJ, Sullivan CE. Effects of short-term NIPPV in the treatment of patients with severe obstructive sleep apnea and hypercapnia. *Chest* 1994; **105**: 434–40.
33. Piper AJ, Wang D, Yee BJ *et al.* Randomised trial of CPAP vs bilevel support in the treatment of obesity hypoventilation syndrome without severe nocturnal desaturation. *Thorax* 2008; **63**: 395–401.
34. Storre JH, Seuthe B, Fiechter R *et al.* Average volume-assured pressure support in obesity hypoventilation: a randomized crossover trial. *Chest* 2006; **130**: 815–21.
35. Hida W, Okabe S, Tatsumi K *et al.* Nasal continuous positive airway pressure improves quality of life in obesity hypoventilation syndrome. *Sleep Breath* 2003; **7**: 3–12.
36. Banerjee D, Yee BJ, Piper AJ *et al.* Obesity hypoventilation syndrome: hypoxemia during continuous positive airway pressure. *Chest* 2007; **131**: 1678–84.
37. Resta O, Guido P, Picca V *et al.* Prescription of nCPAP and nBIPAP in obstructive sleep apnoea syndrome: Italian experience in 105 subjects. A prospective two centre study. *Respir Med* 1998; **92**: 820–7.
38. Rabec C, Merati M, Baudouin N *et al.* Management of obesity and respiratory insufficiency. The value of dual-level pressure nasal ventilation. *Rev Mal Respir* 1998; **15**: 269–78.
39. Schäfer H, Ewig S, Hasper E *et al.* Failure of CPAP therapy in obstructive sleep apnoea syndrome: predictive factors and treatment with bilevel-positive airway pressure. *Respir Med* 1998; **92**: 208–15.
40. Masa JF, Celli BR, Riesco JA *et al.* Noninvasive positive pressure ventilation and not oxygen may prevent overt ventilatory failure in patients with chest wall diseases. *Chest* 1997; **112**: 207–13.
41. Duarte AG, Justino E, Bigler T *et al.* Outcomes of morbidly obese patients requiring mechanical ventilation for acute respiratory failure. *Crit Care Med* 2007; **35**: 732–7.
42. Shivaram U, Cash ME, Beal A. Nasal continuous positive airway pressure in decompensated hypercapnic respiratory failure as a complication of sleep apnea. *Chest* 1993; **104**: 770–4.
43. Ortega A, Peces-Barba G, Fernández I *et al.* Evolution of patients with chronic obstructive pulmonary disease, obesity hypoventilation syndrome or congestive heart failure in a respiratory monitoring unit. *Arch Bronconeumol* 2006; **42**: 423–9.
44. Smith IE, King MA, Siklos PW *et al.* Treatment of ventilatory failure in the Prader-Willi syndrome. *Eur Respir J* 1998; **11**: 1150–2.
45. De Miguel J, De Lucas P, Pérez JJ *et al.* Analysis of withdrawal from noninvasive mechanical ventilation in patients with obesity-hypoventilation syndrome. Medium term results. *Arch Bronconeumol* 2003; **39**: 292–7.
46. Martin TJ, Sanders MH. Chronic alveolar hypoventilation: a review for the clinician. *Sleep* 1995; **18**: 617–34.
47. Mokhlesi B, Tulaimat A, Evans AT *et al.* Impact of adherence with positive airway pressure therapy on hypercapnia in obstructive sleep apnea. *J Clin Sleep Med* 2006; **2**: 57–62.
48. Miljeteig H, Hoffstein V. Determinants of continuous positive airway pressure level for treatment of obstructive sleep apnea. *Am Rev Respir Dis* 1993; **147**: 1526–30.
49. Kushida CA, Chediak A, Berry RB *et al.* Positive airway pressure titration task force; american academy of sleep medicine clinical guidelines for the manual titration of positive airway pressure in patients with obstructive sleep apnea. *J Clin Sleep Med* 2008; **4**: 157–71.
50. Masa JF, Jiménez A, Durán J *et al.* Alternative methods of titrating continuous positive airway pressure: a large multicenter study. *Am J Respir Crit Care Med* 2004; **170**: 1218–24.
51. Schönhofer B, Sonneborn M, Haidl P, Böhrer H, Köhler D. Comparison of two different modes for noninvasive mechanical ventilation in chronic respiratory failure: volume versus pressure controlled device. *Eur Respir J* 1997; **10**: 184–91.
52. Guo YF, Sforza E, Janssens JP. Respiratory patterns during sleep in obesity-hypoventilation patients treated with nocturnal pressure support: a preliminary report. *Chest* 2007; **131**: 1090–9.
53. Mokhlesi B, Tulaimat A. Recent advances in obesity hypoventilation syndrome. *Chest* 2007; **132**: 1322–36.
54. Sanders MH, Kern N. Obstructive sleep apnea treated by independently adjusted inspiratory and expiratory positive airway pressures via nasal mask. Physiologic and clinical implications. *Chest* 1990; **98**: 317–24.
55. Elliott MW. The interface: crucial for successful noninvasive ventilation. *Eur Respir J* 2004; **23**: 7–8.
56. Borel JC, Sabil A, Janssens JP *et al.* Intentional leaks in industrial masks have a significant impact on efficacy of bilevel noninvasive ventilation: a bench test study. *Chest* 2009; **135**: 669–77.
57. Clinical indications for non-invasive positive pressure ventilation in chronic respiratory failure due to restrictive lung disease COPD, and nocturnal hypoventilation – a consensus conference report. *Chest* 1999; **116**: 521–34.

# SECTION J

# Other conditions

# 42

# Bronchiectasis and adult cystic fibrosis

IRENE PERMUT, GERARD J CRINER

## ABSTRACT

Cystic fibrosis is a recessively inherited chronic disease that affects 70 000 people worldwide. Bronchiectasis refers to permanent dilatation of the airways along with parenchymal destruction that results from a variety of pathological processes affecting the respiratory system. Both cystic fibrosis and bronchiectasis are complicated by poor mucus clearance, bacterial colonization and intermittent infections. Both disease processes result in obstructive lung disease and parenchymal destruction causing poor gas exchange and progressive respiratory failure. Treatment of acute respiratory failure often requires endotracheal intubation. The side effects associated with intubation including ventilator-associated pneumonia can be especially dangerous in this population characterized by colonization with virulent and frequently resistant bacteria. In addition, the mortality during and after intubation is high in patients with cystic fibrosis. Non-invasive positive pressure ventilation (NIV) can be a successful alternative to intubation as well as a bridge to transplant. It is an effective means of reversing the acute deterioration in acute respiratory failure and stabilizing pulmonary function in chronic respiratory failure in this population.

## INTRODUCTION

Cystic fibrosis is the most common life-shortening recessively inherited disease in Caucasians. It also affects Hispanics, Native Americans, African Americans and Asian Americans. Cystic fibrosis once was a disease of children, but advances in supportive care and treatment have improved the survival of cystic fibrosis patients such that in 2007 the median survival was 37.4 years.[1]

Bronchiectasis refers to the permanent dilataion of airways associated with destruction of the bronchi or subsegmental bronchioles. Its prevalence is unknown due to the multiple aetiologies that contribute to its development. The syndrome consists of chronic sputum production, recurrent infections and progressive lung damage resulting in a clinical picture similar to cystic fibrosis lung disease.

This chapter will describe the pathophysiology of cystic fibrosis, the indications and evidence base for the use of non-invasive positive pressure ventilation (NIV) for acute and chronic respiratory failure in cystic fibrosis and bronchiectasis, and technical considerations in the use of NIV. A brief discussion of adjunctive therapies and areas for future research in cystic fibrosis concludes the chapter.

## PATHOPHYSIOLOGY

Cystic fibrosis is caused by a mutation in the cystic fibrosis transmembrane conductance regulator (*CFTR*) gene. The protein encoded by the *CFTR* gene belongs to a family of proteins involved in ion transport. It acts at the chloride transport channel and the epithelial sodium channel. Defective transport of sodium and chloride across the respiratory epithelial cell membrane causes dehydration of peri-ciliary liquid and mucous layers resulting in defective mucociliary function and diminished clearance.[2] Impaired mucous clearance results in colonization and infection of the airways. Infected airways attract neutrophils, which release elastase and reactive oxygen species causing cell damage. Over time, neutrophils undergo apoptosis and release their cell contents, further thickening the mucus and impairing mucociliary clearance[3] (Fig. 42.1).

Cystic fibrosis is complicated by periodic infections and exacerbations and the universal development of chronic lung disease. Respiratory failure is the leading cause of death in cystic fibrosis.[3] Acute respiratory failure can be triggered by infection, upper abdominal surgery and disease progression.[4] Pain experienced after upper abdominal surgery causes

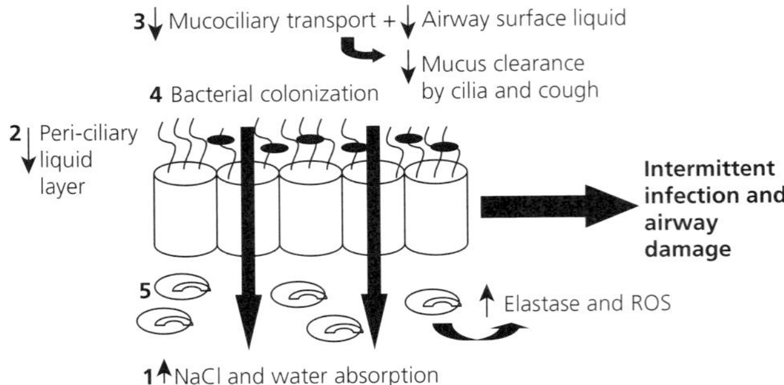


**Figure 42.1** Cystic fibrosis airway dysfunction due to defective transport of sodium and chloride causing dehydration of the peri-ciliary liquid layer. Defective NaCl transport causes defective mucus clearance due to mucociliary dysfunction and decreased clearance.[2] Airways become colonized and infected by bacteria. Infected airways attract neutrophils that release elastase and reactive oxygen species causing cell damage, further thickening mucus and impairing mucociliary clearance.[3]

splinting and impaired cough, worsening the process of mucus plugging and atelectasis. This results in increased ventilation–perfusion ($\dot{V}/Q$) mismatch and decreased functional residual capacity (FRC) and lung compliance, causing increased work of breathing (WOB).[4]

The goal of NIV for respiratory failure in cystic fibrosis and bronchiectasis is to increase FRC, decrease atelectasis, increase compliance, and decrease resistance thereby decreasing $\dot{V}/Q$ mismatch.[4] NIV applies positive pressure during inhalation and exhalation. Positive pressure during exhalation prevents airway and alveolar collapse thereby decreasing atelectasis, maintaining FRC and improving oxygenation. Positive pressure during inspiration increases tidal volume and mean airway pressure, preventing respiratory failure related to neuromuscular fatigue. NIV is an alternative to endotracheal intubation in acute and chronic respiratory failure due to cystic fibrosis and bronchiectasis. Its use limits complications related to intubation such as laryngeal damage, subglottic oedema, tracheal stenosis, and ventilator-associated pneumonia. NIV has the benefits of ease of communication, intermittent use and decreased need for sedation.[4]

## EVIDENCE-BASED USE OF NON-INVASIVE POSITIVE PRESSURE VENTILATION IN ACUTE RESPIRATORY FAILURE

Non-invasive positive pressure ventilation frequently improves the clinical status of patients with acute respiratory failure due to cystic fibrosis. Improvements are observed even when clinical worsening occurs despite therapy with continuous positive airway pressure (CPAP) and oxygen.[4,5] Rapid improvement in gas exchange has been demonstrated in case series of children and young adults with cystic fibrosis.[3–5]

Non-invasive positive pressure ventilation decreases WOB and reports of dyspnoea in cystic fibrosis patients with acute respiratory failure.[3–5] In addition, improved respiratory muscle strength with the use of NIV has been demonstrated.[5] Decreased respiratory muscle use in patients with chronic obstructive pulmonary disease (COPD) with the use of NIV has been studied and may explain its mechanism of action in cystic fibrosis. Ambrosino *et al.* demonstrated decreased surface diaphragm EMG signal during negative pressure ventilation in COPD.[6] Nava *et al.* described decreased diaphragmatic activity in stable COPD patients by measuring transdiaphragmatic pressure prior to and after the use of NIV.[7] By improving gas exchange, NIV may improve the impaired respiratory muscle function in the setting of acidosis.[8]

Chest physiotherapy is a critical component of care for patients with cystic fibrosis and bronchiectasis.[9] Techniques promoting airway clearance decrease the rate of decline of pulmonary function in cystic fibrosis.[10] However, chest physiotherapy may increase energy expenditure and provoke oxygen desaturation, respiratory muscle fatigue and dyspnoea, particularly during acute exacerbations.[11,12] NIV has been shown to decrease respiratory muscle work at rest in stable cystic fibrosis patients and decrease the incidence of acute respiratory failure.[13] Holland *et al.* demonstrated preserved muscle strength and improved oxygenation with the use of NIV in a study of 26 adults with acute cystic fibrosis exacerbations and copious secretions.[14]

## EVIDENCE-BASED USE OF NON-INVASIVE VENTILATION IN CHRONIC RESPIRATORY FAILURE

The major cause of hypoxaemia in cystic fibrosis is $\dot{V}/Q$ mismatch from chronic progressive lung disease. However, hypoventilation also plays a role. Kyphosis, respiratory muscle weakness, central nervous system (CNS) depression, and sleep-disordered breathing (SDB) all participate in the progression to chronic hypoventilation.

Frequent steroid use, the inflammatory state resulting from recurrent infections and concomitant inactivity all contribute to accelerated bone loss in cystic fibrosis.[15] Kyphosis causes decreased chest wall compliance and decreased efficiency of coupling between the respiratory muscles and the chest wall. The result is increased WOB and hypoventilation.[16–18]

Controversy exists regarding whether respiratory muscle weakness in cystic fibrosis patients contributes to chronic hypoventilation. Malnutrition due to pancreatic insufficiency and an increased catabolic state from chronic inflammation and infection may play a role. Chronic airway obstruction resulting in gas trapping and hyperinflation also contribute to respiratory muscle weakness.[19] However, other authors have demonstrated increases in diaphragm strength and diaphragm muscle mass in cystic fibrosis patients with moderate to severe lung dysfunction.[20] Despite these controversial findings, Granton *et al.* found that NIV acutely improved oxygenation and decreased minute ventilation in eight adult cystic fibrosis patients with chronic respiratory failure and stable lung function. The authors hypothesized that the diaphragm in cystic fibrosis patients is at a mechanical disadvantage due to destruction of the lung parenchyma and the presence of airflow obstruction. Despite decreases in minute ventilation in this study, transcutaneous carbon dioxide did not rise due to improved alveolar ventilation or to reduced carbon dioxide production from decreased WOB.[13]

Chronic pain frequently effects patients with cystic fibrosis.[21] Opiates are frequently used to control pain, which may contribute to chronic hypoventilation by causing CNS depression and decreased respiratory drive. Finally, as lung disease advances in cystic fibrosis, SDB may lead to progressive nocturnal hypoxaemia and hypercapnia particularly during rapid eye movement (REM) sleep.[22] Over time, abnormal gas exchange during sleep can contribute to right-sided heart failure as well as an abnormal sleep pattern and diminished quality of life. Nocturnal oxygen therapy often improves oxygenation noted during sleep but does not always prevent desaturation and may worsen hypercapnia.[23,24] Regnis *et al.* demonstrated improved oxygenation with the use of nocturnal CPAP in seven cystic fibrosis patients with severe lung disease. Nocturnal CPAP had no effect on transcutaneous carbon dioxide levels.[24] However, Gozal *et al.* and Young *et al.* both demonstrated a beneficial effect of NIV on gas exchange in six cystic fibrosis subjects with moderate to severe lung disease.[25,26]

Improved sleep quality and daytime functional status have been reported in cystic fibrosis patients treated with nocturnal NIV.[5] Young *et al.* found improvements in quality of life (QoL), exertional dyspnoea and peak exercise capacity with six weeks of nocturnal NIV.[26] Recently, Faroux *et al.* demonstrated stabilization of lung function in cystic fibrosis patients treated for1 year with nocturnal NIV.[27] The initiation of long-term nocturnal NIV should be based on the severity of lung disease and a baseline polysomnogram documenting nocturnal hypercapnia and oxygen desaturation.[4]

Similar to cystic fibrosis, patients with bronchiectasis develop worsening $\dot{V}/Q$ mismatch, hypoxaemia, and hypercapnia as the disease progresses.[28] Although some series have shown poor long-term continuation of NIV in patients with bronchiectasis,[29] others have shown promising results with its continued use. Gacouin *et al.* performed a retrospective review of 16 patients with bronchiectasis and chronic respiratory failure treated with NIV and oxygen.[30] Study subjects had progressive worsening of gas exchange prior to the initiation of NIV, which was successful in improving gas exchange. Although no improvement beyond baseline blood gas levels occurred, stability in gas exchange was observed for up to 24 months. Gacouin *et al.* also demonstrated a mild but significant increase in forced expiratory volume in 1 second ($FEV_1$), improved daytime activity level and QoL. In addition, long-term compliance with NIV was demonstrated.[30]

Benhamou *et al.* conducted a comparative case–control study of 14 patients with diffuse bronchiectasis and chronic respiratory failure to evaluate the effects of NIV compared with long-term oxygen therapy.[31] Oxygenation improved to a greater extent with the use of NIV with oxygen supplementation than oxygen administration alone. Carbon dioxide values were not significantly lower with NIV, and long-term worsening of blood gas values was not prevented with the use of NIV and oxygen supplementation. There was no survival difference between the groups. The group of patients treated with NIV appeared to have more severe disease as evidenced by more frequent episodes of acute respiratory failure and days spent in hospital[31] (Table 42.1).

## TECHNICAL CONSIDERATIONS

The side effects of NIV in patients with cystic fibrosis and bronchiectasis are similar to those in other disease processes. With long-term or chronic use, skin breakdown may occur. Applying a bio-occlusive dressing to the bridge of the nose, intermittently repositioning the mask, and providing breaks as tolerated may diminish the amount of skin breakdown.[4]

Gastric insufflation and aspiration is a risk in cystic fibrosis patients treated with NIV. While in the hospital, intermittent gastric decompression of the stomach with a nasogastric tube may be helpful. Decreasing the inspiratory pressure to the lowest effective level and positioning patients in the upright, seated position while being treated with NIV may decrease the risk of gastric distention.[4]

Discomfort due to the NIV mask and positive pressure is common. Although NIV is ideally administered without the use of CNS-altering medications, the judicious use of pain medications and sedation may be necessary.[4]

## INITIATION AND WEANING OF NON-INVASIVE POSITIVE PRESSURE VENTILATION

The majority of articles evaluating the use of NIV in cystic fibrosis and bronchiectasis initiate NIV at low pressures. Inspiratory and expiratory pressures are then titrated up in increments of 2 cm $H_2O$ pressure until clinical goals are met. Endpoints for titration of NIV include adequate chest excursion, a goal tidal volume of 6–8 mL/kg, decreased WOB or improvement in gas exchange.[4]

Patients can be weaned from NIV in one of two ways. Once clinical stability is achieved, short trials without NIV may be attempted. As the patient recovers, these periods can be lengthened until the patient is free from NIV or is using it only nocturnally. Alternatively, the pressures can be titrated down until minimal pressure is being used and a trial of NIV is warranted.[4]

**Table 42.1** Summary of studies evaluating the use of non-invasive positive pressure ventilation (NIV) in cystic fibrosis and diffuse bronchiectasis

| Authors (year) | No. | Type of study | Acute/chronic respiratory failure | Gas exchange | Additional findings | Adverse events |
|---|---|---|---|---|---|---|
| Piper *et al.*[5] (1992) | 4 | Case series | Acute-on-chronic | Improved | Variable improvement in spirometry<br>Improved WOB and respiratory muscle strength | 1 patient required intubation |
| Regnis *et al.*[24] (1994) | 7 | Prospective crossover study with nocturnal CPAP | Chronic | Improved oxygenation, no effect on $CO_2$ | Decreased nocturnal respiratory disturbance | 2 patients slept poorly with CPAP |
| Gacouin *et al.*[30] (1996) | 16 | Retrospective review DB | Chronic | Stabilization of gas exchange | Reported improved QoL; decreased hospitalization; improved $FEV_1$ | 1 patient with conjunctivitis, chronic sinusitis |
| Benhamou *et al.*[31] (1997) | 14 | Case–control DB | Chronic | Initial improvement of $PaO_2$, minimal effect on $CO_2$ | No survival difference | 3 subjects with poor tolerance to NIV. Short-term improved QoL. Decreased hospitalizations |
| Madden *et al.*[32] (2002) | 113 | Retrospective review | Both | Improved oxygenation, no change in hypercapnia | 28 patients underwent transplant | 72 patients died, 29 while awaiting transplantation |
| Hodson *et al.*[33] (1991) | 6 | Retrospective review | Acute-on-chronic | Improved | Successful bridge to transplant | 1 death while awaiting transplantation |
| Gozal *et al.*[25] (1997) | 6 | Prospective crossover study nocturnal NIV vs oxygen | Chronic | Improved | Increased $T_cCO_2$ with oxygen therapy alone | 2 patients excluded – did not tolerate NIV |
| Sprague *et al.*[4] (2000) | 5 | Retrospective review | Acute | Improved | Improved WOB | 1 patient: skin breakdown |
| Holland *et al.*[14] (2003) | 26 | Randomized crossover NIV with chest PT | Acute | Improved oxygenation | No change in $FEV_1$, forced vital capacity (FVC); improved $FEF_{25-75}$; improved muscle strength, decrease in reported breathlessness | None reported |
| Faroux *et al.*[27] (2008) | 41 | Review | Chronic | NA | Stabilization of lung function | NA |
| Young *et al.*[26] (2008) | 8 | Randomized, placebo-controlled crossover | Chronic | Improved nocturnal $T_cCO_2$ | Improved QoL, exercise performance. No improvement in daytime gas exchange or lung function | 1 patient had aerophagia, which improved with decreased inspiratory pressure by 2 cm $H_2O$ |

CPAP, continuous positive airway pressure; DB, diffuse bronchiectasis; FEF, forced expiratory flow; $FEV_1$, forced expiratory volume in 1 second; QoL, quality of life; $T_cCO_2$, transcutaneous carbon dioxide; WOB, work of breathing.

## ADDITIONAL THERAPEUTIC STRATEGIES AND IDEAS FOR FUTURE RESEARCH

Cornerstones of therapy for cystic fibrosis include chest physiotherapy, nutrition, inhaled medications, and antibiotic prophylaxis. Additional therapies to improve sputum clearance are emerging.

Inflammation, colonization and intermittent infections contribute to lung destruction and respiratory failure in cystic fibrosis. Therapy with macrolides, specifically azithromycin and inhaled tobramycin, have been shown to improve outcomes.[35,36] Cystic fibrosis patients 6 years of age with chronic *Pseudomonas aeruginosa* infections had small but significant improvements in $FEV_1$, decreased exacerbation rates and increased weight gain when treated with azithromycin three days a week compared with placebo.[35] Similarly, cystic fibrosis patients chronically colonized with *Pseudomonas aeruginosa* and treated with inhaled tobramycin had increased $FEV_1$, decreased bacterial density, and decreased hospitalizations compared with placebo.[36]

Dornase alfa is thought to improve mucociliary clearance of sputum in cystic fibrosis and bronchiectasis by hydrolysing extracellular DNA released by airway neutrophils.[37] McCoy *et al.* demonstrated a significant increase in $FEV_1$ and FVC with the use of once-daily inhaled dornase alfa for 12 weeks in adult cystic fibrosis patients. There was no significant difference in the frequency of pulmonary exacerbations, adverse events or overall hospitalizations between the groups.[38]

Nebulized isotonic saline (IS) is frequently used in chronic lung disease to enhance mucus clearance. Sputum in bronchiectasis is hypotonic relative to serum.[39] Administration of hypertonic saline may enhance mucociliary clearance by its osmotic effect, improvements in ciliary function, and decreased viscosity of mucus. Kellett *et al.* evaluated the use of nebulized hypertonic saline (7 per cent) in 17 adults with bronchiectasis not due to cystic fibrosis. Hypertonic and isotonic saline were both superior to active cycle breathing technique in increasing sputum yield, decreasing viscosity, and improving ease of expectoration. There was a significant advantage with hypertonic saline over isotonic saline when evaluating sputum weight, viscosity and ease of expectoration.[40]

Most data presented were from retrospective studies and case reports on NIV in cystic fibrosis. Future research should focus on larger randomized studies to prospectively evaluate the effects of NIV on survival outcomes in cystic fibrosis and bronchiectasis.

## CONCLUSIONS

NIV may reverse hypoxaemia, hypercapnia and respiratory muscle fatigue in patients with cystic fibrosis and bronchiectasis. Unfortunately, the mortality rate in cystic fibrosis patients who require mechanical ventilation is high while intubated as well as 1 year after intubation.[34] Use of NIV may decrease need for intubation. As lung transplantation becomes more prevalent, NIV should be considered in both acute and chronic respiratory failure as a potential bridge to transplantation for patients with cystic fibrosis.[32–34]

## REFERENCES


1. Cystic Fibrosis Foundation Annual Data Report. Baltimore: Cystic Fibrosis Foundation, 2007.
2. Knowles MR, Boucher RC. Mucus clearance as a primary innate defense mechanism for mammalian airways. *J Clin Invest* 2002; **109**: 571–7.
3. Gibson RL, Burns JL, Ramsey BW. Pathophysiology and management of pulmonary infections in cystic fibrosis. *Am J Respir Crit Care Med* 2003; **168**: 918–31.
4. Sprague K, Graff G, Tobias JD. Noninvasive ventilation in respiratory failure due to cystic fibrosis. *South Med J* 2000; **93**: 954–61.
5. Piper AJ, Parker S, Torzillo PJ *et al.* Nocturnal nasal IPPV stabilizes patients with cystic fibrosis and hypercapnic respiratory failure. *Chest* 1992; **102**: 846–50.
6. Ambrosino N, Nava S *et al.* Physiologic evaluation of pressure support ventilation by nasal mask in patients with stable COPD. *Chest* 1992; **101**: 385–91.
7. Nava S, Ambrosino N, Rubini F *et al.* Effect of nasal pressure support ventilation and external PEEP on diaphragmatic activity in patients with severe stable COPD. *Chest* 1993; **103**: 143–50.
8. Juan G, Calverley P, Talamo C *et al.* Effect of carbon dioxide on diaphragm function in human beings. *N Engl J Med* 1984; **310**: 874–9.
9. Orenstein DM, Winnie GB, Altman H. Cystic fibrosis: a 2002 update. *J Pediatr* 2002; **140**: 156–64.
10. Williams M. Chest physiotherapy and cystic fibrosis. Why is the most effective form of treatment still unclear? *Chest* 1994; **106**: 1872–82.
11. Miller S, Hall DO, Clayton CB *et al.* Chest physiotherapy in cystic fibrosis: a comparative study of autogenic drainage and the active cycle of breathing techniques with postural drainage. *Thorax* 1995; **50**: 165–9.
12. Faroux B, Boule M, Lofaso F *et al.* Chest physiotherapy in cystic fibrosis: improved tolerance with nasal pressure support ventilation. *Pediatrics* 1999; **103**: E32.
13. Granton JT, Kesten S. The acute effects of nasal positive pressure ventilation in patients with advanced cystic fibrosis. *Chest* 1998; **113**: 1013–18.
14. Holland AE, Denehy L, Ntoumenopoulos G *et al.* Non-invasive ventilation assists chest physiotherapy in adults with acute exacerbations of cystic fibrosis. *Thorax* 2003; **58**: 880–4.
15. Aris RM, Merkel PA, Bachrach LK *et al.* Guide to bone health and disease in cystic fibrosis. *J Clin Endocrinol Metab* 2005; **90**: 1888–96.

16. Henderson RC, Specter BB. Kyphosis and fractures in children and young adults with cystic fibrosis. *J Pediatr* 1994; **125**: 208–12.
17. Logvinoff MM, Fon GT, Taussig LM *et al.* Kyphosis and pulmonary function in cystic fibrosis. *Clin Pediatr (Phila)* 1984; **23**: 389–92.
18. Mason RJMJ, Nadel JA, Broaddus VC, eds. *Textbook of respiratory medicine*, 4th edn. Philadelphia: Elsevier Saunders, 2005.
19. Lands L, Desmond KJ, Demizio D *et al.* The effects of nutritional status and hyperinflation on respiratory muscle strength in children and young adults. *Am Rev Respir Dis* 1990; **141**: 1506–9.
20. Pinet C, Cassart M, Scillia P *et al.* Function and bulk of respiratory and limb muscles in patients with cystic fibrosis. *Am J Respir Crit Care Med* 2003; **168**: 989–94.
21. Festini F, Ballarin S, Codamo T *et al.* Prevalence of pain in adults with cystic fibrosis. *J Cyst Fibros* 2004; **5**: 51–7.
22. Tepper RS, Skatrud JB, Dempsey JA. Ventilation and oxygenation changes during sleep in cystic fibrosis. *Chest* 1983; **84**: 388–93.
23. Spier S, Rivilin J, Hughes D *et al.* The effect of oxygen on sleep, blood gases, and ventilation in cystic fibrosis. *Am Rev Respir Dis* 1984; **129**: 712–18.
24. Regnis J, Piper AJ, Henke KG *et al.* Benefits of nocturnal nasal CPAP in patients with cystic fibrosis. *Chest* 1994; **106**: 1717–24.
25. Gozal D. Nocturnal ventilatory support in patients with cystic fibrosis: comparison with supplemental oxygen. *Eur Respir J* 1997; **10**: 1999–2003.
26. Young AC, Wilson JW, Kotsimbos *et al.* Randomised placebo controlled trial of non-invasive ventilation for hypercapnia in cystic fibrosis. *Thorax* 2008; **63**: 72–7.
27. Faroux B, Le Roux E, Ravilly S *et al.* Long-term noninvasive ventilation in patients with cystic fibrosis. *Respiration* 2008; **72**: 168–74.
28. Wedzicha JA, Muir JF. Noninvasive ventilation in chronic obstructive pulmonary disease, bronchiectasis and cystic fibrosis. *Eur Respir J* 2002; **30**: 777–84.
29. Simonds AK, Elliott MW. Outcome of domiciliary nasal intermittent positive pressure ventilation in restrictive and obstructive disorders. *Thorax* 1995; **50**: 604–9.
30. Gacouin A, Desrues B, Lena H *et al.* Long-term nasal intermittent positive pressure ventilation (NIV) in sixteen consecutive patients with bronchiectasis: a retrospective study. *Eur Respir J* 1996; **9**: 1246–50.
31. Benhamou D, Muir JF, Raspaud C *et al.* Long-term efficacy of home nasal mask ventilation in patients with diffuse bronchiectasis and severe chronic respiratory failure. *Chest* 1997; **112**: 1259–66.
32. Madden BP, Kariyawasam H, Siddiqi AJ *et al.* Noninvasive ventilation in cystic fibrosis patients with acute or chronic respiratory failure. *Eur Respir J* 2002; **19**: 310–13.
33. Hodson ME, Madden BO, Steven MH *et al.* Non-invasive mechanical ventilation for cystic fibrosis patients: a potential bridge to transplantation. *Eur Respir J* 1991; **4**: 524–7.
34. Davis PB, di Saint'Agnese PA. Assisted ventilation for patients with cystic fibrosis. *JAMA* 1978; **239**: 1851–4.
35. Saiman L, Marshall BC, Mayer-Hamblett NM *et al.* Azithromycin in patients with cystic fibrosis chronically infected with *Pseudomonas aeruginosa*: a randomized controlled trial. *JAMA* 2003; **290**: 1749–56.
36. Ramsey BW, Pepe MS, Quan JM *et al.* Intermittent administration of inhaled tobramycin in patients with cystic fibrosis. *N Engl J Med* 1999; **340**: 23–30.
37. Shah PL, Ingham S, Marriott C *et al.* The *in vitro* effects of two novel drugs on the rheology of cystic fibrosis and bronchiectasis sputum. *Eur Respir J* 1994; **7** Suppl 18: 12S.
38. McCoy K, Hamilton S, Johnson C. Effects of 12-week administration of dornase alfa in patients with advanced cystic fibrosis lung disease. *Chest* 1996; **110**: 889–95.
39. Willis PJ, Hall RL, Chan W *et al.* Sodium chloride increases ciliary transportability of cystic fibrosis and bronchiectasis sputum on the mucus depleted bovine trachea. *J Clin Invest* 1997; **99**: 9–13.
40. Kellett F, Redfern J, Niven RM. Evaluation of nebulised hypertonic saline (7%) as an adjunct to physiotherapy in patients with stable bronchiectasis. *Respir Med* 2005; **99**: 27–31.

# 43

# Non-invasive ventilation in highly infectious conditions: lessons from severe acute respiratory syndrome

DAVID S C HUI

## ABSTRACT

Severe acute respiratory syndrome (SARS) is a highly infectious conditions with significant morbidity and mortality. Bats are natural reservoirs of SARS-like coronaviruses. The human and civet isolates of SARS-coronavirus nestle phylogenetically within the spectrum of SARS-like coronaviruses. SARS has the potential of being converted from droplet to airborne transmission. The presence of SARS-like coronaviruses in horseshoe bats raises the possible role of bats in previous and potentially future SARS outbreaks in humans. Respiratory failure is the major complication in patients hospitalized with SARS, and about 20 per cent of patients may progress rapidly to acute respiratory distress syndrome (ARDS), requiring intensive care support. Due to the rapid progression of the clinical course of SARS, most of the published data have been uncontrolled or based on retrospective review. Non-invasive positive pressure ventilation (NIPPV) may play a limited supportive role for early ARDS/acute lung injury as a bridge to invasive mechanical ventilation in SARS although it is contraindicated in critically ill patients with multiorgan failure and haemodynamic instability. However, healthcare workers should take adequate respiratory protection in addition to strict contact and droplet precautions when managing patients with SARS as the application of NIPPV may disperse potentially infected aerosols. Further research is needed to examine the exhaled air dispersion distances during application of NIPPV via different masks so that the healthcare providers can better protect themselves within the dangerous distances when managing patients in acute respiratory failure (ARF) due to highly infectious diseases. In addition, more research is needed in the technical improvement of the different NIPPV masks/viral-bacterial filters and the design of safer hospital ward environments in order to prevent nosocomial transmission of these infections. Advances will facilitate management of ARF due to future SARS outbreaks and other emerging infectious diseases such as pandemic influenza.

## INTRODUCTION

The rapid emergence of severe acute respiratory syndrome (SARS) in 2003 caught the medical profession by surprise and posed an enormous threat to international health and economies.[1–4] By the end of the epidemic in July 2003, 8098 probable cases were reported in 29 countries and regions, with a mortality of 774 (9.6 per cent).[5] A novel coronavirus (CoV) was responsible for SARS,[6] and the genome sequence of the SARS-CoV was not closely related to any of the previously characterized coronaviruses.[7] SARS re-emerged at small scales in late 2003 and early 2004 in South China after resumption of wild animal trading activities in markets.[8,9] A virus very similar to SARS-CoV has been discovered in Chinese horseshoe bats, bat SARS-CoV,[10] and data suggest that bats are natural reservoirs of SARS-like CoV.[11]

SARS appears to spread by close person-to-person contact via droplet transmission or fomites.[12] The high infectivity of this viral illness is shown by the fact that 138 patients (many of whom were healthcare workers) were hospitalized with SARS within 2 weeks as a result of exposure to one single index patient, who was admitted with community-acquired pneumonia (CAP) to a general medical ward at the Prince of Wales Hospital in Hong Kong.[1,13] This super-spreading event was thought to be related to the use of a nebulized bronchodilator for its mucociliary clearance effect to the index case, together with overcrowding and poor ventilation in the hospital ward.[1,13] In addition, there was evidence to suggest that SARS might have spread by airborne transmission in a major community outbreak in a private residential complex in Hong Kong.[14] There are additional data in support of SARS having the potential of being converted from droplet to airborne transmission.[15,16] Two polymerase chain reaction (PCR)-positive air samples were obtained from a room occupied by a patient with SARS in Canada, indicating the presence of the virus in the air of the room and the possibility of airborne droplet transmission.[15] These data emphasize the need for adequate respiratory protection in addition to strict contact and droplet precautions when managing patients with pneumonia due to highly infectious diseases.

## CLINICAL FEATURES

The estimated mean incubation period of SARS was 4.6 days (95 per cent confidence interval [CI] 3.8 to 5.8 days) whereas the mean time from symptom onset to hospitalization varied between 2 and 8 days, decreasing over the course of the epidemic. The mean time from onset to death was 23.7 days (CI 22.0 to 25.3 days), whereas the mean time from onset to discharge was 26.5 days (CI 25.8 to 27.2 days).[17] The major clinical features on presentation include persistent fever, chills/rigor, myalgia, dry cough, headache, malaise and dyspnoea. Sputum production, sore throat, coryza, nausea and vomiting, dizziness and diarrhoea are relatively less common features.[1,12,18]

The clinical course of SARS generally follows a typical pattern:[19] phase 1 (viral replication) is associated with increasing viral load and clinically characterized by fever, myalgia and other systemic symptoms that generally improve after a few days; phase 2 (immuno-pathological injury) is characterized by recurrence of fever, hypoxaemia, and radiological progression of pneumonia with falls in viral load. The high morbidity of SARS was highlighted by the observation that even when there was only 12 per cent of total lung field involved by consolidation on chest radiographs, 50 per cent of patients would require supplemental oxygen to maintain satisfactory oxygenation above 90 per cent.[20] About 20 per cent of patients would progress into acute respiratory distress syndrome (ARDS) necessitating invasive ventilatory support.[19] Peiris *et al.*[19] have shown progressive decrease in rates of viral shedding from the nasopharynx, stool and urine from day 10 to day 21 after symptom onset in 20 patients who had serial measurements with RT-PCR. Thus clinical worsening during phase 2 is most likely the result of immune-mediated lung injury due to an over-exuberant host response and cannot be explained by uncontrolled viral replication.[19]

The route of entry for SARS-CoV in humans is through the respiratory tract mainly by droplet transmission. Once infection can be established, the mechanisms by which SARS-CoV causes disease can be separated into direct lytic effects on host cells, and indirect consequences resulting from the host immune response. While clinically SARS is characterized by a pronounced systemic illness, the pathology of SARS, as revealed from fatal cases, was mainly confined to lungs where diffuse alveolar damage was the most prominent feature. Multinucleated syncytial giant cells, though characteristic, are rarely seen. In cases without secondary infection, a remarkable lack of immune response was observed at this late terminal stage. Apart from those related to end-stage multiorgan failure, the pathology of gastrointestinal tract, urinary system, liver and other organ systems were unremarkable.[21–23] Lungs and the intestinal tract are the only two organ systems that support a high level of SARS-CoV replication.[24]

When evaluating epidemiologically, high-risk patients with CAP and no immediate alternative diagnosis, a low absolute neutrophil count on presentation, along with poor responses after 72 hours of antibiotic treatment, may raise the index of suspicion for SARS.[25]

## EVIDENCE BASE FOR USE OF NON-INVASIVE VENTILATION

Several uncontrolled studies have shown that single circuit non-invasive positive pressure ventilation (NIPPV) might provide life-saving treatment for patients in respiratory failure as a result of SARS infection.[26–28] Among 120 patients meeting clinical criteria for SARS who were admitted to a hospital for infectious diseases in Beijing, 25 per cent of patients (30/120) had experienced acute respiratory failure (ARF) at $10.7 \pm 3.8$ days after the onset of SARS. Of interest, 16 of these patients (53 per cent) exhibited hypercapnia ($PaCO_2$ >45mm Hg), and 10 hypercapnic events occurred within 1 week of admission. NIPPV was instituted in 28 patients; one was intolerant of NIPPV. In the remaining 27 patients, NIPPV was initiated $1.2 \pm 1.6$ days after ARF onset. An hour of NIPPV therapy led to significant increases in $PaO_2$ and $PaO_2$/fraction of inspired oxygen ($FiO_2$) and a decrease in respiratory rate ($p < 0.01$). Endotracheal intubation was required in a third of the patients (9 of 27) who initially had a favourable response to NIPPV. Remarkable pulmonary barotrauma was noted in 7 of all 120 patients (5.8 per cent) and in 6 of those (22 per cent) on NIPPV. The overall fatality rate at 13 weeks was 6.7 per cent (8/120) but it was higher (26.7 per cent) in those needing NIPPV. No caregiver contracted SARS. The authors concluded that NIPPV was a feasible and appropriate treatment for ARF occurring as a result of SARS infection.[26]

In another study NIPPV was applied via oronasal masks to 20 SARS patients without chronic obstructive pulmonary disease (COPD), who developed severe hypoxaemic respiratory failure in a hospital ward environment in Hong Kong with efficient room air exchange, stringent infection control measures, full personal protective equipment (PPE), and addition of a viral-bacterial filter to the exhalation port of the NIPPV device. The mean age was 51.4 years, and mean acute physiology and chronic health evaluation II score was 5.35. SARS-CoV serology was positive in 95 per cent (19 of 20 patients). NIPPV was started 9.6 days (mean) from symptom onset, and mean duration of NIPPV usage was 84.3 h. Endotracheal intubation was avoided in 14 patients (70 per cent), in whom the length of intensive care unit stay was shorter (3.1 days vs 21.3 days, $p < 0.001$) and the chest radiography score within 24 hours of NIPPV was lower (15.1 vs 22.5, $p = 0.005$) compared with intubated patients. Intubation avoidance was predicted by a marked reduction in respiratory rate (9.2 breaths/min) and supplemental oxygen requirement (3.1 L/min) within 24 hours of NIPPV. Complications were few and reversible. There were no clinical infections among the 105 healthcare workers caring for the patients receiving NIPPV. NIPPV appeared effective in the treatment of ARF in the patients with SARS who were studied, and its use was safe for healthcare workers in this single-centre study.[27]

A retrospective analysis was conducted on all respiratory failure patients identified from the Hong Kong Hospital Authority SARS Database. Intubation rate, mortality and secondary outcome of a hospital utilizing NIPPV under standard infection control conditions (NIPPV hospital) were compared against 13 hospitals using solely invasive mechanical ventilation (IMV hospitals). Both hospital groups had comparable demographics and clinical profiles, but the NIPPV hospital (42 patients) had higher lactate dehydrogenase ratio and worse radiographic score on admission and ribavirin-corticosteroid commencement. Compared with IMV hospitals (451 patients), the NIPPV hospital had lower adjusted odds ratios for intubation (0.36, 95 per cent CI 0.164 to 0.791, $p = 0.011$) and death (0.235, 95 per cent CI 0.077 to 0.716, $p = 0.011$), and improved earlier after pulsed steroid rescue. There were no instances of transmission of SARS among healthcare workers due to the use of NIPPV. Compared with IMV, NIPPV as initial ventilatory support for ARF in the presence of SARS appeared to be associated with reduced intubation need and mortality in this study.[28]

## IMPLICATIONS FOR HEALTHCARE WORKERS

During the global outbreak of SARS, 13–26 per cent of patients developed ARDS necessitating invasive ventilatory support at a time of reaching very high viral load, and thus healthcare workers were particularly prone to infection while caring for their patients.[1,18,19] The relative risk of developing SARS was 13-fold for healthcare workers in Toronto who were involved in intubating SARS patients compared with those who were not, whereas NIPPV was not associated with a statistically significant risk for the healthcare workers (1/6 exposed healthcare workers versus 2/28 non-exposed, risk ratio 2.33, $p = 0.5$).[29] This was probably because tracheal suctioning was not generally performed for patients ventilated with NIPPV and the study sample size was small.[29] However, a retrospective study by Xiao *et al.* described NIPPV exposure as being associated with clinical SARS infection in two healthcare workers in Guangzhou, China.[30]

A major case–control study involving 124 medical wards in 26 hospitals in Guangzhou and Hong Kong has identified NIPPV as one of six independent risk factors of super-spreading nosocomial outbreaks of SARS (Box 43.1).[31]

**Box 43.1 Independent risk factors for super-spreading nosocomial outbreaks of SARS[31]**

- Minimum distance between beds <1 m (OR 6.98, 95 per cent CI 1.68 to 28.75, $p = 0.008$)
- Washing or changing facilities for staff (OR 0.12, 95 per cent CI 0.02 to 0.97, $p = 0.05$)
- Performance of resuscitation (OR 3.81, 95 per cent CI 1.04 to 13.87, $p = 0.04$)
- Staff working while experiencing symptoms (OR 10.55, 95 per cent CI 2.28 to 48.87, $p = 0.003$)
- SARS patients requiring oxygen therapy (OR 4.30, 95 per cent CI 1.00 to 18.43, $p = 0.05$)
- SARS patients requiring non-invasive positive pressure ventilation (OR 11.82, 95 per cent CI 1.97 to 70.80, $p = 0.007$)

NIPPV should be commenced under infection control measures as listed in Box 43.2 for patients with SARS if nasal oxygen above 5 L/min fails to maintain target $SpO_2$ at 93–96 per cent. NIPPV is delivered from a positive airway pressure system with independent positive inspired (IPAP) and expired pressures (EPAP). IPAP is adjusted to achieve respiratory rates below 25 breaths per minute and exhaled tidal volumes above 6 mL/kg. EPAP is adjusted to achieve target oxygenation with minimum carbon dioxide re-breathing. Criteria for intubation are: intolerance to NIPPV; patient fatigue; or when supplemental oxygen at 12 L/min fails to maintain at least 93 per cent $SpO_2$ while on NIPPV.[28]

## TECHNICAL CONSIDERATIONS

Healthcare workers should take precautions when managing patients with CAP of unknown aetiology that is complicated by respiratory failure. Experimental studies based on a sophisticated human patient simulator and

**Box 43.2 Infection control precautions in the ICU[28,32]**

Staff education

- Limit opportunities for exposure: limit aerosol generating procedures and limit number of healthcare workers present
- Effective use of time during patient contact
- How to 'gown up' and 'gown down' without contamination
- Emphasis on importance of vigilance and adherence to all infection control measures in addition to monitoring own health

Personal protection equipment (PPE)

- N95 respirator for airborne and surgical mask for droplet precautions
- Contact precautions: disposable gloves, gown and cap
- Eye protection with non-reusable goggles and face shield
- Powered air purification respirators may be used when performing high-risk procedures
- Pens, paper, other personal items and medical records should not be allowed into or removed from the room
- Immediate removal of grossly contaminated PPE and showering in nearby facility

Environment/equipment

- Conform to Centers for Disease Control (CDC) recommendation for environmental control of tuberculosis: minimum 6 air changes per hour (ACH). Where feasible, increase to 12 ACH or recirculate air through HEPA filter
- Preferred: Negative pressure isolation rooms with antechambers, with doors closed at all times
- Equipment should not be shared among patients
- Alcohol-based hand and equipment disinfectants
- Gloves, gowns, masks and disposal units should be readily available
- Careful and frequent cleaning of surfaces with disposable cloths and alcohol-based detergents
- Use of video camera equipment or windows to monitor patients

Transport

- Avoid patient transport when possible: Balance risks and benefits of investigations which necessitate patient transport

Special precautions for the ICU

- Viral-bacterial filter placed in expiratory port of bag-valve mask
- Two filters per ventilator: between expiratory port and the ventilator, and another on the exhalation outlet of the ventilator
- Closed system in-line suctioning of endotracheal/tracheostomy tubes
- Heat and moisture exchanger (HME) preferred to heated humidifier: Careful handling of contaminated HME required
- Scavenger system for exhalation port of ventilator. Optional if negative pressure with high air exchange (>12/h) is achieved

laser visualization technique have shown that the maximum exhaled air particle dispersion distances from patients receiving oxygen via Hudson mask and NIPPV via the ResMed Ultra Mirage mask were 0.4 m and 0.5 m, respectively, along the exhalation port.[33,34] A more recent study showed that the maximum exhaled air dispersion distance from the Respironics ComfortFull 2 mask was 0.95 m at a predictable direction from the exhalation diffuser perpendicular to the patient, whereas leakage though the Respironics Image 3 mask, connected to the whisper swivel exhalation port, was much more extensive and diffuse.[35] The whisper swivel is an efficient exhalation device to prevent carbon dioxide rebreathing but it would not be advisable to use such an exhalation port in managing patients with febrile respiratory illness of unknown aetiology, especially in the setting of highly infectious conditions such as SARS with high human to human transmission potential, for fear of causing major nosocomial infection. It is also important to avoid the use of higher IPAP, which could lead to wider distribution of exhaled air and substantial room contamination.[35] These data have important clinical implications in preventing any future nosocomial outbreaks of SARS and other highly infectious conditions such as pandemic influenza.

NIPPV should be applied in severe CAP only if there is adequate protection for healthcare workers, because of the potential risk of transmission via deliberate or accidental mask interface leakage and flow compensation causing dispersion of contaminated aerosols.[36] In patients with respiratory failure receiving NIPPV via nasal masks, air leakage through the mouth or other routes besides the exhalation valve can occur.[37] In clinical practice, pressure necrosis often develops at the skin around the nasal bridge if the mask is applied tightly for a prolonged period of time. Many patients loosen the mask strap to relieve discomfort, and air leakage from the nasal bridge is definitely a potential source for transmission of viral infection. Careful mask fitting is important for successful and safe application of NIPPV.[36] Addition of a viral-bacterial filter to the breathing system of NIPPV between the mask and the exhalation port [26–28] or using a dual circuit NIPPV may reduce the risk of nosocomial transmission of viral infection.[34] However, the use of viral-bacterial filters is difficult due to frequent blockage by moist secretions and can be applied only in some cases.[26–28]

In view of the observation that higher ventilator pressures result in a wider dispersion of exhaled air and a higher concentration of air leakage,[34,35] it is advisable to start NIPPV with low IPAP level (8–10 cm $H_2O$) and gradually increase as necessary, instead of starting high and titrating downward if the patient is intolerant.[38] SARS-related ARF responds readily to low positive pressures of CPAP of 4–10 cm $H_2O$ or IPAP of <10 cm $H_2O$ and EPAP of 4–6 cm $H_2O$.[32] Higher pressures should be avoided because of the common finding of spontaneous pneumomediastinum and pneumothorax in SARS.[1,18–20]

The World Health Organization (WHO) interim guidelines on prevention and control of acute respiratory diseases in healthcare has included NIPPV among those aerosol-generating procedures in which there is possibly increased risk of respiratory pathogen transmission. In addition to maintaining contact, droplet and standard precautions among the healthcare workers when providing routine care to such patients, the WHO recommends full PPE for the healthcare worker, covering the torso, arms, eyes, nose and mouth, and this should include long-sleeved gown, single-use gloves, eye protection, and wearing an N95 mask or equivalent as the minimum level of respiratory protection. NIPPV should be provided in an adequately ventilated single room and addition of an expiratory port with a viral-bacterial filter can reduce aerosol emission.[39]

## FUTURE RESEARCH

Emerging infectious diseases such as SARS and influenza are highly infectious conditions with significant morbidity and mortality. NIPPV may play a limited supportive role for early ARDS/acute lung injury as a bridge to IMV in SARS and other emerging respiratory infections, although it is contraindicated in critically ill patients with multiorgan failure and haemodynamic instability.[36] However, as the application of NIPPV may disperse potentially infected aerosols,[34,35] further research is needed to examine the exhaled air dispersion distances during application of NIPPV via different masks so that the healthcare providers can better protect themselves within the dangerous distances when managing patients in ARF due to highly infectious diseases. In addition, more research is needed in the technical improvement of the different NIPPV masks/viral-bacterial filters, and in the design of a safe hospital ward environment in order to prevent nosocomial transmission of these infections. Advances in knowledge will facilitate management of ARF due to future SARS outbreaks and other emerging infectious diseases such as pandemic influenza.

## REFERENCES


1. Lee N, Hui DS, Wu A *et al.* A major outbreak of severe acute respiratory syndrome in Hong Kong. *N Engl J Med* 2003; **348**: 1986–94.
2. Hsu LY, Lee CC, Green JA *et al.* Severe acute respiratory syndrome in Singapore: clinical features of index patient and initial contacts. *Emerg Infect Dis* 2003; **9**: 713–17.
3. Booth CM, Matukas LM, Tomlinson GA *et al.* Clinical features and short-term outcomes of 144 patients with SARS in the greater Toronto area. *JAMA* 2003; **289**: 2801–9.
4. Twu SJ, Chen TJ, Chen CJ *et al.* Control measures for severe acute respiratory syndrome (SARS) in Taiwan. *Emerg Infect Dis* 2003; **9**: 718–20.
5. WHO. Summary of probable SARS cases with onset of illness from 1 November to 31 July 2003. Available at: www.who.int/csr/sars/country/table2003_09_23/en (accessed February 2010).
6. Peiris JS, Lai ST, Poon LL *et al.* Coronavirus as a possible cause of severe acute respiratory syndrome. *Lancet* 2003; **361**: 1319–25.
7. Marra MA, Jones SJ, Astell CR *et al.* The genome sequence of the SARS-associated coronavirus. *Science* 2003; **300**: 1399–404.
8. Wang M, Yan M, Xu H *et al.* SARS-CoV infection in a restaurant from palm civet. *Emerg Infect Dis* 2005; **11**: 1860–5.
9. Che XY, Di B, Zhao GP *et al.* A patient with asymptomatic severe acute respiratory syndrome (SARS) and antigenemia from the 2003–2004 community outbreak of SARS in Guangzhou, China. *Clin Infect Dis* 2006; **43**: e1–5.
10. Lau SK, Woo PC, Li KS *et al.* Severe acute respiratory syndrome coronavirus-like virus in Chinese horseshoe bats. *Proc Natl Acad Sci U S A* 2005; **102**: 14040–5.
11. Li W, Shi Z, Yu M *et al.* Bats are natural reservoirs of SARS-like coronaviruses. *Science* 2005; **310**: 676–9.
12. Peiris JS, Yuen KY, Osterhaus AD *et al.* The severe acute respiratory syndrome. *N Engl J Med* 2003; **349**: 2431–41.
13. Wong RS, Hui DS. Index patient and SARS outbreak in Hong Kong. *Emerg Infect Dis* 2004; **10**: 339–41.
14. Yu IT, Li Y, Wong TW *et al.* Evidence of airborne transmission of the severe acute respiratory syndrome virus. *N Engl J Med* 2004; **350**: 1731–9.
15. Booth TF, Kournikakis B, Bastien N *et al.* Detection of airborne Severe acute respiratory syndrome (SARS) coronavirus and environmental contamination in SARS outbreak units. *J Infect Dis* 2005; **191**: 1472–7.
16. Yu IT, Wong TW, Chiu YL *et al.* Temporal-spatial analysis of severe acute respiratory syndrome among hospital inpatients. *Clin Infect Dis* 2005; **40**: 1237–43.
17. Leung GM, Hedley AJ, Ho LM *et al.* The epidemiology of severe acute respiratory syndrome in the 2003 Hong Kong epidemic: an analysis of all 1755 patients. *Ann Intern Med* 2004; **141**: 662–73.

18. Hui DS, Wong PC, Wang C. Severe acute respiratory syndrome: clinical features and diagnosis. *Respirology* 2003; **8**: S20–S4.
19. Peiris JS, Chu CM, Cheng VC *et al.* Clinical progression and viral load in a community outbreak of coronavirus-associated SARS pneumonia: a prospective study. *Lancet* 2003; **361**: 1767–72.
20. Hui DS, Wong KT, Antonio GE *et al.* Severe Acute Respiratory Syndrome (SARS): Correlation of clinical outcome and radiological features. *Radiology* 2004; **233**: 579–85.
21. Lo AW, Tang NL, To KF. How the SARS coronavirus causes disease: host or organism? *J Pathol* 2006; **208**: 142–51.
22. Ng WF, To KF, Lam WW *et al.* The comparative pathology of severe acute respiratory syndrome and avian influenza A subtype H5N1 – a review. *Hum Pathol* 2006; **37**: 381–90.
23. Gu J, Korteweg C. Pathology and pathogenesis of severe acute respiratory syndrome. *Am J Pathol* 2007; **170**: 1136–47.
24. To KF, Tong JH, Chan PK *et al.* Tissue and cellular tropisms of the coronavirus associated with severe acute respiratory syndrome-an in-situ hybridization study of fatal cases. *J Pathol* 2004; **202**: 157–63.
25. Lee N, Rainer TH, Ip M *et al.* Role of laboratory variables in differentiating SARS-coronavirus from other causes of community-acquired pneumonia within the first 72 hrs of hospitalization. *Eur J Clin Microbiol Infect Dis* 2006; **25**: 765–72.
26. Han F, Jiang YY, Zheng JH *et al.* Noninvasive positive pressure ventilation treatment for acute respiratory failure in SARS. *Sleep Breath* 2004; **8**: 97–106.
27. Cheung TM, Yam LY, So LK *et al.* Effectiveness of noninvasive positive pressure ventilation in the treatment of acute respiratory failure in severe acute respiratory syndrome. *Chest* 2004; **126**: 845–50.
28. Yam LY, Chan AY, Cheung TM *et al.* Hong Kong Hospital Authority SARS Collaborative Group (HASCOG). Non-invasive versus invasive mechanical ventilation for respiratory failure in severe acute respiratory syndrome. *Chin Med J (Engl)* 2005; **118**: 1413–21.
29. Fowler RA, Guest CB, Lapinsky SE *et al.* Transmission of severe acute respiratory syndrome during intubation and mechanical ventilation. *Am J Respir Crit Care Med* 2004; **169**: 1198–202.
30. Xiao Z, Li Y, Chen RC *et al.* A retrospective study of 78 patients with severe acute respiratory syndrome. *Chin Med J* 2003; **116**: 805–10.
31. Yu IT, Xie ZH, Tsoi KK *et al.* Why did outbreaks of severe acute respiratory syndrome occur in some hospital wards but not in others? *Clin Infect Dis* 2007; **44**: 1017–25.
32. Yam LY, Chen RC, Zhong NS. SARS: ventilatory and intensive care. *Respirology* 2003; **8**: S31–S5.
33. Hui DS, Hall SD, Chan MT *et al.* Exhaled air dispersion during oxygen delivery via a simple oxygen mask. *Chest* 2007; **132**: 540–6.
34. Hui DS, Hall SD, Chan MT *et al.* Non-invasive positive pressure ventilation: an experimental model to assess air and particle dispersion. *Chest* 2006; **130**: 730–40.
35. Hui DS, Chow BK, Ng SS *et al.* Exhaled air dispersion distances during noninvasive ventilation via different respironics face masks. *Chest* 2009; **136**: 998–1005.
36. Hui DS, Sung JJ. Editorial: Treatment of severe acute respiratory syndrome. *Chest* 2004; **126**: 670–4.
37. Hill NS, Carlisle C, Kramer NR. Effect of a nonrebreathing exhalation valve on long-term nasal ventilation using a bilevel device. *Chest* 2002; **122**: 84–91.
38. Meduri GU, Turner RE, Abou-Shala N *et al.* Noninvasive positive pressure ventilation via face mask: first-line intervention in patients with acute hypercapnic and hypoxemic respiratory failure. *Chest* 1996; **109**: 179–93.
39. World Health Organization. Infection and control of epidemic- and pandemic-prone acute respiratory diseases in health care. WHO interim Guidelines. World Health Organization, 2007. Available at: www.who.int/csr/resources/publications/WHO_CD_EPR_2007_6/en/ (accessed 19 March 2009).

# 44

# Cancer patients

PIETER DEPUYDT, ELIE AZOULAY, MARCIO SOARES, DOMINIQUE BENOIT

## ABSTRACT

Cancer patients represent a specific category of patients in whom acute respiratory failure (ARF) is a frequent event and one associated with poor, albeit improving, prognosis. It has been recently shown that non-invasive ventilation (NIV) is an efficient way of reversing early stages of ARF in these patients, and that cancer patients receiving NIV have a better outcome than patients treated with invasive mechanical ventilation. However, as failure rates of NIV in cancer patients are high, patients need to be carefully selected for a trial of NIV. In this chapter, we review the evidence on the use of NIV in patients with haematological malignancy or with solid tumours. Data provided by interventional trials and observational reports are integrated into a framework that will help the clinician to identify the cancer patient with ARF who is likely to benefit from NIV, paying attention to indications and contraindications for NIV as well as to predictors of NIV failure. In addition, we address some areas of controversy and identify issues for future research.

## INTRODUCTION

Acute respiratory failure (ARF) is the most frequent reason for intensive care unit (ICU) admission in cancer patients, and more than 60 per cent of patients with haematological cancers or solid tumours require mechanical ventilation during their ICU stay.[1–6] The mortality of mechanically ventilated cancer patients remains high but it has significantly decreased over the past two decades: hospital mortalities have dropped from 80–90 per cent in the 1980s to 65–75 per cent in the 1990s and even less than 50 per cent in specialized centres.[1–5,7,8] This trend has been observed in patients with haematological malignancies,[3,5,7,8] patients with solid tumours,[1,4] as well as in specific categories such as patients with lung cancer.[9] Consequently, the appreciation of the usefulness of mechanical ventilation in cancer patients has fundamentally changed. Whereas the prevailing opinion was to consider mechanical ventilation in cancer patients as futile therapy, most commentaries nowadays advocate no limitations in the use of mechanical ventilation at the earliest phase of the malignancy, and at least a trial of intensive organ support, including mechanical ventilation, in critically ill cancer patients who are likely to achieve extended disease-free survival.[10]

The reasons for the improved outcome in mechanically ventilated cancer patients are probably many-fold, including better and earlier selection of patients for ICU referral as well as advances in organ support. For example, implementation of evidence-based sepsis 'bundle' protocols, which have been shown to reduce mortality among general ICU patients,[11–13] is also feasible in the cancer population.[14] In addition, the rate of ventilator-associated complications may have been reduced through the increasing use of non-invasive modes of ventilatory support.[8] In this chapter, we will focus on the use of non-invasive ventilation (NIV) as a means to treat ARF in cancer patients, summarizing the current evidence and providing recommendations for selection of patients.

## PATHOPHYSIOLOGY

Acute respiratory failure is symptomatic of acute lung injury with alveolar–epithelial aggression and alteration of the alveolar–capillary membrane. It is immediately life-threatening with severe hypoxaemia developing within days to hours. In cancer patients, ARF may result from direct pulmonary involvement by the malignancy, can be induced by infection, or may reflect therapy-induced toxicity. In addition, ARF may be caused by comorbid illness as chronic obstructive pulmonary disease (COPD) or congestive cardiac failure, conditions that are increasingly encountered in ageing cancer patients. This heterogeneity in underlying causes translates into a variable clinical presentation of ARF: as severe hypoxaemia in an otherwise haemodynamically stable patient with diffuse pulmonary infiltrates, as hypercapnic acidosis in patients with respiratory pump failure, or as part of a syndrome of severe sepsis or septic shock. While a good outcome in ARF essentially requires reversal of the underlying mechanisms, correction of hypoxaemia and oxygen delivery as well as hypercapnic acidosis is pivotal to ensure patient survival in the meantime. The primary approach in hypoxaemic patients is to raise alveolar oxygen content by increasing the inspired fraction of oxygen; more profound hypoxaemia can be reversed by pushing up alveolar oxygen pressure and inducing alveolar recruitment with continuous positive airway pressure (CPAP). Correcting hypercarbia on the other hand usually requires increasing alveolar ventilation and unloading of respiratory muscles by positive pressure mechanical ventilation, e.g. by applying pressure support or bi-level positive airway pressure.[15]

While mechanical ventilation supports the failing respiratory system and reverses the physiopathological derangements, the aetiology of ARF should be aggressively investigated to guide therapy and estimate prognosis. The outcome of ARF in cancer patients is still variable, and has been shown to be related to the underlying cause. Some aetiologies such as bacterial sepsis or cardiogenic pulmonary oedema carry a better prognosis than others, such as invasive fungal disease or direct airway invasion by the malignancy.[2,4,5,16,17] The relationship between aetiology and outcome is determined by the availability (or lack) of effective therapies and by the speed at which the underlying disease may be reversed. For instance, outcome in ARF caused by fungal invasion (which responds more slowly to therapy) is worse than that caused by bacterial pneumonia.[16] Similarly, it has been shown that ARF directly caused by haematological malignancy (leukaemic pulmonary infiltrates and leukostasis) can be reversed by aggressive chemotherapy (provided that it is a first presentation of disease in a patient who can tolerate such a treatment);[17] in contrast, pulmonary involvement by solid tumours still carries a grim prognosis.[4] Being able to identify the aetiology of ARF itself appears to be associated with a better outcome, as in patients without a clear diagnosis there is very high mortality.[2]

In summary, ARF is frequent and severe, mostly requiring ventilatory support that can be invasive or non-invasive, and carries a complex diagnosis–prognosis association.

## EVIDENCE BASE

The evidence about the use of NIV in cancer patients consists of two small interventional trials,[18,19] as well as of a larger set of observational studies.

Both interventional studies randomized immunocompromised patients with hypoxaemic ARF (defined as a ratio of $PaO_2$ to the fraction of inspired oxygen [$PaO_2/FiO_2$] of below 200) to either NIV or standard supplemental oxygen only; endpoints were need for intubation, and ICU and hospital mortality. Antonelli *et al.* (40 patients) considered solid organ transplantation patients only: NIV averted intubation in 80 per cent (significantly more than in patients treated without NIV), and was associated with reduced ICU, but not hospital, mortality.[18] Hilbert *et al.* included a heterogeneous population of immunocompromised patients (56 patients), 30 of whom had haematological malignancy: intubation was avoided in 54 per cent, and both ICU and hospital mortality were significantly lower in the NIV-treated arm as compared with the control arm.[19] In both studies, the lower ICU mortality in NIV-treated patients was mainly due to the lower rate of fatal complications following intubation. Moreover, in the study of Hilbert *et al.*, only one cancer patient who required intubation survived, a picture which has nowadays become very unusual.

In addition to these two small interventional trials, several observational studies have related outcome in cancer patients with ARF to the invasiveness of ventilatory support.[2,3,7,8,20–27] Non-invasive ventilation was provided to 4[4]–39[23] per cent of patients and intubation averted in a third[7,26] to half of them,[8,25] although in one early report, 11 of 16 haematological ARF patients (68 per cent) who were treated with NIV avoided intubation and were discharged.[27] In most but not in all studies,[7,22] NIV as compared with invasive ventilation was associated with better survival, but only three studies corrected this for differences in severity-of-illness between invasively and non-invasively ventilated patients. Results were equivocal, with Azoulay *et al.* finding a protective effect associated with the use of NIV,[8] and Depuydt *et al.* finding none.[7,22] Some of these studies reported mortality rates above 90 per cent in patients failing a trial of NIV;[2,7] in one, both intubation following NIV and NIV failure after 24 h were independent predictors of mortality.[2]

The divergence between the results of the interventional and that of observational studies partly stems from differences in study design, and partly may relate to differences in case mix and patient selection. Both interventional studies compared respiratory support by NIV to standard care with supplemental oxygen only, considering intubation as an endpoint.[18,19] On the other hand, as most of the observational studies compared patients treated with NIV as initial mode with patients who were immediately intubated,[7,22,24] inclusion of these more severely ill patients may have biased the results to the disadvantage of invasive ventilation. Similarly, patients recruited to interventional trials were more likely to receive NIV at an earlier stage of ARF than patients included in observational studies. A longer delay to the start of NIV has been shown to be an independent predictor of NIV failure.[25] In addition, the association between ventilatory mode and outcome may have been confounded by case mix of the patient population, as the underlying cause of ARF has been shown to be a strong predictor of outcome. Finally, intubated patients had much higher ICU mortality in the interventional studies (78 per cent[18] and 87 per cent[19]), as compared with the observational reports (50–70 per cent).[2,4,7,22] Of note, it is striking that all these studies were single-centre studies, which not only creates additional bias but also precludes any adjustment on centre effects related either to expertise in managing ARF in cancer patients or to expertise and annual volume of NIV in a given centre.[3]

## CLINICAL APPLICATIONS

Based on the current evidence, NIV can be considered as an effective mode of ventilatory support in cancer patients with ARF. However, the same contraindications that exclude NIV in general ICU patients are to be respected in cancer patients. Guidelines and reviews on the use of NIV in ARF have issued the following absolute contraindications: imminent respiratory arrest, haemodynamic instability or life-threatening arrhythmia, inability to protect the airway or vomiting, or anatomical incompatibility with the patient–ventilator interface. Additional, more relative, contraindications for NIV are excessive respiratory secretions, recent upper gastrointestinal or airway surgery, decreased consciousness or agitation.[28–30]

In the absence of these contraindications, NIV should be considered as the first-line ventilatory mode in cancer patients with hypercapnic ARF due to COPD exacerbation, or with hypoxaemic ARF due to cardiogenic pulmonary oedema.[28–30] In hypoxaemic ARF due to other (or unknown at presentation) causes, early application of NIV may help to avoid intubation as compared with supportive therapy with oxygen only.[18,19] In addition, a trial of NIV in hypoxaemic ARF may be preferred over immediate intubation, provided that the odds for success for NIV are sufficiently high. This, however, implies careful selection of patients and setting clear goals of therapy to guide further management. Indeed, prolonged NIV in hypoxaemic patients may preclude any diagnostic strategy. Moreover, prolonged NIV should be strongly discouraged given the dismal survival associated with late intubation and invasive mechanical ventilation.[2,25] Aside from patient characteristics, tolerance and success of NIV may depend upon the appropriate choice of the type of ventilator, the mode of NIV and the patient–ventilator interface. However, apart from two centres reporting better tolerance of NIV delivered by helmet instead of face mask,[31,32] no studies have compared different NIV ventilators or settings in immunocompromised or cancer patients.

In most studies on NIV in cancer patients, NIV failed in at least half of the cases.[2,4,7,8,18–26] As such, the framework of indications and contraindications used to guide the use of NIV in general ICU patients needs refinement for this specific category of patients. In a retrospective study, failure of NIV in haematological patients was significantly associated with a delay in initiating NIV, a diagnosis of acute respiratory distress syndrome (ARDS), and the presence of extrapulmonary organ failure, i.e. need for vasopressors and for renal replacement therapy. In addition, increasing respiratory rate while receiving NIV was an early predictor for NIV failure.[25] In this study, prolonged dependency on NIV and NIV failure were associated with decreased survival. From other reports, it has been argued that a NIV trial is likely to fail when the underlying cause of ARF is unknown or not rapidly reversible.[2,22] Figure 44.1 provides a flow chart to guide the clinician in choosing the initial mode of ventilatory support in cancer patients with hypoxaemic ARF.

In addition, some authors have described the use of NIV in ARF patients refusing intubation, or considered to be poor candidates for intubation because of severely impaired functional status or advanced stage of malignancy.[33–38] A questionnaire sent to critical care physicians of 20 ICUs in the USA and Canada documented widespread use of NIV in this palliative or near end-of-life setting,[39] and a task force of the Society of Critical Care Medicine developed a framework to guide clinicians in this potential application of NIV.[40] Whereas the subgroup of do-not-intubate patients with advanced cancer experienced 85 per cent failure of NIV in one report,[34] two other studies described successful reversal of ARF and ICU survival in more than half of do-not-intubate patients with cancer.[36,37] However, prognosis beyond ICU appears to be limited in these patients, and NIV may only serve to 'buy awake time' for the patients and their relatives.[38] As such, these reports on palliative NIV raise several issues: Is the ICU the best place for palliative NIV? Is the ICU the best place for dying? How miserable is it to die behind an NIV mask? Therefore, not only quantitative survival data but also qualitative data are needed before palliative NIV should be encouraged.

## FUTURE RESEARCH

Acute respiratory failure in cancer patients is a heterogeneous disease with variable outcome. Failure rates of NIV in the reports published so far are high, and more data are required to identify those patients with ARF who are most likely to benefit from NIV. In addition, some reports have observed that mortality rates in patients intubated after a failed NIV trial were much higher than those in patients who were immediately intubated. At present it is not clear whether the excess mortality in patients failing NIV is due to irreversibility of the underlying disease process (where NIV is more likely to fail than in rapidly reversible ARF) or to harm caused by inappropriate use of NIV. In other words, did intubated patients later die irrespective of the (otherwise adequate) ventilatory strategy (which suggests that they also would have died if they were intubated earlier) or because

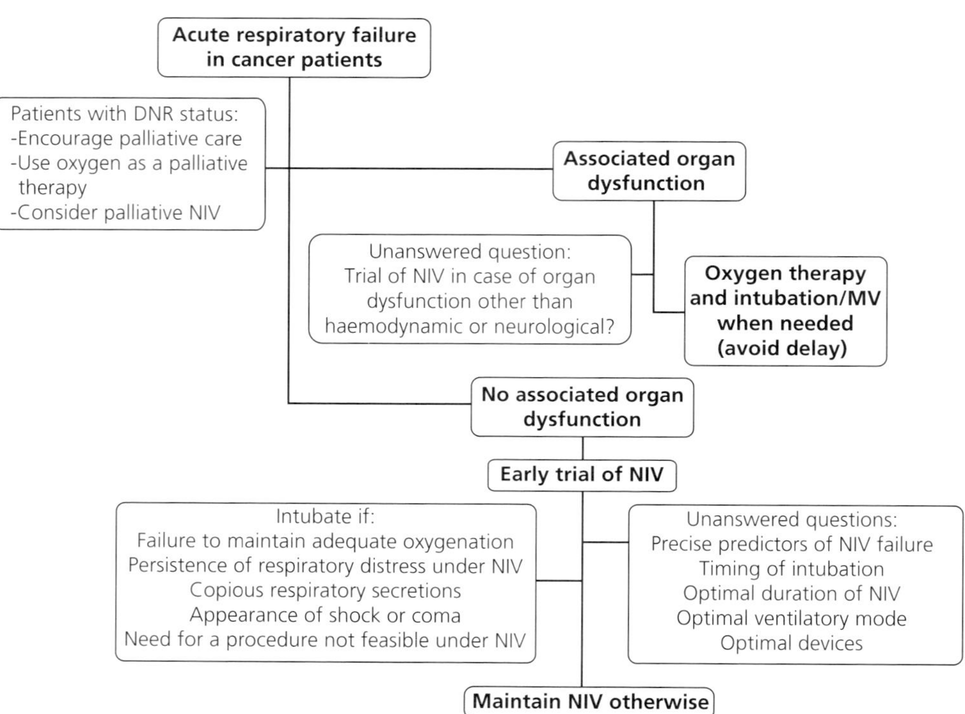


**Figure 44.1** Flow chart to guide the choice of ventilatory strategy in cancer patients with acute respiratory failure. DNR, do not resuscitate; MV, mechanical ventilation; NIV, non-invasive ventilation.

they were managed suboptimally (which suggests that earlier intubation would have been associated with better outcome)? Finally, the timing of NIV is likely to influence the chances for success of NIV, as suggested by the discrepancies between the interventional studies and some of the observational reports. An additional interventional study aiming to achieve early identification of ARF in cancer patients, followed by prompt referral to the ICU for a trial of NIV as compared with standard care, could provide valuable data.

## REFERENCES


1. Taccone F, Artigas A, Sprung C *et al.* Characteristics and outcomes of cancer patients in European ICUs. *Crit Care* 2009; **13**: R15.
2. Azoulay E, Thiéry G, Chevret S *et al.* The prognosis of acute respiratory failure in critically ill cancer patients. *Medicine* 2004; **83**: 360–70.
3. Lecuyer L, Chevret S, Guidet B *et al.* Case volume and mortality in haematological patients with acute respiratory failure. *Eur Respir J* 2008; **32**: 748–54.
4. Soares M, Salluh J, Spector N *et al.* Characteristics and outcomes of cancer patients requiring mechanical ventilatory support for >24 hours. *Crit Care Med* 2005; **33**: 520–6.
5. Benoit D, Vandewoude K, Decruyenaere J *et al.* Outcome and early prognostic indicators in patients with a hematologic malignancy admitted to the intensive care unit for life-threatening complication. *Crit Care Med* 2003; **31**: 104–12.
6. Chaoui D, Legrand O, Roche N *et al.* Incidence and prognostic value of respiratory events in acute leukemia. *Leukemia* 2004; **18**: 670–5.
7. Depuydt PO, Benoit DD, Vandewoude KH *et al.* Outcome in noninvasively and invasively ventilated hematologic patients with acute respiratory failure. *Chest* 2004; **126**: 1299–306.
8. Azoulay E, Alberti C, Bornstain C *et al.* Improved survival in cancer patients requiring mechanical ventilatory support: impact of noninvasive mechanical ventilatory support. *Crit Care Med* 2001; **29**: 519–25.
9. Adam AK, Soubani AO. Outcome and prognostic factors of lung cancer patients admitted to the medical intensive care unit. *Eur Respir J* 2008; **31**: 47–53.
10. Azoulay E, Afessa A. The intensive support of patients with malignancy: do everything that can be done. *Intensive Care Med* 2006; **32**: 3–5.
11. Micek S, Roubinian N, Heuring T *et al.* Before-after-study of a standardized hospital order set for the management of septic shock. *Crit Care Med* 2006; **34**: 2707–13.
12. Ferrer R, Artigas A, Levy M *et al.* Improvement in process of care and outcome after a multicenter severe sepsis educational program in Spain. *JAMA* 2008; **19**: 2294–303.
13. El Solh A, Akinnusi M, Alsawalha L *et al.* Outcome of septic shock in older adults after implementation of the 'sepsis bundle'. *J Am Geriatr Soc* 2008; **56**: 272–8.
14. Pene F, Percheron S, Lemiale V *et al.* Temporal changes in management and outcome of septic shock in patients with malignancies in the intensive care unit. *Crit Care Med* 2008; **36**: 690–6.
15. Rajan T, Hill NS. Noninvasive positive pressure ventilation. In: Fink MP, Abraham E, Vincent JL *et al.*, eds.

*Textbook of critical care*, 5th edn. Philadelphia: Elsevier Saunders, 2005:519–26.

16. Benoit D, Depuydt P, Peleman A *et al.* Documented and clinically suspected bacterial infection precipitating intensive care unit admission in patients with hematological malignancy: impact on outcome. *Intensive Care Med* 2005; **31**: 934–42.
17. Benoit D, Depuydt P, Vandewoude K *et al.* Outcome in severely ill patients with hematological malignancies who received intravenous chemotherapy in the intensive care unit. *Intensive Care Med* 2006; **32**: 93–9.
18. Antonelli M, Conti G, Bufi M *et al.* Noninvasive ventilation for treatment of acute respiratory failure in patients undergoing solid organ transplantation: a randomized trial. *JAMA* 2000; **283**: 235–41.
19. Hilbert G, Gruson D, Vargas D *et al.* Noninvasive ventilation in immunosuppressed patients with pulmonary infiltrates, fever, and acute respiratory failure. *N Engl J Med* 2001; **344**: 481–7.
20. Hilbert G, Gruson D, Vargas D *et al.* Noninvasive positive airway pressure in neutropenic patients with acute respiratory failure requiring intensive care unit admission. *Crit Care Med* 2000; **28**: 3185–90.
21. Varon J, Walsh GL, Fromm RE. Feasibility of noninvasive mechanical ventilation in the treatment of acute respiratory failure in postoperative cancer patients. *J Crit Care* 1998; **13**: 55–7.
22. Depuydt PO, Benoit DD, Roosens CD. The impact of the initial ventilatory strategy on survival in hematological patients with acute hypoxemic respiratory failure. *J Crit Care* 2009; [Epub ahead of print].
23. Rabbat A, Chaoui D, Montani D *et al.* Prognosis of patients with acute myeloid leukemia admitted to intensive care. *Br J Haematol* 2005; **129**: 350–57.
24. Rabitsch W, Staudinger T, Locker G *et al.* Respiratory failure after stem cell transplantation:improved outcome with non-invasive ventilation. *Leuk Lymphoma* 2005; **46**: 1151–7.
25. Adda M, Coquet I, Darmon M *et al.* Predictors of noninvasive ventilation failure in patients with hematologic malignancy and acute respiratory failure. *Crit Care Med* 2008; **36**: 2766–72.
26. Tognet E, Mercatello A, Coronel B *et al.* Treatment of acute respiratory failure with non-invasive positive pressure ventilation in haematological patients. *Clin Intensive Care* 1994; **5**: 282–8.
27. Conti G, Marino P, Cogliati A *et al.* Noninvasive ventilation for the treatment of acute respiratory failure in patients with hematologic malignancies: a pilot study. *Intensive Care Med* 1998; **24**: 1283–8.
28. British Thoracic Society Standards of Care Committee. Non-invasive ventilation in acute respiratory failure. *Thorax* 2002; **57**: 192–211.
29. Nava S, Hill N. Non-invasive ventilation in acute respiratory failure. *Lancet* 2009; **374**: 250–9.
30. Schönhofer B, Kuhlen R, Neumann P *et al.* Nichtinvasive Beatmung als Therapie der akuten respiratorischen Insuffizienz: das Wichtigste der neuen S3-Leitlinie. *Der Anaesthesist* 2008; **11**: 1091–102.
31. Principi T, Pantanetti S, Catani F *et al.* Noninvasive continuous positive airway pressure delivered by helmet in hematological malignancy patients with hypoxemic acute respiratory failure. *Intensive Care Med* 2004; **30**: 147–50.
32. Rocco M, Dell'Utri D, Morelli A *et al.* Noninvasive ventilation by helmet or face mask in immunocompromized patients. *Chest* 2004; **126**: 1508–15.
33. Chu C, Chan V, Wong I *et al.* Noninvasive ventilation in patients with acute hypercapnic exacerbation of chronic obstructive pulmonary disease who refused endotracheal intubation. *Crit Care Med* 2004; **32**: 372–7.
34. Schettino G, Altobelli N, Kacmarek R. Noninvasive positive pressure ventilation reverses acute respiratory failure in select 'do-not-intubate' patients. *Crit Care Med* 2005; **33**: 1976–82.
35. Levy M, Tanios M, Nelson D *et al.* Outcomes of patients with do-not-intubate orders treated with noninvasive ventilation. *Crit Care Med* 2004; **32**: 2002–7.
36. Cuomo A, Delmastro M, Ceriana P *et al.* Noninvasive mechanical ventilation as a palliative treatment of acute respiratory failure in patients with end-stage solid cancer. *Palliat Med* 2004; **18**: 602–10.
37. Meert A, Berghmans T, Hardy M *et al.* Non-invasive ventilation for cancer patients with life-supporting techniques limitation. *Support Care Cancer* 2006; **14**: 167–71.
38. Fernandez R, Baigorri F, Artigas A. Noninvasive ventilation in patients with 'do-not-intubate' orders: medium-term efficacy depends critically on patient selection. *Intensive Care Med* 2007; **33**: 350–4.
39. Sinuff T, Cook D, Keenan S *et al.* Noninvasive ventilation for acute respiratory failure near the end of life. *Crit Care Med* 2008; **36**: 789–94.
40. Curtis J, Cook D, Sinuff T *et al.* Noninvasive positive pressure ventilation in critical and palliative care settings: understanding the goals of therapy. *Crit Care Med* 2007; **5**: 932–9.

45

# Non-invasive ventilation in the elderly

ERWAN L'HER

## ABSTRACT

The definition of elderly is difficult because there is no general agreement on the threshold of 'old age'. The concept of vulnerability taking into account both calendar age and the existence of comorbidities seems much more accurate. Non-invasive ventilation can obviate the need for intubation and thus reduce complications and mortality in adult patients with acute hypercapnic respiratory failure due to chronic obstructive pulmonary disease and for cardiogenic pulmonary oedema. There is very little literature describing its benefit in an elderly population. Several arguments exist to consider that within these specific indications, non-invasive ventilation is as well tolerated and as successful in an older population as it is in a younger population. In addition, it may be used successfully as a treatment of last resort in those patients in whom endotracheal intubation and ventilation in the intensive care unit is not appropriate. It can be initiated in patients who refuse endotracheal intubation, in those with do-not-resuscitate orders or in those on palliative care, but always on an individual basis. In these cases, the clinician should take into account both the patient's and their caregivers' wishes with due regard for ethical standards related to proportionate care. Comfort improvement will be a major goal and non-invasive ventilation should be withdrawn if it fails.

## INTRODUCTION

Non-invasive ventilation (NIV) reduces the need for endotracheal intubation as well the rate of mortality in adult patients with various causes of acute respiratory failure (ARF).[1,2] However, most patients included within randomized controlled trials were deemed to undergo invasive mechanical ventilation if necessary, and few of them would be considered as '*elderly*'. One could therefore argue that such beneficial results cannot be transferred to such a specific population, even if others argued that age by itself does not confer a specific pathological pattern. A number of studies have investigated endotracheal intubation and mechanical ventilation in elderly patients within an intensive care unit, but only a few have looked at NIV administration. Considering this argument, the evidence pertaining to use of NIV in very elderly patients (>75 years) has been given a favourable level 4 ('case series and poor-quality cohort and case–control studies') in a recent systematic review of the literature.[3]

More recently, there has been increased interest in the use of NIV in patients who decline invasive life-support measures,[4] especially in elderly patients with various chronic comorbidities and/or 'do-not-resuscitate' (DNR) orders. However, the utility of NIV in patients with ARF who have declined intubation and resuscitation[5,6] or those who have chosen comfort measures only is rather controversial.[7] While NIV can reverse non-terminal ARF, it may be considered inappropriate when patients have elected to limit life support near the end of their life. Nevertheless, NIV may benefit some patients who have chosen a DNR status, and such an indication could be recommended at a favourable evidence level 2 ('analyses of similar cohort studies or poor-quality randomized controlled trials').[3]

The purpose of this chapter is to review the potential uses of NIV in elderly patients, and to provide clinicians with the indications and determinants of success. It will also discuss NIV endpoints and response to failure in this specific population.

## PATHOPHYSIOLOGY

### Definition of 'elderly'

Most industrialized countries have accepted the chronological age of 65 years as the threshold of 'elderly'. But although there are several commonly used definitions of old age, there is no general agreement on the age at which a person should be considered old.[8] It is important to stress that although the common use of a calendar age to mark the threshold of old age assumes equivalence with biological age, yet it is also generally accepted that these two are not necessarily synonymous. Some authors have focused on the age of 80, considering that octogenarians, as compared with others, are more likely to have impaired functional status before they develop critical illness, and they also have a relatively short remaining lifespan even without a critical illness.[9,10]

Whatever the chosen biological age threshold for being considered 'elderly', the assessment of patients' vulnerability is certainly of more importance. 'Vulnerable elderly patients' could be considered as people aged 65 and older who are at increased risk of functional decline or death over 2 years.[11] These people are more likely to undergo aggressive life-sustaining care, which makes this discussion much more crucial. Indeed, many of these patients will die despite intensive care unit (ICU) admission, raising questions about whether critical care services may have unnecessarily prolonged their dying experience or caused harm to the patient and their family.

### Epidemiology of the ageing population

Around the world, the oldest sector of the population is expected to grow the fastest.[12] The fastest growing age cohort is made up of those aged ≥80 years, increasing at an estimated 3.8 per cent per year and projected to represent one-fifth of all older people by 2050.[13] The ageing population increase is predicted to have a peak in 2011, when the first baby-boom cohort will reach the age of 65 years. A study performed by Rockwood *et al.* in the early 1990s established that patients 65 years and older already accounted for 26–51 per cent of all ICU admissions.[14] According to population ageing statistics, the number of ventilated patients is expected to increase by 31 per cent in 2010 in some regions.[15]

### Incidence and clinical impact of comorbidities

Older age is associated with higher prevalence of chronic illness and functional impairment, contributing to an increased rate of hospitalization. The coexistence of cardiac and respiratory diseases in elderly patients admitted for acute respiratory distress increases the difficulty of making an aetiopathogenic diagnosis.[16,17] In a study of 122 patients admitted for cardiac decompensation, the initial diagnosis was confirmed in only 29 per cent of cases. Chronic obstructive pulmonary disease (COPD) or underlying obesity were considered responsible for 42 per cent of 'false diagnoses'.[18] In a study of 11 000 patients hospitalized for cardiogenic pulmonary oedema, 54 per cent of patients were aged over 70 years and 24 per cent had an associated chronic lung disease.[19] Therefore in elderly people, NIV will have to be often initiated for a symptomatic diagnosis (i.e. hypercarbic vs hypoxaemic ARF) rather than for a precise diagnosis.

### Prognosis and patient preferences

In most industrial countries, the dying experience is nowadays largely a hospital experience with 1 in 5 of these deaths occurring in the ICU.[20,21] Little attention has been paid to the quality of care that vulnerable elders receive, and previous studies exploring the association between age and ICU outcome have yielded conflicting results. A few studies have concluded that age is not a predictor,[22,23] while others have concluded the opposite – that increasing age is associated with increased ICU short-term mortality.[9,24,25] When questioned, most people would prefer to die at home[26,27] and most elderly patients, when provided with a choice, would prefer a less aggressive treatment plan than a technologically supported, institutionalized death.[28] On the contrary, evidence also suggests clinicians may sometimes underestimate the degree of intervention desired by older patients.[29]

In a study of hospitalized elderly patients in the USA, 70 per cent reported that their baseline quality of life was fair or poor and most wanted comfort measures as opposed to life-prolonging treatments.[30] Nevertheless, 54 per cent of these patients were admitted to ICUs. In another American study, at least half of seriously ill patients reported pain and many died after unwanted prolongation of their dying process in an ICU.[31] Such considerations must be put forward when thinking of NIV initiation in an elderly patient, especially when the patient is unconscious or demented and thus cannot give their consent to care.

## CLINICAL APPLICATIONS

Non-invasive ventilation has become a standard therapy for the treatment ARF in selected populations and is increasingly used in many acute care settings.[32,33] This increased utilization has been driven in large part by the desire to avoid complications of invasive mechanical ventilation. Non-invasive ventilation could be considered in elderly people for the same indications as in younger patients, even if the diagnosis may often be imprecise.

## Chronic obstructive pulmonary disease

In the specific case of hypercarbic ARF due to exacerbations of COPD, NIV has been shown to reduce the rates of endotracheal intubation, mortality and length of hospital stay.[1,34,35] But despite the extensive evidence for the use of NIV during acute exacerbations of COPD, its specific use in an elderly population has been little studied, and there is no high level evidence whether elderly patients gain similar benefits from NIV as do younger patients.

Benhamou *et al.*[36] reported the results of NIV in 30 patients with hypercapnic respiratory failure and mean age of 76 years, of whom only 20 had COPD. The rate of treatment failure was 40 per cent in this study, probably because only 68 per cent of patients had COPD. In a prospective cohort study of 36 patients aged 65 years or above hospitalized for acute hypercapnic respiratory failure related to COPD, Balami *et al.* investigated the impact of NIV.[37] Staff were fully trained in the administration of NIV and two beds with high-dependency facilities for the administration of NIV were specifically available within the unit. The mean age of patients in this study was 77.4 years as compared with a mean age of 60 years in most randomized studies. The patients' condition was severe, with a pre-NIV pH of 7.23 ± 0.07 and a $PaCO_2$ of 80 ± 21 mm Hg. In all of these patients, a decision that NIV was to be the treatment of last resort had been made prior to NIV initiation. None of the patients developed complications related to NIV, and a 79 per cent success rate was observed, according to predetermined clinical and biological improvement criteria. All patients who failed NIV died (25 per cent of all NIV trials – two patients had failed initially). In a retrospective cohort of 127 elderly hypercapnic COPD exacerbations, NIV treatment was considered as successful in 78.3 per cent of cases.[38] The patients' condition was also severe, with a mean pH value of 7.26 ± 0.1 and a $PaCO_2$ of 71 ± 20 mm Hg. Cumulative delirium was present in 38 per cent of cases, and almost 28 per cent of these patients were concomitantly disabled and demented. Four patients (3.4 per cent) were intubated and 21 other patients (18.3 per cent) were considered for subsequent treatment limitation; all 25 patients died within the hospital. The authors concluded that, although high, mortality in elderly patients under NIV was probably not worse than that in younger patients, and that the success rate was high. Moreover they also indicated that in such a population, NIV was generally well tolerated.

## Cardiogenic pulmonary oedema

Non-invasive ventilation is beneficial in many patients with cardiogenic pulmonary oedema in the absence of acute coronary ischaemia.[2,39–41] In a prospective randomized study, L'Her *et al.* evaluated the clinical efficacy of continuous positive airway pressure (CPAP) versus standard medical treatment in 89 consecutive elderly patients (≥75 years) admitted to emergency departments, with acute hypoxaemic respiratory failure related to cardiogenic pulmonary oedema.[42] Mean age of the patients was 86 years. Within 1 hour, non-invasive CPAP led to decreased respiratory rate and improved oxygenation as compared with baseline, whereas no differences were observed within the standard treatment group. Early 48-hour mortality was 7 per cent in the non-invasive CPAP group, compared with 24 per cent in the standard treatment group ($p$ = 0.017); however, no sustained benefits were observed during the overall hospital stay, probably because of therapeutic limitations or exacerbations and comorbidities in several patients during their subsequent hospital stay. Although early clinical improvement is a worthy goal by itself, these beneficial results are, however, to be viewed with caution owing to a lack of sustained benefit, which has also been questioned in younger populations. A meaningful benefit should include decreases in both mortality and morbidity, whereas a short-term mortality benefit that is ultimately lost by the time of discharge could just be considered as a way of delaying the inevitable.

## Non-invasive ventilation for elderly patients who refuse endotracheal intubation, and/or with 'do-not-resuscitate' orders

In most NIV trials, if the treatment failed the standard therapy given was intubation and mechanical ventilation. Although NIV is a widely accepted treatment for some patients with ARF, the use of NIV in vulnerable elderly people who may have decided to forego endotracheal intubation is controversial.[43] Given its high success rate in the previously developed indications, NIV appears to be an attractive option to support patients with respiratory failure who refuse intubation. It should therefore be used as the treatment of last resort. Unfortunately, some authors also pointed out the fact that many physicians have been considering NIV to be a routine therapeutic option for patients who have explicitly requested that mechanical ventilation should not be implemented in the event of severe or life-threatening medical illness.[44] This is compounded by the additional observation that patients in such a condition may frequently require either chemical or physical restraints to tolerate this intervention, raising major ethical concerns.

In a prospective observational study about the use of NIV in COPD patients who refused endotracheal intubation, a 1-year survival of ~30 per cent was recorded in COPD patients with the 'do-not-intubate' (DNI) code who developed acute hypercapnic respiratory failure requiring NIV. The majority of survivors developed another life-threatening event in the following year.[45]

## Non-invasive ventilation in palliative care

Some authors have suggested that NIV should be used in palliative care patients on a trial basis, to help alleviate respiratory distress and attempt to provide some additional time to finalize personal affairs.[46] In such a situation, NIV may lessen dyspnoea, preserve patient autonomy, and permit eating and verbal communication, thus improving patients' comfort. But the realistic aspect of such a therapy in terms of palliative measures has also been questioned. Some authors have suggested that it should be inappropriate to use NIV because it is still a form of artificial life support, whatever the type of interface, and that it may therefore cause discomfort while only prolonging the dying process.[5] The answer to that question clearly depends on how the clinician defines *palliation* for a specific patient. If the goal is patient comfort during an inevitable and untreatable dying process, then not only is NIV of *dubious* value, it should be contraindicated. It will only prolong a dying process that is expected and anticipated. However, if the goal is to aggressively treat the patient who has a predetermined stop order (i.e. therapeutic limitation such as 'no intubation and/or mechanical ventilation'), NIV may be of some value as a palliative treatment, to reduce the discomfort of dyspnoea, with no expectation of coincidental prolongation of life.

# TECHNICAL CONSIDERATIONS

Concerning the technical aspects of NIV in elderly people, a very few distinctions arise when compared with a younger population. An empirical therapeutic algorithm for consideration of NIV in the elderly population can be designed, even if it mainly relies on clinical experience and general ethical concerns, rather than on scientific evidence (Fig. 45.1).

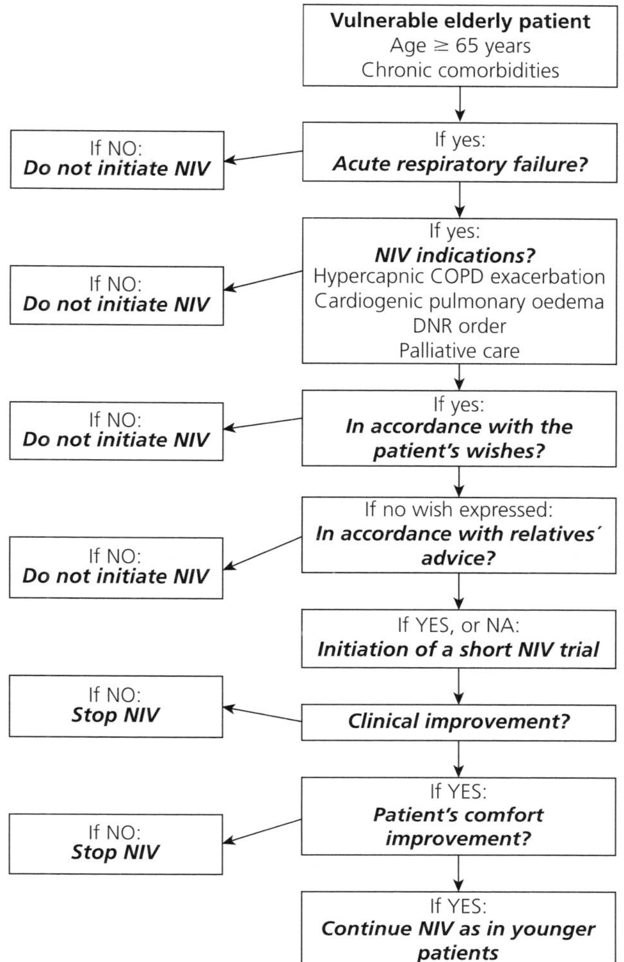


**Figure 45.1** Therapeutic algorithm for consideration of non-invasive ventilation (NIV) in elderly people. This algorithm mainly relies on clinical experience and general ethical concerns, rather than on scientific evidence. Patients with chronic disabilities should be treated with NIV regardless of their age. In the other patients, a time-limited trial of treatment may sometimes be appropriate. The use of NIV should always be discussed on an individual basis, taking into account various factors and the patient's wishes. In most cases, NIV should be used as the treatment of last resort. COPD, chronic obstructive pulmonary disease; DNR, do not resuscitate; NA, not available.

## Should non-invasive ventilation be initiated?

Elderly patients without chronic disabilities should be treated with NIV regardless of their age. However, the use of NIV as the treatment of last resort should always be discussed on an individual basis, taking into account various factors and the patient's wishes.

If patient comfort is to be maintained and the family is supportive, a time-limited trial of treatment for an elderly person with chronic critical illness may sometimes be appropriate. However, continuation of treatment in the chronic phase of critical illness should never be driven by default, i.e. in the absence of conscious medical decisions that are informed by effective communication and that take into account the patient's goals, preferences and values.[47] It will always be necessary to weigh the benefits and burdens of treatment and to re-evaluate this balance as the clinical situation evolves. In ideal circumstances, the patient will participate directly in this process, but the reality of both acute and chronic critical illness is that decision making capacity is typically lacking.

## Taking into account the patient's and their relatives' wishes

Many clinicians seem to interpret a DNI order as an order permitting all forms of treatment except intubation. But is

NIV any different from endotracheal intubation in a practical sense? Except for the presence of a foreign body in the trachea, NIV is essentially the same, in that it uses hardware to achieve an end-stage therapeutic advantage not possible with more conservative methods. Patient preferences regarding end-of-life treatment are usually unknown.[48] In such situations, the family or other caregivers' wishes play a major role. Neither a proxy nor an advance directive is a perfect alternative, but both may help to illuminate decision making from the patient's perspective. Physicians therefore frequently consult relatives regarding the appropriateness of treatment intervention, despite data suggesting that the consulted relatives find this emotionally stressful and do not consistently make decisions that accurately reflect their relative's wishes.[49,50]

## What should be the intensity of care?

Although ICU resources and intensive treatments are often denied to elderly patients, it is clear that age as such is a poor predictor of medical outcome. When confronted with extended mechanical ventilation and associated care, a significant proportion of elderly patients would accept this care only in the event of improved prognosis.[51] However, in patients with chronic critical illness admitted to the ICU, severe brain dysfunction and delirium is very prevalent.[52] If elderly patients with a potential critical illness are questioned about end-of-life decisions, up to 41 per cent choose to limit certain life-sustaining therapies including cardiopulmonary resuscitation, ventilation and ICU admission.[53,54]

**Table 45.1** The three-category approach to the use of non-invasive ventilation (NIV) in acute respiratory failure

| | Category 1 | Category 2 | Category 3 |
|---|---|---|---|
| Definition | Life support without limits | Life support with preset limits (do-not-intubate) | Comfort measures only |
| Primary goals of care | Assist ventilation and/or oxygenation<br>Alleviate dyspnoea<br>Achieve comfort<br>Reduce risk of intubation<br>Reduce risk of mortality<br>Avoid intubation | Include same as category 1 except intubation<br>In some cases to prolong life for specific purposes (e.g. arrival of family member) | Palliation of symptoms (relief of dyspnoea) |
| Goals to communicate with patient and family | To restore health and use intubation if necessary | To restore health without using intubation and without unacceptable discomfort | To maximize comfort<br>To minimize adverse effects of opiates |
| Determinants of success | Improved oxygenation and/or ventilation<br>Tolerance of NIV with minimal discomfort (outweighed by benefit) | Improved oxygenation and/or ventilation<br>Tolerance of NIV with minimal discomfort (outweighed by benefit) | Improved symptoms<br>Tolerance of NIV |
| Endpoints | Unassisted ventilation<br>NIV intolerance | Unassisted ventilation<br>NIV intolerance | Patient is not more comfortable<br>Patient wants NIV to be stopped<br>Patient becomes unable to communicate |
| Response to failure | Intubation and mechanical ventilation | Change to comfort measures and palliate symptoms only | Palliate symptoms without NIV |
| Likely location of NIV | ICU<br>Possible in step-down units or acute care beds with appropriate monitoring and training | ICU in some cases<br>Step-down units or acute care beds with appropriate monitoring and training | Not in the ICU<br>Acute care beds<br>Should also be possible in hospice if trained personnel |

The use of NIV has been conceptualized in three categories by the Society of Critical Care Medicine Palliative Noninvasive Positive Pressure Ventilation Task Force.[45] This table is only an abstract of the original and the reader should refer to the original table and article that are described in more detail in the subsequent categories. Clinicians may take into account this conceptual framework while dealing with vulnerable elderly patients with acute respiratory failure, but they might also wish to consider several variables, and specific factors and characteristics of every individual – the patient or a relative.

ICU, intensive care unit.

Adapted from the Society of Critical Care Medicine Palliative Noninvasive Positive Pressure Ventilation Task Force.[45]

Critical care decision making is an imprecise process. It takes time to see whether therapy works. Aggressive care gives the patient the benefit of the doubt, but this approach increases the possibility of dependence on life support.[55] Accordingly, it soon becomes necessary to consider limiting a critical care plan when a point of diminishing returns is reached.[56] Without limits, 'the potential for warehousing warm cadavers looms large'.[7] That care plan will lead 'to another population, one composed of patients who were left not alive (in the sense of being capable of enjoying life) and not able to die (because technology temporarily arrested a disease process but did not reverse it)'.[57]

The use of NIV has been conceptualized in three categories by the Society of Critical Care Medicine Noninvasive Positive Pressure Ventilation Task Force.[43] This scheme, which also takes into account individual patient characteristics and wishes, provides clinicians with a conceptual framework that may help to provide proportionate care, determine the goals and determinants of success, and set NIV endpoints, response to failure and to discuss the ideal place for NIV initiation (Table 45.1). This scheme is not specifically intended for elderly patients, but it may be applied to institute proportionate care in all vulnerable patients that may require NIV initiation.

Briefly, category 1 patients are those for whom life support without pressure limits has to be applied. In these patients, the response to NIV failure will require intubation and mechanical ventilation. These patients may be treated within ICUs, but also in some specific step-down or acute care units with appropriate monitoring and trained personnel. Category 3 patients are those for whom comfort measures solely are to be applied. In these patients, NIV should be initiated outside the ICU, in specific beds with appropriately trained personnel. NIV failure should be considered if patients are not more comfortable than prior to NIV institution or if they become unable to communicate. The response to failure should be to palliate symptoms without NIV. Category 2 is in between the two other categories, in which the goal should be to restore the patient's health without using endotracheal intubation and without causing unacceptable discomfort.

### Interfaces

There are no specific issues concerning elderly people with regard to these items. A major determinant of success in general is NIV tolerance.[58] The vulnerability of elderly patients, combined with the fact that NIV will often be considered as the treatment of last resort, may increase the necessity to help patients tolerate the interfaces as much as possible. One should therefore focus on the use of more comfortable masks, encourage moving the mask to shift pressure points over the patient's face, and mainly use it intermittently.

## CONCLUSION

Despite scant literature on the topic, NIV seems as efficient in elderly patients as in younger ones. However, the need for proportionate care is much more crucial in the former than in younger patients, and NIV should be used as the treatment of last resort in most elderly patients, especially vulnerable ones. Patients' preferences regarding end-of-life treatment are often unknown as most patients are unconscious and/or demented on admission, which makes such a discussion difficult in an emergency. The relatives' opinions will therefore provide some clues regarding patients' preferences about the intensity of treatment to be applied, but the relative may not be available at the moment of the decision. Goals of NIV should never include the unnecessary prolongation of life, but rather to restore health as much as possible and, if not possible, at least to relieve the dyspnoea. Physicians should be able to accept NIV failure and to cease treatment if the patient is not more comfortable having NIV, if they want NIV to be stopped, or if they become unable to communicate.

## REFERENCES


1. Keenan SP, Sinuff T, Cook DJ *et al.* Which patients with acute exacerbation of chronic obstructive pulmonary disease benefit from noninvasive positive-pressure ventilation? A systematic review of the literature. *Ann Intern Med* 2003; **138**: 861–70.
2. Masip J, Roque M, Sanchez B *et al.* Noninvasive ventilation in acute cardiogenic pulmonary edema: systematic review and metaanalysis. *JAMA* 2005; **294**: 3124–30.
3. Nava S, Hill N. Non-invasive ventilation in acute respiratory failure. *Lancet* 2009; **374**: 250–9.
4. Sinuff T, Cook DJ, Keenan SP *et al.* Noninvasive ventilation for acute respiratory failure near the end of life. *Crit Care Med* 2008; **36**: 789–94.
5. Clarke DE, Vaughan L, Raffin TA. Noninvasive positive pressure ventilation for patients with terminal respiratory failure: the ethical and economic costs of delaying the inevitable are too great. *Am J Crit Care* 1994; **3**: 4–5.
6. Evans TW, Albert RK, Angus DC *et al.* International consensus conferences in intensive care medicine: non-invasive positive pressure ventilation in acute respiratory failure. Organised jointly by the American Thoracic Society, the European Respiratory Society, the European Society of Intensive Care Medicine, and the Société de Réanimation de Langue Française, and approved by the ATS Board of Directors, December 2000. *Am J Respir Crit Care Med* 2001; **163**: 283–91.
7. Crippen DW, Whetstine LM. Noninvasive ventilation and palliative care: unfolding the promise. *Crit Care Med* 2004; **32**: 881–2.

8. Roebuck J. When does old age begin? The evolution of the English definition. *J Soc Hist* 1979; **12**: 416–28.
9. Campion EW, Mulley AG, Goldstein RL *et al.* Medical intensive care for the elderly. A study of current use, costs, and outcomes. *JAMA* 1981; **246**: 2052–6.
10. Bo M, Massaia M, Raspo S *et al.* Predictive factors of in hospital mortality in older patients admitted to a medical intensive care unit. *J Am Geriatr Soc* 2003; **51**: 529–33.
11. Wenger NS, Solomon DS, Roth CP *et al.* The quality of medical care provided to vulnerable community-dwelling older patients. *Ann Intern Med* 2003; **139**: 740–7.
12. Anonymous. World population ageing: 1950–2050. Department of Economic and Social Affairs PD, United States, New York, 2001.
13. Population Division, Department of Economic and Social Affairs, United Nations: World Population Ageing 1950–2050. Available at: www.un.org/esa/population/publications/worldageing19502050/ (accessed February 2010).
14. Rockwood K, Noseworthy TW, Gibney RT *et al.* One year outcomes of elderly and young patients admitted to intensive care units. *Crit Care Med* 1993; **21**: 687–91.
15. Needham DM, Bronskill SE, Sibbald WJ *et al.* Mechanical ventilation in Ontario, 1992–2000: incidence, survival, and hospital bed utilization of noncardiac surgery adult patients. *Crit Care Med* 2004; **32**: 1504–9.
16. Owen A, Cox S. Diagnosis of heart failure in elderly patients in primary care. *Eur J Heart Fail* 2001; **3**: 79–81.
17. Caruana L, Petrie MC, Davie AP *et al.* Do patients with suspected heart failure and preserved left ventricular systolic function suffer from 'diastolic heart failure' or from misdiagnosis? A prospective descriptive study. *BMJ* 2000; **321**: 215–18.
18. Cowie MR, Struthers AD, Wood DA *et al.* Value of natriuretic peptides in assessment of patients with possible new heart failure in primary care. *Lancet* 1997; **350**: 1349–53.
19. Cleland JG, Cohen-Solal A, Aguilar JC *et al.* Management of heart failure in primary care (the improvement of heart failure programme): an international survey. *Lancet* 2002; **360**: 1631–9.
20. Heyland DK, Lavery JV, Tranmer JE *et al.* Dying in Canada: is it an institutionalized, technologically supported experience? *J Palliat Care* 2000; **16**: S10–S16.
21. Cook D, Rocker G, Marshall J *et al.* Withdrawal of mechanical ventilation in anticipation of death in the intensive care unit. *N Engl J Med* 2003; **349**: 1123–32.
22. Torres OH, Francia E, Longobardi V *et al.* Short and long term outcomes of older patients in intermediate care unit. *Intensive Care Med* 2006; **32**: 1052–9.
23. Somme D, Maillet J-M, Gisselbrecht M *et al.* Critically ill old and the oldest-old patients in intensive care: Short- and long-term outcomes. *Intensive Care Med* 2003; **29**: 2137–43.
24. Martin GS, Mannino DM, Moss M. The effect of age on the development and outcome of adult sepsis. *Crit Care Med* 2006; **34**: 15–21.
25. Boumendil A, Aegerter P, Guidet B *et al.* Treatment intensity and outcome of patients aged 80 and older in intensive care units: a multicentre matched-cohort study. *J Am Geriatr Soc* 2005; **53**: 88–93.
26. Townsend J, Frank AO, Fermont D *et al.* Terminal cancer care and patients' preference for place of death: a prospective study. *BMJ* 1990; **301**: 415–17.
27. Stajduhar KI, Allan DE, Cohen SR *et al.* Preferences for location of death of seriously ill hospitalized patients: perspectives from Canadian patients and their family caregivers. *Palliat Med* 2008; **22**: 85–8.
28. Lynn J, Teno JM, Phillips RS *et al.* Perceptions by family members of the dying experiences of older and seriously ill patients. SUPPORT Investigators. *Ann Intern Med* 1997; **126**: 97–106.
29. Hakim RB, Teno JM, Harrell FE Jr *et al.* Factors associated with do-not-resuscitate orders: patients' preferences, prognoses, and judgments. SUPPORT Investigators. Study to Understand Prognoses and Preferences for Outcome and risks of Treatment. *Ann Intern Med* 1996; **125**: 284–93.
30. Somogyi-Zalud E, Zhong Z, Hamel MB *et al.* The use of life-sustaining treatments in hospitalized persons aged 80 and older. *J Am Geriatr Soc* 2002; **50**: 930–4.
31. The SUPPORT Investigators. A controlled trial to improve care for seriously ill hospitalized patients. *JAMA* 1995; **274**: 1591–8.
32. Mehta S, Hill NS. Noninvasive ventilation. *Am J Respir Crit Care Med* 2001; **163**: 540–77.
33. Demoule A, Girou E, Richard JC *et al.* Increased use of noninvasive ventilation in French intensive care units. *Intensive Care Med* 2006; **32**: 1747–55.
34. Peter JV, Moran JL, Phillips-Hughes J *et al.* Noninvasive ventilation in acute respiratory failure: a meta-analysis update. *Crit Care Med* 2002; **30**: 555–62.
35. Lightowler JV, Wedzicha JA, Elliott MW *et al.* Non-invasive positive pressure ventilation to treat respiratory failure resulting from exacerbations of chronic obstructive pulmonary disease: Cochrane systematic review and meta-analysis. *BMJ* 2003; **326**: 185.
36. Benhamou D, Girault C, Faure C *et al.* Nasal mask ventilation in acute respiratory failure: experience in elderly patients. *Chest* 1992; **102**: 912–17.
37. Balami JS, Packham SM, Gosney MA. Non-invasive ventilation for respiratory failure due to acute exacerbations of chronic obstructive pulmonary disease in older patients. *Age Ageing* 2006; **35**: 78–9.
38. Rozzini R, Sabatini T, Trabucchi M. Non-invasive ventilation for respiratory failure in elderly patients. *Age Ageing* 2006; **35**: 546–7.
39. Vital FM, Saconato H, Ladeira MT *et al.* Non-invasive positive pressure ventilation (CPAP or bilevel NPPV) for cardiogenic pulmonary edema. *Cochrane Database Syst Rev* 2008; **3**: CD005351.

40. Collins SP, Mielniczuk LM, Whittingham HA *et al.* The use of noninvasive ventilation in emergency department patients with acute cardiogenic pulmonary edema: a systematic review. *Ann Emerg Med* 2006; **48**: 260–9.
41. Winck JC, Azevedo LF, Costa-Pereira A *et al.* Efficacy and safety of non-invasive ventilation in the treatment of acute cardiogenic pulmonary edema – a systematic review and meta-analysis. *Crit Care* 2006; **10**: R69.
42. L'Her E, Duquesne F, Girou E *et al.* Noninvasive continuous positive airway pressure in elderly cardiogenic pulmonary edema patients. *Intensive Care Med* 2004; **30**: 882–8.
43. Curtis JR, Cook DJ, Sinuff T *et al.* Noninvasive positive pressure ventilation in critical and palliative care settings: understanding the goals of therapy. *Crit Care Med* 2007; **35**: 932–9.
44. Crausman RS. The ethics of bilevel positive airway pressure. *Chest* 1998; **113**: 258.
45. Chu CM, Chan VL, Wong IW *et al.* Noninvasive ventilation in patients with acute hypercapnic exacerbation of chronic obstructive pulmonary disease who refused endotracheal intubation. *Crit Care Med* 2004; **32**: 372–7.
46. Freichels TA. Palliative ventilatory support: use of noninvasive positive pressure ventilation in terminal respiratory insufficiency. *Am J Crit Care* 1994; **3**: 6–10.
47. Camhi SL, Mercado AF, Morrison RS *et al.* Deciding in the dark: advance directives and continuation of treatment in chronic critical illness. *Crit Care Med* 2009; **37**: 919–25.
48. Wunsch H, Harrison DA, Harvey S *et al.* End-of-life decisions: a cohort study of the withdrawal of all active treatment in intensive care units in the United Kingdom. *Intensive Care Med* 2005; **6**: 823–31.
49. Azoulay E, Pochard F, Kentish-Barnes N *et al.* Risk of post-traumatic stress symptoms in family members of intensive care unit patients. *Am J Respir Crit Care Med* 2005, **171**: 987–94.
50. Emmanuel EJ, Emmanuel LL. Proxy decision making for incompetent patients: an ethical and empirical analysis. *JAMA* 1992; **267**: 2067–71.
51. Lloyd CB, Nietert PJ, Silvestri GA. Intensive care decision making in the seriously ill and elderly. *Crit Care Med* 2004; **32**: 649–54.
52. Nelson JE, Tandon N, Mercado AF *et al.* Brain dysfunction: another burden for the chronically critically ill. *Arch Intern Med* 2006; **166**: 1993–9.
53. Reilly BM, Magnussen CR, Ross J *et al.* Can we talk? Inpatient discussions about advance directives in a community hospital. Attending physicians' attitudes, their inpatients' wishes, and reported experience. *Arch Intern Med* 1994; **154**: 2299–308.
54. Essebag V, Cantarovich M, Crelinsten G. Routine advance directive and organ donation questioning on admission to hospital. *Ann R Coll Phys Surg Can* 2002; **35**: 225–31.
55. Crippen D. Terminally weaning awake patients from life sustaining mechanical ventilation: the critical care physician's role in comfort measures during the dying process. *Clin Intensive Care* 1992; **3**: 206–12.
56. Schneiderman LJ, Gilmer T, Teetzel HD. Impact of ethics consultations in the intensive care setting: a randomized, controlled trial. *Crit Care Med* 2000; **28**: 3920–4.
57. Danis M, Federman D, Fins JJ *et al.* Incorporating palliative care into critical care education: principles, challenges, and opportunities. *Crit Care Med* 1999; **27**: 2005–13.
58. Carlucci A, Richard JC, Wysocki M *et al.* Noninvasive versus conventional mechanical ventilation. An epidemiologic survey. *Am J Respir Crit Care Med* 2001; **163**: 874–80.

# 46

# Post-surgery non-invasive ventilation

SAMIR JABER, BORIS JUNG, GERALD CHANQUES

## ABSTRACT

Post-operative non-invasive ventilation (NIV) can be employed in two ways: preventive or 'prophylactic' application to prevent post-operative acute respiratory failure (ARF) from developing in patients at risk; and 'curative' application, once ARF occurs, to ease respiratory failure while avoiding endotracheal intubation, a cause of increased morbidity. Post-surgery hypoxaemia and/or ARF mainly develop following abdominal and/or thoracic surgery. Anaesthesia, post-operative pain and surgery (more so as the site of the surgery approaches the diaphragm) induce respiratory alterations: hypoxaemia, decrease in pulmonary volumes and atelectasis associated with a restrictive syndrome and diaphragm dysfunction. These alterations of respiratory function occur early after surgery and are often transient. Post-operative NIV should be beneficial in patients at high risk for respiratory post-operative complications (elderly, obese, patients with chronic obstructive pulmonary disease, etc.). The rationale for post-operative NIV use is the same as for post-extubation NIV use plus the specific indication due to the respiratory alterations induced by the surgery. Post-operative NIV improves gas exchange, decreases work of breathing and reduces atelectasis. The effectiveness of NIV in decreasing the need for reintubation has been demonstrated in the treatment of ARF following pulmonary surgery and solid organ transplantation, as has continuous positive airway pressure for the treatment of hypoxaemia following abdominal surgery.

## INTRODUCTION

Post-operative pulmonary complications following surgery are common and associated with increased morbidity and mortality and hospital length of stay.[1,2] Post-surgery hypoxaemia and/or acute respiratory failure (ARF) mainly develop following abdominal and/or thoracic surgery.[1–4] Anaesthesia, post-operative pain and surgery (more so as the site of the surgery approaches the diaphragm) induce alterations in respiratory function: hypoxaemia, reduced pulmonary volume and atelectasis,[3] associated with a restrictive syndrome and diaphragm dysfunction.[5] These alterations of respiratory function occur early after surgery and are most often transient. The major objectives for the physician are, first, to prevent the occurrence of post-operative complications and, second, if ARF does occur, to ensure oxygen administration and carbon dioxide removal while avoiding intubation.[1,4] Non-invasive ventilation (NIV) does not require an artificial airway (endotracheal tube or tracheostomy) and its use is well established for ARF prevention (prophylactic treatment) and treatment of ARF to avoid reintubation (curative treatment). Studies demonstrate that patient-related risk factors, such as chronic obstructive pulmonary disease (COPD), age older than 60 years, American Society of Anesthesiologists (ASA) class of II or higher, obesity, functional dependence and congestive heart failure, increase the risk for post-operative pulmonary complications.[1–4] NIV should be beneficial to these patients at high risk, especially after 'aggressive' surgery.

This chapter aims to review the main respiratory alterations induced by surgery and anaesthesia, to justify using post-operative NIV and to present the results of studies on preventive and curative NIV in a surgical context. Some recommendations for the safe application of post-surgery NIV are also proposed.

## SURGERY- AND ANAESTHESIA-INDUCED RESPIRATORY ALTERATIONS AND RATIONALE FOR POST-OPERATIVE NON-INVASIVE VENTILATION USE

Major changes in respiratory function occur in all patients after anaesthesia and surgical incisions, especially on the thorax and upper abdomen, because of a decrease in the functional residual capacity with minimal change in the closing volume leading to airway closure during tidal breathing. Indeed, post-operative ARF is generally observed after abdominal and/or thoracic surgery. Anaesthesia, surgery and post-operative pain[6] lead to respiratory function modifications, mainly hypoxaemia, which results from changes in ventilation/perfusion ratio. The latter is a consequence of both functional residual capacity and vital capacity reductions related to respiratory muscle dysfunction and atelectasis. Moreover, peri-operative related modifications of the ventilatory system and hypoxaemia frequently observed in the early post-operative period may be aggravated by other factors such as excessive peri-operative vascular loading,[7] transfusion-related acute lung injury, inflammation, sepsis and aspiration. The expected benefit of NIV would be to partially compensate for the affected respiratory function by reducing the work of breathing, by improving alveolar ventilation associated with increased gas exchange, by reducing left ventricular afterload with an increase in cardiac output and by reducing atelectasis.[8]

## DEFINITIONS AND PRINCIPLES OF THE TWO MAIN NIV TECHNIQUES: CONTINUOUS POSITIVE AIRWAY PRESSURE AND BI-LEVEL POSITIVE AIRWAY PRESSURE

Two types of NIV are commonly used: continuous positive airway pressure (CPAP) and bi-level positive airway pressure (BiPAP), which refers to the combinations of pressure support ventilation with positive end expiratory pressure (PSV + PEEP).

### Non-invasive ventilation application

Post-operative NIV can be applied in two ways. The first is a preventive or 'prophylactic' application in order to prevent post-operative ARF from developing in patients at risk, and the second consists of a 'curative' application, once ARF occurs, in order to alleviate respiratory failure while avoiding endotracheal intubation, a cause of increased morbidity.

### Setting up NIV and duration of trial

Non-invasive ventilation works best in patients who are relaxed and prepared. Continuous positive airway pressures of 7–10 cm $H_2O$ are required to keep tracheal pressure positive during the entire respiratory cycle and to consistently improve gas exchange. In PSV + PEEP, patient comfort and interface acceptance may be improved by starting with PEEP alone and then slowly increasing the PSV level once the mask is applied. We recommend starting with a PSV of 3–5 cm $H_2O$ and increasing in increments of 2 cm $H_2O$ to achieve a 6–10 mL/kg expiratory tidal volume, a decrease in the patient's respiratory rate and a comfort improvement.[9] The PEEP is started at 3–5 cm $H_2O$ and increased as needed to improve oxygenation without adverse haemodynamic effects up to 10 cm $H_2O$. The insufflation pressure (PSV + PEEP) applied should be less than 25 cm $H_2O$. These setting recommendations are based solely on clinical experience without any formal data to support the superiority of one technique over another.[10] Surgical complications arise in nearly half the cases of ARF. The treatment for these cases is generally a second intervention and the management of the ARF is only a symptomatic treatment, and there is no reason to use NIV to avoid intubation as the patient will be intubated in the operating room for general anaesthesia.

Evidence to guide duration of a NIV trial is lacking, so the recommendations are based largely on practitioner experience. In the post-operative area, we recommend 'sequential' use, wherein periods of use alternate with lengthy ventilator-free periods, and total daily use ranges between 3 hours and 12 hours, depending on the type of application (curative or prophylactic use). In our practice,[9] during the first 24 hours, for the majority of the patients, NIV is applied for approximately 30–45 minutes at 2- to 4-hour intervals (prophylactic), depending on the patient's clinical condition. Some patients are treated during the initial period with NIV for 60–90 minutes at 2- to 3-hour intervals (range, 8–2 h/day; curative). Between the periods of NIV, the patients breathe through a Venturi mask. The length of NIV cycles is progressively reduced and NIV withdrawn completely as blood gas values and the clinical condition improve.

### Interfaces

To date, there is no evidence to support the use of particular patient interface devices in the surgical context. Therefore, practitioners should try different mask sizes and types in an effort to enhance patient comfort.[11,12]

### Contraindications and limitations

Patient cooperation without deteriorating mental status, absence of haemodynamic instability and ability to protect airways are crucial to the application and the success of NIV. The relative and absolute contraindications of NIV use are given in Box 46.1.

### Problems related to digestive tubes and their relationship with NIV

Upper digestive tract stitching necessitates great prudence with the use of early post-operative NIV. Historically, NIV was contraindicated in cases of upper gastrointestinal tract

**Box 46.1 Contraindications for the use of post-operative non-invasive ventilation**

Absolute contraindications

- Cardiac or respiratory arrest
- Multiple organ failure
- Severe agitation or encephalopathy
- Copious secretions
- Uncontrolled vomiting
- Inability to protect airway
- Severe upper gastrointestinal bleeding or haemoptysis
- Immediate endotracheal intubation necessary (except for pre-oxygenation NIV)
- Facial trauma
- Haemodynamic instability or unstable cardiac arrhythmia

Relative contraindications

- Mildly decreased level of consciousness
- Progressive severe respiratory failure
- Uncooperative patient who cannot be calmed or comforted

anastomoses. In fact, there is a risk of intra-digestive air insufflation when high insufflation pressures are applied (PSV + PEEP >25 cm $H_2O$).[10] However, the risk of stitch leakage due to non-optimal NIV settings may be avoided by using CPAP in preference to PSV. If PSV is required, the PSV level must be maintained below 6–8 cm $H_2O$. Moreover, compared with PSV + PEEP, CPAP is easier to perform especially outside the intensive care unit and/or in post-anaesthesia care. One limiting factor in PSV + PEEP implementation might be operator skill. It is known that the more experienced the operator and/or the team, the higher the success rate of PSV + PEEP. However, in some patients, CPAP and PSV + PEEP may be applied alternately, aiming to improve tolerance and/or efficiency.

## RESULTS OF THE USE OF NON-INVASIVE VENTILATION WITH PREVENTIVE OR CURATIVE INTENT IN DIFFERENT TYPES OF SURGERY (TABLE 46.1)

### Cardiac surgery

#### PREVENTIVE NIV

The restrictive syndrome following cardiac surgery is generally less severe than that observed after thoracic or abdominal surgery.[4] However, the incidence of diaphragm dysfunction is higher.[4] Early studies mainly compared CPAP to standard treatment (oxygen + physiotherapy). Most of them reported improved oxygenation and ventilation parameters. None of these studies found any reduction in the incidence of atelectasis in the groups treated by NIV, in fact mainly CPAP, except for Jousela *et al.*[13] and Gust *et al.*,[7] who obtained a reduction in extravascular lung water when NIV was applied with CPAP alone or with PSV (PSV + PEEP). Matte *et al.*,[14] in a study including 96 patients, evaluated 'preventive' NIV in the first 2 days following surgery. Various strategies were compared in three randomized groups. The first group received 1 hour of bi-level NIV every 3 hours with an average assistance level of 12 cm $H_2O$ of PSV and 5 cm $H_2O$ of PEEP. The second group received a 1-hour session of CPAP at 5 cm $H_2O$ every 3 hours and a third group had 20 minutes of incentive spirometry every 2 hours. Using NIV, whether with one or two pressure levels, permitted improved oxygenation and a lower reduction of lung volumes. However, the incidence of atelectasis was similar (12–15 per cent) in all three groups.[14] Pasquina *et al.*[15] compared the effect of systematic application of a 30-minute trial of 5 cm $H_2O$ CPAP with NIV (PSV 10 and PEEP 5) in two groups of 75 patients. The NIV group had improved radiological scores (i.e. less marked atelectasis) on standard chest X-ray. There was no significant difference in oxygenation parameters.[15] Recently, Zarbock *et al.*[16] reported, in a prospective randomized study which included 500 patients scheduled for elective cardiac surgery, the effect of prophylactic nasal CPAP of 10 cm $H_2O$ (study) for at least 6 hours per day following surgery in comparison to standard treatment (control) including 10 minutes of intermittent nasal CPAP at 10 cm $H_2O$ every 4 hours. In the study group, CPAP improved arterial oxygenation, reduced the incidence of pulmonary complications, including pneumonia and reintubation rate, and reduced readmission rate to the intensive or intermediate care unit.

#### CURATIVE NIV

To our knowledge, at the time of writing, no study has been published on the effect of curative NIV in patients who have developed ARF after cardiac surgery.

### Thoracic surgery

#### PREVENTIVE NIV

In a physiological study, Aguilo *et al.*[17] studied the effects of a 1-hour NIV trial after pulmonary resection in 10 patients; NIV was applied without any complications due to the technique and allowed improved oxygenation without increasing leaks around thoracic drains in the study group compared with a control group who did not receive NIV.[17] Perrin *et al.*[18] reported a prospective randomized clinical trial on the benefits of NIV administered pre- and post-operatively. Patients were required to follow standard treatment without or with NIV for 7 days at home before the surgery and 3 days postoperatively. In this study, 2 hours after surgery, oxygenation and lung volumes values were significantly better in the NIV group.[18] On days 1, 2 and 3, oxygenation was significantly improved in the NIV group. The hospital stay was significantly longer in the control group than in the NIV group. This first prospective randomized study has shown that prophylactic use of NIV pre- and post-operatively significantly reduces pulmonary dysfunction after lung resection.[18]

### CURATIVE NIV

In an observational study, Rocco *et al.*[19] described their experience of NIV in 21 patients who developed ARF after lung transplantation. Tolerance of NIV was good in all patients. In 18 patients reintubation was avoided.[19] In a prospective randomized study including 24 patients in each group, Auriant *et al.*[20] showed the efficiency of NIV in ARF after lung resection. In this trial,[20] NIV was delivered by a nasal mask using a single circuit ventilator and compared with standard treatment (oxygen + physiotherapy + bronchodilators). The former reduced the need for invasive mechanical ventilation (21 per cent vs 50 per cent, respectively) and mortality (13 per cent vs 38 per cent, respectively). Lefebvre *et al.*[21] confirmed in an observational prospective survey the feasibility and efficacy of early NIV in ARF following lung resection. During a 4-year period, of 690 patients at risk for severe complications following lung resection, 16 per cent experienced ARF, which was initially managed by NIV. The overall success rate of NIV was 85 per cent.

## Abdominal surgery

### PREVENTIVE NIV

Hypoxaemia complicates the recovery of 30–50 per cent of patients after abdominal surgery, even among those undergoing uneventful procedures. Stock *et al.*[22] showed that applying CPAP in patients having cholecystectomy by laparotomy led to a significant reduction in the incidence of atelectasis compared with treatment by incentive spirometry. After bariatric surgery (gastroplasty) for morbid obesity, Joris *et al.*[23] demonstrated a significant reduction of the occurrence of restrictive syndrome and significant improvement in oxygenation evaluated by oximetry ($SpO_2$) with NIV applied for two-thirds of the first post-operative 24 hours. Compared with the control group, forced vital capacity improved significantly only with a moderately high PSV level of 12 cm $H_2O$, as another group treated with a PSV level of 8 cm $H_2O$ did not have a significant improvement in chronic respiratory failure. This finding remains important today, given the sharp increase in the rate of obesity surgery.[23] Kindgen-Milles *et al.*[24] studied the effect of systematic use of CPAP at 10 cm $H_2O$ for 12–24 hours a day after thoracoabdominal surgery (for treatment of aneurysm of the thoracoabdominal aorta). The group of patients receiving CPAP had significantly improved oxygenation and a shorter intensive care unit and hospital stay compared with the control group. A large Italian study[25] was stopped early due to reduction in intubation related to CPAP therapy in hypoxaemic patients after abdominal surgery. This randomized study[25] included 209 patients in two groups: one group received CPAP and a control group received oxygen via a face mask. The patients receiving CPAP had significantly lower rates of intubation, pneumonia and sepsis compared with the control group.[25]

### CURATIVE NIV

Patients with post-operative ARF have been included with other types of patient in studies evaluating NIV to treat ARF of multiple causes.[10] In these studies, no comparison has been made between patients with ARF resulting from medical causes and those with post-operative ARF, probably because of the heterogeneity and small numbers of patients included. Varon *et al.*[26] reported the feasibility of NIV in post-operative ARF in cancer patients (25 gastrointestinal, 15 urogenital, 6 lung). Intubation was avoided in 70 per cent of patients in this study.[26] Kindgen-Milles *et al.*,[27] in a non-controlled prospective study, showed that CPAP rapidly improved oxygenation and avoided intubation in 18 of 20 patients treated after abdominal and/or thoracic surgery. Jaber *et al.*[9] reported, in an observational study, their experience over a 2-year period using NIV in 72 patients with severe ARF after gastrointestinal surgery. In this prospective trial,[9] intubation was avoided in 66 per cent of patients. This study[9] demonstrated the feasibility, good tolerance and safety of NIV for the treatment of ARF after gastrointestinal surgery. More severe initial hypoxaemia and lower improvement of $PaO_2$ after NIV were predictive of NIV failure.[9] Jaber's results were confirmed in a recent study that included 72 patients who developed ARF after abdominal surgery, whereby intubation was avoided in 42 patients (58 per cent).[28] Conti *et al.*[12] in a match-controlled study compared the efficacy of NIV delivered by a helmet interface and a face mask in patients with ARF after abdominal surgery. These authors reported a NIV success rate of 80 per cent in the helmet group and of 52 per cent in the face mask group.[12] In a controlled randomized trial in organ transplant recipients with hypoxaemic ARF,[29] Antonelli *et al.* showed that NIV reduced the rate of intubation, the incidence of fatal complications and intensive care unit mortality compared with the provision of supplemental oxygenation alone. More recently, Michelet *et al.*[30] compared, in a case–control study, the efficacy of NIV with conventional treatment in 36 patients who developed post-operative ARF after planned oesophagectomy. They showed that the use of NIV was associated with a lower intubation rate, a lower incidence of acute respiratory distress syndrome and anastomotic leakage, and a reduction in length of stay in the intensive care unit.

**Table 46.1** Main studies on post-surgery non-invasive ventilation classified by type of surgery and date

| Authors | Year | Type of surgery | Study design | Indication | Patients | NIV mode and main settings | Interface | Results | Success rate of NIV (%) |
|---|---|---|---|---|---|---|---|---|---|
| Gust *et al.*[7] | 1996 | Cardiac | Physiological | Preventive | $n = 75$ 3 groups | SB; CPAP; PSV + PEEP | Facial CPAP Nasal PSV + PEEP | Extravascular lung water decrease | NA |
| Matte *et al.*[14] | 2000 | Cardiac | Physiological | Preventive | $n = 96$ 3 groups | SB; CPAP + 5; PSV + 12−PEEP + 5 | Facial | Oxygenation and lung volumes improvement, | NA |
| Pasquina *et al.*[15] | 2004 | Cardiac | Physiological | Preventive | $n = 150$ 2 groups | CPAP + 5; PSV + 10−PEEP + 5 | Facial | Atelectasis decrease | 100 |
| Zarbock *et al.*[16] | 2009 | Cardiac | Prospective, randomized | Preventive | $n = 500$ | CPAP | Nasal | Oxygenation improvement, reduced the incidence of pulmonary complications and reduced readmission rate to ICU | 99 |
| Aguilo *et al.*[17] | 1997 | Pulmonary | Physiological | Preventive | $n = 20$ 2 groups | SB; PSV + 10−PEEP + 5 | Nasal | Oxygenation improvement | NA |
| Rocco *et al.*[19] | 2001 | Pulmonary (transplant) | Retrospective, Observational | Curative | $n = 21$ | PSV + 14−PEEP + 5 | Facial | Feasibility, safety. Oxygenation improvement | 86 |
| Auriant *et al.*[20] | 2001 | Pulmonary | Prospective, randomized | Curative | $n = 48$ 2 groups | SB; PSV + 9−PEEP + 4 | Nasal | Intubation and mortality decrease | 79 |
| Lefebvre *et al.*[21] | 2009 | Pulmonary | Prospective, observational | Curative | $n = 89$ | CPAP and/or NIV | Facial Or nasal | Feasibility, safety. Oxygenation improvement | 85 |
| Stock *et al.*[22] | 1985 | Abdominal (cholecystectomy) | Physiological | Preventive | $n = 65$ 2 groups | SB; CPAP + 8 | Facial | Atelectasis decrease, FRC improvement | NA |
| Joris *et al.*[23] | 1997 | Abdominal (obses-gastroplasty) | Physiological | Preventive | $n = 33$ 3 groups | SB; PSV + 8−PEEP + 5 PSV + 12−PEEP + 5 | Nasal | Oxygenation and lung volumes improvement | NA |

| | | | | | | | | | |
|---|---|---|---|---|---|---|---|---|---|
| Kindgen-Miles *et al.*[27] | 2000 | Thoraco-abdominal | Prospective, observational | Curative | $n = 20$ | CPAP + 10 | Nasal | Oxygenation improvement, | 90 |
| Antonelli *et al.*[29] | 2000 | Thoraco-abdominal (liver transplant, renal, lung) | Prospective, randomized | Curative | $n = 40$ 2 groups | SB PSV + 15 PEEP + 6 | Facial | Intubation and mortality decrease | 80 |
| Kindgen-Miles *et al.*[24] | 2005 | Thoraco-abdominal | Prospective, randomized | Preventive | $n = 50$ 2 groups | SB CPAP + 10 | Nasal | Oxygenation improvement, Hospital stay decrease | 96 |
| Jaber *et al.*[9] | 2005 | Abdominal | Prospective, observational | Curative | $n = 72$ | PSV + 14−PEEP + 6 | Facial | Feasibility, safety. Oxygenation improvement | 66 |
| Squadrone[2] *et al.*[5] | 2005 | Abdominal | Prospective, randomized | Curative | $n = 209$ 2 groups | SB CPAP + 7,5 | Facial and helmet | Intubation and sepsis decrease | 99 |
| Michele *et al.*[30] | 2009 | Abdominal and thoracic (oesophagectomy) | Retrospective, Case mix | Curative | $n = 72$ 2 groups | SB PSV + 13-PEEP+5 | Facial | Lower intubation, ARDS rate and lower ICU stay | 75 |
| Wallet *et al.*[28] | 2009 | Abdominal | Prospective, observational | Curative | $n = 72$ | SB PSV + 15−PEEP + 6 | Facial | Feasibility, safety. Oxygenation improvement | 58 |

CPAP, continuous positive airway pressure; NA, not applied; PEEP, positive end expiratory pressure; PSV, pressure support ventilation; ICU, intensive care unit; SB, spontaneous breathing.

## CONCLUSION

Regardless of the presence of complications, thoracic and/or abdominal surgery necessarily and profoundly alters the respiratory system for long periods. Mechanical ventilation through an endotracheal tube may be responsible for increased morbidity (barotraumatic complications, nosocomial pneumonia, etc.). During the past decade, NIV has proven to be an effective strategy to reduce intubation rates, nosocomial infections, intensive care unit and hospital lengths of stay, and morbidity and mortality in patients with either hypercapnic or non-hypercapnic ARF. However, before initiation of NIV in patients with post-operative ARF, surgical complications (anastomosis leakage, intra-abdominal sepsis, etc.) should be treated and eliminated. Then, if the patient is cooperative and able to protect their airway, NIV can be initiated with due regard to safety procedures and contraindications. The application of post-operative NIV by a trained and experienced intensive care unit team, with careful patient selection, should optimize patient outcomes.

## REFERENCES

1. Qaseem A, Snow V, Fitterman N *et al.* Risk assessment for and strategies to reduce perioperative pulmonary complications for patients undergoing noncardiothoracic surgery: a guideline from the American College of Physicians. *Ann Intern Med* 2006; **144**: 575–80.
2. Smetana G. Preoperative pulmonary evaluation. *N Engl J Med* 1999; **340**: 937–45.
3. Duggan M, Kavanagh BP. Pulmonary atelectasis. A pathogenic perioperative entity. *Anesthesiology* 2005; **102**: 838–54.
4. Warner M. Preventing postoperative pulmonary complications. The role of the anesthesiologist. *Anesthesiology* 2000; **92**: 1467–72.
5. Simonneau G, Vivien A, Sartene R *et al.* Diaphragm dysfunction induced by upper abdominal surgery. Role of postoperative pain. *Am Rev Respir Dis* 1983; **128**: 899–903.
6. Vassilakopoulos T, Mastora Z, Katsaounou P *et al.* Contribution of pain to inspiratory muscle dysfunction after upper abdominal surgery: a randomized controlled trial. *Am J Respir Crit Care Med* 2000; **161**: 1372–5.
7. Gust R, Gottschalk A, Schmidt H *et al.* Effects of continuous (CPAP) and bi-level positive airway pressure (BiPAP) on extravascular lung water after extubation of the trachea in patients following coronary artery bypass grafting. *Intensive Care Med* 1996; **22**: 1345–50.
8. Jaber S, Gallix B, Sebbane M *et al.* Noninvasive ventilation improves alveolar recruitment in postoperative patients with acute respiratory failure: a CT-scan study. *Intensive Care Med* 2005; S148.
9. Jaber S, Delay J, Sebbane M *et al.* Outcomes of patients with acute respiratory failure after abdominal surgery treated with noninvasive positive-pressure ventilation. *Chest* 2005; **128**: 2688–95.
10. International consensus conferences in Intensive care medicine. Noninvasive positive pressure ventilation in acute respiratory failure. *Am J Respir Crit Care Med* 2001; **163**: 283–91.
11. Antonelli M, Pennisi MA, Pelosi P *et al.* Noninvasive positive pressure ventilation using a helmet in patients with acute exacerbation of chronic obstructive pulmonary disease: a feasibility study. *Anesthesiology* 2004; **100**: 16–24.
12. Conti G, Cavaliere F, Costa R *et al.* Noninvasive positive pressure ventilation with different interfaces in patients with respiratory failure after abdominal surgery. A match-control study. *Respir Care* 2007; **52**: 1463–71.
13. Jousela I, Rasanen J, Verkkala K *et al.* Continuous positive airway pressure by mask in patients after coronary surgery. *Acta Anaesthesiol Scand* 1994; **38**: 311–16.
14. Matte P, Jacquet M, Vandyck M *et al.* Effects of conventional physiotherapy, continuous positive airway pressure and non-invasive ventilatory support with bilevel positive airway pressure after coronary artery bypass grafting. *Acta Anaesthesiol Scand* 2000; **44**: 75–81.
15. Pasquina P, Merlani P, Granier J *et al.* Continuous positive airway pressure versus noninvasive pressure support ventilation to treat atelectasis after cardiac surgery. *Anesth Analg* 2004; **99**: 1001–8.
16. Zarbock A, Mueller E, Netzer S *et al.* Prophylactic nasal continuous positive airway pressure following cardiac surgery protects from postoperative pulmonary complications. A prospective, randomized, controlled trial in 500 patients. *Chest* 2009; **135**: 1252–9.
17. Aguilo R, Togores B, Pons S *et al.* Noninvasive ventilatory support after lung resectional surgery. *Chest* 1997; **112**: 117–21.
18. Perrin C, Jullien V, Vénissac N *et al.* Prophylactic use of noninvasive ventilation in patients undergoing lung resectional surgery. *Respir Med* 2007; **101**: 1572–8.
19. Rocco M, Conti G, Antonelli M *et al.* Non-invasive pressure support ventilation in patients with acute respiratory failure after bilateral lung transplantation. *Intensive Care Med* 2001; **27**: 1622–6.
20. Auriant I, Jallot A, Hervé P *et al.* Noninvasive ventilation reduces mortality in acute respiratory failure following lung resection. *Am J Respir Crit Care Med* 2001; **164**: 1231–5.
21. Lefebvre A, Lorut C, Alifano M *et al.* Noninvasive ventilation for acute respiratory failure after lung resection. An observational study. *Intensive Care Med* 2009; **35**: 663–70.
22. Stock M, Downs J, Gauer P *et al.* Prevention of postoperative pulmonary complications with CPAP, incentive spirometry, and conservative therapy. *Chest* 1985; **87**: 151–7.

23. Joris J, Sottiaux T, Chiche J *et al.* Effect of bi-level positive airway pressure (BiPAP) on the postoperative pulmonary restrictive syndrome in obese patients undergoing gastroplasty. *Chest* 1997; **111**: 665–70.
24. Kindgen-Milles D, Muller E, Buhl R *et al.* Nasal-continuous positive airway pressure reduces pulmonary morbidity and length of hospital stay following thoracoabdominal aortic surgery. *Chest* 2005; **128**: 821–8.
25. Squadrone V, Coha M, Cerutti E *et al.* Continuous positive airway pressure for treatment of postoperative hypoxemia. A randomized controlled trial. *JAMA* 2005; **293**: 589–95.
26. Varon J, Walsh G, Fromm RJ. Feasibility of noninvasive mechanical ventilation in the treatment of acute respiratory failure in postoperative cancer patients. *J Crit Care* 1998; **13**: 55–7.
27. Kindgen-Milles D, Buhl R, Gabriel A *et al.* Nasal continuous positive airway pressure. A method to avoid endotracheal reintubation in postoperative high-risk patients with severe nonhypercapnic oxygenation failure. *Chest* 2000; **117**: 1106–11.
28. Wallet F, Scoeffler M, Reynaud M *et al.* Factors associated with noninvasive ventilation failure in postoperative acute respiratory insufficiency. An observational study. *Eur J Anaesthesiol* 2009 [Epub ahead of print].
29. Antonelli M, Conti G, Bufi M *et al.* Noninvasive ventilation for treatment of acute respiratory failure in patients undergoing solid organ transpantation. A randomized trial. *JAMA* 2000; **283**: 235–41.
30. Michelet P, D'Journo XB, Seinaye F *et al.* Non-invasive ventilation for treatment of postoperative respiratory failure after oesophagectomy. *Br J Surg* 2009; **96**: 54–60.

# 47

# Trauma

UMBERTO LUCANGELO, MASSIMO FERLUGA

## ABSTRACT

Blunt chest trauma is a frequent finding in multiple trauma patients, and endotracheal intubation and mechanical ventilation are, to date, the treatments of choice. Pulmonary parenchymal contusion represents the most frequent lesion, whereas flail chest is a rare finding in multiple trauma patients, although it has a significant impact on chest wall motion. During the early 1980s, following the ever-increasing evidence of infectious complications caused by invasive ventilation, the use of non-invasive ventilation (NIV) was suggested as conservative treatment in chest trauma patients, with good results. Lately, the application of NIV has also spread outside the intensive care unit (ICU), and the development of protocols including different analgesic techniques together with early respiratory physio-kinesitherapy has allowed for devising increasingly conservative treatment of chest trauma, with lower costs and shorter ICU stays. In the ICU, patients may be treated by NIV, without necessarily needing tracheal intubation during their stay in hospital. In this case, the use of non-invasive positive pressure ventilation is preferable to continuous positive airways pressure (CPAP). In addition, it favours early extubation, and maintenance of gas exchange, avoiding the collapse of the injured lung regions and bacterial suprainfection. Furthermore, ventilatory support sensibly reduces respiratory muscle work, alleviating at the same time the patient's painful symptoms. For all these reasons, NIV represents a valuable alternative to tracheal intubation in chest trauma patients, and the performance of randomized controlled studies will lead to a better positioning of this long-standing ventilation technique in the daily practice of intensivists.

## INTRODUCTION

Blunt chest trauma is a frequent finding in multiple trauma patients, with an incidence of approximately 25 per cent. Furthermore, chest injuries are associated with a mortality rate of up to 10 per cent, and they are responsible for 25 per cent of deaths in multiple trauma patients.[1] The most frequent cause of blunt chest trauma is road accidents, followed by accidents at work, trauma related to falls, and gunshot or side-arm wounds. In general, isolated chest trauma does not require surgical intervention, as it can be managed by chest tube insertion, positive pressure ventilation, pain control and airway clearance.

Tracheal intubation and intermittent positive pressure ventilation (IPPV) is still the gold standard in the treatment of acute respiratory failure (ARF) in trauma patients.[2] However, in patients with pulmonary contusion, when gas exchange is not too severely compromised and, importantly, when there are no additional severe lesions that could lead to alterations in consciousness or haemodynamic instability, tracheal intubation should be avoided to limit the risk of pulmonary barotrauma and ventilator-associated pneumonia (VAP), caused mainly by suprainfection within the injured region. In fact, it has been shown that mechanical ventilation performed for more than 48 hours is the main risk factor for developing VAP; in particular, Antonelli *et al.*[3] demonstrated an increased incidence of pneumonia in intubated chest and abdominal trauma patients. These authors also observed that early intubation may reduce the incidence of early-onset pneumonia, as it guarantees adequate ventilation of atelectatic lung areas and reduces bacterial translocation; on the other hand, intubation for more than 5 days has been associated with an increased risk of developing late-onset pneumonia.

Non-invasive ventilation (NIV) consists of ventilatory support provided through the upper airways using a face mask or other similar devices; hence, it is different from invasive techniques that bypass the upper airways, such as laryngeal mask, endotracheal tube or tracheostomy. Nowadays, NIV has become a common tool in intensive care, and its application in internal medicine is increasingly frequent. The main indications for its use are ARF in patients with relapsing chronic obstructive pulmonary disease (COPD), acute cardiogenic pulmonary oedema, neuromuscular diseases, and asthma.

Of the large number of publications on NIV, only a few deal with its application on trauma patients.[4–6] The first studies on the use of NIV in this field date back to the second world war, when Buford and Burbank showed an improvement in gas exchanges in chest trauma patients using a combination of NIV and intercostal nerve blocks.[7] Later, with innovations in the material used for endotracheal tubes and the development of increasingly reliable ventilators, endotracheal intubation and mechanical ventilation became the first choice of treatment in patients with ARF of any origin. During the early 1980s, following the ever-increasing finding of infectious complications caused by invasive ventilation, the use of continuous positive airway pressure (CPAP) was suggested as conservative treatment in chest trauma patients, with good results;[4,5] later, with the introduction of dedicated ventilators, pressure support ventilation (PSV) also proved to be comparably effective.[8,9] Lately, NIV has also started to be used in out-of-hospital first aid and the development of protocols including different analgesic techniques together with early respiratory physio-kinesitherapy has allowed for increasingly conservative treatment of chest trauma and for lower costs and shorter intensive care unit (ICU) stays.

## PATHOPHYSIOLOGY

Pulmonary parenchymal contusion represents the most common trauma injury, with a 15 per cent incidence in multiple trauma patients and mortality rates up to 35 per cent.[10] This condition is characterized by bleeding and lung oedema, which lead to alveolar collapse, pleural effusion, either reactive or caused by associated pleural lesion, and consolidation of the injured regions. This leads to a decreased lung compliance and to an altered ventilation/perfusion ratio, caused by an arteriovenous shunt through the non-ventilated lung. From a clinical viewpoint, patients present with dyspnoea, tachypnoea and hypoxia; furthermore, a non-productive cough, shallow breathing caused by the increased elastic load and pain may encourage the development of atelectasis and bacterial suprainfection. A chest X-ray generally shows irregular infiltrates or inhomogeneous opacities, caused by alveolar haemorrhage and oedema, beginning within 4–6 hours of the accident, often localized near the rib, sternal or clavicular fractures. The best modality for the diagnosis and staging of pulmonary contusion is chest computed tomography (CT); in fact, in a recent study patients with a contusion >20 per cent of the total lung volume on chest CT were four times more likely to develop adult respiratory distress syndrome (ARDS).[11] The latter develops in 5–20 per cent of cases, with a higher risk within the first 24 hours of the trauma injury, and its onset may also be determined by pulmonary contusion *per se*, without any other predictive factor. In the absence of a progressive reduction of oedema and haemorrhage, pneumonia may develop in 5–50 per cent of pulmonary contusion cases, although if there is a coexisting flail chest the incidence may reach 85 per cent.

Flail chest is a rare finding in multiple trauma patients, although it is one of the most severe in those with chest wall involvement, with mortality rates up to 35 per cent. This condition occurs in the presence of bifocal fractures of three or more adjacent ribs, or combined fractures of the sternum, ribs and cartilages. A loss of continuity with the intact section ensues, and this portion of the chest wall moves inwards during inspiration, retracted by the negative intrathoracic pressure, and outwards during expiration. The presence of a flail chest makes the patient unable to produce a negative pressure sufficient to obtain an adequate tidal volume, leading to the creation of areas of atelectasis. The diagnosis is primarily clinical, and the treatment is usually conservative, consisting of pneumatic stabilization of the region using positive pressure ventilation.[12]

Endotracheal intubation is indicated in chest trauma patients with ARF, airway obstruction, severely compromised awareness, characterized by a Glasgow Coma Scale score of <8, and severe haemodynamic instability.[1] However, it must be pointed out that if there is no indication for it, such as in the absence of severe respiratory failure, tracheal intubation does not improve the prognosis of trauma patients.[13] In fact, using an endotracheal tube makes the tracheal portion above the cuff a constant reservoir for bacteria and germs that may easily migrate into the distal airways. In addition, mucociliary clearance is altered, which significantly decreases the patient's capacity to remove bronchial secretions. Lastly, maintaining patient intubation, and most of the times even sedation, makes the quantification of the patient's respiratory autonomy and the possibility of extubation more difficult.

The effects of the application of positive pressure through non-invasive devices have been widely studied and demonstrated. In fact, positive pressure determines an increased functional residual capacity (FRC) by reopening the collapsed alveoli, an improvement in gas exchange by reducing the arteriovenous shunt, a decrease in respiratory rate, and an increase in tidal volume, leaving the minute volume unchanged. The reduced work of breathing, in particular the diaphragmatic, leads to an increase in $PaO_2$ and $PaCO_2$ and, at the same time, a decrease in pH. In flail chest patients NIV dramatically reduces the severity of the paradoxical motion, helping the intercostal muscles to contract during inspiration.[12]

## EVIDENCE BASE

The main studies on the use of NIV in the treatment of trauma patients were conducted in the 1980s and 1990s. Hurst *et al.* treated 33 patients with CPAP with different levels of air pressure and only two patients then needed tracheal intubation.[5] In a later study, Bollinger *et al.* compared patients treated with CPAP and thoracic epidural analgesia with patients who had been intubated and treated with intravenous analgesia; the results were in favour of the first group, with a significantly reduced length of ICU stay. The drawback of this study was that the intubated patients had a higher injury severity score (ISS) than the NIV patients.[6] Gregoretti and Beltrame proved the effectiveness of NIV using PSV in chest trauma patients in two clinical studies.[8,9] In the first study, 22 patients who were admitted to the ICU with a diagnosis of chest trauma were intubated and mechanically ventilated; after undergoing a brief T-tube trial, they were promptly extubated and ventilated by NIV. At the end of the treatment, nine patients needed reintubation, while the remaining were treated non-invasively during their stay in the ICU. Furthermore, NIV showed comparable effects to invasive ventilation in terms of gas exchange and spirometric values.The second study examined 46 patients who had been admitted to the ICU with spontaneous breathing and had undergone NIV; 33 of them were successfully weaned and maintained spontaneous breathing.

With regard to the evidence-based indication for NIV, in 2002 the British Thoracic Society (BTS) published a comprehensive literature review concerning the use of NIV, and in the section on chest trauma, NIV was recommended, although supported by low evidence, in trauma patients who remained hypoxaemic in spite of adequate analgesia and high oxygen concentrations. Furthermore, due to the risk of developing or worsening of a pneumothorax, chest trauma patients treated by CPAP or NIV required intensive monitoring, which was only possible in an ICU.[14] In the same year, Vidhani *et al.* reached the same conclusions, although they recommended not to delay tracheal intubation in patients who did not respond to NIV treatment.[15]

Lastly, in 2009 the proceedings of a consensus conference on NIV were published, in which experts on the use of this technique basically confirmed the indications provided by the BTS in 2002: NIV in patients with pulmonary contusion represents a valuable alternative to tracheal intubation, even though there is not enough evidence, often due to methodological pitfalls in the studies examined.[16]

As concerns patients admitted to the ICU with a diagnosis of flail chest, the literature recommends internal pneumatic stabilization by tracheal intubation and positive pressure mechanical ventilation as the gold standard.[17] However, owing to the high likelihood of pulmonary contusion in the area below the lesion, in 1975 Trinkle *et al.* had introduced the principle of treating these patients as if they had only pulmonary contusion, thus avoiding tracheal intubation and using NIV in association with an antalgic intercostal nerve block, intravenous administration of morphine, fluid restriction and satisfactory clearance of bronchial secretions.[18] Later, other authors confirmed their findings, and some noticed a reduced incidence of hospital-acquired infections and an increased survival as compared with intubated patients.[4,19]

## CLINICAL APPLICATIONS

Concerning the possible clinical applications of CPAP, it may be used outside the ICU, beginning with out-of-hospital first aid, and in the emergency settings, where chest trauma patients with multiple rib fractures and no major head trauma or other severe lesions that may compromise the level of cooperation or the state of awareness might benefit from the positive pressure generated by a face mask and high-flow oxygen. In this case, the possible presence of a traumatic pneumothorax must be borne in mind, which in the absence of chest drainage might be worsened by extrinsic positive pressure. Hence, if there is suspicion of a possible coexistent pneumothorax, or if after CPAP application the respiratory and haemodynamic functions are progressively compromised, this technique must be abandoned immediately. In the ICU, patients may be treated by NIV, thus reducing the need for intubation.[9] In this case, the use of a ventilator with the same level of pressure support and the same positive end-expiratory pressure (PEEP) that would have been used during invasive ventilation is suggested. If on the other hand the patient needs tracheal intubation, once admitted to the ICU and after undergoing adequate monitoring, early extubation and maintenance of gas exchange by NIV prevents the onset of injured airway bacterial suprainfection and favours lung re-expansion.[8] Recently, bi-level ventilation has proved to be a safe technique; it improved gas exchange in 22 chest trauma patients.[20]

The crucial importance of pain control must be emphasized; according to the patient's specific problems, this can be achieved with different techniques. Usually systemic opioids and non-steroidal anti-inflammatory drugs (NSAIDs) are used, together with epidural catheters, intercostal nerve blocks, thoracic paravertebral blocks and intrapleural analgesia. Furthermore, the patient must be correctly instructed on bronchial secretion removal; patients must be invited to cough repeatedly, and they must be able to remove the mask to allow expectoration. For the same reason, respiratory physio-kinesitherapy must be started as soon as possible.

The most important contraindications to NIV in trauma patients are: confused or clouded consciousness; haemodynamic instability; craniofacial trauma; inability to cough or expectorate; and undrained pneumothorax.

Lastly, trauma patients may also have the usual complications associated with NIV, in particular gastric distension and spontaneous pneumothorax, when the latter is not already present. In addition, particular care must be paid to possible non-invasive treatment failure, either due to the patient's intolerance to the mask or to the positive pressure, or because of the underlying disease. In both cases, tracheal intubation must never be delayed for any reason, as it has been demonstrated that patients in whom invasive ventilation is delayed had a worse outcome.[15,21]

## TECHNICAL CONSIDERATIONS

For NIV administration in chest trauma patients, face as well as nasal masks have been successfully used. The use of a helmet in trauma patients does not seem to be indicated.

With regard to the method of NIV administration, high-flow CPAP is used, which only requires dedicated flow meters that are easy to use in an emergency setting, as well as ventilators that use modalities increasingly dedicated to this ventilation technique. These ventilators are able to compensate for possible leaks and to improve patient–ventilator interaction. In fact, in patients with pulmonary contusion, ventilation modalities such as bi-level or PSV have now become much more common than CPAP. Not only do these two types of assisted ventilation prevent injured lung region collapse, which leads to atelectasis (and this is also ensured by CPAP), but they also permit the recruitment of perfused but non-ventilated lung regions to reduce the shunt, and to improve gas exchange. Furthermore, the support provided by the ventilator significantly reduces inspiratory muscle work, and at the same time alleviates the patient's pain.

An appropriate pressure support with adequate trigger threshold values and ventilator cycling are crucial for minimizing patient–ventilator asynchrony. This phenomenon seems to be the main cause for the increased work of breathing and for NIV failure.[22] Airway humidification is not suggested in non-invasively treated patients with pulmonary contusion, in that it could delay alveolar oedema reabsorption, while it is essential in other lung diseases. The monitoring needed during NIV is basically the same as that commonly performed in intensive care, as it includes peripheral oxygen saturation ($SpO_2$), electrocardiogram (ECG) and arterial blood pressure and, whenever possible, capnography. Blood gas analysis (BGA) monitoring is also equally important, with the recommendation to draw blood 1 hour after each variation in the ventilatory parameters or in the fraction of inspiratory oxygen ($FiO_2$).

The favourable outcome that may be achieved with NIV is not free from side effects: in fact, the increase in intrathoracic pressure leads to an increase in central venous pressure (CVP), which compromises venous return, leading to reduced cardiac output. Hence, the importance of absolutely preventing hypovolaemia must be emphasized, because this is a condition that could possibly affect patients with pulmonary contusion, as they have to undergo fluid restriction as well as needing to maintain normovolaemia, so that the patient may compensate for this effect with an increased heart rate. It must also be remembered that NIV leads to an increase in intracranial pressure which lowers cerebral perfusion pressure; the latter is almost never clinically relevant, although attention must be paid to it when applying NIV to multiple trauma patients.

## FUTURE RESEARCH

As highlighted by the latest literature reviews,[14,19,20] the evidence for using NIV in the place of tracheal intubation in chest trauma patients is still low. Non-invasive ventilation represents an easy-to-learn and easy-to-apply technique. Performance of randomized controlled studies, preferably multicentre, will lead to a better positioning of this long-standing ventilation technique in the daily practice of intensivists, and will promote its inclusion among the guidelines for trauma patient management (ATLS®). Lastly, the recent introduction of innovative ventilation techniques such as neurally adjusted ventilation assistance (NAVA), which uses a modified nasogastric tube to measure diaphragmatic electrical activity, will certainly be widely used in trauma patients, both to improve patient–ventilator interaction, regulating the ventilation support according to the patient's actual need, and to promote early extubation, thus helping the patient to progressively recover respiratory autonomy.[23] The effectiveness of combined and sequential techniques to increase the efficacy and tolerance of each single interface has yet to be demonstrated. This dilemma will be solved after new clinical studies are conducted, which, however, are difficult to design due to the possible ethical concerns involved when caring for trauma patients.

## REFERENCES

1. Allen GS, Coates NE. Pulmonary contusion: a collective review. *Am Surg* 1996; **62**: 895–900.
2. American College of Surgeons. *ATLS Advanced trauma life support program for doctors*, 7th edn. Chicago, 2004.
3. Antonelli M, Moro ML, Capelli O *et al.* Risk factors for early onset pneumonia in trauma patients. *Chest* 1994; **105**: 224–8.
4. Linton DM, Potgieter PD. Conservative management of blunt chest trauma. *S Afr Med J* 1982; **61**: 917–19.
5. Hurst JM, DeHaven CB, Branson RD. Use of CPAP mask as the sole mode of ventilatory support in trauma patients with mild to moderate respiratory insufficiency. *J Trauma* 1985; **25**: 1065–8.
6. Bollinger CT, Van Eeden SF. Treatment of multiple rib fractures. Randomized controlled trial comparing ventilatory with nonventilatory management. *Chest* 1990; **97**: 943–8.
7. Buford TH, Burbank B. Observations on certain physiologic fundamentals of thoracic trauma. *J Thorac Surg* 1945; **14**: 415–24.
8. Gregoretti C, Beltrame F, Lucangelo U *et al.* Physiologic evaluation of non-invasive pressure support ventilation in trauma patients with acute respiratory failure. *Intensive Care Med* 1998; **24**: 785–90.
9. Beltrame F, Lucangelo U, Gregori D *et al.* Noninvasive positive pressure ventilation in trauma patients with

acute respiratory failure. *Monaldi Arch Chest Dis* 1999; **54**: 109–14.

10. Cohn SM. Pulmonary contusion. *J Trauma* 1997; **42**: 973–9.
11. Miller PR, Croce MA, Bee TK *et al.* ARDS after pulmonary contusion: accurate measurement of contusion volume identifies high-risk patients. *J Trauma* 2001; **51**: 223–30.
12. Davignon K, Kwo J, Bigatello LM. Pathophysiology and management of the flail chest. *Minerva Anestesiol* 2004; **70**: 193–9.
13. Ruchholtz S, Waydhas C, Ose C *et al.* Prehospital intubation in severe thoracic trauma without respiratory insufficiency: a matched-pair analysis based on the trauma registry of the german trauma society. *J Trauma* 2002; **52**: 879–86.
14. British Thoracic Society Standards of Care Committee. Non-invasive ventilation in acute respiratory failure. *Thorax* 2002; **57**: 192–211.
15. Vidhani K, Kause J, Parr M. Should we follow ATLS® guidelines for the management of traumatic pulmonary contusion: the role of non-invasive ventilatory support. *Resuscitation* 2002; **52**: 265–8.
16. Keenan SP, Mehta S. Noninvasive ventilation for patients presenting with acute respiratory failure: the randomized controlled trials. *Respir Care* 2009; **54**: 116–24.
17. Rodriguez A. Injuries of the chest wall, the lung and the pleura. In: Turney SZ, Rodriguez A, Cowley RA, (eds.) *Management of cardiothoracic trauma.* Baltimore: Williams and Wilkins, 1990:155–77.
18. Trinkle JK, Richardson JD, Franz JL *et al.* Management of flail chest without mechanical ventilation. *Ann Thorac Surg* 1975; **19**: 355–63.
19. GunduzM, Unlugenc H, Ozalevli M *et al.* A comparative study of continuous positive airway pressure (CPAP) and intermittent positive pressure ventilation (IPPV) in patients with flail chest. *Emerg Med J* 2005; **22**: 325–9.
20. Xirouchaki N, Kondoudaki E, Anastasaki M *et al.* Noninvasive bilevel positive pressure ventilation in patients with blunt thoracic trauma. *Respiration* 2005; **72**: 517–22.
21. Esteban A, Frutos-Vivar F, Ferguson ND *et al.* Noninvasive positive-pressure ventilation for respiratory failure after extubation. *N Engl J Med* 2004; **350**: 2452–60.
22. Georgopoulos D, Prinianakis G, Kondili E. Bedside waveforms interpretation as a tool to identify patient-ventilator asynchronies. *Intensive Care Med* 2006; **32**: 34–47.
23. Navalesi P, Costa R. New modes of mechanical ventilation: proportional assist ventilation, neurally adjusted ventilatory assist, and fractal ventilation. *Curr Opin Crit Care* 2003; **9**: 51–8.

# 48

# Role of non-invasive respiratory support after spinal cord damage

JOHN W H WATT

## ABSTRACT

The respiratory system is affected by motor and autonomic paralysis following spinal cord damage at the higher thoracic and cervical levels. Children are especially vulnerable. Neurological assessment of respiratory muscle sparing is necessary in the different syndromes to help predict respiratory failure. Regular bedside assessments of vital capacity should identify deterioration to avoid unplanned rescue intubations. The onset of respiratory muscle fatigue may be rapid but this may be prevented by judicious use of non-invasive respiratory support in addition to vigorous preventative physiotherapy using available adjuncts as appropriate to compensate for the loss of active cough, the significance of which is less well appreciated in generalist centres. Many patients now have internal fixation which accounts for some reports in which the majority of patients with acute tetraplegia have invasive ventilation. There is scope for more non-invasive support but this needs to be balanced against possible difficult airway management in an emergency. Weaning from ventilatory support usually takes some weeks. Patients with the complete lesion above the phrenic nucleus at C3/4/5 may need life-long respiratory support on either a full-time or part-time basis. There is experience of such patients having non-invasive respiratory support but this needs to be balanced against overall safety, comfort, convenience with management of interfaces, and impact on discharge and care packages. While there is some improvement in spirometry and pressure generating capacity in the majority of cervical cord damage patients after rehabilitation, there remains a life-long risk of atelectasis, pneumonia and respiratory failure. Apart from the range of physiotherapy adjuncts, preventive measures for patients with recurrent chest infections may include part-time non-invasive ventilatory support. Evidence of sleep disordered breathing can be found in up to half of those with tetraplegia in the longer term, but even in the acute phase, obstructive or central sleep apnoea has to be anticipated. Purely obstructive sleep apnoea often responds to simple CPAP if the mask can be managed within the patient's social context, but other patients present in the later stages with irreversible cor pulmonale. Pure obstructive sleep apnoea needs to be differentiated from mixed sleep apnoea, which is observed though not adequately described in the literature.

## INTRODUCTION

Spinal cord damage may follow an acute event such as trauma, transverse myelitis or an epidural abscess and the likelihood of recovery is low after a complete neurological transection. The respiratory consequences depend upon the level of the lesion and the completeness of the transection, i.e. whether there is both motor and sensory as well as autonomic interruption. At levels above the mid-thoracic region, there is respiratory vulnerability due to paralysis of either inspiratory and/or expiratory muscles and respiratory support may be necessary in the short or longer term.

The reported annual incidence of acute traumatic spinal cord injury varies tremendously, ranging from 10 to 80 per million population per annum,[1] and the proportion with tetraplegia compared with paraplegia has increased over the years towards half. Acute ventilation has been reported in over two-thirds of all new cases of mid- and low-level tetraplegia, 87 per cent being associated with pneumonia and nearly half having tracheostomy. Early 'airway control' has been recommended to prevent catastrophic respiratory failure.[2] Around 2 per cent of all new spinal cord injury cases require ventilatory support beyond the immediate period; this may work out around 2 per 10 million per annum.

The estimates of prevalence of spinal cord injury (SCI) range between 11 and 112 per 100 000,[3] and so with a reduced life expectancy compared with paraplegia the prevalence of tetraplegia is likely to be between 50 to 200 per million. The principal cause of death in established SCI identified in a number of studies is respiratory in origin in over 20 per cent of individuals,[4] and among the 134 patients successfully weaned from mechanical ventilation in the author's centre, two-thirds of the later 32 deaths were known to be respiratory in nature. Some countries have centres dedicated to SCI, where staff are familiar with the different neurological presentations and will be familiar with the pathophysiological respiratory consequences of SCI.[5] However many patients are initially admitted to a local hospital where fundamental respiratory vulnerabilities are poorly appreciated: for example, inability to generate an effective cough due to reduced maximum expiratory pressure (PE maximum mean $48 \pm 15$ cm $H_2O$),[6] or a reduced vital capacity in the sitting position.[7] Many generalist staff even initially place a 'do not resuscitate' order for tetraplegic patients in respiratory failure, exercising their own value-judgements on the patient's quality of life, whereas studies of quality of life of people ventilated after spinal cord injury show that professionals underestimate patients' life satisfaction.[8]

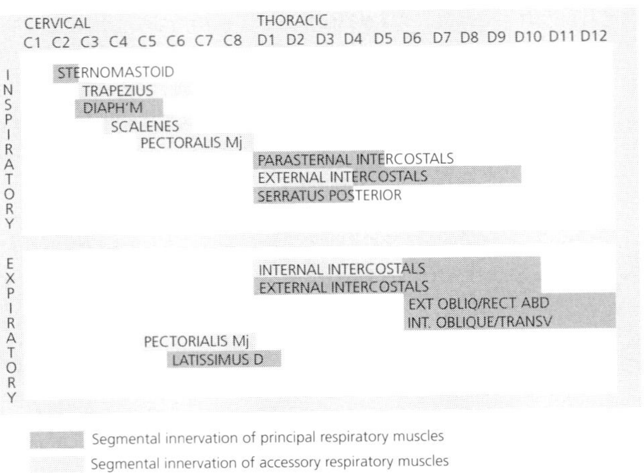


**Figure 48.1** Segmental innervation of principal and accessory inspiratory and expiratory muscles.

## PATHOPHYSIOLOGY

### Neurology

It is vital that in making a respiratory assessment of a patient with spinal cord damage that the neurology be accurately defined with reference to the motor scoring system in accepted use.[9] However, it should be noted that the motor charting for tetraplegia is primarily based upon upper limb function for tetraplegia and does not score for those myotomes above C5. The vital diaphragm takes its innervation from the phrenic motor neurones C3/4/5 and the only respiratory accessory muscles above this level which can be recruited are the sternocleidomastoid muscles, innervated by the spinal accessory nerve, homologous with C2 (Fig. 48.1).

It should also be noted that there may be asymmetry in a complete tetraplegia lesion so that one diaphragm may be paralysed in addition to paralysis of intercostal muscles and this may be unrecognized despite the severe reduction in vital capacity.[10] Even before formal screening or neurophysiological assessments of the right and left diaphragms independent from one another, it is usually possible to gauge their relative function with reference to the ipsilateral deltoid muscle, having a C5 segmental innervation, and the trapezius, supplied by a branch of spinal accessory and homologous with C3. More recent neurorespiratory research reports a decussation of the bulbospinal axons within the spinal cord to provide a crossed phrenic nerve pathway with the potential to support a contralateral diaphragm whose normal phrenic motor neurone has been damaged. Agents such as theophylline in particular may help activate this pathway[11] but the full physiological and clinical potential of this crossed phrenic pathway humans is unknown.

### Patterns of incomplete tetraplegia

These fall into four groups.

- The first is characterized by some long axon preservation but with motor impairment below the level of the lesion, either below or at a Medical Research Council (MRC) grade 3 and graded as ASIA B, C or D. The other three are clinical syndromes in which there may be unusual involvement of the respiratory muscles.
- *Central cord syndrome*: occurs almost exclusively in the cervical region, produces a sacral sensory sparing and typically a more severe motor impairment in the upper limb than the lower limb. Its significance is that there may be diaphragmatic paralysis but preservation of intercostal function.
- *Syndrome of Brown-Séquard*: a unilateral lesion that produces a motor and proprioceptive impairment on the same side as the injury, and a loss of thermal and pain sensitivity on the contralateral side.
- *Anterior cord syndrome:* an injury that produces a variable motor, thermal and pain impairment, but preserves the proprioception.

The *autonomic nervous system* can now also be incorporated into a formal charting system,[12] though in the respiratory domain the abnormal options are: 'Unable to breathe requiring full ventilatory support; impaired voluntary breathing requiring partial ventilatory support; and voluntary respiration impaired does not require ventilatory support'.[12] This does not highlight that paralysis of the sympathetic system does lead to abolition of the nasal cycle and congestion[13] and mild bronchoconstriction[14] as well as the more obvious slowing of heart rate and lowering of blood pressure in those with tetraplegia which is characteristic of spinal shock. This latter term is more strictly applied to the phase of neurological areflexia following an acute spinal cord damage, associated with lower gastrointestinal paresis and distension, which themselves inhibit gastric emptying and may cause respiratory compromise because of abdominal distension.

High level spinal cord damage can extend into the medulla involving the lower cranial nerves, resulting in risks of aspiration or vocal cord paresis which will impact upon options for non-invasive respiratory support.

## CLINICAL ASSESSMENT OF RESPIRATORY MUSCLE FUNCTION AFTER SPINAL CORD INJURY

### Volumes, pressures and diaphragm screening

After acute spinal cord damage, regular bedside spirometry is used to detect the onset of muscle fatigue and respiratory failure, and a downward trend should permit intervention before there is a major deterioration in arterial blood gases. It is usually acceptable for the vital capacity to fall to about 10 mL/kg but a drop in compliance associated with atelectasis or pneumonia will result in rapid deterioration. Patients who retain some diaphragmatic function despite respiratory failure need supported respiration on average for 5 weeks until the diaphragms become strong enough to maintain breathing independently. A small proportion of patients losing diaphragm function altogether may demonstrate a much later diaphragmatic recovery.[15]

If there is uncertainty about diaphragmatic function, fluoroscopy should demonstrate descent of over 3 cm in 77 per cent of the population, with no more difference between left and right than 1 cm.[16] It is not always possible to provide such quantitative accuracy with ultrasound, but there are detailed descriptions of the sonographic assessment of diaphragm motion using the M mode.[10] A further alternative is to record electromyographic activity of the diaphragm with surface electrodes because of the EMG silence of the intercostal muscles,[17] but one should beware of picking up the signal from the contralateral diaphragm.

In the situation of diaphragmatic preservation, the trough in vital capacity seen straight after injury gradually picks up towards the fifth week with a more gradual recovery thereafter to reach about 60 per cent of predicted by 5 months.[18] The vital capacity, as well as other respiratory parameters, bears a negative relationship to the level of cervical cord injury with the neurological level.[19,20] There is minimal expiratory reserve volume above C5 and peak flows are not helpful in this group of patients. A widespread practice is to augment diaphragmatic function in the *sitting* position by the use of an abdominal binder and a recent meta analysis gave a significant increase in vital capacity of 0.32 L even though the overall quality of the 11 studies was stated to be poor.[21] Peak expiratory pressure (see above) in a group of 35 patients with tetraplegia was $42 \pm 22$ cm $H_2O$.[22] A more recent well-controlled longitudinal study confirms universal loss in respiratory pressures and volumes after spinal injury, and while there is some increase between the time of start of active rehabilitation until the time of discharge in all lesion level subgroups, there is little change over the following year. At this time, however, the expiratory volumes in the higher level tetraplegics, and the peak expiratory flows in patients at all neurological levels, remained subnormal.[21]

### Differences and management in children

Unfortunately, SCI in children occurs proportionately more often in the upper spine, especially the upper cervical spine because of the relatively large head.[23] The respiratory system in children is already more vulnerable than in adults in illness even without SCI, and Table 48.1 highlights some salient differences.

Thus while the high level apnoeic cases would need tracheal intubation for assisted ventilation, for those with mid-cervical lesions there is a strong case for regular sessions of non-invasive respiratory support for the maintenance of lung expansion and for chest physiotherapy in the attempt to avoid invasive ventilation. Very young children are likely to tolerate this better, but with good support it can be managed in other selected cases.

Following SCI in childhood, many go on to develop severe kyphoscoliosis which has the potential to result in respiratory failure. A number of such children have surgical correction later and will need some days of assisted ventilation to prevent frank respiratory failure. The more mature children can usually learn the technique of non-invasive respiratory support in the pre-operative period in readiness for elective respiratory support post-operatively.

## EVIDENCE BASE FOR NON-INVASIVE RESPIRATORY SUPPORT AFTER ACUTE SPINAL CORD DAMAGE

### Non-invasive ventilatory support with orofacial interfaces

With long experience of non-invasive ventilation in established SCI, Bach has advocated the use of non-invasive support during the acute phase, citing success in a single case reportedly with profound loss of vital capacity.[29] Moreover, he has issued a challenge to the 'model' spinal injury centres in the USA to use the non-invasive options more widely.[30] That it has not widely been taken up in the acute phase may be understood when it is considered that delivering

**Table 48.1** Differences between children and adults contributing to vulnerability to respiratory failure

| Physiological vulnerability of children for respiratory failure | |
|---|---|
| **Anatomico-physiological difference from adult** | **Pathophysiological consequence** |
| Ribs aligned more horizontally | Lack of 'bucket-handle' action |
| Diaphragms less domed | Lower rib cage pulled inwards by diaphragmatic contraction |
| High chest wall compliance up to age 2 | 'Wasted' respiratory effort from chest wall distortion |
| Closing volume exceeds functional residual capacity to age 6[24] | Shunting of blood and hypoxaemia, especially in supine position |
| Low % type I fatigue resistant muscle fibres in diaphragm[25] | Diaphragm more prone to fatigue |
| More time spent in rapid eye movement (REM) sleep[26] | Inward movement of rib cage on inspiration |
| Lower ratio of functional residual capacity to minute volume ventilation[27] | Apnoeic time to 90% $SpO_2$ 20 seconds (half adult); time to 40% $SpO_2$ 40 seconds |
| Facial skeleton growing up to age 12[28] | Risk of mid-face hypoplasia from prolonged use of mask non-invasive ventilation |

full-time non-invasive respiratory support to an otherwise apnoeic patient presents a major risk of acute desaturations with even the shortest interruption of ventilation. These patients will be nursed in a supine position, often with an external fixator in position, limiting choice of NIV interface, and are likely to have abdominal ileus and distension. This impacts also on gastric function and the positive pressure risks distending the stomach with air with possible sudden vomiting and risk of aspiration of gastric contents. Furthermore, many patients undergo internal fixation surgery and the rates of post-operative tracheal ventilation approach 100 per cent for at least a period of time.[2] Finally, a major cautionary note relates to the likelihood of difficult tracheal intubation in most of these patients, which makes unplanned rescue intubations or reintubations hazardous.

A more reasonable proposition is to identify the signs of incipient fatigue in the patient with diaphragmatic breathing and to reduce its workload by means of intermittent non-invasive respiratory support. This approach is followed in our centre for cases with unilateral diaphragm paralysis, bilateral diaphragm weakness and bilateral diaphragm paralysis with intercostal preservation.

Tromans *et al.* reviewed their experience in providing bi-level positive airways pressure (BiPAP) successfully in 10 out of 17 cases, when the mean vital capacity had fallen to 0.9 L and the patients were showing signs of fatigue and respiratory distress.[31] Reasons for failure in the other seven included ascending neurology (two cases), chronic obstructive pulmonary disease (one case), inadequate pressure range available on the early BiPAP machine, and mask pressure problems. This group also weaned 13 patients using BiPAP in a mean time of 33 days. Weaning using invasive ventilation in a case series of difficult-to-wean patients after admission to the Southport spinal centre took a mean time of 39.5 days,[32] though one patient required nocturnal BiPAP for a further 8 months due to central hypoventilation.

It is not self-evident that BiPAP hastens weaning in this group, and the use of a well-selected plain tracheostomy tube[33,34] may be less of a hindrance for the patient in accessing and using the services of rehabilitation departments.

## Alternative non-invasive techniques

Brief reference may be made to diaphragmatic pacing since there may be a role for non-invasive respiratory support to complement pacing: either to provide a period of diaphragmatic rest every 24 hours to avoid fatigue, or to treat the severe obstructive sleep-disordered breathing that results from closure of the tracheostomy.

In common with other conditions, non-invasive respiratory support comprises: various orofacial masks and mouthpieces for delivery of pressure supported respiration; negative pressure ventilation by means of external cuirasses or pneumosuit; intermittent positive abdominal pressure by the pneumobelt; and glossopharyngeal breathing. There are enthusiasts for some of these various approaches and it may be the case that some techniques, such as glossopharyngeal breathing (GPB) are underused for reasons of unfamiliarity by the staff. However, it is probably more difficult for acutely severely paralysed patients to learn GPB during the time the tracheostomy is plugged off. However, one patient has been described after a C2 injury, who was able to extend his ventilator-free time to 30 minutes.[35] The largest report of GPB in SCI in 1967 described self-ventilating tetraplegic patients increasing their vital capacity and pulmonary health by this means,[36] and these findings were replicated in a recent study, though a fifth of participants could not master the technique.[37]

The pneumobelt has been used sporadically for some time to support the respiration of the tetraplegic patient in the sitting position; pressures of up to 30–40 cm $H_2O$ have to be delivered by a large capacity pump capable of being mounted on a wheelchair. The report by Miller[38] reviews 19 patients over the course of the decade from 1976 but there was no discussion of possible development of hydronephrosis, and since this development is often silent in the first instance, this risk would be a major drawback to this technique. The review of tetraplegic weaning from invasive ventilation by Sortor[39] included 9 out of 15 using a pneumobelt, but other techniques such as negative pressure ventilation (NPV) were also used in five patients.

Negative pressure ventilation may increase the tendency to obstructive sleep breathing and needs to be used with the patient in the recumbent position, but frequently the spinal patient must lie with a pelvic tilt for pressure relief purposes which poses problems in applying the cuirass. More than one care attendant may be required to apply a pneumosuit to the paralysed patient and if the patient requires respiratory support during sleep with a tendency to nod off during the day – common in many with spinal cord injury perhaps because of the deafferentation – this method of support is not convenient.

Mouthpiece delivered positive pressure ventilation was used in our own centre for a patient with hemidiaphragm paralysis back in 1985, though this proved insufficiently secure when he died later that year at home during a chest infection. The main advocates of mouthpiece ventilation describe their results for the weaning and long-term support of 70 high-level quadriplegic patients.[40] Of the 43 who remained dependent on ventilatory support, 28 were discharged with tracheostomy ventilation for all or part of the time. Fifteen patients were discharged on non-invasive respiratory support, of whom seven were full time dependent and with negligible vital capacity. Three NIV patients died later of respiratory failure but it has to be acknowledged that it is difficult to deduce meaningful and comparative survival data from this paper.

## Sleep-disturbed breathing and spinal cord injury

After acute, neurologically complete, spinal cord damage at a high level, there is marked deafferentation with corresponding reduction of input to the ascending reticular activating system. This in itself leads to sleepiness, may contribute to central sleep apnoea,[41] and may be more likely when increased respiratory load induces central fatigue.[42] More common is the obstructive sleep breathing during the weeks of enforced supine position after spinal column trauma.

Another reason for acute central sleep apnoea is seen in high incomplete central cord syndrome in which the patient maintains voluntary respiration by means of the spared intercostal muscles but with the onset of sleep, apnoea supervenes because of the underlying diaphragm paralysis. Sudden respiratory arrest in the second week of injury has been reported in over a fifth of patients with cervical injury despite absence of premonitory symptoms, and they were especially vulnerable during sleep.[43] More usually one should anticipate that there may be an ascent of level of lesion within the first 48 hours which can progress to apnoea in a self-ventilating C4 patient.

There is increasing recognition that over half of persons with tetraplegia can be shown to have obstructive sleep apnoea, the rate increasing from the second to the fourth week of injury.[44] Other studies, however, have found that the incidence increases with the passage of years[45] and this may be related to the high incidence of the metabolic syndrome and obesity and the use of medications, though the antispasmodic drug baclofen has been reported to contribute either in a negative[46] or positive manner.[47] Most of the sleep-disordered breathing is obstructive in type and could respond to CPAP therapy, but there is a proportion in whom there is significant central hypoventilation and in whom significant central sleep apnoeic episodes remain with hypercapnia after stabilization on CPAP. In these patients BiPAP would be more appropriate, with or without timed respirations delivered by the machine, as appropriate.

## Central sleep apnoea and established spinal cord injury

The experience of the North West Regional Spinal Injuries Centre (NWRSIC) in Southport, UK, in common with many centres, is that sleep-disordered breathing can arise in tetraplegic patients some time after the initial injury, perhaps after some gain in both years and weight. Most of the subjects are found to have obstructive sleep apnoea and yet there appear to be a significant minority with a degree of central hypoventilation. We are not aware of any study to address this, but in our own patient group of about 1500 patients on follow-up within the regional population of 6 million, and with 55 discharged with invasive ventilatory support, we have had six patients requiring CPAP, and five patients have required non-invasive BiPAP. Earlier on most of these patients could not be assessed by full polysomnography either in the NWRSIC or in local sleep laboratories because of difficulties in access and assistance, but with the more recent availability of limited polysomnography in our centre it has been possible to identify more closely those with true central hypoventilation, bearing in mind that underlying chronic or acute diaphragmatic fatigue may lead to a decrease in central drive and reduced phrenic nerve activity.[42]

There are undoubtedly more patients with sleep apnoea in our own population of spinal cord damaged, but the diagnosis in itself raises as many questions and problems as it solves. Many patients with tetraplegia rely on an assistant to remove the mask even if a quick release mechanism is incorporated. This can work well for a couple in an established relationship where the wife (usually) is able to share the bed and easily manage the partner's NIV. This becomes problematic for a single person, and a healthcare needs assessment would point to high priority for a healthcare attendant during the night. Although in England there is now a decision-support tool for an equable assessment for ongoing healthcare needs (Table 48.2), negotiation for the funding for this in itself is often quite protracted and sometimes the patient may have to relocate from their own home or settlement hostel in order that the appropriate healthcare assistance for management of the NIV can be met, which caused one patient with severe OSA to reject the offer of CPAP.

**Table 48.2** Decision-support tool for National Health Service (NHS) continuing healthcare

| Description | Level of need |
|---|---|
| Normal breathing, no issues with shortness of breath | No needs |
| Shortness of breath which may require the use of inhalers or a nebuliser and had no impact on daily living activities | Low |
| Episodes of breathlessness which do not respond to management and limit some activities<br>Or requires any of the following:<br>• low level oxygen therapy (24%)<br>• room air ventilators via a facial or nasal mask<br>• other therapeutic appliances to maintain airflow | Moderate |
| Is able to breathe independently through a tracheotomy, that they can manage themselves, or with the support of carers or care workers<br>Or<br>CPAP (continuous positive airways pressure)<br>Or<br>Breathlessness due to symptoms of chest infections which are not responding to therapeutic treatment and limit all activities of daily living | High |
| Difficulty in breathing, even through a tracheotomy, which requires suction to maintain airway<br>Or<br>Demonstrates severe breathing difficulties at rest, in spite of maximum medical therapy | Severe |
| Unable to breathe independently, requires invasive mechanical ventilation | Priority |

1. Circle the assessed level above.
2. Describe below the actual needs of the individual providing the evidence why that level has been chosen, including the frequency and intensity of need, unpredictability, deterioration and any instability.

Reproduced from Department of Health (2009).[48]

Having identified severe nocturnal oxygen desaturation, the clinician might reasonably wonder if it is safe to discharge the patient until such provisions are in place, in case, for instance, of sudden hypoxia-associated bradycardia which is characteristic of acute tetraplegia. Considering the possible impact of all this for the patient, the simpler solution of a mandibular advancement device can be tried in selected cases and we have had success with this in a small number of cases. Another alternative is a long-term tracheostomy or tracheal stent,[49] which can be safer or more acceptable for the patient even though in the UK they may also require continuing healthcare provision. Long-term oxygen therapy is not likely to prevent the development of hypercapnia or pulmonary hypertension. While invoking continuing healthcare eligibility has a financial impact on the limited budget of the primary care trust, and ultimately the tax payer, the prescribing clinician must primarily look at the clinical and social implications for the patient. Sometimes the prospect of a change in home life circumstances and obtrusive presence of caregivers in the home has actually led some patients with tetraplegia in this centre to turn down a recommendation for CPAP or NIV support. Other cases might face the necessity of moving to a nursing home with elderly residents and at some distance.

Other countries have different constraints. In Japan for example, there is a greater incentive to convert a high-level tetraplegic patient from invasive ventilation to non-invasive support for the opportunity for community reintegration.[50]

## The role of physiotherapy in maintaining patients with spinal injury off the ventilator

Non-invasive respiratory support of the patient with high tetraplegia in whom there is a weak cough and no access for clearance of tracheo-bronchial secretions will require a soundly based back-up by application of some of the array of physiotherapy-based techniques, some of which are suitable for community care.

## FUTURE RESEARCH

The respiratory failure that accompanies acute SCI has a time course ranging from the instantaneous to the more insidious with a spectrum of respiratory muscle paralyses. It is not possible or probably ethical to submit these patients to a randomized research protocol for even the larger centres have relatively small numbers. What is apparent is that there is an increasing role for provision of non-invasive respiratory support for these patients whether in the short or longer term, and professionals must take advantage of the opportunity to utilize the improved NIV technology while maintaining a broad overview of the needs of the patient and the family and friends.

There is a need for more descriptive studies of management of non-invasive ventilatory support in the setting of acute spinal cord damage, as well as in established SCI. This in turn might facilitate a wider understanding by intensivists of the profoundly weak cough and need for physiotherapy in the intensive care unit to prevent failure of NIV and progression to invasive ventilation.

There is a need for more research into the part played by central hypoventilation in sleep-disordered breathing and the extent to which this may reflect long-standing fatigue and low chest wall compliance characteristic of chronic tetraplegia. There is also a need to identify the extent of insidious pulmonary hypertension in the long-standing tetraplegic patient associated with sleep-disordered breathing which may present first as a late terminal event.

## ACKNOWLEDGEMENT

The author wishes to acknowledge Sue Pieri-Davies, Consultant AHP in Ventilatory Support, for her expertise in NIV management and in downloading and analysing sleep study records.

## REFERENCES


1. Wyndaele M, Wyndaele J-J. Incidence, prevalence and epidemiology of spinal cord injury. *Spinal Cord* 2008; **44**: 523–9.
2. Hassid VJ, Schinco MA, Tepas JJ *et al.* Definitive establishment of airway control is critical for optimal outcome in lower cervical spinal cord injury. *J Trauma* 2008; **65**: 1328–32.
3. Blumer CE, Quine S. Prevalence of spinal cord injury. An international comparison. *Neuroepidemiology* 1995; **14**: 258–68.
4. Garshick E, Kelley A, Cohen SA *et al.* A prospective assessment of mortality in chronic spinal cord injury. *Spinal Cord* 2005; **43**: 408–16.
5. Winslow C, Rozovsky J. Effect of spinal cord injury on the respiratory system. *Am J Phys Med Rehabil* 2003; **82**: 803–14.
6. Gounden P. Static respiratory pressures in patients with post-traumatic tetraplegia. *Spinal Cord* 1997; **35**: 43–7.
7. Baydour A, Adkins RH, Milic-Emili J. Lung mechanics in individuals with spinal cord injury: effects of injury level and posture. *J Appl Physiol* 2001; **90**: 405–11.
8. Bach JR, Tilton MC. Life satisfaction and well-being measures in ventilator assisted individuals with traumatic tetraplegic. *Arch Phys Med Rehabil* 1994; **75**: 262–32.
9. Maynard FM, Bracken MB, Creasey G. International standards for neurological classifcation of spinal cord injury. *Spinal Cord* 1997; **35**: 266–74.
10. Lloyd T, Tang Y-M, Benson MD *et al.* Diaphramatic paralysis: the use of M mode ultrasound for diagnosis in adults. *Spinal Cord* 2006; **44**: 505–8.
11. Zimmer MB, Nantwi K, Goshgarian HG. Effect of spinal cord injury on the respiratory system: basic research and current clinical treatment options. *J Spinal Cord Med* 2007; **30**: 319–30.
12. Alexander MS, Beiring-Sorenson F, Bodner D *et al.* International Standards to document remaining autonomic function after spinal cord injury. *Spinal Cord* 2009; **47**: 36–63.
13. Saroha D, Botrill A, Saif M *et al.* Is the nasal cycle ablated in patients with high spinal cord trauma? *Clin Otolaryngol Allied Sci* 2003; **28**: 142–5.
14. Mateus SRM, Beraldo PSS, Hroan TA. Cholinergic bronchomotor tone and airway calibre in tetraplegic patients. *Spinal Cord* 2006; **44**: 269–74.
15. Oo T, Watt JWH, Soni MB *et al.* Delayed diaphragm recovery in 12 patients after high spinal cervical cord injury. A retrospective review of the diaphragm status of 107 patients ventilated after acute spinal cord injury. *Spinal Cord* 1999; **37**: 117–22.
16. Simon G, Bonnell J, Kazantzis G *et al.* Some radiological observations on the range of movement of the diaphragm. *Clin Radiol* 1969; **20**: 231–3.
17. Normand J, Brulé JF, Cotrel A *et al.* Les paralysies diaphragmatiques. Disagnostic, pronostic, perspectives thérapeutiques. *Annal Réadap Mèd Phys* 1990; **33**: 151–7.
18. Ledsome JR, Sharp JM. Pulmonary function in acute cervical spinal cord injury. *Am Rev Respir Dis* 1981; **124**: 41–4.
19. Anke A, Aksnes AK, Stanghelle JK *et al.* Lung Volumes in tetraplegic patients according to cervical spinal cord injury level. *Scand J Rehabil Med* 1993; **25**: 73–7.
20. Müller G, de Groot S, van der Woude L *et al.* Time-courses of lung function and respiratory muscle pressure generating capacity after spinal cord injury: a prospective cohort study. *J Rehabil Med* 2008; **40**: 269–76.
21. Wadsworth BM, Haines TP, Cornwell PL *et al.* Abdominal binder use in people with spinal cord injuries; a systematic review and meta-analysis. *Spinal Cord* 2009; **47**: 274–85.
22. Huldtgren AC, Fugl-Meyer AR, Johansson E *et al.* Ventilatory dysfunction and respiratory rehabilitation in post-traumatic quadriplegia. *Eur J Respir Dis* 1980; **61**: 347–56.
23. Vogel LC, Anderson CJ, Betz RR *et al.* The child with a high tetraplegic spinal cord injury. *Top Spinal Cord Inj Rehabil* 2004; **10**: 19–29.
24. Morton NS, ed. *Paediatric intensive care.* Oxford: Oxford University Press, 1997:109–12.
25. Keens TG, Bryan AC, Levison H *et al.* Developmental pattern of muscle fibre types in human ventilatory muscles. *J Appl Phys* 1978; **44**: 909–13.
26. Ohayon NM, Carskadon MA, Guilleminaulot C *et al.* Meta-analysis of quantitative sleep parameters from

childhood to old age in healthy individuals. *Sleep* 2004; **27:** 1255–73.

27. Hardman JG, Willis JS. The development of hypoxaemia during apnoes in children: a computational modelling investigation. *Br J Anaesth* 2006; **97**: 564–70.
28. Faroux B, Lavis J-F, Nicot F *et al.* Facial side effects during non-invasive positive pressure ventilation in children. *Intensive Care Med* 2005; **31**: 965–9.
29. Bach JR, Hunt D, Horton JA. Traumatic tetraplegia: non-invasive management in the acute setting. *Am J Phys Med Rehabil* 2002; **81**: 792–7.
30. Bach JR. Prevention of respiratory complications of spinal cord injury: a challenge to 'model' spinal injury units. *J Spinal Cord Med* 2006; **29**: 3–4.
31. Tromans AM, Mecci M, Barrett FH *et al.* The use of the BiPAP biphasic positive pressure airway system in acute spinal cord injury. *Spinal Cord* 1998; **38**: 481–4.
32. Atito-Narh E, Pieri-Davies S, Watt JWH. Slow ventilator weaning after cervical spinal cord injury. *Br J Intensive Care* 2008; **18:** 13–19.
33. Björling G, Johansson U-B, Andersson G *et al.* A retrospective survey of outpatients with long-term tracheostomy. *Acta Anaesthesiolog Scand* 2006; **50**: 399–406.
34. Singaravelu S, Watt JWH. The choice of plain tracheostomy tube: 22 years of domiciliary ventilation for high tetraplegia. *Br J Intensive Care* 2010; **20**: 13–17.
35. Warren VC. Glossopharyngeal and neck accessory muscle breathing in a young adult with C2 complete tetraplegia resulting in ventilator dependency. *Phys Ther* 2002; **82**: 590–600.
36. Montero JC, Feldman DJ, Montero D. Effects of glossopharyngeal breathing on respiratory function after cervical cord transaction. *Arch Phys Med Rehabil* 1967; **48**: 650–3.
37. Nygren-Bonnier M, Wahman K, Lindhom P *et al.* Glossopharyngeal pistoning for lung insufflation in patients with cervical spinal cord injury. *Spinal Cord* 2009; **47**: 418–22.
38. Miller HJ, Thomas E, Wilmot CB. Pneumobelt use among high quadriplegic population. *Arch Phys Med Rehabil* 1988; **69**: 369–72.
39. Sortor S. Pulmonary issues in quadriplegia. *Eur Respir Rev* 1992; **2**: 330–4.
40. Bach JR, Alba AS. Noninvasive options for ventilatory support of the traumatic high level quadriplegic patient. *Chest* 1990; **98**: 613–19.
41. Wang D. Reticular formation and spinal cord injury. *Spinal Cord* 2009; **47**: 204–12.
42. Aleksandrova NP, Isaev GG. Central and peripheral components of diaphragm fatigue during inspiratory resistive loads in cats. *Acta Physiol Scand* 2003; **161**: 355–60.
43. Lu K, Lee T-C, Liang C-L *et al.* Delayed apnoea in patients with mid- to lower cervical spinal cord injury. *Spine* 2000; **25**: 1332–8.
44. Berlowitz DJ, Brown DJ, Campbell DA *et al.* A longitudinal evaluation of sleep and breathing in the first year after cervical spinal cord injury. *Arch Phys Med Rehabil* 2005; **86**: 1193–9.
45. Bach JR, Wang T-G. Pulmonary function and sleep disordered breathing in patients with traumatic tetraplegia. A longitudinal study. *Arch Phys Med Rehabil* 1994; **75**: 279–84.
46. Bensmail D, Quera Salva Ma, Roche N *et al.* Effect of intrathecal baclofen on sleep and respiratory function in patients with spasticity. *Neurology* 2006; **67**: 1432–6.
47. Finnimore AJ, Roebuck M, Sajkov d *et al.* The effects of the GABA agonist, baclofen, on sleep and breathing. *Eur Respir J* 1995; **8**: 230–4.
48. Department of Health. *Decision support tool for NHS continuing care.* London: Department of Health, 2009. Available at: www.dh.gov.uk/dr_consum_dh/groups/dh_digitalassets/documents/digitalasset/dh_103329.pdf (accessed 15 February 2010).
49. Hall AM, Watt JWH. The use of tracheal stents in high spinal cord injury: a patient-friendly alternative to long-term tracheostomy tubes. *Spinal Cord* 2008; **46**: 753–5.
50. Toki A, Tamura R, Sumida M. Long-term ventilation for high-level tetraplegia: A report of 2 cases of non-invasive positive pressure ventilation. *Arch Phys Med Rehabil* 2008: **89**: 779–83.

# SECTION K

# Paediatric ventilatory failure

49

# Equipment and interfaces in children

BRIGITTE FAUROUX, BRUNO LOUIS, FRÉDÉRIC LOFASO

## ABSTRACT

Non-invasive positive pressure ventilation (NIPPV) is increasingly used in children, in both the acute and the chronic settings. Indeed, acute or chronic respiratory failure of various origins may be improved or cured by means of NIPPV. Respiratory mechanics and maxillofacial development are different in children as compared with adults, which justifies age-adapted equipment. However, the number of children treated with NIPPV is extremely small as compared with the adult population. This may explain the lack of ventilators and interfaces specifically designed for children, especially for the youngest ones. This lack of paediatric equipment limits the wider use of NIPPV in this group of patients, in whom the use of a non-invasive mode of ventilatory assistance clearly represents great progress. Bench studies and clinical trials comparing different ventilators and interfaces in children are warranted.

## INTRODUCTION

Non-invasive positive pressure ventilation (NIPPV) is increasingly used in children, in both the acute and the chronic settings. Indeed, acute or chronic respiratory failure of various origins may be improved or cured by means of NIPPV, which is now recommended as a first-line therapy in the paediatric intensive care unit (PICU) for bronchiolitis,[1–4] acute respiratory exacerbations caused by neuromuscular disease, cystic fibrosis,[5–7] pneumonia,[8,9] or sickle cell disease,[10] and upper airway obstruction.[11,12] The number of children treated at home with long-term NIPPV for neuromuscular or lung disease, or various causes of upper airway obstruction, is also growing rapidly.[13]

Respiratory mechanics and maxillofacial development are different in children as compared with adults, which justifies age-adapted ventilators and interfaces. There is, however, a paucity of ventilators and interfaces available for young children. In the paediatric intensive care unit (PICU), ICU ventilators may be used for NIPPV, but the lack of commercial interfaces which may be used instantly in the acute setting represents a major limitation for a wider use of NIPPV. In the chronic setting, a growing number of young patients are treated with NIPPV. These patients represent a heterogeneous group, not only with regard to the underlying disease, but also with regard to age, weight and maxillofacial physiognomy.[13] Numerous children have genetic diseases associated with facial deformities, such as Treacher Collins syndrome, Goldenhar syndrome, Pierre Robin syndrome, achondroplasia, or osteogenesis imperfecta. Individually adapted interfaces are thus mandatory for these patients.

In this review, the pathophysiology, clinical applications and technical considerations for NIPPV in acute and chronic respiratory failure will be discussed, with the exception of neonates.

## PATHOPHYSIOLOGY

### Respiratory pattern

As compared with adults, breathing patterns in children are characterized by a smaller tidal volume and a higher respiratory rate. In children, normal tidal volume is approximately 10 mL/kg, with a respiratory rate of 40 breaths/min at birth and 20 breaths/min at the age of 2 years. In respiratory failure the tidal volume decreases, together with an increase in respiratory rate. A ventilator should thus be able to deliver small tidal volumes with a relatively high frequency. Also, when a spontaneous mode is used, the ventilator should be able to detect the onset of the patient's inspiratory effort (by means of a change in pressure or flow) and deliver a preset pressure or volume within a time delay compatible with the patient's respiratory rate. As such, trigger time delays exceeding 100 ms for young children are too long and inadequate because the patients will have terminated their inspiration before the delivery of the pressure or volume by the ventilator.[14]

The respiratory effort, i.e. the negative intrathoracic pressure that the patient has to generate during inspiration, varies according to the underlying condition. This inspiratory effort may be extremely high in cases of upper airway obstruction or lung disease such as cystic fibrosis,[11,12,15,16] but very low in cases of neuromuscular disease, because of the weakness of the respiratory muscles. It will be extremely difficult for a ventilator to detect the onset of the inspiration in a patient who has a very low inspiratory effort because the change in airway pressure or flow will be too small.[14] NIPPV in young children with an 'extreme' breathing pattern may thus be very challenging, requiring a ventilator able to detect minor changes in airway pressure or flow, and capable of an adapted response within a tight time frame, i.e. 100–150 ms. Such requirements are further challenged by leaks, which are unavoidable during NIPPV. Leaks are the main cause of ineffective ventilation with persistent hypercapnia, patient–ventilator asynchrony and NIPPV failure.[17] The detrimental effects of leaks will be more pronounced in the youngest patients in whom the volume of leaks may represent a greater percentage of their tidal volume. The ratio between the tidal volume and the volume of the interface is important with regard to rebreathing. Indeed, a large volume of interface, with respect to the patient's tidal volume, will increase the risk of rebreathing.

### Maxillofacial development

The anatomy of the facial bones and the proportions between the facial elements are different in children and adults. The anatomy of the maxillofacial structures changes continuously during growth, which is particularly rapid during the two first years of life. Interfaces for NIPPV thus need to be adapted specifically to the facial anatomy and physiognomy of children. They need to be changed frequently, especially within the first months of life. The soft tissue beneath the skin is thinner in children than in adults. They are thus at greater risk of skin injury during NIPPV. Skin injury occurs as a consequence of pressure sores which are defined as a lesion on any skin surface that occurs as a result of pressure. The principal causative factor is the application of localized pressure to an area of skin not adapted to the magnitude and duration of such external forces. Tissue damage will occur if both a critical pressure threshold and a critical time are exceeded. Because young children may need NIPPV during extended periods including nocturnal sleep and daytime naps, they are at increased risk of skin injury.[18] Also of importance is the effect of repetitive loading on skin and bone tissue, which is the case during NIPPV. Facial growth occurs predominantly in an anterior and sagittal axis in children. NIPPV hinders this normal facial growth and may cause facial deformity. Facial flattening and maxilla retrusion are commonly observed in children receiving long-term NIPPV and justify a systematic evaluation and follow-up by a paediatric maxillofacial surgeon before and during NIPPV.[18]

## CLINICAL APPLICATIONS

### Choice of the ventilatory mode

Several ventilatory modes may be effective for a particular disease or condition. Ventilators are generally classified as pressure or volume targeted devices, although some ventilators may deliver both modes.

The simplest mode is continuous positive airway pressure (CPAP). Upper airway patency is maintained with CPAP by a pneumatic splinting effect to prevent dynamic collapse during the breathing cycle. CPAP has become the treatment of choice for the treatment of obstructive events during sleep and has been used in children with upper airway obstruction for decades.[19–21] In addition, CPAP reduces the work of breathing in patients with flow limitation by overcoming the inspiratory threshold imposed by intrinsic positive end-expiratory pressure (PEEP). Thus, if the main indication of CPAP is obstructive sleep apnoea (OSA), it is also advocated in obstructive lung disease, when intrinsic PEEP increases the work of breathing. But this mode may be insufficient in patients with respiratory function abnormalities. Indeed, this mode has been evaluated in patients with cystic fibrosis, in whom it was associated with an improvement in exercise tolerance and gas exchange during sleep.[22,23] However, because of their associated lung disease, this mode is not sufficient to correct hypoventilation in cases of advanced lung disease.

Volume targeted ventilation is characterized by the delivery of a fixed, predetermined tidal volume. The main advantage of this mode is that a guaranteed minimum tidal volume is delivered, but this can result in detrimentally high inspiratory airway pressures causing discomfort and poor tolerability. Despite many of the volume targeted ventilators having no leak compensation mechanisms, this mode is suited for patients with neuromuscular diseases where the ventilator acts as a substitute for the weakened respiratory muscles. However, a relatively high back-up rate (2–3 breaths lower than the spontaneous respiratory rate of the patient) is required when these patients become unable to trigger the ventilator, to avoid nocturnal desaturations. As a consequence, many patients adopt a controlled mode without triggering the ventilator. Because these devices were the first to be used for NIPPV, their inspiratory triggers are generally not very sensitive, which is another factor justifying the use of a relatively high back-up rate.[14,24] These ventilators designed for home use are relatively portable. They are not as technologically sophisticated as hospital ventilators. Furthermore, few of them are able to operate within certain limits (i.e. tidal volume <50–100 mL).

Pressure support is a pressure targeted mode during which each breath is triggered and terminated by the patient and supported by the ventilator; the patient can control his respiratory rate, inspiratory duration and tidal volume.[25] This explains the relative ease in adapting to the device, and the greater comfort and patient–ventilator synchrony of this mode. In contrast to volume targeted ventilation, tidal volume is not predetermined but depends on the level of pressure support, the inspiratory effort of the patient and the mechanical properties of the patient's respiratory system. During this mode, since there are no mandatory breaths present, an in-built low frequency back-up rate is used to prevent episodes of apnoea. Furthermore, because the breaths are triggered by the patient, the sensitivity of the trigger is crucial.[16] The sensitivity of the inspiratory triggers of the different ventilators designed for the home is variable but some are as sensitive as those of intensive care devices.[26] Because during pressure support, inspiratory muscle activity may influence respiratory frequency and tidal volume, this ventilatory mode is generally proposed in patients who can breathe spontaneously for substantial periods of time and require mainly nocturnal ventilation.

Bi-level positive pressure ventilation combines pressure support with PEEP, permitting an independent adjustment of expiratory (EPAP) and inspiratory positive airway pressure (IPAP). With this mode, upper airway obstruction and/or work of breathing induced by intrinsic PEEP are prevented by EPAP and thus pressure support can be triggered easily by the patient. This ventilatory mode has been used in children with OSA,[27] cystic fibrosis[28] and neuromuscular disease.[29]

## Interfaces for children

Non-invasive interfaces can be classified as full face masks (which enclose mouth and nose), nasal masks, nasal pillows or plugs (which insert directly into the nostrils), mouthpieces and the helmet (Table 49.1, Fig. 49.1). Nasal pillows and plugs are too large for young children and mouthpieces require good cooperation and are difficult to use in neuromuscular patients. In young children, nasal masks are preferred because they have less static dead space, are less claustrophobic and allow communication and expectoration more easily than full face masks. Nasal masks allow also the use of a pacifier in infants, which contributes to the

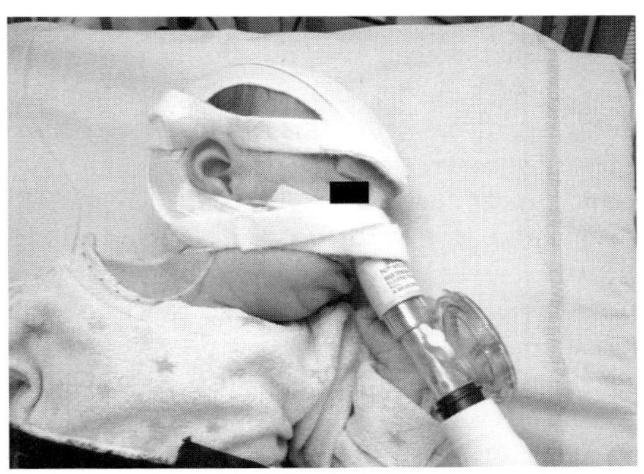

**Figure 49.1** Custom-made nasal mask for an infant.

**Table 49.1** Interfaces for non-invasive positive pressure ventilation (NIPPV) in children

| | Nasal mask | Face mask | Nasal prongs | Mouthpiece | Helmet |
|---|---|---|---|---|---|
| Age | All ages | All ages | Adolescent | Child, adolescent | All ages |
| Contraindications | Inability to close the mouth | Oesogastric reflux, patient without autonomy | | | Not for home NIPPV |
| Advantages | Small volume, comfortable, allows eating and speaking, allows the use of a pacifier in infants | No mouth leaks | No facial contact | Use *ad libitum* (neuromuscular patients) | No facial contact |
| Limitations | Mouth leaks | Large volume (risk of rebreathing) | | Ability to seal lips around the mouthpiece (leaks) | Large volume (risk of rebreathing), changes ventilator performance |

better acceptance of NIPPV and the reduction of mouth leaks. More recently, the use of a cephalic plastic helmet has been evaluated during acute exacerbations of neuromuscular disease in children in the paediatric intensive care unit (Fig. 49.2).[30,31] This interface has proved to be an efficient alternative to a nasal or a face mask but its high dead space and the risk of asphyxia in case of power failure or other technical problems restricts its use to the PICU. Also, the quality of the ventilatory support may be less optimal with this interface than with a face mask or a tracheal cannula.[32]

Interfaces are classified as vented and non-vented. Vented interfaces are used for PEEP, with generally a minimal level of 4 cm $H_2O$. In adult patients, the severity of the manufacturer's intentional leaks on the mask may influence the quality of NIPPV. Indeed, a first bench study showed that the type of interface and the severity of the leaks did not influence trigger performances.[33] However, the ability to achieve and maintain IPAP was significantly decreased with all ventilators and in all simulated lung conditions when intentional leaks increased (especially with leaks >40 L min). A second study showed that the severity of the manufacturer's intentional leaks on the mask may modify the patient–ventilator synchronization, the ventilator performance, and the risk of reabreathing.[34] Such studies have not been performed in children. However, a systematic clinical evaluation of every mask change is recommended to check, and eventually adjust, the inspiratory trigger sensitivity and pressurization, and to check the absence of rebreathing.[35]

Few industrial masks are available for children. This shortcoming is even more important for infants. In an acute situation, the interface should be immediately available. In the PICU, due to the shortage of adequate nasal interfaces for young children, nasal masks designed for older children are sometimes used as face masks for infants. For home NIPPV, time is available to try different interfaces or to prepare a custom-made mask for infants and children who cannot use industrial masks (Fig. 49.1).[18]

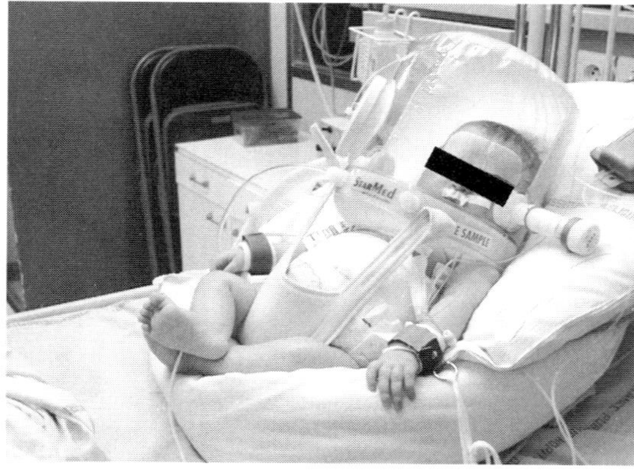

**Figure 49.2** Helmet on an infant with bronchiolitis in the paediatric intensive care unit.

The interface represents a crucial determinant of the success of NIPPV. The patient will be unable to tolerate NIPPV when there is facial discomfort, skin injury, or significant air leaks. The evaluation of the short-term tolerance of the nasal mask is thus an essential component of NIPPV.[18] NIPPV is generally used during sleep, which can represent the major part of the day in young infants. In these young patients, there is thus a potential risk of skin injury and facial deformity, such as facial flattening and maxilla retrusion, caused by the pressure applied by the mask on growing facial structures.

## TECHNICAL CONSIDERATIONS

Continuous positive airway pressure is the simplest ventilatory mode. During CPAP, the device should be able to maintain a constant positive airway pressure during various conditions including 'extreme' patient profiles (such as an obese adult patient) or leaks.[36] We have shown in a bench study using an adult profile that devices that are able to measure the pressure loss in the circuitry and are able to adjust the pressure under dynamic conditions outperform the other devices.[36] However, these observations have to be validated also in the paediatric population.

Concerning pressure and volume targeted ventilation, the quality of the inspiratory and expiratory triggers are of major importance for children when a spontaneous mode is used. As discussed above, the quality of the triggers varies greatly among the different ventilators but also for a specific ventilator, according to the type of circuit, the interface, and the patient profile.[14,24] Another important technical requisite is the ability of the ventilator to reach the preset pressure or volume within a timeframe and to maintain a constant airway pressure during the whole duration of the inspiration for pressure support.[14] This also varies significantly between the different ventilators.[14,24] The choice of the best ventilator for a particular patient is a real challenge for the physician.

Home ventilators are becoming more sophisticated and tend to integrate continuously new options and measures. A large number of ventilators are now able to deliver different ventilatory modes, such as pressure support, with or without PEEP, as well as volume targeted ventilation. Different circuits (simple, double or leak circuit) and triggers (pressure or flow triggers) may be available on the same ventilator.

We have recently shown that the performance of a ventilator may vary according to the ventilatory mode or the type of trigger and circuit, but also according to the patient profile.[14] Indeed, when we evaluated the performance of 17 home ventilators with six different paediatric patient profiles, our conclusions were: no ventilator is perfect and was able to adequately ventilate all the six different patient profiles; the performance of the ventilators was heterogeneous and depended on the type of trigger and circuit, and most importantly, on the characteristics of the patient; and the sensitivity of the inspiratory triggers of most of the ventilators was insufficient for infants. A systematic paediatric bench and clinical evaluation is thus recommended before use of a ventilator in clinical practice.

For all ventilatory modes, alarms must be correctly set. When positive pressure ventilators are used, low pressure or disconnect alarms are classically present. Alarms for high pressure, incorrect timing and power failure are also warranted. The alarm of a minimal tidal volume is very useful in children. A back-up frequency is generally set on the ventilator. All these alarms must be carefully checked before the discharge of the patient for home NIPPV.

## FUTURE RESEARCH

Future research should combine the development of equipment specifically designed for children in collaboration with the industry, with clinical studies evaluating and comparing different interfaces, ventilatory modes and ventilators for children, in both the acute and the chronic setting. The 'ideal' ventilator, which will be able to ventilate every patient, from the infant to the adolescent, with different diseases, probably does not exist. An important area of research will thus be to determine the optimal (and minimal) technical requirements for a ventilator for a specific condition or disease. Ergonomic characteristics such as weight and autonomy are also important aspects for home NIPPV. For the interfaces, the development of interfaces adapted for infants is urgently waited for by all physicians involved in paediatric NIPPV. Research should also include the assessment of short-term (with regard to skin injury) and long-term (facial deformity) tolerance of these new interfaces. Improvements in ventilator performances and paediatric interfaces will certainly boost the use of NIPPV in the acute and chronic settings.

## REFERENCES


1. Pirret AM, Sherring CL, Tai JA *et al.* Local experience with the use of nasal bubble CPAP in infants with bronchiolitis admitted to a combined adult/paediatric intensive care unit. *Intensive Crit Care Nurs* 2005; **21**: 314–19.
2. Shah PS, Ohlsson A, Shah JP. Continuous negative extrathoracic pressure or continuous positive airway pressure for acute hypoxemic respiratory failure in children. *Cochrane Database Syst Rev* 2008; **1**: CD003699.
3. Javouhey E, Barats A, Richard N *et al.* Non-invasive ventilation as primary ventilatory support for infants with severe bronchiolitis. *Intensive Care Med* 2008; **34**: 1608–14.
4. Thia LP, McKenzie SA, Blyth TP *et al.* Randomised controlled trial of nasal continuous positive airways pressure (CPAP) in bronchiolitis. *Arch Dis Child* 2008; **93**: 45–7.
5. Ellafi M, Vinsonneau C, Coste J *et al.* One-year outcome after severe pulmonary exacerbation in adults with cystic fibrosis. *Am J Respir Crit Care Med* 2005; **171**: 158–64.
6. Sood N, Paradowski LJ, Yankaskas JR. Outcomes of intensive care unit care in adults with cystic fibrosis. *Am J Respir Crit Care Med* 2001; **163**: 335–8.
7. Texereau J, Jamal D, Choukroun G *et al.* Determinants of mortality for adults with cystic fibrosis admitted in intensive care unit: a multicenter study. *Respir Res* 2006; **7**: 14–24.
8. Fortenberry JD, Del Toro J, Jefferson LS *et al.* Management of pediatric acute hypoxemic respiratory insufficiency with bilevel positive pressure ($B_iPAP$) nasal mask ventilation. *Chest* 1995; **108**: 1059–64.
9. Padman R, Lawless S, Von Nessen S. Use of $B_iPAP$ by nasal mask in the treatment of respiratory insufficiency in pediatric patients: preliminary investigation. *Pediatr Pulmonol* 1994; **17**: 119–23.
10. Essouri S, Durand P, Chevret L *et al.* Physiological effects of noninvasive positive ventilation during acute moderate hypercapnic respiratory insufficiency in children. *Intensive Care Med* 2008; **34**: 2248–55.
11. Fauroux B, Pigeot J, Polkey MI *et al.* Chronic stridor caused by laryngomalacia in children. Work of breathing and effects of noninvasive ventilatory assistance. *Am J Respir Crit Care Med* 2001; **164**: 1874–8.
12. Essouri S, Nicot F, Clement A *et al.* Noninvasive positive pressure ventilation in infants with upper airway obstruction: comparison of continuous and bilevel positive pressure. *Intensive Care Med* 2005; **31**: 574–80.
13. Fauroux B, Boffa C, Desguerre I *et al.* Long-term noninvasive mechanical ventilation for children at home: a national survey. *Pediatr Pulmonol* 2003; **35**: 119–25.
14. Fauroux B, Leroux K, Desmarais G *et al.* Performance of ventilators for noninvasive positive-pressure ventilation in children. *Eur Respir J* 2008; **31**: 1300–7.
15. Fauroux B, Pigeot J, Isabey D *et al.* In vivo physiological comparison of two ventilators used for domiciliary ventilation in children with cystic fibrosis. *Crit Care Med* 2001; **29**: 2097–105.
16. Fauroux B, Nicot F, Essouri S *et al.* Setting of pressure support in young patients with cystic fibrosis. *Eur Respir J* 2004; **24**: 624–30.
17. Gonzalez J, Sharshar T, Hart N *et al.* Air leaks during mechanical ventilation as a cause of persistent hypercapnia in neuromuscular disorders. *Intensive Care Med* 2003; **29**: 596–602.
18. Fauroux B, Lavis JF, Nicot F *et al.* Facial side effects during noninvasive positive pressure ventilation in children. *Intensive Care Med* 2005; **31**: 965–9.
19. Guilleminault C, Nino-Murcia G, Heldt G *et al.* Alternative treatment to tracheostomy in obstructive sleep apnea syndrome: nasal continuous positive airway pressure in young children. *Pediatrics* 1986; **78**: 797–802.

20. Guilleminault C, Pelayo R, Clerk A *et al.* Home nasal continuous positive airway pressure in infants with sleep-disordered breathing. *J Pediatr* 1995; **127**: 905–12.
21. Waters WA, Everett FM, Bruderer JW *et al.* Obstructive sleep apnea: the use of nasal CPAP in 80 children. *Am J Respir Crit Care Med* 1995; **152**: 780–5.
22. Henke KG, Regnis JA, Bye PTP. Benefits of continuous positive airway pressure during exercise in cystic fibrosis and relationship to disease severity. *Am Rev Respir Dis* 1993; **148**: 1272–6.
23. Regnis JA, Piper AJ, Henke KG *et al.* Benefits of nocturnal nasal CPAP in patients with cystic fibrosis. *Chest* 1994; **106**: 1717–24.
24. Fauroux B, Louis B, Hart N *et al.* The effect of back-up rate during non-invasive ventilation in young patients with cystic fibrosis. *Intensive Care Med* 2004; **30**: 673–81.
25. Brochard L, Pluskwa F, Lemaire F. Improved efficacy of spontaneous breathing with inspiratory pressure support. *Am Rev Respir Dis* 1987; **136**: 411–15.
26. Lofaso F, Brochard L, Hang T *et al.* Home versus intensive care pressure support devices. Experimental and clinical comparison. *Am J Respir Crit Care Med* 1996; **153**: 1591–9.
27. Marcus CL, Rosen G, Ward SL *et al.* Adherence to and effectiveness of positive airway pressure therapy in children with obstructive sleep apnea. *Pediatrics* 2006; **117**: e442–51.
28. Milross MA, Piper AJ, Norman M *et al.* Low-flow oxygen and bilevel ventilatory support. Effects on ventilation during sleep in cystic fibrosis. *Am J Respir Crit Care Med* 2001; **163**: 129–34.
29. Simonds A, Muntoni F, Heather S *et al.* Impact of nasal ventilation on survival in hypercapnic Duchenne muscular dystrophy. *Thorax* 1998; **53**: 949–52.
30. Piastra M, Antonelli M, Chiaretti A *et al.* Treatment of acute respiratory failure by helmet-delivered non-invasive pressure support ventilation in children with acute leukemia: a pilot study. *Intensive Care Med* 2004; **30**: 472–6.
31. Piastra M, Antonelli M, Caresta E *et al.* Noninvasive ventilation in childhood acute neuromuscular respiratory failure: a pilot study. *Respiration* 2006; **73**: 791–8.
32. Moerer O, Fischer S, Hartelt M *et al.* Influence of two different interfaces for noninvasive ventilation compared to invasive ventilation on the mechanical properties and performance of a respiratory system: a lung model study. *Chest* 2006; **129**: 1424–31.
33. Borel JC, Sabil A, Janssens JP *et al.* Intentional leaks in industrial masks have a significant impact on efficacy of bilevel noninvasive ventilation: a bench test study. *Chest* 2009; **135**: 669–77.
34. Louis B, Leroux K, Fauroux B *et al.* Effect of manufacturer-inserted mask leaks on ventilator performance. *Eur Respir J* 2010; **35**: 627–36.
35. Paiva R, Krivec U, Aubertin G *et al.* Carbon dioxide monitoring during long-term noninvasive respiratory support in children. *Intensive Care Med* 2009; **35**: 1068–74.
36. Louis B, Leroux K, Boucherie M *et al.* Pressure stability with CPAP devices: a bench evaluation. *Sleep Med* 2010; **11**: 96–9.

# 50

# Chronic non-invasive ventilation for children

BRIGITTE FAUROUX


## ABSTRACT

Chronic non-invasive positive pressure ventilation (NIPPV) is increasingly used in children and has become a first-line treatment for children with severe chronic alveolar hypoventilation caused by various disorders such as neuromuscular diseases and skeletal deformities, obstructive sleep apnoea (OSA), and lung diseases. NIPPV improves alveolar ventilation by replacing or assisting the respiratory muscles in neuromuscular or lung diseases, or by maintaining airway patency during the breathing cycle in OSA. The optimal criteria to start NIPPV in children according to the underlying disease have not been defined by prospective, controlled studies and are mainly based on consensus conferences or clinical experience. The benefits of NIPPV vary according to the underlying disease. The correction of nocturnal hypoventilation has been demonstrated for all diseases. The increase in survival is a major issue for patients with neuromuscular disease and cystic fibrosis but evidence-based data are lacking. Other benefits, such as the slowing of the decline in lung function and the improvement in quality of life, have been observed in some diseases but not in others. Technical aspects are of major importance. Few ventilators and interfaces have been designed for young children, which limits a larger use of NIPPV in this age group. Long-term side effects, such as facial deformities, are commonly observed and justify a systematic paediatric maxillofacial follow-up. In conclusion, NIPPV is probably underused in children because of underestimation or under-diagnosis of nocturnal hypoventilation in some children and the shortage of paediatric-adapted equipment. The greater accuracy of alveolar hypoventilation diagnosis and the improvement in paediatric ventilators and interfaces will contribute to a larger use of NIPPV in children.


## INTRODUCTION

A growing population of children have chronic respiratory failure due to neuromuscular disease, abnormalities of the airways, the chest wall and/or the lungs, or disorders of ventilatory control. These disorders are fundamentally hypoventilation disorders. As such, oxygen therapy *alone* is not only usually ineffective in relieving symptoms, but has also been shown to be dangerous and may lead to a marked acceleration of carbon dioxide retention.[1,2] Non-invasive positive pressure ventilation (NIPPV), by replacing or assisting the respiratory muscles in neuromuscular or lung diseases, or by maintaining airway patency during the breathing cycle in obstructive sleep apnoea (OSA), improves alveolar ventilation. The benefits for other consequences of alveolar hypoventilation, such as sleep quality or quality of life, or on the evolution of the underlying disease, is less clear. The indications and contraindications of NIPPV change according to clinical experience and improvements in technology.

This chapter focuses on chronic NIPPV for children, with a special focus on indications and contraindications, before commenting on possible future developments.

## PATHOPHYSIOLOGY

The ability to sustain spontaneous ventilation can be viewed as a balance between neurological mechanisms controlling ventilation together with respiratory muscle power, and the respiratory load, determined by lung, thoracic and airway mechanics (Fig. 50.1). Significant dysfunction of any of these components of the respiratory system may impair the ability to spontaneously generate efficacious breaths. In normal individuals, central respiratory drive and ventilatory muscle power exceed the

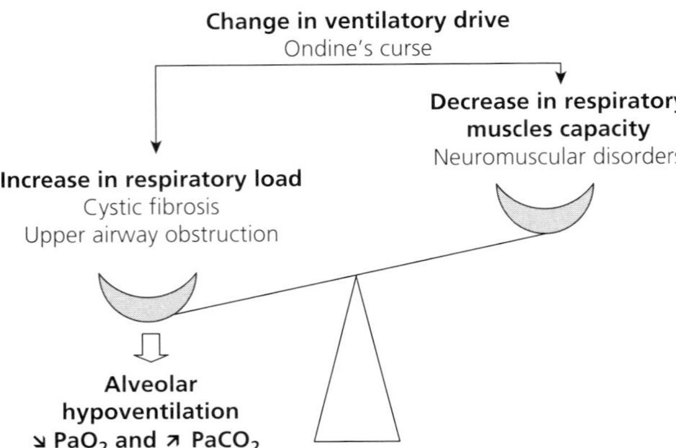


**Figure 50.1** Spontaneous ventilation is the result of a balance between neurological mechanisms controlling ventilation together with ventilatory muscle power, on one side, and the respiratory load, determined by lung, thoracic and airway mechanics, on the other. If the respiratory load is too high and/or ventilatory muscle power or central respiratory drive is too low, ventilation may be inadequate, resulting in alveolar hypoventilation with hypercapnia and hypoxaemia.

respiratory load, enabling them to sustain adequate spontaneous ventilation. However, if the respiratory load is too high and/or respiratory muscle power or central respiratory drive is too low, ventilation may be inadequate, resulting in hypercapnia. Chronic ventilatory failure, then, is the result of an imbalance in the respiratory system, in which respiratory muscle power and central respiratory drive are inadequate to overcome the respiratory load. If this imbalance cannot be corrected with medical treatment, long-term ventilatory support may be indicated. This ventilatory support will be delivered preferentially by means of a non-invasive interface, which is associated with a greater comfort and less morbidity than a tracheostomy.

Three categories of respiratory system dysfunction may thus be treated with NIPPV: an increase in respiratory load (due to intrinsic cardiopulmonary disorders, upper airway abnormalities, or skeletal deformities), respiratory muscle weakness (due to neuromuscular diseases or spinal cord injury), or failure of neurological control of ventilation (with central hypoventilation syndrome being the most common presentation).

## Increase in respiratory load

Upper or lower airway obstruction and chest wall deformity are disorders characterized by an increase in respiratory load. Obstructive sleep apnoea is less common in children than in adults. The pathophysiology is also different with the predominant role of enlarged tonsils and adenoids.[3] If adenotonsillectomy is not able to relieve upper airway obstruction, then non-invasive continuous positive airway pressure (CPAP) ventilation is proposed as a first therapeutic option.[4–6] Indeed, the maintenance of airway patency by means of a continuous positive airway pressure reduces the respiratory muscle output, which translates into an improvement in alveolar ventilation.

An increase in respiratory load is also observed in children and young adults with advanced pulmonary cystic fibrosis disease. Indeed, as lung disease progresses, indices reflecting the respiratory muscle output, such as the oesophageal ($PTP_{oes}$) and diaphragmatic pressure time product ($PTP_{di}$) and the elastic work of breathing, increase dramatically.[7] As a result, the patients develop a compensatory mechanism of rapid shallow breathing pattern in an attempt to reduce the increase in load, which translates into a rise in partial arterial carbon dioxide pressure ($PaCO_2$). Short-term physiological studies, during wakefulness and sleep, have demonstrated that NIPPV reduces respiratory muscle load and work of breathing,[8–10] which improves alveolar ventilation and gas exchange.

## Respiratory muscle weakness

Respiratory muscles are rarely spared in neuromuscular diseases.[11] In general, respiratory muscle weakness includes inspiratory muscle weakness which limits inspiration, resulting in atelectasis, as well as expiratory muscle weakness, causing inability to cough, predisposing to pulmonary infection; and hypoventilation, resulting in inadequate gas exchange. Respiratory muscle weakness, dysfunction or paralysis can occur because of neuromuscular disease, or as a result of spinal cord injury.

The most common neuromuscular diseases requiring NIPPV during childhood are Duchenne muscular dystrophy (DMD) and spinal muscular atrophy (SMA). Duchenne is a progressive disorder and ventilatory failure is inevitable in the course of the disease, although the time course of progression to it varies between individuals. Home NIPPV counteracts the hypoventilation and can improve survival.[12–14] Respiratory failure is also common in children with SMA type I or II. Respiratory failure is less frequent in other muscular dystrophies, such as Becker, limb girdle and facioscapulohumeral dystrophies. Congenital myopathies are often static.[11] However, the conditions of children may deteriorate functionally with growth because weakened muscles are unable to cope with increasing body mass.

The likelihood of respiratory failure with spinal cord injury depends on the level of the injury. High spinal cord injury, above C-3, causes diaphragm paralysis. In patients with lower cervical cord injury, expiratory muscle function is compromised, impairing cough and the clearance of bronchial secretions. As a result, retention of secretions leading to atelectasis and bronchopneumonia frequently occurs. All these children with respiratory muscle weakness often do not have severe intrinsic or parenchymal lung disease, being thus good candidates for home NIPPV.

**Table 50.1** Potential benefits of long-term non-invasive positive pressure ventilation in children according to the underlying disease

| | Neuromuscular disorders | Obstructive sleep apnoea | Cystic fibrosis |
|---|---|---|---|
| Improvement in nocturnal hypoventilation and gas exchange | Yes | Yes | Yes |
| Increase in survival | Yes (in patients with Duchenne muscular dystrophy) | Not applicable (tracheostomy is an alternative) | Not proven |
| Improvement in lung function | Not proven | Not applicable | Limited data |
| Improvement in respiratory muscle performance | Not proven | Not applicable | Limited data |
| Improvement in exercise tolerance | Not proven | Not applicable | Limited data |
| Preservation of normal pulmonary mechanics and lung growth | Not proven | Not applicable | Not applicable |
| Improvement of quality of life | Yes | Yes (as an alternative to tracheostomy) | Not proven |

### Failure of the neurological control of ventilation

Disorders of neurological control of breathing that are severe enough to cause chronic respiratory failure are uncommon to rare. Congenital central hypoventilation syndrome (Ondine's curse) is the most common presentation in childhood and is characterized by failure of autonomic control of breathing occurring predominantly during sleep.[15] A tracheostomy is nearly always mandatory in infants and young children but older children may be switched to NIPPV when ventilatory assistance may be restricted to sleep.[16,17]

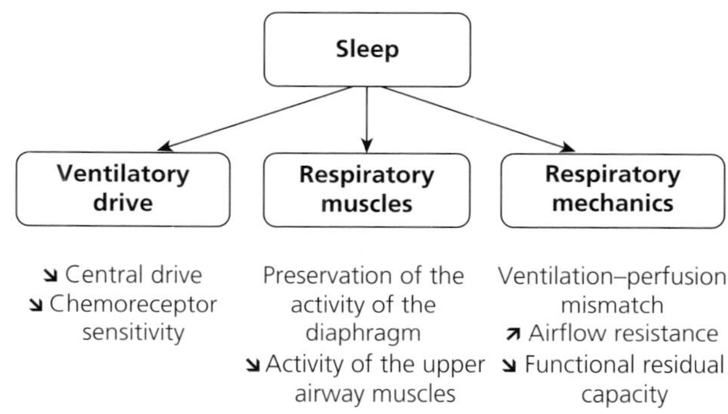


**Figure 50.2** Physiological alterations during sleep explaining the worsening of respiratory failure during sleep.

## EVIDENCE BASE

The benefits of NIPPV vary according to the underlying disease. Some beneficial effects, such as the correction of nocturnal alveolar hypoventilation, are common to the different diagnostic groups, whereas other effects, such as the increase in survival, may be specific for some disorders (Table 50.1). Evidence-based studies in children on chronic NIPPV are scarce. This may be explained by the limited number of NIPPV centres, the heterogeneity of the underlying diseases and ethical issues.

### Correction of nocturnal hypoventilation and gas exchange

The correction of nocturnal hypoventilation with NIPPV has been documented for all causes of alveolar hypoventilation in children. Sleep is associated with changes in respiratory mechanics, such as an increase in ventilation–perfusion mismatch and in airflow resistance and a fall in functional residual capacity (Fig. 50.2). Although the activity of the diaphragm is preserved, that of the intercostal and the upper airway muscles is decreased significantly. Finally, central drive and chemoreceptor sensitivity are less efficient during sleep than during wakefulness. All these abnormalities explain a physiological degree of nocturnal hypoventilation causing a rise in $PaCO_2$ of up 3 mm Hg (0.4 kPa) in healthy adults.[18] This decrease in alveolar ventilation predominates during rapid eye movement (REM) sleep and explains why patients with chronic respiratory failure are more vulnerable during this sleep stage.

NIPPV has been shown to correct nocturnal hypoventilation in children with OSA,[4–6,19] neuromuscular disease[20–23] and cystic fibrosis.[24–27]

### Increase in survival

The improvement in survival represents a major expectation of NIPPV in patients with progressive neuromuscular or lung disease. But this benefit has only been observed in patients with DMD in a case series[13] and in one nationwide study; indeed, the analysis of the national DMD register in Denmark showed that mortality fell significantly between 1977 and 2001 due to the large increase in ventilator users.[14] NIPPV, associated with nutritional support and cough-assisted techniques, has also been shown to increase survival in infants with SMA type I.[28] An increase in survival has not been demonstrated in patients with cystic fibrosis. In patients with OSA, survival is not an issue, because a tracheostomy may constitute an alternative to NIPPV.

## Improvement in lung function, respiratory muscle performance and exercise tolerance

The stabilization or the slowing of the decline in lung function by NIPPV in patients whose disease course is characterized by a decline in lung function, such as patients with neuromuscular disease or cystic fibrosis, represents a major expectation of long-term NIPPV. No data are presently available to support this hypothesis for patients with neuromuscular disease.[23,29] Data from the French Cystic Fibrosis Observatory have shown that NIPPV may be associated with a stabilization of the decline in lung function in patients with advanced lung disease.[30] However, no change in lung function was observed after 6 weeks of NIPPV in eight adult patients with cystic fibrosis.[27]

Only three studies have analysed the effect of NIPPV on respiratory muscle function in patients with cystic fibrosis. An increase in maximal expiratory pressure (MEP) and inspiratory pressure (MIP) has been observed in four adults with cystic fibrosis after 1 month of NIPPV.[31] But because of the very small number of patients and the possibility of a learning effect or a better motivation, these results should be interpreted with caution. More interestingly, significant increases in MIP and MEP have been observed in children and adults with cystic fibrosis after a physiotherapy session performed with NIPPV as compared with standard physiotherapy session.[32,33]

NIPPV seems to improve exercise tolerance in patients with cystic fibrosis. Indeed, use of nasal CPAP was associated with an improvement in exercise tolerance in 33 patients with cystic fibrosis[34] and a significant improvement in the Modified Shuttle Test was observed in eight adult patients with cystic fibrosis after 6 weeks of nocturnal NIPPV.[27]

Patients with chronic respiratory insufficiency are at risk of acute exacerbations, which are mainly triggered by respiratory tract infections. Although no prospective randomized trial is available (and would be ethically questionable), the use of NIPPV in patients with cystic fibrosis hospitalized for an acute respiratory exacerbation was associated with a more rapid recovery.[35–37] Within the same context, long-term NIPPV was associated with a decrease in hospitalizations for respiratory tract infection in children with neuromuscular disease.[22,38]

## Preservation of normal pulmonary mechanics and lung growth

A major concern in children is the effect of chronic hypoventilation on lung and chest wall growth, and, as a logical consequence, the effect of NIPPV in promoting or preserving physiologic lung growth in the developing child. To the author's knowledge, no clinical study is available, but animal models have shown that congenital absence of the diaphragm or the intercostal muscles is associated with lung hypoplasia and a lack of lung differentiation.[39,40]

## Improvement of quality of life

Studies are scarce in children but NIPPV has not been shown to be associated with deterioration in quality of life in children with neuromuscular disease. In a small group of children with SMA and other neuromuscular diseases, NIPPV was associated with an improvement in symptoms of nocturnal hypoventilation and with maintenance of the different domains of quality of life measures, with the exception of the physical domain, which reflects the progression of the underlying neuromuscular disease.[29] NIPPV was also associated with an improvement in quality of life in boys with DMD.[13] Such a benefit has not been demonstrated yet in patients with cystic fibrosis. However, NIPPV has been shown to reduce dyspnoea during physiotherapy[33] and also in the long term.[27] In patients with OSA, the alternative for NIPPV is tracheostomy, which clearly puts the balance in favour of NIPPV.

# CLINICAL APPLICATIONS

## Indications

Validated criteria for starting long-term NIPPV are lacking in children.[41] These criteria may vary according to the underlying disease. For patients with neuromuscular disease, consensus conferences agree on the value of daytime hypercapnia and acute respiratory exacerbations to initiate NIPPV because these criteria are the signature of established ventilatory failure.[42–45] These criteria may also be applied for patients with lung disease such as cystic fibrosis. But these classical criteria are preceded by a variable period of nocturnal hypoventilation during which treatable symptoms, such as frequent arousals, poor sleep quality, severe orthopnoea, daytime fatigue and alterations in cognitive function, may worsen the daily life of the patient. A major issue is thus to detect symptoms suggestive of alveolar hypoventilation in children. Sleep-disordered breathing may be difficult to establish in children because of reliance on parents and other caregivers who have a different perception of the child's disease.[29] Patients with chronic disorders tend to underestimate symptoms such as fatigue before using NIPPV because onset is generally insidious. A major issue is thus to determine the optimal timing of a sleep study to document nocturnal hypoventilation. A polysomnography should be organized without delay when the patient recognizes symptoms related to sleep-disordered breathing. Lung function parameters are poor indicators of nocturnal hypoventilation. In patients with neuromuscular disease, vital capacity and inspiratory vital capacity (IVC) have been shown to have some correlation with daytime and nocturnal gas exchange.[45,46] Daytime predictors of nocturnal hypoventilation have mainly been identified for patients with DMD, who represent a more homogeneous group. As such, the forced expiratory volume in one second ($FEV_1$), daytime $PaO_2$ and $PaCO_2$, base excess, and the rapid shallow breathing index are all significantly correlated to nocturnal hypoventilation in patients with DMD.[47–50] A recent study showed that the initiation of NIPPV at the stage of nocturnal hypercapnia without daytime hypercapnia in children and adults with neuromuscular disorders and chest wall disease was associated with an improvement in nocturnal gas exchange.[51] Larger prospective studies, in homogeneous groups of patients, are warranted to confirm the benefit of this 'early' initiation of NIPPV.

No predictors for nocturnal hypoventilation have been identified for patients with CF or other lung diseases. Studies analysing the correlation between sleep parameters and daytime lung function are thus mandatory. Abundant recent data have underpinned the importance of neuro-cognitive dysfunction in children with OSA.[52,53] These attention, memory and developmental deficits and behavioural disturbances have been demonstrated even in children with mild or moderate OSA. The demonstration of a disequilibrium in some neural metabolites in children with severe untreated OSA may suggest that some of these effects may be definitive.[54] Thus, future studies are mandatory to establish, for every diagnostic group, first the most pertinent criteria for a sleep study, and second, those which may require the initiation of NIPPV.

## Contraindications, side effects and limits of NIPPV

The general point of view is that NIPPV is preferred over invasive mechanical ventilation as the first therapy of chronic respiratory failure. However, NIPPV is contraindicated in some circumstances which, however, evolve continuously[55] (Box 50.1). These contraindications depend also on the local experience of the medical team, the child's medical condition, and the quality of the family training, structure and reliability. Discharge to home care requires a motivated family, with adequate and appropriate training of the family and caregivers, a suitable home environment, and adequate funding and healthcare resources.

NIPPV may be temporarily contraindicated in cases of recent pneumothorax, which may occur in patients with advanced cystic fibrosis lung disease. An ear, nose and throat (ENT) examination of the upper airways is systematically recommended before the initiation of NIPPV. Indeed, in patients with cystic fibrosis, nasal polyps are common and should be treated before the initiating of NIPPV. In children with OSA, adenotonsillectomy is the first-line treatment and may be sufficient to correct the sleep-disordered breathing.

**Box 50.1 Contraindications to non-invasive positive pressure ventilation**

Relative contraindications

- Severe swallowing impairment
- Inadequate family/caregiver support
- Need for full-time ventilatory assistance

Absolute contraindications

- Complete persistent upper airway obstruction during NIPPV
- Uncontrollable secretion retention
- Inability to cooperate
- Inability to achieve adequate peak cough flow, even with assistance
- Inability to fit any non-invasive interface

Adapted from Hill.[55]

Side effects of NIPPV are more often due to the interface than to NIPPV itself. In our experience, skin injury, from transient erythema to permanent skin necrosis, due to the nasal mask, was observed in 53 per cent of the 40 patients during their routine 6 months follow-up.[56] In young children, there is also a potential risk of facial deformity, such as facial flattening and maxilla retrusion, caused by the pressure applied by the mask on growing facial structures. These potential side effects justify the systematic evaluation before the initiation and during the follow-up of children receiving NIPPV by a paediatric maxillofacial specialist. Abdominal distension caused by NIPPV is an uncommon problem which can be lessened by switching to a pressure support mode or decreasing the tidal volume on a volume targeted ventilator. Sleep quality should be logically improved with NIPPV but some studies in adult patients have shown that this is not always the case.[57] NIPPV is not always successful in adequately relieving hypoventilation.[58] Air leaks have been shown to be an important cause of persistent hypercapnia in both invasively and non-invasively ventilated neuromuscular patients.[59] Simple practical measures such as changing the mask, using a chin strap, increasing minute ventilation and changing the type of the ventilator, are able to reduce the volume of air leaks and improve the efficacy of ventilation.[58,59]

In patients with neuromuscular disease, cough-assisted techniques are useful when ventilatory dependence is increasing. Several techniques are available such as manual physiotherapy, intermittent positive pressure breathing, and mechanical insufflation–exsufflation.[60,61] These techniques, associated with daytime ventilation by means of a mouthpiece,[62] extend the use of NIPPV in patients having increasing ventilatory dependency.

However, despite these measures, in progressive diseases such as some neuromuscular diseases a tracheostomy may become necessary at a certain moment. Close monitoring of the patient's physiological status and disease progression, together with clear information for the family, are essential before a tracheostomy. It is essential that the child, if the age permits it, and the parents should have the opportunity to discuss the tracheostomy in advance. Discussion should start long enough before the anticipated need to allow the child and the family to evaluate options thoroughly and to discuss their feelings. Because non-invasive ventilation leaves airway protection, those with copious secretions or severe swallowing dysfunction may respond poorly, requiring discussion of a tracheostomy with the patient and his or her family.

## TECHNICAL CONSIDERATIONS

### Ventilatory modes and ventilators

The type of equipment and the specific ventilator settings that should be chosen for an individual patient remain a matter of debate. The specific equipment available for therapy evolves more rapidly with industry capability rather than with clear indications available from scientific studies. A description of the different ventilatory modes and ventilators is given in Chapter 49.

### Interfaces

The necessity of interfaces specifically designed for children represents an important technical limitation of NIPPV in paediatric patients. Few industrial masks are available for children. This shortcoming is even more important for infants. Most often, NIPPV is thus limited to some highly specialized paediatric centres which have the possibility to manufacture custom-made masks for infants and children who cannot use industrial masks.[56] The interface is a crucial determinant of the success of NIPPV. The patient will be unable to tolerate and accept NIPPV when there is facial discomfort, skin injury or significant air leaks. The evaluation of the tolerance of the interface is thus an essential component of NIPPV.[56]

## FUTURE RESEARCH

Future studies should aim at defining the most pertinent criteria to schedule a sleep study in a child suspected of having alveolar hypoventilation. Then, the clinical, respiratory and polysomnographic criteria that should lead to the initiation of NIPPV should be defined, as well as the clinical and physiological benefits, including the quality of life of the child and his or her family. Because of the heterogeneity of the diseases that may cause chronic alveolar hypoventilation in children, these criteria should ideally be adapted for each disease or group of diseases.

## CONCLUSION

NIPPV is increasingly used in children and infants. Unfortunately, in this age group, this therapy is generally initiated on an empirical basis. Further studies are urgently warranted to determine the most pertinent criteria to initiate NIPPV according to the disease and the age of the patient, to evaluate the long-term benefits with regard to the increase in survival, stabilization in the decline in lung function and respiratory muscle performance, promotion of lung growth and respiratory mechanics, and most importantly, the quality of life of the child and his or her family.

## REFERENCES


1. Gay P, Edmonds L. Severe hypercapnia after low-flow oxygen therapy in patients with neuromuscular disease and diaphragmatic dysfunction. *Mayo Clin Proc* 1995; **70**: 327–30.
2. Masa J, Celli B, Riesco J *et al.* Noninvasive positive pressure ventilation and not oxygen may prevent overt ventilatory failure in patients with chest wall disease. *Chest* 1997; **112**: 207–13.
3. Croft CB, Brockbank MJ, Wright A *et al.* Obstructive sleep apnea in children undergoing routine tonsillectomy and adenoidectomy. *Clin Otolaryngol* 1990; **15**: 307–14.
4. Waters WA, Everett FM, Bruderer JW *et al.* Obstructive sleep apnea: the use of nasal CPAP in 80 children. *Am J Respir Crit Care Med* 1995; **152**: 780–5.
5. Guilleminault C, Nino-Murcia G, Heldt G *et al.* Alternative treatment to tracheostomy in obstructive sleep apnea syndrome:nasal continuous positive airway pressure in young children. *Pediatrics* 1986; **78**: 797–802.
6. Guilleminault C, Pelayo R, Clerk A *et al.* Home nasal continuous positive airway pressure in infants with sleep-disordered breathing. *J Pediatr* 1995; **127**: 905–12.
7. Hart N, Polkey MI, Clément A *et al.* Changes in pulmonary mechanics with increasing disease severity in children and young adults with cystic fibrosis. *Am J Respir Crit Care Med* 2002; **166**: 61–6.
8. Fauroux B, Pigeot J, Isabey D *et al.* In vivo physiological comparison of two ventilators used for domiciliary ventilation in children with cystic fibrosis. *Crit Care Med* 2001; **29**: 2097–105.
9. Fauroux B, Louis B, Hart N *et al.* The effect of back-up rate during non-invasive ventilation in young patients with cystic fibrosis. *Intensive Care Med* 2004; **30**: 673–81.
10. Fauroux B, Nicot F, Essouri S *et al.* Setting of pressure support in young patients with cystic fibrosis. *Eur Resp J* 2004; **24**: 624–30.

11. Nicot F, Hart N, Forin V *et al.* Respiratory muscle testing: a valuable tool for children with neuromuscular disorders. *Am J Respir Crit Care Med* 2006; **174**: 67–74.
12. Vianello A, Bevilacqua M, Salvador V *et al.* Long-term nasal intermittent positive pressure ventilation in advanced Duchenne's muscular dystrophy. *Chest* 1994; **105**: 445–8.
13. Simonds A, Muntoni F, Heather S *et al.* Impact of nasal ventilation on survival in hypercapnic Duchenne muscular dystrophy. *Thorax* 1998; **53**: 949–52.
14. Jeppesen J, Green A, Steffensen BF *et al.* The Duchenne muscular dystrophy population in Denmark, 1977–2001: prevalence, incidence and survival in relation to the introduction of ventilator use. *Neuromuscul Disord* 2003; **13**: 804–12.
15. Gozal D. Congenital central hypoventilation syndrome:an update. *Pediatr Pulmonol* 1998; **26**: 273–82.
16. Nielson DW, Black PG. Mask ventilation in congenital central alveolar hypoventilation syndrome. *Pediatr Pulmonol* 1990; **9**: 44–5.
17. Zaccaria S, Braghiroli A, Sacco C *et al.* Central hypoventilation in a seven year old boy. Long-term treatment by nasal mask ventilation. *Monaldi Arch Chest Dis* 1993; **48**: 37–8.
18. Gothe B, Altose MD, Goldman MD *et al.* Effect of quiet sleep on resting and CO2 stimulated breathing in humans. *J Appl Physiol* 1981; **50**: 724–30.
19. Fauroux B, Pigeot J, Polkey MI *et al.* Chronic stridor caused by laryngomalacia in children. Work of breathing and effects of noninvasive ventilatory assistance. *Am J Respir Crit Care Med* 2001; **164**: 1874–8.
20. Simonds AK, Ward S, Heather S *et al.* Outcome of paediatric domiciliary mask ventilation in neuromuscular and skeletal disease. *Eur Respir J* 2000; **16**: 476–81.
21. Mellies U, Ragette R, Dohna Schwake C *et al.* Long-term noninvasive ventilation in children and adolescents with neuromuscular disorders. *Eur Respir J* 2003; **22**: 631–6.
22. Katz S, Selvadurai H, Keilty K *et al.* Outcome of non-invasive positive pressure ventilation in paediatric neuromuscular disease. *Arch Dis Child* 2004; **89**: 121–4.
23. Annane D, Orlikowski D, Chevret S *et al.* Nocturnal mechanical ventilation for chronic hypoventilation in patients with neuromuscular and chest wall disorders. *Cochrane Database Syst Rev* 2007; **4**: CD001941.
24. Regnis JA, Piper AJ, Henke KG *et al.* Benefits of nocturnal nasal CPAP in patients with cystic fibrosis. *Chest* 1994; **106**: 1717–24.
25. Gozal D. Nocturnal ventilatory support in patients with cystic fibrosis: comparison with supplemental oxygen. *Eur Resp J* 1997; **10**: 1999–2003.
26. Milross MA, Piper AJ, Norman M *et al.* Low-flow oxygen and bilevel ventilatory support. Effects on ventilation during sleep in cystic fibrosis. *Am J Respir Crit Care Med* 2001; **163**: 129–34.
27. Young AC, Wilson JW, Kotsimbos TC *et al.* Randomised placebo controlled trial of non-invasive ventilation for hypercapnia in cystic fibrosis. *Thorax* 2008; **63**: 72–7.
28. Oskoui M, Levy G, Garland CJ *et al.* The changing natural history of spinal muscular atrophy type 1. *Neurology* 2007; **69**: 1931–6.
29. Young HK, Lowe A, Fitzgerald DA *et al.* Outcome of noninvasive ventilation in children with neuromuscular disease. *Neurology* 2007; **68**: 198–201.
30. Fauroux B, Le Roux E, Ravilly S *et al.* Long-term noninvasive ventilation in patients with cystic fibrosis. *Respiration* 2008; **76**: 168–74.
31. Piper AJ, Parker S, Torzillo PJ *et al.* Nocturnal nasal IPPV stabilizes patients with cystic fibrosis and hypercapnic respiratory failure. *Chest* 1992; **102**: 846–50.
32. Fauroux B, Boulé M, Lofaso F *et al.* Chest physiotherapy in cystic fibrosis:improved tolerance with nasal pressure support ventilation. *Pediatrics* 1999; **103**: e32–e40.
33. Holland AE, Denehy L, Ntoumenopoulos G *et al.* Non-invasive ventilation assists chest physiotherapy in adults with acute exacerbations of cystic fibrosis. *Thorax* 2003; **58**: 880–4.
34. Henke KG, Regnis JA, Bye PTP. Benefits of continuous positive airway pressure during exercise in cystic fibrosis and relationship to disease severity. *Am Rev Respir Dis* 1993; **148**: 1272–6.
35. Sood N, Paradowski LJ, Yankaskas JR. Outcomes of intensive care unit care in adults with cystic fibrosis. *Am J Respir Crit Care Med* 2001; **163**: 335–8.
36. Ellafi M, Vinsonneau C, Coste J *et al.* One-year outcome after severe pulmonary exacerbation in adults with cystic fibrosis. *Am J Respir Crit Care Med* 2005; **171**: 158–64.
37. Texereau J, Jamal D, Choukroun G *et al.* Determinants of mortality for adults with cystic fibrosis admitted in intensive care unit: a multicenter study. *Respir Res* 2006; **7**: 14–24.
38. Dohna-Schwake C, Podlewski P, Voit T *et al.* Non-invasive ventilation reduces respiratory tract infections in children with neuromuscular disorders. *Pediatr Pulmonol* 2008; **43**: 67–71.
39. Inanlou MR, Kablar B. Abnormal development of the diaphragm in mdx:Myo-/-9th embryos leads to pulmonary hypoplasia. *Int J Dev Biol* 2003; **47**: 363–71.
40. Inanlou MR, Kablar B. Abnormal development of the intercostal muscles and the rib cage in Myf5-/- embryos leads to pulmonary hypoplasia. *Dev Dyn* 2005; **232**: 43–54.
41. Management of pediatric patients requiring long-term intubation. *Chest* 1998; **113**: S332–36.
42. Robert D, Willig TN, Paulus J. Long-term nasal ventilation in neuromuscular disorders: report of a Consensus Conference. *Eur Respir J* 1993; **6**: 599–606.
43. Rutgers M, Lucassen H, Kesteren RV *et al.* Respiratory insufficiency and ventilatory support. 39th European Neuromuscular Centre International Workshop. *Neuromuscul Disord* 1996; **6**: 431–5.
44. A Consensus Conference Report. Clinical indications for noninvasive positive pressure ventilation in chronic respiratory failure due to restrictive lung disease, COPD, and nocturnal hypoventilation. *Chest* 1999; **116**: 521–34.

45. Ragette R, Mellies U, Schwake C *et al.* Patterns and predictors of sleep disordered breathing in primary myopathies. *Thorax* 2002; **57**: 724–8.
46. Mellies U, Ragette R, Schwake C *et al.* Daytime predictors of sleep disordered breathing in children and adolescents with neuromuscular disorders. *Neuromuscul Disord* 2003; **13**: 123–8.
47. Barbé F, Quera-Salva MA, McCann C *et al.* Sleep-related respiratory disturbances in patients with Duchenne muscular dystrophy. *Eur Respir J* 1994; **7**: 1403–8.
48. Lyager S, Steffensen B, Juhl B. Indicators of need for mechanical ventilation in Duchenne muscular dystrophy and spinal muscular atrophy. *Chest* 1995; **108**: 779–85.
49. Hukins CA, Hillman DR. Daytime predictors of sleep hypoventilation in Duchenne muscular dystrophy. *Am J Respir Crit Care Med* 2000; **161**: 166–70.
50. Toussaint M, Steens M, Soudon P. Lung function accurately predicts hypercapnia in patients with Duchenne muscular dystrophy. *Chest* 2007; **131**: 368–75.
51. Ward S, Chatwin M, Heather S *et al.* Randomised controlled trial of non-invasive ventilation (NIV) for nocturnal hypoventilation in neuromuscular and chest wall disease patients with daytime normocapnia. *Thorax* 2005; **60**: 1019–24.
52. Kheirandish L, Gozal D. Neurocognitive dysfunction in children with sleep disorders. *Dev Sci* 2006; **9**: 388–99.
53. Montgomery-Downs HE, Gozal D. Snore-associated sleep fragmentation in infancy:mental development effects and contribution of secondhand cigarette smoke exposure. *Pediatrics* 2006; **117**: e496–502.
54. Halbower AC, Degaonkar M, Barker PB *et al.* Childhood obstructive sleep apnea associates with neuropsychological deficits and neuronal brain injury. *PLoS Med* 2006; **3**: e301.
55. Hill NS. Ventilator management for neuromuscular disease. *Semin Respir Crit Care Med* 2002; **23**: 293–305.
56. Fauroux B, Lavis JF, Nicot F *et al.* Facial side effects during noninvasive positive pressure ventilation in children. *Intensive Care Med* 2005; **31**: 965–9.
57. Parthasarathy S, Tobin MJ. Effect of ventilator mode on sleep quality in critically ill patients. *Am J Respir Crit Care Med* 2002; **166**: 1423–9.
58. Paiva R, Krivec U, Aubertin G *et al.* Carbon dioxide monitoring during long-term noninvasive respiratory support in children. *Intensive Care Med* 2009; **35**: 1068–74.
59. Gonzalez J, Sharshar T, Hart N *et al.* Air leaks during mechanical ventilation as a cause of persistent hypercapnia in neuromuscular disorders. *Intensive Care Med* 2003; **29**: 596–602.
60. Chatwin M, Ross E, Hart N *et al.* Cough augmentation with mechanical insufflation/exsufflation in patients with neuromuscular weakness. *Eur Respir J* 2003; **21**: 502–8.
61. Fauroux B, Guillemot N, Aubertin G *et al.* Physiologic benefits of mechanical insufflation-exsufflation in children with neuromuscular diseases. *Chest* 2008; **133**: 161–8.
62. Toussaint M, Steens M, Wasteels G *et al.* Diurnal ventilation via mouthpiece: survival in end-stage Duchenne patients. *Eur Resp J* 2006; **28**: 549–55.

# 51

# Non-invasive positive pressure ventilation in children with acute respiratory failure

GIORGIO CONTI, MARCO PIASTRA, SILVIA PULITANÒ

## ABSTRACT

The aim of this chapter is to briefly review the main indications and the clinical results obtained with non-invasive positive pressure ventilation (NIPPV) in the paediatric population. In contrast with the large body of evidence available for the adult population, there are relatively few published observational studies and only a single randomized controlled trial in support of NIPPV in paediatric patients with acute respiratory distress. Despite this paucity of data from large prospective clinical trials in the paediatric population, which does not mean that benefits described in adults can be assumed to be present in children, several case series and at least two large studies published in the past decade have suggested that NIPPV also has great potential as an alternative to standard treatment in infants and children with acute respiratory distress. The main results obtained with NIPPV in a specific subset of patients are also described.

## INTRODUCTION

The term 'non-invasive positive pressure ventilation' (NIPPV) refers to the application of inspiratory positive airway pressure to the airways, usually in combination with positive end-expiratory pressure (PEEP), in order to increase tidal volume, augment alveolar ventilation and decrease the work of breathing in patients with acute respiratory insufficiency.

In a large subset of patients, NIPPV avoids the need for an invasive interface (typically an endotracheal tube) and uses an external interface, a nasal, a face mask or a helmet usually in conjunction with a pressure targeted ventilator. The aim of this chapter is to briefly review the possible indications and advantages of NIPPV application in children with acute respiratory failure (ARF); we will not address other non-conventional forms of non-invasive ventilation, such as assistance with negative (subatmospheric) pressure devices or the use of NIPPV for children with chronic respiratory failure (see Chapter 50).

The major advantage of NIPPV over invasive mechanical ventilation is the capacity to treat disorders associated with hypoventilation and/or increased respiratory workload without an indwelling artificial airway. In adults, treatment with NIPPV has been associated with a dramatic reduction of the need for endotracheal intubation and ventilator-associated pneumonia,[1,2] and in acute exacerbations of chronic obstructive pulmonary disease (COPD) or in hypoxaemic immunocompetent and immunocompromised patients, a significantly improved survival has been reported, compared with that observed in patients treated with conventional treatment and invasive mechanical ventilation.[3–5]

Conversely, the number of prospective and controlled clinical trials comparing NIPPV with standard treatments or conventional ventilation in paediatric patients is still extremely low, but several case series, including a large single-centre study[6] and a recent randomized controlled trial (RCT) in children with acute hypoxaemic respiratory failure, strongly support the use of NIPPV in children with ARF.[7]

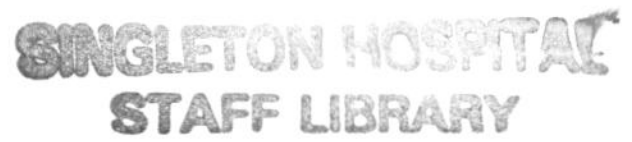

## EVIDENCE BASE

A large body of evidence, including several RCTs, support the early administration of NIPPV in adults with ARF of various aetiologies. In such patients, NIPPV has been shown to significantly decrease the need for endotracheal intubation, improve survival compared with standard care and decrease the incidence of ventilator-associated pneumonia.[2] Conversely, there are relatively few published studies in support of NIPPV in paediatric patients with acute respiratory distress.[6–8] Despite the paucity of data from large prospective clinical trials in the paediatric population, which does not allow assuming the above-described benefits also occur in children, several case series and at least two large studies published in the past decade have suggested that NIPPV also has great potential as an alternative to standard treatment in infants and children with acute respiratory distress.

In the early case reports and small series, NIPPV was used in children with acute respiratory distress caused by pneumonia, advanced cystic fibrosis, non-cardiogenic pulmonary oedema and aspiration lung injury, generally showing its safety and effectiveness.[9–12] More recently we reported the safe and successful use of NIPPV in patients with acute respiratory distress caused by pneumonia in neuromuscular infants,[13] in children with haematological malignancies complicated by ARF,[14] in children with myasthenia gravis[15] and with post-operative acute respiratory insufficiency after thoracic surgery for malignancy.[16]

The largest published experience on NIPPV application in the paediatric population was reported by Essouri *et al.*;[6] 114 consecutive, unselected patients were treated with NIPPV during 5 consecutive years (including infants/children with pneumonia, bronchiolitis, acute lung injury (ALI)/acute respiratory distress syndrome (ARDS), post-extubation ARF, and acute chest syndrome complicating sickle cell disease). Of the 114 patients, 83 (77 per cent) were successfully treated by NIPPV and avoided intubation (NIPPV success group). Interestingly, the success rate of NIPPV was significantly lower (22 per cent) in the patients with ARDS than in the other patients. The Pediatric Risk of Mortality II and Pediatric Logistic Organ Dysfunction scores at admission were significantly higher in patients who were unsuccessfully treated with NIPPV (NIPPV failure group). Baseline values of $PCO_2$, pulse oximetry and respiratory rate did not differ between the two groups. Multivariate analysis showed that a diagnosis of ARDS and a high Pediatric Logistic Organ Dysfunction score were independent predictive factors for NIPPV failure. Only 11 patients (9.6 per cent), all belonging to the NIPPV failure group, died during the study. The authors concluded that their study demonstrated the feasibility and efficacy of NIPPV in the daily practice of a paediatric ICU and that NIPPV could be proposed as a first-line treatment in children with acute respiratory distress, except in those with a diagnosis of ARDS.[6]

Recently, the first prospective randomized multicentre trial in the paediatric population was published by Yanez *et al.*[7], comparing the benefits of non-invasive ventilation (NIPPV) plus standard therapy with standard therapy alone in children with acute respiratory failure. Fifty patients with acute respiratory failure (mainly from RSV bronchiolitis) admitted to paediatric intensive care units were recruited: 25 patients were randomly allocated to NIPPV plus standard therapy (study group); the remaining 25 were given standard therapy (control group). Both groups were comparable in demographic terms. The study group received NIPPV under inspiratory positive airway pressure ranging between 12 cm $H_2O$ and 18 cm $H_2O$ and PEEP between 6 cm $H_2O$ and 12 cm $H_2O$. Heart rate and respiratory rate improved significantly with NIPPV. Detailed analysis revealed that both heart and respiratory rate were significantly lower after 1 hour of treatment compared with admission and this trend continued over time. With NIPPV, $PO_2/FIO_2$ improved significantly from the first hour. The endotracheal intubation rate was significantly lower (28 per cent) in the non-invasive ventilation group than in the control group (60 per cent). The authors concluded that NIPPV reduces hypoxaemia and the signs and symptoms of acute respiratory failure, thus avoiding endotracheal intubation and related complications in these patients.

A useful tool for the clinical use of NIPPV in the paediatric population should be the identification of predictive factors for NIPPV failure and success: this aspect has been recently evaluated in a prospective paper by Bernet *et al.*[17] Unfortunately the study included both NIPPV and CPAP given in a large age range (from newborns to children) making it difficult to interpret the results. More recently Mayordomo-Colunga *et al.*[18] published a prospective observational study including 116 episodes of ARF. The clinical data collected were respiratory rate (RR), heart rate and $FiO_2$ before NIPPV. The same data and expiratory and support pressures were collected at 1, 6, 12, 24 and 48 hours. Conditions precipitating ARF were classified into two groups: type 1 hypoxaemic ARF (38 episodes) and type 2 hypercapnic ARF (78 episodes). Factors predicting NIV failure were determined by multivariate analysis. Most common admission diagnoses were pneumonia (81.6 per cent) in type 1, and bronchiolitis (39.7 per cent) and asthma (42.3 per cent) in type 2. Complications secondary to NIPPV were detected in 23 episodes (20.2 per cent). NIPPV success rate was 84.5 per cent (68.4 per cent in type 1 and 92.3 per cent in type 2). Type 1 patients showed a higher risk of NIPPV failure compared with type 2 (odds ratio [OR] 11.108, 95 per cent confidence interval [CI] 2.578 to 47.863). A higher PRISM score (OR 1.138, 95 per cent CI 1.022 to 1.267), and a lower RR decrease at 1 hour and at 6 hours (OR 0.926, 95 per cent CI 0.860 to 0.997; and OR 0.911, 95 per cent CI 0.837 to 0.991, respectively) were also independently associated with NIPPV failure. The authors concluded that NIPPV is a useful respiratory support

**Table 51.1** Main clinical studies on non-invasive positive pressure ventilation in paediatric patients

| Authors | No. of patients | Diagnosis | No. intubated (per cent) | Comments |
|---|---|---|---|---|
| Akingbola *et al.*[19] | 2 | Down's, leukaemia, ARDS | 0 | Used post-extubation |
| Marino *et al.*[11] | 1 | Leukaemia | 0 | Avoided intubation |
| Piastra *et al.*[14] | 4 | Leukaemia, ARDS | 2 (50) | Helmet-delivered NIPPV, prevented intubation |
| Fortenberry *et al.*[10] | 28 | Pneumonia, neurological disorders | 3 (11) | Retrospective chart review. NIPPV improved oxygenation in hypoxaemic ARF |
| Padman *et al.*[20] | 34 | Neuromuscular disease, encephalopathy | 3 (9) | Prospective clinical study. NIPPV avoided intubation |
| Bernet *et al.*[17] | 42 | Pneumonia, viral respiratory infection, post-operative congenital heart disease, miscellaneous | 18 (43) | Prospective clinical study. Level $FiO_2$ after 1 hour of NIPPV may be a predictive factor for the outcome of NIPPV |
| Essouri *et al.*[6] | 114 | Community-acquired pneumonia, acute lung injury/ARDS, acute chest syndrome, post-extubation ARF | 31 (27) | Observational retrospective cohort study. NIPPV first-line treatment in children with ARF |
| Pancera *et al.*[21] | 120 | Haematological malignancy, solid tumours | 31 (25,8) | Retrospective cohort study mechanical ventilation vs NIPPV: mortality rate lower in the non-invasive ventilation group |
| Yanez *et al.*[7] | 50 | Status asthmaticus, viral/bacterial infection, respiratory syncytial virus, pneumoniae/bronchiolitis, influenza A, pneumonia | 7 NIV (28)<br>15 ST (60) | Prospective randomized study. NIPPV vs standard therapy: NIPPV reduced the need for intubation |
| Mayordomo-Colunga *et al.*[18] | 116 | Pneumonia, bronchiolitis, asthma | 18 (16) | Prospective observational study; mixed children treated with NIPPV or continuous positive airway pressure |
| Piastra *et al.*[8] | 23 | ARDS in immunocompromised children | 10 (44) | Observational clinical study; lower incidence of septic complications in non-invasive ventilation group |

ARDS, acute respiratory distress syndrome; ARF, acute respiratory failure.

technique in paediatric patients. Type 1 group classification, higher PRISM score, and lower RR decrease during NIV were independent risk factors for NIV failure. This is a very interesting study, including the large sample: however, unfortunately, the authors combined the data on children treated with NIPPV with those of children treated with CPAP alone, making the results more difficult to interpret: a large study on the prediction of NIPPV failure in the paediatric population is therefore still needed. Table 51.1 summarizes the main clinical studies on non-invasive positive pressure ventilation in paediatric patients, and Box 51.1 lists the advantages of using NIPPV in children.

More controversial is the use of NIPPV in children with severe hypoxaemia due to status asthmaticus.[22,23] Despite NIPPV being effective in improving oxygenation and the clinical picture in a subset of children admitted to a paediatric ICU with acute asthma, agitation that required treatment with intravenous sedatives was often reported.[23] Moreover in the same study, NIPPV did not prevent endotracheal intubation in a subset of children with hypercarbia and acute asthma.

**Box 51.1 Advantages of applying non-invasive positive pressure ventilation in children**

- Avoids local trauma due to endotracheal intubation
- No interference with swallowing and airway clearance mechanisms
- Offsets additional work of breathing due to the small endotracheal tube
- Possibility of intermittent use

Recent paediatric experience seems to confirm the role of NIPPV in immunocompromised patients affected by early ARDS, as has been demonstrated in adults.[4,24–26] In our feasibility study we reported that 13/23 (56 per cent) of immunocompromised children with ARDS, deemed to require mechanical ventilation, were successfully managed with NIPPV, avoiding endotracheal intubation.[8] Children successfully ventilated with NIPPV also had a shorter paediatric intensive care unit (PICU) and hospital stay, a lower incidence of septic complications (including VAP and septic shock) and lower respiratory and heart rate at the end of treatment, suggesting better haemodynamic and respiratory stability. Notably, at PICU admission severity scores and organ failure did not differ between the group treated successfully with NIPPV and that in which NIPPV failed. Our data suggest that a NIPPV trial could be considered in immunocompromised children with early ARDS. Moreover, extensive application of NIV in a paediatric oncology setting has been reported, independent of the severity and grade of the respiratory condition.[21] Box 51.2 lists the optimal timing of application of NIPPV in children.

## CLINICAL MANAGEMENT OF NIPPV IN THE PAEDIATRIC POPULATION

An important technical aspect still unsolved is the selection of the optimal interface in children with acute respiratory distress treated with NIPPV. Whereas NIPPV for long-term use is typically well tolerated by paediatric patients using a nasal mask, this interface presents major problems with air leaks and inability to attain the set inspiratory pressure in the acute setting. Thus face masks are generally considered the first choice in critically ill children with acute respiratory failure. However, some disadvantages have been reported also for the face masks, mainly due to the natural fear in children of any device that 'closes' their upper airways.

Although this problem can be partly relieved by an experienced team, it is quite common to use sedatives in the paediatric ICU setting. It is important to remember that (differently from the adult setting), due to their immature gastro-oesophageal sphincter function, children with respiratory distress are relatively prone to the development of gastro-oesophageal reflux; moreover gastric distension with gas is very common during NIPPV and can induce regurgitation of the gastric contents into the face mask. In order to increase tolerance, in older children a new interface, the helmet,[13,14] has been proposed for NIPPV administration. This innovative interface is associated with better tolerance than the face masks, but, due to its large internal volume and dead space, it increases the risk for carbon dioxide rebreathing and patient–ventilator asynchronies. In our experience the use of the helmet should therefore be reserved for children weighing more than 20–25 kg.

Minor complications are commonly reported in children treated with NIPPV and include dermal abrasion at the nasal bridge, eye irritation and gastric distension with air. Conversely, major complications have been rarely reported in the PICU setting where optimal monitoring, caregiver expertise and careful device choice are the norm. Children treated with NIPPV must be observed by expert staff using cardiovascular and respiratory monitors, pulse oximetry and frequent assessment of blood gases.

Important variables that need to be carefully analysed before starting NIPPV in paediatric patients are the age and the dimensions of the child, the kind of respiratory system dysfunction, and the level of cardiovascular stability. Usually NIPPV is considered difficult to apply in young infants with severe respiratory distress (Box 51.3). NIPPV is also absolutely contraindicated in children with significant cardiovascular/rhythm instability, in children with facial/cervical trauma and in patients with seizures or coma.

Conventional ICU ventilators can be used to administer NIPPV with inspiratory pressure support and PEEP in the PICU setting. Previous generation bi-level ventilators were not equipped for air leak compensation or limitation of the inspiratory time. In the presence of significant air leaks, as commonly observed in paediatric patients, the preset inspiratory cycling-off criteria are often not reached, thus inspiratory flow is maintained and the device does not cycle to expiration (hang-up phenomenon). This problem is a frequent cause of ineffective NIPPV administration, gas exchange deterioration and agitation. The only solution is to minimize air leaks: this can be achieved either by using a better fitting mask, or by reducing the pressure applied to

### Box 51.2 Timing of therapy in children

- **Early**: to prevent endotracheal intubation (+++)
- **Established**: as an alternative to intubation (++)
- **Resolving**: as a bridge to wean from ventilation (rarely evaluated)
- **Post-extubation**: to prevent reintubation (++)

### Box 51.3 Indications for conversion to intubation and conventional ventilation

- Cardiovascular/rhythm instability
- $SaO_2$ below 90 per cent with $FiO_2$ 0.5 or higher
- pH stable below 7.30 after 2 hours of NIPPV
- Mental deterioration/seizures
- Absent cough or gag reflex
- Mask intolerance
- Need for heavy sedation

the airways, or, mainly in infants and smaller children, by obtaining a more correct position of neck and chin, eventually also with a cervical collar.

NIPPV is usually started with 8–10 cm $H_2O$ of inspiratory pressure support and 5 cm $H_2O$ of PEEP, with subsequent increase in increments of the pressure support to obtain an optimal reduction of respiratory rate and inspiratory efforts, with optimal gas exchange. The PEEP level should be set to achieve two objectives: increase FRC and maintain the patency of the upper airway at end-expiration. Usually PEEP levels between 5 cm $H_2O$ and 10 cm $H_2O$ are sufficient in the paediatric clinical applications of NIPPV.

## CONCLUSIONS

Despite the publication of a single multicentre prospective randomized study, a growing body of evidence, including several large studies, support the usefulness of NIPPV in the paediatric setting. Despite these encouraging results, there is still large scope for improvement on several aspects, including new interfaces specifically designed for paediatric use and new assisted modes for optimizing child–ventilator interaction.

## REFERENCES


1. Bencault N, Boulair T. Mortality rate attributed to ventilator-associated nosocomial pneumonia in an adult intensive care unit: a prospective case-control study. *Crit Care Med* 2001; **29**: 2303–9.
2. Girou E, Brun-Buisson C, Taille S *et al.* Secular trends in nosocomial infections and mortality associated with noninvasive ventilation in patients with exacerbation of COPD and pulmonary edema. *JAMA* 2003; **290**: 2985–91.
3. Brochard L, Isabey D, Piquet J *et al.* Reversal of acute exacerbations of chronic obstructive lung disease by inspiratory pressure assistance with a face mask. *N Engl J Med* 1990; **323**: 1523–30.
4. Hilbert G, Gruson D, Vargas F *et al.* Noninvasive ventilation in immunosuppressed patients with pulmonary infiltrates, fever, and acute respiratory failure. *N Engl J Med* 2001; **344**: 481–7.
5. Antonelli M, Conti G, Rocco M *et al.* A comparison of noninvasive positive-pressure ventilation and conventional mechanical ventilation in patients with acute respiratory failure. *N Engl J Med* 1998; **339**: 429–35.
6. Essouri S, Chevret L, Durand P *et al.* Noninvasive positive pressure ventilation: five years of experience in a pediatric intensive care unit. *Pediatr Crit Care Med* 2006; **7**: 329–34.
7. Yanez L, Yunge M, Emilfork M *et al.* A prospective, randomized, controlled trial of noninvasive ventilation in pediatric acute respiratory failure. *Pediatr Crit Care Med* 2008; **9**: 484–9.
8. Piastra M, De Luca D, Pietrini D *et al.* Noninvasive pressure support ventilation in immuno-compromised children with ARDS: a feasibility study. *Intensive Care Med* 2009; **35**: 1420–7.
9. Padman R, Nadkarmi V, Von Nessen S *et al.* Noninvasive positive pressure ventilation in end-stage cystic fibrosis: a report of seven cases. *Respir Care* 1994; **39**: 736–9.
10. Fortenberry JD, Del Toro J, Jefferson LS *et al.* Management of pediatric acute hypoxemic respiratory insufficiency with bilevel positive pressure ($B_iPAP$) nasal mask ventilation. *Chest* 1995; **108**: 1059–64.
11. Marino P, Rosa G, Conti G *et al.* Treatment of acute respiratory failure by prolonged non-invasive ventilation in a child. *Can J Anaesth* 1997; **44**: 727–31.
12. Akingbola O, Palmisano J, Servant G *et al.* Bi-PAP mask ventilation in pediatric patients with acute respiratory failure. *Crit Care Med* 1994; **22**: A144.
13. Piastra M, Antonelli M, Caresta E *et al.* Noninvasive ventilation in childhood acute neuromuscular respiratory failure: a pilot study. *Respiration* 2006; **73**: 791–8.
14. Piastra M, Antonelli M, Chiaretti A *et al.* Treatment of acute respiratory failure by helmet-delivered non-invasive pressure support ventilation in children with acute leukemia: a pilot study. *Intensive Care Med* 2004; **30**: 472–6.
15. Piastra M, Conti G, Caresta E *et al.* Noninvasive ventilation options in pediatric myasthenia gravis. *Pediatr Anaesth* 2005; **15**: 699–702.
16. Piastra M, De Luca D, Zorzi G *et al.* Noninvasive ventilation in large postoperative flail chest. *Pediatr Blood Cancer* 2008; **51**: 831–3.
17. Bernet V, Hug MI, Frey B. Predictive factors for the success of noninvasive mask ventilation in infants and children with acute respiratory failure. *Pediatr Crit Care Med* 2005; **6**: 660–4.
18. Mayordomo-Colunga J, Medina A, Rey C *et al.* Predictive factors of non invasive ventilation failure in critically ill children: a prospective epidemiological study. *Intensive Care Med* 2009; **35**: 527–36.
19. Akingbola OA, Servant GM, Custer JR *et al.* Non-invasive Bi-level positive airway pressure in the management of pediatric lung disease. *Respir Care* 1993; **38**: 1092–8.
20. Padman R, Lawless ST, Kettrick RG. Noninvasive ventilation via bilevel positive airway pressure support in pediatric practice. *Crit Care Med* 1998; **26**: 169–73.
21. Pancera CF, Hayashi M, Fregnani JH *et al.* Noninvasive ventilation in immunocompromised pediatric patients: eight years of experience in a pediatric oncology intensive care unit. *J Pediatr Hematol Oncol* 2008; **30**: 533–8.
22. Teague WG. Noninvasive ventilation in the pediatric intensive care unit for children with acute respiratory failure. *Pediatr Pulmonol* 2003; **35**: 418–26.
23. Teague WG, Lowe E, Dominick J *et al.* Non-invasive positive pressure ventilation (NPPV) in critically ill children with status asthmaticus. *Am J Respir Crit Care Med* 1998; **157**: A542.

24. Antonelli M, Conti G, Bufi M *et al.* Noninvasive ventilation for the treatment of acute respiratory failure in patients undergoing solid organ transplantation: a randomized trial. *JAMA* 2000; **283**: 235–41.
25. Conti G, Marino P, Cogliati A *et al.* Noninvasive ventilation for the treatment of acute respiratory failure in patients with hematological malignancies: a pilot study. *Intensive Care Med* 1998; **24**: 1283–8.
26. Rocco M, Conti G, Antonelli M *et al.* Noninvasive pressure support ventilation in patients with acute respiratory failure after bilateral lung transplantation. *Intensive Care Med* 2001; **27**: 1622–6.

# SECTION L

# Special situations

# 52

# Bronchoscopy during non-invasive ventilation

MASSIMO ANTONELLI, GIUSEPPE BELLO

## ABSTRACT

Fibreoptic bronchoscopy is associated with transient alterations in pulmonary mechanics and gas exchange. Arterial oxygen tension may fall significantly below its baseline value during the procedure and remain low for a few minutes to several hours after removal of the bronchoscope. Placing the bronchoscope into the major airways decreases the area available for air flow and consequently increases airway resistance. This very quickly results in the development of an auto-positive end-expiratory pressure and, therefore, in an increase in the work of breathing. Non-intubated, spontaneously breathing patients with hypoxaemia should not undergo fibreoptic bronchoscopy because of their high risk for developing respiratory failure or serious cardiac arrhythmias. In these hypoxaemic patients, non-invasive ventilation (NIV) has been demonstrated to be a valuable tool for prevention of gas-exchange deterioration accompanying fibreoptic bronchoscopy, and for compensating for the increased work of breathing occurring during the procedure, thus avoiding endotracheal intubation and its associated complications. Performing fibreoptic bronchoscopy during NIV has been described either in at-risk patients who were initially breathing spontaneously and who started NIV to assist the procedure, or in patients who were already receiving NIV and who were scheduled for fibreoptic bronchoscopy while on NIV. When NIV is delivered through a face mask, a T-adapter is attached to the mask for insertion of the bronchoscope through the nose. Conversely, if a helmet is being used, the bronchoscope is passed through the specific seal connector placed in the plastic ring of the helmet. The internal adjustable diaphragm of the seal connection can prevent loss of the respiratory gases, maintaining ventilation throughout fibreoptic bronchoscopy.

## INTRODUCTION

Fibreoptic bronchoscopy with broncheoalveolar lavage (BAL) has a central role in the diagnosis of pneumonia in critically ill patients. Prompt identification of the responsible pathogens is crucial for starting appropriate antimicrobial therapy and avoiding the empirical administration of unnecessary and often toxic antibiotics. Non-intubated, spontaneously breathing patients with hypoxaemia (defined as inability to maintain an arterial oxygen partial pressure ($PaO_2$) <75 mm Hg or an oxygen saturation >90 per cent despite oxygen supplementation) should not undergo fibreoptic bronchoscopy because of their high risk for developing respiratory failure or serious cardiac arrhythmias.[1] Until a few years ago, the available options in hypoxaemic patients suspected of having pneumonia were to avoid fibreoptic bronchoscopy and institute empirical treatment, or to perform endotracheal intubation and administer mechanical ventilation for ensuring adequate gas exchange during the procedure. Non-invasive ventilation (NIV) has been demonstrated to be a valuable tool for assisting spontaneous breathing during diagnostic bronchoscopy, successfully avoiding the need for endotracheal intubation in high-risk patients.[2–6] This chapter covers the rationale for using NIV to assist patients undergoing fibreoptic bronchoscopy, a review of the available literature supporting this method, and some procedural considerations.

In this chapter, the term CPAP refers to non-invasive constant continuous positive airway pressure delivered to spontaneously breathing patients, whereas NIPPV refers to non-invasive intermittent positive pressure ventilation with or without positive end-expiratory pressure (PEEP). NIV is considered to include either CPAP or NIPPV.

## RATIONALE

Fibreoptic bronchoscopy is associated with transient alterations in pulmonary mechanics and gas exchange.[7,8]

$PaO_2$ may fall significantly below its baseline value during the procedure and remain decreased for a few minutes to several hours after removing the bronchoscope.[7,8] In a large group of critically ill mechanically ventilated patients undergoing fibreoptic bronchoscopy, the mean drop in $PaO_2$ at the end of the procedure was of 26 per cent compared with the control value.[9] Hypoxaemia may be more pronounced when BAL is performed because of ventilation and perfusion abnormalities resulting from the instillation of saline solution.[10]

In a non-intubated adult male, a 5.7 mm outside diameter flexible bronchoscope has been calculated to occupy about 10 per cent of the tracheal cross-sectional area and about 15 per cent of the cross-sectional area at the cricoid ring.[7] Placing the bronchoscope into the major airways decreases the area available for air flow and, consequently, increases airway resistance.[7] Transnasal insertion of a 5.2 mm bronchoscope into a trachea with an inside diameter of 11 mm would increase airway resistance approximately twofold.[8] The high exhalation resistance very quickly results in an increase in functional residual capacity (FRC) and, therefore, in the development of an intrinsic PEEP mechanism.[8] This may have deleterious consequences, such as requiring additional work of breathing and the risk of barotrauma, especially during coughing.

Besides the physical presence of the bronchoscope in the airway, ongoing suction through the instrument working channel is another cause of the alterations in pulmonary mechanics and gas exchange during fibreoptic bronchoscopy. Removal of tracheobronchial gas by excessive use of suction evacuates respiratory gas from the lungs and decreases FRC with consequent hypoxaemia.[7]

In the 1990s, the encouraging results obtained in the treatment of acute respiratory failure with NIV[11–13] stimulated investigations of various applications of NIV in the acute care setting. In hypoxaemic patients needing fibreoptic bronchoscopy with BAL, NIV has been employed to prevent gas-exchange deterioration accompanying the procedure, and to compensate for the increase in work of breathing during the procedure, thus avoiding endotracheal intubation and its associated complications.

## EVIDENCE BASE

Several investigators have evaluated the use of NIV in hypoxaemic patients needing a diagnostic procedure. Antonelli *et al.*[2] originally described the application of face mask NIPPV during fibreoptic bronchoscopy in eight immunocompromised hypoxaemic (i.e. $PaO_2$ to inspired oxygen fraction [$FiO_2$] ratio <100) patients with suspected pneumonia. NIPPV was associated with a significant improvement in $PaO_2/FiO_2$ during the procedure. The technique was well tolerated, and no patient required endotracheal intubation.

The successful application of NIPPV during fibreoptic bronchoscopy was also reported in patients with chronic obstructive pulmonary disease (COPD). Da Conceiçao *et al.*[3] investigated 10 consecutive COPD patients with pneumonia who were admitted to the intensive care unit with hypercapnia (i.e. arterial carbon dioxide tension [$PaCO_2$] 67 ± 11 mm Hg) and hypoxaemia (i.e. $PaO_2$, 53 ± 13 mm Hg). During fibreoptic bronchoscopy with NIPPV, arterial oxygen saturation of haemoglobin measured by pulse oximetry ($SpO_2$) increased from 91 ± 4.7 per cent at baseline to 97 ± 1.7 per cent. There were no changes in $PaCO_2$ and $PaO_2$ in the hour following the end of the procedure, and no patients were intubated within 24 hours.

Maitre *et al.*[4] conducted a randomized double-blind study of 30 patients with $PaO_2/FiO_2$ <300 to compare a new CPAP treatment with oxygen administration in maintaining oxygenation during fibreoptic bronchoscopy. The face mask CPAP device was based on four funnel-shaped microchannels connected to an oxygen source and generating high-velocity microjets, and thus positive pressure; CPAP allowed minimal alterations in gas exchange and prevented subsequent respiratory failure. During fibreoptic bronchoscopy and 30 minutes thereafter, $SpO_2$ was significantly higher in the CPAP group than the oxygen group. Arterial blood gas measurements 15 minutes after termination of fibreoptic bronchoscopy showed that the $PaO_2$ had increased by 10.5 ± 16.9 per cent in the CPAP group and decreased by 15 ± 16.6 per cent in the oxygen group ($p = 0.01$).[4] Five patients in the oxygen group, but none in the CPAP group, developed respiratory failure and required intubation in the 6 hours following the procedure.

In a subsequent trial, Antonelli *et al.*[5] randomized 26 hypoxaemic (i.e. $PaO_2/FiO_2$ <200) patients needing diagnostic fibreoptic bronchoscopy to receive an $FiO_2$ of 0.9 via face mask, or NIV via oronasal mask with pressure support ventilation of 15–17 cm $H_2O$, expiratory pressure of 5 cm $H_2O$, and $FiO_2$ of 0.9. The $PaO_2/FiO_2$ was substantially higher both during fibreoptic bronchoscopy (261 mm Hg versus 139 mm Hg) and 1 hour after (176 mm Hg versus 140 mm Hg), although both groups started at essentially the same $PaO_2/FiO_2$ at baseline (143 mm Hg versus 155 mm Hg). After undergoing the procedure, three patients required non-emergent intubation, one patient in the NIPPV group (7 hours after the procedure) and two patients in the control group (9 and 5 hours after the procedure). In all three cases, the intubation was not apparently related to fibreoptic bronchoscopy.

A more recent study[6] has shown that in patients with hypoxaemic acute respiratory failure receiving NIPPV through the helmet, fibreoptic bronchoscopy with BAL is a safe and feasible technique, capable of avoiding endotracheal intubation and discontinuation of assisted ventilation.

## CLINICAL APPLICATIONS

Performing fibreoptic bronchoscopy during the delivery of NIV has been used either to assist spontaneous breathing in patients at risk for developing acute respiratory failure during the procedure or to avoid the discontinuation of NIV in patients scheduled to undergo fibreoptic bronchoscopy.

The risks associated with either the NIV application or bronchoscopic examination should be weighed against the benefits in the patient who needs the procedure. The criteria for excluding patients from NIV treatment include severe central neurological disturbances, the inability to protect the airway, unstable haemodynamic conditions, vomiting, facial deformities and recent oral, oesophageal or gastric surgery. However, even if the patient has no contraindications to NIV, fibreoptic bronchoscopy should not be carried out in the following circumstances: absence of consent from the patient; lack of trained personnel; refractory hypoxaemia even during NIV; inability to normalize platelet count and coagulation if biopsy or brushing are anticipated; unstable cardiac disease (the risks of fibreoptic bronchoscopy are thought to be reduced four to six weeks after myocardial infarction);[14] and uncontrolled bronchospasm.[15]

The complication rate of fibreoptic bronchoscopy has been shown to be increased in COPD patients.[16] In these patients, oxygen supplementation as well as intravenous sedation should be avoided or given with extreme caution to prevent dangerous increases in $PaCO_2$.

## TECHNICAL CONSIDERATIONS

The bronchoscopic technique is slightly different depending on the type of interface that is used to deliver NIV. When NIV is delivered through a face mask, a T-adapter is attached to the mask for insertion of the bronchoscope through the nose or the mouth (Fig. 52.1). Conversely, if a helmet is used, the bronchoscope is passed through the specific seal connector placed in the plastic ring of the helmet. This connector can also be used to spray local anaesthetic into the nostrils and pharynx of the patient. The internal adjustable diaphragm of the seal connection can prevent loss of the respiratory gases, maintaining ventilation and PEEP throughout fibreoptic bronchoscopy.[6]

Prior to performing fibreoptic bronchoscopy, NIV is administered (if not yet started) for at least 5 minutes in order to obtain an adequate patient–ventilator interaction. Non-invasive ventilation is maintained during fibreoptic bronchoscopy and for at least 30 minutes after termination of the procedure, after which it is discontinued if the patient is not showing respiratory difficulties or significant gas exchange deterioration. The $FiO_2$ is kept at 0.9–1 while the patient adjusts to the ventilator and during the examination. Over the first 30 minutes after the completion of FB, the applied $FiO_2$ is gradually reduced to the pre-FB requirements as long as the patient is able to maintain $SpO_2$ at >92 per cent.

Topical anaesthesia of the nose and pharynx can be obtained by spraying 10 per cent lidocaine solution. Topical anaesthesia of the larynx and vocal cords can be performed by injecting 2 per cent lidocaine through the working channel of the bronchoscope. When fibreoptic bronchoscopy is used to obtain samples from the lower respiratory tract for the diagnosis of pneumonia, the sampling area is selected by localizing new or progressive infiltrates on chest radiograph or the segment visualized

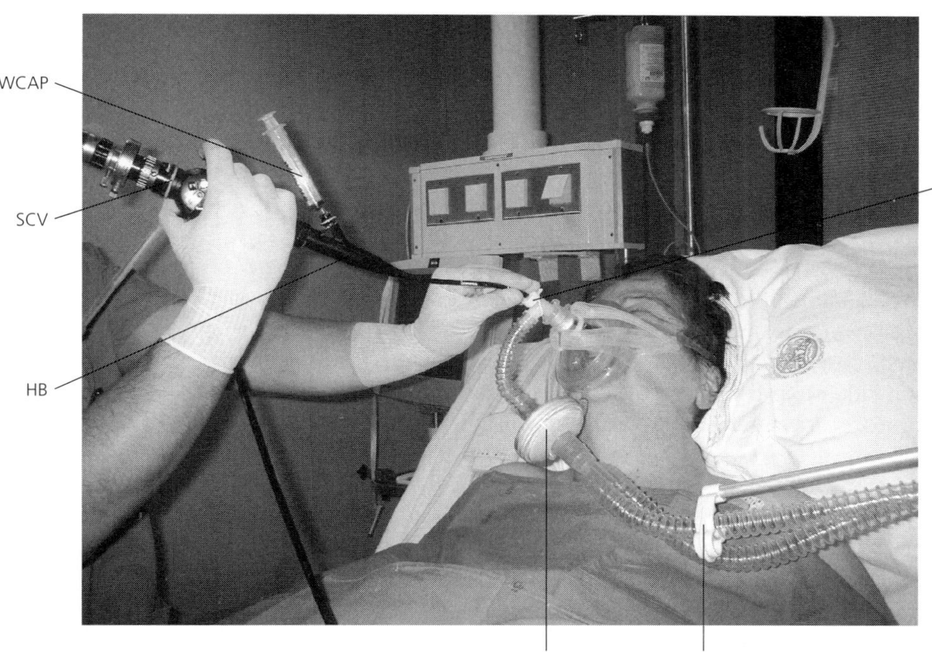


**Figure 52.1** Fibreoptic bronchoscopy being performed with non-invasive ventilation delivered through an oronasal mask. HB, handle of the bronchoscope; HME, heat and moisture exchanger; RC, respiratory circuit; SC, seal connection; SCV, suction control valve; WCAP, working channel access port.

during the procedure as having purulent secretions.[17] Information is unclear about the sampling site in patients with diffuse lung infiltrates. In the supine patient, BAL fluid recovery is best from the right middle lobe or the lingula. When BAL is performed, the tip of the bronchoscope is wedged as far as possible into a distal airway, generally the fourth to fifth order bronchi, and sterile saline solution is instilled through the bronchoscope and then aspirated into a sterile trap. Additional aliquots of 20–60 mL are injected and aspirated back after each instillation. The total amount of fluid used to obtain BAL ranges from 140 mL to 240 mL.[17] Bacterial pneumonia is diagnosed when at least 10 000 colony-forming units per millilitre of bacteria are measured in the BAL fluid.[18]

It is necessary for the patient to have no oral feeding (or enteral nutrition) for 4 hours and no clear oral fluids for 2 hours before fibreoptic bronchoscopy.[15] Subjects with a history of asthma should be premedicated with a bronchodilator before the procedure. Accurate cardiorespiratory monitoring is necessary during the procedure, including continuous electrocardiogram and $SpO_2$, continuous intra-arterial blood pressure or intermittent cuff blood pressure measurement at least every 5 minutes, tidal volume, minute ventilation and airway pressure.

Finally, the type of NIV interface may affect the feasibility of the technique. When the helmet is used, fibreoptic bronchoscopy could be difficult if there is a large distance between the plastic ring of the helmet and the patient's nose or mouth. This problem is easily solved by reducing this distance by gently pushing the plastic ring toward the face of the patient. Also, the specific seal connector placed in the plastic ring of the helmet, which is used to pass the cord of the bronchoscope, may be too much out of line with the mouth or the nose of some patients, thus increasing the difficulty of the technique. In this case, the plastic ring of the helmet should be gently shifted in order to make the cord of the bronchoscope as straight as possible. Removal of the screw cap of the patient access port of the helmet for just a few seconds can facilitate the procedure, by allowing the operator to hold the insertion cord of the bronchoscope with one hand inside the helmet and rapidly introduce it into the patient's nose or mouth. Soon after, the patient access port is closed and NIV is resumed.

Transnasal fibreoptic bronchoscopy in patients undergoing face mask NIV may involve some technical difficulties if the opening of the face mask, which is attached to the ventilator circuit, is not positioned above the patient's nose. When it occurs, it may be difficult either to introduce the bronchoscope into the nose, or to manoeuvre the instrument through the airways. Replacing the face mask with another model can overcome this problem.

## FUTURE RESEARCH

Performing fibreoptic bronchoscopy during NIV has been described both in at-risk patients who were initially breathing spontaneously and who started NIV to assist fibreoptic bronchoscopy, and an patients who were already receiving NIV and who were scheduled to undergo fibreoptic bronchoscopy during NIV. In all cases, fibreoptic bronchoscopy was needed to obtain BAL specimens for the diagnosis of pneumonia. It would be interesting to investigate the safety and usefulness of fibreoptic bronchoscopy during NIV in at-risk patients who need a bronchoscopic examination for diagnostic purposes other than BAL, such as biopsies, or for therapeutic procedures, such as laser treatment and removal of retained secretions.

## REFERENCES


1. Goldstein RA, Rohatgi PK, Bergofsky EH *et al.* Clinical role of bronchoalveolar lavage in adults with pulmonary disease. *Am Rev Respir Dis* 1990; **142**: 481–6.
2. Antonelli M, Conti G, Riccioni L *et al.* Noninvasive positive-pressure ventilation via face mask during bronchoscopy with BAL in high-risk hypoxemic patients. *Chest* 1996; **110**: 724–8.
3. Da Conceiçao M, Genco G, Favier JC *et al.* Fiberoptic bronchoscopy during noninvasive positive-pressure ventilation in patients with chronic obstructive lung disease with hypoxemia and hypercapnia. *Ann Fr Anesth Reanim* 2000; **19**: 231–6.
4. Maitre B, Jaber S, Maggiore SM *et al.* Continuous positive airway pressure during fiberoptic bronchoscopy in hypoxemic patients: a randomized double-blind study using a new device. *Am J Respir Crit Care Med* 2000; **162**: 1063–7.
5. Antonelli M, Conti G, Rocco M *et al.* Noninvasive positive-pressure ventilation vs. conventional oxygen supplementation in hypoxemic patients undergoing diagnostic bronchoscopy. *Chest* 2002; **121**: 1149–54.
6. Antonelli M, Pennisi MA, Conti G *et al.* Fiberoptic bronchoscopy during noninvasive positive pressure ventilation delivered by helmet. *Intensive Care Med* 2003; **29**: 126–9.
7. Lindholm CE, Ollman B, Snyder JV *et al.* Cardiorespiratory effects of flexible fiberoptic bronchoscopy in critically ill patients. *Chest* 1978; **74**: 362–8.
8. Matsushima Y, Jones RL, King EG *et al.* Alterations in pulmonary mechanics and gas exchange during routine fiberoptic bronchoscopy. *Chest.* 1984; **86**: 184–8.
9. Trouillet JL, Guiguet M, Gibert C *et al.* Fiberoptic bronchoscopy in ventilated patients: evaluation of cardiopulmonary risk under midazolam sedation. *Chest* 1990; **97**: 927–33.
10. Lin CC, Wu JL, Huang WC. Pulmonary function in normal subjects after bronchoalveolar lavage. *Chest* 1988; **93**: 1049–53.

11. Meduri GU, Conoscenti CC, Menashe P *et al.* Noninvasive face mask ventilation in patients with acute respiratory failure. *Chest* 1989; **95**: 865–70.
12. Brochard L, Isabey D, Piquet J *et al.* Reversal of acute exacerbations of chronic obstructive lung disease by inspiratory assistance with a face mask. *N Engl J Med* 1990; **323**: 1523–30.
13. Elliott MW, Steven MH, Phillips GD *et al.* Non-invasive mechanical ventilation for acute respiratory failure. *BMJ* 1990; **300**: 358–60.
14. Eagle KA, Brundage BH, Chaitman BR *et al.* Guidelines for perioperative cardiovascular evaluation for noncardiac surgery. Report of the American College of Cardiology/American Heart Association Task Force on Practice Guidelines. Committee on Perioperative Cardiovascular Evaluation for Noncardiac Surgery. *Circulation* 1996; **93**: 1278–317.
15. British Thoracic Society Bronchoscopy Guidelines Committee, a Subcommittee of Standards of Care Committee of British Thoracic Society. British Thoracic Society guidelines on diagnostic flexible bronchoscopy. *Thorax* 2001; **56** Suppl 1: i1–21.
16. Peacock MD, Johnson JE, Blanton HM. Complications of flexible bronchoscopy in patients with severe obstructive pulmonary disease. *J Bronchol* 1994; **1**: 181–6.
17. Meduri GU, Chastre J. The standardization of bronchoscopic techniques for ventilator-associated pneumonia. *Chest* 1992; **102**: 557S–64S.
18. American Thoracic Society; Infectious Diseases Society of America. Guidelines for the management of adults with hospital-acquired, ventilator-associated, and healthcare-associated pneumonia. *Am J Respir Crit Care Med* 2005; **171**: 388–416.

53

# Non-invasive ventilation in pregnancy

JOHN M SHNEERSON

## ABSTRACT

The respiratory drive increases in pregnancy, but as the arterial $PCO_2$ falls, physiological central sleep apnoeas appear. The upper airway resistance increases and the diaphragm becomes elevated. A restrictive defect appears mainly due to the enlarged uterus and intra-abdominal hypertension. The reduction in lung volume also leads to ventilation–perfusion mismatching and hypoxia. Ventilatory failure is most commonly seen in neuromuscular and skeletal disorders and obesity hypoventilation. It is important to identify high-risk patients before or early in pregnancy and to monitor their progress, particularly with respiratory sleep studies. There is limited clinical experience of non-invasive ventilation (NIV) in this situation but it is capable of relieving ventilatory failure and enabling the foetus to be successfully delivered. There is insufficient evidence to compare different ventilatory modalities.

## INTRODUCTION

The physiological effects of pregnancy on respiratory function have been extensively studied,[1] but their implications for the development of ventilatory failure and the use of NIV is largely confined to case reports and short series. The older literature indicates that, in neuromuscular and skeletal disorders, maternal mortality ranges from 2.6 per cent to 3.8 per cent and foetal mortality from 4 per cent to 10 per cent.[2,3] Very often, however, both pregnancy and delivery occur uneventfully.[4,5] The reasons for this variability and the implications for treatment with NIV will be discussed in this chapter.

## PATHOPHYSIOLOGY

The respiratory system is significantly modified during pregnancy (Table 53.1). Upper airway resistance increases because of hyperaemia, mucosal oedema and hypersecretion due to increased oestrogen secretion, particularly in the third trimester. Snoring is more common in pregnancy, and obstructive sleep apnoea (OSA) may develop.[6] The presence of OSA is associated with gestational hypertension[7] and the foetal outcome in pre-eclampsia is worse if OSA is present. In addition, in neuromuscular disorders there may be weakness of the upper airway stabilizing dilator muscles, and congenital mandibular abnormalities also increase the risk of OSA.

The respiratory drive increases during pregnancy[8] due to increased progesterone secretion and the $PCO_2$ often falls to around 4 kPa. This leads to physiological central sleep apnoeas but, together with the increased metabolic rate during pregnancy, imposes extra demands on the respiratory system.

The enlarging uterus increases the intra-abdominal pressure in an analogous way to the abdominal compartment syndrome.[9] The functional residual capacity and residual volume are reduced with an increase in ventilation–perfusion mismatching and elevation of the diaphragm. Movement of the rib cage becomes relatively more important than abdominal expansion[10] and this is particularly important if rib cage expansion is limited as in, for instance, ankylosing spondylitis. The mechanical effects on the diaphragm and the rib cage are similar, but more complex, when the chest wall is asymmetrical as in scoliosis.

The worsening ventilation–perfusion matching leads to hypoxia. This is particularly marked during sleep.

**Table 53.1** Pathophysiological changes in pregnancy

| Physiological changes | Consequences |
|---|---|
| Increased respiratory drive | Low $PCO_2$<br>Central sleep apnoeas |
| Increased nasal resistance | Snoring<br>Obstructive sleep apnoeas |
| Increased intra-abdominal pressure | Restrictive defect |
| Increased rib cage movement | Abnormal respiratory mechanics |
| Elevation of diaphragm | Ventilatory failure |
| Impaired ventilation–perfusion matching | Hypoxia |

Hypercapnia is seen initially in rapid eye movement (REM) sleep when inspiration is almost entirely dependent on diaphragmatic function. The fall in $PO_2$ also causes pulmonary vasoconstriction leading to pulmonary hypertension. The increase in blood volume and cardiac output of around 30 per cent by mid-pregnancy also contributes to this and to right heart failure, which is seem particularly late in pregnancy or shortly after delivery.[11,12]

The combination of increasing upper airway resistance, a worsening restrictive defect, hypoxia and sleep-related changes in respiratory drive all contribute to the risk of developing ventilatory failure during pregnancy if there is an underlying neuromuscular or skeletal disorder, OSA or obesity. Ventilatory failure usually appears late in pregnancy when the intra-abdominal pressure is increasing rapidly as the foetus and uterus enlarge.

The foetus extracts oxygen readily from the maternal blood because its oxyhaemoglobin dissociation curve is displaced to the left. The foetal lung is able to develop in a low oxygen environment[13] and maternal acidosis associated with ventilatory failure increases the oxygen available to the foetus. Severe maternal hypoxia is, however, probably associated with increased risk of intra-uterine foetal death, premature labour and low birth weight of the foetus.

## CLINICAL APPLICATIONS

### Pre-pregnancy planning

This is important to identify those women who are at risk of developing respiratory complications or right heart failure during pregnancy. In general, pregnancy should not be advised if the vital capacity is less than 1 L, if significant pulmonary hypertension is present, or if the arterial $PCO_2$ is raised while awake. In these situations it may be best to consider contraception or sterilization.

### Assessment during pregnancy

It is essential to monitor those at high risk of ventilatory or right heart failure during pregnancy. Respiratory sleep studies with, ideally, both oxygen saturation and transcutaneous $PCO_2$ monitoring are advisable, although $PCO_2$ monitoring is not required if only OSA is suspected. It is also important to monitor the foetus during pregnancy in order to assess any impact of cardiorespiratory problems on foetal development.

### Non-invasive ventilation

This is usually required for those with neuromuscular or skeletal disorders and when obesity hypoventilation is suspected.[14] The rise in progesterone increases the laxity of ligaments and may worsen spinal deformities, especially scoliosis. Chronic obstructive pulmonary disease (COPD) and cystic fibrosis are uncommon causes of respiratory failure in pregnancy and if there is extensive diffuse lung disease, supplemental oxygen rather than ventilatory support is likely to be required. Occasionally acute severe asthma requires ventilatory support and, while non-invasive ventilation may be useful in some patients, intubation and if necessary emergency delivery of the foetus by caesarean section[15] should be considered if the patient or foetus deteriorates. Nasal continuous positive airway pressure treatment is effective in relieving OSA induced by pregnancy and may also reduce the hypertension in pre-eclampsia when this occurs in association with OSA.[16]

There are few data about the management of obesity hypoventilation in pregnancy, but in principle this should be similar to neuromuscular and skeletal disorders. In the latter, termination of pregnancy is occasionally the best option in ventilatory failure,[17] although it should be possible to avoid this in most patients by providing non-invasive ventilatory support.[18–24] This can support ventilation both during the day and at night and may be required for increasing durations later in pregnancy, and to control ventilatory failure before elective caesarean section.[25] Bi-level pressure preset ventilation has been used most frequently, but there are no data to indicate whether this is preferable to other ventilatory modalities.

In both obesity hypoventilation and neuromuscular and skeletal disorders respiratory failure may be detected only when it is severe, and intubation may be urgently required. Pre-oxygenation, cricoid pressure and avoidance of a nasotracheal tube (because of the risk of damage to the nose) are all important. If the patient cannot be resuscitated promptly, emergency delivery of the foetus should be attempted. Once ventilatory failure is controlled it is best to wean the patient in the sitting or lateral decubitus position to avoid obstruction of the inferior vena cava and to substitute non-invasive for invasive ventilatory support.

## FUTURE RESEARCH

Further research is required in the following areas:

- better understanding of the development of abnormal respiratory mechanics during pregnancy
- better understanding of ventilation–perfusion matching within the lungs in pregnancy, particularly the interaction of the physiological changes with the hypoxia and acidosis of ventilatory failure
- clearer identification of patients at risk of developing ventilatory failure during pregnancy
- better understanding of why some women develop OSA during pregnancy and why only some of these, and some without OSA, develop obesity hypoventilation
- clearer evidence about the indications for and timings of sleep studies during pregnancy
- research into the value of prophylactic non-invasive ventilation in those at risk of ventilatory failure, but who have not yet developed it during pregnancy
- better understanding of the value of foetal monitoring in assessing the indications for NIV in pregnancy.

## SUMMARY

- Physiological changes during pregnancy increase the respiratory drive and upper airway resistance and lead to a restrictive defect due primarily to the enlarging uterus. The arterial $PCO_2$ falls, but so may the $PO_2$ due to worsening ventilation–perfusion matching.
- Ventilatory failure during pregnancy can be avoided by pre-pregnancy planning and monitoring of high-risk patients at an early stage in pregnancy by repeated sleep studies.
- Non-invasive ventilation is required most frequently in neuromuscular and skeletal disorders and obesity hypoventilation and is often effective in controlling ventilatory failure and enabling successful delivery.
- OSA can be treated with nasal CPAP and this may also improve gestational hypertension.

## REFERENCES


1. Fishburne JL. Physiology and disease of the respiratory system in pregnancy. A review. *J Reprod Med* 1979; **22**: 177–89.
2. Phelan JP, Dainer MJ, Cowherd DW *et al.* Pregnancy complicated by thoracolumbar scoliosis. *South J Med* 1978; **71**: 76–8.
3. Kopenhager T. A review of 50 pregnant patients with kyphoscoliosis. *Br J Obstet Gynaecol* 1977; **84**: 585–7.
4. Chau W, Lee KH. Kyphosis complicating pregnancy. *Obstet Gynaecol Br Commonw* 1970; **77**: 1098–102.
5. Manning CW, Prime FJ, Zorab PA. Pregnancy and scoliosis. *Lancet* 1967; **ii**: 792–5.
6. Santiago JR, Nolledo MS, Kinzler W *et al.* Sleep and sleep disorders in pregnancy. *Ann Intern Med* 2001; **134**: 396–408.
7. Champagne K, Schwartzman K, Opatrny L *et al.* Obstructive sleep apnoea and its association with gestational hypertension. *Eur Respir J* 2009; **33**: 559–65.
8. Contreras G, Gutierrez M, Berioza T *et al.* Ventilatory drive and respiratory muscle function in pregnancy. *Am Rev Respir Dis* 1991; **144**: 837–41.
9. Malbrain MLNG. A new concept: the polycompartment syndrome – Part 2. *Int J Intensive Care* 2009; **Spring**: 24–31.
10. Gilroy RJ, Mangura BT, Lavietes MH. Rib cage and abdominal volume displacements during breathing in pregnancy. *Am Rev Respir Dis* 1988; **137**: 668–72.
11. Berge JE. Pregnancy associated with severe kyphoscoliosis of the thoracic spine. *J Obstet Gynaecol Br Commonw* 1962; **69**: 81–98.
12. Jones DH. Kyphoscoliosis complicating pregnancy. *Lancet* 1964; **1**: 517–20.
13. Groenman F, Rutter M, Caniggia I *et al.* Hypoxia-inducible factors in the first trimester human lung. *J Histochem Cytochem* 2007; **55**: 355–63.
14. Shneerson JM. Pregnancy in neuro-muscular and skeletal disorders. *Monaldi Arch Chest Dis* 1994; **49**: 227–30.
15. Tomlinson MW, Caruthers TJ, Whitty JE *et al.* Does delivery improve maternal condition in the respiratory-compromised gravida? *Obstet Gynecol* 1998; **91**:108–11.
16. Edwards N, Blyton DM, Kirjavainen T *et al.* Nasal continuous positive airway pressure reduces sleep-induced blood pressure increments in pre-eclampsia. *Am J Respir Crit Care Med* 2000; **162**: 252–7.
17. Bender S. Pregnancy in a 31 in (77.5 cm) dwarf. *Br Med J* 1965; **ii**: 1166.
18. Nilsson ED. The delivery of a quadriplegic patient confined to a respirator. *Am J Obstet Gynecol* 1953; **65**: 1334–7.
19. Sawicka EH, Spencer GT, Branthwaite MA. Management of respiratory failure complicating pregnancy in severe kyphoscoliosis: a new use for an old technique? *Br J Dis Chest* 1986; **80**: 191–6.
20. Woollam CHM, Houlton MCC. Respiratory failure in pregnancy. *Anaesthesia* 1976; **31**: 1217–20.
21. Restrick LJ, Clapp BR, Mikelsons C *et al.* Nasal ventilation in pregnancy: treatment of nocturnal hypoventilation in a patient with kyphoscoliosis. *Eur Respir J* 1997; **10**: 2657–8.
22. Yim R, Kirschner K, Murphy E *et al.* Successful pregnancy in a patient with spinal muscular atrophy and severe kyphoscoliosis. *Am J Phys Med Rehabil* 2003; **82**: 222–5.
23. Diaz-Lobato S, Mendieta MAG, Garcia MSM *et al.* Two full-term pregnancies in a patient with mitochondrial myopathy and chronic ventilatory insufficiency. *Respiration* 2005; **72**: 654–6.
24. Warren J, Sharma SK. Ventilatory support using bilevel positive airway pressure during neuraxial blockade in a patient with severe respiratory compromise. *Anesth Analg* 2006; **102**: 910–11.
25. Greenwood JJ, Scott WE. Charcot-Marie-tooth disease: peripartum management of two contrasting clinical cases. *Int J Obstet Anesth* 2007; **16**: 149–54.

# 54

# Tracheostomy

PIERO CERIANA, PAOLO PELOSI

## ABSTRACT

Tracheostomy is one of the most common procedures carried out in critically ill patients. It has several theoretical advantages compared with translaryngeal endotracheal intubation, such as reduced laryngeal injury, better patient tolerance, reduced inspiratory load, and easier nursing care. Tracheostomy is indicated for prolonged ventilatory support and long-term airway maintenance, and makes easier the process of weaning from mechanical ventilation and discharge from the intensive care unit. In recent years percutaneous dilational tracheostomy has gained popularity as an alternative to the conventional surgical technique, allowing the procedure to be performed at the bedside without moving the patient to the operating theatre. The long-term management of tracheostomy requires consideration of several factors such as tube selection, recognition of displacement, tube change, cuff management, swallowing, speech, etc. A multidisciplinary team can improve the care of tracheostomized patients and should include doctors, nurses, speech therapists, physiotherapists and dietetic staff; these personnel have to work in a coordinated manner to ensure that all of the patient's needs are met and outcomes are optimized.

## INTRODUCTION

Cases of respiratory failure in which non-invasive mechanical ventilation is contraindicated or fails[1] require translaryngeal intubation and invasive mechanical ventilation (IMV). Approximately 35–50 per cent of patients admitted to the intensive care unit (ICU) for respiratory failure, regardless of origin, require IMV.[2] While in about 75 per cent of patients the cause of respiratory failure resolves within a few days, thus allowing extubation, the remaining 25 per cent of patients require respiratory assistance for a longer period. Almost half of these patients can then be definitely weaned from IMV within the third week of respiratory assistance, while the remaining patients (about 5–13 per cent of the overall number) cannot be weaned from the respiratory prosthesis and require prolonged mechanical ventilation.[3] The persistent need for ventilatory support, however, implies *in situ* maintenance of the translaryngeal tube and this can cause pressure necrosis and laryngeal mucosal abrasion, mainly through a mechanism of tube movement and friction.[4] While in most cases these lesions are fully reversible and heal within a few weeks,[5] persistent posterior commissure stenosis and vocal cord paresis have been described.[6] In order to prevent laryngeal damage, it is common and accepted practice to convert the interface for IMV from translaryngeal intubation into tracheostomy in those patients who require prolonged mechanical ventilation.

The term 'tracheostomy' is derived from Greek and means 'to cut the trachea'. It can be considered one of the most ancient surgical procedures, since the first reports about an intervention very similar to modern tracheostomy can be found in books of Hindu and Egyptian medicine written about 3500–4000 years ago.[7] Over the course of centuries, tracheostomy was considered, at times, as a life-saving technique or a sort of 'barbaric' procedure, so that after periods of great success there were periods of obsolescence. This alternation lasted approximately until the nineteenth century, when, thanks to the work of Trousseau and Chevalier Jackson, clearer rules about indications and techniques were set. But the present popularity of this technique has been boosted by developments in the past 60 years: first, the poliomyelitis epidemics in the 1950s contributed to the inclusion of prolonged mechanical ventilation among the main indications for tracheostomy, which was until then mainly employed for upper airway obstruction; and second and third, respectively, the development of tracheostomy tubes specifically designed to minimize tracheal injury and percutaneous dilational techniques that made this procedure simpler and feasible at the bedside. Despite their frequent interchangeable use, the terms tracheostomy and tracheotomy are distinct and indicate an opening in the trachea with or without a surgical attachment to the skin, respectively.[8]

## PATHOPHYSIOLOGY

### Tracheostomy and humidification

Placement of a tracheostomy tube (as well as a translaryngeal tube) diverts the flow of air from the upper native airways, thus bypassing the anatomical site where inspired air is normally warmed and humidified. Tracheostomized patients, in the absence of artificial humidification, can develop chronic inflammation in the tracheal mucosa as well as squamous metaplasia[9] and dehydration of the tracheobronchial tree, with subsequent reduced ciliary function and thickened secretions. With these predisposing factors, especially in the presence of a weak cough mechanism, the patient can suffer lung atelectasis or obstruction of the cannula by mucous plugs and respiratory tract infections.

### Dead space and airflow resistance

Breathing through a tracheal cannula shortens the distance covered by air from the atmosphere to the alveolar spaces, reducing dead space by about 80–100 mL,[10] and bypasses the upper native airways, i.e. the site with the greatest share of total airway resistance: 80 per cent and 50 per cent in case of, respectively, nose or mouth breathing.[11] Based on these assumptions, it could be argued that after tracheostomy the resistive load of breathing is reduced, but other issues must be taken into account. First, while the native tracheal diameter is about 20 mm, the diameter of a standard tracheostomy cannula ranges from 7 mm to 8 mm, so that the true lumen available for the passage of air is significantly reduced after tracheostomy. Besides, flow through artificial conduits obeys Poiseuille's law, according to which resistance is directly proportional to the tube length and inversely proportional to the fourth or fifth power of the tube radius for, respectively, laminar or turbulent flow. Therefore, in every case in which the airflow is increased (high inspiratory demand) or the tube radius is reduced (small and long cannula, apposition of secretions) the patient has to cope with a higher resistive load. Tube design and features, however, allow the clinician to minimize the increased resistive load imposed by the tracheostomy cannula: presence of fenestration,[12] removal of the inner cannula[13] and deflation of the cuff[14,15] are all means of decreasing the airflow resistance and the inspiratory work of breathing.

### Tracheostomy and weaning from mechanical ventilation

Poiseuille's laws give further theoretical support to the importance of converting a translaryngeal tube into a tracheostomy one, besides the reasons already mentioned above regarding the prevention of laryngeal injury. Switching to a shorter and sometime larger tube, in fact, reduces airflow resistance and this can also increase expiratory flow and reduce dynamic hyperinflation; the decreased resistive and threshold load could facilitate the process of weaning from IMV in patients with marginal respiratory reserve. This has been confirmed both *in vitro* and *in vivo*: in a lung model with intubation manikin and artificial trachea[16] it was demonstrated that, for every experimental setting, the imposed work of breathing was lower with the tracheostomy cannula than with the translaryngeal tube. Even in a physiological study conducted on a group of difficult-to-wean patients,[17] the conversion from translaryngeal intubation to tracheostomy decreased ventilatory demand, respiratory drive, work of breathing and intrinsic positive end-expiratory pressure.

Other physiological advantages of tracheostomy include easier airway suctioning, better patient comfort and oral care, easier and more secure airway fastening, less need for sedation, enhanced ability to communicate, greater mobility and the possibility of transferring the patient from the ICU. Despite the lack of scientific demonstration, the relevance of these last factors is supported by a shared clinical practice and caregivers' experience and opinions.[18]

### Tracheostomy and swallowing

The human larynx serves three main functions: respiration, lower airway protection from inhalation of foreign material and phonation. Proper coordination between respiration and swallowing requires perfect integration of the pharyngolaryngeal muscles and reflex mechanisms. During the swallowing act, the larynx is elevated by contraction of the geniohyoid, hyoglossus and thyrohyoid muscles, the epiglottis is displaced downwards, the false cords approximate in the midline and the true vocal cords adduct. Respiration through a tracheostomy, spontaneously or mechanically assisted, implies the diversion of air from the natural laryngeal passage. Moreover, if one considers that the patient is frequently artificially tube-fed, has impaired phonation and can still be suffering from the after-effects of previous intubation, one can understand how the overall glottic function comes to a state of temporary standstill. This does not necessarily mean that the larynx undergoes a process of disuse atrophy, after tracheostomy, but simply that resumption of swallowing and phonation during the post-acute phase can be delayed and problematic. The presence of a tracheostomy tube, *per se*, can impair the process of swallowing through the following mechanisms: reduced laryngeal elevation, hindered glottic closure, decreased larynx sensitivity to the penetration of foreign material, reduced efficiency of protective cough[19] and impaired coordination between respiration and swallowing.[20] Then, the leak created by tracheostomy in the normally closed subglottic system causes the loss of subglottic pressure, a mechanism normally important for the protection of airways from aspiration[21] and for the preservation of the physiological benefit of so-called pursed-lips breathing, a mechanism which, generating physiological positive end-expiratory pressure, is a useful compensatory mechanism in cases of intrathoracic airflow obstruction.[22] The presence of an inflated tracheostomy cuff represents a worsening situation, since it favours anchoring of the larynx to the anterior neck, which limits the process of elevation, delays the onset of the swallowing reflex, and increases the amount of bolus retention in the pharyngeal valleculae.[23]

## EVIDENCE BASE

There is little evidence-based literature serving as a guide for the management of the tracheostomized patient.[24] Clinicians caring for these patients generally achieve a certain degree of skill and experience based on recommendations derived from shared clinical procedures, commonsense and accepted routine practice. We will briefly review some debated points on which a sufficient degree of agreement can be found.

### Indications

Until the mid-twentieth century the main indication for tracheostomy was upper airway obstruction due to a foreign body, trauma or infection, especially diphtheria. However, at present, indications in the critically ill patient are as follows:

- access to the airway in patients requiring long-term mechanical ventilation
- removal of airway secretions in cases of a weak cough mechanism or failure, to protect the lower airways against the risk of aspiration of oral or gastric material
- relief of upper airway obstruction, generally not as a first choice, but after an initial translaryngeal intubation or emergency cricothyroidotomy.[25]

### Timing

Despite the absence of clear guidelines, current and generally accepted recommendations suggest considering the performance of tracheostomy when IMV is expected to last longer than 3 weeks.[26] The procedure, however, should not follow strict rules regarding time, but should be tailored to the individual patient, taking into account the underlying cause of respiratory failure and the clinical course. A simple approach to the problem is to allow the patient at least 1 week after the acute onset of respiratory failure in order to achieve clinical stabilization and possible resolution; at the end of this period the patient is re-evaluated and, if extubation is considered likely within the following week, translaryngeal intubation could be prolonged, otherwise tracheostomy can be planned and carried out even earlier than the third week of IMV. Another strategy, not alternative but complementary to the previous one, takes into account the underlying disease: if the cause of respiratory failure is an acute lung injury or a postoperative critical state, intubation can be protracted, since the resolution of the disease within the first week can be expected. In cases of acute respiratory distress syndrome or exacerbation of chronic lung disease a wait-and-watch strategy can be the best choice, allowing a longer time for the resolution while maintaining the patient under close observation on a day-to-day basis. Last, when respiratory failure is the consequence of a neuromuscular disease, severe head or spinal trauma, then the caring team can plan a tracheostomy even within the first week.

According to the most relevant published trials, clinicians refer to as 'early' tracheostomy the performance of the procedure within the first week of ICU admission, even as early as the second day of IMV, while 'late' tracheostomy is commonly carried out after 2 weeks of IMV. A recent systematic review on this topic[27] concluded that timing of tracheostomy did not alter mortality and the risk of pneumonia, but patients undergoing early tracheostomy had a shorter duration of IMV and of ICU stay.

## CLINICAL APPLICATIONS

### Choice of cannula

Metal tubes, formerly used for permanent placement after laryngectomy, are seldom used nowadays due to their high cost and design limitations. Plastic tubes, on the other hand, are currently available in a huge variety of models, size and design, and can fit almost any kind of patient and any individual need and peculiarity. The choice of the cannula depends on several factors:

- need for IMV
- ability to protect the lower airways
- temporary or permanent use
- specific anatomical problems (neck size and length, deformities)
- presence of tracheal or glottic stenosis.

The ideal tracheostomy tube should meet all the above requirements, should facilitate proper speech and swallowing function and should minimize complications. One of the first features to consider is the size: this should be a compromise between the size of stoma, in order to allow an easy introduction, and the size of the native airway, in order to achieve a proper airway seal without the need to overinflate the cuff. Tubes are identified by three measurements: inner diameter (ID), outer diameter (OD) and length: as a simple rule, a 10 mm OD and an 11 mm OD are generally adequate for women and men, respectively. Tubes can be angled or curved and can be available in standard size as well as with the proximal or the distal segment longer, in order to adjust to different anatomical variants.[28] Some tubes are made of silicone and are reinforced by an inner spiral wire so that they never kink or collapse: they are specially helpful for tracheal stenosis, tracheomalacia and thoracic deformities; the presence of an adjustable flange allows the clinician to easily advance or withdraw the cannula up to the desired length. Note that these tubes are incompatible with magnetic resonance imaging, lasers and electrosurgical devices.

Other specially designed tubes have a suction port just above the cuff, in order to facilitate the aspiration of subglottic secretions, whose role in the onset of early ventilator-associated pneumonia has been evidenced in recent years;[29] the extra suction channel requires a tube with a greater OD and great care to avoid obstruction from mucus plugs.

## Fenestration

Fenestrated tubes are similar to non-fenestrated ones, but have an opening in the posterior curved portion above the cuff, which can be single or multiple. These cannulas have a disposal inner cannula available with and without fenestration: only when the fenestrated inner cannula is in place, the opening is complete and effective. During expiration, air passes through the fenestration and crosses the glottis, thus facilitating phonation; this process can be enhanced by the deflation of the cuff and by capping the cannula, and requires, of course, optimal adaptation to the patient's anatomy, so that the fenestration is properly positioned in the middle of the tracheal lumen. Our suggestion is to leave the fenestration open only temporarily; if the fenestration is left open permanently, the posterior tracheal wall can be drawn inwards by suction, leading to adherence and granulation inside the cannula with problems during airway clearance and serious risks during cannula replacement.

## Inner cannula

The presence of an inner cannula, in the so-called dual-cannula tubes, prevents the deposition of thickened secretions into the internal lumen, thus maintaining its full patency and postponing the time of replacement: the reusable inner cannula is removed and cleaned while the new one is positioned. The presence of an inner cannula, however, reduces the true ID and this can have an influence on the inspiratory resistive load[13] and the imposed work of breathing. The advantages of the inner cannula are better appreciated in long-term domiciliary management, where delayed replacement and the possibility of relieving a sudden obstruction by simply pulling out the inner cannula are highly desirable.

## Cuff management

Tracheostomy tubes may or may not have an inflatable cuff, which is designed to seal the residual natural airspace between the cannula and the tracheal wall. The maintenance of a closed system is desirable for those patients who cannot protect their lower airways from spillage of nose and mouth secretions, in order to prevent respiratory tract infections, but it is mainly indicated during IMV to avoid leaks and to achieve full control and easier manipulation of gas exchange. This is not mandatory, since 'open' ventilation using cuffless tubes can be effectively performed by experienced teams[30,31] in patients with preserved glottic function and adequate pulmonary compliance. The cuff should be inflated with air up to a pressure not higher than the tracheal capillary perfusion pressure, to avoid mucosal ischaemia: to this purpose it is generally agreed that a maximum intracuff pressure of 25 mm Hg (or 35 cm $H_2O$) is acceptable.[28] Monitoring cuff pressure with only manual appreciation of the pilot balloon tension can be misleading, therefore the manoeuvre should be done with a manometer every time that the cuff is inflated or deflated, in case of leaks, or when the cannula is repositioned or replaced.

Cuffs are available in three different kinds:

- Low-volume high-pressure cuffs, also called tight-to-shaft cuffs, when deflated, perfectly adhere to the tube surface without forming wrinkles. They are silicone-made and permeable to gas, so that they must be filled with sterile water instead of air. The only advantage of these tubes is the easier insertion through the stoma, and the better air passage when the cuff is deflated, but, apart from these, they are seldom used due to the higher risk of mucosal ischaemia.
- High-volume low-pressure cuffs are most commonly used for the specific design that reduces the risk of tracheal damage. Compared with tight-to-shaft tubes, the cuff has a larger volume and, when deflated, forms protruding wrinkles and folds (Fig. 54.1); if the cuff requires overinflation to achieve a good airway seal, it is likely that the chosen cannula is too small in diameter.
- Foam-cuffed tubes have a large cuff made of polyurethane foam lined on the outer surface by a sheath of silicone. Before insertion, the cuff is evacuated, then it is allowed to re-expand without manual syringe inflation: the pilot conduit remains open to the atmosphere, so that the intra-cuff pressure equals ambient pressure. This cannula is specifically designed to avoid mucosal ischaemia and to minimize tracheal injury, but, despite this sound rationale, it has not gained widespread use.

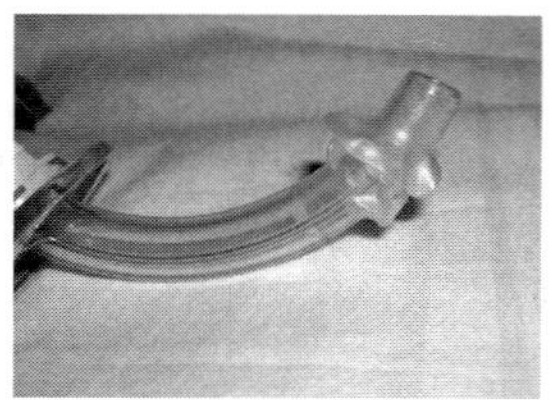

**Figure 54.1** A high-volume low-pressure cuff. When deflated, the cuff tends to get wrinkled with folds.

## Weaning from tracheostomy

When the initial cause of respiratory failure that required tracheostomy has resolved, the patient can be evaluated for possible decannulation, taking into account age, past history and baseline disease. If upper airway obstruction was the cause (e.g. epiglottitis), restoration of adequate upper airspace must be carefully evaluated by means of endoscopy; if tracheostomy was indicated for secretions clearance and for protecting the airways, then cough function and strength must be adequately evaluated, as well as swallowing function. Last, in patients tracheostomized for prolonged IMV, the persisting need for ventilatory support must be carefully evaluated: about 50–60 per cent of patients admitted to weaning centres are definitely weaned from mechanical ventilation or require it only during the night;[32] therefore, a possible conversion to non-invasive ventilation and subsequent decannulation can be considered. In summary, the baseline checklist for screening candidates for tracheostomy removal should include the following items:

- clinical stability
- mental alertness and integrity, including the capacity to understand benefits and risks of decannulation
- consent of both patient and relatives
- sufficient pulmonary reserve and stability of blood gas values
- absence of tracheal or glottic stenosis
- limited volume of airway secretions and proper cough efficiency
- adequate airway protection and swallowing mechanisms.

Cough efficiency can be evaluated by measuring peak cough flow and maximal expiratory pressure; this can be reliably measured by connecting the manometer directly to the cuffed tracheostomy tube.[33] Values as high as 160 L/min[34] and 40 cm $H_2O$[35] for, respectively, peak cough flow and maximal expiratory pressure have been indicated as desirable during the process of decannulation. In the presence of most favourable factors or in the absence of absolute contraindications, the team can proceed to the operative phase. The first step is to cap the tube for gradually longer periods in order to assess the adequacy of native airways; if the patient can comfortably breath around a capped 8 mm ID tube with deflated cuff, it is likely that his or her native airways are intact and they have sufficient pulmonary reserve. The following step can be straightforward tube removal without the intermediate phases if all the required criteria are met, otherwise gradual downsizing must be done, with the patient under close observation. Borderline cases (residual swallowing problems, abundant secretions, etc.) can be managed even with a temporary discharge with a small cannula still in place and subsequent new evaluation 2–3 months later. Among the available devices, the stomal button (Olympic Medical) enables airway access, prevents stoma closure and frees the tracheal space from the tube:[36] great care, however, must be paid when this device is in place, due to the possible risk of dislodgement and migration to the distal airways. After tube removal the stoma generally closes within a few days, especially after percutaneous dilational technique; only in very rare cases is there circumferential skin growth and lining over the mucosal edge, which prevents stoma closure and requires surgical closure.

# TECHNICAL CONSIDERATIONS

## Percutaneous dilational tracheostomy (PDT)

The percutaneous dilatational technique was proposed by Ciaglia *et al.* in 1985.[37] Those authors carried out progressive dilatation with blunt tipped dilators; since then, several other methods have been proposed to perform percutaneous tracheostomy at the bedside.[38–41] Some of them are characterized by the insertion of the tracheostomy cannula from outside the trachea: the modified original Ciaglia technique ('single step' Blue-Rhino);[38] the guidewire dilator forceps technique proposed by Griggs *et al.*;[39] and the Percu-twist as proposed by Frova and Quintel.[40] Another one is characterized by the fact that the tracheostomy cannula is inserted from inside the trachea: the translaryngeal technique proposed by Fantoni and Ripamonti.[41]

The Blue-Rhino is characterized by a modification of the original Ciaglia technique simplified with only one single dilator. An initial skin incision and blunt preparation of the pretracheal tissue may be helpful in identifying the tracheal rings, thus avoiding either too high or too low tracheal puncture. After dilatation with the maximal available dilator, a tracheal cannula (inner diameter up to 9 mm) can be inserted while mounted on a corresponding dilator. The main problems related to this technique are difficult ventilation, bleeding, and rupture or dislocation of the tracheal rings.

The Grigg technique is characterized by the use of forceps for blunt dilatation of the pretracheal and intercartilagineous tissue after insertion of the guide wire into the trachea and skin incision. Applying this method on patients with a short and or thick neck may be difficult, if not dangerous, particularly while attempting to perform intercartilagineous dilation. The main problems of this technique are that dilation with forceps is not easily calibrated with the cannula diameter, rupture or dislocation of tracheal rings, and difficult ventilation. The Percu-twist technique is characterized by a controlled rotating dilation performed by an external spiral, which should reduce tracheal wall collapse during the manoeuvre. One problem encountered with this technique is the rupture or dislocation of tracheal rings. All these percutaneous techniques are characterized by the dilation of the tissues with the forces being applied from the outside to the inside of the tracheal wall.

The translaryngeal technique is different from the previous ones because the cannula is stripped from inside to outside. In contrast with other techniques the initial puncture of the trachea is carried out with the needle directed cranially and the tracheal cannula inserted with a pull-through technique along the orotracheal route. This modification in the direction of the forces should favour: much less injury of the tissues and tracheal wall itself, both in the anterior and posterior wall; reduced bleeding; the possibility to ventilate during the manoeuvre; and possible application of this technique in paediatric patients in which all other techniques are contraindicated. The major problems related to this technique are: difficulty in intubating the patients with a rigid fibrescope; need for several intubations and extubations (thus this technique is contraindicated in patients with difficult intubation and in those in whom the extension of the neck has to be avoided); difficulties in ventilation during the manoeuvre; and not suitable in an emergency.

While performing percutaneous tracheostomy, independently from the technique, several tools have been suggested to improve the safety of the manoeuvre:

- bronchoscopy with simple endoscopy or video-assisted endoscopy to facilitate and reduce possible complications[42]
- previous evaluation by chest radiography, magnetic resonance imaging (MRI) and ultrasound assessment prior to percutaneous dilational tracheostomy in patients with altered neck and tracheal anatomy[43]
- chest X-ray following dilatational percutaneous tracheostomy after procedures noted to be difficult by the physician.[44]

In particular clinical situations the usefulness of ultrasound-guided control and the use of a laryngeal mask has also been reported.[45,46]

Finally, the following must be standardized: correct ventilatory procedure in pressure control, inspired oxygen fraction of 1.0 and positive end-expiratory pressure of 0 cm $H_2O$; although some authors have demonstrated that the procedure is safe even with the use of high positive end-expiratory pressures in patients with severe respiratory failure.[47]

### Surgical tracheostomy

Surgical tracheostomy is usually carried out in the operating theatre, despite similar outcomes being achievable in the ICU, provided that proper equipment and adequate staff are available. After a horizontal incision, superficial vessels are ligated and the thyroid isthmus is transected or moved away from the incision. The second or third tracheal ring is identified and cut about 1.5–2 cm below the cricoid membrane; it is in fact important to create the stoma far from the cricoid cartilage to avoid damaging this structure, as it is the only complete cartilagineous ring in the upper airway. Subglottic stenosis is a likely occurrence after cricoid cartilage injury, due to the loss of laryngeal integrity. The stoma is made through the anterior tracheal wall by means of an incision that can be horizontal, vertical or cruciate, although most surgeons seem to prefer the horizontal incision.

### Comparison of percutaneous dilatational technique with surgical tracheostomy

Percutaneous tracheostomy can be performed immediately, once the decision has been made, whereas surgical tracheostomy requires more organization and, if it is to be done in the operating theatre, time scheduling. The time required for percutaneous tracheostomy is generally shorter than that for the surgical route, and implies less stress to the patient and better use of resources. Although a cost comparison between percutaneous and surgical tracheostomies is not easy because of varying reimbursment systems and hospital structures, available studies show that percutaneous tracheostomy is considerably cheaper than the surgical route: it is in fact commonsense that if fewer personnel and no operating theatre are required, the overall cost of percutaneous tracheostomy will be lower than that of surgical tracheostomy.[48] In Table 54.1 we present the randomized trials comparing percutaneous and surgical tracheostomies. The majority of the prospective randomized trials reported that the potential advantages of percutaneous technique relative to surgical tracheostomy include ease of performance, lower incidence of peristomal bleeding and post-operative infection associated with lower costs, although the real clinical impact of these study results is limited by the heterogeneity of the samples and percutaneous techniques employed.

## FUTURE RESEARCH

In conclusion, tracheostomy can offer several advantages in the management of critically ill patients who need mechanical ventilation and/or control of airways. The right timing of tracheostomy remains controversial, but it appears that early tracheostomy in selected patients, such as in severe trauma and neurological patients, could be effective in reducing intensive care stay and associated costs. Percutaneous tracheostomy techniques are becoming the procedure of choice in the majority of cases, because these are safe, easy, quick to do, and the complications and costs, compared with surgical tracheostomies, seem to be lower.

**Table 54.1** Comparison between surgical (ST) and percutaneous (PDT) tracheostomy techniques: randomized trials

| Study | Type | No. of patients | Type of patients | Intubation/ tracheostomy length* (days) | Bleeding (no. of patients) | Infections (no. of patients) | Intraoperative complications† (no. of patients) | Postoperative complications‡ (no. of patients) | ICU deaths (no. of patients) |
|---|---|---|---|---|---|---|---|---|---|
| Holdgaard *et al.*[49] | ST/PDT | 60 | Medical/trauma | 6.7/9.9 | 36/9 | 19/3 | 26/19 | 30/7 | N/A |
| Heikkinen *et al.*[50] | ST/PDT | 56 | Medical/trauma | N/A | 1/5 | 0/0 | 0/1 | N/A | 0/0 |
| Freeman *et al.*[51] | ST/PDT | 80 | Medical/surgical | 14.1/N/A | 2/0 | N/A | N/A | 1/0 | 1/0 |
| Friedman *et al.*[52] | ST/PDT | 53 | Medical | 19.2/21.5 | 7/5 | 4/0 | 11/9 | 12/3 | 9/10 |
| Massick *et al.*[53] | ST/PDT | 164 | Miscellaneous | 9.7/N/A | 11/4 | 3/1 | 8/2 | 30/5 | 0/1 |
| Crofts *et al.*[54] | ST/PDT | 53 | Medical/trauma | 11.5/N/A | 3/3 | 1/0 | N/A | 10/6 | 14/8 |
| Hazard *et al.*[55] | ST/PDT | 46 | Medical/trauma | 8.4/19.4 | 4/1 | 8/1 | N/A | 11/3 | 18/10 |
| Porter *et al.*[56] | ST/PDT | 53 | Medical/trauma | 11.1/N/A | 0/0 | 0/0 | 1/5 | 0/0 | 0/1 |
| Gysin *et al.*[57] | ST/PDT | 70 | N/A | 6.6/N/A | 4/4 | 3/4 | 4/14 | 1/6 | 0/0 |
| Antonelli *et al.*[58] | ST/PDT | 139 | Medical/trauma | 10/N/A | 2/1 | 2/5 | 2/2 | 1/1 | 0/0 |
| Silvester *et al.*[59] | ST/PDT | 200 | Medical/surgical | 6/N/A | 2/7 | 1/1 | 14/13 | 9/6 | |

*Intubation and tracheostomy length: means days of translaryngeal intubations/days of tracheostomy.
†Hypotension; hypoxia; subcutaneous emphysema; cuff puncture; difficulties in tube placement.
‡Accidental decannulation; cannula obstruction; tracheitis; tracheal stenosis; pneumothorax.
NA, not available.

The surgical technique should be considered when contraindications to percutaneous techniques are present, such as anatomical difficulties or previously failed percutaneous technique. No one percutaneous technique seems superior in comparison with the rest, but the experience of the operator and clinical, individual, anatomical and physiopathological characteristics of the patient should always be considered.

## REFERENCES


1. Metha S, Hill NS. Noninvasive ventilation. *Am J Respir Crit Care Med* 2001; **163**: 540–77.
2. Esteban A, Anzueto A, Frutos F *et al.* Characteristics and outcomes in adult patients receiving mechanical ventilation. *JAMA* 2002; **287**: 345–55.
3. Nevins ML, Epstein SK. Weaning from prolonged mechanical ventilation. *Clin Chest Med* 2001; **22**: 13–33.
4. Bishop MJ. Mechanism of laryngotracheal injury following prolonged tracheal intubation. *Chest* 1989; **96**: 185–6.
5. Whited RE. Laryngeal disfunction following prolonged intubation. *Ann Otol Rhinol Laryngol* 1979; **88**: 474–8.
6. Whited RE. A prospective study of laryngotracheal sequelae in long-term intubation. *Laryngoscope* 1984; **94**: 367–77.
7. Szmuk P, Ezri T, Evron S *et al.* A brief history of tracheostomy and tracheal intubation from the bronze age to the space age. *Int Care Med* 2008; **34**: 222–8.
8. Reibel JF. Tracheotomy/tracheostomy. *Respir Care* 1999; **44**: 820–3.
9. Motoyama E. Physiologic alterations in tracheostomy. In: Myers E, Stool SE, Johnson JT, eds. *Tracheotomy.* New York: Churchill Livingstone, 1985:177–200.
10. Chadda K, Louis B, Benaissa L *et al.* Physiological effects of decannulation in tracheotomised patients. *Intensive Care Med* 2002; **28**: 1761–7.
11. Epstein SK. Anatomy and physiology of tracheotomy. *Respir Care* 2005; **50**: 476–82.
12. Hussey JD, Bishop MJ. Pressures required to move gas through the native airway in the presence of a fenestrated vs a nonfenestrated tracheostomy tube. *Chest* 1996; **110**: 494–7.
13. Cowan T, Op't Holt TB, Gegenheimer C *et al.* Effect of inner cannula removal on the work of breathing imposed by tracheotomy tubes: a bench study. *Respir Care* 2001; **46**: 460–5.
14. Beard B, Monaco MJ. Tracheostomy discontinuation: impact of tube selection on resistance during tube occlusion. *Respir Care* 1993; **38**: 267–70.
15. Ceriana P, Carlucci A, Navalesi P *et al.* Physiological responses during a T-piece weaning trial with a deflated tube. *Intensive Care Med* 2006; **32**: 1399–403.
16. Davis K Jr, Branson RD, Porembka D. A comparison of the imposed work of breathing with endotracheal and tracheostomy tubes in a lung model. *Respir Care* 1994; **39**: 611–16.
17. Diehl JL, Atrous S, Touchard D *et al.* Changes in the work of breathing induced by tracheotomy in ventilator-dependent patients. *Am J Respir Crit Care Med* 1999; **159**: 383–8.
18. Astrachan DI, Kirchner JC, Goodwin WJJ. Prolonged intubation vs tracheotomy: complications, practical and psychological consideration. *Laryngoscope* 1988; **98**: 1165–9.
19. Nash M. Swallowing problems in the tracheotomized patient. *Otolaryngol Clin North Am* 1988; **21**: 701–9.
20. Shaker R, Dodds WJ, Dantas RO *et al.* Coordination of deglutitive glottic closure with oropharyngeal swallowing. *Gastroenterology* 1990; **98**: 1478–84.
21. Eibling DE, Diez Gross R. Subglottic air pressure: a key component of swallowing efficiency. *Ann Otol Rhinol Laryngol* 1996; **105**: 253–8.
22. Higenbottam T, Payne J. Glottis narrowing in lung disease. *Am Rev Respir Dis* 1982; **125**: 746–50.
23. Devita MA, Spierer-Rundback MS. Swallowing disorders in patients with prolonged intubation or tracheostomy tubes. *Crit Care Med* 1990; **18**: 1328–32.
24. Littlewood KE. Evidence-based management of tracheotomies in hospitalized patients. *Respir Care* 2005; **50**: 516–18.
25. Heffner JE. Tracheotomy application and timing. *Clin Chest Med* 2003; **24**: 389–98.
26. Make BJ, Hill NS, Goldberg AI *et al.* Mechanical ventilation beyond the intensive care unit. Report of a consensus conference of the American College of Chest Physicians. *Chest* 1998; **113**: 289S–344S.
27. Griffiths J, Barber VS, Morgan L *et al.* Systematic review and meta-analysis of studies of the timing of tracheostomy in adult patients undergoing artificial ventilation. *BMJ* 2005; **330**: 1243.
28. Hess DR. Tracheostomy tubes and related appliances. *Respir Care* 2005; **50**: 497–510.
29. Depew CL, McCarthy MS. Subglottic secretion drainage: a literature review. *AACN Adv Crit Care* 2007; **18**: 366–79.
30. Bach JR, Alba AS. Tracheostomy ventilation: a study of efficacy with deflated cuffs and cuffless tubes. *Chest* 1990; **97**: 679–83.
31. Gregoretti C, Squadrone V, Fogliati C *et al.* Transtracheal open ventilation in acute respiratory failure secondary to severe chronic obstructive pulmonary disease exacerbation. *Am J Respir Crit Care Med* 2006; **173**: 877–81.
32. Ceriana P, Delmastro M, Rampulla C *et al.* Demographics and clinical outcomes of patients admitted to a respiratory intensive care unit located in a rehabilitation center. *Respir Care* 2003; **48**: 670–6.
33. Vitacca M, Paneroni M, Bianchi L *et al.* Maximal inspiratory and expiratory pressures measurement in tracheotomised patients. *Eur Respir J* 2006; **27**: 343–9.
34. Bach JR, Saporito LR. Criteria for extubation and tracheotomy tube removal for patients with ventilatory failure. *Chest* 1996; **110**: 1566–71.

35. Ceriana P, Carlucci A, Navalesi P *et al.* Weaning from tracheotomy in long-term mechanically ventilated patients: feasibility of a decisional flowchart and clinical outcome. *Intensive Care Med* 2003; **29**: 845–8.
36. Long J, West G. Evaluation of the Olympic Trach-Button as a precursor to tracheotomy tube removal. *Respir Care Clin North Am* 1980; **25**: 1242–3.
37. Ciaglia P, Firshing R, Syniec C. Elective percutaneous dilatational tracheostomy: a new simple bedside procedure: preliminary report. *Chest* 1985; **87**: 715–19.
38. Byhahn C, Wilke HJ, Halbig S *et al.* Percutaneous tracheostomy: Ciaglia Blue Rhino versus the basic Ciaglia technique of percutaneous dilatational tracheostomy. *Anesth Analg* 2000; **91**: 882–6.
39. Griggs WM, Worthley LIG, Gilligan JE *et al.* A simple percutaneous tracheostomy technique. *Surg Gynec Obstet* 1990; **170**: 543–5.
40. Frova G, Quintel M. A new simple method for percutaneous tracheostomy: controlled rotating dilating. A preliminary report. *Intensive Care Med* 2002; **28**: 299–303.
41. Fantoni A, Ripamonti D. A non derivative, non-surgical tracheostomy: the translaryngeal method. *Intensive Care Med* 1997; **23**: 386–92.
42. Oberwalser M, Weis H, Nehoda H *et al.* Videobronchoscopic guidance makes percutaneous dilational tracheostomy safer. *Surg Endosc* 2004; **18**: 839–42.
43. Muhammad JK, Major E, Patton DW. Evaluating the neck for percutaneous dilatational tracheostomy. *J Craniomaxillofac Surg* 2000; **28**: 336–42.
44. Datta D, Onyirimba F, McNamee MJ. The utility of chest radiographs following percutaneous dilatational tracheostomy. *Chest* 2003; **123**: 1603–6.
45. Rustic A, Zupan Z, Antoncic I. Ultrasound-guided percutaneous dilatational tracheostomy with laryngeal mask airway control in a morbidly obese patients. *J Clin Anesth* 2004; **16**: 121–3.
46. Dosemeci L, Yilmaz M, Gurpinar F *et al.* The use of the laryngeal mask airway as an alternative to the endotracheal tube during percutaneous dilatational tracheostomy. *Intensive Care Med* 2002; **28**: 63–7.
47. Beiderlinden M, Groeben H, Peters J. Safety of percutaneous dilatational tracheostomy in patients ventilated with high positive end expiratory pressure (PEEP). *Intensive Care Med* 2003; **29**: 944–8.
48. Kaylie DM, Andersen PE, Wax MK. An analysis of time and staff utilization for open versus percutaneous tracheostomies. *Otolaryngol Head Neck Surg* 2003; **128**: 109–14.
49. Holdgaard HO, Pedersen J, Jensen RH *et al.* Percutaneous dilatational tracheostomy versus conventional surgical tracheostomy: a clinical randomized trial. *Acta Anesthesiol Scand* 1998; **42**: 545–50.
50. Heikkinen M, Aarnio P, Hannukainen J. Percutaneous dilatational tracheostomy or conventional surgical tracheostomy? *Crit Care Med* 2000; **28**: 1399–402.
51. Freeman BD, Isabella K, Cobb JP *et al.* A prospective, randomized study comparing percutaneous with surgical tracheostomy in critically ill patients. *Crit Care Med* 2001; **29**: 926–30.
52. Friedman Y, Fildes J, Mizock B *et al.* Comparison of percutaneous and surgical tracheostomies. *Chest* 1996; **110**: 480–5.
53. Massick DD, Yao S, Powell DM *et al.* Bedside tracheostomy in the intensive care unit: a prospective randomized trial comparing open surgical tracheostomy with endoscopically guided percutaneous dilatational tracheotomy. *Laryngoscope* 2001; **111**: 494–500.
54. Crofts SL, Alzeer A, McGuire M *et al.* A comparison of percutaneous and operative tracheostomies in intensive care patients. *Can J Anaesth* 1999; **42**: 775–9.
55. Hazard P, Jones C, Benitone J. Comparative clinical trial of standard operative tracheostomy. *Crit Care Med* 1991; **19**: 1018–24.
56. Porter JM, Ivatury RR. Preferred route of tracheostomy-percutaneous versus open at the bedside: a randomized, prospective study in the surgical intensive care unit. *Am Surg* 1999; **65**: 142–6.
57. Gysin C, Dulguerov P, Guyot JP *et al.* Percutaneous versus surgical tracheostomy: a double blind randomized trial. *Ann Surg* 1990; **230**: 708–14.
58. Antonelli M, Michetti V, Di Palma A *et al.* Percutaneous translaryngeal versus surgical tracheostomy: a randomized trial with 1-yr double blind follow-up. *Crit Care Med* 2005; **33**: 1015–20.
59. Silvester W, Goldsmith D, Uchino S *et al.* Percutaneous versus surgical tracheostomy: a randomized controlled study with long-term follow-up. *Crit Care Med* 2006; **34**: 2145–52.

55

# Non-invasive ventilation in end-of-life care

LAURA EVANS, MITCHELL M LEVY

## ABSTRACT

Non-invasive ventilation (NIV) is frequently used in the management of acute respiratory failure; however the use of NIV at the end of life remains controversial. In selected patients with acute respiratory failure and a do-not-intubate (DNI) order, the use of NIV may improve survival. In this patient population, it is critical that the patient, family and clinicians have a clear understanding of the risks, benefits and expected outcomes of NIV as well as the alternatives to NIV prior to its initiation. The mechanism by which the success of NIV will be gauged should be clearly stated, as should the plan of care if NIV fails to achieve the stated goals of therapy. Frequent reassessment of patient tolerance of NIV is essential. At the end of life, patients who do not desire life-prolonging treatment may potentially benefit from NIV. NIV may alleviate dyspnoea while preserving the ability to communicate, decreasing the need for opiates or benzodiazepines, or extending life for a period of time sufficient to complete end-of-life tasks. However, NIV is a form of life support and its use may be inappropriate in patients who have decided to limit life-sustaining treatments because of their current quality of life or other personal reasons. In patients who do not want life-sustaining measures, use of NIV may reduce the clarity of patients', families' and clinicians' understanding of the goals of care. All members of the multidisciplinary team should be involved in decisions regarding NIV at the end of life in order to minimize ambiguity for patients and families. During clinician–patient or clinician–family meetings in which information is conveyed about patient status, prognosis and preferences, discussion of NIV is essential when discussing life-sustaining therapies. Clinicians should provide patients/families a clear description of NIV, the potential risks, benefits and alternatives, and elicit information about the patient's preferences.

## INTRODUCTION

Non-invasive ventilation (NIV) is commonly and increasingly used in acute and critical care settings as a part of standard management of acute respiratory failure in certain patient populations.[1] Non-invasive ventilation has been demonstrated to decrease the need for endotracheal intubation, hospital length of stay and mortality among certain subsets of patients. Patient populations that have benefited include those with hypercapnic respiratory failure from chronic obstructive pulmonary disease (COPD), immunocompromised patients with hypoxaemic respiratory failure and patients with acute cardiogenic pulmonary oedema without active cardiac ischaemia.[2–11] In these clinical conditions use of NIV is widely accepted. However, the use of NIV for acute respiratory failure in patients who have declined intubation (do not intubate [DNI]), and for palliation of dyspnoea at the end of life remains controversial.[12–14] In patients at the end of life who have a stated desire to survive hospitalization, NIV may be of benefit. Some observational data suggest that DNI patients with acute respiratory failure may have improved outcomes compared with those who are not treated with NIV. Also, NIV may potentially offer benefit to patients at the end of life, even those who do not desire life-prolonging treatment. NIV alleviates respiratory distress while preserving the ability to communicate, by decreasing the need for opiates or benzodiazepines and by providing a form of life support for a period of time sufficient to complete end-of-life tasks and finalize personal affairs. Conversely NIV is a form of life support and its use may be inappropriate in patients who have decided to limit life-sustaining treatments because of their current quality of life or other personal reasons.[15] Additionally, use of NIV in DNR/DNI patients may lead to a lack of clarity about the goals of care among patients, families and clinicians with potential negative effects on patient/family and clinician communication.

Deaths in the intensive care unit (ICU) frequently occur in the context of withholding or withdrawal of life-sustaining treatment.[16–18] Epidemiologic data have found that approximately 20 per cent of Americans will die in an ICU or shortly after an ICU stay. In this context, ICU clinicians are very likely to face decisions of whether to offer or initiate NIV at the end of life. Some data suggest that decisions about NIV at the end of life already occur frequently. In a recent survey of Canadian intensivists, pulmonologists and respiratory therapists, clinicians reported that NIV is very frequently offered to or initiated in patients with a DNR order when the cause of acute respiratory failure is reversible. In these circumstances, over 80 per cent of respondents reported they offer or initiate NIV 'at least sometimes' in DNR patients with acute respiratory failure due to COPD or cardiogenic pulmonary oedema. Furthermore, 40 per cent of physicians and 50.5 per cent of respiratory therapists reported that they 'at least sometimes' offered or initiated NIV in patients receiving comfort measures only.[19] In this study, clinicians reported they were more likely to use NIV for patients with COPD or cardiogenic pulmonary oedema and less likely to use NIV for patients with an underlying malignancy. Of interest, respiratory therapists reported they were most commonly asked to initiate NIV to help families come to terms with the patients' end of life, and less commonly in order to allow patients to finalize personal affairs. In contrast, physicians reported they were most likely to use NIV to relieve dyspnoea or to provide time for patients to get their affairs in order. Additionally, a recent survey conducted in European respiratory intermediate care and high dependency units reported use of NIV as the limit of ventilatory care in 402/1292 (31 per cent) patients.[17] Since clinicians in ICUs and those who treat patients with advanced respiratory diseases are very likely to participate in decisions regarding the use of NIV at the end of life, the goal of this chapter is to provide a discussion of patient and clinician factors that should be considered in the decision-making process surrounding the use of NIV at the end of life.

## PATIENT FACTORS

### Use of non-invasive ventilation as the limit of ventilatory assistance in patients with DNR/DNI orders

Observational studies have suggested that use of NIV in DNI patients with acute respiratory failure may lead to decreased hospital mortality. A study of 114 consecutive patients with acute respiratory failure treated with NIV reported 43 per cent of patients survived to hospital discharge. In the same study, patients with COPD and cardiogenic pulmonary oedema had rates of survival to hospital discharge of 50 per cent and 70 per cent, respectively, with patients with a diagnosed malignancy faring less well.[20] Another observational study reported similar findings, with 35 per cent of DNI patients treated with NIV surviving to hospital discharge. In the subgroup of patients with advanced malignancy and acute respiratory failure, only 15 per cent survived to hospital discharge.[21] However, in a study of 23 patients with advanced stage solid cancer and acute respiratory failure treated with NIV, 61 per cent survived to hospital discharge and 39 per cent survived to 6 months.[22] Pneumonia and COPD exacerbation were the most common precipitants of acute respiratory failure in this study.

In patients with acute respiratory failure who have decided to forego intubation and mechanical ventilation after consideration of the risks/benefits and expected outcomes of therapy, NIV may be a therapeutic option if it is in keeping with the established goals of care. Prior to initiation of NIV, it is critical that the patient, family and clinicians have a clear understanding of the possible outcomes of NIV. Their discussion should include the wishes of the patient for survival, as well as possible time limits of NIV. Potential use of NIV, including the risks, benefits and alternatives, should be incorporated into discussions of other life-sustaining treatments. The intended effect of NIV in this situation should be to restore the patient to their previous state of health (if so desired by the patient) or to prolong life for a sufficient period of time to accomplish a predefined goal (i.e. arrival of a family member). It should also provide comfort through the relief of dyspnoea. Frequent reassessment of the success or failure of NIV, including patient tolerance, should be performed. If NIV fails to accomplish the previously defined goals or the patient cannot tolerate NIV, these aspects of care should be reviewed with the patient or family and careful consideration should be given to changing the goals of care and withdrawing NIV.

### Use of non-invasive ventilation as palliative therapy in patients receiving comfort measures only

Dyspnoea is a common and distressing symptom for patients and families at the end of life.[23] Medications used to alleviate dyspnoea at the end of life, usually opiates and benzodiazepines, may result in sedation as a side effect. While relieving distressing symptoms, such sedation and resultant hypoventilation may potentially hasten death. Clinicians recognize and accept this 'double effect' because the intended effects are relief of burdensome symptoms and the provision of comfort at the end of life in patients who have decided to forego life-extending treatments.[24] While patients and families place great value on maintaining comfort at the end of life, they also find value in maintaining the ability to communicate.[25,26] NIV may potentially alleviate dyspnoea while preserving cognition and the patients' ability to communicate although data regarding this effect at the end of life are scant. In patients with neuromuscular diseases not specifically at the end of life, studies have shown that NIV reduces dyspnoea and improves quality of life.[27–29] Additionally NIV may relieve dyspnoea in patients with acute respiratory failure from COPD[30,31] and advanced cancer.[22] It is unknown how use of NIV for palliation of dyspnoea compares with pharmacological therapies, nor is it known if any additional benefit is derived from the use of NIV in combination with pharmacological treatment. No studies to date have addressed the overall risk/benefit relationship of NIV in patients who want only comfort measures. Potential negative effects of NIV in this patient population include discomfort and skin breakdown associated with a tight fitting mask, prolongation of the dying process, and reducing the clarity of goals of care. Indeed, the use of NIV may be perceived as an escalation in the level of care.[14] A request for NIV when the goal of care is comfort may represent ambiguity or uneasiness with the plan of care. This should be explored during discussions with the patient and/or family.

Communication between the patient/family and clinician is of utmost importance when considering use of NIV as a palliative therapy in patients who want comfort measures only. As mentioned, the goal of NIV in this setting is to maximize comfort through relief of dyspnoea while minimizing adverse effects of opiates and benzodiazepines, without causing significant discomfort from the NIV mask. This intention must be emphasized to patients and their loved ones, as the ability to tolerate NIV varies across patient populations. Patients should not be encouraged to tolerate discomfort from the NIV mask if the goal of care is comfort. Furthermore, patients and families should understand that they may choose to discontinue NIV if it is too burdensome. This aspect of care is particularly true for families, for whom discontinuation may evoke ambivalence and distress. Since one of the theoretical benefits of NIV as a palliative therapy is maintenance of the patient's ability to communicate, the burden of NIV at the end of life for patients who cannot communicate probably outweighs any potential benefit, and use of NIV in this setting should be discouraged. Frequent reassessment of the success or failure of NIV, as well as patient tolerance, should be performed. If NIV fails to improve patient comfort, it should be discontinued and symptoms should be palliated with pharmacological measures without the use of NIV.

## CLINICIAN FACTORS

Multiple studies have identified communication between patients/families and clinicians as an aspect of care needing improvement.[32–34] Patients and families report that talking with doctors and other clinicians who are comfortable talking about death is an important part of preparation for the end of life.[25] Unfortunately, many clinicians find caring for dying patients to be emotionally and psychologically stressful.[35,36] Establishing goals of care during end-of-life discussions can contribute to the stress associated with caring for dying patients.[37] However clinician comfort and skill with communication regarding end-of-life issues are essential and can have long-lasting impact on families after the death of their loved one.[38,39]

Different members of the multidisciplinary care team may have varied opinions and expectations about the use of NIV at the end of life. Sinuff reported that physicians were more likely than respiratory therapists to believe that NIV has additive benefit as a supplement to pharmacological management of dyspnoea and facilitates verbal communication with families and clinicians for patients who have opted for DNR status or comfort measures only.[19] In the same study, pulmonologists were more likely than intensivists to believe that NIV offers additive benefit for relief of dyspnoea. The observed difference between physicians and respiratory therapists' opinions about the utility of NIV in relieving dyspnoea and improving the patient's ability to communicate suggests a potential area of concern about communication among members of the multidisciplinary team. It is important to recognize the possibility of giving mixed-messages to patients and their families. No studies to date have examined nurses' perception of the efficacy of NIV in relieving dyspnoea and facilitating communication at the end of life. As nurses and respiratory therapists are likely to spend more time at the bedside of patients on NIV than physicians do, understanding their perceptions of the utility of NIV at the end of life is essential to providing the best possible end-of-life care for critically ill patients and their families. We suggest that all members of the multidisciplinary team should be involved in decisions regarding NIV at the end of life in order to provide consistent recommendations and minimize ambiguity for patients and families. Additionally, in a 'shared decision-making' model, discussion of NIV is appropriate when discussing other life-sustaining therapies. Such discussion should take place during clinician–patient or clinician–family meetings, in which information is conveyed about patient status, prognosis and preferences. Clinicians should provide patients/families with a clear description of NIV, its potential risks, benefits and alternatives, and the methods by which success or failure of NIV will be assessed. Information about the patient's preferences should also be elicited. Clinicians should not assume that the wish to avoid endotracheal intubation routinely implies that NIV is an acceptable alternative. Clinicians should bear in mind that the goals of care may change based on the success or failure of NIV in achieving its stated goals.

## WITHDRAWING NON-INVASIVE VENTILATION

Some authors have suggested that when a decision has been reached to withdraw life-sustaining treatments, mechanical ventilation should be weaned rather than abruptly discontinued.[40,41] Weaning invasive mechanical ventilation over a period of 15–20 minutes while titrating medications for treatment of dyspnoea, pain or anxiety may improve patient comfort during the process of withdrawal of mechanical ventilation and ensure that the patient's symptoms are adequately controlled prior to removal of the endotracheal tube.[42] No data exist about the withdrawal of NIV at the end of life. However, if a patient has been receiving a substantial level of ventilatory assistance, weaning the level of support over 15–30 minutes with anticipatory dosing of opiates and/or benzodiazepines as appropriate may make the transition from NIV to spontaneous breathing smoother with less dyspnoea, anxiety or discomfort for the patient.

## FUTURE RESEARCH

Additional research is needed on the effects of NIV on palliation of dyspnoea at the end of life, as well as the relationship of benefit to burden in this patient population. Clearly, NIV may have different benefit to burden relationships in different subset of patients. Identifying and clarifying the factors that determine this balance – for families, patients and caregivers alike – is an important area of future research. Regardless of the results of future studies, the most important tools for guiding the use of non-invasive ventilation in end-of-life care are the caring and attentive communication skills of caregivers.

## REFERENCES


1. Mehta S, Hill NS. Noninvasive ventilation. *Am J Respir Crit Care Med* 2001; **163**: 540–77.
2. Crippen DW, Whetstine LM. Noninvasive ventilation and palliative care: Unfolding the promise. *Crit Care Med* 2004; **32**: 881–2.
3. Hilbert G, Gruson D, Vargas F *et al.* Noninvasive ventilation in immunosuppressed patients with pulmonary infiltrates, fever, and acute respiratory failure. *N Engl J Med* 2001; **344**: 481–7.
4. Keenan SP, Sinuff T, Cook DJ *et al.* Which patients with acute exacerbation of chronic obstructive pulmonary disease benefit from noninvasive positive-pressure ventilation? A systematic review of the literature. *Ann Intern Med* 2003; **138**: 861–70.
5. Masip J, Betbese AJ, Paez J *et al.* Non-invasive pressure support ventilation versus conventional oxygen therapy in acute cardiogenic pulmonary oedema: a randomised trial. *Lancet* 2000; **356**: 2126–32.
6. Masip J, Roque M, Sanchez B *et al.* Noninvasive ventilation in acute cardiogenic pulmonary edema: systematic review and meta-analysis. *JAMA* 2005; **294**: 3124–30.
7. Mehta S, Hill NS. Noninvasive ventilation in acute respiratory failure. *Respir Care Clin N Am* 1996; **2**: 267–92.
8. Peter JV, Moran JL. Noninvasive ventilation in exacerbations of chronic obstructive pulmonary disease: implications of different meta-analytic strategies. *Ann Intern Med* 2004; **141**: W78–9.
9. Peter JV, Moran JL, Phillips-Hughes J *et al.* Noninvasive ventilation in acute respiratory failure – a meta-analysis update. *Crit Care Med* 2002; **30**: 555–62.
10. Rusterholtz T, Kempf J, Berton C *et al.* Noninvasive pressure support ventilation (NIPSV) with face mask in patients with acute cardiogenic pulmonary edema (ACPE). *Intensive Care Med* 1999; **25**: 21–8.
11. Schettino G, Altobelli N, Kacmarek RM. Noninvasive positive-pressure ventilation in acute respiratory failure outside clinical trials: experience at the Massachusetts General Hospital. *Crit Care Med* 2008; **36**: 441–7.
12. Bach JR. Palliative care becomes 'uninformed euthanasia' when patients are not offered noninvasive life preserving options. *J Palliat Care* 2007; **23**: 181–4.
13. Benditt JO. Noninvasive ventilation at the end of life. *Respir Care* 2000; **45**: 1376–81; discussion 81–4.
14. Curtis JR, Cook DJ, Sinuff T *et al.* Noninvasive positive pressure ventilation in critical and palliative care settings: understanding the goals of therapy. *Crit Care Med* 2007; **35**: 932–9.
15. Clarke DE, Vaughan L, Raffin TA. Noninvasive positive pressure ventilation for patients with terminal respiratory failure: the ethical and economic costs of delaying the inevitable are too great. *Am J Crit Care* 1994; **3**: 4–5.
16. Cook D, Rocker G, Marshall J *et al.* Withdrawal of mechanical ventilation in anticipation of death in the intensive care unit. *N Engl J Med* 2003; **349**: 1123–32.
17. Nava S, Sturani C, Hartl S *et al.* End-of-life decision-making in respiratory intermediate care units: a European survey. *Eur Respir J* 2007; **30**: 156–64.
18. Sprung CL, Cohen SL, Sjokvist P *et al.* End-of-life practices in European intensive care units: the Ethicus Study. *JAMA* 2003; **290**: 790–7.
19. Sinuff T, Cook DJ, Keenan SP *et al.* Noninvasive ventilation for acute respiratory failure near the end of life. *Crit Care Med* 2008; **36**: 789–94.
20. Levy M, Tanios MA, Nelson D *et al.* Outcomes of patients with do-not-intubate orders treated with noninvasive ventilation. *Crit Care Med* 2004; **32**: 2002–7.
21. Schettino G, Altobelli N, Kacmarek RM. Noninvasive positive pressure ventilation reverses acute respiratory failure in select 'do-not-intubate' patients. *Crit Care Med* 2005; **33**: 1976–82.
22. Cuomo A, Delmastro M, Ceriana P *et al.* Noninvasive mechanical ventilation as a palliative treatment of acute respiratory failure in patients with end-stage solid cancer. *Palliat Med* 2004; **18**: 602–10.
23. Carlet J, Thijs LG, Antonelli M *et al.* Challenges in end-of-life care in the ICU. Statement of the 5th

International Consensus Conference in Critical Care: Brussels, Belgium, April 2003. *Intensive Care Med* 2004; **30**: 770–84.
24. Quill TE, Dresser R, Brock DW. The rule of double effect – a critique of its role in end-of-life decision making. *N Engl J Med* 1997; **337**: 1768–71.
25. Steinhauser KE, Christakis NA, Clipp EC *et al.* Preparing for the end of life: preferences of patients, families, physicians, and other care providers. *J Pain Symptom Manage* 2001; **22**: 727–37.
26. Steinhauser KE, Christakis NA, Clipp EC *et al.* Factors considered important at the end of life by patients, family, physicians, and other care providers. *JAMA* 2000; **284**: 2476–82.
27. Hill NS, Eveloff SE, Carlisle CC *et al.* Efficacy of nocturnal nasal ventilation in patients with restrictive thoracic disease. *Am Rev Respir Dis* 1992; **145**: 365–71.
28. Bourke SC, Bullock RE, Williams TL *et al.* Noninvasive ventilation in ALS: indications and effect on quality of life. *Neurology* 2003; **61**: 171–7.
29. Thibodeaux LS, Gutierrez A. Management of symptoms in amyotrophic lateral sclerosis. *Curr Treat Options Neurol* 2008; **10**: 77–85.
30. Bott J, Carroll MP, Conway JH *et al.* Randomised controlled trial of nasal ventilation in acute ventilatory failure due to chronic obstructive airways disease. *Lancet* 1993; **341**: 1555–7.
31. Meduri GU, Fox RC, Abou-Shala N *et al.* Noninvasive mechanical ventilation via face mask in patients with acute respiratory failure who refused endotracheal intubation. *Crit Care Med* 1994; **22**: 1584–90.
32. Curtis JR, Engelberg RA, Wenrich MD *et al.* Missed opportunities during family conferences about end-of-life care in the intensive care unit. *Am J Respir Crit Care Med* 2005; **171**: 844–9.
33. Levy CR, Ely EW, Payne K *et al.* Quality of dying and death in two medical ICUs: perceptions of family and clinicians. *Chest* 2005; **127**: 1775–83.
34. Stapleton RD, Engelberg RA, Wenrich MD *et al.* Clinician statements and family satisfaction with family conferences in the intensive care unit. *Crit Care Med* 2006; **34**: 1679–85.
35. Poncet MC, Toullic P, Papazian L *et al.* Burnout syndrome in critical care nursing staff. *Am J Respir Crit Care Med* 2007; **175**: 698–704.
36. Yang MH, McIlfatrick S. Intensive care nurses' experiences of caring for dying patients: a phenomenological study. *Int J Palliat Nurs* 2001; **7**: 435–41.
37. Redinbaugh EM, Sullivan AM, Block SD *et al.* Doctors' emotional reactions to recent death of a patient: cross sectional study of hospital doctors. *BMJ* 2003; **327**: 185.
38. McDonagh JR, Elliott TB, Engelberg RA *et al.* Family satisfaction with family conferences about end-of-life care in the intensive care unit: increased proportion of family speech is associated with increased satisfaction. *Crit Care Med* 2004; **32**: 1484–8.
39. Lautrette A, Darmon M, Megarbane B *et al.* A communication strategy and brochure for relatives of patients dying in the ICU. *N Engl J Med* 2007; **356**: 469–78.
40. Curtis JR, Rubenfeld GD. *Managing death in the intensive care unit: The transition from cure to comfort.* New York: Oxford University Press, 2001.
41. Rubenfeld GD. Principles and practice of withdrawing life-sustaining treatments. *Crit Care Clin* 2004; **20**: 435–51, ix.
42. Treece PD, Engelberg RA, Crowley L *et al.* Evaluation of a standardized order form for the withdrawal of life support in the intensive care unit. *Crit Care Med* 2004; **32**: 1141–8.

# SECTION M

# Prolonged weaning

# 56

# Epidemiology and cost of weaning failure

WILLIAM B HALL, SHANNON S CARSON

## ABSTRACT

Weaning failure has significant implications for patient outcome and healthcare resource utilization, especially when it leads to prolonged mechanical ventilation and chronic critical illness. Population-based studies indicate that the incidence of prolonged mechanical ventilation has more than doubled in the previous decade, and it will double again by 2020. Patients who experience prolonged weaning failure are at high risk for short-term and long-term mortality, and this has improved little over the past 30 years. Most survivors experience significant physical or cognitive limitations, and prolonged institutional care and hospital readmission are common after initial hospital discharge. Risk factors for mortality include advanced age, number of concomitant organ failures, and underlying diagnosis, especially chronic obstructive pulmonary disease (COPD). Hospital costs of weaning failure can be estimated from cost associated with mechanical ventilation, which is approximately US$1500 per day. However this may overestimate hospital costs since the daily cost of ICU care decreases as patients near successful weaning, and fixed costs are not affected by fewer ventilator days for a given patient. Cost-effectiveness analysis, which measures costs relative to a utility based outcome such as quality-adjusted life-years, is a more comprehensive approach to assessing the costs of weaning failure. Cost-effectiveness analyses indicate that the provision of prolonged mechanical ventilation is cost-effective for many patients, with exceptions being patients with predicted 1-year survival of less than 50 per cent. The most useful approaches to control costs include measures to decrease the likelihood of intubation and mechanical ventilation including the appropriate use of non-invasive ventilation, interventions and practices that shorten the time to successful extubation, and possibly the utilization of lower intensity post-acute care weaning units. Comparative effectiveness studies designed to assess innovative interventions in these areas will be needed to improve outcomes and reduce costs for these resource intensive patients.

## INTRODUCTION

Based upon definitions established at the Sixth International Consensus Conference on Intensive Care Medicine in 2005, the process of weaning begins at the time of the first spontaneous breathing trial (SBT) for a mechanically ventilated patient. Difficult weaning is defined as patients who fail initial weaning and require up to three SBTs or as long as 7 days from the first SBT to achieve successful weaning. Patients who fail more than three weaning attempts or require greater than 7 days of weaning after the first SBT are categorized as prolonged weaning.[1] Depending on how long it takes for patients to meet initial weaning criteria, this clinical definition can represent a range of time that often extends into periods of prolonged mechanical ventilation (PMV), defined as ≥21 consecutive days of mechanical ventilation for ≥6 hours per day.[2] Patients who experience weaning failure and PMV constitute a large portion of the patients considered to be chronically critically ill. In addition to prolonged ventilation, chronically critically ill patients are often characterized by substantial deficits in muscle mass and strength, volume overload, frequent delirium or coma, tracheostomy and gastrostomy, recurrent infections with resistant organisms, and endocrine derangements including hyperglycaemia, loss of bone mineral density, and relative adrenal insufficiency.[3] As is obvious from this clinical characterization, weaning failure has significant implications for patient outcome and healthcare resource utilization, especially when it leads to chronic critical illness. This chapter will focus on the epidemiology and costs of weaning failure, including trends in incidence, risk factors, mortality outcomes, technical considerations for cost-effectiveness analysis, evidence base for costs, and clinical approaches to reduce costs.

## THE COST OF WEANING FAILURE

The cost of weaning failure can be viewed from different perspectives. The simplest perspective involves determining the cost of a day of mechanical ventilation. Dasta and colleagues attempted to answer this question in a large retrospective cohort study of over 51 000 medical and surgical intensive care unit (ICU) admissions.[27] Of these, 35 per cent were mechanically ventilated during their ICU stay. Cost was estimated by hospital charges multiplied by cost-to-charge ratios. Over the entire cohort, mechanically ventilated patients cost on average US$1500/day more than non-ventilated ICU patients.

Based upon the data above, it could then be assumed that any day associated with a failed weaning trial costs US$1500. An important study by Kahn *et al.* used different logic that suggests that this approach may be too simplistic and may overestimate the hospital cost of weaning failure.[28] When a patient is successfully liberated from mechanical ventilation, the actual cost savings to the medical system is in the form of decreased ICU length of stay. This savings is the difference between the cost of the last ICU day compared to the first day on the medical/surgical ward. Since the last ICU day is usually the least expensive, the saving is marginal. Furthermore, the actual saving is not the entire cost of an ICU day, but rather the difference between variable costs of the ICU compared to the ward, since fixed costs are not affected by early discharge. In their study, the direct-variable costs for an ICU stay were estimated to be 19.3 per cent of total costs, and the difference between the costs of the last ICU day compared with the first ward day were determined to be US$118, or 0.2 per cent of hospital expenditures. In another recent analysis, Milbrandt *et al.* showed that the difference between ICU and ward costs have been steadily decreasing from a factor of 3 to 1.73 as patients with increasing levels of illness severity are being managed on medical and surgical wards.[29]

A more comprehensive way to estimate the cost of weaning failure is to examine cost-effectiveness of mechanical ventilation in different populations with and without weaning failure. This approach examines the question from society's perspective rather than just hospital costs. Hamel and colleagues examined 1005 patients enrolled in the Study to Understand Prognoses and Preferences for Outcomes and Risks of Treatments (SUPPORT) trial, who required ventilatory support for pneumonia or acute respiratory distress syndrome (ARDS) to determine the cost-effectiveness of mechanical ventilation.[30] They found that patients with a greater than 70 per cent probability of surviving 2 months cost US$29 000/QALY. Those with 50–70 per cent likelihood of surviving 2 months cost US$44 000/QALY, and those with a <50 per cent probability of surviving cost US$100 000/QALY. These data suggest that mechanical ventilation is cost-effective in all but the sickest patients.

A cost-effectiveness analysis by Cox and colleagues focused specifically on patients with prolonged weaning failure.[25] Using the perspective of a healthcare payer and a one-year time horizon, they estimated the cost-effectiveness of prolonged mechanical ventilation compared to withdrawal of support before day 21 of ventilation. For the base case of a 65-year-old patient with two comorbidities, they found that the incremental cost-effectiveness of ventilation was US$82 411/QALY. Costs increased to greater than US$100 000/QALY for patients with age greater than 68 or predicted 1-year survival <50 per cent. Cox reinforced Hamel's findings that prolonged mechanical ventilation is cost-effective in most patients, but the cost-effectiveness worsens with increasing age or worsening prognosis. Cox's analysis also determined that cost-effectiveness was most sensitive to the time spent in the acute hospital setting rather than costs associated with care after hospital discharge.

## CONTROLLING COSTS OF WEANING FAILURE

Controlling the costs of mechanical ventilation in the hospital broadly involves three strategies: prevention of intubation, liberation from mechanical ventilation as efficiently and safely as possible, and when available, early discharge to post-acute weaning facilities. Figure 56.2 is a schematic diagram representing approaches to limit the hospital costs for mechanical ventilation. It should first be established that initial or prolonged mechanical ventilation is consistent with a patient's wishes in the context of their chronic and acute conditions and likely outcome. If not, appropriate palliative interventions should be provided, and withholding or withdrawal of unwanted life sustaining therapies should be considered. Shared decision making around these questions should not be driven by cost-considerations but by patient autonomy in regard to preferences for life-sustaining therapies.[31,32]

Non-invasive ventilation (NIV) can be successfully employed in many disease states to prevent intubation and invasive ventilation. This is associated with a reduced length of stay, fewer hospital acquired pneumonias, and reduced mortality. Disease states which clearly benefit from NIV are COPD, cardiogenic pulmonary oedema, and hypoxia associated with immunosupression.[33] Non-invasive ventilation can also facilitate early extubation in patients with COPD. Keenan and colleagues showed that appropriate use of NIV for respiratory failure due to COPD exacerbations instead of invasive ventilation saves CAN$3244 per patient.[34] These cost-savings are reduced considerably if patients are managed in an ICU while receiving NIV rather than an intermediate care unit.

Specialized weaning units were originally developed to concentrate multidisciplinary expertise in settings devoted to the unique needs of chronically critically ill patients.[35] The number of the free-standing weaning facilities have increased dramatically in the USA, largely due to mutually beneficial economic circumstances of acute care and post-acute care hospitals. Long-term acute care hospitals

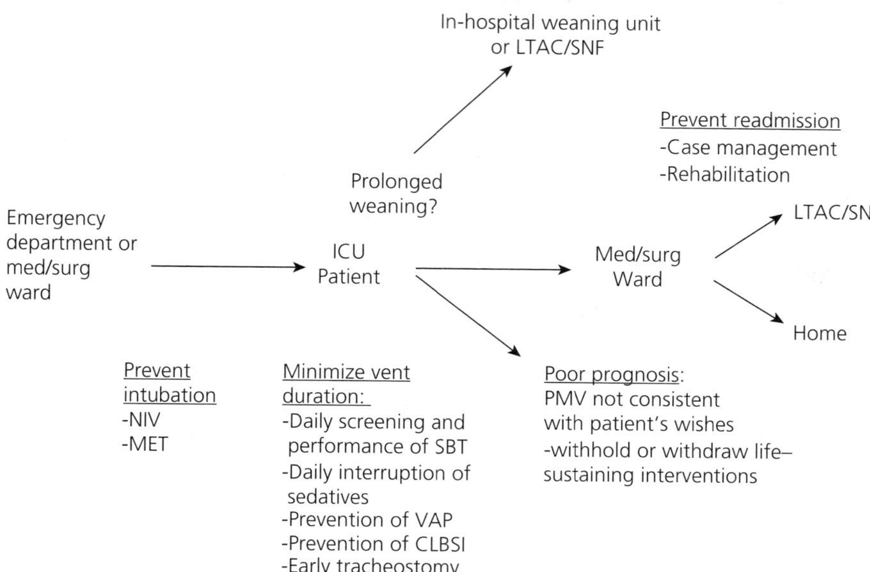


**Figure 56.2** Approaches to controlling costs of mechanical ventilation and weaning failure. Med/Surg, medical or surgical; CLBSI, central line-related bloodstream infection; LTAC, long-term acute care hospital; MET, medical emergency team; NIV, non-invasive ventilation; PMV, prolonged mechanical ventilation; SBT, spontaneous breathing trial; SNF, skilled nursing facility; VAP, ventilator-associated pneumonia.

(LTACs) have proven to be profitable under multiple reimbursement schemes, and referring hospitals have strong incentives to transfer costly mechanically ventilated patients as soon as possible in order to maximize fixed reimbursements that are based upon diagnosis rather than actual costs. One study indicated that LTACs can reduce the costs of care for the entire episode of illness for patients who have failed weaning,[36] but no studies have been performed to assess the cost-effectiveness of transferring patients to these facilities. Dedicated weaning units for stable patients with prolonged weaning failure should be established within acute hospitals without access to LTACs. By utilizing lower nurse to patient ratios but more specialized multidisciplinary care, hospital costs can be reduced without affecting patient outcome.

## FUTURE RESEARCH

Rising healthcare costs and ageing populations worldwide will place a strain on ICU resources in the near future. The number of patients requiring PMV will continue to rise over the foreseeable future in developed countries. Cost-effectiveness analyses suggest that mechanical ventilation is expensive, but even prolonged ventilation is a worthwhile venture in patients with a reasonable prognosis. Future research should be dedicated to new interventions and organizational changes that can prevent mechanical ventilation and improve efficiency of extubation for ventilated patients. New weaning modes and closed-loop systems with feedback enhancements may improve efficiency of weaning. New short-acting sedatives should be assessed in comparative effectiveness studies. Further research into early animation to improve functional outcomes is very important. Finally, the comparative effectiveness of in-hospital and free-standing weaning units in reducing costs and improving long-term outcomes in weaning failure should be conducted within different healthcare systems.

## REFERENCES


1. Boles JM, Bion J, Connors A *et al.* Weaning from mechanical ventilation. *Eur Respir J* 2007; **29**: 1033–56.
2. MacIntyre NR, Epstein SK, Carson S *et al.* Management of patients requiring prolonged mechanical ventilation: report of a NAMDRC consensus conference. *Chest* 2005; **128**: 3937–54.
3. Nierman DM, Nelson JE. Chronic critical illness. *Crit Care Clin* 2002; **18**: xi–xii.
4. Zilberberg MD, de Wit M, Pirone JR *et al.* Growth in adult prolonged acute mechanical ventilation: implications for healthcare delivery. *Crit Care Med* 2008; **36**: 1451–5.
5. Cox CE, Carson SS, Holmes GM *et al.* Increase in tracheostomy for prolonged mechanical ventilation in North Carolina, 1993–2002. *Crit Care Med* 2004; **32**: 2219–26.
6. Carson SS. Outcomes of prolonged mechanical ventilation. *Curr Opin Crit Care* 2006; **12**: 405–11.
7. Schonhofer B, Euteneuer S, Nava S *et al.* Survival of mechanically ventilated patients admitted to a specialised weaning centre. *Intensive Care Med* 2002; **28**: 908–16.
8. Spicher JE, White DP. Outcome and function following prolonged mechanical ventilation. *Arch Intern Med* 1987; **147**: 421–5.
9. Gracey DR, Naessens JM, Krishan I *et al.* Hospital and posthospital survival in patients mechanically ventilated for more than 29 days. *Chest* 1992; **101**: 211–14.


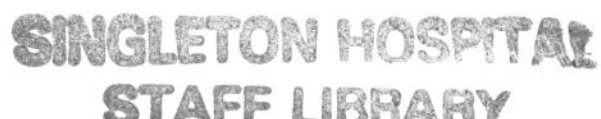

10. Combes A, Costa MA, Trouillet JL *et al.* Morbidity, mortality, and quality-of-life outcomes of patients requiring >or=14 days of mechanical ventilation. *Crit Care Med* 2003; **31**: 1373–81.
11. Engoren M, Arslanian-Engoren C, Fenn-Buderer N. Hospital and long-term outcome after tracheostomy for respiratory failure. *Chest* 2004; **125**: 220–7.
12. Cox CE, Carson SS, Lindquist JAH *et al.* Differences in one-year health outcomes and resource utilization by definition of prolonged mechanical ventilation: a prospective cohort study. *Crit Care* 2007; **11**: R9.
13. Carson SS, Garrett J, Hanson LC *et al.* A prognostic model for one-year mortality in patients requiring prolonged mechanical ventilation. *Crit Care Med* 2008; **36**: 2061–9.
14. Douglas SL, Daly BJ, Brennan PF *et al.* Hospital readmission among long-term ventilator patients. *Chest* 2001; **120**: 1278–86.
15. Nelson JE, Tandon N, Mercado AF *et al.* Brain dysfunction. Another burden for the chronically critically ill. *Arch Intern Med* 2006; **166**: 1993–9.
16. Carson SS, Bach PB, Brzozowski L *et al.* Outcomes after long-term acute care. An analysis of 133 mechanically ventilated patients. *Am J Respir Crit Care Med* 1999; **159**: 1568–73.
17. Engoren M, Arslanian-Engoren C. Hospital and long-term outcome of trauma patients with tracheostomy for respiratory failure. *Am Surg* 2005; **71**: 123–7.
18. Rubenfeld GD. Cost-effectiveness considerations in critical care. *New Horiz* 1998; **6**: 33–40.
19. Shorr AF. An update on cost-effectiveness analysis in critical care. *Curr Opin Crit Care* 2002; **8**: 337–43.
20. Roberts RR, Frutos PW, Ciavarella GG *et al.* Distribution of variable vs fixed costs of hospital care. *JAMA* 1999; **281**: 644–9.
21. Kahn JM. Understanding economic outcomes in critical care. *Curr Opin Crit Care* 2006; **12**: 399–404.
22. Bacchetta MD, Girardi LN, Southard EJ *et al.* Comparison of open versus bedside percutaneous dilatational tracheostomy in the cardiothoracic surgical patient: outcomes and financial analysis. *Ann Thorac Surg* 2005; **79**: 1879–85.
23. Shorr AF, Zilberberg MD, Kollef M. Cost-effectiveness analysis of a silver-coated endotracheal tube to reduce the incidence of ventilator-associated pneumonia. *Infect Control Hosp Epidemiol* 2009; **30**: 759–63.
24. Alolabi B, Bajammal S, Shirali J *et al.* Treatment of displaced femoral neck fractures in the elderly: a cost-benefit analysis. *J Orthop Trauma* 2009; **23**: 442–6.
25. Cox CE, Carson SS, Govert JA *et al.* An economic evaluation of prolonged mechanical ventilation. *Crit Care Med* 2007; **35**: 1918–27.
26. Weinstein MC, Siegel JE, Gold MR *et al.* Recommendations of the Panel on Cost-effectiveness in Health and Medicine. *JAMA* 1996; **276**: 1253–8.
27. Dasta JF, McLaughlin TP, Mody SH *et al.* Daily cost of an intensive care unit day: the contribution of mechanical ventilation. *Crit Care Med* 2005; **33**: 1266–71.
28. Kahn JM, Rubenfeld GD, Rohrbach J *et al.* Cost savings attributable to reductions in intensive care unit length of stay for mechanically ventilated patients. *Med Care* 2008; **46**: 1226–33.
29. Milbrandt EB, Kersten A, Rahim MT *et al.* Growth of intensive care unit resource use and its estimated cost in Medicare. *Crit Care Med* 2008; **36**: 2504–10.
30. Hamel MB, Phillips RS, Davis RB *et al.* Outcomes and cost-effectiveness of ventilator support and aggressive care for patients with acute respiratory failure due to pneumonia or acute respiratory distress syndrome. *Am J Med* 2000; **109**: 614–20.
31. Luce JM, Rubenfeld GD. Can health care costs be reduced by limiting intensive care at the end of life? *Am J Respir Crit Care Med* 2002; **165**: 750–4.
32. White DB, Engelberg RA, Wenrich MD *et al.* Prognostication during physician–family discussions about limiting life support in intensive care units. *Crit Care Med* 2007; **35**: 442–8.
33. Nava S, Hill N. Non-invasive ventilation in acute respiratory failure. *Lancet* 2009; **374**: 250–9.
34. Keenan SP, Gregor J, Sibbald WJ *et al.* Noninvasive positive pressure ventilation in the setting of severe, acute exacerbations of chronic obstructive pulmonary disease: more effective and less expensive. *Crit Care Med* 2000; **28**: 2094–102.
35. Scheinhorn DJ, Chao DC, Hassenpflug MS *et al.* Post-ICU weaning from mechanical ventilation: the role of long-term facilities. *Chest* 2001; **120** Suppl 6: 482S–4S.
36. Medicare Payment Advisory Commission. Defining long-term care hospitals (Chapter 5, June 2004 report). Available at: www.medpac.gov/publications (accessed November 2009).

# 57

# Pathophysiology of weaning failure

ELENI ISCHAKI, THEODOROS VASSILAKOPOULOS

ABSTRACT

Weaning failure is caused mainly by an imbalance between ventilatory needs and neurocardiorespiratory capacity. This can happen if there is an increase in the load faced by the respiratory muscles, a decrease in their capacity, increased energy demands, and/or decreased energy supplies. Less frequently the ventilatory pump impedes the circulatory pump, leading to heart failure or ischaemia, or hypoxaemia or dyspnoea and anxiety develop during weaning trials.

## INTRODUCTION

For most mechanically ventilated patients resumption of spontaneous ventilation can be a rapid and uneventful process. However, there is a substantial number of mechanically ventilated patients (20–30 per cent) in whom weaning is difficult and likely to fail, posing a great challenge for clinicians because the pathophysiology of weaning failure is complex.[1–3]

Failure to sustain spontaneous breathing is usually due to incomplete resolution of the illness requiring ventilatory support or to a new pathological condition that has developed. In either case, weaning failure is usually caused by the inability of the respiratory muscle pump to tolerate the load imposed upon it. Consequently, weaning a patient from the ventilator will be successful whenever an appropriate relationship exists between ventilatory needs and neuromuscular capacity of the respiratory muscles and will ultimately fail whenever this relationship becomes imbalanced. Less often, failure to wean is due to cardiovascular dysfunction, hypoxaemia or dyspnoea/anxiety that develops on transition to spontaneous breathing.

## VENTILATORY NEEDS AND NEUROMUSCULAR CAPACITY

To take a spontaneous breath, the inspiratory muscles must generate sufficient force to overcome the elastic loads of the lungs and chest wall as well as the resistive load of the airways and tissue (Fig. 57.1). This requires an adequate central respiratory drive, functional nerve integrity, unimpaired neuromuscular transmission, an intact chest wall and adequate muscle strength. Under normal conditions there are reserves that permit a considerable increase in load. The ability of the respiratory muscles to sustain this load without the appearance of fatigue is called 'endurance' and is determined by the balance between energy supplies (Us) and energy demands (Ud)[4] (Fig. 57.2).

On the one hand, energy supplies depend on the inspiratory muscle blood flow, the blood substrate concentration and arterial oxygen content, the ability to extract and utilize energy sources and the muscle's energy stores. On the other hand, energy demands increase proportionally with the mean tidal pressure developed by the inspiratory muscles ($P_I$), expressed as a fraction of the maximum inspiratory pressure ($P_I/P_{I,max}$), the minute ventilation (V'E), the inspiratory duty cycle ($T_I/T_{TOT}$) and the mean inspiratory flow rate ($V_t/T_I$) and are inversely related to the efficiency of the muscles.[5,6]

Bellemare and Grassino[7] have suggested the 'tension-time index' ($TTI_{di}$) that is related to the endurance time and is determined by the $T_I/T_{TOT}$ and the mean transdiaphragmatic pressure expressed as a fraction of maximal ($P_{di}/P_{di,max}$):

$$TTI = (P_I/P_{I,max}) \times (T_I/T_{TOT})$$

Whenever TTI is smaller than the critical value of 0.15 the load can be sustained indefinitely, but when it exceeds the

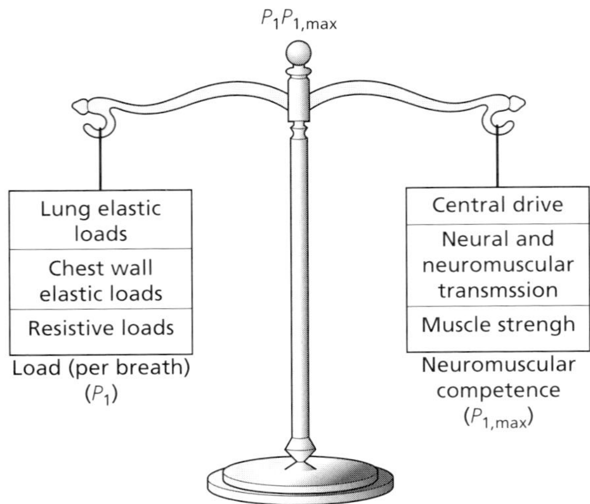


**Figure 57.1** The balance between load and neuromuscular competence. Adapted from Vassilakopoulos *et al.*[4]

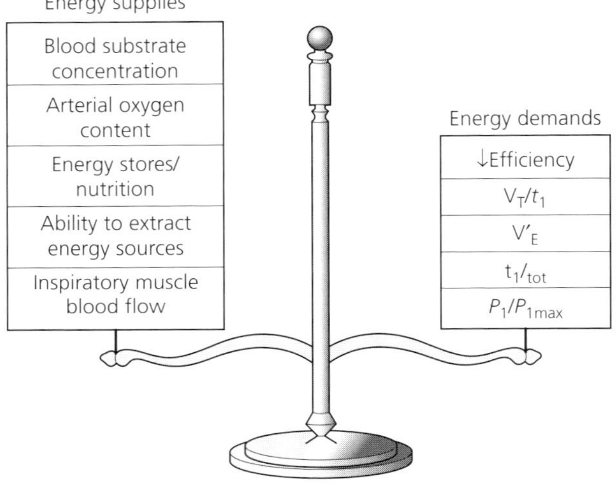


**Figure 57.2** The balance between energy supplies and demands. Adapted from Vassilakopoulos *et al.*[4]

critical zone of 0.15–0.18 the load can be sustained only for a limited time period (endurance time). Given that $T_I/T_{TOT}$ and $P_I/P_{I,max}$ are among the determinants of energy demands, an increase in either will also increase the energy demands, which might not be met by the energy supplies.

Roussos *et al.*[8] have directly related $P_I/P_{I,max}$ with the endurance time. The critical value of $P_I/P_{I,max}$ that could be generated indefinitely at functional residual capacity (FRC) was around 0.60. Greater values of $P_I/P_{I,max}$ were inversely related to the endurance time in a curvilinear fashion.

But what determines the ratio $P_I/P_{I,max}$? The numerator is determined by the elastic and resistive loads imposed on the inspiratory muscles. The denominator is determined by the neuromuscular competence. It follows that the value of $P_I/P_{I,max}$ is determined by the balance between load and competence (see Fig. 57.1). But $P_I/P_{I,max}$ is also one of the determinants of energy demands (see Fig. 57.2), so the two balances, i.e. between load and competence and energy supply and demand, are in essence linked, creating a system. This can be schematically represented by two linked balances (Fig. 57.3) in which the $P_I/P_{I'max}$, one of the determinants of energy demands, is replaced by its equivalent, the balance between load and neuromuscular competence. When the central hinge of the system is at the horizontal level or moves upwards, the neurorespiratory capacity exceeds the ventilatory needs and spontaneous ventilation can be sustained. When the central hinge of the system moves downwards spontaneous breathing cannot be sustained and weaning will ultimately fail.[4]

Table 57.1 on page 524 summarizes all possible factors that can lead to an inappropriate relationship between ventilator needs and neurorespiratory capacity and thus to weaning failure.

## VENTILATOR-INDUCED DIAPHRAGMATIC DYSFUNCTION

Controlled mechanical ventilation (CMV) is a mode of ventilator support where the ventilator takes full responsibility for inflating the respiratory system using the minute ventilation set by the clinician. It is traditionally used in severely ill patients who cannot tolerate partial ventilator support. Sometimes it is used when weaning fails to rest the respiratory muscles.

However, CMV can induce dysfunction of the diaphragm, resulting in decreased diaphragmatic force generating capacity and diaphragmatic injury, also called ventilator-induced diaphragmatic dysfunction (VIDD).[9] After a period of CMV, the pressure generating capacity of the diaphragm declines by 35–50 per cent[10–12] and this is an early and progressive phenomenon.[13,14] The endurance of the diaphragm is also significantly compromised.[10] This is not due to changes in lung volume[15] or abdominal compliance.[10,11] Neural and neuromuscular transmissions remain intact, as evidenced by the lack of changes in phrenic nerve conduction (latency) and the stable response to repetitive stimulation of the phrenic nerve.[11]

*In vitro* results suggest that impairment in the diaphragmatic force-generating capacity appears to reside within the myofibres and the main known mechanisms of VIDD are muscle atrophy, oxidative stress and structural injury.[9]

- CMV decreases protein synthesis and increases proteolysis in the diaphragm resulting in atrophy.[16] Six hours of CMV in rats decreased the *in vivo* rate of mixed protein synthesis by 30 per cent and the rate of myosin heavy chain protein synthesis by 65 per cent, both of which persisted throughout 18 hours of CMV.[17] After 24 hours of CMV, the mRNA levels of insulin-like growth factor which stimulates protein synthesis are depressed.[18] Also all three intracellular proteolytic systems of mammalian cells, calpains, lysosomal proteins and proteasomes, are activated during CMV.[19]

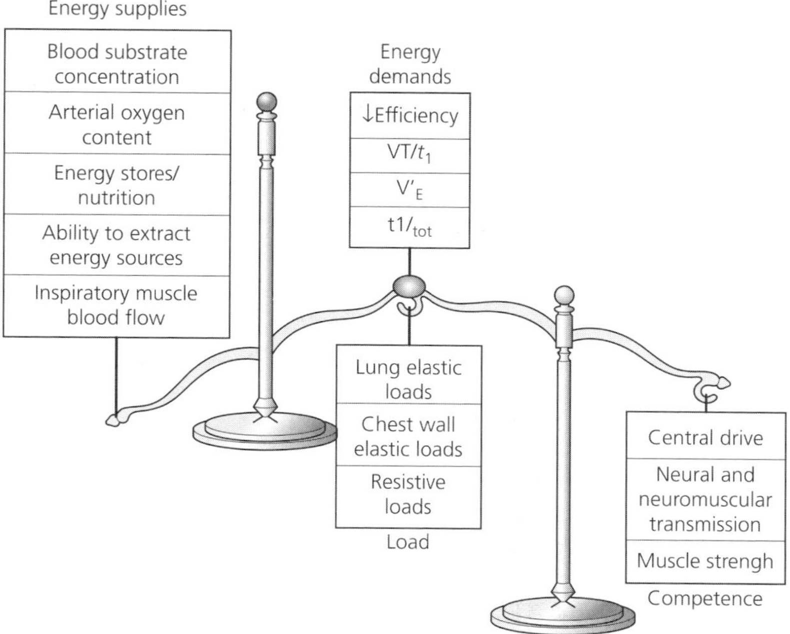


**Figure 57.3** The system of two balances, incorporating the various determinants of load, competence, energy supplies and demands (see text). Adapted from Vassilakopoulos *et al.*[4]

- The onset of oxidative stress occurs within the first 6 hours of the institution of CMV,[20] as indicated by the increased protein oxidation and lipid peroxidation by-products[19,20] and is long-lasting.[15] This was evident in insoluble proteins with molecular masses of about 200, 128, 85 and 40 kDa and raises the possibility that actin (40 kDa) and myosin (200 kDa) undergo oxidative modification during CMV, which would be expected to compromise diaphragm contractility.[20]
- Structural abnormalities such as disrupted myofibrils, increased numbers of lipid vacuoles in the sarcoplasm and abnormally small mitochondria containing focal membrane disruptions have been found after 2–3 days of CMV.[12,14,21] These alterations have detrimental effects on diaphragmatic force-generating capacity.[12]

The documentation of VIDD in patients is difficult because of the presence of confounding factors such as disease state (e.g. sepsis) and drug therapy (e.g. corticosteroids)[9] and the difficulties in assessing diaphragmatic function in the ICU. However, atrophy secondary to CMV was documented in human brain-dead organ donors[22] after a few hours of CMV.

VIDD should be suspected in patients who fail to wean after a period of CMV and when other known causes of respiratory muscle weakness have been ruled out.[9] CMV should be curtailed as much as possible, especially in older patients, given that the results of animal studies suggest that the effects of ageing and mechanical ventilation are additive.[23] Assisted modes should be used whenever possible, although further studies are needed to determine the amount of activity the respiratory muscles should have to prevent VIDD.[24] There is no established therapy for VIDD. In theory, resumption of spontaneous breathing should retrain the respiratory muscles, but the time course of recovery is unknown.

## RESPIRATORY MUSCLE FATIGUE

Consideration of the imbalance between energy supply and demand of the respiratory muscles suggests that inspiratory muscle fatigue is frequently a final common pathway leading to weaning failure.

During weaning trials patients who fail to wean show electromyographic evidence of excessive inspiratory muscle load, which is prevented by the application of pressure support.[25,26] The load that the respiratory muscles of patients who fail to wean are facing (assessed as the TTI) is increased to the range that would predictably produce fatigue of the respiratory muscles,[27] if patients were allowed to continue spontaneous breathing without ventilator assistance. When these same patients wean successfully the load is reduced below the fatiguing threshold.[27,28]

It is common in daily practice to use CMV in cases of weaning failure after a spontaneous breathing trial or after extubation, based on the premise that respiratory muscle fatigue (requiring rest to recover) is the cause of weaning failure.[4,29] Recent evidence, however, does not support the existence of low frequency fatigue (the type of fatigue that is long-lasting, taking more than 24 hours to recover) in patients who fail to wean despite the excessive respiratory muscle load.[30] The twitch transdiaphragmatic pressure elicited by magnetic stimulation of the phrenic nerve was not altered before and after the failing weaning trials.[30] The tension–time index of the diaphragm ($TT_{di}$) was 0.17–0.22 during failing weaning trials.[30] Bellemare and Grassino[7] reported that the relationship between the $TT_{di}$ and time to task failure in healthy subjects follows an inverse power function: time to task failure = 0.1 $(TT_{di})^{-3.6}$. Based on this formula, the expected times to task failure would be 28–59 minutes. The average value of the $TT_{Idi}$ during the last minute of the trial was 0.26, and the weaning failure

**Table 57.1** Various factors that can lead to an inappropriate relationship between ventilator needs and neurorespiratory capacity

| Energy supplies | Energy demands | Load (per breath) | | | Neuromuscular competence | | |
|---|---|---|---|---|---|---|---|
| ↓Energy stores<br>1. Poor nutrition<br>2. Catabolic states<br>3. Prolonged submaximal breathing<br><br>↓Blood fuel<br>1. Extreme inanition<br><br>Inability to utilize energy<br>1. Sepsis<br>2. Cyanide poisoning<br><br>↓$CaO_2$<br>1. Sepsis<br>2. Anaemia<br><br>↓Inspiratory muscle Q<br>1. ↓CO(shock LVF)<br>2. ↑force of contraction<br>3. ↑$tI/t_{TOT}$ | ↓Efficiency<br><br>↑ Minute ventilation<br>a. ↑$\dot{V}CO_2$<br>1. Fever<br>2. Sepsis<br>3. Shivering<br>4. Tetanus<br>5. Pain/agitation<br>6. Trauma/ burns<br>7. Excess carbohydrates<br><br>b. ↑$V_D/V_T$<br>1. Pulmonary embolism<br>2. Emphysema<br>3. ARDS<br>4. Hypovolaemia<br>5. Endotracheal tube connectors and filters<br>6. ↑FRC<br>↑$V_T/tI$<br>↑$tI/t_{TOT}$ | ↑Resistive loads<br>1. Bronchospasm<br>2. Airway oedema and secretions<br>3. Upper airway obstruction<br>4. Endotracheal tube kinking and secretion encrustation<br>5. Obstructive sleep apnoea<br>6. Ventilatory circuit resistance | ↑Lung elastic loads<br>1. Hyperinflation (PEEPi)<br>2. Alveolar oedema<br>3. Infection<br>4. Atelectasis<br>5. Interstitial inflammation and/or oedema<br>6. Lung tumour | ↑Chest wall elastic loads<br>1. Pleural effusion<br>2. Pneumothorax<br>3. Flail chest<br>4. Tumour<br>5. Obesity<br>6. Ascites<br>7. Abdominal distention | ↓Drive<br>1. Drug overdose<br>2. Brain stem lesion<br>3. Sleep deprivation<br>4. Hypothyroidism<br>5. Starvation/ malnutrition<br>6. Metabolic alkalosis<br>7. Toxic metabolite<br>8. Bulbar poliomyelitis<br>9. Acid maltase deficiency<br>10. Myotonic dystrophy<br>11. Sleep-induced hypoventilation | Impaired nerve/neuromuscular transmission<br>1. Phrenic nerve injury<br>2. Spinal cord lesion<br>3. Neuromuscular blockers<br>4. Myasthenia gravis<br>5. Aminoglycosides<br>6. Guillain–Barré<br>7. Botulism<br>8. Critical illness polyneuropathy<br>9. Poliomyelitis | Muscle weakness<br>1. Electrolyte derangement<br>2. Malnutrition<br>3. Myopathy<br>4. Hyperinflation<br>5. Drugs, corticosteroids<br>6. Diffuse atrophy<br>7. Sepsis |

↓, reduced; ↑, increased; ARDS, adult respiratory distress syndrome; $CaO_2$, arterial oxygen content; CO, cardiac output; $CO_2$, carbon dioxide elimination; LVF, left ventricular failure; PEEPi, intrinsic positive end-expiratory pressure; Q′, perfusion; V′ $V_D/V_T$, physiologic dead space/tidal volume ratio.

patients would be predicted to sustain this effort for another 13 minutes before developing diaphragmatic fatigue.[30] Thus, the lack of development of low frequency respiratory muscle fatigue despite the excessive load is due to the fact that physicians have adopted criteria for the definition of spontaneous breathing trial failure which lead them to put patients back on the ventilator before the development of low frequency respiratory muscle fatigue. Thus, no reason exists to completely unload the respiratory muscles with CMV for low frequency fatigue reversal if weaning is terminated based on widely accepted predefined criteria.

## CRITICAL ILLNESS POLYNEUROPATHY (CIP) AND MYOPATHY (CIM)

Critical illness polyneuropathy and myopathy are major complications of severe critical illness and its management. CIP is an acute axonal sensorimotor polyneuropathy usually suspected in ICU patients who, after a period of days or weeks, cannot be weaned from the ventilator despite the absence of pulmonary or cardiac causes of respiratory failure, or because they suffer from various degrees of limb weakness.[31] Critical illness myopathy is an acute primary myopathy with a continuum of myopathic findings, from myopathies with pure functional impairment and normal histology to myopathies with atrophy and necrosis. Among many risk factors implicated, sepsis, systemic inflammatory response syndrome, multiple organ failure and possibly hyperglycaemia appear to play a crucial role in CIP/CIM.[32]

## CARDIOVASCULAR DYSFUNCTION

Approximately, 20–30 per cent of weaning failures resulted from congestive heart failure.[4,33] This is supported by the increase of brain natriuretic peptide (BNP) during the course of failed weaning trials.[34,35] Patients with underlying ventricular dysfunction may increase their pulmonary artery occlusion pressure and sometimes ultimately decrease their cardiac output on removal from positive pressure mechanical ventilation.[36] Several factors may be responsible[37,38] (Table 57.2). During spontaneous breathing the increase in respiratory muscle work load as well as anxiety and sympathetic discharge result in an abrupt increase in oxygen and cardiac demands. The failing left ventricle is unable to respond normally and left ventricular end-diastolic pressure (LVEDP) rises, causing interstitial, peribronchial and alveolar oedema, which reduces lung compliance, increases airway resistance and worsens

**Table 57.2** Factors increasing pulmonary capillary wedge pressure during unsuccessful weaning from mechanical ventilation

| Increased preload | Reduced contractility | Increased afterload |
|---|---|---|
| A. Increased venous return<br>Decreased pleural pressure<br>Sympathetic discharge (stress, hypercapnia)<br>Increased abdominal pressure | Myocardial ischaemia<br>Myocardial hypoxia<br>Myocardial acidosis, especially due to hypercapnia<br>Ionized hypocalcaemia | ↑Systolic blood pressure (hypercapnia, catecholamine discharge)<br>↓Pleural pressure |
| B. Reduced LV compliance (diastolic stiffness)<br>Myocardial ischaemia<br>↓$O_2$ supply<br>↓$PaO_2$<br>↑LVEDP and ↑HR<br>↓Mean arterial pressure<br>↑$O_2$ demands<br>↑Catecholamines<br>↑HR<br>↑Systolic blood pressure<br>LV enlargement<br>RV enlargement (ventricular interdependence)<br>↑Venous return<br>↑Pulmonary artery pressure (acute)<br>RV ischaemia leading to reduced RV contractility<br>Compression of heart chambers by regionally hyperinflated lung | Drugs | |

↓, reduced; ↑, increased; LV, left ventricle; LVEDP, left ventricular end-diastolic pressure; HR, heart rate; $PaO_2$, arterial oxygen tension; RV, right ventricle.

ventilation–perfusion mismatching, leading to hypoxaemia. Energy demands of the respiratory muscles are increased, whereas energy supplies are either diminished or not sufficiently increased (inadequate cardiac output, hypoxaemia). This eventually leads to the inability to sustain spontaneous ventilation at a level adequate to achieve normocapnia and $PCO_2$ rises. The abnormal blood gasses depress cardiac contractility and, at the same time, respiratory muscle function. This worsens blood gasses more and creates a vicious circle that may culminate in failure to wean.[36]

Several factors may be responsible,[37,38] the most important being the changes in intrathoracic and intra-abdominal pressures on initiation of spontaneous breathing. Normally, spontaneous inspiration increases abdominal pressure at the same time it decreases pleural pressure due to diaphragmatic contraction and descent. The role of the decreased pleural pressure or venous return is already known. An increase in abdominal pressure would compress the abdominal venous system, through which two-thirds of the venous return passes,[39] and this would increase the amount of blood returning to the heart.[40] At the same time, the negative intrathoracic pressure increases the afterload of both ventricles, and this, combined with the increased venous return, may lead to right ventricular distention. Because the two ventricles are constrained by a common pericardial sac and share the interventricular septum, changes in the volume of one ventricle may affect the function of the other; thus, right ventricular distention impedes the filling of the left ventricle.[41] This occurs both through a generalized increase in pericardial pressure and also because of a shift of the interventricular septum toward the left. Left ventricular filling impediment increases its diastolic stiffness at the same time that its afterload is elevated due to the decreased pleural pressure. These combined effects lead to the elevation of LVEDP, culminating in weaning failure.

Lemaire *et al.*[36] studied the haemodynamic effects of changing from positive pressure to spontaneous ventilation in 15 patients with combined COPD and coronary artery disease. Spontaneous breathing increased cardiac output and right and left ventricular filling pressures, leading rapidly to respiratory failure. Although no patient had clinical evidence of volume overload, all were subsequently forced into diuresis for 1 week, losing an average of 5 kg. After that, 8 of the 15 patients were successfully weaned. These patients now had cardiac output and filling pressures during spontaneous breathing essentially unaltered from their values during mechanical ventilation. An interesting explanation for these findings could be that, before diuresis, these patients' abdominal capacitance vessels were congested. During spontaneous breathing, their mean abdominal pressure rose leading to increased venous return, which along with elevation of the left ventricular afterload caused by the lowered pleural pressure precipitated heart failure and, in turn, respiratory failure. After diuresis, the abdominal capacitance vessels were less congested and thus more compressible; increased abdominal pressure did not increase venous return as much, due to the compression of the abdominal inferior vena cava; thus the deterioration of heart function was prevented, leading these patients into successful weaning.[42,43]

Jubran *et al.*[44] reported that patients who fail to wean develop a relative decrease in oxygen delivery associated with an increase in oxygen extraction, leading to a substantial decrease in mixed venous oxygen saturation ($ScvO_2$). However, this response is actually not observed in all patients who fail to wean. Accordingly, in a mixed population of patients who fail to wean, two distinct patterns of haemodynamic and global tissue oxygenation response are observed.[45] In patients who fail without increasing their oxygen consumption the increase in oxygen delivery is accompanied by a decrease in oxygen extraction. In patients who fail and increase their oxygen consumption (by >10 per cent) this increase is met mainly by an increase in oxygen extraction. $ScvO_2$ slightly increases in the former patients, whereas it decreases in the latter. Thus, the fall in $ScvO_2$ is not observed in all patients who fail to wean. Furthermore, this fall of $ScvO_2$ is not specific for weaning failure. In patients who weaned successfully after cardiovascular surgery in whom oxygen consumption increased by more than 10 per cent, oxygen extraction remained stable in patients after aortic surgery, increased slightly after cardiac surgery and significantly after cardiac transplantation, with corresponding decreases in $ScvO_2$.[46] Hence, the haemodynamic response to weaning from mechanical ventilation is complex,[4,45,47] and a fall in $ScvO_2$ is observed in some but not all patients who fail to wean and may also be observed in patients who wean successfully.

## MYOCARDIAL ISCHAEMIA

Another cardiovascular cause of weaning failure is myocardial ischaemia due to the increased cardiac workload on resumption of spontaneous breathing.[48–52] In the literature, many studies have found either electrocardiographic evidence of myocardial ischaemia[48,51,52] or evidence from myocardial scintigraphy with thallium 201 during discontinuation of mechanical ventilation.[49] However, ischaemia was detected more frequently (10 per cent) in patients with a history of coronary artery disease (CAD) and was associated with weaning failure in 22 per cent of these patients.[52]

The haemodynamic and ventilatory changes associated with resumption of spontaneous breathing may increase myocardial oxygen demands to such an extent that they cannot be met by the available coronary oxygen supply, probably due to coronary atherosclerosis or spasm, thus leading to ischaemia. The incidence of myocardial ischaemia might be underestimated because the methods usually used (electrocardiographic criteria) to detect it are inherently faced with the weakness of false-negative findings. The available data suggest that myocardial ischaemia is relatively infrequent in the usual ICU population although its incidence increases in susceptible patient populations, such as those with coronary artery disease, where it is more likely associated with weaning failure. Myocardial ischaemia should be suspected in the susceptible patient who fails to wean, even in the absence of electrocardiogram changes.[29]

## HYPOXAEMIA

Mechanical ventilation may improve oxygen transfer across the lung for a variety of reasons:

- by preventing atelectasis and improving ventilation–perfusion mismatching[53]
- in cases of congestive heart failure, by reducing lung oedema formation[41]
- by putting the respiratory muscles at rest, thus decreasing their oxygen consumption.

Hypoxaemia is rarely a cause of weaning failure, largely because weaning is not contemplated in patients who display significant problems with oxygenation. However, during weaning, the beneficial effects of mechanical ventilation on oxygenation are no longer exerted. If the underlying lung pathology that led to hypoxaemic respiratory failure necessitating mechanical ventilation has not resolved completely, withdrawal of machine support may lead to the development of severe hypoxaemia and thus to weaning failure. Furthermore, mechanical ventilation may mask a complication that developed during the period of machine support.[29]

## DYSPNOEA AND ANXIETY

During weaning trials, patients display fearfulness and apprehension related to the anticipation of dyspnoea,[54–56] rather than the stress of the activity *per se*.[57] This sense is frequently underestimated by their physicians.[54]

Dyspnoea is closely associated with anxiety,[54,58] which has four physiological consequences:

- Muscle tone is increased and this leads to increased $\dot{V}O_2$ at the same time that the respiratory muscles also increase their $\dot{V}O_2$. Increased muscle tone also elevates the chest wall elastic load *via* its effect on the intercostals,[59] which in turn makes inspiration more difficult, since they are expiratory muscles.
- Anxiety causes muscle deconditioning and this leads to uncoordinated breathing, again increasing the load.[59]
- Anxiety increases the concentration of circulating catecholamines. This increases the heart's afterload (by increasing systemic vascular resistance), its preload (by constricting the great veins and forcing blood towards the heart) and the myocardial oxygen demands.
- Breathing frequency may increase, which in turn would increase the energy demands of the respiratory muscles, and generate dynamic hyperinflation.

The beneficial effect of biofeedback and/or hypnosis in successfully weaning patients who had previously failed[60–62] may be attributed mainly to the reduction of anxiety.

Certainly, the pathways presented that lead to weaning failure are not mutually exclusive and are very difficult to separate. However, keeping these in mind helps the clinician to understand the underlying physiology and plan therapeutic strategies.

## REFERENCES


1. Brochard L, Rauss A, Benito S *et al.* Comparison of three methods of gradual withdrawal from ventilatory support during weaning from mechanical ventilation. *Am J Respir Crit Care Med* 1994; **150**: 896–903.
2. Esteban A, Frutos F, Tobin MJ *et al.* A comparison of four methods of weaning patients from mechanical ventilation. *N Engl J Med* 1995; **332**: 345–50.
3. Esteban A, Alia I, Gordo F *et al.* Extubation outcome after spontaneous breathing trials withT-tube or pressure support ventilation. *Am J Respir Crit Care Med* 1997; **156**: 459–65.
4. Vassilakopoulos T, Zakynthinos S, Roussos CH. Respiratory muscles and weaning failure. *Eur Respir J* 1996; **9**: 2383–400.
5. Roussos CH, Macklem PT. The respiratory muscles. *N Engl J Med* 1982; **307**: 786–97.
6. Macklem PT. Respiratory muscle dysfunction. *Hosp Pract* 1986; **2**: 83–96.
7. Bellemare F, Grassino A. Effect of pressure and timing of contraction on human diaphragm fatigue. *J Appl Physiol* 1982; **53**: 1190–5.
8. Roussos CH, Fixley D, Gross D *et al.* Fatigue of inspiratory muscles and their synergic behavior. *J Appl Physiol* 1979; **46**: 897–904.
9. Vassilakopoulos T, Petrof BJ. Ventilator-induced diaphragmatic dysfunction. *Am J Respir Crit Care Med* 2004; **169**: 336–41.
10. Anzueto A, Peters JI, Tobin MJ *et al.* Effects of prolonged controlled mechanical ventilation on diaphragmatic function in healthy adult baboons. *Crit Care Med* 1997; **25**: 1187–90.
11. Radell PJ, Remahl S, Nichols DG *et al.* Effects of prolonged mechanical ventilation and inactivity on piglet diaphragm function. *Intensive Care Med* 2002; **28**: 358–64.
12. Sassoon CS, Caiozzo VJ, Manka A *et al.* Altered diaphragm contractile properties with controlled mechanical ventilation. *J Appl Physiol* 2002; **92**: 2585–95.

13. Powers SK, Shanely RA, Coombes JS *et al.* Mechanical ventilation results in progressive contractile dysfunction in the diaphragm. *J Appl Physiol* 2002; **92**: 1851–8.
14. Zhu E, Sassoon CS, Nelson R *et al.* Early effects of mechanical ventilation on isotonic contractile properties and MAF-box gene expression in the diaphragm. *J Appl Physiol* 2005; **99**: 747–56.
15. Jaber S, Sebbane M, Koechlin C *et al.* Effects of short vs. prolonged mechanical ventilation on antioxidant systems in piglet diaphragm. *Intensive Care Med* 2005; **31**: 1427–33.
16. Hussain SN, Vassilakopoulos T. Ventilator-induced cachexia. *Am J Respir Crit Care Med* 2002; **166**: 1307–8.
17. Shanely RA, Van Gammeren D, Deruisseau KC *et al.* Mechanical ventilation depresses protein synthesis in the rat diaphragm. *Am J Respir Crit Care Med* 2004; **170**: 994–9.
18. Gayan-Ramirez G, De Paepe K, Cadot P *et al.* Detrimental effects of short-term mechanical ventilation on diaphragm function and IGF-I mRNA in rats. *Intensive Care Med* 2003; **29**: 825–33.
19. Shanely RA, Zergeroglu MA, Lennon SL *et al.* Mechanical ventilation induced diaphragmatic atrophy is associated with oxidative injury and increased proteolytic activity. *Am J Respir Crit Care Med* 2002; **166**: 1369–74.
20. Zergeroglu MA, McKenzie MJ, Shanely RA *et al.* Mechanical ventilation-induced oxidative stress in the diaphragm. *J Appl Physiol* 2003; **95**: 1116–24.
21. Bernard N, Matecki S, Py G *et al.* Effects of prolonged mechanical ventilation on respiratory muscle ultrastructure and mitochondrial respiration in rabbits. *Intensive Care Med* 2003; **29**: 111–18.
22. Levine S, Nguyen T, Taylor N *et al.* Rapid disuse atrophy of diaphragm fibers in mechanically ventilated humans. *N Engl J Med* 2008; **358**: 1327–35.
23. Criswell DS, Shanely RA, Betters JJ *et al.* Cumulative effects of aging and mechanical ventilation on in vitro diaphragm function. *Chest* 2003; **124**: 2302–8.
24. Sassoon CS, Zhu E, Caiozzo VJ. Assist-control mechanical ventilation attenuates ventilator-induced diaphragmatic dysfunction. *Am J Respir Crit Care Med* 2004; **170**: 626–32.
25. Cohen CA, Zagelbaum G, Gross D *et al.* Clinical manifestations of inspiratory muscle fatigue. *Am J Med* 1982; **73**: 308–16.
26. Brochard L, Hart A, Lorino H *et al.* Inspiratory pressure support prevents diaphragmatic fatigue during weaning from mechanical ventilation. *Am Rev Respir Dis* 1989; **139**: 513–21.
27. Vassilakopoulos T, Zakynthinos S, Roussos C. The tension-time index and the frequency/tidal volume ratio are the major pathophysiologic determinants of weaning failure and success. *Am J Respir Crit Care Med* 1998; **158**: 378–85.
28. Carlucci A, Ceriana P, Prinianakis G *et al.* Determinants of weaning success in patients with prolonged mechanical ventilation. *Crit Care* 2009; **13**: R97.
29. Vassilakopoulos T, Roussos C, Zakynthinos S. Weaning from mechanical ventilation. *J Crit Care* 1999; **14**: 39–62.
30. Laghi F, Cattapan SE, Jubran A *et al.* Is weaning failure caused by low-frequency fatigue of the diaphragm? *Am J Respir Crit Care Med* 2003; **167**: 120–7.
31. De Jonghe B, Bastuji-Garin S, Sharshar T *et al.* Does ICU-acquired paresis lengthen weaning from mechanical ventilation? *Intensive Care Med* 2004; **30**: 1117–21.
32. Bolton CF. Neuromuscular manifestations of critical illness. *Muscle Nerve* 2005; **32**: 140–63.
33. Epstein SK. Etiology of extubation failure and the predictive value of the rapid shallow breathing index. *Am J Respir Crit Care Med* 1995; **152**: 545–9.
34. Chien JY, Lin MS, Huang YC *et al.* Changes in B-type natriuretic peptide improve weaning outcome predicted by spontaneous breathing trial. *Crit Care Med* 2008; **36**: 1421–6.
35. Grasso S, Leone A, De Michele M *et al.* Use of N-terminal pro-brain natriuretic peptide to detect acute cardiac dysfunction during weaning failure in difficult-to-wean patients with chronic obstructive pulmonary disease. *Crit Care Med* 2007; **35**: 96–105t.
36. Lemaire F, Teboul JL, Cinotti L *et al.* Acute left ventricular dysfunction during unsuccessful weaning from mechanical ventilation. *Anesthesiology* 1988; **69**: 171–9.
37. Lemaire F. Difficult weaning. *Intensive Care Med* 1993; **19**: 69–73.
38. Richard Ch, Teboul J-L, Archanbaud F *et al.* Left ventricular function during weaning of patients with chronic obstructive pulmonary disease. *Intensive Care Med* 1994; **20**: 181–6.
39. Robotham JL, Becker LC: The cardiovascular effects of weaning: Stratifying patient populations. *Intensive Care Med* 1994; **20**: 171–2.
40. Permutt S. Circulatory effects of weaning from mechanical ventilation: The importance of transdiaphragmatic pressure. *Anesthesiology* 1988; **69**: 157–60.
41. Biondi JW, Schulman DS, Matthay RA. Effects of mechanical ventilation on right and left ventricular function. *Clin Chest Med* 1988; **9**: 55–74.
42. Takata M, Robotham JL. Effects of inspiratory diaphragmatic descent on inferior vena caval venous return. *J Appl Physiol* 1992; **72**: 597–607.
43. Takata M, Wise RA, Robotham JL. Effects of abdominal pressure on venous return. *J Appl Physiol* 1990; **69**: 1961–72.
44. Jubran A, Mathru M, Dries D *et al.* Continuous recordings of mixed venous oxygen saturation during weaning from mechanical ventilation and the ramifications thereof. *Am J Respir Crit Care Med* 1998; **158**: 1763–9.
45. Zakynthinos S, Routsi CH, Vassilakopoulos T *et al.* Differential cardiovascular responses during weaning failure: effects on tissue oxygenation and lactate. *Intensive Care Med* 2005; **31**: 1634–42.
46. De Backer D, El Haddad P, Preiser JC *et al.* Hemodynamic responses to successful weaning from mechanical ventilation after cardiovascular surgery. *Intensive Care Med* 2000; **26**: 1201–6.

47. Richard C, Teboul JL. Weaning failure from cardiovascular origin. *Intensive Care Med* 2005; **31**: 1605–7.
48. Räsänen I, Nikki P, Heikkila J. Acute myocardial infarction complicated by respiratory failure: the effects of mechanical ventilation. *Chest* 1984; **85**: 21–8.
49. Hurford WE, Lynch KE, Strauss WH *et al.* Myocardial perfusion as assessed by thallium 201 scintigraphy during the discontinuation of mechanical ventilation in ventilator dependent patients. *Anesthesiology* 1991; **74**: 1007–16.
50. Hurford WE, Favorito F. Association of myocardial ischemia with failure to wean from mechanical ventilation. *Crit Care Med* 1995; **23**: 1475–80.
51. Abalos A, Leibowitz AB, Distefano D *et al.* Myocardial ischemia during the weaning period. *Am J Crit Care* 1992; **3**: 32–6.
52. Chatila W, Ani S, Guaglianone D *et al.* Cardiac ischemia during weaning from mechanical ventilation. *Chest* 1996; **109**: 1577–83.
53. Kreit JW, Eschenbacher WL. The physiology of spontaneous and mechanical ventilation. *Clin Chest Med* 1998; **9**: 55–74.
54. Knebel AR, Janson-Bjerklie SL, Malley JD *et al.* Comparison of breathing comfort during weaning with two ventilatory modes. *Am J Respir Crit Care Med* 1994; **149**: 14–18.
55. Petrof BJ, Legare M, Goldberg P *et al.* Continuous positive airway pressure reduces work of breathing and dyspnea during weaning from mechanical ventilation in severe chronic obstructive pulmonary disease. *Am Rev Respir Dis* 1990; **141**: 281–9.
56. Stroetz RW, Hubmayr RD. Tidal volume maintenance during weaning with pressure support. *Am J Respir Crit Care Med* 1995; **152**: 1034–40.
57. Criner GJ, Isaac L. Psychological problems in the ventilator dependent patient. In: Tobin J, ed. *Principles and practice of mechanical ventilation.* New York: McGraw Hill, 1994:1163–75.
58. LaFond L, Horner J. Psychological issues related to long-term ventilatory support. *Prob Respir Care* 1988; **1**: 241–56.
59. Holliday JE, Hyers TM. The reduction of weaning time from mechanical ventilation using tidal volume and relaxation biofeedback. *Am Rev Respir Dis* 1990; **141**: 1214–20.
60. La Riccia PJ, Katz RH, Peters JW *et al.* Biofeedback and hypnosis in weaning from mechanical ventilators. *Chest* 1985; **87**: 267–9.
61. Gorson JA, Grant JL, Moulton DP *et al.* Use of biofeedback in weaning paralyzed patients from respirators. *Chest* 1979; **76**: 543–5.
62. Yarnal JR, Herrel DW, Sivak ED. Routine use of biofeedback in weaning patients from mechanical ventilation. *Chest* 1981; **79**: 127–9.

58

# Non-invasive ventilation for weaning and extubation failure

SCOTT K EPSTEIN

## ABSTRACT

Non-invasive ventilation (NIV) has become a standard therapeutic intervention for many forms of acute respiratory failure, with a goal of improving outcome by avoiding intubation and its attendant complications. With increasing skill in application clinicians have extended the use of NIV in an effort to shorten the duration of mechanical ventilation. Difficult weaning prolongs mechanical ventilation and is associated with increased complications and mortality. Similarly, patients who fail extubation and require reintubation experience significantly increased duration of intubation and a substantial increase in mortality. Therefore, increasingly NIV has been used to facilitate weaning in patients failing spontaneous breathing trials and for patients after planned extubation. Randomized controlled trials and meta-analyses indicate that NIV is an effective tool for facilitating weaning but only in a very select group of patients, those with acute exacerbation of chronic obstructive pulmonary disease (COPD) (e.g. acute-on-chronic respiratory failure). In this setting NIV reduces the duration of intubation, need for reintubation, shortens length of stay in the intensive care unit and hospital, decreases risk for pneumonia and need for tracheostomy, and improves survival. At present using NIV to facilitate weaning cannot be recommended for patients without COPD. Randomized controlled trials indicate that NIV is not effective as treatment for established post-extubation respiratory distress and may be harmful if reintubation is required but unnecessarily delayed. This may not be true for COPD patients because these trials contained few COPD patients and a well-performed case–control study showed benefit in reducing the need for reintubation. Routine use of NIV, applied very soon after extubation, cannot be recommended except for patients assessed to be at significantly increased risk for extubation failure. Indeed, two randomized trials show that immediate application of NIV in high-risk patients reduces the need for reintubation.

## INTRODUCTION

Non-invasive ventilation (NIV) has become a standard therapeutic intervention for many forms of acute respiratory failure, with a goal of improving outcome by avoiding intubation and its attendant complications.[1] With increasing skill in application, clinicians have extended the use of NIV to shorten the duration of mechanical ventilation by facilitating weaning (earlier extubation),[2–4] preventing reintubation in surgical patients in the post-operative period,[5,6] and for patients after planned extubation.[7–10] In the latter instance, NIV is used as a preventive strategy with application immediately post-extubation in patients predicted to be at increased risk for extubation failure.[9,10] On the other hand, NIV has been used in patients who develop clear signs of respiratory failure after extubation.[7,8] The use of NIV for these applications has increased significantly. An observational study found that 30 per cent of applications of NIV for acute respiratory failure were for facilitating weaning or after extubation.[11] In another observational study, 21 per cent of NIV applications were for post-extubation respiratory failure.[12] In this chapter, the rationale for using NIV to facilitate weaning and to prevent extubation failure will first be discussed. Subsequently, a detailed review of randomized controlled trials (RCTs) will lead to recommendations for effective use.

## RATIONALE: THE IMPORTANCE OF FACILITATING WEANING AND EXTUBATION

Mechanical ventilation, delivered via an endotracheal tube, provides essential and life-saving support for patients intubated with various forms of acute respiratory failure. Invasive delivery of ventilatory support is predictably associated with clinically significant complications including injury to the upper airway (vocal cord dysfunction, tracheal stenosis, tracheomalacia), increase risk for gastrointestinal bleeding and for thromboembolism (consequences of increased stress and immobility), injury to lung parenchyma (e.g. volutrauma, barotrauma), and infection (e.g. sepsis, sinusitis, ventilator-associated pneumonia).[13] In general, the risk for complications increases with duration of mechanical ventilation. Approximately 25 per cent intubated for acute respiratory failure will require 7 or more days of mechanical ventilation and 10 per cent require greater than 3 weeks.[14] Up to 40–60 per cent of mechanical ventilation time is spent weaning the patient, a procedure that is dependent on the process of care.[15] Weaning patients as soon as possible is crucial because mortality increases with duration of intubation.[14]

Once ventilatory support is no longer required, attention shifts to removing the endotracheal tube (i.e. extubation). Both delayed extubation and failed extubation (reintubation) are associated with poor outcomes. The importance of timely extubation was demonstrated in a study of 136 mechanically ventilated brain-injured patients.[16] These patients were screened daily to ascertain readiness for extubation. The 27 per cent of patients with delayed extubation (failure to extubate within 48 hours of achieving readiness criteria) experienced more pneumonia, longer intensive care unit (ICU) and hospital stay and increased mortality when compared with the patients extubated without delay.

Extubation failure is defined as respiratory failure necessitating reinstitution of mechanical ventilatory support (reintubation or NIV), within 48–72 hours of endotracheal tube removal.[17] In one multicentre study, 25 per cent of 980 extubated patients developed, within 48 hours of extubation, signs of respiratory distress with at least two of the following: hypercapnia ($PaCO_2$ >45 mm Hg or ≥20 per cent increase from pre-extubation), respiratory acidosis (pH <7.35 with $PaCO_2$ >45 mm Hg), clinical signs of respiratory muscle fatigue or increased work of breathing, respiratory rate >25 breaths/min for two consecutive hours, and hypoxaemia ($SpO_2$ <90 per cent or $PaO_2$ <80 mm Hg on $FiO_2$ ≥0.50).[7] Fifty per cent of these patients required reintubation. Rates of extubation failure depend on many factors (Box 58.1). Extubation failure is more common in paediatric, medical, multidisciplinary and neurological ICU patients with rates averaging 13–17 per cent.[17,18]

Extubation failure markedly prolongs the duration of invasive mechanical ventilation. In medical ICU patients, extubation failure led to 12 additional days on mechanical ventilation, three additional weeks in the ICU, and 30 additional days in the hospital.[19] Patients experiencing extubation failure are significantly more likely to require tracheostomy.[19–26]

**Box 58.1 Factors associated with increased risk for extubation failure**

Patient factors

- Type of patient (medical, paediatric, multidisciplinary, ICU)
- Older age
- Pneumonia as cause for mechanical ventilation
- Higher severity of illness at the time of extubation
- Abnormal mental status, delirium

Process of care factors

- Use of continuous intravenous sedation (versus bolus dosing)
- Semi-recumbent positioning
- Transport out of ICU for procedures
- Reduced physician and nurse staffing in the ICU

Extubation failure is associated with increased mortality; univariate analyses show mortality rates 2–10 times that experienced by successfully extubated patients.[19,23,25,27–33] Mortality rates of 40–50 per cent were observed in general surgical, medical, multidisciplinary and paediatric patients with extubation failure. In contrast, trauma and cardiothoracic surgical patients experience mortality rates of approximately 10 per cent. With multivariate analyses adjusted for severity of illness and comorbid conditions, most studies found extubation failure to be independently associated with mortality.[19,25,27] Mortality rates are lower when reintubation results from upper airway obstruction, aspiration or excess pulmonary secretions compared with reintubation from respiratory or cardiac failure.[19,32] A number of explanations have been offered for the association of extubation failure and mortality. Extubation failure may be another marker for increased severity of illness. Reintubation, especially when performed emergently, may result in direct complications (e.g. haemodynamic instability, pneumonia) that contribute to poor outcome. Once reintubated, patients experience more prolonged intubation and are subject to the risks mentioned earlier. Lastly, clinical deterioration can occur between extubation and reintubation, especially when there are delays in re-establishing ventilatory support in the patient with post-extubation respiratory distress. This hypothesis is supported by the observation that mortality is lowest in patients who are relatively rapidly reintubated. As an example, patients reintubated after self-extubation do not have excess hospital mortality, perhaps because the vast majority are reintubated within 1 hour of extubation.[21,34] In a study that controlled for cause of extubation failure, increased time from planned extubation to reintubation was independently associated with mortality.[22] Four additional studies found more delayed reintubation associated with poor outcome.[23,30,35,36] A potential mechanism was suggested by a study that found a lower incidence of pneumonia in patients immediately reintubated compared to patients with more delayed reintubation.[36] This relationship between time to reintubation and outcome suggests that earlier re-establishment of ventilatory support, using NIV, may improve outcome.

## PATHOPHYSIOLOGY

The pathophysiology of weaning failure has been extensively investigated by comparing patients who fail with those who pass a trial of spontaneous breathing (SBT). Alternatively a cohort of patients serves as their own controls, studied first at the time of weaning failure, then again at the time of weaning success. Patients intolerant of spontaneous breathing demonstrate rapid shallow breathing, increased elastic and resistive work of breathing, increased intrinsic PEEP, abnormal gas exchange, respiratory muscle weakness, and increased tension–time index.[37,38] The latter finding suggests that weaning failure is characterized by a potentially fatiguing set of conditions. Fortunately, overt respiratory muscle fatigue may be avoided by careful monitoring during the SBT. Returning the patient to full ventilator support at the earliest sign of trouble during the trial avoids the development of respiratory muscle fatigue.[39] Weaning failure is also characterized by an abnormal cardiovascular response manifested as a failure to increase oxygen transport to the respiratory muscles.[40] Studies indicate a range of additional cardiovascular abnormalities during weaning failure including an increased transmural pulmonary artery occlusion pressure, decreased left ventricular ejection fraction, ischaemia detected by electrocardiogram, and an elevated brain natriuretic peptide (BNP) or pro-BNP.[41–45]

The physiologic effects of NIV can reverse many of the abnormalities seen with weaning failure (Box 58.2). Non-invasive ventilation is associated with decreased rapid shallow breathing, improved gas exchange, improved alveolar ventilation and decreased work of breathing.[46,47] Pressure–time product, an indicator of work of breathing, is consistently reduced by NIV in proportion to the level of non-invasive pressure support applied.[48] This effect results in a 17–93 per cent reduction in the diaphragmatic electromyography (EMG) signal.[48] NIV can deliver extrinsic positive end-expiratory pressure (PEEP) to counterbalance intrinsic PEEP, decreasing work of breathing and reducing the inspiratory threshold load that results from dynamic hyperinflation.[46,47] The positive intrathoracic pressure associated with NIV reduces both cardiac preload and afterload, improving cardiovascular function.

A number of additional potential benefits occur when NIV permits removal of the endotracheal tube (Box 58.3). These benefits must be weighed against the fact that, unlike mechanical ventilation delivered via an endotracheal tube, there is no guaranteed minute ventilation with NIV. NIV does not enhance airway clearance and does not provide the convenient access of an endotracheal tube to suction copious airway secretions. Sedating the agitated patient on mechanical ventilation can be challenging without the airway protection of an endotracheal tube. Fortunately, agitation usually decreases when the endotracheal tube is removed and therefore sedation requirements should diminish as a result.

**Box 58.2 Physiological effects of NIV that favourably counterbalance pathophysiological causes of weaning failure**

- Reduces work of breathing
- Counterbalances intrinsic PEEP
- Increases dynamic compliance
- Unloads diaphragm (reduces EMG signal of diaphragm)
- Decreases respiratory rate
- Increases tidal volume
- Reduces rapid shallow breathing
- Increases $PaO_2$
- Decreases $PaCO_2$
- Increases pH
- Decreases cardiac preload
- Decreases cardiac afterload

**Box 58.3 Advantages of removing an endotracheal tube**

- Eliminates imposed work of breathing that can occur with a narrow endotracheal tube
- Decreases risk for nosocomial infection and pneumonia
- Improves communication
- Improves patient comfort and may reduce need for sedation
- Allows for effective cough
- Improves mucociliary secretion clearance
- Improves sinus drainage

## NON-INVASIVE VENTILATION TO FACILITATE WEANING

### Evidence base

Uncontrolled studies published in the 1990s indicated that NIV could be used to wean patients from mechanical ventilation. The earliest reports used NIV in patients with prolonged mechanical ventilation with a tracheostomy.[49–51] In this way, these studies differ substantially from the RCTs discussed subsequently. The initial three reports suggested a success rate approaching 90 per cent with weaning by NIV.[49–51] The lack of controls makes it impossible to determine the actual effectiveness of the technique.

Subsequently, enthusiasm was tempered by a study where NIV was used in 22 intubated trauma patients.[52] After a T-piece trial to assess the patient's capacity for spontaneous breathing, all 22 patients were extubated to NIV. The authors found no difference in blood gases and respiratory parameters when comparing measurements made with equivalent settings of either invasive or non-invasive pressure support. Of concern, nine patients (36 per cent) required reintubation and six eventually died on mechanical ventilation.

One additional observational study used NIV in 15 patients intubated for acute respiratory failure.[53] Patients were extubated after satisfying the following criteria: $PaO_2 \geq 40$ mm Hg (on $FiO_2$ 0.21), $PaCO_2 \leq 55$ mm Hg, pH >7.32, respiratory rate ≤40 breaths/ min, tidal volume ≥3 mL/kg, frequency/tidal volume ratio ≤190 breaths/L/ min and negative inspiratory force ≥20 cm $H_2O$. These criteria are substantially more liberal than usual and would not typically indicate readiness for weaning and extubation. Non-invasive ventilation (continuous positive airway pressure [CPAP] of 5 cm $H_2O$ and PSV of 15 cm $H_2O$) was applied after extubation and maintained for a median of 2 days. Both modes of NIV resulted in physiological benefits including improved oxygenation, increased tidal volume and decreased respiratory rate. Non-invasive pressure support ventilation reduced $PaCO_2$, increased minute ventilation, and increased pH. Thirteen of 15 patients were successfully extubated. Although this success rate appears impressive we cannot be certain that all 15 patients were true weaning failure patients.

Eight randomized controlled trials using NIV to facilitate weaning (versus weaning in those who remain intubated) in patients failing at least one SBT have been reported, including three abstracts and one published in the Chinese language literature[2–4,54–58] (Table 58.1). Four more trials, published in Chinese and summarized in a meta-analysis, studied COPD patients with pneumonia randomized to NIV versus continued invasive mechanical ventilation after pulmonary infection was thought to be under control.[59] These four studies fundamentally differ from the studies listed in Table 58.1 in that patients did not fail a SBT before randomization.

The first randomized trial, by Nava *et al.*, screened 68 COPD patients intubated with severe acute-on-chronic respiratory failure.[4] Patients had an average $PaCO_2$ of 90 mm Hg prior to intubation and approximately 40 per cent failed NIV prior to intubation. Once intubated, patients were ventilated in volume-assist control mode facilitated by heavy sedation and neuromuscular blockade (Fig. 58.1). Patients were then changed, after approximately 12 hours, to pressure support. A two-hour SBT was then performed, approximately 48 hours after intubation. The 50 patients (74 per cent) failing the T-piece trial were randomized. Twenty-five patients remained intubated and underwent weaning by gradual reduction in the level of pressure support with a goal respiratory rate <25 breaths/ min. They also received twice daily SBTs on either CPAP or T-tube. The remaining 25 patients were extubated to NIV via an oronasal mask using an ICU ventilator in pressure support mode. Patients extubated to NIV underwent a weaning protocol similar to that for the invasive group. When compared to patients who remained intubated those randomized to NIV experienced significantly better outcomes including a reduction in duration of mechanical ventilation, shorter length of ICU stay, increased weaning success, and improved 60-day survival (Table 58.2). Complications associated with NIV were common but not severe with the most frequent being nasal bridge abrasions. No NIV patient developed pneumonia compared with 25 per cent of those remaining intubated, suggesting a possible mechanism for improved outcome with NIV. This study is also notable for demonstrating that failure of NIV as primary therapy did not preclude successful use of NIV at a later time.

Girault and colleagues published a randomized controlled trial with a design similar to that of Nava. Thirty-three patients with acute-on-chronic respiratory failure who failed a 2-hour T-tube trial were randomized to extubation to NIV or continued invasive weaning using pressure support mode.[3] In contrast to Nava, in the Girault study NIV was delivered either by nasal or oronasal mask and with either pressure support or volume-assist control modes. Using this approach, weaning using NIV resulted in a 3-day reduction in duration of intubation (4.6 vs 7.7 days). Yet, no significant differences were noted in rate of weaning success (77 per cent vs 75 per cent), ICU (12 vs 14 days) or hospital length of stay (27 vs 28 days), reintubation (23 per cent vs 25 per cent) or mortality at 3 months (0 per cent vs 12 per cent). The total duration of mechanical ventilation (combining intubated and NIV time) was longer with NIV (16 vs 8 days), a result of seven patients still requiring nocturnal NIV at discharge.

Ferrer *et al.* studied 43 patients (77 per cent with chronic lung disease) randomized after failing at least *three* trials of spontaneous breathing.[2] NIV was applied for a minimum of 24 hours using a bi-level mode (initial settings: inspiratory positive airway pressure [IPAP] 10–20 cm $H_2O$, expiratory positive airway pressure [EPAP] 4–5 cm $H_2O$) delivered with a nasal or oronasal mask. The study was halted early after the first interim analysis. Compared to invasive weaning, weaning facilitated by extubation with NIV was associated with significant decreases in duration of invasive mechanical ventilation, duration of ICU and hospital stay, incidence of septic shock and pneumonia (Table 58.3). Weaning using NIV was associated with decreased ICU and 90-day mortality. This investigation is notable for the dramatic benefits seen with NIV despite the relatively small cohort studied.

**Table 58.1** Randomized controlled trials using non-invasive ventilation (NIV) to facilitate weaning from mechanical ventilation

| Study, year (enrolment criteria) | Per cent with chronic obstructive pulmonary disease | No. of patients | Effects of NIV versus control group weaning with endotracheal tube in place |
|---|---|---|---|
| Ferrer *et al.* (2003)[2] (failed at least 3 SBTs) | 58 | 43 | ↓ Duration of intubation<br>↓ ICU length of stay<br>↓ Hospital length of stay<br>↓ Septic shock<br>↓ Pneumonia<br>↓ Need for tracheostomy<br>↑ ICU survival<br>↑ 90-day survival |
| Girault *et al.* (1999)[3] (failed single 2-hour SBT) | 76 | 33 | ↓ Duration of intubation<br>↑ Total duration of mechanical ventilation (invasive plus non-invasive) |
| Nava *et al.* (1998)[4] (failed single 2-hour SBT) | 100 | 50 | ↓ Duration of mechanical ventilation<br>↓ ICU length of stay<br>↓ Hospital length of stay<br>↓ 60-day survival<br>↓ Pneumonia |
| Chen *et al.* (2001)[54] | 100 | 24 | ↓ Duration of intubation<br>↓ Hospital length of stay<br>↓ Pneumonia |
| Hill *et al.* (2000)[55] (failed single 30-minute SBT) | 33 | 21 | ↓ Duration of intubation |
| Trevisan and Vieira (2008)[56] (failed single 30-minute SBT) | 35* | 65 | ↓ Complications<br>↓ Need for tracheostomy |
| Rabie (2004)[57] *et al.* (failed single 2-hour SBT) | 100 | 37 | ↓ Duration of intubation<br>↓ ICU length of stay<br>↓ Hospital length of stay<br>↓ Pneumonia<br>↑ Weaning success |
| Girault *et al.* (2009)[†58] (Failed single 5–120-minute SBT) | 100 | 208 | None |

*Includes patients with chronic obstructive pulmonary disease (COPD) and asthma.
†Includes third randomization group that was extubated to oxygen alone.
ICU, intensive care unit; SBT, spontaneous breathing trial.

In a trial published in abstract form, 303 patients with acute respiratory failure were screened including 45 who failed a 30-minute T-piece trial.[55] Sixteen patients met exclusion criteria because of either excessive secretions or the presence of abnormal mental status. Of the remaining patients, 21 of 29 were enrolled and randomized, with nine remaining intubated and 12 extubated to NIV. Four of 12 NIV patients failed and required reintubation, while eight of nine controls weaned successfully. No difference was observed in hospital survival (NIV, 92 per cent; intubation, 89 per cent). NIV was associated with decreased duration of intubation (6.6 vs 15.2 days). Full appraisal of this study is difficult as only limited details have been reported. The study demonstrates that of all patients intubated for acute respiratory failure, NIV for weaning is applicable for fewer than 10 per cent.

Another study used a quasi-randomized design (allocation to groups based on order rather than blind randomization) in 24 COPD patients intubated for 3 days or more for an acute exacerbation.[54] Non-invasive ventilation was associated with a significant decrease in the incidence of pneumonia (0/12 vs 7/12, $p = 0.027$), reduced duration of invasive ventilation (7 vs 15 days, $p > 0.05$) and length of hospitalization after randomization (16 vs 25 days, $p < 0.05$). No difference was found in mortality but the study was underpowered to adequately examine this outcome (NIV, 0/12 vs control, 3/12, $p = 0.2$).

Burns *et al.* performed a meta-analysis of these five RCTs (totalling 171 patients, 81 per cent with COPD) comparing weaning via NIV versus weaning in intubated patients.[60] The investigators were quick to note that the five trials were characterized by design weaknesses.

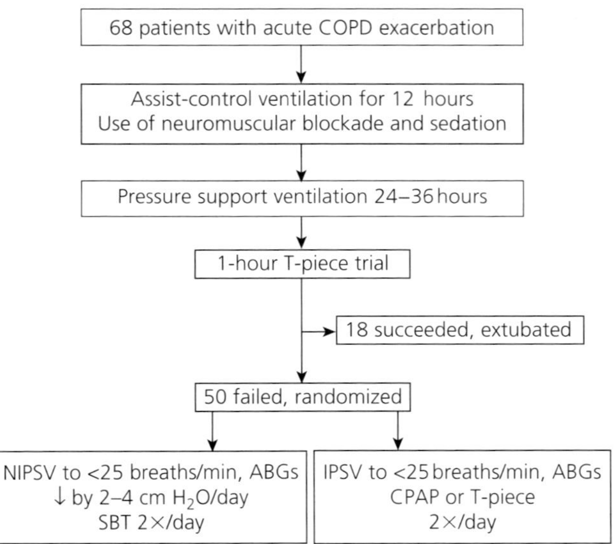


**Figure 58.1** Design of a randomized controlled trial using non-invasive ventilation (NIV) to wean patients with acute-on-chronic respiratory failure secondary to chronic obstructive pulmonary disease (COPD).[4] Patients failing a T-piece trial were randomized to continued intubation with pressure support weaning (IPSV) or weaning with NIV (NIPSV). ABG, arterial blood gas; ACV, volume assist control ventilation; CPAP, continuous positive airway pressure; PSV, pressure support ventilation; SBT, spontaneous breathing trial.

**Table 58.2** Results from the randomized controlled trial by Nava *et al.* comparing weaning with non-invasive ventilation (NIV) versus continued intubation[4]

| | NIV | Intubation | *p* Value |
|---|---|---|---|
| Duration of mechanical ventilation (days) | 10 | 17 | <0.05 |
| ICU length of stay (days) | 15 | 25 | <0.05 |
| Weaning success at 60 days (%) | 88 | 68 | <0.05 |
| Survival at 60 days (%) | 92 | 72 | <0.05 |
| Pneumonia after randomization (%) | 0 | 25 | <0.05 |

For example, four of five studies failed to use blinded assessment of outcome and did not fully control for important co-interventions that may influence outcome. Two studies did not use a weaning protocol and two did not have predefined reintubation criteria, thus raising the potential for bias. With these limitations noted, the meta-analysis found NIV was associated with decreased mortality (relative risk [RR], 0.41), decreased risk for pneumonia (RR 0.28), shorter duration of mechanical ventilation (–7.33 days), shorter ICU (–6.88 days) and hospital length

**Table 58.3** Results from the randomized controlled trial by Ferrer *et al.* comparing weaning with non-invasive ventilation (NIV) versus continued intubation[2]

| | NIV | Intubation |
|---|---|---|
| Duration of intubation (days) | 9.5 | 20.1 |
| ICU length of stay (days) | 14 | 25 |
| Hospital length of stay (days) | 28 | 49 |
| Tracheostomy (%) | 5 | 59 |
| ICU mortality (%) | 10 | 41 |
| 90-day mortality (%) | 29 | 59 |
| Nosocomial pneumonia (%) | 24 | 59 |
| Septic shock (%) | 10 | 41 |
| Reintubation (%) | 14 | 27 |

All comparisons were statistically significant except for reintubation.

of stay (–7.33 days). Weaning using NIV was not associated with a higher probability of weaning success.

Rabie and co-workers enrolled 37 COPD patients, intubated for acute-on-chronic respiratory failure, who failed a 2-hour SBT.[57] When compared with patients who remained intubated those weaned using NIV were more likely to experience successful weaning and extubation and had a shorter duration of intubation, decreased ICU and hospital length of stay, and fewer pneumonias. As with the study of Hill *et al.*, this study, published only in abstract form, is difficult to fully appraise.

Trevisan and Vieira randomized 65 patients, ventilated for at least 48 hours, who failed a 30-minute SBT.[56] The patients differed substantially from those discussed earlier where 58–100 per cent had COPD. In contrast, this study population was heterogeneous and consisted of patients with obstructive lung disease (35 per cent, COPD or asthma), post-surgery/thoracic trauma (28 per cent), pneumonia/tuberculosis/other respiratory disease (18 per cent), and heart disease (16 per cent). Thirty-seven patients remained intubated and underwent weaning with daily SBTs. The remaining 28 patients were extubated to NIV (bi-level positive airway pressure) using an IPAP from 10–30 cm $H_2O$ delivered via a face mask. NIV weaning was carried out by systematically decreasing the level of pressure support. Weaning with NIV produced similar results to that performed in intubated patients: ICU length of stay (18.9 vs 20.8 days), hospital length of stay (34.5 vs 42.4 days), hospital survival (68 per cent vs 73 per cent), and duration of time on mechanical ventilation (14.9 vs 17.3 days). NIV weaning was associated with a reduction in complications (pneumonia, sepsis, congestive heart failure) and fewer patients required tracheostomy (29 per cent vs 76 per cent). Six of 28 (21 per cent) extubated to NIV required reintubation.

Burns and colleagues published an updated meta-analysis including the seven studies discussed above, an unpublished dissertation, and four Chinese studies that differed significantly in study design. These latter

52. Gregoretti C, Beltrame F, Lucangelo U *et al.* Physiologic evaluation of non-invasive pressure support ventilation in trauma patients with acute respiratory failure. *Intensive Care Med* 1998; **24**: 785–90.
53. Kilger E, Briegel J, Haller M *et al.* Effects of noninvasive positive pressure ventilatory support in non-COPD patients with acute respiratory insufficiency after early extubation. *Intensive Care Med* 1999; **25**: 1374–80.
54. Chen J, Qiu D, Tao D. Time for extubation and sequential noninvasive mechanical ventilation in COPD patients with exacerbated respiratory failure who received invasive ventilation. *Zhonghua Jie He He Hu Xi Za Zhi* 2001; **24**: 99–100.
55. Hill N, Lin D, Levy M *et al.* Noninvasive positive pressure ventilation (NPPV) to facilitate extubation after acute respiratory failure: a feasibility study. *Am J Respir Crit Care Med* 2000; **161**: A263.
56. Trevisan CE, Vieira SR. Noninvasive mechanical ventilation may be useful in treating patients who fail weaning from invasive mechanical ventilation: a randomized clinical trial. *Crit Care* 2008; **12**: R51.
57. Rabie G, Mohamed A, Mohamed R. Noninvasive ventilation in the weaning of patients with acute-on-chronic respiratory failure due to COPD. *Chest* 2004; **126**: 755S.
58. Girault C, Bubenheim M, Benichou J *et al.* Non invasive ventilation (NIV) and weaning from mechanical ventilation (MV) in chronic respiratory failure (CRF) patients: The VENISE study preliminary results. *Proc Am Thorac Soc* 2009; A2165.
59. Burns KE, Adhikari NK, Keenan SP *et al.* Use of non-invasive ventilation to wean critically ill adults off invasive ventilation: meta-analysis and systematic review. *BMJ* 2009; **338**: b1574.
60. Burns KE, Adhikari NK, Meade MO. A meta-analysis of noninvasive weaning to facilitate liberation from mechanical ventilation. *Can J Anaesth* 2006; **53**: 305–15.
61. Girou E, Brun-Buisson C, Taille S *et al.* Secular trends in nosocomial infections and mortality associated with noninvasive ventilation in patients with exacerbation of COPD and pulmonary edema. *JAMA* 2003; **290**: 2985–91.
62. Girou E, Schortgen F, Delclaux C *et al.* Association of noninvasive ventilation with nosocomial infections and survival in critically ill patients. *JAMA* 2000; **284**: 2361–7.
63. Brook AD, Ahrens TS, Schaiff R *et al.* Effect of a nursing-implemented sedation protocol on the duration of mechanical ventilation. *Crit Care Med* 1999; **27**: 2609–15.
64. Kollef MH, Levy NT, Ahrens TS *et al.* The use of continuous i.v. sedation is associated with prolongation of mechanical ventilation. *Chest* 1998; **114**: 541–8.
65. Kress JP, Pohlman AS, O'Connor MF *et al.* Daily interruption of sedative infusions in critically ill patients undergoing mechanical ventilation. *N Engl J Med* 2000; **342**: 1471–7.
66. Kirton OC, DeHaven CB, Morgan JP *et al.* Elevated imposed work of breathing masquerading as ventilator weaning intolerance. *Chest* 1995; **108**: 1021–5.
67. Keenan SP, Sinuff T, Cook DJ *et al.* Which patients with acute exacerbation of chronic obstructive pulmonary disease benefit from noninvasive positive-pressure ventilation? A systematic review of the literature. *Ann Intern Med* 2003; **138**: 861–70.
68. Hilbert G, Gruson D, Portel L *et al.* Noninvasive pressure support ventilation in COPD patients with postextubation hypercapnic respiratory insufficiency. *Eur Respir J* 1998; **11**: 1349–53.
69. Meduri GU, Turner RE, Abou-Shala N *et al.* Noninvasive positive pressure ventilation via face mask. First-line intervention in patients with acute hypercapnic and hypoxemic respiratory failure. *Chest* 1996; **109**: 179–93.
70. Chiang AA, Lee KC. Use of noninvasive positive pressure ventilation via nasal mask in patients with respiratory distress after extubation. *Zhonghua Yi Xue Za Zhi (Taipei)* 1995; **56**: 94–101.
71. Epstein SK. Noninvasive ventilation to shorten the duration of mechanical ventilation. *Respir Care* 2009; **54**: 198–208; discussion 11.
72. Jiang JS, Kao SJ, Wang SN. Effect of early application of biphasic positive airway pressure on the outcome of extubation in ventilator weaning. *Respirology* 1999; **4**: 161–5.
73. El-Solh AA, Aquilina A, Pineda L *et al.* Noninvasive ventilation for prevention of post-extubation respiratory failure in obese patients. *Eur Respir J* 2006; **28**: 588–95.
74. Agarwal R, Aggarwal AN, Gupta D *et al.* Role of noninvasive positive-pressure ventilation in postextubation respiratory failure: a meta-analysis. *Respir Care* 2007; **52**: 1472–9.

59

# Weaning strategies and protocols

MICHELE VITACCA

## ABSTRACT

The chapter presents the state of the art of the weaning process including use of protocols derived from mechanical ventilation in patients with chronic obstructive pulmonary disease or those who experienced acute respiratory failure. The weaning process is a delicate time in the medical history of a patient who survives an acute episode of respiratory failure and spends a period of time under mechanical ventilation. In fact, during the period of mechanical ventilation, there are a lot of implications that are currently somehow underestimated in daily medical practice: occupation of beds, healthcare costs, burden for the families and for the patients themselves. Although these occurrences are quite common and critical, there are no clear guidelines on the minimal criteria required for assessing the correct weaning time for different diseases, or on the need for a screening test prior to a spontaneous breathing test. It is also crucial to identify the patients who can be considered possible successful responders to the weaning process. A careful review of the literature shows the crucial role of the respiratory therapist in the multidisciplinary team (physician, nurse, respiratory therapist and family as well), who should be involved in such a delicate process. In general, weaning should start early in patients under mechanical ventilation and it has been observed that the majority of patients can be successfully weaned on the first attempt. The spontaneous breathing test is the major diagnostic test to determine if patients can be successfully extubated. However, there are too many aspects that still need to be investigated. Therefore, the specific need of availability of clear weaning protocols is stressed and recommended.

## INTRODUCTION

In the past 10 years, the availability of beds in intensive care units (ICU), new technologies and improved levels of care have increased the population of patients defined as 'survivors of catastrophic illness', often requirng prolonged weaning procedures.[1] About 80 per cent of patients admitted to an ICU and mechanically ventilated because of acute respiratory failure (ARF) resume spontaneous breathing quite easily after a few days of ventilation.[2] The weaning success rate differs among studies depending on the case mix and referrals to an individual ICU. The 20 per cent unsuccessful cases are mainly concentrated in specific populations, in which age, residual or premorbidity impairment of the cardiorespiratory or neuromuscular systems render the discontinuation from mechanical ventilation particularly difficult.[2] These patients represent <10 per cent of ICU admissions but account for a huge demand on financial resources.[1] In addition, from a financial point of view, prolonged mechanical ventilation (>30 days) in the ICU results in high costs for the healthcare system.[3]

To this end, new strategies and protocols for weaning from mechanical ventilation are clearly needed in the daily practice of healthcare.

## EVIDENCE BASE

### Weaning from mechanical ventilation: rarely early, often too late

While unnecessary delays in withdrawing mechanical ventilation can increase the risk of complications, prolong ICU stay and significantly amplify healthcare costs, premature attempts at withdrawal of mechanical ventilation might lead to development of severe distress, hamper the recovery process and further delay weaning.[4] Physicians often fail to recognize patients who may already be ready for extubation. Studies among patients who are

**Box 59.2 Advice on implementation of a weaning protocol**

- Identify the issues related to the patient's care
- Test your institution's lengths of stay and complication rates
- Design protocols (evidence-based methods, local experts, review of protocols)
- Change of 'weaning culture'
- Create a team approach (hospital administrator, physicians, nurses, respiratory therapists, ethicists)
- Define the main local goals, successful and unsuccessful
- Avoid changing personnel (dedicated personnel)
- Education, timely feedback, compliance monitoring, appropriate outcomes: be pragmatic and improve your protocol over time
- Avoid rigid interpretation of the rules
- Clinical judgment remains important
- Periodic updating of implementation processes

## CLINICAL APPLICATIONS: NON-INVASIVE VENTILATION PROTOCOLS

### Nurse/respiratory therapist protocol during non-invasive ventilation

An important guide to NIV use was published by Knebel *et al*,[37] providing background information and illustrating key aspects of each type of support before, during and after the use of NIV. A specialized trained nurse is usually crucial in the first hours of NIV care (10 hours), usually closely supported by the other ICU nurses familiar with NIV.[38] This approach has not been found to be easy and is time consuming for nurses, and, even if possible in a general non-specialized ICU, it requires some expertise and reasonable co-operation on the part the patient.[38] In a later publication, Nava *et al.*[39] showed that, in the first 48 hours of mechanical ventilation, both human and economic resources needed to ventilate COPD patients either invasively or non-invasively are very similar and that, after this period, there is a significant reduction in medical and paramedical time spent only in the NIV group. Even in the acute period (first 48 hours), the combined time spent by nurses, doctors and respiratory therapists was <45 per cent of that in the first 48 hours. In this study,[39] the patients undergoing NIV with a face mask were periodically disconnected from the machine to allow them to drink, eat or talk with relatives for periods of time not exceeding 1 hour. While disconnected, the patients breathed spontaneously with oxygen supplementation delivered via nasal cannulas to achieve an arterial oxygen saturation >90 per cent. Hilbert showed that the time spent by the nurse per session was 25 per cent of the ventilatory time during the first 24 hours after initiation, and dropped significantly to 15 per cent of the ventilatory time after the first 24 hours.[40,41] In the Hilbert protocol, NIV is delivered with a full face mask, strict evaluation of side effects and use of a wound care dressing. Non-invasive ventilation was used in a sequential mode consisting of periods of ventilation alternating with periods of spontaneous breathing. The ventilation periods lasted for 30 minutes, and were performed at very regular intervals, i.e. every 3 or 4 hours.

### Non-invasive ventilation as a weaning technique

In a multicentre Italian study,[42] after intubation because of emergency situations, 50 chronic obstructive pulmonary disease (COPD) patients were randomized to either extubation with immediate application of NIV or to continued weaning with endotracheal tube in place. Mean duration of mechanical ventilation, ICU stay, nosocomial pneumonia and 60-day mortality were significantly reduced in the NIV group.[42] Similar results were found by Ferrer *et al.*[43] in patients with persistent weaning failure and by Squadrone *et al.*[44] in patients who developed hypoxaemia after elective major abdominal surgery. In contrast with previous experience, a more recent study by Esteban *et al.*[45] showed that NIV does not prevent the need for reintubation or reduce mortality in unselected patients who have respiratory failure after extubation.

A retrospective analysis conducted in COPD patients admitted for weaning from invasive ventilation[46] showed that NIV was associated with better long-term survival, independent of age and length of stay.

### Weaning from non-invasive ventilation use

Long-term dependency (LTD) on NIV is not an uncommon situation after resolution of a hypercapnic ARF episode, especially in patients with non-COPD causes of respiratory failure. At the same time, the predictive factors for LTD on NIV immediately after hypercapnic ARF have not been identified. Data about progressive periods of withdrawal from NIV are lacking. It is logical to assume that the restoration of arterial blood gases, patient comfort, and the absence of dyspnoea achieved with mechanical ventilation are prerequisites for weaning from NIV. It is not easy to decide if NIV withdrawal needs to be immediate or progressive and if the support needs to be maintained at night time or not.

A weaning protocol based on progressive periods of NIV withdrawal has been proposed by Damas *et al.* and demonstrated to have a high success rate.[47] Weaning was performed as follows: on the first day, every 3 hours, 1 hour without NIV (except during the night); on the second day, every 3 hours, 2 hours without NIV (except during the night); and on the third day, NIV was used only during the night.

Cuvelier *et al.*[48] studied 42 COPD patients and 58 non-COPD patients successfully treated with NIV for a hypercapnic ARF episode. The incidence of LTD-NIV was 39 per cent and 19 per cent in non-COPD and COPD patients, respectively. A multivariate analysis with stepwise logistic regression showed that lower baseline pH values and non-infectious causes of hypercapnic ARF were independently associated with LTD-NIV.[48] Outcome after 1 year was poor in COPD patients. The need for prospective validation of a weaning protocol in patients managed by NIV for an episode of hypercapnic ARF remains.

### Non-invasive ventilation protocols and outcome

According to the various controlled trials that have been published, NIV success rates range between 75 per cent to 100 per cent for COPD and 20–70 per cent for non-COPD patients. The use of NIV outside the ICU allows the clinicians performing early intervention to prevent further respiratory deterioration, gives access to respiratory support in patients who would not otherwise be admitted to ICU, and gives ventilatory support in a friendlier environment. During the past decades, several factors have been suggested to explain this variability in outcome, such as the severity of encephalopathy, the level of the arterial blood gases or respiratory rate. In addition, all these variables might be influenced by the patient's tolerance, which is directly related to staff training, experience of NIV, location of the patients receiving NIV and adequate monitoring.[49–51] Regular attendance at training programmes for medical and paramedical staff is mandatory for staff working with ventilated patients. Medical and paramedical staff expertise is a variable difficult to measure although it directly influences outcome and has been poorly studied. The study by Carlucci *et al.*[52] showed that, over time, better staff training allows the treatment of more severe, and a greater number of, patients without significantly changing the rate of success. These authors suggested that, with better staff training and experience, more severely ill patients may be treated with a lower risk of failure.

## FUTURE RESEARCH

Future studies should define: the minimal criteria required for assessing the correct weaning time in view of the different underlying diseases; the need for a screening test prior to the SBT; identification of patients who are successful on a spontaneous breathing trial but who fail extubation; the role of constant positive airway pressure (CPAP)/PEEP in the COPD patient undergoing an SBT; required duration of the SBT in patients who failed the initial trial; and which specific aspects improve the weaning outcome.

## CONCLUSIONS

- Weaning should be considered in the early stages in patients receiving mechanical ventilation.
- The majority of patients can be successfully weaned at the first attempt.
- For the majority of patients, the spontaneous breathing trial is the major diagnostic test to determine if they can be successfully extubated.
- The initial spontaneous breathing trial should last 30 minutes and consist of either T-tube breathing or low levels of PSV with or without 5 cm $H_2O$ positive end-expiratory pressure.
- Synchronized intermittent mechanical ventilation should be avoided as a weaning modality.
- The major limitation of protocols is the lack of generalizability in different diseases and conditions: different diseases require different physiopathological approaches and thus require different weaning protocols.
- A protocol to start weaning or to decide the extubation time is mandatory. Conversely, less evidence is available about the need for a rigid protocol to perform weaning in terms of the modality chosen or the time dedicated for each step of weaning.
- Weaning protocols are necessary as feedback for young doctors, for ICUs with a high turnover, for units with a rapid change in expertise, for better cooperation between the different members of a weaning team and to better document the clinical activity.
- Weaning protocols are most valuable in hospitals where physicians otherwise do not adhere to standardized weaning guidelines.
- Weaning protocols seem advantageous for COPD patients and for prolonged or difficult to wean patients: the generalized use could result only in a few hours reduction of intubation.
- How the weaning is conducted and the patient's underlying condition may be more influential than the ventilator modality *per se* when considering weaning outcomes (days of mechanical ventilation, rate of success but not survival).
- The potential role of NIV and synergic effect of cough assistance devices during weaning needs further clarification.

See Appendix B: Weaning strategies and protocols in the Vitalsource ebook edition.

## REFERENCES

1. Nava S, Vitacca M. Chronic ventilator facilities. In: Tobin M, ed. *Principles and practice of mechanical ventilation.* New York: McGraw-Hill, 2006: 691–704.
2. Carlet J, Artigas A, Bihari D *et al.* The first European Consensus Conference in Intensive Care Medicine: introductory remarks. *Intensive Care Med* 1992; **18**: 180–1.

3. Halpern NA, Bettes L, Greenstein R. Federal and nationwide intensive care units and healthcare costs: 1986–1992. *Crit Care Med* 1994; **22**: 2001–7.
4. Boles JM, Bion J, Connors A *et al.* TASK FORCE weaning from mechanical ventilation statement of the Sixth International Consensus Conference on intensive care medicine. *Eur Respir J* 2007; **29**: 1033–56.
5. Epstein SK, Nevins ML, Chung J. Effect of unplanned extubation on outcome of mechanical ventilation. *Am J Respir Crit Care Med* 2000; **161**: 1912–16.
6. Betbese AJ, Perez M, Bak E *et al.* A prospective study of unplanned endotracheal extubation in intensive care unit patients. *Crit Care Med* 1998; **26**: 1180–6.
7. Nevins ML, Chung J. Effect of unplanned extubation on outcome of mechanical ventilation. *Am J Respir Crit Care Med* 2000; **161**: 1912–16.
8. Vitacca M, Vianello A, Colombo D *et al.* Comparison of two methods for weaning patients with chronic obstructive pulmonary disease requiring mechanical ventilation for more than 15 days. *Am J Respir Crit Care Med* 2001;**164**: 225–30.
9. Esteban A, Alia I, Ibanez J *et al.* Modes of mechanical ventilation and weaning. A national survey of Spanish hospitals. The Spanish Lung Failure Collaborative Group. *Chest* 1994; **106**: 1188–93.
10. Brochard L, Rauss A, Benito S *et al.* Comparison of three methods of gradual withdrawal from ventilatory support during weaning from mechanical ventilation. *Am J Respir Crit Care Med* 1994: **150**: 896–903.
11. Esteban A, Frutos F, Tobin MJ *et al.* A comparison of four methods of weaning patients from mechanical ventilation. *N Engl J Med* 1995; **332**: 345–50.
12. Esteban A, Alia I, Tobin MJ *et al.* Effect of spontaneous breathing trial duration on outcome of attempts to discontinue mechanical ventilation. *Am J Respir Crit Care Med* 1999; **159**: 512–18.
13. Ely EW, Meade MO, Haponik EF *et al.* Mechanical ventilator weaning protocols driven by non physician health-care professionals: evidence-based clinical practice guidelines. *Chest* 2001; **120**: 454S–63S.
14. Ely EW, Baker AM, Dunagan DP *et al.* Effect of the duration of mechanical ventilation of identifying patients capable of breathing spontaneously. *N Engl J Med* 1996; **335**: 1864–9.
15. Kollef MH, Shapiro SD, Silver P *et al.* A randomized, controlled trial of protocol-directed versus physician-directed weaning from mechanical ventilation. *Crit Care Med* 1997; **25**: 567–74.
16. Saura P, Blanch L, Mestre J *et al.* Clinical consequences of the implementation of a weaning protocol. *Intensive Care Med* 1996**; 22**: 1052–6.
17. Marelich GP, Murin S, Battistella F *et al.* Protocol weaning of mechanical ventilation in medical and surgical patients by respiratory care practitioners and nurses: effect on weaning time and incidence of VAP. *Chest* 2000; **118**: 459–67.
18. Durbin C. Therapist driven protocols in adult intensive care unit patients. In: Stoller JK, Kester L, eds. *Therapist driven protocols.* Philadelphia: Saunders Company, 1996.
19. ACCP, AARC, ACCCM task force. Evidence based guidelines for weaning and discontinuing ventilatory support. *Chest* 2001; **120**: 375s–95s.
20. Norrenberg M, Vincent JL. A profile of European intensive care unit physiotherapists. European Society of Intensive Care Medicine. *Intensive Care Med* 2000; **26**: 988–94.
21. Horst HM, Mouro D, Hall-Jenssens RA *et al.* Decrease in ventilation time with a standardized weaning process. *Arch Surg* 1998; **133**: 483–9.
22. Kollef MH, Levy NT, Ahrens TS *et al.* The use of continuous IV sedation is associated with prolongation of mechanical ventilation. *Chest* 1998; **114**: 541–8.
23. Dries DJ, McGonigal MD, Malian MS *et al.* Protocol-driven ventilator weaning reduces use of mechanical ventilation, rate of early reintubation, and ventilator-associated pneumonia. *J Trauma* 2004; **56**: 943–51.
24. Henneman E, Dracup K, Ganz T *et al.* Effect of a collaborative weaning plan on patient outcome in the critical care setting. *Crit Care Med* 2001; **29**: 297–303.
25. Chan PK, Fischer S, Stewart TE *et al.* Practising evidence-based medicine: the design and implementation of multidisciplinary team-driven extubation protocol. *Crit Care* 2001: **5**: 349–54.
26. Iregui M, Ward S, Clinikscale D *et al.* Use of handheld computer by respiratory care practitioners to improve the efficacy of weaning patients from MV. *Crit Care Med* 2002; **30**: 2038–204.
27. Namen AM, Ely W, Tatter SB *et al.* Predictors of succesful extubation in neurological patients. *Am J Respir Crit Care Med* 2001; **163**: 658–64.
28. Randolph AG, Wypij D, Venkataraman ST *et al.* Effect of mechanical ventilator weaning protocols on respiratory outcomes in infants and children. A randomised controlled trial. *JAMA* 2002; **288**: 2561–8.
29. Duane TM, Riblet JL, Golay D *et al.* Protocol driven ventilator management in a trauma Intensive care unit population. *Arch Surg* 2002; **137**: 1223–7.
30. Krishan JA, Moore D, Robeson C *et al.* A prospective controlled trial of a protocol-based strategy to discontinue mechanical ventilation. *Am J Respir Crit Care Med* 2004; **169**: 673–8.
31. Bach JR, Gonçalves MR, Hamdani I, Winck JC. Extubation of patients with neuromuscular weakness: a new management paradigm. Prepublished online 29 December 2009, DOI 10.1378.Chest.09-2144.
32. Brook AD, Ahrens TS, Schaiff R *et al.* Effect of a nursing-implemented sedation protocol on the duration of mechanical ventilation. *Crit Care Med* 1999; **27**: 2609–15.
33. Kress JP, Pohlman AS, O'Connor MF *et al.* Daily interruption of sedative infusions in critically ill patients undergoing mechanical ventilation. *N Engl J Med* 2000; **342**: 1471–7.

34. Schweickert WD, Gehlbach BK, Pohlman AS *et al.* Daily interruption of sedative infusions and complications of critical illness in mechanically ventilated patients. *Crit Care Med* 2004; **32**: 1272–6.
35. Ely EW, Bennett PA, Bowton DL *et al.* Large scale implementation of a respiratory therapist-driven protocol for ventilator weaning. *Am J Respir Crit Care Med* 1999; **159**: 439–46.
36. Scheinhorn D, Chao DC, Stearn-Hassenpflug M *et al.* Outcome in post-ICU mechanical ventilation. A therapist implemented weaning protocol. *Chest* 2001; **119**: 236–42.
37. Knebel A, Allen M, McNemar A *et al.* A guide to noninvasive intermittent ventilatory support. *Heart Lung* 1997; **26**: 307–16.
38. Chevrolet JC, Jolliet P, Abajo B *et al.* Time-consuming procedure for nurses with acute respiratory failure. Difficult and time-consuming procedure for nurses. *Chest* 1991; **100**: 775–82.
39. Nava S, Evangelisti I, Rampulla C *et al.* Human and financial costs of noninvasive mechanical ventilation in patients affected by COPD and acute respiratory failure. *Chest* 1997; **111**: 1631–8.
40. Hilbert G, Gruson D, Gbikpi-Benissan G *et al.* Sequential use of noninvasive pressure support ventilation for acute exacerbations of COPD. *Intensive Care Med* 1997; **23**: 955–61.
41. Hilbert G, Gruson D, Vargas F *et al.* Noninvasive ventilation for acute respiratory failure. Quite low time consumption for nurses. *Eur Respir J* 2000; **16**: 710–16.
42. Nava S, Ambrosino N, Clini E *et al.* Non invasive mechanical ventilation in the weaning of patients with respiratory failure due to chronic obstructive pulmonary disease. A randomized controlled trial. *Ann Intern Med* 1998; **128**: 721–8.
43. Ferrer M, Esquinas A, Arancibia F *et al.* Non-invasive ventilation during persistent weaning failure: a randomized controlled trial. *Am J Respir Crit Care Med* 2003; **168**: 70–6.
44. Squadrone V, Coha M, Cerutti E *et al.* Continuous positive airway pressure for treatment of postoperative hypoxemia. A randomized controlled trial. *JAMA* 2005; **293**: 589–95.
45. Esteban A, Frutos-Vivar F, Ferguson ND *et al.* Non invasive positive pressure ventilation for respiratory failure after extubation. *N Engl J Med* 2004; **350**: 2452–60.
46. Quinnell TG, Pilsworth S, Shneerson JM *et al.* Prolonged invasive ventilation following acute ventilatory failure in COPD weaning results, survival, and the role of noninvasive ventilation. *Chest* 2006; **129**: 133–9.
47. Damas C, Andrade C, Araujo JP *et al.* Weaning from non-invasive positive pressure ventilation: experience with progressive periods of withdraw. *Rev Port Pneumol* 2008; **14**: 49–53.
48. Cuvelier A, Viacroze C, Benichou J *et al.* Dependency on mask ventilation after acute respiratory failure in the intermediate care unit. *Eur Respir J* 2005; **26**: 289–97.
49. Nava S, Ceriana P. Causes of failure of non-invasive mechanical ventilation. *Respir Care* 2004; **49**: 295–303.
50. Soo Hoo GW, Santiago S, Williams AJ. Nasal mechanical ventilation for hypercapnic respiratory failure in chronic obstructive pulmonary disease: determinants of success and failure. *Crit Care Med* 1994; **22**: 1253–61.
51. Plant PK, Owen JL, Elliott MW. Early use of non-invasive ventilation for acute exacerbations of chronic obstructive pulmonary disease on general respiratory wards: a multicentre randomised controlled trial. *Lancet* 2000; **355**: 1931–5.
52. Carlucci A, Delmastro M, Rubini F *et al.* Changes in the practice of non-invasive ventilation in treating COPD patients over 8 years. *Intensive Care Med* 2003; **29**: 419–25.

# 60

# Specialized weaning units

ADITI SATTI, GERARD J CRINER, BERND SCHÖNHOFER

## ABSTRACT

The improved survival of critically ill patients and the increased demand for intensive care unit beds has made the development of specialized weaning units vital to the care of these patients. The patient on prolonged mechanical ventilation experiences significant muscle weakness which can lead to secondary complications and increased time on the ventilator. The care of these patients should be multidisciplinary, focusing on early mobility, rehabilitation, speech, swallowing, nutrition and overall psychological wellbeing. Specialized weaning units can provide effective medical care to patients on prolonged mechanical ventilation.

## INTRODUCTION

The advancement of care on the intensive care unit (ICU) has improved survival in the catastrophically ill patient. The improvement in medical technology and a greater understanding of many disease states has led to an increased demand for intensive care beds and has created an increased strain on our current healthcare system. It is projected that by 2017, healthcare spending will reach over US$4.3 trillion dollars. Forty per cent of healthcare resources are consumed by critical care medicine; critical care costs account for 1 per cent of the US gross domestic product. It is generally accepted that the cost of a critical care bed is three times the cost of a non-critical care bed.[1] Critical care costs have increased by 190 per cent from 1985 to 2000.[2] Chronic ventilated patients require expensive care that is inadequately reimbursed. In a study of 70 Medicare patients, a net loss of US$16 600 per ventilated patient was reported.[3] Moreover, the increased demands for ICU care have led to competing demands for the use of a relatively small number of ICU beds. Efforts to decrease ICU length of stay for chronic ventilated patients are desperately needed to contain the costs associated with critical care medicine and also to free up ICU beds for other types of critically ill patients who do not require chronic ventilation.

A prolonged ICU stay and the presence of a chronic critical illness are associated with muscle weakness, deconditioning, decreased mental and physical functioning and an impaired quality of life. Acute respiratory distress syndrome (ARDS), a common condition encountered in the ICU, is an example of an illness that requires prolonged ventilation and is associated with long-term psychological and functional dysfunction. In a study reviewing 109 survivors of ARDS, muscle fatigue, weakness and weight loss were the major reasons given for the patient's persistent functional limitations. These functional limitations were evident in the lower than predicted distance walked in 6 minutes at 1 year after ICU discharge.[4] We found that survivors of prolonged ventilation also experienced a marked impairment in their physical quality of life, even though their mental health was preserved.[5]

There is an increased need for mobility in the ICU because of the harmful consequences of prolonged bed rest. A prolonged ICU stay and chronic critical illness is not only associated with weakness, deconditioning, decreased whole-body function and quality of life, but also increases the risk for hospital-acquired pneumonia, venous thromboembolism and the development of decubitus ulcers. The goal of specialized weaning units is to improve weaning potential of the chronic ventilated patient, as well as their overall physical, psychological and social function to avoid the complications associated with immobility through whole-body and respiratory rehabilitation, aggressive nutritional support, and speech and swallowing therapy.

## MUSCULAR WEAKNESS IN THE INTENSIVE CARE UNIT

The effects of limb muscle deconditioning are known primarily from studies done in healthy people placed on bed rest in space programmes constructed to evaluate the effects of low-gravity environments on skeletal muscle structure and function in normal healthy volunteers.[6] Muscle atrophy, loss of force generation and changes in muscle fibre types occur rapidly with bed rest alone and even more so in hypercatabolic ICU patients who have increased oxidant stress. It has been found that even short periods of bed rest adversely affect skeletal muscle performance. After 14 and 35 days, muscle force decreases by 15 per cent and 25 per cent, and thigh and calf muscle volumes also significantly decrease.[6] Limb skeletal muscle atrophy that occurs with disuse also occurs in the diaphragm; diaphragm atrophy occurs even in normal subjects more rapidly than previously believed. Diaphragm biopsy specimens from previously normal brain-dead thoracic organ donors who were placed on mechanical ventilation for only 18–69 hours showed significant atrophy of both the slow- and fast-twitch diaphragm muscle fibres.[7] This indicates that diaphragm muscle weakness can occur very rapidly in patients receiving controlled ventilation even in previously normal hosts and indicates the profound effects that rest and catabolic illness (e.g. oxidant injury) may have on skeletal muscle in the ICU patients, even the diaphragm. Obviously these changes could markedly impair weaning from mechanical ventilation and worsen the patients' overall functional status.

## EARLY MOBILITY

Prior studies have demonstrated the benefits of rehabilitation in respiratory failure. We previously evaluated and reported the efficacy of aggressive whole-body rehabilitation in 49 chronically ventilated patients.[8] All patients had been ventilated for at least 14 days and none had underlying neuromuscular disorders. Physical therapy was started on admission to our ventilator rehabilitation unit after transfer from the ICU. The rehab programme consisted of trunk control, active and passive upper and lower extremity resistance training, ambulation and inspiratory muscle training. Deconditioning was assessed daily using a five-point motor score looking at strength and range of motion of all muscle groups. Improvements in patient strength was seen after a whole-body rehabilitation programme. All patients, initially bed bound, were able to sit and stand; and the majority (81 per cent) were able to ambulate prior to discharge. Increased upper motor strength decreased the amount of time spent on the ventilator. This may have been due to strengthening of the pectoralis muscles and an improvement in inspiratory and expiratory function.

Past studies in different patient populations have shown an improvement in ventilatory mechanics (increased mean inspiratory pressure and expiratory reserve volume) with pectoralis muscle training.[9] Table 60.1 summarizes the results of upper extremity training and the effect on ventilatory muscle strength and endurance. It can be concluded from our study that whole-body rehabilitation should be an integral part of the care of a chronically ventilated patient, and if started earlier may have additional benefit.

An early mobility programme, consisting of sitting, standing and ambulation, can be done safely in the majority of ICU patients. A study that examined the safety of early activity showed that the majority of respiratory patients were able to participate in a physical therapy programme in the ICU, even while orally intubated, without adverse events (1 per cent).[12] A similar study in 31 patients showed an increased heart rate and blood pressure response to early mobilization, but these haemodynamic effects were not significant and did not require any specific interventions. From this study we can conclude that, with adequate screening measures, patients can be safely and effectively mobilized.[13] The European Respiratory Society and European Society of Intensive Care Medicine Task Force suggests that rehabilitation can begin when certain stability criteria have been met (Fig. 60.1).[14]

**Table 60.1** Summary of studies of upper extremity training on ventilatory muscle strength and endurance

| Authors (year) | Subject | Results |
|---|---|---|
| Keens *et al.* (1977)[9] | Cystic fibrosis | 57 per cent increase in ventilatory muscle endurance |
| Clanton *et al.* (1987)[10] | Female swimmers | 25 per cent increase in MIP, 100 per cent in ventilatory endurance |
| Estenne *et al.* (1989)[11] | C8–C8 quads | Six weeks of isometric pectoralis major training increased ERV by 47 per cent |

ERV, expiratory reserve volume; MIP, maximum inspiratory pressure.

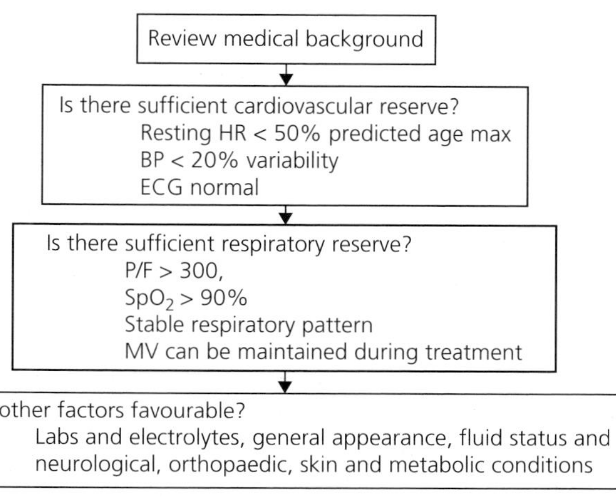


**Figure 60.1** European Respiratory Society and European Society of Intensive Care Medicine Task Force guidelines for mobilization of the critically ill patient. Adapted from Stiller *et al.*[14]

Portable ventilators now allow patients to be mobilized earlier in their hospital course despite higher needs for oxygenation or even continuous mechanical ventilation. Invasive ventilation can be provided by 'laptop'-sized ventilators that are suspended from wheelchairs or walkers to allow standing and ambulation despite the requirements for full ventilation. Additionally, other new respiratory therapy techniques provide methods to unload the respiratory work in the non-intubated ICU patient and include continuous positive airway pressure (CPAP), bi-level positive airway pressure, helium–oxygen administration and high-flow oxygen. All of these methods can also be organized to be made portable and provided non-invasively to unload the patient's work of breathing during periods of ambulation or higher levels of whole-body rehabilitation.

ICU patients are a special population who benefit from early mobility. The ability to sit, stand and ambulate not only improves their quality of life and functional status, but also mitigates the complications of immobility, such as deep venous thrombosis, pulmonary embolism and decubitus ulcers.

## RESPIRATORY MUSCLE TRAINING

Spontaneous breathing provides ventilatory muscle endurance training but inspiratory muscle strength training may also be beneficial to increase respiratory muscle strength and improve weaning outcome. A substantial body of literature demonstrates the ability of loaded inspiratory breathing training on increasing respiratory muscle strength in quadriplegics, normal controls and patients with COPD. Martin *et al.*[15] demonstrated that daily inspiratory muscle training in 10 chronically ventilated patients resulted in an increase in inspiratory muscle strength and success in weaning nine out of 10 patients from mechanical ventilation after its implementation. In order to provide inspiratory muscle strength training, at our facilities, we routinely institute inspiratory muscle training at one-third the maximum inspiratory pressure for 10 minutes daily, or twice daily in patients able to spontaneously breathe by tracheal collar.[15]

## SPEECH AND SWALLOWING

The ability to speak and eat also has a benefit on overall psychological wellbeing. These issues are extremely important and therapy should be instituted as early as feasible when caring for chronically ventilated patients. Most patients report that their inability to communicate is the most important factor contributing to the sense of fear and isolation. Speech therapists are an integral part of the multidisciplinary rehabilitation team. The use of an electrolarynx, one-way speaking valve, or even periods of cuff deflation with finger occlusion of the tracheostomy tube can be individualized to assist in their speech.

Reinstitution of eating is also a primary concern for chronically ventilated patients and their families. Although conversion of an endotracheal to tracheostomy tube may allow resumption of oral intake, patients receiving chronic ventilation may have a significant incidence of swallowing abnormalities.

When we evaluated the effects of chronic mechanical ventilation on swallowing function, we found that 43 per cent of patients who received prolonged mechanical ventilation had evidence of aspiration on a modified barium swallow study with videoflouroscopy.[16] A modified barium swallow study is particularly important because it helps to point out the mechanism(s) responsible for the high incidence of aspiration detected on bedside examination in the patient with tracheostomy and mechanical ventilation. Scintigraphy is another method to evaluate early aspiration after oral feeding in patients receiving prolonged ventilation via tracheostomy.[17]

Neuromuscular disorders, medications, underlying medical illness, weakness of the oropharyngeal muscles and laryngeal oedema are all factors that may contribute to swallowing dysfunction. Speech therapists should evaluate swallowing, oral motor strength and adequate cough and gag reflexes. The initial goal in a patient with swallowing dysfunction is to prevent aspiration. Proper patient positioning, alternative routes of nutrition, and assessment for other neurological conditions contributing to swallowing dysfunction should be included in the management of these patients. The ability to eat, speak and socially interact re-engages the patient in normal human behaviour, which is vital to their overall wellbeing. After appropriate swallowing evaluation and training, most patients receiving chronic ventilation without obvious severe neuromuscular diseases can successfully resume normal oral intake.

## SLEEP

Other issues that contribute to psychological dysfunction in the ventilated patient are sleep deprivation, the inability to communicate and social isolation. Patients admitted to the ICU are susceptible to sleep deprivation due to underlying illnesses, medications and the ICU environment itself; the ICU is a noisy environment that provides the patient with continuous, meaningless sensory input. Normal sleep architecture is disturbed in the ICU and can lead to ICU-related delirium. Sleep has a role in healing and deprivation may impair immunity and tissue repair. Steps to improve sleep such as creating a diurnal environment and minimizing interruptions should be taken.[18] Some steps that may be beneficial are placing patients in individual rooms with a window, regular orientation with a clock and calendar, early mobilization and uninterrupted sleep.

## PSYCHOLOGICAL DYSFUNCTION

Psychological disorders such as delirium and anxiety are commonly seen in the ICU. The incidence of delirium in the ICU is 30–40 per cent with an increased incidence in the elderly population.[19] Delirium is associated with poor outcomes such as prolonged hospitalization, functional decline, and increased use of chemical and physical restraints and an increased mortality (>30 per cent). Risk factors for delirium include older age, prior cognitive impairment, the presence of infection, multiple comorbidities, dehydration and psychotropic medication use. Individuals at high risk for delirium should be assessed daily using a standardized tool to facilitate prompt identification and management. The Confusion Assessment Method (CAM; see Fig. 11.1) is a simple validated tool used for the detection of delirium in both the clinical and research settings. The CAM-ICU uses four key delirium criteria to rapidly assess the patient's cognition; acute change in mental status, inattention, disordered thinking and an altered level of consciousness, to determine the presence of delirium. The CAM-ICU uses picture recognition and non-verbal responses to assess delirium. The CAM assessment has been shown to be useful and reproducible in ventilated and non-ventilated patients.[19] Non-pharmacologic interventions to improve delirium include the use of assistive devices to facilitate speech, the ability to eat, improved mobility and the promotion of good sleep. Creating a diurnal environment and normalizing a patient's daily routine by getting a patient out of bed and ambulating may minimize confusion and delirium. Haloperidol and atypical antipsychotics are also used in the treatment of delirium.

## EXPERIENCE WORLDWIDE

The process of weaning from mechanical ventilation support may be long and frustrating and time consuming for patients, their families and the healthcare team. The financial and medical implications of caring for these patients has led to the development of intermediate and specialized weaning facilities. These facilities often utilize a multidisciplinary team approach and emphasize the rehabilitation, medical and psychosocial issues of the patient and their family. Caring for an increased population of patients on prolonged mechanical ventilation in an optimal and cost-effective manner has become a global challenge.

### The North American perspective

Unlike in Europe, intensive care medicine in the USA has always been closely linked to respiratory medicine. Specialized weaning facilities are much more common in the USA and play an important role in patients on prolonged mechanical ventilation. The number of facilities has increased due to the improved reimbursement and diagnosis-related group (DRG) exemption. These long-term facilities often have differing admission and discharge criteria, patient care staffing ratios and weaning approaches. One of the first specialized units was a 24-bed prolonged respiratory care unit started at Bethesda Lutheran Medical Center in 1979.[20] Their 18-month trial showed cost savings when compared to an acute care centre. Elpern *et al.* showed a decrease in the daily cost of care of US$2000 per patient in those transferred to the weaning facility.[21]

Temple University Hospital was one of the four original sites selected to participate in a study funded by the Health Care Financing Administration (HCFA) Chronic Ventilator Dependent Unit Demonstration Project.[22] The ventilator rehabilitation unit (VRU) at Temple is an 18-bed non-invasive respiratory care unit in a tertiary care hospital and has provided care to over 2500 patients with prolonged respiratory failure. One of the goals in the VRU is to achieve maximum functional status despite the ongoing need of the patient for mechanical ventilation. The VRU is composed of a multidisciplinary team, each with a unique role. The team is composed of a pulmonary attending, pulmonary fellow, nurse coordinator, speech therapist, pharmacist, respiratory therapists, physical and occupational therapists and a nutritionist. Appropriate consultations are made to otolaryngologists and psychiatrists on an as-needed basis. The purpose of the study was to examine the effect of a multidisciplinary rehabilitation programme, costs, survival and quality of life in patients requiring prolonged mechanical ventilation. The study showed that patients in a specialized ventilator-dependent unit (VDU) were more likely to be weaned from the ventilator and be discharged to home. These patients were also found to be more functionally independent at the time of discharge. Patients treated in the VDU generated lower costs/day compared with matched patients who received conventional care in the ICU. The success of the Temple VRU was dependent on the organization of the treatment team and quality of the rehabilitation programme. Similar experiences have been documented at other institutions.

The experience of the respiratory special care unit (ReSCU) at the Cleveland Clinic showed that of 212 patients, 60 per cent were weaned successfully from the ventilator. There was a mortality rate of 18 per cent. A cost analysis was done comparing the charges for patients in the special weaning unit versus in the ICU. To make the comparison, it was assumed that those patients who were transferred to the weaning unit would have stayed in the ICU for the entire length of stay. The difference in daily cost per bed between the ICU and ReSCU is US$585. This is a cost savings of US$13 339 per patient for those transferred to ReSCU.[23] Though lacking prospective supportive data, specialized weaning units may provide a clinically and cost effective alternative to ICU care.

## The European perspective

There has been a growing interest in specialized weaning facilities in Europe over the past decade.[24] RICUs (respiratory intensive care units) specialize in non-invasive and prolonged mechanical ventilation and provide a step-down unit from the ICU to the general ward. There is a nurse:patient ratio of 1:4 or 1:5, accounting for some of the cost savings. Germany and Italy have the largest number of RICUs of all European countries. The management of the RICU by a respiratory specialist is a new and emerging trend.

In a nationwide German survey the contemporary status of weaning centres driven by chest physicians was evaluated in the year 2006. Thirty-eight centres participated in the survey, which was divided into 10 sections, covering properties of the clinic, weaning strategies, patients and outcomes. The survey represents a total number of 2718 patients with difficult or prolonged weaning. Almost three-quarters of patients were transferred to the weaning centre from an external ICU. The weaning success rate was 66.4 per cent. In 31.9 per cent, home mechanical ventilation was started after weaning. The overall hospital mortality rate was 20.8 per cent. Major differences between individual centres were found concerning the number of patients, setting of the weaning unit and weaning strategies.[25]

A 3-month prospective, cohort study done of 26 Italian RICUs provides insight into the prevalence and description of these units.[26] The study showed that the presence of RICUs contributed to increased ICU bed availability. Of the 756 patients, 61 per cent had tracheostomies and were considered ventilator dependent. The predicted mortality according to the APACHE 2 score was 22 per cent with an actual mortality of 16 per cent The study showed that patients admitted to the Italian RICU achieved ventilator independence rates similar to the studies done in the USA and were able to successfully manage patients with acute-on-chronic respiratory failure.

## OUTCOMES

Multiple studies have evaluated the outcomes and survival of patients transferred to a weaning facility. The evidence is mainly limited to observational, retrospective, single-centre, non-randomized studies. The patient population, outcome reporting and weaning methods often differ between studies. Despite these confounding variables, there has been documented success in weaning and a proven financial benefit in these specialized units. Scheinhorn *et al.* studied 1123 ventilator-dependent patients transferred to a regional weaning facility over an 8-year period.[27] Patients were transferred earlier to a weaning facility; 55 per cent of patients were successfully weaned and 29 per cent died in the unit. During the time period, the survival rate 1 year after discharge had improved from 29 per cent to 37 per cent. Differences in patient population can be clearly seen when comparing the prior study with Gracey *et al.* in 2000.[28] In this study, 60 per cent of patients were successfully weaned and 6 per cent died. The patient population was predominately post-surgical, younger and had fewer comorbidities.

Despite the substantial differences in patient makeup between the studies, these studies do demonstrate the safety and success of weaning patients in a less costly environment than the intensive care unit with the use of specialized weaning units. The major studies and their findings are given in Table 60.2.

**Table 60.2** Studies of weaning outcomes

| | Pilcher *et al.*[33] | Schönhofer *et al.*[32] | Gracey *et al.*[30] | Scheinhorn *et al.*[29] | Bagley and Cooney[31] |
|---|---|---|---|---|---|
| Patients | 153 | 232 | 132 | 421 | 278 |
| Mean age (y) | 62 | 65 | 67 | 70 | 67 |
| Diagnosis | | | | | |
| COPD (per cent) | 27 | 54 | 13 | 24 | 30 |
| Surgery (per cent) | 24 | 7 | 63 | 24 | 11 |
| ALS (per cent) | – | 5 | 1 | 32 | 28 |
| Neuromuscular (per cent) | 31* | 16 | – | 8 | 19 |
| Miscellaneous (per cent) | 18 | 18 | 23 | 12 | 12 |
| Weaning | | | | | |
| Ventilation days | 26 | 44 | 14 | 49 | – |
| Days to wean | 19 | 7.5 | 16 | 39 | – |
| Weaning success (per cent) | 38 | 65 | 70 | 53 | 38 |
| Survival | | | | | |
| At discharge (per cent) | 73 | 72 | 90 | 71 | 53 |
| Long-term (per cent) | 73 | 64– (3 months) | – | 28– (1 year) | – |

ALS, amyotrophic lateral sclerosis; COPD, chronic obstructive pulmonary disease.

## SUMMARY

Multiple retrospective and observational studies have shown that specialized weaning units can provide effective care to the patient on prolonged mechanical ventilation, both financially and medically. The multidisciplinary approach to care, with an emphasis on rehabilitation, nutrition and speech, has improved patients' overall psychological wellbeing and facilitated weaning from the ventilator. Prospective, randomized controlled trials are still needed to improve the care and utility of these specialized units.

## REFERENCES


1. Hopkins RO, Spuhler VJ, Thomsen GE. Transforming ICU culture to facilitate early mobility. *Crit Care Clin* 2007; **23**: 81–96.
2. Halpern NA, Pastores SM, Greenstein RJ. Critical care medicine in the United States: 1985–2000. An analysis of bed numbers, use and cost. *Crit Care Med* 2004; **32**: 1254–9.
3. Frienchels T. Financial implications and recommendations for care of ventilator-dependent patients. *J Nurs Adm* 1993; **23**: 16–20.
4. Herridge MS, Cheung AM, Tansey CM *et al.* One-year outcomes in survivors of the acute respiratory distress syndrome. *N Engl J Med* 2003; **348**: 683–93.
5. Euteneuer S, Windisch W, Suchi S *et al.* Health-related quality of life in patients with chronic respiratory failure after long-term mechanical ventilation. *Respir Med* 2006; **100**: 477–86.
6. Adams GR, Caiozzo VJ, Baldwin KM. Skeletal muscle unweighting: space flight and ground based models. *J Appl Physiol* 2003; **95**: 2185–201.
7. Levine S, Nguyen T, Taylor N *et al.* Rapid disuse atrophy of diaphragm fibers in mechanically ventilated humans. *N Engl J Med* 2008; **358**: 1327–35.
8. Martin U, Hincapie L, Nimchuk M *et al.* Impact of whole-body rehabilitation in patients receiving chronic mechanical ventilation. *Crit Care Med* 2005; **33**: 2259–65.
9. Keens TG, Krastins IR, Wannamaker EM *et al.* Ventilatory muscle endurance training in normal subjects and patients with cystic fibrosis. *Am Rev Respir Dis* 1977; **116**: 853–60.
10. Clanton TL, Dixon GF, Drake J *et al.* Effects of swim training on lung volumes and inspiratory muscle conditioning. *J Appl Physiol* 1987; **62**: 39–46.
11. Estenne M, Knoop C, Vanvaerenbergh J *et al.* The effect of pectoralis muscle training in training tetraplegic subjects. *Am Rev Respir Dis* 1989; **139**: 1218–22.
12. Bailey P, Thomsen GE, Spuhler VJ *et al.* Early activity is feasible and safe in respiratory failure patients. *Crit Care Med* 2007; **35**: 139–45.
13. Stiller K, Phillips A, Lambert P. The safety of mobilization and its effects on haemodynamic and respiratory status of intensive care patients. *Physiother Theory Pract* 2004; **20**: 175–85.
14. Stiller K, Phillips A, Lambert P. Safety aspects of mobilising acutely ill inpatients. *Physiother Theory Pract* 2003; **19**: 239–57.
15. Martin DA, Davenport PD, Franceschi AC *et al.* Use of inspiratory muscle strength training to facilitate ventilator weaning. *Chest* 2002; **122**: 192–6.
16. Tolep K, Getch CL, Criner GJ *et al.* Swallowing dysfunction in patients receiving prolonged mechanical ventilation. *Chest* 1996; **109**: 167–72.
17. Schönhofer B, Barchfeld T, Haidl P *et al.* Scintigraphy for evaluation of early aspiration after oral feeding in patients receiving prolonged ventilation via tracheotomy. *Intensive Care Med* 1999; **25**: 311–14.
18. Krachman SL, D'Alonzo GE, Criner CJ *et al.* Sleep in the intensive care unit. *Chest* 1995; **107**: 1713–20.
19. Criner G. *Psychological disturbances in the ICU.* Critical Care Study Guide. New York, Springer, 2002.
20. Indihar FJ, Forsberg DP. Experience with a prolonged respiratory care unit. *Chest* 1982; **81**: 189–92.
21. Elpern EH, Silver MR, Rosen RL *et al.* The noninvasive respiratory care unit. *Chest* 1999; **1**: 205–8.
22. Criner G. Long term ventilation: introduction and perspectives. *Respir Care Clin* 2002; **8**: 345–53.
23. Dasgupta A, Rice R, Mascha E *et al.* Four year experience with a unit for long-term ventilation at the Cleveland Clinic Foundation. *Chest* 1999; **116**: 447–55.
24. Corrado A, Roussos C, Ambrosino N *et al.* Respiratory intermediate care units: a European survey. *Eur Respir J* 2002; **20**: 1343–50.
25. Schönhofer B, Berndt C, Achtzehn U *et al.* Weaning from mechanical ventilation. A survey of the situation in pneumologic respiratory facilities in Germany. *Dtsch Med Wochenschr* 2008; **133**: 700–4.
26. Confalonieri M, Cuvelier A, Elliott M *et al.* Respiratory intensive care units in Italy: a national census and prospective cohort study. *Thorax* 2001; **56**: 373–8.
27. Scheinhorn DJ, Chao DC, Stearn-Hassenpflug MA *et al.* Post ICU mechanical ventilation: treatment of 1123 patients at a regional weaning center. *Chest* 1997; **11**: 1654–9.
28. Gracey DR, Hardy DC, Koenig GE. The chronic ventilator-dependent unit: a lower cost alternative to intensive care. *Mayo Clin Proc* 2000; **75**: 445–9.
29. Scheinhorn DJ, Artinian BM, Catlin JL. Weaning from prolonged mechanical ventilation. *Chest* 1994; **105**: 534–9.
30. Gracey DR, Naessens JM, Viggiano RW *et al.* Outcomes of patients cared for in a ventilator-dependent unit in a general hospital. *Chest* 1995; **107**: 494–9.
31. Bagley PH, Cooney E. A community-based regional ventilator weaning unit: development and outcomes. *Chest* 1997; **111**: 1024–9.

32. Schönhofer B, Haidl P, Kemper P *et al.* Withdrawal from the respirator (weaning) in long-term ventilation. The results in patients in a weaning centre. *Dtsch Med Wochenschr* 1999; **124**: 1022–8.

33. Pilcher DV, Bailey MJ, Treacher DF *et al.* Outcomes, cost and long term survival of patients referred to a regional weaning centre. *Thorax* 2005; **60**: 187–92.

# SECTION N

# The physiotherapist and assisted ventilation

# 61

# Respiratory physiotherapy (including cough assistance techniques and glossopharyngeal breathing)

MIGUEL R GONÇALVES, JOÃO CARLOS WINCK

## ABSTRACT

Respiratory physiotherapy techniques for augmenting normal mucociliary clearance, lung expansion and cough efficacy have been used for many years to treat patients with respiratory disorders. Both inspiratory and, indirectly, expiratory muscle function can be assisted by glossopharyngeal breathing. Airway clearance refers to two separate, but connected, mechanisms: mucociliary clearance and cough efficacy. This chapter describes comprehensive and practical aspects of respiratory physiotherapy interventions in patients under mechanical ventilation. The goal of this chapter is to explore the potential of updated respiratory physiotherapy techniques in both acute and chronic settings as a complementary therapy to non-invasive ventilation to promote a better quality of life in respiratory patients.

## INTRODUCTION

Techniques for augmenting normal mucociliary clearance and cough efficacy have been used for many years in the treatment of patients with respiratory disorders of different aetiologies. In recent years, new technologies and more advanced techniques have been developed, which are more comfortable and effective in the majority of patients. Postural drainage with manual chest percussion and shaking has, in most parts of the world, been replaced by more independent and effective techniques.

The evidence in support of these techniques is variable and the literature is not always clear, and is sometimes conflicting, regarding the clinical indication for each technique.[1] Moreover, it can be confusing for healthcare professionals, patients and their caregivers when it comes to choosing and utilizing the most appropriate airway clearance techniques and products.

Although the use of respiratory muscle aids is an important intervention for eliminating airway secretions in patients with muscle weakness, as for normal coughing these aids may not adequately eliminate secretions that are obstructing the smaller airways.[2] In these situations, it is important to consider techniques to gradually loosen and mobilize secretions to assist mucociliary clearance from the lower airway into the upper airway to avoid the risk of atelectasis and pneumonia, which can often lead to numerous hospitalizations and even premature death.

One of the techniques that may be helpful in patients with ventilatory impairment is glossopharyngeal breathing (GFB). This technique was commonly used in the 1950s in poliomyelitis patients to enhance their breathing capabilities.[3] This same technique can be used in patients with neuromuscular disease[4] and those with high spinal cord injury (SCI).[5]

A great majority of the episodes of secretion encumbrance develop in acute respiratory failure and it has been demonstrated that morbidity and mortality can be avoided without hospitalization, with a correct and effective secretion management protocol.[6] Moreover conventional chest physical therapy for secretion management does not increase the chances of weaning and extubation success in critical ill patients.[7] However, some of these patients may have normal mucociliary clearance but ineffective peak cough flows (PCF), which itself has been associated with extubation failure.[8,9] A protocol that includes assisting coughing techniques as adjunct to an efficient non-invasive ventilation (NIV) application may increase the success rates of extubation in patients who are difficult to wean.

## CLINICAL INDICATIONS FOR AIRWAY CLEARANCE PHYSIOTHERAPY TECHNIQUES

For patients with chronic airways disease, mucus stasis can contribute to bronchial obstruction and chronic expectoration can be a physically and socially disabling problem. Mucus retention can also cause pathological changes in the lungs and is thought to contribute to the progression of airways disease. It is, therefore, not surprising that, for patients with chronic airways disease, mucus hypersecretion has been associated with increased mortality,[10] and it is thought to contribute to the development of respiratory tract infections.

Mucus clearance and bronchial hygiene is often decreased in patients with airways disease, as well as in both paediatric and adult patients with neuromuscular disorders and consequent dysfunctional cough or glottic control.

### Patients with airways disease

Hypersecretion is usually present in the acute episodes of asthma and normal mucus transport is impaired due to reduction of ciliary activity.[11] In these patients, mucus transport can recover or remain reduced, despite favourable changes in mucus viscoelasticity, after an exacerbation.

In patients with chronic obstructive pulmonary disease (COPD) there is a persistent and permanent dyspnoea and airway obstruction, with incomplete reversibility with therapy. Usually in these patients, the mucociliary transport is not seriously impaired until an acute exacerbation occurs. Secretion encumbrance has been associated with failure of NIV in COPD, where endotracheal intubation and mechanical ventilation may become necessary during acute exacerbations.

Cystic fibrosis is a relatively common, inherited, life-limiting disorder. The genetic defect causes abnormal mucus secretion in the airways, potentially leading to airway obstruction and mucus plugging. Treatment methods that improve mucus clearance are considered essential in optimizing respiratory status and reducing the progression of lung disease in these patient populations. The goal is to reduce disease progression by augmenting the normal mucociliary clearance mechanism of the lungs and facilitating expectoration.[12]

### Patients with neuromuscular disorders

The effectiveness in eliminating secretions is determined by the amount of flow generated in the expulsive phase. These factors depend on the linear velocity of gas flow, the diameter of the segment, and dynamic compression, and they are manifested basically in the value of PCF.[13]

In neuromuscular disorders (NMDs) there is a progressive decrease in vital capacity, which is mainly related to the combination of muscle weakness and alterations of the mechanical properties of the lungs and chest wall.[14] Changes in the ability to cough, understood as the inability to expel secretions effectively or finding it difficult to do so, may precede alterations in alveolar ventilation and places patients at risk for atelectasis, mucus plugging and pneumonia. Such alterations are the main cause of morbidity and mortality in patients with NMDs.[6] Along with hypoventilation, these alterations represent the most important problem from the patient's point of view.[15]

Severe bulbar and glottic dysfunction most commonly occur in patients with amyotrophic lateral sclerosis (ALS), spinal muscle atrophy (SMA) type 1, and the pseudobulbar palsy of central nervous system aetiology.[16] Inability to close the glottis and vocal cords results in complete loss of the ability to cough and swallow.

## CONTROL OF MUCUS AND AIRWAY CLEARANCE TECHNIQUES

Airway clearance refers to two separate, but connected, mechanisms: mucociliary clearance and cough clearance. Approaches to preventing airway secretion retention include pharmacotherapy to reduce mucus hypersecretion or to liquefy secretions, and the application of chest physiotherapy techniques. These techniques do not appear to benefit patients during recovery from acute exacerbations of COPD or pneumonia. These conditions are characterized by interstitial pathology, which cannot be influenced by physical interventions in the airways.[17–19] Further studies are needed to identify the patients and circumstances that are at risk from complications or adverse effects of manual chest physiotherapy.

### Positioning, breathing control techniques and chest physiotherapy

Positioning the patient to enable gravity to assist the flow of bronchial secretions from the airways has been a standard treatment for some time in patients with retained secretions.[20] The combination of positioning with breathing techniques and manual chest physiotherapy increases the effectiveness of airway clearance in patients with diferent aetiologies (Fig. 61.1). Positioning can also place the patient at risk for skin and cardiac complications, cerebral blood flow or intracranial pressure changes, and for gastroesophageal reflux.[21]

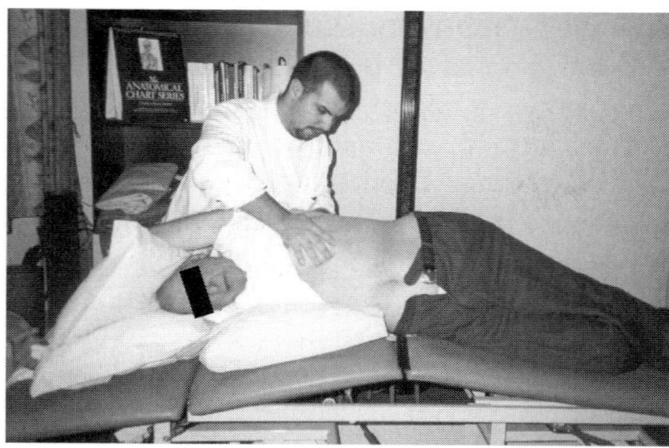

**Figure 61.1** Manual chest physiotherapy applied in a patient with airway disease.

Breathing control techniques include autonomous breathing exercises such as forced and deep expirations, and diaphragmatic breathing to optimize airway mucus clearance. One of the techniques described as most efficient in mucus clearance is the active cycle of breathing technique (ACBT),[20] which consists of repeated cycles of three ventilatory phases: breathing control, thoracic expansion exercises and the forced expiration technique.

Another breathing control technique that is widely used is autogenic drainage.[20,22] This technique is based on breathing at different lung volumes (low volume, tidal volume and high volume) and expiration is used to move the mucus. The aim is to maximize expiratory flow. When sufficient mucus has reached the upper airways, it may be cleared by a cough.

Both ACBT and autogenic drainage are not indicated in severe ventilator dependent patients, however, it may be used during weaning protocols.

Approaches to preventing retention of airway secretions include the use of medication to reduce mucus hypersecretion or to liquefy secretions, and the facilitation of mucus mobilization. To complement this objective, chest physiotherapy techniques can be very effective in preventing pulmonary complications in infant and adult patients with secretion accumulation.

Manual chest percussion (clapping) and chest vibration have been shown to increase in airflow obstruction[23] and hypoxaemia.[20] On the basis of three randomized controlled trials, manual chest physiotherapy is ineffective and perhaps even detrimental in the treatment of patients with acute exacerbations of COPD.[24]

Guidebooks of manual thoracic techniques are available demonstrating the hand placements and thrusting techniques in children and adults.[25]

## Instrumental techniques for mucus mobilization

Methods of promoting airway clearance using specific devices have been included in most respiratory therapy programmes. Positive expiratory pressure (PEP) breathing is usually applied by breathing through a face mask or mouthpiece with an inspiratory tube containing a one-way valve, and an expiratory tube containing a variable expiratory resistance. It results in positive expiratory pressure throughout expiration.[20,21,26,27]

A combination of PEP and air column oscillation applied at the mouth can be obtained when the patient expires through a small pipe-shaped device called Flutter VRP1. The expiratory opening of the pipe is closed by a small stainless steel ball. The mucus mobilizing effect is thought to be due to both the widening of the airways due to the increased expiratory pressure and the occurrence of airflow oscillations due to the oscillating ball.[28] Another similar device is the RC Cornet. This device is a curved plastic tube containing a flexible latex-free valve-hose. Just as with the flutter, secretions mobilized to the central airways are cleared by coughing or huffing.

## Manual assisted coughing techniques

Manually assisted cough is the external application of pressure to the thoracic cage or epigastric area, coordinated with a forced exhalation. The combination of deep lung insufflations to the maximum insufflation capacity (MIC)[29] (Fig. 61.2) followed by manual assisted cough with abdominal thrust (Fig. 61.3) has been shown to increase significantly PCF values in NMD patients.[30,31]

Although an optimal insufflation followed by an abdominal thrust provides the greatest increase in PCF, it can also be significantly increased by providing only maximal insufflation or providing only an abdominal thrust. Interestingly, PCFs are increased significantly more by the maximal insufflation than by the abdominal thrust.[32,33] Manually assisted coughing and the MIC manoeuvre requires a cooperative patient and good coordination between the patient and caregiver (Fig. 61.4).

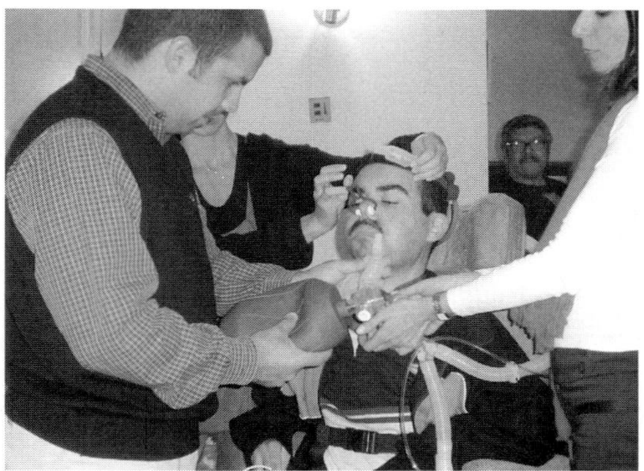

**Figure 61.2** Air stacking with manual resuscitator via a mouthpiece in a patient with Duchenne muscular dystrophy with low vital capacity and suboptimal peak cough flow.

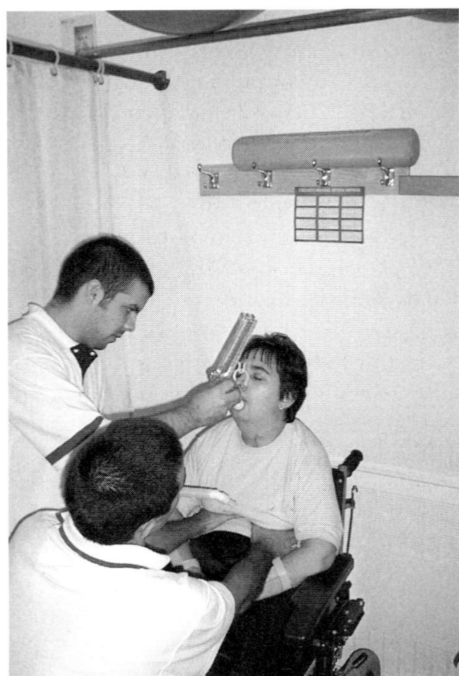

**Figure 61.3** Manual assisted cough with abdominal thrust to measure peak cough flows in the sitting position in a patient with a neuromuscular disorder.

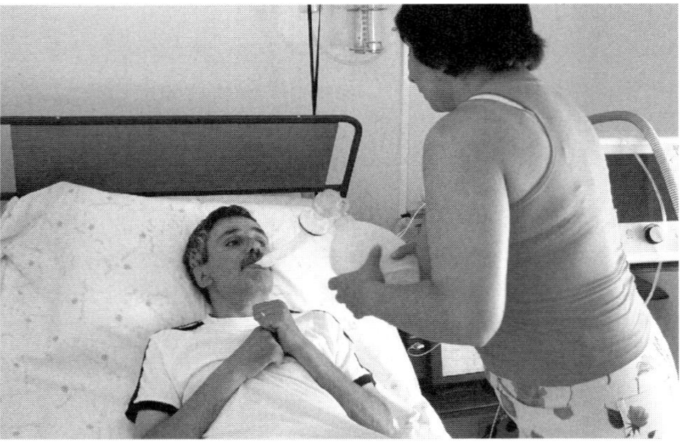

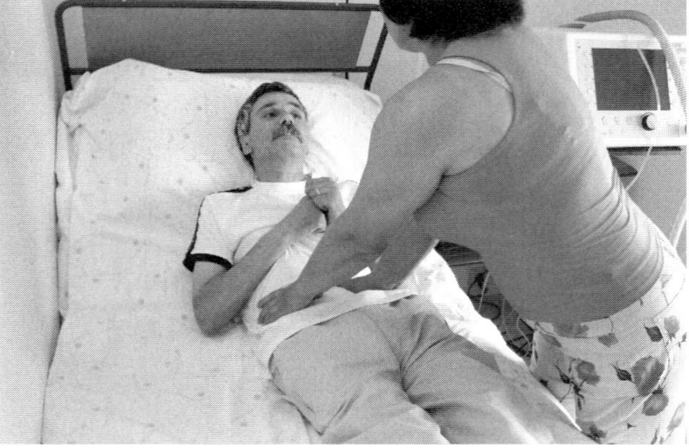

**Figure 61.4** Air stacking and manual assisted cough in a patient with neuromuscular disease, performed by the family caregiver.

Abdominal compressions should not be used for 1–1.5 hours following a meal, but chest compressions can be used to augment PCF. Chest thrusting techniques must be performed with caution in the presence of an osteoporotic rib cage. Unfortunately, since it is not widely taught to healthcare professionals, manually assisted coughing is underutilized.[34]

## GLOSSOPHARYNGEAL BREATHING

Both inspiratory and, indirectly, expiratory muscle function can be assisted by GPB. The technique involves the use of the glottis to add to an inspiratory effort by projecting (gulping) boluses of air into the lungs. The glottis closes with each 'gulp'. One breath usually consists of six to nine gulps of 40–200 mL each.[3] During the training period the efficiency of GPB can be monitored by spirometrically measuring the millilitres of air per gulp, gulps per breath, and breaths per minute.

Glossopharyngeal breathing (or 'frog' breathing) uses the muscles of the tongue (the glossa) and the throat (pharyngeal muscles) to force air into the trachea and lungs through a repetitious process. Neuromuscular and SCI patients are perfect candidates because of their intact bulbar function, but most of them need considerable instruction and encouragement to learn this technique, as well as hours of practice to master it. Approximately 60 per cent of ventilator users with no autonomous ability to breathe and good bulbar muscle function can use GPB for autonomous breathing for periods of minutes to up to all day.[35,36] Several daily activities can interfere with an individual's ability to perform GPB. The reason is because these daily activities involve the mouth and throat muscles, thus causing interference. With plenty of practice and confidence patients can learn to master these daily requirements and still be able to effectively perform GFB.[37]

Although extremely useful, GPB is rarely taught since there are few healthcare professionals familiar with the technique. This technique is also rarely useful in the presence of an indwelling tracheostomy tube. It cannot be used when the tube is uncapped, as it is during tracheostomy or invasive positive pressure support (IPPV), and even when capped, the gulped air tends to leak around the outer walls of the tube and out of the stoma. The safety and versatility afforded by GPB is one reason to avoid tracheostomy in favour of non-invasive aids.

## MECHANICAL RESPIRATORY MUSCLE AIDS FOR SECRETION MANAGEMENT

Respiratory muscle aids for secretion management are devices and techniques that involve mechanical application of forces to the body or intermittent pressure changes to the airway to assist expiratory muscle function and airway mucus clearance.

## Intrapulmonary percussive ventilation

The intrapulmonary percussive ventilator is an airway clearance device that simultaneously delivers aerosolized solution and intrathoracic percussion. This modified method of intermittent positive pressure breathing superimposes high-frequency minibursts of gas (at 50–550 cycles/min) on the patient's own respiration. This creates a global effect of internal percussion of the lungs, which can promote clearance of the peripheral bronchial tree. The high-frequency gas pulses expand the lungs, vibrate and enlarge the airways, and deliver gas into distal lung units, beyond the accumulated mucus.[22,38,39]

This technique has been shown to be as effective as standard chest physiotherapy and to assist mucus clearance in patients with secretion encumbrance due to different aetiologies, such as cystic fibrosis,[40] acute exacerbations of COPD[41] and Duchenne muscle dystrophy.[38] In cystic fibrosis, intrapulmonary percussive ventilation (IPV) was found to be as effective as the other methods of airway clearance in sputum mobilization, when the amount of sputum produced was assessed by dry weight.[42]

Intrapulmonary percussive ventilation can be delivered through a mouthpiece, a face mask and also through endotracheal and tracheostomy tubes. The primary aims of this technique are to reduce secretion viscosity, promote deep lung recruitment, improve gas exchange, deliver a vascular 'massage', and protect the airway against barotrauma. The main contraindication is the presence of diffuse alveolar haemorrhage with haemodynamic instability. Relative contraindications include active or recent gross haemoptysis, pulmonary embolism, subcutaneous emphysema, bronchopleural fistula, oesophageal surgery, recent spinal infusion, spinal anaesthesia or acute spinal injury, presence of a transvenous or subcutaneous pacemaker, increased intracranial pressures, uncontrolled hypertension, suspected or confirmed pulmonary tuberculosis, bronchospasm, empyema or large pleural effusion and acute cardiogenic pulmonary oedema.[43]

## High-frequency chest wall oscillation

During high-frequency chest wall oscillation (HFCWO), positive pressure air pulses are applied to the chest wall through a vest or under a chest shell. This technique provides oscillation at 5–25 Hz. Mechanical vibration is performed at frequencies up to 40 Hz. Vibration is applied during the entire breathing cycle or during expiration only. The adjustable inspiratory/expiratory ratio permits asymmetrical inspiratory and expiratory pressure changes (for example +3–6 cm $H_2O$), which favour higher exsufflation flow velocities to mobilize secretions. The average length of time spent in each treatment session will vary according to patient tolerance, amount and consistency of secretions, and the phase of the patient's illness (acute or chronic).[39] Simultaneous use of an aerosolized medication or saline is recommended throughout the treatment. This humidifies the air to counteract the drying effect of the increased airflow.[46] HFCWO may act like a physical mucolytic, reducing both the spinnability and viscoelasticity of mucus and enhancing clearance by coughing.[21,22,44] HFCWO has demonstrated efficacy in assisting mucus clearance in patients with cystic fibrosis.[44–47]

These beneficial effects on both mucus clearance and clinical parameters are not so evident in other groups of patients, such as COPD. Moreover, side effects of percussion and vibration include increasing obstruction to airflow for patients with COPD.[19,48,49] The value of HFCWO in patients with relatively normal mucus composition and characteristics but neuromuscular weakness is still under investigation, especially as a long-term treatment modality. In one study, the addition of HFCWO to randomly selected patients with ALS failed to achieve any significant clinical benefits in relation to the time of death (survival days). In addition, HFCWO failed to modify the rate of decline in forced vital capacity (FVC), given the progressive nature of this chronic neurodegenerative disease process.[50] On the other hand, Lange *et al.*[51] also compared lung function parameters in ALS patients who were randomized to 12 weeks of HFCWO or no treatment. Results showed maintenance of FVC and decreased fatigue and dyspnoea in the HFCWO group compared with the untreated group.

Contraindications for HFCWO are mostly the same as for IPV, plus head or unstable neck injury, burns, open wounds, infection or recent thoracic skin grafts, osteoporosis, osteomyelitis, coagulopathy, rib fracture, lung contusion, distended abdomen and chest wall pain.[21,46]

## Mechanical insufflation–exsufflation

A mechanical insufflator-exsufflator (CoughAssist, Philips Respironics) delivers deep insufflations (at positive pressures of 30–60 cm $H_2O$) followed immediately by deep exsufflations (at negative pressures of –30 to –60 cm $H_2O$). The insufflation and exsufflation pressures and delivery times are independently adjustable.[52] With a correct inspiratory and expiratory time, there is a very good correlation between the pressures used and the flows obtained.[53,54]

Except after a meal, an abdominal thrust is applied in conjunction with the exsufflation.[33] Mechanical in-exsufflation can be provided via an oronasal mask, a simple mouthpiece or a translaryngeal or tracheostomy tube. When delivered via the latter, the cuff, when present, should be inflated.[55]

Mechanical insufflation–exsufflation applied with an oronasal mask (Fig. 61.5) can generate PCFs greater than 2.7 L/s in motor neuron disease patients, with the exception of those with very acute bulbar dysfunction,[56] in whom there may be great instability of the upper airways.[57]

The CoughAssist can be manually or automatically cycled. Manual cycling facilitates caregiver–patient coordination of

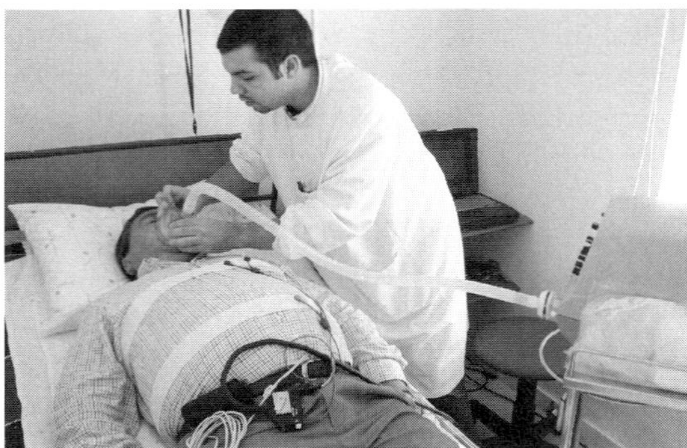

**Figure 61.5** Mechanical in-exsufflation provided via an oronasal mask in a monitored patient with neuromuscular disease.

inspiration and expiration with insufflation and exsufflation, but it requires assistance to deliver an abdominal thrust, to hold the mask on the patient, and to cycle the machine. One treatment consists of about five cycles followed by a short period of normal breathing or ventilator use to avoid hyperventilation.[58] Insufflation and exsufflation pressures are almost always from +35 to +60 cm $H_2O$ to –35 to –60 cm $H_2O$. Most patients use pressures between 35 and 45 cm $H_2O$ for both insufflations and exsufflations. In experimental models, +40 to –40 cm $H_2O$ pressures have been shown to provide maximum forced deflation vital capacities and flows.[32,54,59] Multiple treatments are given until no further secretions are expulsed and any secretion or mucus-induced desaturations are reversed.[60]

The use of MIE via the upper airway can be effective for children as long as they permit its effective use by not crying or closing their glottis. Between 2 and 5 years of age most children become able to cooperate and cough with MIE.[61] Whether via the upper airway or via indwelling airway tubes, routine airway suctioning misses the left main stem bronchus about 90 per cent of the time. MIE, on the other hand, provides the same exsufflation flows in both left and right airways without the discomfort or airway trauma of tracheal suctioning and it can be effective when suctioning is not. Patients almost invariably prefer MIE to suctioning for comfort and effectiveness and they find it less tiring.[62,63]

Contraindications of the technique include previous barotrauma, the existence of bullae, emphysema and bronchial hyper-reactivity.[64] Even when used following abdominal surgery and following extensive chest wall surgery no disruption of recently sutured wounds was noted.[65,66] As patients with spinal shock can develop bradycardias, MIE should be carried out with caution, with gradual increase in pressures or premedication with anticholinergics.[67] In patients with very low vital capacity who have not previously received maximum insufflations, the use of high pressures may cause thoracic muscle discomfort; thus, progressive increase is indicated.

The use of MIE has been demonstrated to be very important in extubating NMD patients following general anaesthesia despite their lack of spontaneous breathing, and to manage them with NIV.[5,6,68] It has also facilitated avoidance of intubation or rapid extubation of NMD and high SCI patients (Fig. 61.6) in acute ventilatory failure with no spontaneous breathing and profuse airway secretions due to intercurrent chest infections.[69–71] MIE in a protocol with manually assisted coughing, oximetry feedback, and home use of NIV was shown to effectively decrease hospitalizations and respiratory complications and mortality for patients with NMD.[72,73]

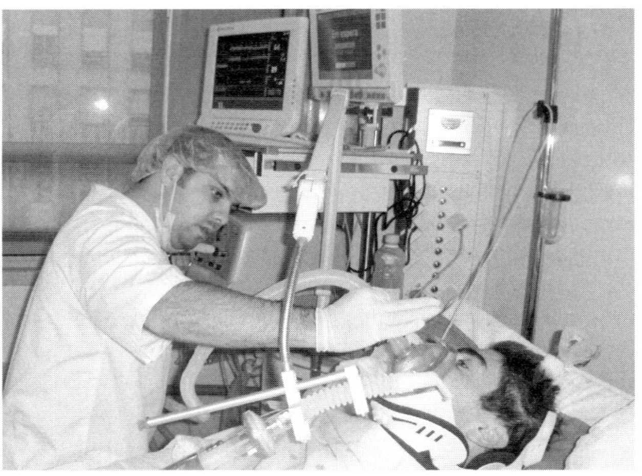

**Figure 61.6** 21-year-old man with a high level spinal cord injury (C2), extubated with a vital capacity of 120 mL and a peak cough flow of 125 L/min, using mechanically assisted coughing with CoughAssist (Phillips Respironics) via an oronasal interface at pressures of 40 to −40 cm $H_2O$, after extubation to continuous non-invasive ventilation. Mechanically assisted coughing was performed by a trained respiratory therapist.

## CONCLUSION

There continues to be widespread debate as to which airway clearance regimen should be used and when. In most comparisons, bronchial hygiene physical therapy produced no significant effects on pulmonary function, apart from clearing sputum in chronic obstructive pulmonary disease and in bronchiectasis.[19] However there is strong evidence that supports the use of respiratory physical therapy techniques for secretion clearance in neuromuscular disease to improve quality of life and survival.[6,68]

So, in patients with ventilatory impairment, NIV is a very efficient technique in respiratory management, but in the majority of the cases secretions are excessive and NIV alone is likely to fail. The role of respiratory physiotherapy is important and should be based on evidence and directed to the goals of intervention described in this chapter to permit efficient treatment while the patient is hospitalized, and prevent hospitalizations when the patient is at home, where family members must be trained to provide the treatments and maintain the achievement of the goals, and therefore maximize the potential of pulmonary rehabilitation.

## REFERENCES


1. van der Schans CP, Postma DS, Koeter GH *et al.* Physiotherapy and bronchial mucus transport. *Eur Respir J* 1999; **13**: 1477–86.
2. Gomez-Merino E, Bach JR. Duchenne muscular dystrophy: prolongation of life by noninvasive respiratory muscle aids. *Am J Phys Med Rehabil* 2002; **81**: 411–15.
3. Dail CW. Glossopharyngeal breathing by paralyzed patients: a preliminary report. *California Medicine* 1951; **75**: 217–18.
4. Bach J, Bianchi C, Lopes M *et al.* Lung Inflation by glossopharyngeal breathing and 'air stacking' in Duchenne muscular dystrophy. *Am J Phys Med Rehabil* 2007; **86**: 295–300.
5. Nygren-Bonnier M, Wahman K, Lindholm P *et al.* Glossopharyngeal pistoning for lung insufflation in patients with cervical spinal cord injury. *Spinal Cord* 2009; **47**: 418–22.
6. Tzeng AC, Bach JR. Prevention of pulmonary morbidity for patients with neurosmucular disease. *Chest* 2000; **118**: 1390–96.
7. Templeton M, Palazzo MG. Chest physiotherapy prolongs duration of ventilation in the critically ill ventilated for more than 48 hours. *Intensive Care Med* 2007; **33**: 1938–45.
8. Smina M, Salam A, Khamiees M *et al.* Cough peak flows and extubation outcomes. *Chest* 2003; **124**: 262–8.
9. Bach JR, Saporito LR. Criteria for extubation and tracheostomy tube removal for patients with ventilatory failure. A different approach to weaning. *Chest* 1996; **110**: 1566–71.
10. American Thoracic Society. Standards for the diagnosis and care of patients with chronic obstructive pulmonary disease. *Am J Respir Crit Care Med* 1995; **152**: S77–S120.
11. Hondras MA, Linde K, Jones AP. Manual therapy for asthma. *Cochrane Database Syst Rev* 2000; **2**: CD001002.
12. Bradley JM, Moran FM, Elborn JS. Evidence for physical therapies (airway clearance and physical training) in cystic fibrosis: an overview of five Cochrane systematic reviews. *Respir Med* 2006; **100**: 191–201.
13. Sancho J, Servera E, Diaz J *et al.* Comparison of peak cough flows measured by pneumotachograph and a portable peak flow meter. *Am J Phys Med Rehabil* 2004; **83**: 608–12.
14. Schneerson JM. Noninvasive ventilation for chest wall and neuromuscular disorders. *Eur Respir J* 2002; **20**: 480–7.
15. Bach JR, Campagnolo DI, Hoeman S. Life satisfaction of individuals with Duchenne muscular dystrophy using long-term mechanical ventilatory support. *Am J Phys Med Rehabil* 1991; **70**: 129–35.
16. Chaudri MB, Liu C, Hubbard R *et al.* Relationship between supramaximal flow during cough and mortality in motor neurone disease. *Eur Respir J* 2002; **19**: 434–8.
17. Plant PK, Owen JL, Elliot MW. Non-invasive ventilation in acute exacerbations of chronic obstructive pulmonary disease: long term survival and predictors of in-hospital outcome. *Thorax* 2001; **56**: 708–12.
18. van der Schans CP, Piers DA, Beekhuis H *et al.* Effect of forced expirations on mucus clearance in patients with chronic airflow obstruction: effect of lung recoil pressure. *Thorax* 1990; **45**: 623–7.
19. Jones AP, Rowe BH. Bronchopulmonary hygiene physical therapy for chronic obstructive pulmonary disease and bronchiectasis. *Cochrane Database Syst Rev* 2000; **2**: CD000045.
20. Pryor JA. Physiotherapy for airway clearance in adults. *Eur Respir J* 1999; **14**: 1418–24.
21. Van der Schans C, Bach J, Rubin BK. Chest physical therapy: mucus-mobilization techniques. In: Bach JR, ed. *Noninvasive mechanical ventilation*, 1st edn. Philadelphia: Hanley & Belfus, Inc, 2002:259–84.
22. Hess DR. The evidence for secretion clearance techniques. *Respir Care* 2001; **46**: 1276–93.
23. Wolmer P, Ursing K, Midgren B *et al.* Ineficiency of chest percussion in the physical therapy of chronic bronchitis. *Eur J Respir Dis* 1985; **66**: 233–39.
24. Bach PB, Brown C, Gelfand SE *et al.* Management of acute exacerbations of chronic obstructive pulmonary disease: a summary and appraisal of published evidence. *Ann Intern Med* 2001; **134**: 600–20.
25. Hubert J. Mobilisations du Thorax. *Les edicions Medicales et Paramedicales de Charleroi, Montignies-sur-Sambre.* Belgium 1989.
26. Lannefors L, Wollmer P. Mucus clearance with three chest physiotherapy regimes in cystic fibrosis: a comparison between postural drainage, PEP and physical exercise. *Eur Respir J* 1992; **5**: 748–53.
27. Bellone A, Spagnolatti L, Massobrio M *et al.* Short-term effects of expiration under positive pressure in patients with acute exacerbation of chronic obstructive pulmonary disease and mild acidosis requiring non-invasive positive pressure ventilation. *Intensive Care Med* 2002; **28**: 581–5.
28. Konstan MW, Stern RC, Doershuk CF. Efficacy of the Flutter device for airway mucus clearance in patients with cystic fibrosis. *J Pediatr* 1994; **124**: 689–93.
29. Kang SW, Bach JR. Maximum insufflation capacity. *Chest* 2000; **118**: 61–5.
30. Sivasothy P, Brown L, Smith IE *et al.* Effects of manually assisted cough and mechanical insufflation on cough flow of normal subjects, patients with chronic obstructive pulmonary disease (COPD), and patients with respiratory muscle weakness. *Thorax* 2001; **56**: 438–44.
31. Bach JR, Goncalves MR, Paez S *et al.* Expiratory flow maneuvers in patients with neuromuscular diseases. *Am J Phys Med Rehabil* 2006; **85**: 105–11.
32. Bach JR. Mechanical Insufflation-exsufflation: comparison of peak expiratory flows with manually assisted and unassisted coughing techniques. *Chest* 1993; **104**: 1553–62.

33. Bach JR. Don't forget the abdominal thrust. *Chest* 2004; **126**: 1388–9; author reply 89–90.
34. Bach JR, Chaudhry SS. Standards of care in MDA clinics. Muscular Dystrophy Association. *Am J Phys Med Rehabil* 2000; **79**: 193–6.
35. Bach JR, Alba AS. Noninvasive options for ventilatory support of the traumatic high level quadriplegic patient. *Chest* 1990; **98**: 613–19.
36. Bianchi C, Grandi M, Felisari G. Efficacy of glossopharyngeal breathing for a ventilator-dependent, high-level tetraplegic patient after cervical cord tumor resection and tracheotomy. *Am J Phys Med Rehabil* 2004; **83**: 216–19.
37. Nygren-Bonnier M, Markstrom A, Lindholm P *et al.* Glossopharyngeal pistoning for lung insufflation in children with spinal muscular atrophy type II. *Acta Paediatr* 2009; **98**: 1324–8.
38. Toussaint M, De Win H, Steens M *et al.* Effect of intrapulmonary percussive ventilation on mucus clearance in duchenne muscular dystrophy patients: a preliminary report. *Respir Care* 2003; **48**: 940–7.
39. Langenderfer B. Alternatives to percussion and postural drainage. A review of mucus clearance therapies: percussion and postural drainage, autogenic drainage, positive expiratory pressure, flutter valve, intrapulmonary percussive ventilation, and high-frequency chest compression with the ThAIRapy Vest. *J Cardiopulm Rehabil* 1998; **18**: 283–9.
40. Varekojis SM, Douce FH, Flucke RL *et al.* A comparison of the therapeutic effectiveness of and preference for postural drainage and percussion, intrapulmonary percussive ventilation, and high-frequency chest wall compression in hospitalized cystic fibrosis patients. *Respir Care* 2003; **48**: 24–8.
41. Vargas F, Bui HN, Boyer A *et al.* Intrapulmonary percussive ventilation in acute exacerbations of COPD patients with mild respiratory acidosis: a randomized controlled trial [ISRCTN17802078]. *Crit Care* 2005; **9**: R382–9.
42. Newhouse PA, White F, Marks JH *et al.* The intrapulmonary percussive ventilator and flutter device compared to standard chest physiotherapy in patients with cystic fibrosis. *Clin Pediatr (Phila)* 1998; **37**: 427–32.
43. Nava S, Barbarito N, Piaggi G *et al.* Physiological response to intrapulmonary percussive ventilation in stable COPD patients. *Respir Med* 2006; **100**: 1526–33.
44. Hansen LG, Warwick WJ, Hansen KL. Mucus transport mechanisms in relation to the effect of high frequency chest compression (HFCC) on mucus clearance. *Pediatr Pulmonol* 1994; **17**: 113–18.
45. van der Schans C, Prasad A, Main E. Chest physiotherapy compared to no chest physiotherapy for cystic fibrosis. *Cochrane Database Syst Rev* 2000; **2**: CD001401.
46. Scherer TA, Barandun J, Martinez E *et al.* Effect of high-frequency oral airway and chest wall oscillation and conventional chest physical therapy on expectoration in patients with stable cystic fibrosis. *Chest* 1998; **113**: 1019–27.
47. Darbee JC, Kanga JF, Ohtake PJ. Physiologic evidence for high-frequency chest wall oscillation and positive expiratory pressure breathing in hospitalized subjects with cystic fibrosis. *Phys Ther* 2005; **85**: 1278–89.
48. Hansen LG, Warwick WJ. High-frequency chest compression system to aid in clearance of mucus from the lung. *Biomed Instrum Technol* 1990; **24**: 289–94.
49. Jones A, Rowe BH. Bronchopulmonary hygiene physical therapy in bronchiectasis and chronic obstructive pulmonary disease: a systematic review. *Heart Lung* 2000; **29**: 125–35.
50. Chaisson KM, Walsh S, Simmons Z *et al.* A clinical pilot study: high frequency chest wall oscillation airway clearance in patients with amyotrophic lateral sclerosis. *Amyotroph Lateral Scler* 2006; **7**: 107–11.
51. Lange DJ, Lechtzin N, Davey C *et al.* High-frequency chest wall oscillation in ALS: an exploratory randomized, controlled trial. *Neurology* 2006; **67**: 991–7.
52. Chatwin M. How to use a mechanical insufflator-exsufflator 'cough assist machine'. *Breathe* 2008; **4**: 321–5.
53. Chatwin M, Ross E, Hart N *et al.* Cough augmentation with mechanical insufflation/exsufflation in patients with neuromuscular weakness. *Eur Respir J* 2003; **21**: 502–8.
54. Gomez-Merino E, Sancho J, Marin J *et al.* Mechanical insufflation-exsufflation: pressure, volume, and flow relationships and the adequacy of the manufacturer's guidelines. *Am J Phys Med Rehabil* 2002; **81**: 579–83.
55. Bach JR, Smith WH, Michaels J *et al.* Airway secretion clearance by mechanical exsufflation for post-poliomyelitis ventilator-assisted individuals. *Arch Phys Med Rehabil* 1993; **74**: 170–7.
56. Farrero E, Prats E, Povedano M *et al.* Survival in amyotrophic lateral sclerosis with home mechanical ventilation: the impact of systematic respiratory assessment and bulbar involvement. *Chest* 2005; **127**: 2132–8.
57. Sancho J, Servera E, Diaz J *et al.* Efficacy of mechanical insufflation-exsufflation in medically stable patients with amyotrophic lateral sclerosis. *Chest* 2004; **125**: 1400–5.
58. Winck JC, Goncalves MR, Lourenco C *et al.* Effects of mechanical insufflation-exsufflation on respiratory parameters for patients with chronic airway secretion encumbrance. *Chest* 2004; **126**: 774–80.
59. Sancho J, Servera E, Marin J *et al.* Effect of lung mechanics on mechanically assisted flows and volumes. *Am J Phys Med Rehabil* 2004; **83**: 698–703.
60. Goncalves M, Winck J. Exploring the potential of mechanical insufflation-exsufflation. *Breathe* 2008; **4**: 326–9.
61. Bach JR, Niranjan V, Weaver B. Spinal muscular atrophy type 1: a noninvasive respiratory management approach. *Chest* 2000; **117**: 1100–5.

62. Garstang SV, Kirshblum SC, Wood KE. Patient preference for in-exsufflation for secretion management with spinal cord injury. *J Spinal Cord Med* 2000; **23**: 80–5.
63. Sancho J, Servera E, Vergara P *et al.* Mechanical insufflation-exsufflation vs. tracheal suctioning via traqueostomy tubes for patients with amyotrophic lateral sclerosis: a pilot study. *Am J Phys Med Rehabil* 2003; **82**: 750–3.
64. Whitney J, Harden B, Keilty S. Assisted cough: a new technique. *Physiotherapy* 2002; **88**: 201–7.
65. Williams EK, Holaday DA. The use of exsufflation with negative pressure in postoperative patients. *Am J Surg* 1955; **90**: 637–40.
66. Marchant WAF. Postoperative use of a CoughAssist device in avoiding prolonged intubation. *Br J Anaesth* 2002; **89**: 644–7.
67. Bach JR. Cough in SCI patients. *Arch Phys Med Rehabil* 1994; **75**: 610.
68. Bach JR, Ishikawa Y, Kim H. Prevention of the pulmonary morbidity for patients with duchenne muscular dystrophy. *Chest* 1997; **112**: 1024–8.
69. Vianello AC, Arcaro G, Gallan F *et al.* Mechanical insufflation-exsufflation improves outcomes for neuromuscular disease patients with respiratory tract infenctions. *Am J Phys Med Rehabil* 2005; **84**: 83–8; discussion 89–91.
70. Servera E, Sancho J, Zafra MJ *et al.* Alternatives to endotracheal intubation for patients with neuromuscular diseases. *Am J Phys Med Rehabil* 2005; **84**: 851–7.
71. Bach JR, Gonçalves MR, Hamdani I, Winck JC. Extubation of patients with neuromuscular weakness: a new management paradigm. *Chest* 29 December 2009 [Epub ahead of print].
72. Bach J, Goncalves M. Ventilatory weaning by lung expansion and decanulation. *Am J Phys Med Rehabil* 2004; **83**: 560–8.
73. Bach JR. Prevention of morbidity and mortality with the use of physical medicine aids: The obstructive and paralytic conditions. In: Bach JR, ed. *Pulmonary rehabilitation.* Philadelphia: Hanley & Belfus, Inc, 1996:303–29.

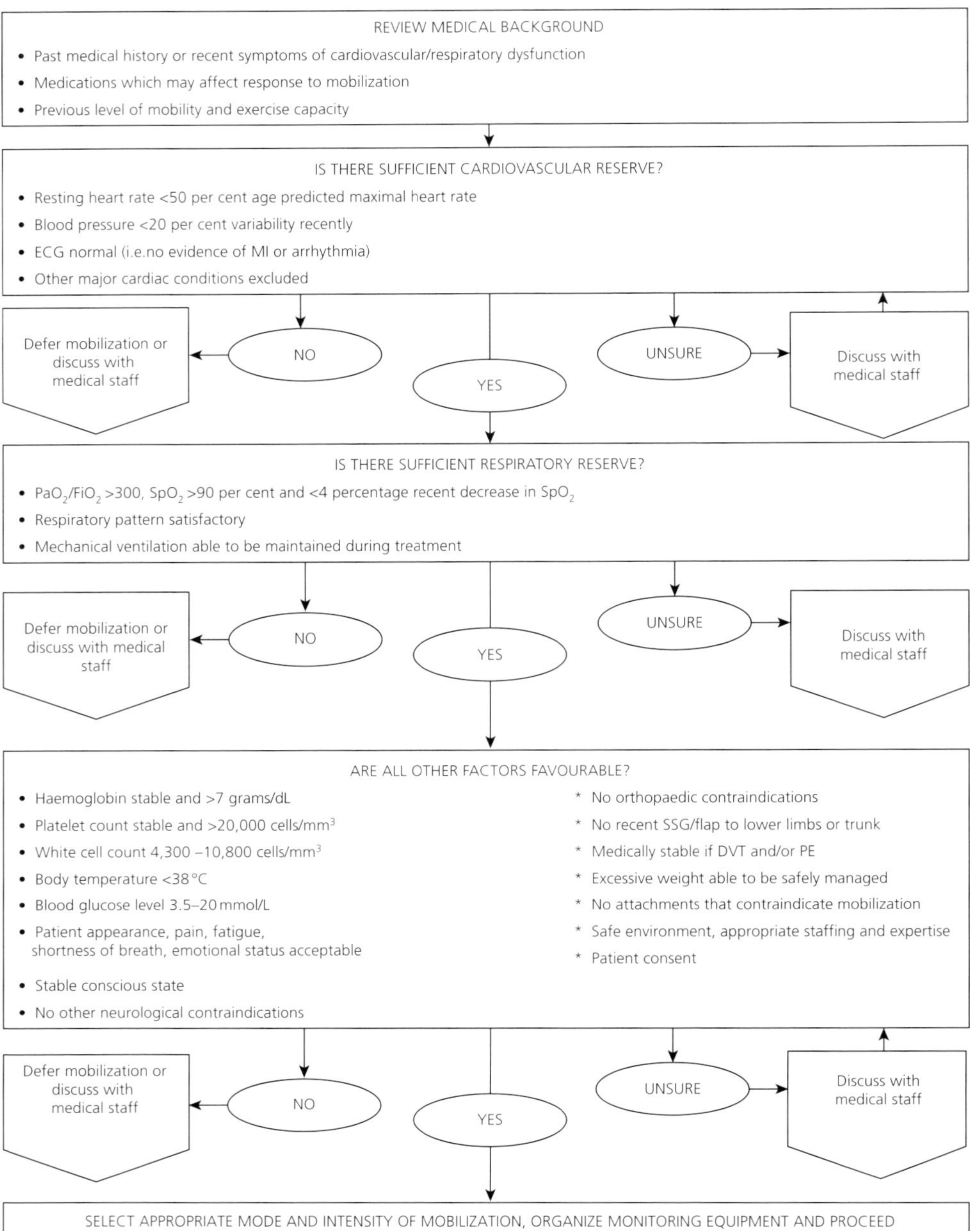


**Figure 62.1** Overview of safety issues before mobilizing critically ill patients. DVT, deep vein thrombosis; ECG, electrocardiogram; MI, myocardial infarction; PE, pulmonary embolism; SSG, split skin graft. Reproduced with permission from Stiller and Phillips.[14]

(leg flexors, knee extensors and dorsal flexors of the foot). De Jonghe *et al.* have proposed that a sum score less than 48 reflects significant ICU-acquired weakness.[6] However, manual muscle testing seems to be insensitive to differences in muscle strength of values above grade 3 (active movement against gravity over the full range of motion).[29] Therefore, several systems have been developed to measure muscle strength more accurately.

Dynamometry with mechanical or electrical equipment is used to measure isometric muscle force. Handgrip dynamometry has been shown to be reliable, and reference values are available.[30] For other upper and lower extremity muscle groups, handheld electrical devices have been developed. Two methods of isometric testing have been described: the make-test and the break-test. In the make-test, the maximum force the subject can exert is equal to the force of the assessor. In the break-test, the force of the assessor exceeds the force of the patient slightly. Both tests are reproducible, but higher values have been found during break-tests.

Hand-held dynamometry is a viable alternative to more costly modes of isometric strength measurements, provided the assessor's strength is greater than that of the specific muscle group being measured. Reference values are available, also for elderly healthy subjects.[31] The limitation of the use of maximal voluntary contractions is the potential for submaximal contractions due to submaximal cortical drive.[32] The use of superimposed electric or magnetic twitch contractions anticipates this potential variation in voluntary activation.[32] Magnetic stimulation is less painful than electrical stimulation, and the 'twitch' stimulations are relatively reproducible. Ultrasound measurement of muscle thickness of the quadriceps, which was introduced and validated against MRI (the gold standard for muscle cross-sectional area), has recently been validated in ICU patients.[7] This allows non-invasive and accurate assessment of muscle size in critically ill and often uncooperative patients.

### Respiratory muscle testing

In clinical practice, respiratory muscle strength is measured as maximum inspiratory and expiratory mouth pressures (MIP and MEP, respectively). These pressure measurements are made via a small cylinder attached to the mouth with a circular mouthpiece. The American Thoracic Society (ATS)/ERS statement describes respiratory muscle testing in more detail.[33] In ventilated patients inspiratory muscle strength is estimated by temporary occlusion of the airway. The procedure involves use of a unidirectional expiratory valve to allow the patient to expire while inspiration is blocked. Optimal length of occlusion time is considered 25–30 seconds in adults.[34] Other techniques have also been developed to assess global respiratory muscle function, such as sniff manoeuvres. More invasive techniques such as electric or magnetic diaphragm stimulation provide more accurate information on diaphragm function and are useful in the diagnosis of diaphragmatic paresis and weakness. Several groups have developed normal values; however, regardless of which set of normal values is used, the standard deviation is large. The presence of inspiratory weakness is accepted when MIP is lower than 50 per cent of the predicted value.

### Functional status

The assessment of functional status may seem to be inapplicable for acutely ill ICU patients but can be implemented in long-term weaning facilities and after ICU discharge. Functional assessment tools are also successfully used to monitor progress of patients in several studies.[12,15,18,23] Furthermore they can play a role in reconstructing the patient's functionality before ICU admission. The Barthel Index, Functional Independence Measure (FIM) and Katz ADL Scale are commonly used and valid tools to score the patient's ability to independently perform a range of activities, mostly related to mobility (e.g. transfers from bed to chair, walking, stair climbing) and self-care (e.g. bathing, grooming, toileting, dressing, feeding). The Berg Balance Scale quantifies impairment in balance function by scoring the performance of simple functional tasks (e.g. sitting, standing, transfers, reaching forward, turning). Walking ability can also be simply assessed using the Functional Ambulation Categories. In patients who are able to walk, the 6-minute walking test can be used to evaluate functional exercise capacity.

### Quality of life

As health-related quality of life is often reduced after prolonged ICU stay,[2] appropriate evaluation of physical and mental health components is necessary. The SF-36 is a widely used generic quality of life questionnaire which includes eight multiple-item scales that assess physical functioning, social functioning, physical role, emotional role, mental health, pain, vitality and general health. An alternative tool is the Nottingham Health Profile, which covers six different quality of life areas: pain, energy, physical mobility, sleep, social isolation and emotional interaction. Both questionnaires have been used frequently in post-ICU quality of life studies.[2] In patients with underlying chronic respiratory diseases, disease-specific questionnaires such as the Chronic Respiratory Disease Questionnaire or the St George's Respiratory Questionnaire can provide more specific information on the impact of the ICU stay on disease perception.

## TREATMENT: WHAT, WHEN AND HOW?

Exercise training is considered a cornerstone component of each rehabilitation programme, in addition to psychosocial interventions. To avoid or minimize physical deconditioning and other complications, short duration mechanical ventilation with early extubation is a prime goal of the critical care team. Early mobilization was shown to reduce the time to wean from mechanical ventilation 30 years ago and is the basis for long-term functional recovery. Evidence for the benefits of body positioning, mobilization, exercise and muscle training, on the prevention and treatment of deconditioning in other patient groups as well as in healthy subjects, lends support for the use of these interventions in the management of critically ill patients. In addition to safety issues, exercise should also be targeted at the appropriate intensity and exercise modality. These are dependent on the stability and cooperation of the patient.

Acutely ill, uncooperative patients are treated with modalities that do not depend on patient compliance and do not put stress on the cardiorespiratory system, such as passive range of motion, muscle stretching, splinting, body positioning, passive cycling with a bed cycle or electrical muscle stimulation. On the other hand, the stable cooperative patient, beyond the acute illness phase but still on mechanical ventilation, should be mobilized on the edge of the bed, transferred to a chair, and perform resistance muscle training or active cycling with a bed cycle

| LEVEL 0 | LEVEL 1 | LEVEL 2 | LEVEL 3 | LEVEL 4 | LEVEL 5 |
|---|---|---|---|---|---|
| UNCOOPERATIVE | UNCOOPERATIVE | COOPERATIVE | COOPERATIVE | COOPERATIVE | COOPERATIVE |
| **ASSESSMENT:**<br>Cardiorespiratory unstable<br>MAP <60mmHg<br>$FiO_2$ >60%<br>$PaO_2/FiO_2$ <200<br>Neurological unstable<br>Acute surgery<br>Temp >40°C<br>S5Q = 0 | **ASSESSMENT:**<br>Cardiorespiratory stable<br>Neurological – Surgical – Trauma condition does not allow transfer to chair<br>S5Q <3 | **ASSESSMENT:**<br>Obesity<br>Neurological – Surgical – Trauma condition does not allow active transfer to chair<br>S5Q >3<br>MRCsum legs <18 | **ASSESSMENT:**<br>S5Q = 4/5<br>MRCsum legs 18<br>BBS Sit to stand = 0<br>BBS Standing = 0<br>BBS Sitting = 1 | **ASSESSMENT:**<br>S5Q = 5<br>MRCsum legs 24<br>BBS Sit to stand >0<br>BBS Standing = 1<br>BBS Sitting = 2 | **ASSESSMENT:**<br>S5Q = 5<br>MRCsum legs 24<br>BBS Sit to stand >0<br>BBS Standing >2<br>BBS Sitting = 3 |
| **BODY POSITIONING:**<br>2hr turning | **BODY POSITIONING:**<br>2hr turning<br>Fowler's position<br>Splinting | **BODY POSITIONING:**<br>2hr turning<br>Splinting<br>Upright sitting position in bed<br>Passive transfer bed to chair | **BODY POSITIONING:**<br>2hr turning<br>Passive transfer bed to chair<br>Sitting out of bed<br>Standing with assist (>2pers) | **BODY POSITIONING:**<br>Active transfer bed to chair<br>Sitting out of bed<br>Standing with assist (>1pers) | **BODY POSITIONING:**<br>Active transfer bed to chair<br>Sitting out of bed<br>Standing |
| **PHYSIOTHERAPY:**<br>No treatment | **PHYSIOTHERAPY:**<br>Passive range of motion<br>Passive bed cycling<br>NMES | **PHYSIOTHERAPY:**<br>Passive/Active range of motion<br>Resistance training arms and legs<br>Passive/Active leg and/or cycling in bed or chair<br>NMES | **PHYSIOTHERAPY:**<br>Active range of motion<br>Resistance training arms and legs<br>Active leg and/or arm cycling in bed or chair<br>NMES<br>ADL | **PHYSIOTHERAPY:**<br>Active range of motion<br>Resistance training arms and legs<br>Active leg and/or arm cycling in chair<br>Walking (with assistance/frame)<br>NMES<br>ADL | **PHYSIOTHERAPY:**<br>Active range of motion<br>Resistance training arms and legs<br>Active leg and arm cycling in chair<br>Walking (with assistance)<br>ADL |

**Figure 62.2** Leuven 'Start to Move' protocol: a step approach to progressive mobilization and physical activity. See Appendix 62.1 on page 575 for S5Q (Standardized 5 Questions) and BBS (Berg Balance Score). NMES, neuromuscular electrical stimulation; ADL, activities of daily living.

or chair cycle and walk with or without assistance. The flow diagram developed in the authors' centre, inspired by the flow diagram produced by Morris *et al.*[17] (Fig. 62.2), has face validity and is an example of such step-up approach. A similar approach was followed by Schweickert *et al.*[15]

The following sections deal with modalities of exercise training with progressive intensity and increasing need of cooperation of the patient. The risk of moving a critically ill patient is weighed against the risk of immobility and recumbency and when employed requires stringent monitoring to ensure the mobilization is instituted appropriately and safely.[14]

## The uncooperative, critically ill patient

The importance of body positioning ('stirring up' patients) was reported as early as the 1940s.[20] Since that time, positioning has been used prescriptively to remediate oxygen transport deficits such as impaired gas exchange by altering the distribution of ventilation ($\dot{V}$) and perfusion (Q), $\dot{V}$/Q matching, airway closure, work of breathing, and work of the heart, as well as mucociliary transport (postural drainage). Recumbency during bed rest in patients who are critically ill exposes them to risk because the vertical gravitational gradient is eliminated, and exercise stress is restricted. To simulate the normal perturbations that the human body experiences in health, the patient who is critically ill needs to be positioned upright (well supported), and rotated when recumbent. These perturbations need to be scheduled frequently to avoid the adverse effects of prolonged static positioning on respiratory, cardiac and circulatory function. The potent and direct physiological effects of changing body position on oxygen transport and oxygenation are exploited when mobilization is contraindicated. This evidence comes primarily from the space science literature in which bed rest has been used as a model of weightlessness. The prone position has been of particular interest in the management of the critically ill patient, but is underused. Knowledge of the physiological effects of body position enables the physiotherapist to prescribe a positioning regimen to exploit its beneficial effects as well as minimize the effects of deleterious body positions. Other indications for active and passive positioning include the management of soft tissue contracture, protection of flaccid limbs and lax joints, nerve impingement and skin breakdown.

Although a specific body position may be indicated for a patient, varied positions and frequent body position changes, particularly extreme body positions, are based on the assessment findings. The efficacy of 2-hourly patient rotation, which is common in clinical practice, has not been verified scientifically. A rotation schedule that is more frequent and promotes turning from one extreme position to another, approximates more normal heart–lung function than a standardized 2-hourly turning regimen. Medically unstable patients who require a rotating or kinetic bed benefit from continuous side-to-side perturbation, which supports the hypothesis that patients may benefit from frequent and extreme position changes rather than fixed, prolonged periods in given positions.[35]

Bed design features in critical care should include hip and knee breaks so the patient can approximate upright sitting as much as can be tolerated. Patients who are sedated, heavy or overweight may need chairs with greater support such as stretcher chairs. Lifts may be needed to change a patient's position safely.

Passive stretching or range of motion exercises may have a particularly important role in the management of patients who are unable to move spontaneously. Studies in healthy subjects have shown that passive stretching decreases stiffness and increases extensibility of the muscle. Passive stretching for at least 30 minutes a day prevented loss of joint mobility and muscle mass in an animal model.[36] Passive movement has been shown to enhance ventilation in neurological patients in high-dependency units.[37] Evidence for using continuous dynamic stretching is based on the observation in other patient groups that continuous passive motion (CPM) prevents contractures and promotes function. CPM has been assessed in patients with critical illness subjected to prolonged inactivity. Three hours of CPM three times per day reduced fibre atrophy and protein loss compared with passive stretching for 5 minutes twice daily.[38]

For patients who cannot be actively mobilized and are at high risk of soft tissue contracture, such as following severe burns, trauma and some neurological conditions, splinting may be indicated. Splinting of the periarticular structures in the stretched position for more than 11 hours a day has been shown to have a beneficial effect on the range of motion in an animal model. In burns patients, fixing the position of joints reduces muscle and skin contraction.[39] In patients with neurological dysfunction, splinting may reduce muscle tone.[40]

The application of exercise training in the early phase of ICU admission is often more complicated due to lack of cooperation and the clinical status of the patient. Recent technological developments have resulted in a bedside cycle ergometer for (active or passive) leg cycling during bed rest (Fig. 62.3). The application of this training modality has been shown to be a safe and feasible exercise tool in patients with severe COPD who are confined to bed and during haemodialysis in patients with end-stage renal disease. The bedside cycle ergometer can facilitate prolonged continuous mobilization, allowing rigorous control of exercise intensity and duration. Furthermore, training intensity can be continuously adjusted to the patient's health status and the physiological responses to exercise. A recent randomized controlled trial of early application of daily bedside leg cycling in critically ill patients showed improved functional status, muscle function and exercise performance at hospital discharge compared with patients receiving standard physiotherapy without leg cycling.[23]

In patients unable to perform voluntary muscle contractions, electrical muscle stimulation (EMS) has been used to prevent disuse muscle atrophy. Applying EMS

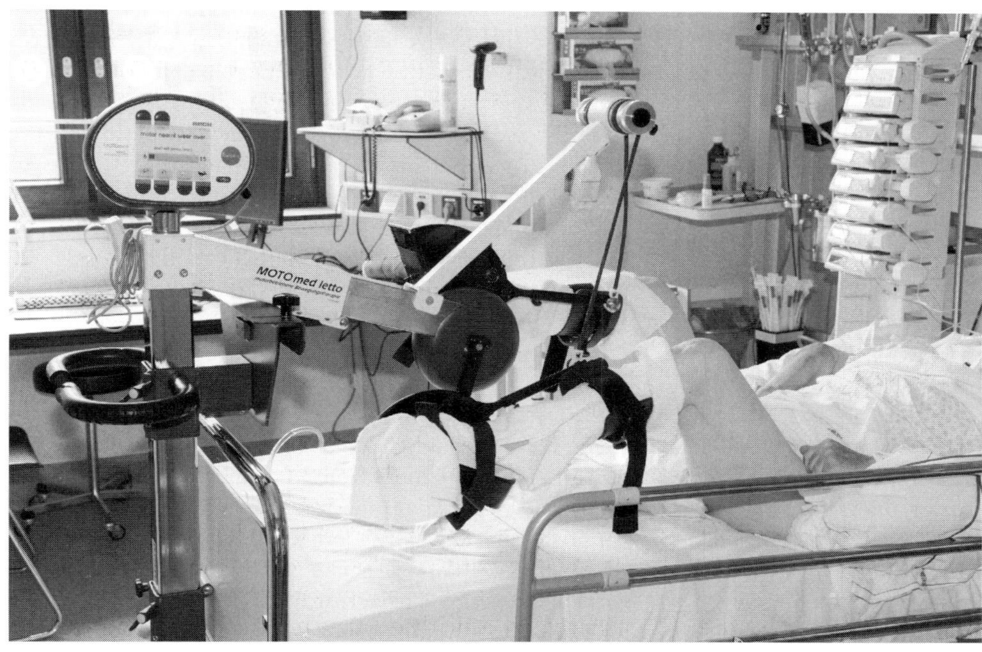


**Figure 62.3** Device for active and passive cycling in a bedridden patient in the intensive care unit.

during an immobilization period prevented the reduction in strength and muscle mass to a substantial extent.[41] In patients with lower limb fractures and cast immobilization for 6 weeks, daily EMS for at least 1-hour reduced the decrease in cross-sectional area of the quadriceps and enhanced normal muscle protein synthesis.[42] Electrical muscle stimulation is also being used in patients with impaired muscle function, e.g. spinal cord lesions, hemi- or quadriplegia and COPD. Slower muscle protein catabolism and increase in total RNA content were also seen after EMS in patients with major abdominal surgery.[43] In patients in the ICU not able to move actively, a reduction of muscle protein breakdown is seen when using EMS, while EMS of the quadriceps, in addition to active limb mobilization, enhanced muscle strength and hastened independent transfer from bed to chair.[44]

## Cooperative patients

Mobilization and ambulation have been part of the physiotherapy management of acutely ill patients for several decades.[20] Mobilization refers to physical activity sufficient to elicit acute physiological effects that enhance ventilation, central and peripheral perfusion, circulation, muscle metabolism and alertness. Strategies – in order of intensity – include sitting over the edge of the bed, standing, stepping in place, transferring in bed and from bed to chair, and walking with or without support. Although the approach of early mobilization has face validity, only recently was the concept studied in two randomized controlled trials.[15,17] Morris *et al.* demonstrated that patients receiving early mobility therapy had reduced ICU stay and hospital stay with no differences in weaning time. No differences were observed in discharge location or in hospital costs of the usual care and early mobility patients. Schweickert *et al.* observed that early physical and occupational therapy improved functional status at hospital discharge, shortened duration of delirium and increased ventilator-free days. These findings did not result in differences in length of ICU or hospital stay.[15]

The team approach (doctor, nurse, physiotherapist and occupational therapist) is important in establishing an early ambulation programme. The early intervention approach is, although not easy, specifically in patients still in need of supportive devices (mechanical ventilation, cardiac assists) or unable to stand without support of personnel or standing aids, a worthwhile experience for the patient.[17,22] The difference in the mentality of the team was elegantly demonstrated by Thomsen *et al.*[11] They studied 104 respiratory failure patients who required mechanical ventilation for more than 4 days. After correction for confounders, transferring a patient from the acute intensive care to the RICU substantially increased the number of patients ambulating threefold compared with pre-transfer rates. Improvements in ambulation with transfer to the RICU were attributed to the differences in the team approach towards ambulating the patients.[11]

Standing and walking frames enable the patient to mobilize safely with attachments for bags, lines and leads that cannot be disconnected. The arm support on a frame or rollator has been shown to increase ventilatory capacity in patients with severe chronic obstructive pulmonary disease (COPD).[45] The frame either needs to be able to accommodate a portable oxygen tank, or a portable mechanical ventilator and seat, or a suitable trolley for equipment can be used. Walking and standing aids, and tilt tables, enhance physiological responses[46] and promote early mobilization of critically ill patients. The tilt table may be used when the patient is unable to move the legs to counter dependent fluid displacement, and may be at risk of orthostatic intolerance. Abdominal belts need to be carefully positioned to support, not restrict, respiration during mobilization. In patients with spinal cord injury this improves vital capacity.[47] Transfer belts facilitate heavy lifts and protect both the patient and the physiotherapist. Non-invasive ventilation (NIV) during mobilization may improve exercise tolerance for non-intubated patients, similar to that demonstrated in patients with stable COPD.[48] However, no randomized trials have been performed in this setting. In ventilated patients, the ventilator settings may require adjustment to the patient's needs (i.e. increased minute ventilation).

Aerobic training and muscle strengthening, in addition to routine mobilization, improved walking distance more than mobilization alone in patients with chronic critical illness on long-term mechanical ventilation.[13] A randomized controlled trial showed that a 6-week upper and lower limb training programme improved limb muscle strength, ventilator-free time and functional outcomes in patients requiring long-term mechanical ventilation compared with a control group.[18] These results are in line with a retrospective analysis of patients on long-term mechanical ventilation who participated in whole-body training and respiratory muscle training.[12] In patients recently weaned from mechanical ventilation,[49] the addition of upper-limb exercise enhanced the effects of general mobilization on exercise endurance performance and dyspnoea. Low-resistance multiple repetitions of resistive muscle training can augment muscle mass, force generation, and oxidative enzymes. Sets of repetitions (three sets of 8–10 repetitions at 50–70 per cent of one repetition maximum [1RM]) within the patient's tolerance can be scheduled daily, commensurate with their goals. Resistive muscle training can include the use of pulleys, elastic bands and weight belts. Patients with cardiovascular dysfunction may benefit from resistance training, although high resistance of large muscle masses may have detrimental cardiovascular effects in elderly subjects with cardiovascular disease. The chair cycle and the above-mentioned bed cycle allow patients to perform an individualized exercise training programme. The intensity of cycling can be adjusted to the individual patient's capacity, ranging from passive cycling via assisted cycling to cycling against increasing resistance.

The prescription of exercise intensity, duration and frequency is response-dependent rather than time-dependent and is based on clinical challenge tests, such as the response to a nursing or investigative procedure, or to a specific mobilization challenge. Exercise should be safely tolerated in any treatment session and if the patient responds positively, greater intensity and duration can be applied. For acutely ill patients, frequent short sessions (analogous to interval training) allow for greater recovery than the less frequent, longer sessions prescribed for patients with chronic stable conditions.[50] Patients with haemodynamic instability, or with little to no oxygen transport reserve capacity (e.g. those on high concentrations of oxygen and high levels of ventilatory support, or those with anaemia or cardiovascular instability), are not candidates for aggressive mobilization. The risk of moving a critically ill patient is weighed against the risk of immobility and recumbency, and when employed requires stringent monitoring to ensure that the mobilization is instituted appropriately and safely.[14]

## Weaning and respiratory muscle training

Only a small proportion of patients fail to wean from mechanical ventilation, but they require a disproportionate amount of resources. Weaning failure has been extensively studied in the clinical literature, and several factors are likely to contribute to it, including inadequate ventilatory drive, respiratory muscle weakness, respiratory muscle fatigue, increased work of breathing or cardiac failure. There is accumulating evidence that weaning problems are associated with failure of the respiratory muscles to resume ventilation.[51,52] Respiratory muscle weakness is often observed in patients with weaning failure. Patients who had received mechanical ventilation for more than 48 hours had reduced inspiratory muscle endurance that worsened with the duration of mechanical ventilation and was present following successful weaning. These data suggest that patients needing prolonged mechanical ventilation are at risk of respiratory muscle fatigue.[52] Indeed, a high ratio of respiratory muscle workload to muscle capacity ($P_I$/MIP) is a major cause of ventilator dependency and predictive of the outcome of successful weaning.[51] Since inactivity ('ventilator induced diaphragm dysfunction') has been suggested as an important cause of respiratory muscle failure and intermittent loading of the respiratory muscles has been shown to attenuate respiratory muscle deconditioning, inspiratory muscle training might be beneficial in patients with weaning failure. Some investigators might argue against the application of loaded breathing in the treatment of weaning failure, based on studies showing subcellular diaphragm muscle damage after loaded breathing.[53] However, these changes were observed after *continuous* loading instead of *intermittent* loading, as applied during inspiratory muscle training (six to eight contractions repeated in three to four series). More recent uncontrolled trials of inspiratory muscle training (threshold loading) observed an improvement in inspiratory muscle function and a reduction in duration of mechanical ventilation and weaning time.[54] Interim analysis of a randomized controlled trial comparing inspiratory muscle training at moderate intensity (~50 per cent MIP) versus sham training in patients with weaning failure showed that a significantly larger proportion of the training group (76 per cent) could be weaned compared with the sham group (35 per cent).[55] Alternatively, in patients unable to cooperate with respiratory muscle training, intermittent electrical stimulation of the diaphragm through phrenic nerve pacing might be applied.[56] So far only studies in patients with spinal cord injury support this concept.[57]

# APPENDIX 62.1

## S5Q: Standardized 5 Questions for cooperation:

- Open and close your eyes.
- Look at me.
- Open your mouth and stick out your tongue.
- Shake yes and no (nod your head).
- I will count to 5, frown your eyebrows afterwards.

## BBS: Berg Balance Score

### SITTING TO STANDING

4 able to stand without using hands and stabilize independently
3 able to stand independently using hands
2 able to stand using hands after several tries
1 needs minimal aid to stand or stabilize
0 needs moderate or maximal assist to stand

### STANDING UNSUPPORTED

4 able to stand safely for 2 minutes
3 able to stand 2 minutes with supervision
2 able to stand 30 seconds unsupported
1 needs several tries to stand 30 seconds unsupported
0 unable to stand 30 seconds unsupported

### SITTING WITH BACK UNSUPPORTED BUT FEET SUPPORTED ON FLOOR OR ON A STOOL

4 able to sit safely and securely for 2 minutes
3 able to sit 2 minutes under supervision
2 able to able to sit 30 seconds
1 able to sit 10 seconds
0 unable to sit without support 10 seconds

## REFERENCES


1. Eisner MD, Thompson T, Hudson LD *et al.* Efficacy of low tidal volume ventilation in patients with different clinical risk factors for acute lung injury and the acute respiratory distress syndrome. *Am J Respir Crit Care Med* 2001; **164**: 231–6.
2. Herridge MS, Cheung AM, Tansey CM *et al.* One-year outcomes in survivors of the acute respiratory distress syndrome. *N Engl J Med* 2003; **348**: 683–93.
3. Convertino VA. Value of orthostatic stress in maintaining functional status soon after myocardial infarction or cardiac artery bypass grafting. *J Cardiovasc Nurs* 2003; **18**: 124–30.
4. Dittmer DK, Teasell R. Complications of immobilization and bed rest. Part 1: Musculoskeletal and cardiovascular complications. *Can Fam Physician* 1993; **39**: 1428–7.
5. Teasell R, Dittmer DK. Complications of immobilization and bed rest. Part 2: Other complications. *Can Fam Physician* 1993; **39**: 1440–6.
6. De Jonghe B, Sharshar T, Lefaucheur JP *et al.* Paresis acquired in the intensive care unit: a prospective multicenter study. *JAMA* 2002; **288**: 2859–67.
7. Gruther W, Benesch T, Zorn C *et al.* Muscle wasting in intensive care patients: Ultrasound observation of the M. quadriceps femoris muscle layer. *J Rehabil Med* 2008; **40**: 185–9.
8. Ali NA, O'Brien JM Jr, Hoffmann SP *et al.* Acquired weakness, handgrip strength, and mortality in critically ill patients. *Am J Respir Crit Care Med* 2008; **178**: 261–8.
9. National Institute for Health and Clinical Excellence. *Rehabilitation after critical illness.* London: NICE Clinical Guidelines, 2009:1–91.
10. Corrado A, Roussos C, Ambrosino N *et al.* Respiratory intermediate care units: a European survey. *Eur Respir J* 2002; **20**: 1343–50.
11. Thomsen GE, Snow GL, Rodriguez L *et al.* Patients with respiratory failure increase ambulation after transfer to an intensive care unit where early activity is a priority. *Crit Care Med* 2008; **36**: 1119–24.
12. Martin UJ, Hincapie L, Nimchuk M *et al.* Impact of whole-body rehabilitation in patients receiving chronic mechanical ventilation. *Crit Care Med* 2005; **33**: 2259–65.
13. Nava S. Rehabilitation of patients admitted to a respiratory intensive care unit. *Arch Phys Med Rehabil* 1998; **79**: 849–54.
14. Stiller K, Philips A. Safety aspects of mobilising acutely ill patients. *Physiother Theory Pract* 2003; **19**: 239–57.
15. Schweickert WD, Pohlman MC, Pohlman AS *et al.* Early physical and occupational therapy in mechanically ventilated, critically ill patients: a randomised controlled trial. *Lancet* 2009; **373**: 1874–82.
16. Bailey P, Thomsen GE, Spuhler VJ *et al.* Early activity is feasible and safe in respiratory failure patients. *Crit Care Med* 2007; **35**: 139–45.
17. Morris PE, Goad A, Thompson C *et al.* Early intensive care unit mobility therapy in the treatment of acute respiratory failure. *Crit Care Med* 2008; **36**: 2238–43.
18. Chiang LL, Wang LY, Wu CP *et al.* Effects of physical training on functional status in patients with prolonged mechanical ventilation. *Phys Ther* 2006; **86**: 1271–81.
19. Dock W. The evil sequelae of complete bed rest. *JAMA* 1944; **125**: 1083–5.
20. Dripps RD, Waters RM. Nursing care of surgical patients. *Am J Nurs* 1941; **41**: 530–4.
21. Gosselink R, Bott J, Johnson M *et al.* Physiotherapy for adult patients with critical illness: recommendations of the European Respiratory Society and European Society of Intensive Care Medicine Task Force on Physiotherapy for Critically Ill Patients. *Intensive Care Med* 2008; **34**: 1188–99.
22. Needham DM. Mobilizing patients in the intensive care unit: improving neuromuscular weakness and physical function. *JAMA* 2008; **300**: 1685–90.
23. Burtin C, Clerckx B, Robbeets C *et al.* Early exercise in critically ill patients enhances short-term functional recovery. *Crit Care Med* 2009; **37**: 2499–505.
24. Morris PE. Moving our critically ill patients: mobility barriers and benefits. *Crit Care Clin* 2007; **23**: 1–20.
25. Stiller K. Safety issues that should be considered when mobilizing critically ill patients. *Crit Care Clin* 2007; **23**: 35–53.
26. Fergusson D, Hutton B, Drodge A. The epidemiology of major joint contractures: a systematic review of the literature. *Clin Orthop Relat Res* 2007; **456**: 22–9.
27. Clavet H, Hebert PC, Fergusson D *et al.* Joint contracture following prolonged stay in the intensive care unit. *CMAJ* 2008; **178**: 691–7.
28. Kleyweg RP, van der Meche FG, Schmitz PI. Interobserver agreement in the assessment of muscle strength and functional abilities in Guillain-Barré syndrome. *Muscle Nerve* 1991; **14**: 1103–9.
29. Bohannon RW. Norm references are essential if therapists are to correctly identify individuals who have physical limitations. *J Orthop Sports Phys Ther* 2005; **35**: 388.
30. Mathiowetz V, Dove M, Kashman N *et al.* Grip and pinch strength: normative data for adults. *Arch Phys Med Rehabil* 1985; **66**: 69–72.
31. Bohannon RW. Reference values for extremity muscle strength obtained by hand-held dynamometry from adults aged 20 to 79 years. *Arch Phys Med Rehabil* 1997; **78**: 26–32.
32. Allen GM, Gandevia SC, McKenzie DK. Reliability of measurements of muscle strength and voluntary activation using twitch interpolation. *Muscle Nerve* 1995; **18**: 593–600.
33. ATS/ERS statement on respiratory muscle testing. *Am J Respir Crit Care Med* 2002; **166**: 518–624.
34. Marini JJ, Smith TC, Lamb V. Estimation of inspiratory muscle strength in mechanically ventilated patients: the measurement of maximal inspiratory pressure. *J Crit Care* 1986; **1**: 32–8.

35. Fink MP, Helsmoortel CM, Stein KL *et al.* The efficacy of an oscillating bed in the prevention of lower respiratory tract infection in critically ill victims of blunt trauma. A prospective study. *Chest* 1990; **97**: 132–7.
36. Williams PE. Use of intermittent stretch in the prevention of serial sarcomere loss in immobilised muscle. *Ann Rheum Dis* 1990; **49**: 316–17.
37. Chang A, Paratz J, Rollston J. Ventilatory effects of neurophysiological facilitation and passive movement in patients with neurological injury. *Aust J Physiother* 2002; **48**: 305–10.
38. Griffiths RD, Palmer A, Helliwell T *et al.* Effect of passive stretching on the wasting of muscle in the critically ill. *Nutrition* 1995; **11**: 428–32.
39. Kwan MW, Ha KW. Splinting programme for patients with burnt hand. *Hand Surg* 2002; **7**: 231–41.
40. Hinderer SR, Dixon K. Physiologic and clinical monitoring of spastic hypertonia. *Phys Med Rehabil Clin N Am* 2001; **12**: 733–46.
41. Gould N, Donnermeyer D, Pope M *et al.* Transcutaneous muscle stimulation as a method to retard disuse atrophy. *Clin Orthop* 1982; **164**: 215–20.
42. Gibson JNA, Smith K, Rennie MJ. Prevention of disuse muscle atrophy by means of electrical stimulation: maintenance of protein synthesis. *Lancet* 1988; **2**: 767–70.
43. Strasser EM, Stattner S, Karner J *et al.* Neuromuscular electrical stimulation reduces skeletal muscle protein degradation and stimulates insulin-like growth factors in an age- and current-dependent manner: a randomized, controlled clinical trial in major abdominal surgical patients. *Ann Surg* 2009; **249**: 738–43.
44. Zanotti E, Felicetti G, Maini M *et al.* Peripheral muscle strength training in bed-bound patients with COPD receiving mechanical ventilation. Effect of electrical stimulation. *Chest* 2003; **124**: 292–6.
45. Probst VS, Troosters T, Coosemans I *et al.* Mechanisms of improvement in exercise capacity using a rollator in patients with COPD. *Chest* 2004; **126**: 1102–7.
46. Chang AT, Boots RJ, Hodges PW *et al.* Standing with the assistance of a tilt table improves minute ventilation in chronic critically ill patients. *Arch Phys Med Rehabil* 2004; **85**: 1972–6.
47. Goldman JM, Rose LS, Williams SJ *et al.* Effect of abdominal binders on breathing in tetraplegic patients. *Thorax* 1986; **41**: 940–5.
48. Van 't Hul A, Kwakkel G, Gosselink R. The acute effects of noninvasive ventilatory support during exercise on exercise endurance and dyspnea in patients with chronic obstructive pulmonary disease: a systematic review. *J Cardiopulm Rehabil* 2002; **22**: 290–7.
49. Porta R, Vitacca M, Gile LS *et al.* Supported arm training in patients recently weaned from mechanical ventilation. *Chest* 2005; **128**: 2511–20.
50. Vogiatzis I, Nanas S, Roussos C. Interval training as an alternative modality to continuous exercise in patients with COPD. *Eur Respir J* 2002; **20**: 12–19.
51. Vassilakopoulos T, Zakynthinos S, Roussos C. The tension-time index and the frequency/tidal volume ratio are the major pathophysiologic determinants of weaning failure and success. *Am J Respir Crit Care Med* 1998; **158**: 378–85.
52. Chang AT, Boots RJ, Brown MG *et al.* Reduced inspiratory muscle endurance following successful weaning from prolonged mechanical ventilation. *Chest* 2005; **128**: 553–9.
53. Orozco-Levi M, Lloreta J, Minguella J *et al.* Injury of the human diaphragm associated with exertion and chronic obstructive pulmonary disease. *Am J Respir Crit Care Med* 2001; **164**: 1734–9.
54. Martin AD, Davenport PD, Franceschi AC *et al.* Use of inspiratory muscle strength training to facilitate ventilator weaning: a series of 10 consecutive patients. *Chest* 2002; **122**: 192–6.
55. Martin D, Davenport PW, Gonzalez-Rothi J *et al.* Inspiratory muscle strength training improves outcome in failure to wean patients. *Eur Respir J* 2006; **28**: 369s.
56. Pavlovic D, Wendt M. Diaphragm pacing during prolonged mechanical ventilation of the lungs could prevent from respiratory muscle fatigue. *Med Hypotheses* 2003; **60**: 398–403.
57. DiMarco AF, Onders RP, Ignagni A *et al.* Inspiratory muscle pacing in spinal cord injury: case report and clinical commentary. *J Spinal Cord Med* 2006; **29**: 95–108.

# SECTION O

# Outcome measures

# 63

# Health status and quality of life

WOLFRAM WINDISCH

## ABSTRACT

Health status and health-related quality of life (HRQoL) evaluation is becoming increasingly important in healthcare practice and research, particularly for patients with chronic, incurable disorders, such as those with chronic respiratory failure (CRF) requiring home mechanical ventilation (HMV). The term HRQoL summarizes different components of health including physical state, psychological wellbeing, social relations and functional capacities. HRQoL assessment in HMV patients has been performed in clinical trials using either generic instruments, which are not specific to any particular disease or condition, or disease/condition-specific instruments, with the latter instruments known to be most capable of reliably assessing changes in HRQoL following treatment intervention. In particular, the Maugeri Foundation Respiratory Failure item set (MRF-28) and the Severe Respiratory Insufficiency (SRI) questionnaire have been specifically designed to measure HRQoL in patients with CRF. Accordingly, the MRF-28 was initially validated in a group of patients with chronic obstructive pulmonary disease (COPD) and kyphoscoliosis receiving long-term oxygen therapy or HMV, while the SRI was primarily validated for a broad spectrum of conditions producing CRF, including COPD, different restrictive thoracic disorders, neuromuscular diseases, and obesity hypoventilation syndrome, with all patients being dependent on long-term non-invasive ventilation used as HMV. However, subsequent validation of the SRI has also specifically targeted COPD. The application of these instruments has revealed substantial improvements in HRQoL following HMV commencement in CRF patients. Thereby, overall HRQoL is reportedly improved in all different diagnostic groups of CRF patients. However, results from the subscales of the questionnaires have demonstrated that improvements in the specific sub-domains of HRQoL depend on the underlying disease. Importantly, COPD patients have also been shown to substantially benefit from HMV when using the new specific instruments, which contrasts with some previous findings, where instruments specifically designed to measure HRQoL in CRF were not available.

## INTRODUCTION

During the last century, enormous progress was made in improving health standards, bringing with it an increase in life expectancy. Between 1900 and 2000 the average life expectancy at birth in the USA increased by nearly 30 years.[1] While the largest gains were made in the first two-thirds of the century, life expectancy still increased significantly by 6 years between 1970 and 2000. However, many of the patients who benefit from modern medicine in terms of increased life expectancy also have chronic, incurable disease; thus, survival is increased in these patients without amelioration of the underlying condition. In this scenario, information about the health status of each patient is needed to better understand the impact of chronic disease on subjective disease perception. For this reason, health-related quality of life (HRQoL) evaluation is becoming increasingly important in healthcare practice and research. HRQoL provides an important means of evaluating the human and financial costs and benefits of modern medical treatment modalities, which is particularly pertinent to patients with chronic and incurable disorders.[2–4] The definition of HRQoL is based on different components of subjectively reported health including physical state, psychological wellbeing, social relations and functional capacities that are influenced by a person's experience, beliefs, expectations and perceptions.[2–4]

There is particular interest to learn more about the limitations of HRQoL in the most severely ill and obviously most severely disabled patients such as those with chronic respiratory failure (CRF). Moreover, it is essential to know if treatment strategies such as home mechanical ventilation (HMV), delivered either non-invasively by a face mask or invasively by the use of a tracheostomy, are capable of enhancing HRQoL. Patients with CRF usually have severe dyspnoea, a medical history of several years or even decades, and end-stage disease with severe limitations of daily living. In addition, HMV is a time-consuming and cost-intensive therapy and can produce significant side effects. Therefore, it needs to be addressed whether prolongation of life achieved by long-term HMV is associated with a subjectively acceptable health status and HRQoL. Importantly, if HMV does increase the burden without producing an acceptable HRQoL this would raise ethical concerns. On the other hand, prolongation of life is not necessarily the primary goal of HMV, since improvements in HRQoL after the commencement of HMV could still occur without actually improving survival.

## METHODOLOGY FOR ASSESSMENT OF HEALTH-RELATED QUALITY OF LIFE

Questionnaires are the most frequently used tool for HRQoL assessment. There are, however, important psychometric properties which need to be established before these instruments can serve as tools for HRQoL assessment in clinical trials.[2] First and foremost, the questionnaire must be objective, i.e. independent from the investigator. This refers to data assessment, data calculation and interpretation of the findings. Next, reliability needs to be established. This term describes the random error for data assessment, where the questionnaire must yield scale scores that are consistent or remain similar under constant conditions. Most importantly, validity needs to be established. In this regard, the question should be addressed as to whether a questionnaire postulating to measure HRQoL actually *does* measure HRQoL. For this reason it must be guaranteed that the targets and measurements of the questionnaire are in accordance with its claims. In addition, changes in HRQoL, such as those observed following treatment intervention, should be sufficiently assessed (responsiveness), and finally, changes in HRQoL should be assessed as sensitively and accurately as possible (sensitivity).

Basically, there are two different types of questionnaire.[2] Generic questionnaires, which are unspecific to any particular disease, can be broadly applied to different diseases in a feasible manner. Another advantage is that these questionnaires are often standardized if reference values for a normal population are available. However, the non-specific nature of such a generic instrument can lead to failing – or at least insufficient – responsiveness and sensitivity, particularly in the evaluation of specific treatment strategies. In contrast, disease – or condition – specific questionnaires are postulated to be most sensitive to HRQoL changes, for example following treatment interventions. However, as a consequence, only limited application according to the specific disease or condition is reasonable.

## HEALTH-RELATED QUALITY OF LIFE QUESTIONNAIRES USED FOR PATIENTS ON HOME MECHANICAL VENTILATION

Several well-validated questionnaires have been repeatedly used for the assessment of HRQoL in patients receiving HMV (Table 63.1).

### Medical Outcome Survey 36-Item Short-Form Health Status Survey

The most commonly used instrument is the Medical Outcome Survey 36-Item Short-Form Health Status Survey (SF-36), a well-validated and widely used multipurpose survey of general health status, in which the results from both the healthy reference population and different disease groups are available.[9–11] In addition, the SF-36 has been shown to be eligible for HRQoL assessment in intensive

**Table 63.1** Instruments used for health-related quality of life assessment in patients receiving home mechanical ventilation

| Instrument | | First author | Scales (n) | Items (n) | Target |
|---|---|---|---|---|---|
| Sickness Impact Profile[5,6] | SIP | Bergner | 12 | 136 | Generic |
| Nottingham Health Profile[7] | NHP | Hunt | 6 | 38 | Generic |
| Hospital Anxiety and Depression Scale[8] | HAD | Zigmond | 2 | 14 | Generic |
| MOS 36-Item Short-Form Health Survey[9–11] | SF-36 | Ware | 8 | 36 | Generic |
| Chronic Respiratory Disease Questionnaire[12] | CRQ | Gyatt | 4 | 20 | COPD |
| St George's Respiratory Questionnaire[13] | SGRQ | Jones | 3 | 76 | COPD |
| Maugeri Foundation Respiratory Failure item set[14] | MRF-28 | Carone | 3 | 28 | CRF |
| Severe Respiratory Insufficiency Questionnaire[15,16] | SRI | Windisch | 7 | 49 | HMV |

COPD, chronic obstructive pulmonary disease; CRF, chronic respiratory failure; HMV, home mechanical ventilation.

care unit populations.[17–21] It consists of eight subscales measuring different aspects of health status. Each subscale produces a standardized score between 0 and 100, with lower scores indicating poorer health or higher disability. The scales can be aggregated into two summary measures (PCS = Physical Component Summary, MCS = Mental Component Summary). Recently, benchmark values were assessed specifically for patients receiving HMV, thus allowing comparisons to other disease categories.[22] In addition, patients with different underlying conditions causing CRF have been included in this study, whereby the SF-36 has been shown capable of discriminating between different underlying conditions of CRF.[22] Although the SF-36 has also been shown to assess changes in HRQoL following treatment interventions in patients with CRF, i.e. the institution of HMV, the generic nature of the SF-36 might not provide a complete picture of HRQoL impairments in CRF patients receiving HMV.

## Chronic obstructive pulmonary disease-specific questionnaires

There are two well-validated questionnaires that specifically focus on HRQoL impairments in patients with chronic obstructive pulmonary disease (COPD), namely the Chronic Respiratory Disease Questionnaire (CRQ)[12] and the St George's Respiratory Questionnaire (SGRQ).[13] Both questionnaires have been successfully used in COPD patients with different levels of disease severity, and have become standard in HRQoL assessment of COPD patients. The CRQ and the SGRQ have also been used in the most severe COPD and CRF patients who require HMV.[23–26] However, it has been argued that both questionnaires were developed based on patients who, on average, had a more moderate form of the disease, when to be useful they should have been based on those with the most severe level of COPD.[14] In addition, it was pointed out that the most severe COPD patients lie at the extremes of the usable scoring range of these questionnaires, which means that in long-term follow-up studies the questionnaires may not be able to detect deterioration over time in these patients.[14] Moreover, although the CRQ and SGRQ have only been validated for COPD patients, these questionnaires have also been used in patients with CRF secondary to diseases other than COPD.[27] However, specific determinants of HRQoL in patients who require HMV because of CRF caused by restrictive thoracic deformities or neuromuscular diseases are not primarily targeted by the CRQ and the SGRQ. Therefore, despite the specific nature of the CRQ and the SGRQ their suitability for patients with CRF is limited. This clearly calls for new instruments which specifically target the sphere of CRF patients who need HMV. Accordingly, two specific questionnaires have recently been developed for assessing HRQoL in patients with CRF, the Maugeri Foundation Respiratory Failure item set (MRF-28) and the Severe Respiratory Insufficiency (SRI) Questionnaire (Table 63.1).

## The Maugeri Foundation Respiratory Failure item set

The MRF-28 is the first questionnaire developed for patients with CRF. It covers 28 items, some of which were drawn from previously developed and validated questionnaires including the Sickness Impact Profile (SIP)[5,6] and the SGRQ.[13] Three different subscales could be identified following validation: Daily Activity, Cognitive Function and Invalidity. Two of the subscales (Cognitive Function and Invalidity) had not been identified by previously developed questionnaires. This clearly indicates the significance of condition-specific questionnaires when assessing HRQoL in patients with CRF. In addition, in the initial validation study on patients with CRF only 39 per cent of the possible scaling range was covered by the generic questionnaire (SIP). While the COPD-specific instrument (SGRQ) already produced a broader range of 76 per cent, nearly the entire scaling range was covered by the MRF-28 alone.[14] This indicates the greater potential of discriminating between different levels of subjectively impaired health in patients with CRF when using the condition-specific questionnaire. Moreover, improvements in HRQoL following initiation of HMV were not evident in COPD patients when the SGRQ was used, but were evident when the MRF-28 was used, again reflecting the superiority of condition-specific questionnaires when condition-related treatment interventions are being evaluated.[26] However, the MRF-28 has only been developed and validated for patients with COPD and kyphoscoliosis, but its suitability in patients with different restrictive thoracic disorders (RTD), obesity hypoventilation syndrome (OHS) or neuromuscular diseases (NMD) still needs to be established. In addition, CRF in patients from the initial validation study was treated either by long-term oxygen therapy (LTOT) alone, invasive (tracheostomy) or non-invasive HMV (nasal mask).[14] Therefore, the MRF-28 is somewhat non-specific in regard to the treatment modality of CRF.

During the validation process, items were initially generated in English, translated into Italian and then back translated into English to ensure that the original meaning of the items had been conveyed correctly in Italian.[14] A French translation of the MRF-28 has also recently been published.[28]

## Severe Respiratory Insufficiency questionnaire[15,16]

In contrast to the MRF-28, the second questionnaire, the SRI, has been specifically developed for a broad spectrum of patients with CRF (including those with COPD, RTD, obesity hyperventilation syndrome [OHS] and neuromuscular disorders [NMDs]) who exclusively receive non-invasive HMV.[15] Therefore, this questionnaire is with RTD and long-term HMV (mean 50 months). Overall, HRQoL was acceptable, given the severe objective limitations, and HRQoL was no worse than that of patients with other chronic disorders such as chronic back pain or rheumatoid arthritis. However, only selected patients with long-term compliance and mild disease progression (mean daily duration of 7.7 hours per day after on average 50 months of HMV) were included in the study, while patients with COPD and rapidly progressive neuromuscular diseases such as ALS were excluded. In a similar, seminal study Simonds and co-workers investigated 136 patients with various disorders including COPD.[39] In this study the SF-36 was filled in by 105 out of 116 patients, confirming the hypothesis that HRQoL was impaired compared to the normal population, and also showing that HRQoL was no worse than that of patients with other chronic medical conditions, such as diabetes, hypertension, recent myocardial infarction or cardiac failure. There were, however, some differences amongst the different underlying disorders, with COPD reportedly having the most HRQoL impairments compared with patients with restrictive disorders.

The largest multicentric cross-sectional trial to date included 226 patients with HMV.[22] Patients with COPD ($n$ = 78) and kyphoscoliosis ($n$ = 57) formed the largest homogeneous subgroups that allowed comparative statistical analysis. The remaining patients had post-tuberculosis sequelae, OHS and both rapid- and slowly-progressive neuromuscular disorders. The analysis of the SF-36 revealed that the overall HRQoL was worse compared to a normal reference population, especially for the physical health parameter, but less so for mental health. In addition, when compared with a historical cohort of chronic lung diseases without CRF, physical health was still significantly impaired, whereas mental health was no worse in HMV patients compared to patients with less severe chronic lung disease. Comparison of COPD and kyphoscoliosis patients revealed no difference in physical health; however, mental health was more impaired in COPD, while kyphoscoliosis patients had no mental impairments at all compared to the normal reference population, according to the results of the SF-36. Patients with Duchenne muscular dystrophy appeared to have even better mental health compared with the normal reference population, although the number of cases was too low to allow further statistical analysis. Another study also indicated that more severe limitations were only evident in Physical Functioning compared to other diseases, while other domains of HRQoL related to mental health (SF-36) did not significantly differ even from age-matched male controls.[40] Therefore, robust data are now available to support the notion that even severe physical handicaps do not necessarily lead to mental limitation, at least in restrictive patients with CRF, once HMV has been successfully instituted. Finally, neither lung function parameters nor blood gases were reported predictors for HRQoL.[22]

Specific instruments have also been used in cross-sectional trials. In a large Spanish trial, the SRI was employed to describe predictors of HRQoL in a cohort of 115 patients who used HMV to treat CRF due to various underlying disorders including RTD, OHS, NMD and COPD.[41] In this study the main predictors of HRQoL domains were dyspnoea, the number of hospitalizations, and the number of emergency room admissions in the preceding year. An obstructive pattern revealed by pulmonary function testing also predicted impairments in HRQoL. In another large study that used the SRI, domains of HRQoL in 231 CRF patients were reportedly predictive for long-term survival, in addition to established risk factors such as low body mass index, impairments in pulmonary function testing and elevated numbers of leukocytes.[42] This was particularly true for non COPD-patients (RTD, OHS, NMD), but not COPD patients. In contrast, according to another trial HRQoL was strongly and independently related to respiratory muscle function in patients with ALS.[43,44] These findings emphasize the impact of the underlying disease on HRQoL.

## Longitudinal trials

Early trials prospectively studied HRQoL in small groups of COPD patients.[23–25,45] Thereby, the impact of HMV on HRQoL changes has been addressed. The methodology of HRQoL assessment varied considerably among these studies. In two studies using the CRQ[23] and the SF-36,[45] respectively, HRQoL did not improve following HMV commencement, but when using the SGRQ HRQoL was shown to improve following HMV.[24,25] However, none of these COPD studies used condition-specific questionnaires that specifically targeted the sphere of patients with CRF, as these instruments were not available at the time the studies were performed.

In the Italian multicentre study of non-invasive ventilation in COPD patients, the addition of HMV to LTOT, but not LTOT alone, resulted in improvements in HRQL, although survival benefits could not be achieved by the addition of HMV to LTOT.[26] However, improvements in HRQoL were only detected using the condition-specific questionnaire MRF-28, whereas even the COPD-specific instrument, the SGRQ, failed to show any significant benefit. This clearly points out the impact of HRQoL measurement methodology on the results, and underlines the importance of using even the most specific HRQoL measurement tools available when specific treatment interventions are being evaluated. Thus, in CRF patients requiring HMV, the instruments specific to CRF appear superior even to the disease-specific instruments developed in patients with milder forms of their disease, i.e. no presence of CRF (see also above). In the most recent randomized controlled trial non-invasive positive pressure ventilation (NIPPV) produced mild survival benefits in stable hypercapnic COPD patients, but this appeared to be at the cost of worsening HRQoL. However, worsening HRQoL was only detectable by generic instruments, but not by the SGRQ.[46] This again emphasizes that HRQoL results are depending on the instruments being used for assessment.

In a recent randomized controlled trial, the addition of non-invasive ventilation to pulmonary rehabilitation reportedly augmented the benefits of pulmonary rehabilitation in COPD patients, with greater improvements in HRQL.[32] In this study both COPD-specific (CRQ) and condition-specific questionnaires (MRF-28 and SRI) were used. Therefore, this study again demonstrates that when specific instruments for HRQoL assessment are used, non-invasive ventilation is shown to impact positively on HRQoL, even in COPD patients.

HRQoL benefits have also been established in non-COPD patients. Early studies again used unspecific questionnaires, with the SF-36 being the most frequently used. Thereby, HRQoL improvements in both RTD and NMD patients were established.[47,48] However, in patients with more rapid NMD, particularly those with ALS, the evaluation of HRQoL is far more difficult. Early studies lacked consistency as they reported both non-significant[49] and significant[44,50,51] improvements following HMV commencement. For example, application of the SF-36 showed that HMV improved the Vitality domain score by as much as 25 per cent for periods of up to 15 months, despite disease progression.[50] Although the other scores did not improve, a decline in HRQoL was not observed despite disease progression.[50] However, more significant changes in either direction could have been missed as the SF-36 is suggested to be too non-specific for the problems unique to ALS patients. Recently, in the largest study of 92 ALS patients, 22 patients were randomized to HMV and 19 patients were randomized to standard care without HMV, while 51 patients did not meet the criteria for randomization during the surveillance period.[52] In this study patients with no or moderate bulbar involvement had large HMV-associated benefits in survival and HRQoL, as measured by a battery of instruments including the sleep apnoea quality-of-life index (SAQLI),[53] the SF-36 and the CRQ. In particular, the duration that HRQoL was maintained above 75 per cent of baseline was substantially longer in patients treated with HMV, compared to those with best supportive care alone. In contrast, there were no benefits in survival and only sparse HRQoL benefits in patients with severe bulbar impairment.

There have also been several prospective trials in which the SRI served as the primary instrument of HRQoL assessment. In the initial study, HRQoL measured by the SRI significantly improved following HMV commencement, both in COPD and restrictive patients, and these improvements were correlated to the decline of $PaCO_2$ that resulted from HMV.[28] In another trial the SRI Summary Score substantially improved following HMV in patients with OHS.[30] In this randomized cross-over trial these improvements were comparable in patients receiving bi-level pressure ventilation with or without the addition of target volume setting.

The largest prospective study using the SRI included 135 patients with different aetiologies of CRF from nine German HMV centres.[31] In this study both short- and long-term effects of HMV were investigated. Interestingly, the overall HRQoL improved after 1 month of HMV treatment, and these improvements could be maintained over the subsequent year during which HMV was continued, despite disease deterioration. Importantly, overall HRQoL as measured by the SRI Summary Scale revealed comparable improvements in patients with COPD, RTD and NMD. This is remarkable, since COPD patients are believed to have less HRQoL benefits when HMV is instituted, with previous cross-sectional trials having indicated a worse HRQoL in COPD patients compared to restrictive patients.[15,22,35] In addition, the positive results in COPD patients obviously contrasts with the more pessimistic view derived from previous trials that used less specific tools for HRQoL assessment. In particular, in the most recent Australian randomized controlled trial NIPPV produced worsening of HRQL, but this was only detectable by generic instruments (see also above).[46] Since the methodology of HRQoL assessment is crucial, findings of studies, in which instruments specifically designed for severe respiratory failure have not been used, should be interpreted with caution. In the German multicentre trial,[35] however, a possible selection bias cannot be excluded with certainty, although patients in this trial were consecutively enrolled, as this was an uncontrolled prospective study. Nevertheless, this study clearly demonstrates that HRQoL in COPD patients can substantially improve when HRQoL is most specifically assessed.

Furthermore, it is also conceivable that HRQoL improvement is dependent on the effectiveness of ventilatory support, and, therefore, on the ability of HMV to improve alveolar ventilation as estimated from $PaCO_2$ levels. In the indicated study $PaCO_2$ could be significantly reduced, and this could also explain improvements in HRQL. This could also explain why HRQoL was not improved in the Australian study.[46] However, the impact of ventilatory strategies needs further investigation.

Finally, subscale scores identified clear differences between patients with differing underlying aetiologies of CRF, indicating that HRQoL benefits in particular domains of HRQoL are disease related. For example, improvements in the subscale Respiratory Complaints were evident in all groups of patients, but this led to improvements in the subscale Physical Functioning only in patients with COPD, RTD and OHS, but not in those with NMD; this is conceivable as the latter group of patients is also substantially impaired by the weakness of the limbs. On the contrary, patients with NMD as well as those with OHS had the most remarkable improvements in the subscale Attendant Symptoms and Sleep, although patients with COPD and RTD also improved. In addition, improvements in the subscale Anxiety were most evident in OHS patients, although all other groups of patients significantly improved as well.

## FUTURE RESEARCH

There is now a rich body of data to suggest that HMV positively impacts on HRQoL in CRF patients. The application of new HRQoL measurement tools specifically addressing the sphere of patients with CRF has recently shown that the HRQoL benefit gained from HMV is even greater than that estimated by more non-specific or generic instruments. These highly specific instruments, namely the MRF-28 and the SRI, are also postulated to be capable of discriminating between different treatment strategies. As an example, high-intensity NIPPV aimed at maximally reducing $PaCO_2$ by using controlled modes of ventilation and inspiratory pressures around 30 cm $H_2O$ has recently been introduced, with favourable results in COPD patients.[54–56] This type of treatment forgoes the more conventional approach of using assisted forms of ventilation and, on average, half the amount of inspiratory pressures.[54–56] More positive physiological results gained by high-intensity NIPPV – particularly regarding the control of nocturnal hypoventilation, improved breathing pattern and lung function – must be balanced against the potential for more frequent side effects related to the increased airflow and mask pressures. A very recent short-term randomized cross-over trial has clearly demonstrated the superiority of high-intensity over the more conventional low-intensity NIPPV, with particular reference to the capability of controlling nocturnal hypoventilation.[57] In this study, there is also a clear trend of more-improved HRQoL as assessed by the SRI in patients who received high-intensity NIPPV; it is important to note, however, that the study was not powered to address this outcome measure. Further studies with higher numbers of patients and long-term follow-up periods are required to verify whether the application technique of HMV impacts on HRQoL, and not just in COPD patients. Ultimately, these therapeutic refinements should always be guided towards improving patient comfort and HRQoL. Finally, the international availability of specific instruments and multilingual questionnaires is highly desirable.

## REFERENCES


1. Lefant C. Clinical research to clinical practice – lost in translation? *N Engl J Med* 2003; **349**: 868–74.
2. Testa MA, Simonson DC. Assessment of quality-of-life outcomes. *N Engl J Med* 1996; **334**: 835–40.
3. Wood-Dauphinee S. Assessing quality of life in clinical research: from where have we come and where are we going? *J Clin Epidemiol* 1999; **52**: 355–63.
4. Higginson IJ, Carr AJ. Measuring quality of life: using quality of life measures in the clinical setting. *BMJ* 2001; **322**: 1297–300.
5. Bergner M, Bobbitt RA, Pollard WE *et al.* The sickness impact profile: validation of a health status measure. *Med Care* 1976; **14**: 57–67.
6. Bergner M, Bobbitt RA, Carter WB *et al.* The sickness impact profile: development and final revision of a health status measure. *Med Care* 1981; **19**: 787–805.
7. Hunt SM, McKenna SP, McEwen J *et al.* The Nottingham Health Profile: subjective health status and medical consultations. *Soc Sci Med A* 1981; **15**: 221–9.
8. Zigmond AS, Snaith RP. The hospital anxiety and depression scale. *Acta Psychiatr Scand* 1983; **67**: 361–70.
9. Ware JE Jr, Sherbourne CD. The MOS 36-item short-form health survey (SF-36). I. Conceptual framework and item selection. *Med Care* 1992; **30**: 473–83.
10. Ware JE Jr, Kosinski M, Bayliss MS *et al.* Comparison of methods for the scoring and statistical analysis of SF-36 health profile and summary measures: summary of results from the medical outcomes study. *Med Care* 1995; **33** Suppl 4: AS264–79.
11. Ware JE Jr. The SF-36 health survey. In: Spilker B (Hrsg), ed. *Quality of life and pharmacoeconomics in clinical trials.* Philadelphia, PA, 1996:337–45.
12. Guyatt GH, Berman LB, Townsend M *et al.* A measure of quality of life for clinical trials in chronic lung disease. *Thorax* 1987; **42**: 773–8.
13. Jones PW, Quirk FH, Baveystock CM. The St George's respiratory questionnaire. *Respir Med* 1991; **85** Suppl B: 25–31.
14. Carone M, Bertolotti G, Anchisi F *et al.* Analysis of factors that characterize health impairment in patients with chronic respiratory failure. Quality of life in chronic respiratory failure group. *Eur Respir J* 1999; **13**: 1293–300.
15. Windisch W, Freidel K, Schucher B *et al.* The Severe Respiratory Insufficiency (SRI) Questionnaire: a specific measure of health-related quality of life in patients receiving home mechanical ventilation. *J Clin Epidemiol* 2003; **56**: 752–9.
16. Windisch W, Budweiser S, Heinemann F *et al.* The Severe Respiratory Insufficiency (SRI) Questionnaire was valid for patients with COPD. *J Clin Epidemiol* 2008; **61**: 848–53.
17. Chrispin PS, Scotton H, Rogers J *et al.* Short Form 36 in the intensive care unit: assessment of acceptability, reliability and validity of the questionnaire. *Anaesthesia* 1997; **52**: 15–23.
18. Ridley SA, Chrispin PS, Scotton H *et al.* Changes in quality of life after intensive care: comparison with normal data. *Anaesthesia* 1997; **52**: 195–202.
19. Welsh CH, Thompson K, Long-Krug S. Evaluation of patient-perceived health status using the Medical Outcomes Survey Short-Form 36 in an intensive care unit population. *Crit Care Med* 1999; **27**: 1466–71.
20. Eddleston JM, White P, Guthrie E. Survival, morbidity, and quality of life after discharge from intensive care. *Crit Care Med* 2000; **28**: 2293–9.
21. Flaatten H, Kvale R. Survival and quality of life 12 years after ICU. A comparison with the general Norwegian population. *Intensive Care Med* 2001; **27**: 1005–11.
22. Windisch W, Freidel K, Schucher B *et al.* Evaluation of health-related quality of life using the MOS 36-Item

Short-Form Health Status Survey in patients receiving noninvasive positive pressure ventilation. *Intensive Care Med* 2003; **29**: 615–21.

23. Elliott MW, Simonds AK, Carroll MP *et al.* Domiciliary nocturnal nasal intermittent positive pressure ventilation in hypercapnic respiratory failure due to chronic obstructive lung disease: effects on sleep and quality of life. *Thorax* 1992; **47**: 342–8.
24. Meecham Jones DJ, Paul EA, Jones PW *et al.* Nasal pressure support ventilation plus oxygen compared with oxygen therapy alone in hypercapnic COPD. *Am J Respir Crit Care Med* 1995; **152**: 538–44.
25. Perrin C, El Far Y, Vandenbos F *et al.* Domiciliary nasal intermittent positive pressure ventilation in severe COPD: effects on lung function and quality of life. *Eur Respir J* 1997; **10**: 2835–9.
26. Clini E, Sturani C, Rossi A *et al.* The Italian multicentre study on noninvasive ventilation in chronic obstructive pulmonary disease patients. *Eur Respir J* 2002; **20**: 529–38.
27. Euteneuer S, Windisch W, Suchi S *et al.* Health-related quality of life in patients with chronic respiratory failure after long-term mechanical ventilation. *Respir Med* 2006; **100**: 477–86.
28. Janssens JP, Héritier-Praz A, Carone M *et al.* Validity and reliability of a French version of the MRF-28 health-related quality of life questionnaire. *Respiration* 2004; **71**: 567–74.
29. Windisch W, Dreher M, Storre JH *et al.* Nocturnal non-invasive positive pressure ventilation: physiological effects on spontaneous breathing. *Respir Physiol Neurobiol* 2006; **150**: 251–60.
30. Storre JH, Seuthe B, Fiechter R *et al.* Average volume assured pressure support in obesity hypoventilation: a randomized cross-over trial. *Chest* 2006; **130**: 815–21.
31. Windisch W. Impact of home mechanical ventilation on health-related quality of life. *Eur Respir J* 2008; **32**: 1328–36.
32. Duiverman ML, Wempe JB, Bladder G *et al.* Nocturnal non-invasive ventilation in addition to rehabilitation in hypercapnic patients with COPD. *Thorax* 2008; **63**: 1052–7.
33. Lopez-Campos JL, Failde I, Jimenez AL *et al.* Health-related quality of life of patients receiving home mechanical ventilation: the Spanish version of the severe respiratory insufficiency questionnaire. *Arch Bronconeumol* 2006; **42**: 588–93.
34. López-Campos JL, Failde I, Masa JF *et al.* Transculturally adapted Spanish SRI questionnaire for home mechanically ventilated patients was viable, valid, and reliable. *J Clin Epidemiol* 2008; **61**: 1061–6.
35. Duiverman ML, Wempe JB, Bladder G *et al.* Health-related quality of life in COPD patients with chronic respiratory failure. *Eur Respir J* 2008; **32**: 379–86.
36. Mehta S, Hill NS. Noninvasive ventilation. *Am J Respir Crit Care Med* 2001; **163**: 540–77.
37. Windisch W, Storre JH, Sorichter S *et al.* Comparison of volume- and pressure-limited NPPV at night: a prospective randomized cross-over trial. *Respir Med* 2005; **99**: 52–9.
38. Pehrsson K, Olofson J, Larsson S *et al.* Quality of life of patients treated by home mechanical ventilation due to restrictive ventilatory disorders. *Respir Med* 1994; **88**: 21–6.
39. Simonds AK, Elliott MW. Outcome of domiciliary nasal intermittent positive pressure ventilation in restrictive and obstructive disorders. *Thorax* 1995; **50**: 604–9.
40. Simonds AK, Muntoni F, Heather S *et al.* Impact of nasal ventilation on survival in hypercapnic Duchenne muscular dystrophy. *Thorax* 1998; **53**: 949–52.
41. López-Campos JL, Failde I, Masa JF *et al.* Factors related to quality of life in patients receiving home mechanical ventilation. *Respir Med* 2008; **102**: 605–12.
42. Budweiser S, Hitzl AP, Jörres RA *et al.* Health-related quality of life and long-term prognosis in chronic hypercapnic respiratory failure: a prospective survival analysis. *Respir Res* 2007; **17**(8): 92.
43. Bourke SC, Shaw PJ, Gibson GJ. Respiratory function vs sleep-disordered breathing as predictors of QOL in ALS. *Neurology* 2001; **57**: 2040–4.
44. Mustfa N, Walsh E, Bryant V *et al.* The effect of noninvasive ventilation on ALS patients and their caregivers. *Neurology* 2006; **66**: 1211–17.
45. Sivasothy P, Smith IE, Shneerson JM. Mask intermittent positive pressure ventilation in chronic hypercapnic respiratory failure due to chronic obstructive pulmonary disease. *Eur Respir J* 1998; **11**: 34–40.
46. McEvoy RD, Pierce RJ, Hillman D *et al.* Australian trial of non-invasive ventilation in chronic airflow limitation (AVCAL) study group. Nocturnal non-invasive nasal ventilation in stable hypercapnic COPD: a randomised controlled trial. *Thorax* 2009; **64**: 561–6.
47. Nauffal D, Doménech R, Martínez García MA *et al.* Noninvasive positive pressure home ventilation in restrictive disorders: outcome and impact on health-related quality of life. *Respir Med* 2002; **96**: 777–83.
48. Doménech-Clar R, Nauffal-Manzur D, Perpiñá-Tordera M *et al.* Home mechanical ventilation for restrictive thoracic diseases: effects on patient quality-of-life and hospitalizations. *Respir Med* 2003; **97**: 1320–7.
49. Pinto AC, Evangelista T, Carvalho M *et al.* Respiratory assistance with a non-invasive ventilator (Bipap) in MND/ALS patients: survival rates in a controlled trial. *J Neurol Sci* 1995; **129** Suppl: 19–26.
50. Lyall RA, Donaldson N, Fleming T *et al.* A prospective study of quality of life in ALS patients treated with noninvasive ventilation. *Neurology* 2001; **57**: 153–6.
51. Bourke SC, Bullock RE, Williams RE *et al.* Non-invasive ventilation in ALS: indications and effect on quality of life. *Neurology* 2003; **61**: 171–7.
52. Bourke SC, Tomlinson M, Williams TL *et al.* Effects of non-invasive ventilation on survival and quality of life in patients with amyotrophic lateral sclerosis: a randomised controlled trial. *Lancet Neurol* 2006; **5**: 140–7.

53. Flemons WW, Reimer MA. Development of a disease-specific health related quality of life questionnaire for sleep apnoea. *Am J Respir Crit Care Med* 1998; **158**: 494–503.
54. Windisch W, Vogel M, Sorichter S *et al.* JC Normocapnia during nIPPV in chronic hypercapnic COPD reduces subsequent spontaneous $PaCO_2$. *Respir Med* 2002; **96**: 572–9.
55. Windisch W, Kostié S, Dreher M *et al.* Outcome of patients with stable COPD receiving controlled NPPV aimed at maximal reduction of $PaCO_2$. *Chest* 2005; **128**: 657–63.
56. Windisch W, Haenel M, Storre JH *et al.* High-intensity non-invasive positive pressure ventilation for stable hypercapnic COPD. *Int J Med Sci* 2009; **6**: 72–6.
57. Dreher M, Storre JH, C. Schmoor *et al.* High-intensity versus low-intensity non-invasive ventilation in stable hypercapnic COPD patients: a randomized cross-over trial. *Thorax* 2010; **65**: 303–8.

# SECTION P

# The patient experience of non-invasive ventilation

# 64

# Psychological issues for the mechanically ventilated patient

LINDA L BIENIEK, DANIEL F DILLING, BERND SCHÖNHOFER

## ABSTRACT

Patients who require mechanical ventilation, whether non-invasive ventilation (NIV) or via tracheostomy, frequently develop psychological complications. In this chapter, we learn from the experiences and insights of an individual who has used various forms of mechanical ventilation for more than 25 years. We identify causes of ventilator users' distress, which results in depressive, anxiety-related, and somatic symptoms, and provide readers with strategies for supporting patients' psychological health. Emphasis is placed on proactive assessment with a stress on patient empowerment and autonomy. Appendices C and D in the Vitalsource ebook edition contain guidelines to copy and give to patients.

## INTRODUCTION

This chapter describes many of the psychological and emotional burdens that NIV users experience. It illustrates how to improve ventilator users' lives by acting on an understanding of psychological health and its value to wellbeing.

Co-author Linda Bieniek has a wealth of experience using both non-invasive (NIV) and invasive mechanical ventilation, and her psychological insights have enhanced the value of this chapter. She is a 58-year-old woman who contracted polio after childhood polio vaccination. She survived the disease, but it weakened her respiratory muscles. Severe kyphoscoliosis and post-polio syndrome compounded her respiratory problems resulting in initiation of NIV later in life. For more than 20 years, she successfully used various forms of NIV and appreciates its attendant complications and frustrations. Unfortunately, emergency surgery prompted the need for invasive mechanical ventilation; and in recovering from that operation she was unable to wean from the ventilator, prompting placement of a tracheostomy. She remains on volume ventilation at night and during parts of each day. Her professional background includes more than 20 years of psychological training often with leading experts. During her 20-year career in a major corporation, she managed its employee assistance programme, assessing and referring individuals with psychological issues to appropriate resources. Since retiring, she has written and lectured at international conferences on psychological issues.

In addition to Ms Bieniek's first-hand experiences, we include findings and examples from the literature, and insights of Joan Headley, Executive Director of International Ventilator Users Network.

The more aware providers are of the psychological challenges that ventilator users face, the more they can employ the strategies identified in this chapter. Professionals will learn how to screen patients to identify symptoms and patterns that can adversely affect ventilator users' psychological, and potentially, physical health. When patients' symptoms indicate the need for professional assistance, providers should urge patients to pursue psychotherapy or other available behavioural health resources.

## EMPOWER PATIENTS

The more patients depend on a ventilator to breathe, the greater the psychological challenges they may face. Loss of autonomy is among the most serious. It is extremely important that providers grasp the potential impact of this loss on patients' lives. With this understanding, providers can empower ventilator users in a number of ways. The key to empowerment is: whenever choices exist, give the individuals information and control over decisions affecting their lives.

Empowerment requires presenting patients with clear information about treatment options, with attendant benefits and risks. Taking time to answer patients' questions and communicating honestly, directly, calmly and compassionately further equips patients to make informed decisions.

> What appears especially important to individuals is that providers show they believe their lives are worthwhile. (Headley JL 2009, interview, June)

Acknowledging the complexities that patients face, encouraging them to be resourceful in assessing options, and then honouring their choices, demonstrates respect for ventilator users' capabilities and rights.

## RECOGNIZE AND EDUCATE PATIENTS ABOUT THE IMPORTANCE OF PSYCHOLOGICAL HEALTH

Psychological health encompasses how one thinks, expresses thoughts and feelings, makes decisions, and chooses to act. A psychologically healthy person is rational and open-minded, solves problems proactively, seeks to gain positive results, and expresses feelings constructively. Spirituality – including both spiritual values and religious beliefs – is extremely important to the psychological health of many individuals.[1] Spirituality can provide a sense of meaning and purpose to life and support individuals in adapting to health changes. Any or all of these factors may influence an individual's choices and responses to pain, suffering, loss and distress.

Ventilator users' responses to distress can affect emotional state, physical symptoms, and quality of life. Providers empower patients first by educating them about the interrelationship of their minds, emotions, behaviours, spirituality and bodies, and then about factors affecting psychological health, as described above. This education includes helping patients understand the value of reducing distress and also of fulfilling emotional needs for support and assistance.

Several studies illustrate potential benefits of good psychological health. One demonstrated that individuals' beliefs, emotions, relationships and problem-solving skills can affect their physical health.[2] It concluded that individuals who use effective approaches to manage anxiety and depressive symptoms can reduce the frequency and intensity of somatic symptoms.[2] This is important for ventilator users to understand, as anxiety can increase shortness of breath, depression can exacerbate fatigue and distress may weaken physical resilience, increasing susceptibility to respiratory illness.

> For much of my life, I resented my body's limitations. In my 30s, work distress and relationship problems prompted me to seek psychotherapy. In the process, I discovered that significant past experiences were affecting my psychological and physical health. When my health forced me to leave my career, I entered a programme for depression. I learned how unresolved traumas triggered anxiety, depression, irritable bowel attacks and other somatic reactions. Most importantly, I learned how to transform negative beliefs and feelings and face myself with compassion. These skills continue to support me in adapting to the progression of post-polio syndrome and my respiratory condition. (Bieniek LL, personal quote, 2009)

A study of patients with motor neurone disease (MND) indicated that individuals who were proactive in confronting problems experienced lower levels of anxiety and depression while adjusting to physical and lifestyle changes.[1] This research revealed that levels of depression and loss of autonomy were determining factors affecting survival times of individuals with MND even when age, disease severity, and time since diagnosis were controlled for.[1]

Generally, psychologically healthy people are better equipped to cultivate supportive relationships. Their connections can increase their emotional resilience, providing a buffer against psychological pain and reducing the risks of depression.[2]

## RESPOND TO THE PSYCHOLOGICAL CHALLENGES VENTILATOR USERS FACE

Ventilator users contend with diverse psychological challenges from their medical conditions, external factors, and unrelated life issues. External impediments and psychological effects of living with a neuromuscular condition appear more distressing to some individuals than their actual physical limitations.[1,3] The following publications contain valuable information about the psychological risks and obstacles they face:

- *What psychotherapists should know about disability*[4]
- University of Toronto's research on *Ventilator users' perspectives on the important elements of health-related quality of life*[3]
- Post-Polio Health International's articles on resolving the effects of traumatic experiences related to childhood medical conditions and disabilities.[5–7]

The following sections describe potential causes of distress that may affect ventilator users' psychological health and wellbeing.

## Difficulties adjusting to non-invasive ventilation

When introducing patients to NIV, communication is paramount. Providers need to explain potential problems, what to do and who to contact. The most effective approach requires collaboration of patient, home health provider and the pulmonologist experimenting with different interfaces and settings until the patient can breathe comfortably on the ventilator.

Difficulties with equipment include, but are not limited to, leaking masks, finding suitable interfaces and synchronizing settings.

> I cried the first few nights I used a ventilator. I recognized that I was entering a new stage of life. My tears also stemmed from my struggle to get in and out of the chest cuirass alone since I have weak hand muscles. Yet, after a few days, I was grateful for being able to breathe better on the ventilator. Once an orthotist made me a custom-fitted polypropylene cuirass, my ventilator became my best friend. (Bieniek LL, personal quote, 2009)

Anxiety or claustrophobia related to a past trauma can resurface when using a face mask or mouthpiece. Individuals with history of trauma involving pressure on the face or in the mouth may develop post-traumatic symptoms while starting NIV. Examples of such traumas include near-drowning, domestic violence, war, assault, a medical experience, and physical or sexual abuse.

Lack of self-acceptance may cause psychological struggles when individuals face the reality of how their medical conditions will impact the rest of their lives.

#### STRATEGIES FOR HEALTHCARE PROFESSIONALS

- Suggest that patients communicate with other ventilator users through disability and disease-related organizations (www.ventusers.org) and listservs (access at www.ventusers.org/net/VentDIR.pdf).
- Encourage patients to pursue resources to manage their anxieties. Refer them to 'Treatment Approach Options' at www.post-polio.org/edu/pphnews/pph19-1p9.pdf.
- Urge patients to seek professional assistance for ongoing distress.

## Refusal to use non-invasive ventilation

Patients with conditions such as MND may decline ventilatory support because they cannot bear living with such a debilitating disease.[1] When they develop intense hopelessness about their future, dying may seem more acceptable than feeling like a 'burden' to their families, 'out of control', 'trapped', or dependent on others.[1]

#### STRATEGIES FOR HEALTHCARE PROFESSIONALS

- Acknowledge the complexities of patients' decisions; express compassion. Ask them to examine decisions with a behavioural health professional or spiritual director to ensure that they are grounded in the reality of their circumstances rather than despair from feelings of fear, grief, anger, or shame – often resolvable through psychotherapy.
- Encourage patients to consider spiritual values and religious beliefs in making final decisions.
- Ask patients to talk with another person who navigates life with a ventilator successfully.
- Respect patients' rights to decline mechanical ventilation and life-sustaining therapies. Discuss options for comfortable end-of-life transitions.

## Progression of neuromuscular conditions

As neuromuscular conditions progress, individuals often need to increase the time spent using NIV and mobility devices. Inaccessibility to external places impedes mobility, independence, and travelling[3] – with significant loss of autonomy and development of dependencies. Losing basic abilities such as talking, seeing and eating may result from using a mouthpiece or mask with NIV during the day. Losing the ability to speak is especially traumatizing. Consequently, it is imperative to find a means for the person to communicate needs and feelings, perhaps even through use of a communication assist device.

Adjusting to loss may include loss of employment and income, relationships, living arrangements, professional and occupational identities, and the ability to participate in social, recreational and spiritual activities.

> It took me five years to accept my need to go on full-time disability. I valued my career and feared losing income and the ability to live independently. When I left work, I became depressed. I realized that I had lost part of my identity. (Bieniek LL, personal quote, 2009)

Accepting dependencies is one of the greatest challenges of living with physical limitations. Asking for and accepting help is difficult regardless of whether one has a disability and is especially challenging for people from families that believe in stoic self-reliance (Headley JL, interview, June 2009).

As patients lose the ability to function independently, they may encounter episodes of anxiety, depression and loss of control. Additionally, their dependencies may trigger fears of abandonment, resentment or avoidance by friends and loved ones. Likewise, when individuals think of themselves as 'a burden' or are treated that way, they feel 'trapped' by their illnesses and can become hopeless and develop despair.[1]

> A friend played chess with her neighbour who had MND and used NIV. She witnessed his wife's demeaning remarks to him which would understandably cause him to feel like a 'burden'. (Bieniek LL, personal quote, 2009)

Even the hiring of care attendants can be a source of anxiety, especially when government programmes or individuals themselves cannot afford to pay them very well. This often hinders the hiring of reliable, trustworthy, competent attendants who will not neglect ventilator users' needs, abuse them, or steal from them (Headley JL, interview, June 2009).

Experiencing chronic pain or fatigue can lead to sadness, anger, isolation or hopelessness, resulting in clinical depression. Emotional distress and spiritual emptiness can exacerbate physical pain.[4] Participating in sexual experiences creates anxiety for individuals when it causes dyspnoea. A pioneering study showed that initiation of NIV markedly reduced patients' sexual activity; however, having a spouse or partner contributed to increases in ventilator use during sexual activities.[8] Another study cited positioning, fatigue and weakness as reasons for reducing sexual activities.[9]

#### STRATEGIES FOR HEALTHCARE PROFESSIONALS

- Urge patients to explore resources for strengthening emotional support. Refer them to 'Treatment Approach Options' chart at www.post-polio.org/edu/pphnews/pph19-1p9.pdf.
- Emphasize the inter-relationship of body, mind, emotions, spirituality and behaviours.
- Refer to specialists to help patients understand causes of pain and fatigue, exacerbating factors, and strategies to reduce their impact.[4]
- Offer to discuss sexual activities with patients, including alternatives for expressing intimacy. Refer them to physical or occupational therapists for options on positioning and movement.

## Medical emergencies

Providers should establish that patients understand their options in case of emergency. They should encourage patients to make autonomous decisions, and to inform surrogate decision makers of their wishes should they become incapacitated. Providers should avoid paternalistic attitudes, such as suggesting that chronic ventilator assistance is an undesirable way to live or that such individuals are a burden to society (Headley JL, interview, June 2009). If one becomes incapacitated, the patient's written instructions or designated surrogate should determine whether to employ or decline medical interventions during an emergency.

Ideally, providers should discuss patients' wishes before an emergency occurs and ask that patients document them in writing. Would they want to be tracheostomized to be kept alive? Are they willing and able to live with a tracheostomy? Do they have adequate verbal and written information about this option in order to make an informed decision?

Patients may become emotionally traumatized by a medical crisis. One study reported that 84 per cent of patients with myasthenia gravis were diagnosed with an anxiety disorder and 69 per cent developed a depressive disorder after unexpected respiratory failure and intubation.[10]

> My experience provides an example of the psychological impact of a medical crisis. While out of town without family, I needed emergency surgery. After recovering, I was shocked to learn I was conscious and in ICU, because I had no memory of this. Knowing my high risk for not surviving surgery, I must have been terrified and blocked out these memories. Trauma experts identify this phenomenon as 'dissociation', a coping strategy for managing overwhelming feelings. (Bieniek LL 2009, personal quote, 2009)

Sometimes ventilator users panic if they sense that emergency personnel or providers do not understand their neuromuscular respiratory needs or other pre-existing conditions. It is imperative that providers become informed about a patient's particular conditions and special needs, consulting an expert to determine the most effective treatment options, if needed.

#### STRATEGIES FOR HEALTHCARE PROFESSIONALS

- Ensure that patients have emergency medical information in place to provide health professionals with key information. Ask them to complete the 'Take Charge, Not Chances' forms and carry them (stating their ventilator settings and special needs) when travelling and going to hospital. Access the forms at www.ventusers.org/vume/index.html.
- Ask patients to document emergency wishes and to designate surrogate decision makers.
- Provide patients with a copy of Appendix C: Exploring the Option of a Trach, available in the Vitalsource ebook edition.
- Insert pertinent documents into the medical record.
- Encourage patients to consider personal values, spiritual and religious beliefs, and available support and resources when deciding about emergency interventions and future options.
- Implement stress reduction techniques such as patient education, music therapy, relaxation exercises and supportive touch while patients are in the intensive care unit (ICU) and transitioning to NIV.[11,12]
- Provide patients with psychological assistance to resolve psychological effects of a medical crisis.[11]
- Consult experts for advice on emergency interventions and treatment options. International Ventilator Users Network at +1-314-534-0475 provides referrals.

## Lack of access to services and equipment

A lack of access to ventilator services causes significant distress for individuals who desire life-sustaining treatment and may lead to premature deaths. Patients in developing countries and remote areas often lack access to specialists who are knowledgeable about treating neuromuscular respiratory problems. Vent users report that government programmes and insurance companies limit their choices of equipment, excluding more effective options (Headley JL, interview, June 2009).

#### STRATEGIES FOR HEALTHCARE PROFESSIONALS

- Encourage government programmes and insurance companies to ensure ventilator services are available in areas lacking them.
- Submit professional service information to International Ventilator Users Network for inclusion in the directory, a source of referrals for patients and professionals internationally. Contact info@ventusers.org. Access the directory at www.ventusers.org/net/vdirhm.html.

## Emotional reactions

Until the actor Christopher Reeve used a ventilator in public, society did not understand mechanical ventilation as a part of some people's lives, and ventilator users were often avoided. Fortunately, Reeve reduced the stigma of using a ventilator by demonstrating that a ventilator-assisted person could live an active life (Headley JL, interview, June 2009). However, individuals still experience demeaning attitudes – and in some cultures and families, having a disability is still considered shameful.

Emotional reactions to living with progressive conditions include grief, fear, loneliness, hopelessness and anger. Individuals experiencing such reactions are especially susceptible to depression, substance abuse and self-destructive behaviours.[4] Shame and anxiety manifest as avoidance of public places and social events and descriptions of feeling 'embarrassed' about being seen with a ventilator.[3] These reactions increase isolation and, in turn, worsen anxiety symptoms.

> I tried to hide the fact that I used the machine, I put a tablecloth over it and then eventually I named it to make it more acceptable to my kids.[3]

Loneliness is a significant challenge for ventilator users who lack adequate support or cannot travel or communicate easily. Loneliness can lead to hopelessness, irrational beliefs and feelings of loss of control – precursors to anxiety and depression.[1] Unresolved anger can impair a person's ability to gain support and assistance when anger is suppressed or expressed destructively (directly or passive-aggressively).

#### STRATEGIES FOR HEALTHCARE PROFESSIONALS

- Encourage patients to learn constructive strategies for expressing feelings and for seeking support. Refer them to 'Treatment Approach Options' chart at www.post-polio.org/edu/pphnews/pph19-1p9.pdf.
- Screen for dependency on alcohol and other substances and self-destructive patterns as advised below.

# GENERAL STRATEGIES FOR HEALTH PROFESSIONALS

## Use psychological screening tools

Individuals with disabilities are at high risk for substance abuse, addictions, and for physical and sexual abuse.[4] Screen for self-destructive behaviours and for anxiety, depressive, and somatic symptoms. These can interfere with patients' health and functioning and exacerbate pain and fatigue. Use of substances to numb emotions (e.g. anxiety, grief, anger, loneliness) or physical pain also may increase breathing problems.

Studies report high rates of suicidal ideation in males with MND and patients with multiple sclerosis.[1,13] If concern for self-harm or harm to another person exists, obtain immediate psychiatric assistance for the patient.

Ask open-ended questions to identify needs for psychological assistance:

- 'How is your mood or spirits?'
- 'What is your attitude towards life these days?'
- 'What do you spend most of your time doing?'
- 'How well do you sleep? Are you eating enough or too much?'
- 'What kind of support do you have? Do you feel safe?'
- 'How are you dealing with your health changes and loss of independence and control?'
- 'Do you have adequate assistance? How well do you communicate your needs?'
- 'If spirituality is important to you, how do you nurture your spiritual needs?'
- 'What do you do to relax when you get frustrated or you're stressed out?'
- 'What are any concerns or behaviours that family or friends see as problems?'
- 'How do you manage pain? What do you take?'
- 'What do you do when you get angry, sad or lonely?'
- 'What do you wish you would do differently to take better care of your health?'
- 'Have you thought about wanting to die or to harm to yourself? Do you have a plan? When? How?'

## Recommend proactive strategies

Encourage patients to pursue resources to reduce distress and fulfil their emotional needs. Refer them to 'Treatment

Approach Options' chart at www.post-polio.org/edu/pphnews/pph19-1p9.pdf and give them a copy of Appendix D: Ventilator User Guidelines for Emotional Health, available in the Vitalsource ebook edition. Patients can explore many of these options independently.

Prescribe psychotherapy or behavioural health resources when you identify:

- ongoing or severe symptoms of anxiety, depression or other psychological conditions
- distress that impairs cognitive or physical functioning
- somatic symptoms, frequent illnesses
- abuse or dependency on alcohol, other substances
- addictions or other self-destructive behaviours
- neglect of healthcare needs
- inability to seek adequate personal care assistance.

Refer patients to resources or therapists you know of; also offer them the choice of finding their own therapist. Finally, respect individuals' rights to decline psychological treatment unless they are at risk of harming self or others or of being harmed.

## SUMMARY

This chapter has illustrated how professionals can raise their patient care to another level by acting on an understanding of psychological health to empower patients. Awareness of the psychological challenges that may interfere with patients' wellbeing provides opportunities to employ the strategies identified within this chapter. Providers can make significant differences to patients' lives by discussing treatment options, emphasizing the importance of psychological health, and honouring their choices. These perspectives indicate a need for further discussion and research of these critical issues.

Providers are encouraged to consult Appendices C and D in the Vitalsource ebook edition and to give copies to patients. They are written by a ventilator user with psychological training and expertise for other ventilator users. One effers a wealth of strategies for deciding on the question of tracheostomy and another for pursuing resources, including psychotherapy, to manage anxieties and other psychological challenges related to using mechanical ventilation.

## ACKNOWLEDGEMENTS

We are indebted to Veronica Cook, Laura Dowdle, Joan Headley, Audrey King, Nicole Lighthouse, Brigid Rafferty, Sarah Perz and Julie Truong for their assistance.

See Appendix C: Exploring the option of a trach and Appendix D: Ventilator guidelines for emotional health in the Vitalsource ebook edition.

## REFERENCES

1. McLeod JE, Clarke DM. A review of psychosocial aspects of motor neurone disease. *J Neurol Sci* 2007; **258**: 4–10.
2. Salovey P, Rothman AJ. Emotional states and physical health. *Am Psychol* 2000; **55**: 110–21.
3. Brooks D, Tonack M, King A. *Ventilator users' perspectives on important elements of health-related quality of life.* A Canadian Quality Study. Toronto: University of Toronto, 2002:1–124.
4. Olkin R. *What psychotherapists should know about disability.* New York: Guilford Press, 1999.
5. Bieniek L, Kennedy K. Improving quality of life: healing polio memories. *Polio Network News* Winter 2002; **18**: 1–7.
6. Bieniek L, Kennedy K. A guide for exploring polio memories. *Polio Network News* Summer 2002; **18**: 3–7.
7. Bieniek L, Kennedy K. Pursuing therapeutic resources to improve your health. *Polio Network News* Fall 2002; **18**: 3–8.
8. Schönhofer B, Von Sydow K, Bucher T *et al.* Sexuality in patients with noninvasive mechanical ventilation due to chronic respiratory failure. *Am J Respir Crit Care Med* 2001; **164**: 1612–17.
9. Lott D. IVUN joins those studying sexual activity and chronic illness. *Ventilator-Assisted Living* 2006; **20**: 4–9.
10. Kulaksizoglu IB. Mood and anxiety disorders in patients with myasthenia gravis: aetiology, diagnosis and treatment. *CNS Drugs* 2007; **21**: 473–81.
11. Thomas LA. Clinical management of stressors perceived by patients on mechanical ventilation. *AACN Clin Issues* 2003; **14**: 73–81.
12. Chlan LL. Music therapy as a nursing intervention for patients supported by mechanical ventilation. *AACN Clin Issues* 2000; **11**: 128–38.
13. Ziemssen T. Multiple sclerosis beyond EDSS: depression and fatigue. *J Neurol Sci* 2009; **277** Suppl 1: S37–41.

# 65

# Reflection on our times with a resident 'Nippy' ventilator

MICHAEL AND ALYSON LINDLEY

Michael Lindley was one of the first patients with motor neurone disease (amyotrophic lateral sclerosis) established on home non-invasive ventilation in Leeds. In this chapter, his wife Alyson reflects on that time. Their story also highlights the challenges to family, friends and home.

When I look back at the photographs, and re-visit this period of time in my memories, I see again the great difference domiciliary ventilation can make. It offers an opportunity for a vast improvement in wellbeing, gives longer life, greater freedom and a means of being able to experience things which would not otherwise be possible. Examples are going to the seaside, our daughter Amy's school play or a day out or in with friends.

The ventilator could be transported to wherever he/we wished to go, provided there was a power point to plug it in, and once his work colleague and friend Richard had developed a 'converter', it could be run in any vehicle that had a cigarette lighter (at the time this was most vehicles, but excluded standard or specialist ambulances as we discovered during several of our more stressful experiences!).

During this acquired extra 'time', in our case 2.5 years, the enrichment to quality of life for Michael was immense. Along with the versatile and mobile 'Nippy', he spent days out with 'the lads', a Saturday here and there on a friend's narrowboat, sailing in a tranquil environment on a sunny day along the canals. He was able to enjoy family breaks at the seaside in a caravan or chalet and gatherings at relatives' houses. He continued to enjoy the arts; a visit to the Lawrence Batley Theatre where our daughter Helen was performing, and being part of 'his band', in which he had been singer and guitarist for many years. The band met fortnightly at our house, and while he could not actively engage in the performance he could continue to 'manage' them. He was able to attend the hospice day-care centre on a Thursday, and enjoyed the friendship and activities there. This was where his book *Hey Up God* was conceived and written. The production of the book gave him something to focus on; it was published and has sold many copies. These are just a few of the possibilities which the Nippy gave us.

Our first introduction to this extraordinary device, which looked like a standard tool box with a pipe coming from it, was at Killingbeck Hospital – a wonderful place, where Michael was sent to see a consultant with 'more experience of this sort of thing,' by a very caring and professional doctor in Huddersfield Infirmary. He had reached a state where he could not stay awake for more than 10 minutes, even after a night's sleep. He didn't want to eat, as everything tasted and smelled bad, and had lost interest in all things. He appeared to be slipping in and out of consciousness and we could not always wake him. His breathing was very shallow, hardly present during these extended periods of sleep. It appeared to be the 'end of the road'.

The team at Killingbeck recommended that I should go with him and stay in the adjoining room, to be able to help with additional needs such as lifting and handling, and helping to calm stressful situations which Michael had experienced during his stay in Huddersfield Hospital and also to learn about the ventilator. It was here, along with the 'Nippy', that we met his new respiratory consultant, Mark Elliott, and Martin his 'specialist nurse'. After an explanation of what was to happen, and Michael's initial resistance to this, the results after one night of using this machine were simply amazing! The following morning, his appetite returned, along with his interest in the world around him, and a much greater state of health and wellbeing were present within him. Although of course it was not a cure for motor neurone disease and its effects, it was a means of 'living with it', rather than dying from it at that point in time.

I was trained how to adjust settings on the machine, clean filters, etc.; and off we went home. This was our first experience of seeing 'near death' becoming very much the opposite in a very short space of time. Every time we arrived at Killingbeck, and then St James's after Killingbeck's closure, the wonderful and dynamic Dr Elliott appeared, along with his team and their expertise, and I knew that everything that could be done would be done.

I feel that we were 'pioneers' in taking this home, in benefiting from, and working with it. I use the term 'we' as it is not something that one individual could take on without the support of a small team. In our case, under the guidance, training and expertise of Dr Elliott and his crew, I was the leader, and our immediate 'ventilation and suction' team consisted of: my sister-in-law Kathryn; our nurse Marlene, who became a family friend; our neighbour Susan who, once the needs had become greater, was willing to go along to St James's hospital for training, so that she could help and support at short notice, should I be struggling; our lovely general practitioner, Dr Orme, who gave constant support and help if needed, and issued me with my own stethoscope; and our physiotherapist Richard, who also became a family friend, and taught me good skills in chest physio, besides administering them himself on his weekly visits to our house. All of this could not have happened without our equally important extended team of many family members, friends and neighbours who also gave much encouragement and help, with the children, cooking, shopping, gardening, etc., and of course, help with the dog. They also gave inspiration, kindness and brought humour, companionship and on-going care. Bigger tasks, such as rewiring the house, was done by my brother Martin and a group of his friends, as our need for more power points increased due to all of the electrical/medical items in use. Meanwhile some 'design and technology' challenges were met by Michael's brother Terry, who with his engineering background was able to convert the only comfortable cottage armchair that Michael could settle in, into a wheel chair, and devise a unique cigarette holder, making smoking, without singeing the straps of his mask too badly, as safe as it possibly could be!

Kirkwood Hospice played an important role, in the earlier stages offering day-care once per week; and the inspiration that came with this, also came the opportunity for making new friendships. As time went on, also offering some support with medical needs during the times of being admitted to their bed area. During the final five weeks of his life Michael was unable to leave the hospice, so I would not have been able to manage without their help.

I hope that our experiences are able to help others, and that some of the initial challenges which come usually with all new systems have been 'ironed out'. Stressful as well as happy times are encountered. I have memories of dashing through the main entrance of St James's on a Saturday afternoon (the busiest time possible) with Michael in the converted armchair on wheels, attempting to get him to the ninth floor before he stopped breathing, running through the many visiting relatives, with Dr Elliott, and our friends running along with the necessary equipment. We were unable to be transported in a normal ambulance as at that time in our area they could not provide mains electricity, and batteries available to power domiciliary ventilators were very rudimentary. So we either borrowed the hospice ambulance and a volunteer driver (usually Ivan, who had become a close friend of Michael), or we went by car with my sister-in law driving. Whichever method, I would be administering oxygen, ventilation and a bit of chest physio as we went along the M1 and through Leeds.

As the caregiver I think you have to be willing to take on the challenge of learning, adapting, of being proactive, of being and staying strong inside, and with this, aiming to keep balance within yourself and for others around you. You have to be dynamic, quick thinking, and willing to tackle the obstacles that occur on the way, certainly not settling in any 'comfort zones'. After Michael's diagnosis, and while on an extended family break, I went for early morning runs along the beach, including doing a few cart-wheels which, being 40 years old, I had not done for many years. Looking back I think this was perhaps one of the first stages in boosting energy levels, developing resilience, and 'breaking through' to a place where difficult and new challenges could be met with a positive attitude. I follow with interest research on motor neurone disease, and support the organization. I am equally passionate about supporting the 'Assisted Ventilation Unit' in Leeds, and am keen to hear of success and progress with this.

After Michael's death, I felt that everything had been done that possibly could be done. Although it was and still is very sad, I felt able to move forwards and free to continue, and enjoy time – with my children, to make up as much as possible for the things that I had inevitably missed out on during the time as Michael's caregiver. Also, to enjoy time with my family and my friends old and new. I returned to work and love my job, and my life as it now is.

Seeing all of this first hand, I think, gives reason to love and enjoy your life, to value your health and to embrace opportunities as they arise.

Alyson Lindley
Huddersfield 2009

See Appendix E: Michael and Alyson Lindley's photo album in the Vitalsource ebook edition.

# Index

Abbreviations: ARF, acute respiratory failure; CPAP, continuous positive airway pressure; CRF, chronic respiratory failure; HMV, home mechanical ventilation.